SECOND EDITION

CARDIOTHORACIC
SURGICAL NURSING

Betsy A. Finkelmeier, RN, MS, MM

Division Administrator and Manager of Clinical Services
Division of Cardiothoracic Surgery
Northwestern Medical Faculty Foundation

Clinical Appointment
Department of Nursing
Northwestern Memorial Hospital
Chicago, Illinois

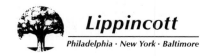

Lippincott
Philadelphia · New York · Baltimore

Acquisitions Editor: Susan M. Glover, RN, MSN
Editorial Assistant: Hilarie M. Surrena
Project Editor: Debra Schiff
Senior Production Manager: Helen Ewan
Senior Production Coordinator: Nannette Winski
Design Coordinator: Brett MacNaughton
Indexer: Katherine Pitcoff
Manufacturing Manager: William Alberti
Compositor: Peirce Graphic Services, Inc.
Printer & Binder: Courier Westford

2nd Edition

9 8 7 6 5 4 3 2 1

Library of Congress Cataloging-in-Publication Data

Finkelmeier, Betsy A.
    Cardiothoracic surgical nursing / Betsy A. Finkelmeier.—2nd ed.
      p. ; cm.
    Includes bibliographical references and index.
    ISBN 0-7817-1713-2 (alk. paper)
    1. Chest—Surgery —Nursing. 2. Heart—Surgery—Nursing. I. Title.
    [DNLM: 1. Perioperative Nursing—methods. 2. Cardiovascular Diseases—
nursing. 3. Cardiovascular Diseases—surgery. 4. Thoracic Diseases—nursing.
5. Thoracic Diseases—surgery. WY 161 F499c 2000]
    RD536 .F465 2000
    610. 73′677—dc21
                                                                    00-022473

Care has been taken to confirm the accuracy of the information presented and to describe generally accepted practices. However, the authors, editors, and publisher are not responsible for errors or omissions or for any consequences from application of the information in this book and make no warranty, express or implied, with respect to the contents of the publication.

The authors, editors, and publisher have exerted every effort to ensure that drug selection and dosage set forth in this text are in accordance with current recommendations and practice at the time of publication. However, in view of ongoing research, changes in government regulations, and the constant flow of information relating to drug therapy and drug reactions, the reader is urged to check the package insert for each drug for any change in indications and dosage and for added warnings and precautions. This is particularly important when the recommended agent is a new or infrequently employed drug.

Some drugs and medical devices presented in this publication have Food and Drug Administration (FDA) clearance for limited use in restricted research settings. It is the responsibility of the health care provider to ascertain the FDA status of each drug or device planned for use in their clinical practice.

To my mother, Marjorie Thompson Finkelmeier,
and my late father, Louis John Finkelmeier, MD,
for their steadfast love and guidance.

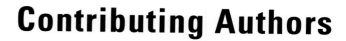

Contributing Authors

Jane Kruse, RN, BSN
Nurse Clinician, Electrophysiology
Department of Nursing
Northwestern Memorial Hospital
Chicago, Illinois

Diane Marolda, RN, MSN, ACNP
Nurse Practitioner
DOCS—Physicians affiliated with Beth Israel Medical Center
Bronx, New York

Kimberly Wilder, RN, MSN, ACNP
Nurse Practitioner, Cardiothoracic Surgery
Department of Nursing
Northwestern Memorial Hospital
Chicago, Illinois

Reviewers: Second Edition

Robert O. Bonow, MD
Goldberg Professor of Medicine and Chief
Division of Cardiology
Northwestern University Medical School
Chicago, Illinois

Kathleen Chaimberg, MD
Assistant Professor of Anesthesiology
Department of Anesthesiology
Dartmouth-Hitchcock Medical Center
Lebanon, New Hampshire

Hao Kenith Fang, MD
Chief Resident, Cardiothoracic Surgery
Division of Cardiothoracic Surgery
Northwestern University Medical School
Chicago, Illinois

David A. Fullerton, MD
Professor of Surgery and Chief
Division of Cardiothoracic Surgery
Northwestern University Medical School
Chicago, Illinois

Mihai Gheorghiade, MD
Professor of Medicine
Division of Cardiology
Northwestern University Medical School
Chicago, Illinois

Linda Hellstedt, RN, MSN
Advanced Practice Nurse, Cardiac Nursing
Department of Nursing
Northwestern Memorial Hospital
Chicago, Illinois

Neal D. Hillman, MD
Instructor of Surgery
Division of Cardiothoracic Surgery
Northwestern University Medical School
Chicago, Illinois

Keith A. Horvath, MD
Assistant Professor of Surgery
Division of Cardiothoracic Surgery
Northwestern University Medical School
Chicago, Illinois

Peter E. Jensen, MD
Resident, Cardiothoracic Surgery
Division of Cardiothoracic Surgery
Northwestern University Medical School
Chicago, Illinois

Maryl Johnson, MD
Associate Professor of Medicine
Division of Cardiology
Northwestern University Medical School
Chicago, Illinois

Jane Kruse, RN, BSN
Nurse Clinician, Electrophysiology
Department of Nursing
Northwestern Memorial Hospital
Chicago, Illinois

Diane Marolda, RN, MSN, ACNP
Nurse Practitioner
DOCS—Physicians affiliated with Beth Israel Medical Center
Bronx, New York

Mary Beth Menduni, RN, CCRN, BSN
Clinical Coordinator, ICU
Department of Nursing
Dartmouth-Hitchcock Medical Center
Lebanon, New Hampshire

Robert M. Mentzer Jr., MD
Frank C. Spencer Professor and Chairman
Director, UK Transplant Center
Department of Surgery
University of Kentucky
Lexington, Kentucky

Pam Pfeifer, RN, MS
Advanced Practice Nurse, Heart Failure
Department of Nursing
Northwestern Memorial Hospital
Chicago, Illinois

John H. Sanders Jr., MD
Professor of Surgery
Division of Cardiothoracic Surgery
Dartmouth-Hitchcock Medical Center
Lebanon, New Hampshire

R. Sudhir Sundaresan, MD
Associate Professor and Head of Thoracic Surgery
Division of Cardiothoracic Surgery
Northwestern University Medical School
Chicago, Illinois

Vicky L. Turner, RN, CCRN
Patient Care Coordinator
Division of Cardiovascular and Thoracic Surgery
University of Kentucky
Lexington, Kentucky

Robert M. Vanecko, MD
Professor of Surgery
Division of Cardiothoracic Surgery
Northwestern University Medical School
Chicago, Illinois

Richard Wade, CCP
Chief Perfusionist
Department of Surgical Services
Northwestern Memorial Hospital
Chicago, Illinois

Kimberly Wilder, RN, MSN, ACNP
Nurse Practitioner, Cardiothoracic Surgery
Department of Nursing
Northwestern Memorial Hospital
Chicago, Illinois

Reviewers: First Edition

Robert W. Anderson, MD
David C. Sabiston Jr. Professor and Chairman
Department of Surgery
Duke University Medical School
Durham, North Carolina

Carl E. Arentzen, MD
Attending Surgeon
Prairie Thoracic and Cardiovascular Surgery
Springfield, Illinois

Carl L. Backer, MD
Associate Professor of Surgery
Division of Cardiothoracic Surgery
Northwestern University Medical School
Chicago, Illinois

Susan Bailey Black, RN, MHA
Augusta, Georgia

Ivan K. Crosby, MD
Chief of Cardiac Surgery
Forsyth Memorial Hospital
Winston-Salem, North Carolina

Catherine S. Dunnington, RN, MS
Clinical Nurse Specialist
Clinical Cardiac Electrophysiology Department
Illinois Masonic Hospital
Chicago, Illinois

John E. Fetter, MD
Attending Cardiothoracic Surgeon
St. Mary's Diluth Clinic
Diluth, Minnesota

James W. Frederiksen, MD
Associate Professor of Surgery
Division of Cardiothoracic Surgery
Northwestern University Medical School
Chicago, Illinois

Willard Fry, MD
Professor of Surgery
Division of Cardiothoracic Surgery
Northwestern University Medical School
Chicago, Illinois

Kathleen L. Grady, RN, MS, PhD
Nursing Director
Heart Failure and Cardiac Transplant Program
Rush Presbyterian St. Luke's Medical Center
Chicago, Illinois

I. Martin Grais, MD
Assistant Professor of Clinical Medicine
Division of Cardiology
Northwestern University Medical School
Chicago, Illinois

Renee S. Hartz, MD
Professor of Surgery
Division of Cardiothoracic Surgery
Tulane University
New Orleans, Louisiana

Mary H. Hawthorne, PhD, RN
Assistant Professor
School of Nursing
Duke University
Durham, North Carolina

Linda F. Hellstedt, MS, RN, CCRN
Advanced Practice Nurse, Cardiac Nursing
Department of Nursing
Northwestern Memorial Hospital
Chicago, Illinois

Axel W. Joob, MD
Attending Surgeon
Cardiovascular and Thoracic Surgery
Lutheran General Hospital
Park Ridge, Illinois

Irving L. Kron, MD
William H. Mueller Jr. Professor and Chief
Division of Cardiothoracic Surgery
Co-Chairman, Department of Surgery
University of Virginia Medical School
Charlottesville, Virginia

Carol Lake, MD
Professor and Chair
Department of Anesthesiology
University of Louisville
Louisville, Kentucky

Joseph LoCicero III, MD
Associate Professor of Surgery
Division of Cardiothoracic Surgery
Harvard University Medical School
Boston, Massachusetts

C. Gregory Lockhart, MD
Attending Surgeon
Surgical Associates of Richmond
Richmond, Virginia

Robert G. Matheny, MD
Attending Cardiothoracic Surgeon
Atlanta Cardiology Group
Atlanta, Georgia

Jane S. McMurray, RN, MSN
Madison, Wisconsin

David D. McPherson, MD
Professor of Medicine
Division of Cardiology
Northwestern University Medical School
Chicago, Illinois

David Mehlman, MD
Associate Professor of Medicine
Division of Cardiology
Northwestern University Medical School
Chicago, Illinois

Robert M. Mentzer, Jr., MD
Frank C. Spencer Professor and Chairman
Director, UK Transplant Center
Department of Surgery
University of Kentucky
Lexington, Kentucky

Lawrence L. Michaelis, MD
Professor of Surgery
Division of Cardiothoracic Surgery
Northwestern University Medical School
Chicago, Illinois

Stanton P. Nolan, MD
Professor of Surgery
Division of Cardiothoracic Surgery
University of Virginia Medical School
Charlottesville, Virginia

Arthur S. Palmer, MD
Assistant Professor of Surgery
Division of Cardiothoracic Surgery
Northwestern University Medical School
Chicago, Illinois

John R. Pellet, MD
Professor of Surgery
Department of Surgery
University of Wisconsin Medical School
Madison, Wisconsin

Pamela B. Pfeifer, MS., RN, CCRN
Advanced Practice Nurse, Heart Failure
Department of Nursing
Northwestern Memorial Hospital
Chicago, Illinois

Jane E. Reedy, RN, BSN
Director of Clinical Services
Thoratec Laboratories
Pleasanton, CA

Robert J. Robison, MD
Attending Surgeon
Division of Cardiovascular Surgery
St. Vincent's Hospital
Indianapolis, Indiana

James E. Rosenthal, MD
Associate Professor of Medicine
Division of Cardiology
Northwestern University Medical School
Chicago, Illinois

Michael H. Salinger, MD
Associate Professor of Clinical Medicine
Division of Cardiology
Northwestern University Medical School
Chicago, Illinois

John H. Sanders, Jr., MD
Professor of Surgery
Division of Cardiothoracic Surgery
Dartmouth-Hitchcock Medical Center
Lebanon, New Hampshire

Thomas W. Shields, MD
Professor Emeritus of Surgery
Department of Surgery
Northwestern University Medical School
Chicago, Illinois

Neil Stone, MD
Associate Professor of Medicine
Division of Cardiology
Northwestern University Medical School
Chicago, Illinois

Medhat Takla, MD
Attending Surgeon
Northeast Cardiovascular
Concord, North Carolina

Robert M. Vanecko, MD
Professor of Surgery
Division of Cardiothoracic Surgery
Northwestern University Medical School
Chicago, Illinois

Timothy V. Votapka, MD
Assistant Professor of Surgery
Division of Cardiothoracic Surgery
Northwestern University
Chicago, Illinois

Leonard D. Wade, MS
Assistant Professor of Anesthesia
Department of Anesthesia
Northwestern University Medical School
Chicago, Illinois

Anne P. Weiland, MSN, MBA
Assistant Vice President, Washington Managed Care Operations
MedStar Health
Washington, DC

Gayle R. Whitman, MSN, RN, FAAN
Director, Cardiothoracic Nursing
Cleveland Clinic Foundation
Cleveland, Ohio

Edward Winslow, MD
Associate Professor of Clinical Medicine
Division of Cardiology
Northwestern University Medical School
Chicago, Illinois

Terry A. Zheutlin, MD
Director, Progressive Coronary Care Unit
Clinical Cardiac Electrophysiology Department
Illinois Masonic Hospital
Chicago, Illinois

Preface

Extraordinary progress has been achieved during the past several decades in the surgical treatment of cardiac and thoracic diseases. Opportunities for surgical therapy have expanded tremendously as a result of improvements in cardiopulmonary bypass and myocardial protection and the development of sophisticated perioperative monitoring capabilities. Concurrent with these advances, cardiothoracic surgical nursing has emerged as an important and challenging area of specialty practice, encompassing the care of patients who have a wide variety of acute, chronic, malignant, and life-threatening cardiac and thoracic diseases of the chest.

Cardiothoracic Surgical Nursing is intended to provide a comprehensive reference for nurses specializing in the care of adult patients with cardiac and thoracic surgical diseases. The second edition includes updated information about specific diseases, surgical therapy, and all aspects of pre- and postoperative nursing care in both routine and complex patient care situations. Unit I, which addresses cardiac surgery, is divided into five parts: cardiovascular diseases, preoperative evaluation and preparation, intraoperative considerations, cardiovascular operations, and postoperative management. In Unit II, cardiothoracic transplantation and trauma are discussed. Unit III covers thoracic surgery, including surgical diseases of the chest, preoperative evaluation and preparation, thoracic operations, and postoperative management.

Since publication of the first edition of *Cardiothoracic Surgical Nursing,* remarkable advances have oc-

curred in the field of cardiothoracic surgery. Minimally invasive techniques have been developed that allow performance of selected valve and coronary artery bypass operations through smaller incisions. In some centers, coronary bypass grafting is being performed without cardiopulmonary bypass. Video-assisted thoracoscopy now obviates the need for thoracotomy in many patients who require general thoracic operations, such as pleurodesis and wedge resection.

Several new operations have been added to the surgical armamentarium, including transmyocardial laser revascularization for patients with end-stage coronary artery disease and lung volume reduction surgery for patients with severe emphysema. For patients with end-stage pulmonary disease, lung transplantation has evolved from a largely experimental form of therapy to a standard treatment modality. Technologic advances also have resulted in increasingly sophisticated implantable devices. Wearable ventricular assist devices now make it possible for selected patients with end-stage heart failure to receive mechanical ventricular support at home. For patients with life-threatening cardiac rhythm disorders, multiprogrammable devices have been developed that provide both pacing and defibrillating therapies with a single device. All of these innovations and developments are addressed in the second edition of *Cardiothoracic Surgical Nursing.* Cardiothoracic surgical nurses will find in the contents a broad foundation of relevant information upon which to base their clinical practice.

Acknowledgments

Many individuals contributed to the first and second editions of *Cardiothoracic Surgical Nursing*. Countless patients and families through the years have taught me much of what is contained in the text. Many nursing and physician colleagues have tolerated endless requests for advice and information and have provided invaluable support in shaping the book. I would particularly like to thank my wonderful family and friends, the surgeons and staff in the Northwestern University Division of Cardiothoracic Surgery, my nursing colleagues at Northwestern Memorial Hospital, and the reviewers of the text.

I would also like to acknowledge the following mentors and colleagues who have contributed greatly to my professional growth. Louis J. Finkelmeier, MD, who practiced as a general surgeon for nearly fifty years in rural Ohio, profoundly influenced my deep commitment to the care of patients. Stanton P. Nolan, MD, and Helen Ripple, RN, MS, had a major impact on my career development during my years at the University of Virginia. John H. Sanders, Jr., MD, Lawrence L. Michaelis, MD, Robert W. Anderson, MD, and David A. Fullerton, MD, have made it possible for me to continue to achieve professional growth and satisfaction during my tenure at Northwestern Memorial Hospital. These individuals share in common a strong commitment to patients and the ability to promote excellence in the people around them.

Contents

Cardiac Surgery

CARDIOVASCULAR DISEASES

1

Coronary Artery Disease

Coronary artery disease (CAD) is one of the most common diseases affecting the adult population. It causes more deaths, disability, and economic loss in industrialized nations than any other group of diseases (Gersh et al., 1997). The United States has the second highest incidence of CAD, exceeded only by Finland; Japan has the lowest incidence (Spencer et al., 1995). Although the death rate from CAD has declined since the late 1970s in the United States and, to a lesser degree, in Europe, the prevalence of CAD-related morbidity and mortality in Asia, with almost half of the world population, has been increasing steadily (Mehta et al., 1998).

Coronary artery disease affects approximately 12 million Americans, and more than 1 million experience a myocardial infarction (MI) each year (American Heart Association, 1998). In addition, CAD accounts for one half of the nearly 1 million annual deaths due to cardiovascular diseases and is the leading cause of death in both men and women (American Heart Association, 1998). CAD also is now recognized as the underlying etiology in most patients with chronic heart failure in the United States, a population that has been increasing steadily, particularly among the elderly (Gheorghiade & Bonow, 1998).

▶ Etiology

Pathogenesis of Atherosclerosis

The major cause of CAD is *atherosclerosis*, a pathologic process that causes irregularity and thickening of artery walls. Atherosclerosis is a chronic, progressive, multifocal disease of the vessel wall intima (innermost layer) whose characteristic lesion is the atheroma or plaque (Schoen, 1997) (Fig. 1-1). The earliest lesions of atherosclerosis can be found in young children in the form of lipid-rich lesions (fatty streaks) composed of macrophages and smooth muscle cells. Fatty streaks are present in almost all people after 20 years of age. In those in whom the lesions progress, fibrous plaques appear around the third decade, and more complicated lesions and their clinical consequences typically begin to develop in the fourth decade (Fuster et al., 1992).

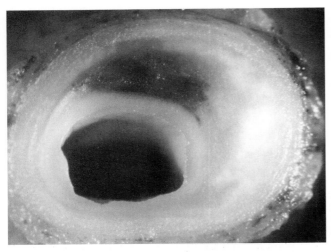

FIGURE 1-1. Cross-section of coronary artery demonstrating eccentric fibrofatty atherosclerotic plaque. (Courtesy of Cornelius Davis, MD)

Advanced lesions of atherosclerosis develop as the result of three biologic processes: (1) accumulation of intimal smooth muscle cells; (2) formation by the proliferated smooth muscle cells of large amounts of connective tissue matrix; and (3) accumulation of lipid, primarily in the form of cholesteryl esters and free cholesterol within the cells as well as in the surrounding connective tissues (Ross, 1997). Small blood vessels grow into the plaque and may rupture, resulting in areas of subintimal hemorrhage that increase the plaque's size. Thrombus formation and ulceration and calcification of the lesion are common.

Atherosclerosis primarily affects large elastic arteries and large and medium-sized muscular arteries of the systemic circulation, particularly at points of branches, sharp curvatures, and bifurcations (Schoen, 1997). In the coronary arterial system, atherosclerotic lesions usually occur as localized narrowings in proximal portions of the major coronary arteries and their branches. As a lesion increasingly occupies an arterial lumen, blood supply to the myocardium can be impeded by one of several mechanisms: (1) the lesion creates a fixed obstruction so that blood flow through the artery cannot increase in response to increased demand; (2) the vessel lumen becomes completely occluded with atheromatous material or thrombus; or (3) portions of clot or plaque embolize, occluding the distal portion of the vessel. The slow growth of obstructive lesions in the coronary arteries causes formation of collateral blood vessels that provide alternative routes of blood flow to the myocardium. However, when one or more of the major arteries becomes significantly obstructed (ie, the arterial lumen is reduced to a small proportion of its normal circumference), myocardial ischemia is likely to occur.

Under normal conditions, coronary arterial flow provides adequate myocardial perfusion at rest and compensatory vasodilatation provides sufficient flow reserve to accommodate increased myocardial demand during vigorous exercise (Schoen, 1997). Atherosclerotic lesions usually do not significantly obstruct blood flow until the coronary artery cross-sectional lumen is more than 75% narrowed. Even with that degree of narrowing, blood flow often is sufficient to meet baseline myocardial oxygen demands except when precipitating factors produce a demand–supply imbalance. However, with 90% or greater reduction in luminal cross-sectional area, coronary flow may be inadequate to meet myocardial demand at rest (Schoen, 1997).

Risk Factors

Atherosclerosis is a multifaceted disease process that is unexplained by a single pathogenic process (Mehta et al., 1998). Although fatty streaks are present in almost all adults, their evolution into clinically relevant fibrous plaques and more complicated lesions varies in incidence and extent among different geographic and ethnic groups (Fuster et al., 1992). Characteristics of an individual or a population that predict the chances for development of coronary atherosclerosis are termed *risk factors* (LaRosa, 1998). Risk factors linked with the occurrence and progression of CAD are displayed in Table 1-1. Perhaps of greatest significance are three major modifiable risk factors for CAD: hypercholesterolemia, hypertension, and cigarette smoking. Elimination or control of these factors offers the most hope of preventing disease and slowing its progression.

Hypercholesterolemia is the dyslipidemia most clearly associated with increased risk of CAD (Farmer & Gotto, 1997). A cholesterol level greater than 200 mg/dL is associated with increased risk for CAD, and the risk increases exponentially with serum cholesterol levels above 240 mg/dL. More than 98 million American adults have blood cholesterol levels of at least 200 mg/dL, and over 39 million have levels of 240 mg/dL or greater (American

---

TABLE 1-1

Risk Factors for Coronary Artery Disease

MAJOR MODIFIABLE RISK FACTORS
Hypercholesterolemia
Hypertension
Cigarette smoking

NONMODIFIABLE RISK FACTORS
Heredity
Increasing age
Male sex

CONTRIBUTING RISK FACTORS
Diabetes
Obesity
Sedentary lifestyle
Cocaine

Heart Association, 1998). The predictive value of serum cholesterol is more powerful in people who have other associated risk factors (Stone, 1997).

Two lipoproteins (ie, complex molecules that transport cholesterol in the bloodstream) also have prognostic significance for development and progression of CAD: low-density lipoprotein cholesterol (LDL-C) and high-density lipoprotein cholesterol (HDL-C). Elevated LDL-C levels are known to accelerate atherogenesis, thereby increasing risk. Significant lowering of LDL-C in patients with CAD not only slows progression but can cause regression of existing atherosclerotic plaques and is associated with a reduction in adverse cardiac events (Stone, 1997; Brown et al., 1990).

In contrast to LDL-C, HDL-C levels are inversely related to risk of cardiovascular disease. In fact, elevated HDL-C appears to slow atherosclerosis. Accordingly, HDL-C levels are considered an important predictor of CAD, independent of serum cholesterol levels. Also, other risk factors for CAD, such as cigarette smoking, obesity, and a sedentary lifestyle, are known to decrease HDL-C (Goe, 1995). Conversely, exercise, postmenopausal estrogens, and moderate alcohol consumption increase HDL-C. Alcohol consumption as a means of increasing HDL-C is not encouraged, however, because of the adverse effects of excess usage, particularly in women and younger people (Stone, 1997). The role of triglycerides as a risk factor for CAD remains controversial. Although hypertriglyceridemia is not an independent risk factor for CAD, triglycerides are a useful indicator that associated metabolic abnormalities may be present (Stone, 1997).

Hypertension affects approximately 50 million Americans; it is more prevalent in African Americans and people living in the southeastern United States (American Heart Association, 1998). The incidence of hypertension also increases in prevalence with advancing age to the point where approximately two thirds of people 65 years of age or older in the United States are hypertensive (Levy & Wilson, 1998). Both systolic and diastolic hypertension independently increase the risk for development of CAD as well as other forms of cardiovascular disease. In addition, absolute risk associated with systolic and diastolic hypertension is higher in older people at corresponding levels of blood pressure and is higher in men than in women (Vokonas & Kannel, 1997). Hypertension acts as an additive risk factor when superimposed on cigarette smoking, cholesterol elevation, glucose intolerance, and other risk factors (Rackley & Schlant, 1994).

Cigarette smoking is the third major modifiable risk factor for CAD. There is strong evidence that smoking accelerates atherosclerosis in already susceptible individuals, lowers HDL-C levels, and increases risk for MI and sudden cardiac death in people with CAD (Stone & Green, 1980). The carbon monoxide contained in cigarettes reduces the oxygen-carrying capacity of hemoglobin, and the nicotine and other substances exert potent effects on vascular smooth muscle, possibly initiating thrombotic events in persons with atherosclerosis (Vokonas & Kannel, 1997). Continuation of smoking after MI is associated with the highest mortality rate of any

of the other associated risk factors, and an increased frequency of restenosis after angioplasty is reported in patients who continue to smoke (Rackley & Schlant, 1994).

Although smoking among adults has declined in the United States since the late 1960s, recent data indicate that this downward trend may have leveled off. More than 48 million adult Americans (27% of men and 23% of women) continue to smoke, as well as 4.1 million adolescents between the ages of 12 and 17 years (American Heart Association, 1998). Nonsmokers exposed to environmental tobacco smoke also face an increased risk of CAD. The risk of death from CAD increases by up to 30% among those exposed to environmental tobacco smoke at home or at work (American Heart Association, 1998). The American Heart Association Council on Cardiopulmonary and Critical Care has concluded that environmental tobacco smoke is a major preventable cause of cardiovascular disease and death (Taylor et al., 1992).

Risk factors for CAD that cannot be modified include heredity, older age, and male sex. A propensity clearly exists in some family groups for the development of CAD at a younger age. This increased familial risk may be mediated by genetic effects on other risk factors such as obesity, hypertension, dyslipidemia, and diabetes (Farmer & Gotto, 1997). Because of increased longevity in the United States and the progressive nature of atherosclerosis, increased age is a risk factor for CAD. By 70 years of age, approximately 15% of men and 9% of women have clinically diagnosable coronary atherosclerosis, and by 80 years of age, the incidence is 20% in both sexes (Loop, 1998). Also, the frequency of death from CAD increases two to four times with each decade of life (Spencer et al., 1995). Approximately 85% of people who die from CAD are 65 years of age or older, and more than half of people older than 65 years of age die from the effects of CAD (American Heart Association, 1998; Nixon, 1997). MI also is much more common in the elderly.

Throughout early and middle adulthood, CAD affects men much more commonly than women. The onset of symptomatic CAD typically is approximately 10 years earlier in men than in women (Farmer & Gotto, 1997). As women approach menopause, however, the protective effects of estrogen may be lost; the risk of heart disease begins to rise and continues to increase with age (American Heart Association, 1998). Women with the combined risk factors of smoking and high cholesterol are at even greater risk. Also, use of oral contraceptives increases risk in women older than 35 years of age, especially if other risk factors are present (Peberdy & Ornato, 1992).

Other important risk factors for CAD include diabetes, obesity, a sedentary lifestyle, and the illicit use of cocaine. Diabetes affects approximately 10 million Americans, and two thirds of diabetic individuals die from some form of heart or blood vessel disease (American Heart Association, 1998). Patients with diabetes mellitus have a significantly increased risk for development of atherosclerosis, and CAD in diabetic patients tends to be more severe than in nondiabetic patients. The risk of MI and the mortality associated with coronary ischemic events are increased significantly in diabetic patients (Weintraub et al., 1998). Diabetes is a more potent contributing risk factor in women than in men. The incidence of CAD is five times higher in women with diabetes compared with nondiabetic women, and affected women have a much greater likelihood of dying from the disease than do women without diabetes (Rosen, 1997). Those women affected before menopause effectively lose the protective effects of estrogen (American Heart Association, 1998).

Progressive weight gain resulting in obesity is a risk factor for CAD in both men and women. According to the American Heart Association (1998), nearly 147 million adults and 5 million children in the United States are overweight or obese. Increases in weight cause increases in several risk factors more directly related to atherogenesis, including blood pressure, serum cholesterol, triglycerides, and blood glucose (Vokonas & Kannel, 1997). Increases in weight also lower HDL-C, thereby removing the protective effect of a low total cholesterol–HDL-C cholesterol ratio. The pattern of fat distribution also appears significant. Abdominal or truncal obesity is associated with hypertension, hyperlipidemia, and glucose intolerance (Vokonas & Kannel, 1997). Obese people who smoke have a tenfold increased risk of cardiovascular events compared with nonobese, nonsmoking people (Gottlieb, 1992).

A sedentary lifestyle also increases risk for coronary atherosclerosis. Physically inactive people face a 1.5 to 2.4 times greater risk for development of CAD (American Heart Association, 1998). Conversely, regular physical exercise is known to lessen the risk of CAD and its adverse consequences. In the United States, physical inactivity is more prevalent among women, African Americans, Hispanics, older adults, less affluent people, and those with less than a 12th grade education (American Heart Association, 1998).

Cocaine abuse can cause myocardial ischemia and MI, even in young adults without other risk factors and in the absence of obstructive CAD. Cardiovascular effects of cocaine include coronary artery vasoconstriction, accelerated atherosclerosis, increased platelet aggregation, and arterial thrombosis (Wynne & Braunwald, 1997).

The role of personality type and emotional stress in risk stratification for CAD remains controversial (Farmer & Gotto, 1997). Much remains to be learned about the pathogenesis of CAD and a number of other potential risk factors are under investigation. These include homocysteinemia, elevated plasma levels of lipoprotein(a), excessive iron load in the body, imbalance between oxidant and antioxidant species, hypercoagulability, and infection leading to inflammation (Mehta et al., 1998).

Mechanisms of Ischemia

Myocardial ischemia represents an imbalance between myocardial oxygen supply and demand. Because the heart depends almost exclusively on aerobic metabolism for the generation of energy, it can develop only a small oxygen debt (Ganz & Braunwald, 1997). Either an in-

creased demand in the presence of fixed obstruction to flow, a reduced supply, or a combination of both rapidly produces ischemia. Ischemia differs from hypoxia (reduced oxygen content with adequate perfusion) in that oxygen deprivation is accompanied by inadequate removal of metabolites consequent to reduced perfusion (Ganz & Braunwald, 1997).

Myocardial demand is affected by changes in heart rate, contractility, and systolic wall tension; among these, increased heart rate is believed to be the single most important determinant of increased myocardial oxygen consumption (Simandl & Cohn, 1997). Most episodes of chronic stable angina are thought to be caused by an increase of myocardial oxygen requirements by exercise, tachycardia, or emotion in the presence of coronary artery obstruction (Ganz & Braunwald, 1997). The presence of fixed atherosclerotic lesions prevents the normal physiologic increase in coronary blood flow to meet increased demand.

Conversely, "supply ischemia," or a reduction in oxygen supply secondary to increased coronary vascular tone, platelet aggregates, or thrombi, is responsible for MI and most episodes of unstable angina (Ganz & Braunwald, 1997). In patients with CAD, oxygen supply may be reduced by the formation of thrombus on atherosclerotic lesions or by factors that cause vasoconstriction, such as smoking, exercise, or exposure to cold.

► Clinical Manifestations

Significant clinical symptoms of CAD typically do not develop until late middle age. Myocardial oxygen deprivation can produce a continuum of events in the muscle ranging from intermittent symptoms of ischemia to irreversible muscle necrosis or MI. In addition, acute pulmonary edema or ventricular tachyarrhythmias can occur. The type and severity of event are quite unpredictable. In many cases, a fatal MI or sudden cardiac death is the first manifestation of CAD. In the United States, at least 250,000 people annually die of CAD within 1 hour of the onset of symptoms and before reaching a hospital (American Heart Association, 1998).

Myocardial Ischemia

Myocardial ischemia may be manifest as anginal discomfort, deviation of the ST segment on the electrocardiogram (ECG), reduced uptake of thallium-201 in myocardial perfusion images, or regional or global impairment of ventricular function (Ganz & Braunwald, 1997). Angina, representing transient myocardial ischemia, is the cardinal recurring symptom of CAD. It afflicts more than six million people in the United States (American Heart Association, 1998).

The terms *angina* and *chest pain* often are used interchangeably. Although myocardial ischemia usually is manifest as chest pain, it alternatively can cause a variety of other somatic sensations. Angina, therefore, describes not only chest pain but any somatic manifestation of myocardial ischemia. The term *anginal equivalent* sometimes is used to denote ischemic symptoms other than typical chest pain. Conversely, chest pain can occur with conditions other than myocardial ischemia, such as gastroesophageal reflux or pleuritis.

Anginal pain is usually substernal, lasts less than 5 minutes, and is relieved by rest or nitrates (Paraskos, 1997). It is described classically as squeezing chest discomfort or pressure. Because of its similarity to epigastric distress, it frequently is mistaken for heartburn. Angina also may occur as an abnormal sensation in the chest, epigastric region, neck, back, or arms. Often patients deny chest pain but describe a long history of tightness, fullness, numbness, or heaviness. Occasionally, the abnormal sensation is entirely outside the thorax (eg, numbness in the wrist, elbows, throat, or jaw). Because of the wide variance in presentation, it is quite common for angina to continue unrecognized or ignored for long periods before its cardiac etiology is diagnosed and appropriate therapy is initiated. The most characteristic feature of angina is that the pattern usually is consistent for a particular person—that is, the nature of the discomfort is similar each time.

Typically, angina is precipitated by exercise, stressful situations, overeating, or exposure to cold (ie, the "four Es"—exercise, emotion, eating, exposure). The Canadian Cardiovascular Society Classification System is useful in categorizing angina according to conditions under which it occurs (Table 1-2). *Exertional angina* and *rest angina* are terms used to describe whether the discomfort occurs in the presence or absence, respectively, of physical effort. The term *angina threshold* describes the level of metabolic activity that precipitates myocardial ischemia. The threshold may be fixed (ie, consistently provoked by the same amount of exertion) or variable, occurring sometimes with minimal exertion and at other times only with vigorous exertion (Simandl & Cohn, 1997).

A variety of other terms are used to further categorize angina. Chronic stable angina is defined as angina that is precipitated by exertion and that has a reasonably stable pattern over weeks to months (Roberts & Pratt, 1991). Unstable angina is angina with the following fea-

tures: (1) new onset or occurring at rest; (2) an accelerating pattern (ie, occurs more frequently or at lower workloads); (3) wakes the patient from sleep; (4) of prolonged duration or unresponsive to nitrates; or (5) associated with symptoms, such as nausea, weakness, dyspnea, diaphoresis, palpitations, syncope, or pulmonary edema (Paraskos, 1997). Unstable angina develops in approximately 750,000 Americans each year and is associated with subsequent MI in 10% of these (Smith & Gersh, 1997). Unstable angina that occurs despite maximal medical therapy, yet without enzymatic evidence of MI, often is termed *preinfarction* or *crescendo angina*. The terms *unstable, preinfarction,* and *crescendo angina* all describe an acute coronary syndrome and are discussed in further detail later in this chapter.

Variant or Prinzmetal's angina is myocardial ischemia that occurs due to spasm of the coronary arteries. The specific mechanisms that produce coronary artery spasm are not well defined. However, both smoking and use of cocaine have been implicated as etiologic factors. Although many patients with variant angina have severe proximal atherosclerotic lesions involving one or more major coronary arteries, others with the same clinical features have angiographically normal arteries (Hillis et al., 1995a). In contrast to other forms of angina, variant angina typically occurs at rest and is unrelated to exertion. The natural history in patients with Prinzmetal's angina varies and spontaneous remission sometimes occurs. Many patients experience an acute active phase with frequent episodes of angina and cardiac events during the first 6 months after presentation, but the long-term prognosis for survival at 5 years ranges from 89% to 97% (Gersh et al., 1997).

Myocardial Infarction

Myocardial infarction is irreversible necrosis of cardiac muscle. It occurs when sudden cessation or prolonged reduction of blood flow severely compromises the supply of oxygenated blood to a portion of the myocardium. Acute reduction in blood flow through a coronary artery may be due to thrombus superimposed on an atherosclerotic lesion, hemorrhage under or rupture into an atherosclerotic plaque, prolonged vasospasm, embolus to the artery, or vasculitis (Goldschlager, 1988). Intracoronary thrombus is by far the most common cause of acute MI. Thrombosis occurs when an atherosclerotic plaque undergoes an abrupt and catastrophic transition, characterized by plaque rupture and exposure of substances that promote platelet activation and thrombin generation (Antman & Braunwald, 1997).

The onset of acute MI appears to demonstrate a marked circadian periodicity and seasonal variation; the peak incidence of MI is in the early to late morning hours and during the winter months (Spencer et al., 1998). Most MIs damage a significant portion of ventricular muscle, and many are fatal. The subendocardium is the most distal region supplied by the coronary arterial system and is the portion of muscle most vulnerable to in-

---

TABLE 1-2

Canadian Cardiovascular Society Classification System for Angina Pectoris

Class	Description
I	Angina occurs with strenuous or rapid or prolonged exertion at work or recreation
II	Slight limitation of ordinary activities by angina
III	Marked limitation of ordinary activities by angina
IV	Angina with any physical activity or at rest

Adapted from Campeau L, 1976: Grading of angina pectoris. Circulation 54:522.

farction. An MI limited to the subendocardial layer is termed *subendocardial* or *nontransmural*. An infarction that extends through all layers of muscle is termed *transmural*. Most MIs involve primarily the left ventricle. Although approximately 50% of patients with inferior wall MI have some degree of right ventricular infarction, isolated right ventricular infarction is observed in only 3% to 5% of autopsy-proven cases of MI (Antman & Braunwald, 1997).

Infarct location corresponds to the occluded coronary artery from which the affected muscle receives its blood supply (Fig. 1-2). The left anterior descending artery supplies the anterior wall of the left ventricle, the anterior portion of the interventricular septum, and most of the bundle branches (Hudak et al., 1998a). Because of the anterior wall's crucial importance to effective left ventricular contraction, an anterior wall MI is particularly damaging. The left circumflex artery supplies the posterior and lateral walls of the left ventricle. Lateral or inferoposterior infarctions result from circumflex artery occlusion. Left main coronary artery occlusion damages all muscle supplied by both the left anterior descending and circumflex arteries, producing global infarction that is invariably fatal. The inferior wall of the left ventricle, the right ventricle, and, usually, sinus and atrioventricular (AV) nodal tissue are supplied by the right coronary artery. Right coronary artery occlusion produces an inferior or diaphragmatic MI of the left ventricle, or a right ventricular infarction.

Myocardial infarction commonly is associated with severe chest pain unrelieved by rest or oral medications and lasting 30 minutes or more. The pain, often described as crushing, usually is substernal and may radiate to the arms, neck, jaw, or back. Shortness of breath, diaphoresis, anxiety, nausea, and vomiting often accompany the pain. Less common manifestations include pulmonary edema, heart block, and ventricular tachycardia. Between 20% to 30% of patients experience what is termed a silent MI, in that they are completely asymptomatic at the onset of coronary occlusion (Schwarz et al., 1997). People with diabetes mellitus are particularly susceptible to silent MI.

The clinical sequelae and prognosis after MI depend not only on location of the infarct but on the amount of muscle damage. Small infarcts may produce no symptoms and may not be detected until an ECG is obtained or the heart is visually inspected during a cardiac operation or postmortem examination. On the other hand, large amounts of muscle necrosis or multiple infarcts may produce significant segmental wall motion abnormalities or global hypokinesis.

Arrhythmias are quite common after acute MI. Ventricular arrhythmias of some type occur in nearly 100% of patients, bradycardia in up to one third (especially with inferior wall MI), and atrial arrhythmias in 10% to 15% (Goldschlager, 1988). First-, second-, or third-degree heart block also is common, occurring in 15% to 25% of patients hospitalized with acute MI (Hillis et al., 1995b). AV block that follows an inferior wall MI usually occurs transiently as a result of AV nodal ischemia, may require temporary pacing, and resolves after a few days. AV block after an anterior wall MI, on the other hand, usually denotes extensive myocardial necrosis that involves conducting tissue below the AV node (Kessler, 1991; Hillis et

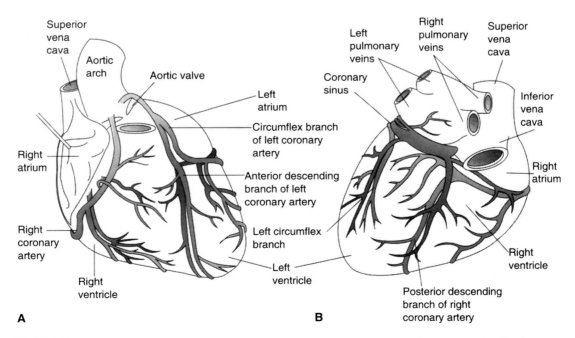

FIGURE 1-2. Anterior **(A)** and posterior **(B)** view of the heart displaying normal distribution of coronary arteries. (Porth CM, 1998: Alterations in cardiac function. In Pathophysiology: Concepts of Altered Health States, ed. 5, p. 390. Philadelphia Lippincott Williams & Wilkins.)

al., 1995b). It is more likely to be permanent and necessitate pacemaker implantation. Because AV block after anterior MI signifies damage to a large amount of myocardium, it is associated with a poor prognosis.

Pericarditis (inflammation of the pericardial sac) or pericardial effusion sometimes occurs in the early post-MI period but usually abates without sequelae. Dressler's syndrome is a more pronounced form of pericarditis that develops in some patients weeks or months after MI. It is characterized by pericarditic chest pain, fever, pericardial friction rub, and pericardial or pleural effusion (Roberts et al., 1994).

Survivors of acute MI face significant risk for future cardiovascular events, including subsequent MI, sudden cardiac death, and heart failure (Rapaport & Gheorghiade, 1996). Twenty-four percent of men and 42% of women die within 1 year after MI; within 6 years, a significant number of MI survivors have another MI (21% of men and 33% of women) or become disabled with congestive heart failure (21% of men and 30% of women; American Heart Association, 1998). Acute MI also can cause a number of serious and potentially lethal complications, discussed later in the chapter and including cardiogenic shock, ventricular aneurysm, systemic or pulmonary embolization, acute mitral regurgitation, and ventricular rupture.

▶ Diagnosis

Because the first symptom of CAD is often a fatal MI or sudden cardiac death, preventive therapy, screening of people in high-risk categories, and early diagnosis and treatment are essential to reduce mortality and morbidity. People with known risk factors require a thorough review of clinical history and a physical examination, chest roentgenogram, and ECG. Unfortunately, severe CAD may be present despite normal physical and roentgenographic findings. The ECG also remains normal, except during episodes of angina and after MI has occurred. Angina often, but not always, produces ST segment depression in leads reflective of ischemic myocardium. Variant angina and myocardial injury produce ST segment elevation. ST-T wave abnormalities, however, also are common in the general population, particularly in people with hypertension or diabetes mellitus, cigarette smokers, and women (Gersh et al., 1997).

Exercise stress testing is the most useful noninvasive screening method for diagnosis of CAD. The study consists of exercising the patient in a controlled setting while monitoring ECG, blood pressure, and heart rate. Although both false-negative and false-positive responses limit the conclusiveness of exercise stress testing, most people with hemodynamically significant atherosclerotic lesions manifest signs or symptoms of myocardial ischemia during the study. Exercise testing is not always performed as part of the diagnostic evaluation. Because coronary angiography provides accurate definition of coronary anatomy and is associated with minimal morbidity, the physician may omit exercise testing and proceed directly to catheterization in patients with suggestive symptoms. Exercise stress testing is specifically avoided if the nature of symptoms or electrocardiographic findings is suspect for high-grade lesions, because the study may precipitate life-threatening myocardial ischemia.

Two radionuclide imaging techniques (ie, myocardial scintigraphy) are useful in the diagnostic evaluation of selected patients with CAD. First, myocardial perfusion imaging is useful in patients with baseline ST segment abnormalities and in those with an inadequate heart rate response to routine exercise testing. In patients unable to exercise, a dipyridamole thallium stress test typically is performed. In this radionuclide study, dipyridamole acts as a pharmacologic stress agent to simulate the increased oxygen demand of exercise. The second radionuclide imaging technique, radionuclide angiography, is used to assess ventricular contractility and estimate ejection fraction.

Cardiac catheterization is the definitive diagnostic study for CAD. The procedure usually includes coronary angiography and left ventriculography. Unless coexisting cardiac disease is suspected, a full catheterization (with catheterization of the right chambers and measurement of intracardiac pressures) is not necessary. During coronary angiography, contrast material is injected selectively into the ostia of the right and left coronary arteries, the coronary anatomy is outlined, and areas of narrowing are identified. A contrast injection of the left ventricle (left ventriculography) is performed to demonstrate the contractile status of the left ventricle and to obtain an estimation of left ventricular ejection fraction. Areas of akinesis (lack of movement), hypokinesis (diminished movement), dyskinesis (abnormal movement), or aneurysmal dilatation also are identified with this portion of the study.

Myocardial infarction often is diagnosed and definitively distinguished from angina by its electrocardiographic manifestations and its effect on cardiac isoenzyme levels. The evolution of a transmural MI produces specific changes in the ECG tracing. The earliest findings, representative of transmural ischemia, occur within minutes. The tracings in leads facing the area of injury display abnormal T waves (prolonged, increased in magnitude, and either upright or inverted) followed by ST segment elevation (Fisch, 1997). Reciprocal ST segment depression occurs in leads opposite those of injured myocardium. As myocardial injury evolves into transmural necrosis, affected leads develop subsequent changes over a period of hours or days, including loss of R wave voltage and appearance of Q waves, normalization of ST segments, and inversion of T waves (Schwarz, 1997; Hillis et al., 1995c). Although transmural MIs usually are associated with Q waves, the presence or absence of Q waves on the ECG does not reliably distinguish between transmural and subendocardial infarction. Patients with transmural infarction do not always have Q waves and, conversely, Q waves are sometimes documented in patients with autopsy evidence of a subendocardial (nontransmural) MI (Antman & Braunwald, 1997).

Measurement of blood enzymes also contributes to diagnosis of MI. When myocardial cells are irreversibly damaged, intracellular enzymes leak through the cell membranes and are detectable in the blood. The enzymes most often used to diagnose acute MI are creatine kinase (CK) and creatine kinase-MB (CK-MB). The amount of muscle damage can be estimated by calculating the percentage of CK-MB isoenzyme (CK-MB/CK). With acute MI, the total CK level rises and the percentage of CK-MB is greater than 5%. The CK level becomes abnormal 4 to 8 hours after the onset of infarction and peaks at approximately 24 hours, although peak levels occur earlier in patients who have had reperfusion as a result of thrombolytic therapy or percutaneous coronary intervention (Antman & Braunwald, 1997). CK-MB levels rise within 3 to 12 hours but may remain elevated longer than the CK level (Table 1-3).

If more than 24 hours has elapsed since an episode of prolonged pain, the CK level may already have returned to normal. In such cases, the MB fraction may still be elevated, or a lactate dehydrogenase level may prove helpful in establishing the diagnosis of a non–Q-wave MI (Schroeder, 1997). More recently, two other enzymes specific for injured myocardial tissue have been used to provide additional data. Troponin I and troponin T levels are very specific and very sensitive to myocardial damage. Levels rise as early as 3.5 hours after the onset of chest pain, peak at 6 to 8 hours, and remain detectable for 5 to 6 days (Schwarz et al., 1997).

► Treatment

Coronary artery disease is a chronic disease. Its presence mandates consistent medical supervision and periodic evaluation for the duration of the patient's life. There is no known cure for CAD. Thus, goals of available therapy are primarily palliative: to slow progression or cause regression of atherosclerosis, to control symptoms effectively, to prevent MI and its potential consequences, and to prolong life. Treatment must be individualized, based on the presence of modifiable risk factors, location and severity of existing lesions, type and severity of symptoms, and the patient's age and lifestyle. Often a combination of medical (risk factor modification and medications) and revascularization therapies is used. With the

many advances that have occurred in the treatment of CAD, the death rate from CAD in the United States has declined by 27% in the decade between 1986 and 1996 (American Heart Association, 1998).

Medical Therapy

Attempts to slow progression or cause regression of atherosclerosis are focused on modification of identified risk factors. Important lifestyle modifications include sustained adherence to a low-fat diet, aerobic exercise, stress reduction, and smoking cessation. Angiographic evidence of coronary atherosclerosis regression has been demonstrated after a period of 5 years in patients able to make and sustain such comprehensive lifestyle changes (Ornish et al., 1998).

A diet with a low percentage of calories derived from total fat and saturated fat and low in dietary cholesterol is recommended. The American Heart Association/American College of Cardiology guidelines for modifying cholesterol levels in people with documented CAD indicate that the goal of therapy should be to lower LDL-C levels to 100 mg/dL or below (LaRosa, 1998). If necessary, cholesterol-lowering medications, such as cholestyramine, cholestipol, niacin, gemfibrozil, or lovastatin, may be prescribed to slow disease progression and cause regression of existing lesions. A surgical procedure, partial ileal bypass, may be performed to achieve sustained lowering of LDL-C in severely affected patients in whom drug therapy has failed or caused toxic effects (Buchwald, 1999).

Cessation of smoking is imperative because of the injurious effects of cigarettes. Smoking cessation substantially decreases the risk of future coronary events and, after MI, is associated with an approximately 50% reduction in mortality rates (Vogel, 1998). Weight reduction in obese patients and a consistent exercise program are prescribed to improve cardiac function. The Surgeon General's report on physical activity and health and the National Institutes of Health Consensus Conference on Physical Activity and Cardiovascular Health both recommend regular, moderate physical activity of at least 30 to 45 minutes on most days for all people, including the elderly (Jue & Cunningham, 1998). Regular exercise promotes decreases in body weight, fat stores, blood pressure, total blood cholesterol, serum triglycerides, and LDL-C, and an increase in HDL-C (Franklin & Fletcher, 1997). Cardiac rehabilitation programs provide a structured setting for consistent exercise and ongoing counseling about lifestyle modification to facilitate risk factor reduction.

Pharmacologic treatment of hypertension is a major component of risk reduction in affected people. Antihypertensive agents, including diuretics, beta-adrenergic blocking agents, angiotensin-converting enzyme inhibitors, or calcium channel blocking agents, are used as necessary to achieve a target blood pressure of 140/90 mm Hg. Interventions, such as weight loss, salt restriction, increased dietary potassium, and exercise also have documented beneficial and independent effects on blood pressure (Luke, 1997).

In postmenopausal women, estrogen replacement ther-

TABLE 1-3

Enzyme Elevations After Myocardial Infarction

Finding	Creatine Kinase	Creatine Kinase-MB	Lactate Dehydrogenase
Rises (hours)	4–8	3–12	10
Peaks (hours)	24	24	24–48
Returns to normal (days)	2–3	2–3	10–14

Adapted from Antman EM, Braunwald E, 1997: Acute myocardial infarction. In Braunwald E (ed): Heart Disease: A Textbook of Cardiovascular Medicine, ed. 5. Philadelphia, WB Saunders.

apy may be recommended. Estrogen increases serum HDL-C and decreases LDL-C, thereby reversing the menopausal changes of raised LDL-C and lowered HDL-C (Stone, 1997). Women most likely to benefit from estrogen therapy are those with a history of CAD and with multiple risk factors (Pitt, 1998). The beneficial effects of estrogen, however, must be weighed against a potential increased risk of breast cancer. Long-term data are being collected to assess the benefits and risks of estrogen therapy.

Three major categories of medications are used to reduce frequency of angina and improve exercise tolerance: nitrates, beta-adrenergic blocking agents, and calcium channel blocking agents. Nitrates dilate coronary arteries and decrease cardiac preload. Short-acting nitrates (sublingual, topical, or intravenous nitroglycerin) are used for acute relief of angina. Long-acting oral nitrates (eg, isosorbide dinitrate) are used to provide sustained drug effects and to prevent myocardial ischemia. Because nitrate use is associated with reflex tachycardia that may increase myocardial oxygen demand, a beta-blocking agent is given concomitantly (Simandl & Cohn, 1997).

Beta-blocking medications decrease both heart rate and contractility, thus lowering myocardial oxygen demand so that it does not exceed the fixed supply available through obstructed coronary arteries. Beta-blocking agents have been shown to decrease significantly the risk of cardiovascular mortality in patients who have experienced an MI (Frishman et al., 1984). Calcium channel blocking medications are effective in patients with CAD principally due to vasodilatation that increases coronary blood flow. To differing degrees, individual calcium channel blocking agents also decrease myocardial oxygen consumption by reducing blood pressure, afterload, and contractility (Kutcher, 1991).

Antiplatelet therapy also is recommended in all patients with established CAD (Vogel, 1998). Aspirin irreversibly inactivates platelet cyclooxygenase, thereby impairing platelet aggregation and reducing the release of platelet-derived vasoconstrictors (Passen & Schaer, 1991). The beneficial effects of aspirin have been demonstrated in patients with unstable angina, and after MI and coronary artery bypass grafting (CABG) (Simandl & Cohn, 1997). Antiarrhythmic agents and medications to treat congestive heart failure are necessary in selected patients. In those with variant angina, nitrates and calcium channel antagonists are the most effective agents. Thrombolytic therapy, used in treatment of acute MI, is discussed later in this chapter.

Revascularization Therapy

Revascularization therapy eventually may be necessary to restore blood supply to cardiac muscle that is jeopardized by acute or chronic obstruction of one or more coronary arteries. Current revascularization therapies include catheter-based revascularization (percutaneous coronary intervention [PCI]) and surgical revascularization (ie, CABG). While percutaneous transluminal coronary angioplasty (PTCA) is the standard catheter-based revascularization technique, the term PCI has been

adopted recently to reflect that the procedure often includes other techniques as well (eg, stent placement). The choice of initial invasive therapy, that is, PCI versus CABG, is based primarily on the anatomic appearance, location, number, and severity of coronary artery lesions. However, quality of ventricular function, associated medical problems, and age and lifestyle of the patient also must be considered. In general, PCI is more suitable for many patients with discrete stenosis in one or two major coronary artery branches (ie, single- or double-vessel CAD), whereas CABG is preferable for those with triple-vessel disease or left main coronary artery stenosis (Kirklin & Barratt-Boyes, 1993a).

In some situations, either PCI or CABG is obviously preferable. For example, single-vessel disease almost never is treated with surgical revascularization unless the lesion is in the left anterior descending artery, proximal to the first septal perforator or other branches, or the patient has experienced recurring restenosis after PCI. Conversely, significant left main coronary artery stenosis is almost always treated with CABG because of the large amount of jeopardized left ventricular myocardium. Because of the significant restenosis rate after PCI and the progressive nature of CAD, many patients treated with PCI eventually require CABG.

Percutaneous coronary intervention is a major therapeutic modality in the treatment of CAD. First performed by Gruentzig in 1977, more than 480,000 PCIs are performed each year in the United States (Gruentzig, 1978; American Heart Association, 1998). PCI is performed in a cardiac catheterization laboratory. Vascular access is achieved by percutaneous femoral artery puncture or, less commonly, brachial artery puncture or cutdown (Lincoff & Topol, 1997). A guide catheter is advanced in a retrograde fashion into the target coronary artery and angiographic views of the stenotic lesion are obtained. A balloon-tipped catheter is then inserted over a steerable coronary guidewire and positioned with the balloon across the stenotic lesion. One or more balloon inflations is performed to dilate the atheromatous segment (Fig. 1-3). The duration of balloon inflation may vary from 15 seconds to 2 to 3 minutes or more at the cardiologist's discretion; duration of balloon inflation usually is limited primarily by the development of ischemic signs or symptoms due to interruption of distal coronary blood flow (Lincoff & Topol, 1997). In approximately 70% of patients, conventional balloon angioplasty is accompanied by placement of an intracoronary stent or atherectomy (Johnson et al., 1997) (Fig. 1-4).

Improvements in angioplasty catheters and in the skills of interventional cardiologists, along with the development of intracoronary stenting devices, have made it possible to dilate more complex coronary artery lesions. The procedure is suited to a particular subset of patients, however, and cannot always substitute for CABG. Candidates most appropriate for angioplasty are symptomatic patients with single-vessel disease or single lesions producing the ischemia, that can be effectively dilated (King, 1996). Balloon angioplasty also is useful in dilating distal anastomoses in vein grafts, particularly in those who have undergone recent CABG. Data regarding value of PCI in

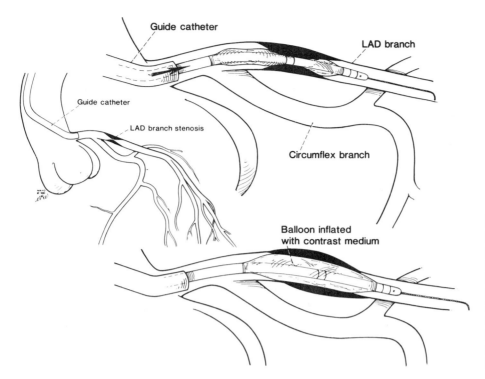

FIGURE 1-3. Diagram of percutaneous transluminal coronary angioplasty. A guide catheter is positioned at left coronary artery ostium; the deflated balloon catheter is advanced over a guidewire through the stenosis in the left anterior descending artery (LAD); the balloon is then inflated. (Vlietstra RE, Holmes DR, 1988: Percutaneous transluminal coronary angioplasty. J Cardiac Surg 3:55)

patients with multivessel disease are being evaluated. Multivessel PCI is known to be associated with a higher initial risk and a greater probability of restenosis (King, 1996). PCI is not advisable in patients with left main coronary artery obstruction or in vessels with less than critical stenoses.

Several alternative techniques for reopening obstructed coronary arteries are available in some catheterization laboratories for primary or adjunctive use. Laser therapy appears to be effective in treating chronic, total occlusions and long-length lesions; its use is limited by a significant incidence of arterial dissection. Atherectomy devices (high-speed rotational, low-speed rotational, and direc-

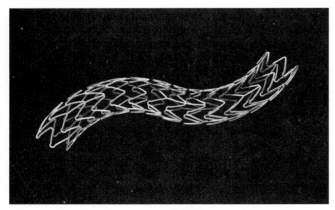

FIGURE 1-4. The ACS Multilink Duet™ Stent, one example of a commercially available device used for stenting the coronary artery during PCI to decrease incidence of restenosis. (Courtesy of Guidant Corporation, Santa Clara, CA)

tional) are available for debulking plaque from coronary artery lesions not well treated by standard balloon dilatation. Long-term data are not yet available about these techniques, and thus their efficacy remains undetermined.

Cardiothoracic surgeons, an operating room, support personnel, and equipment for rapid institution of cardiopulmonary bypass should be readily available in any setting in which PCI is performed. Balloon dilatation of a coronary artery can cause acute occlusion of blood flow due to spasm, dissection, or embolization of thrombotic material. Acute ischemia, infarction, cardiogenic shock, or cardiac arrest may result. In these unusual cases, emergency CABG may be necessary to restore blood flow to jeopardized muscle.

In extreme cases it may be necessary to perform cardiopulmonary resuscitation while transporting a patient from the catheterization laboratory to the operating room. In this situation, every effort is made to place the patient on cardiopulmonary bypass as quickly as possible to protect jeopardized myocardium. Portable cardiopulmonary bypass, using percutaneous femoral cannulation, may be instituted in the catheterization laboratory to stabilize the patient before transportation to the operating room. The operative mortality rate in this group of patients is high and optimal revascularization may be compromised if internal thoracic artery harvest is sacrificed in the interest of expedient revascularization.

In selected high-risk situations, PCI may be performed with arterial and venous cannulae in place for rapid institution of portable cardiopulmonary bypass or with prophylactic institution of percutaneous bypass during the procedure. Such maneuvers help protect the patient in those situations in which iatrogenic arterial occlusion jeopardizes a significant amount of myocardium and is likely to have lethal consequences. However, the practice of using percutaneous cardiopulmonary bypass for this purpose remains controversial because of its potential complications. Although PCI most often is performed as an elective procedure, it also is being performed increasingly as an emergent treatment for acute MI. The use of PCI in the treatment of acute coronary syndromes is discussed later in the chapter.

Death occurs in approximately 1.0% of patients who undergo PCI, nonfatal MI occurs in 4.3%, and emergency surgical revascularization is necessary in 3.4% (Lincoff & Topol, 1997). Most patients who undergo PCI experience substantial, immediate relief of symptoms of myocardial ischemia; angina is decreased or eliminated in 88% and 76% of patients, respectively (Lincoff & Topol, 1997). The most significant long-term limitation of PCI is a restenosis rate of approximately 30% within 6 months. In patients who receive an intracoronary stent during PCI, the restenosis rate is somewhat lower (Han et al., 1996). The major pathologic process leading to restenosis is excessive medial and plaque smooth muscle proliferation as an exaggerated response to angioplasty-induced injury (Schoen, 1997).

Recurrence of ischemic signs or symptoms is most likely during the first year after PCI (Lincoff & Topol, 1997). A number of patients who undergo PCI require subsequent PCI or CABG during this period. For this reason, some cardiologists recommend surveillance coronary angiography 6 months after PCI. Predictors of the need for early CABG after PCI include the number of critical lesions at the time of initial PCI and their location (Johnson et al., 1997).

Surgical revascularization of the coronary arteries, or CABG, is the other major form of revascularization therapy, and has been performed in the United States since the late 1960s. Nearly 370,000 Americans undergo CABG operations each year (American Heart Association, 1998). CABG consists of using internal thoracic arteries or saphenous veins as conduit material to bypass obstructed coronary arteries. Surgical revascularization is discussed in detail in Chapter 15, Surgical Treatment of Coronary Artery Disease.

For patients with diffuse CAD not amenable to catheter or surgical revascularization, transmyocardial and percutaneous laser revascularization techniques are being evaluated as a means of promoting angiogenesis (development of new blood vessels) in the myocardium. In addition, cardiologists and cardiac surgeons are investigating the efficacy of percutaneous and transmyocardial administration of growth factors to promote angiogenesis.

▶ Acute Coronary Syndrome

Definitions and Pathogenesis

Acute coronary syndrome is uncontrolled exacerbation of cardiac muscle ischemia or injury, during which portions of ventricular myocardium are jeopardized but not yet

damaged irreversibly. The syndrome represents a continuum of myocardial pathophysiology, ranging from reversible ischemia to partial- or full-thickness MI with bordering areas of ischemic tissue. Acute coronary syndrome includes the following conditions: (1) unstable angina, defined earlier, and including anginal equivalents such as acute pulmonary edema or ventricular tachycardia; (2) evolving MI; and (3) completed MI with unstable, postinfarction angina.

Evolving MI is defined as prolonged ischemia, usually lasting more than 20 minutes but less than 4 to 6 hours (Roberts et al., 1994). It occurs because of the dynamic nature of myocardial necrosis. After abrupt coronary occlusion, the center of the perfusion defect near the endocardium becomes necrotic first; as uninterrupted ischemia progresses, a wave-front of cell death evolves outward from the mid-subendocardial region toward and eventually encompassing the lateral borders and subepicardial and peripheral regions (Schoen, 1997). The temporal evolution of necrosis and resulting extent of infarct size are influenced by alterations in myocardial oxygen supply and demand during the first several hours after the onset of blood flow occlusion (Roberts et al., 1994) (Fig. 1-5). Although injury becomes irreversible when blood flow occlusion is sustained for 4 to 6 hours of ischemia, most of the damage occurs in the first 2 to 3 hours (Roberts et al., 1994).

Postinfarction angina is unstable angina that occurs after a completed MI. It indicates the presence of reversibly ischemic muscle surrounding the infarct. Approximately 40% to 50% of patients with non–Q-wave MI and 15% of patients with Q-wave MI have early postinfarction angina (Franco & Hammond, 1996).

An acute coronary syndrome usually is precipitated by

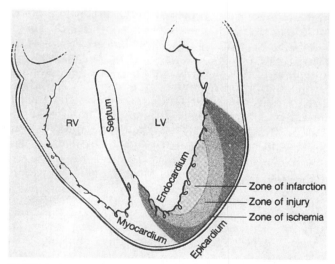

FIGURE 1-5. Diagram demonstrating dynamic nature of myocardial infarction with the potential for spread of muscle necrosis from the subendocardium through the ventricular myocardium. RV, right ventricle; LV, left ventricle. (Woods SL, Underhill SL, Cowan M, 1991: Coronary heart disease. In Patrick ML, Woods SL, Craven RF, et al. [eds]: Medical-Surgical Nursing: Pathophysiological Concepts, ed. 2, p. 695, JB Lippincott)

atherosclerotic plaque disruption with hemorrhage, fissuring, or ulceration (Schoen, 1997). Factors contributing to vessel occlusion include thrombosis, embolization, coronary artery spasm, and platelet aggregation. These factors may act in isolation or in combination with one another. In fact, interactions probably occur among the factors whereby the presence of one triggers the activation of another (Epstein & Palmeri, 1984).

The distinction between the clinical entities that make up acute coronary syndrome is not always clear. However, the common factor among them is the presence of jeopardized, ischemic myocardium. The delivery of oxygen and nutrients to cells in the ischemic area of muscle is compromised, altering cell metabolism and impairing both electrical conduction and ventricular contractility (Black et al., 1990). An acute coronary syndrome that is not reversed leads either to a completed MI or, in the case of postinfarction angina, to extension of the infarct with increased muscle loss.

Treatment

Prompt diagnostic and therapeutic interventions during the period of acute myocardial ischemia greatly increase the probability of salvaging myocardium (preventing infarct or limiting infarct size) and, in many cases, of saving the patient's life. Also, differentiation of ischemia from infarction and identification of the approximate onset of MI have profound implications for timing of therapies that reestablish blood flow. Restoring perfusion to newly infarcted muscle more than 6 hours but within 24 hours after onset of MI can cause a complex pathophysiologic process called *reperfusion injury*. The cascade of biochemical cellular events that results from reperfusion of recently infarcted myocardium increases cell damage and produces significant ventricular dysfunction.

The patient with acute myocardial ischemia must be monitored carefully in a coronary intensive care setting for episodes of angina. Duration of anginal episodes and any associated electrocardiographic changes or symptoms are carefully noted. Severity of discomfort is usually measured using a 1 to 10 rating scale (1 = minimal, 10 = maximal discomfort). ECGs are obtained daily and during episodes of suspected ischemia. CK-MB evaluation is performed after each presumed episode of angina to determine if muscle necrosis (MI) has occurred. Complete bed rest and, if necessary, sedation is used to reduce myocardial oxygen consumption. Narcotic analgesia (morphine sulfate or meperidine) is administered for pain relief. If acute invasive therapy is likely, oral nourishment may be withheld.

Increased understanding of the roles that spasm, thrombosis, and platelet aggregation play in precipitating acute coronary syndromes has broadened therapeutic options to include additional strategies. Thus, therapy is directed not only toward preventing myocardial oxygen demand from exceeding coronary blood supply, but toward limiting coronary vasoconstriction and platelet thrombus formation (Schroeder, 1997). A combination of anti-platelet, vasodilating, thrombolytic, and anticoagulant pharmacologic agents is used commonly in the treatment of acute coronary syndromes. The specific therapy or combination of therapies depends on a number of factors, the most important of which are the extent and severity of CAD, occurrence and timing of MI, and ability to palliate ischemic symptoms.

Aspirin (160 mg of chewable tablets or 325 mg oral tablet) is administered as soon as possible after the onset of an acute coronary syndrome, and aspirin therapy is continued indefinitely (Topol & Van de Werf, 1998). Aspirin decreases both mortality and subsequent MI when given immediately to patients with unstable angina (Schroeder, 1997; ISIS-2 Collaborative Group, 1988). Because beta-adrenergic blocking medications are effective in reducing cardiovascular risk after acute MI, they are initiated or maintained during an acute coronary syndrome. Beneficial effects of angiotensin-converting enzyme inhibitors also are being increasingly recognized (Rapaport & Gheorghiade, 1996).

Heparin usually is administered to prevent further intracoronary thrombosis because nonoccluding thrombus is present in most patients with acute myocardial ischemia (Roberts & Pratt, 1991). Clinical trials investigating the use of heparin for treatment of unstable angina have demonstrated an 85% reduction in the risk of fatal or nonfatal MI (Theroux, 1991). Intravenous nitroglycerin is another standard component of therapy for acute coronary syndrome. It improves coronary artery blood flow and also relieves coronary artery spasm, which may be a contributing factor (Epstein & Palmeri, 1984). Administered as a continuous infusion, nitroglycerin is titrated to suppress anginal episodes and maintain systolic blood pressure in the range of 100 to 110 mm Hg.

Although calcium channel blocking agents have an anti-ischemic effect, their efficacy in the treatment of acute ischemia has not been demonstrated and they may in fact increase mortality when prescribed routinely to patients with acute MI (Antman & Braunwald, 1997). Nifedipine, formerly recommended for acute ischemia, now is specifically contraindicated because of reports of associated acute MI or stroke (Schroeder, 1997). Angina that persists despite maximal pharmacologic therapy may be treated with intra-aortic balloon counterpulsation (IABC). IABC is beneficial in reducing ischemia because it improves coronary blood flow and reduces afterload.

In patients with unstable angina, coronary angiography is performed urgently to identify the severity and extent of coronary artery lesions. Catheter and revascularization PCI or CABG is performed if myocardial ischemia is refractory to medical interventions and if suitable target vessels for revascularization are demonstrated angiographically. If an evolving MI is in progress, it is most likely due to acute thrombotic artery occlusion. Reopening the occluded vessel with thrombolytic therapy or PCI greatly increases the probability of preventing necrosis of jeopardized myocardium, thereby limiting infarct size.

Thrombolytic therapy is the most commonly used

reperfusion therapy for patients with evolving MI. Thrombolytic drugs convert plasminogen to plasmin, causing the degradation of fibrin and fibrinogen, and resulting in clot lysis (Hudak et al., 1998b). If administered during a critical window of time after thrombotic occlusion, thrombolytic agents can produce rapid recanalization of the occluded artery. Numerous clinical trials have shown that timely administration of thrombolytic agents reduces infarct size, preserves left ventricular function, and improves short- and long-term survival rates (Willerson, 1996).

Intravenous thrombolytic agents commonly used in the United States include streptokinase, anisoylated plasminogen streptokinase activator complex, and tissue plasminogen activator (t-PA). Because enzymatic elevation cannot be detected during the critical period of MI evolution, the decision to administer one of these thrombolytic agents is based on a clinical and electrocardiographic diagnosis of MI.

Thrombolytic agents almost always are administered intravenously, often in the emergency department as soon as electrocardiographic evidence of acute MI is obtained. Prompt intravenous administration of thrombolytic therapy is recommended for all patients without contraindications who present within 12 hours of symptom onset and who have ST segment elevation or new-onset left bundle branch block (White & Van de Werf, 1998). Intravenous infusion is more practical because it can be initiated earlier after onset of infarction and emergency coronary angiography is not necessary. Because of the delay involved in initiating cardiac catheterization in patients with acute MI, intracoronary administration is reserved for those in whom coronary thrombosis develops during an angiographic procedure and in whom a coronary catheter is already in place or can be rapidly placed (Antman & Braunwald, 1997).

Successful recanalization is manifest by the combined occurrence of relief of chest pain, resolution of ST segment elevation, and appearance of reperfusion arrhythmias (Black et al., 1990). An intravenous heparin infusion is initiated after administration of thrombolytic therapy to help prevent reocclusion. If the thrombolytic agent is successful in restoring blood flow to jeopardized myocardium and if the patient remains hemodynamically stable, coronary angiography and a definitive plan of therapy for residual disease can be delayed 2 to 3 weeks. However, thrombolytic therapy is effective only in eradicating fresh thrombus and has no effect on underlying atherosclerotic lesions. PCI or CABG to treat underlying disease frequently is necessary once the risk of reperfusion injury is no longer present.

Patients with acute MI who receive early intravenous administration of thrombolytic agents demonstrate improved survival (Antman & Braunwald, 1997). Vessel recanalization is achieved in 60% to 90% of patients; highest efficacy is associated with earliest time of infusion of the thrombolytic agent (Schoen, 1997). The Global Utilization of Streptokinase and Tissue Plasminogen Activator for Occluded Coronary Arteries (GUSTO) trial established intravenous t-PA used in combination with intravenous heparin as the most effective thrombolytic agent (Gersh, 1998). However, timeliness of thrombolytic therapy administration is probably a more important factor in efficacy than is the particular thrombolytic agent. Although considerably more expensive than streptokinase, t-PA is the agent administered to most patients receiving thrombolytic therapy in the United States (Topol & Van de Werf, 1998).

Successful reperfusion is not achieved in all patients and vessel reocclusion can occur. The major complication of thrombolytic medications is bleeding. Patients at increased risk for bleeding complications include those older than 75 years of age or with a history of significant hypertension, recent trauma or surgery, bleeding ulcer or bleeding diathesis, aneurysm, or cerebral vascular accident (Andrien & Lemberg, 1990; Black et al., 1990). Bleeding occurs most commonly at the insertion site of an invasive catheter, but also can occur during median sternotomy when urgent surgical revascularization is necessary. Intracranial hemorrhage, the most serious form of bleeding complication, occurs in less than 1% of patients treated with thrombolytic agents (Becker, 1996).

The other primary reperfusion therapy for restoring blood supply to jeopardized myocardium during evolving MI is PCI. Patients with acute MI who can be brought to a catheterization laboratory within 1 hour of hospital admission may be treated with PCI of the infarct vessel. Immediate PCI provides an alternative therapeutic modality for acute MI, appears to provide morbidity and mortality outcomes comparable with those of thrombolytic therapy, and offers the advantage of early definition of coronary anatomy. The superiority of thrombolytic therapy versus primary PCI remains controversial. Primary PCI is associated with higher rates of Thrombolysis in Myocardial Infarction (TIMI) grade 3 blood flow, and lower rates of reocclusion and recurrent MI, but utilization and outcomes of PCI are more variable among institutions, and benefits of PCI have not been consistently maintained at 6 months (Gersh, 1998). Primary PCI may be a preferable treatment for selected subgroups of patients, such as those with a contraindication to thrombolytic therapy, those with hemodynamic instability, and those at high risk for intracranial bleeding, such as elderly patients (Tiefenbrunn et al., 1998). Emergent CABG as a primary intervention for evolving MI usually is reserved for patients with significant left main coronary artery stenosis or in whom thrombolytic therapy or immediate PCI is contraindicated or unsuccessful. CABG performed in the presence of acute symptoms, particularly with ischemic electrocardiographic change, is associated with a significantly higher risk of perioperative MI (Loop, 1998).

After a completed transmural MI (ie, more than 6 hours after onset), PCI or CABG ideally is delayed at least 48 hours to avoid possible reperfusion injury. Postinfarction angina is treated with medications and IABC to relieve ischemia. However, if the patient continues to have severe postinfarction angina that is unrelieved by medical therapy and IABC, emergent CABG may be necessary to prevent extension of the MI.

► Complications of Myocardial Infarction

Ventricular Dysfunction

Myocardial infarction can be associated with serious, sometimes fatal, complications. If a significant amount of myocardium is damaged by MI, a dysfunctional portion of ventricular muscle, called a *wall motion abnormality,* remains. Either hypokinesis, dyskinesis, or akinesis of the affected segment may be present, compromising the ability of the ventricle to eject an adequate stroke volume. Global or diffuse hypokinesis may be present after massive MI or after MI in a ventricle already damaged by previous infarction. The ventricular dysfunction can result in congestive heart failure, pulmonary edema, or cardiogenic shock. In addition, scarred endocardial tissue associated with a major wall motion abnormality can act as a focus for recurrent ventricular tachycardia or fibrillation. These patients are at increased risk for recurring, symptomatic ventricular tachyarrhythmias or sudden cardiac death.

Cardiogenic shock, or inability of the myocardium to maintain cardiac output at a level necessary for adequate organ perfusion, occurs in 5% to 15% of patients with acute MI and is the leading cause of in-hospital death (Lee & Wechsler, 1996). It occurs after MI when at least 40% of left ventricular muscle mass has been damaged (Ashton et al., 1997). Cardiogenic shock is characterized by a cardiac index less than 2.0 L/min/m^2, systolic blood pressure less than 90 mm Hg, and urine output less than 20 mL/h. It may represent massive, acute damage or a smaller amount of acute damage in association with myocardial necrosis from a prior MI.

Cardiogenic shock after MI causes infarct extension for two reasons. First, ventricular function is compromised to such a degree that coronary blood flow is inadequate to meet myocardial oxygen demands. Second, the reduction in coronary blood flow promotes coronary artery thrombosis. Consequently, cardiogenic shock often is fatal and is almost certain to be so unless aggressive supportive therapy is instituted promptly. Cardiogenic shock after acute MI is associated with a mortality rate of 80% to 100% when treated conservatively and with a mortality rate of 10% to 50% when rapid revascularization to salvage ischemic myocardium is performed (Lee & Wechsler, 1996). IABC is a major component of therapy in almost all patients, along with inotropic and, if tolerated, vasodilating agents. If the patient cannot be stabilized with these interventions, coronary angiography may be undertaken to determine if areas of reversible ischemia are present. If so, emergency PCI or CABG may be performed with the goal of improving ventricular function by relieving ischemia.

Ventricular Aneurysm

Myocardial infarction also can cause formation of *ventricular aneurysm,* a discrete area of necrosed, thinned myocardium that is noncontractile or that contracts paradoxically from the rest of the ventricular muscle. The precise incidence of left ventricular aneurysm formation after acute MI is unknown; data generated before availability of acute interventional therapy indicate an incidence of 10% to 15% (Gay, 1997). Approximately 90% of ventricular aneurysms occur because of occlusion of the left anterior descending artery, which supplies the anterior and apical regions of the left ventricular free wall and the distal portion of the ventricular septum (Cox, 1997). Consequently, most aneurysms involve the anterolateral wall near the apex after a large transmural infarction (Kirklin & Barratt-Boyes, 1993b) (Fig. 1-6).

The presence of a ventricular aneurysm after trans-

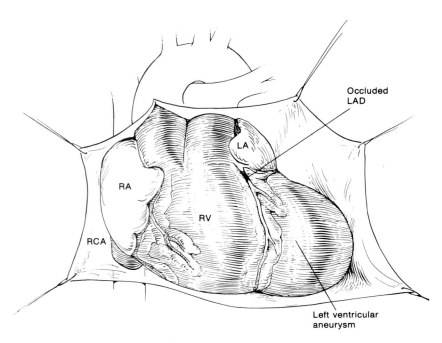

FIGURE 1-6. Typical presentation of a post-infarction left ventricular aneurysm involving the anterolateral left ventricular wall and apex. The illustration depicts the commonly associated finding of occlusion of the proximal left anterior descending (LAD) artery. LA, left atrium; RA, right atrium; RCA, right coronary artery; RV, right ventricle. (With permission from Mundth ED, 1979: Left ventricular aneurysmectomy. In Cohn LH [ed]: Modern Technics in Surgery, p 11–4. Mount Kisco, NY, Futura)

mural MI is suggested by an abnormal cardiac impulse at the apex, a ventricular gallop (S_3), left ventricular enlargement and pulmonary congestion on the chest roentgenogram, and persistent ST segment elevation on the ECG (Gay, 1997). The diagnosis is confirmed with left ventriculography during cardiac catheterization. In some cases, a ventricular aneurysm does not produce symptoms and may not require surgical therapy. It can, however, cause congestive heart failure, angina, or arrhythmias. Because ventricular aneurysms often contain thrombus, they also provide a source of recurrent systemic emboli and may lead to stroke, subsequent MI, or peripheral arterial occlusion. Surgical treatment of ventricular aneurysm is discussed in Chapter 15, Surgical Treatment of Coronary Artery Disease.

Thromboembolism

The incidence of *deep venous thrombosis* and *pulmonary embolism* has decreased owing to the frequent use of intravenous heparin and thrombolytic therapy and the trend toward early ambulation after MI (Hochmann & Gersh, 1998). It is most likely in patients with congestive heart failure, cardiogenic shock, or preexisting venous disease, and in elderly patients (Chung, 1988). In addition to deep venous thrombosis, thrombotic material is likely to collect along endocardial surfaces of akinetic or dyskinetic infarcted ventricular muscle. Portions of this thrombotic material, known as mural thrombus, can embolize to one of the vital organs or to the extremities. The risk for systemic embolization from mural thrombus continues, not just in the immediate postinfarction period, but indefinitely (Stratton & Resnick, 1987).

Acute Mechanical Defects

Acute mechanical complications of MI include mitral valve regurgitation and rupture of the left ventricular free wall or septum. All three of these complications usually produce significant hemodynamic instability and often necessitate emergency operative intervention. As a group, mechanical defects caused by rupture of acutely infarcted tissue are estimated to account for approximately 15% of deaths resulting from acute MI (Antman & Braunwald, 1997).

Acute *mitral regurgitation* can develop because of one of several different pathophysiologic mechanisms, including papillary muscle dysfunction, papillary muscle rupture, or annular dilatation. Two papillary muscles (posteromedial and anterolateral) support the mitral valve. Because both have chordal attachments to each of the mitral valve leaflets, dysfunction or rupture of either papillary muscle can affect function of both valve leaflets (Roberts, 1980). Mitral regurgitation secondary to papillary muscle dysfunction may represent transient muscle ischemia or necrosis. Papillary muscle ischemia sometimes is reversed successfully by reestablishing blood flow to the papillary muscle with thrombolytic therapy,

PCI, or CABG. If so, valve competence is likely to be restored and surgical valve repair or replacement may be avoided.

Actual rupture of a papillary muscle also can occur. In 75% of cases, rupture occurs in the posteromedial papillary muscle; in 25%, the anterolateral papillary muscle is ruptured (Kirklin & Barratt-Boyes, 1993c). Most commonly, rupture involves only one or two of the apical heads of a papillary muscle. Less often, one of the papillary muscles is completely disrupted, resulting in flailing of both valve leaflets (Kirklin & Barratt-Boyes, 1993c). Acute annular dilatation of the mitral valve occurs less commonly for several reasons: (1) the surface area of the valve leaflets is approximately twice that of the orifice size and is adequate to maintain valvular competence despite some degree of annular dilatation; (2) the mitral valve annulus contracts during ventricular systole; and (3) the fibrous skeleton surrounding the annulus makes dilatation at the base of the left ventricle less than in its midportion (Roberts, 1980).

Acute mitral regurgitation is suggested by a new holosystolic murmur and progressive congestive heart failure after MI. These findings also occur with acute rupture of the ventricular septum, and further diagnostic testing is necessary to differentiate the two conditions. Because of the high degree of diagnostic accuracy possible with color-flow Doppler imaging, Doppler echocardiography usually is performed to differentiate acute mitral regurgitation and ventricular septal rupture. The procedure can be rapidly performed at the bedside.

Diagnosis also can be achieved with oxygen saturation measurements using a pulmonary artery catheter. Oxygen saturation levels from the proximal and distal ports of the catheter are measured to detect a "step-up" or increase in oxygen saturation between the right atrium and pulmonary artery. Oxygen saturation levels are normally the same until blood travels through the pulmonary vasculature. In patients with acute mitral regurgitation, pulmonary artery blood samples reveal no step-up in oxygen saturation. A step-up indicates left-to-right shunting of oxygenated blood at the ventricular level (ie, a ventricular septal defect). Patients with mitral regurgitation also demonstrate large "v" waves on the pulmonary capillary wedge and pulmonary artery tracings. However, v waves indicative of mitral regurgitation do not eliminate the diagnosis of ventricular septal defect. Mitral regurgitation due to left ventricular dysfunction also is present in as many as 33% of patients with acute ventricular septal rupture (Madsen & Daggett, 1997).

Depending on the severity of valvular incompetence, IABC may be necessary to support cardiac function until the mitral valve is surgically repaired or replaced. Before surgical intervention, it is preferable to perform coronary angiography for identification of coexisting coronary artery lesions. However, patients with acute ischemic mitral regurgitation may be too critically ill to withstand cardiac catheterization. In rare cases, emergency mitral valve replacement may be performed without preoperative definition of the coronary artery anatomy.

Rupture of the ventricular myocardium is an unusual

complication that occurs when necrotic tissue in the area of infarction becomes too weakened to withstand intraventricular pressure. Myocardial rupture occurs more frequently in women than in men, in older than in younger people, after recurrent MI, and in patients with multivessel disease (Loop, 1998). Depending on the area of infarct, either the free wall or ventricular septum may rupture. Rupture in either location occurs only with transmural infarction, usually within 1 week of acute MI, and classically in the periphery of the infarct, at the junction of necrotic and healthy tissue (Roberts, 1980).

Rupture of the free wall of infarcted ventricle occurs in as many as 10% of patients who die in the hospital of acute MI (Antman & Braunwald, 1997). It nearly always is fatal. Ventricular wall rupture is treated with immediate operative intervention. Portable cardiopulmonary bypass may be necessary to support the patient during transport to the operating room and until standard cardiopulmonary bypass is instituted. Rarely, the rupture is small and bleeding is contained by pericardium. Such a contained rupture forms a pseudoaneurysm (ie, false aneurysm). The term *pseudoaneurysm* denotes that the aneurysm wall consists of pericardium and not myocardium, as would be the case with a true ventricular aneurysm. The presence of a pseudoaneurysm is established with left ventriculography (Frances et al., 1998). Pseudoaneurysm also is treated with surgical resection because delayed rupture can occur at any time.

Rupture of the interventricular septum is estimated to occur in approximately 2% of patients with acute MI (Antman & Braunwald, 1997). However, survival from septal rupture is more likely than after free wall rupture if recognition and treatment are prompt. *Acute septal rupture* usually is associated with complete occlusion of a coronary artery and extensive transmural infarction in a patient with less diffuse CAD and thus less well developed collateral vessels (Madsen & Daggett, 1996). The resulting acute ventricular septal defect most commonly occurs in the apical septum after an anterior MI. Inferior infarctions are associated with rupture of the basal septum. Ventricular septal rupture usually occurs within 2 weeks of MI (Rosengart & Isom, 1998).

The diagnosis of ventricular septal defect is suggested by a new holosystolic murmur, particularly in the presence of hypotension, congestive heart failure, or cardiogenic shock after acute MI. Chest pain may be noted in as many as one third of patients (Rosengart & Isom, 1998). Acute mitral regurgitation secondary to left ventricular dysfunction also may be present, particularly in patients with rupture of the posterior septum (Madsen & Daggett, 1996). The diagnosis of ventricular septal defect is confirmed by Doppler echocardiography or by measurement of pulmonary artery oxygen saturation, as previously described.

An intra-aortic balloon catheter almost always is placed on detection of the defect. Counterpulsation is important in maintaining hemodynamic stability until surgical repair is undertaken. It decreases afterload, thereby increasing forward flow and reducing left-to-right shunting through the defect. Intravenous pharmacologic support of cardiac function usually is required as well. Mortality associated with acute ventricular septal defect is high; without surgical intervention, 25% of patients die within 24 hours, 50% die within 1 week, and only 20% survive more than 4 weeks (Madsen & Daggett, 1997; Kirklin & Barratt-Boyes, 1993d).

In most patients with acute ventricular septal defects, hemodynamic instability develops rapidly. Surgical closure of the defect is performed immediately in hemodynamically unstable patients. However, timing of operation in relation to MI greatly affects operative mortality and remains controversial in hemodynamically stable patients. Some surgeons favor emergency operative repair as soon as the defect is diagnosed because precipitous, fatal hemodynamic deterioration can occur at any time. Other surgeons believe that operative repair should be delayed for several weeks unless hemodynamic deterioration occurs. Delay of the operation allows time for the myocardium to recover from the infarct and for the defect edges to strengthen, making the procedure technically easier. Waiting several weeks improves the likelihood of surviving the operation, but precipitous hemodynamic deterioration can occur at any time. Patients who might have survived with early surgical repair may die during the waiting period (Komeda et al., 1990). In addition, in the presence of cardiogenic shock, operative mortality for ventricular septal defect repair rises to 40% to 50%, in contrast to a 10% to 20% mortality rate when cardiogenic shock is not present (Rosengart & Isom, 1998).

The traditional method for repair of an acute ventricular septal defect includes infarctectomy (ie, resection of infarcted muscle) and closure of the septal defect using a Dacron patch. A newer operative technique consists of suturing glutaraldehyde-fixed bovine pericardium to endocardium around the infarcted muscle and simple ventricular closure; the necrotic muscle is not excised. This type of repair with a bioprosthetic endocardial patch is technically easier and is associated with a lower operative mortality rate (Loop, 1998).

REFERENCES

American Heart Association, 1998: 1999 Heart and Stroke Statistical Update. Dallas, American Heart Association

Andrien P, Lemberg L, 1990: Thrombolytic therapy in acute myocardial infarction. Heart Lung 19:1

Antman EM, Braunwald E, 1997: Acute myocardial infarction. In Braunwald E (ed): Heart Disease: A Textbook of Cardiovascular Medicine, ed. 5. Philadelphia, WB Saunders

Ashton RC, Oz MC, Rose EA, 1997: Surgery for acute myocardial infarction-cardiogenic shock. In Edmunds LH Jr (ed): Cardiac Surgery in the Adult. New York, McGraw-Hill

Becker RC, 1996: Hematologic and coagulation considerations in patients with cardiac disease. In Kvetan V, Dantzker DR (eds): The Critically Ill Cardiac Patient: Multisystem Dysfunction and Management. Philadelphia, Lippincott-Raven

Black L, Coombs VJ, Townsend SN, 1990: Reperfusion and reperfusion injury in acute myocardial infarction. Heart Lung 19:3

Brown G, Albers JJ, Fisher LD, et al., 1990: Regression of coronary artery disease as a result of intensive lipid-lowering therapy in men with high levels of apolipoprotein B. N Engl J Med 323:1289

Buchwald H, 1999: Role of the surgeon in managing hypercholesterolemia. Surgery 125:465

Chung EK, 1988: Coronary artery disease. In Chung EK: Manual of Acute Cardiac Disorders. Boston, Butterworths

Cox JL, 1997. Surgical management of left ventricular aneurysms: A clarification of the similarities and differences between the Jatene and Dor techniques. Semin Thorac Cardiovasc Surg 9:131

Epstein SE, Palmeri ST, 1984: Mechanisms contributing to precipitation of unstable angina and acute myocardial infarction: Implications regarding therapy. Am J Cardiol 54:1245

Farmer JA, Gotto AM Jr, 1997: Dyslipidemia and other risk factors for coronary artery disease. In Braunwald E (ed): Heart Disease: A Textbook of Cardiovascular Medicine, ed. 5. Philadelphia, WB Saunders

Fisch C, 1997: Electrocardiography. In Braunwald E (ed): Heart Disease: A Textbook of Cardiovascular Medicine, ed. 5. Philadelphia, WB Saunders

Frances C, Romero A, Grady D, 1998: Left ventricular pseudoaneurysm. J Am Coll Cardiol 32:557

Franco KL, Hammond GL, 1996: Surgical indications for coronary revascularization. In Baue AE, Geha AS, Hammond GL, et al. (eds): Glenn's Thoracic and Cardiovascular Surgery, ed. 6. Stamford, CT, Appleton & Lange

Franklin BA, Fletcher GF, 1997: The effect of exercise on the heart and the athlete's heart. In Alpert JS (ed): Cardiology for the Primary Care Physician, ed. 2. Philadelphia, Current Medicine

Frishman WH, Furberg CD, Friedewald WT, 1984: β-Adrenergic blockade for survivors of acute myocardial infarction. N Engl J Med 310:830

Fuster V, Badimon JJ, Badimon L, 1992: Clinical-pathological correlations of coronary disease progression and regression. Circulation 86(Suppl III):III-1

Ganz P, Braunwald E, 1997: Coronary blood flow and myocardial ischemia. In Braunwald E (ed): Heart Disease: A Textbook of Cardiovascular Medicine, ed. 5. Philadelphia, WB Saunders

Gay WA Jr, 1997: Ventricular aneurysm. In Sabiston DC Jr (ed): Textbook of Surgery: The Biological Basis of Modern Surgical Practice, ed. 15. Philadelphia, WB Saunders

Gersh BJ, 1998: Current issues in reperfusion therapy. Am J Cardiol 82(8B):3P

Gersh BJ, Braunwald E, Rutherford JD, 1997: Chronic coronary artery disease. In Braunwald E (ed): Heart Disease: A Textbook of Cardiovascular Medicine, ed. 5. Philadelphia, WB Saunders

Gheorghiade M, Bonow RO, 1998: Chronic heart failure in the United States: A manifestation of coronary artery disease. Circulation 97:282

Goe MR, 1995: Laboratory tests using blood. In Woods SL, Froelicher ES, Halpenny CJ, Motzer SU, (eds): Cardiac Nursing, ed. 3. Philadelphia, JB Lippincott

Goldschlager NF, 1988: Acute myocardial infarction. In Luce JM, Pierson DJ (eds): Critical Care Medicine. Philadelphia, WB Saunders

Gottlieb SO, 1992: Cardiovascular benefits of smoking cessation. Heart Dis Stroke 1:173

Gruentzig A, 1978: Transluminal dilatation of coronary artery stenosis. Lancet 1:263

Han JJ, Ayres S, Hess ML, 1996: Pathophysiology of cardiac insufficiency and failure. In Kvetan V, Dantzker DR (eds): The Critically Ill Cardiac Patient. Philadelphia, Lippincott-Raven

Hillis LD, Lange RA, Winniford MD, Page RL, 1995a: Coronary arterial spasm. In Manual of Clinical Problems in Cardiology, ed. 5. Boston, Little, Brown

Hillis LD, Lange RA, Winniford MD, Page RL, 1995b: Atrioventricular block complicating myocardial infarction. In Manual of Clinical Problems in Cardiology, ed. 5. Boston, Little, Brown

Hillis LD, Lange RA, Winniford MD, Page RL, 1995c: Detection and quantitation of myocardial infarction. In Manual of Clinical Problems in Cardiology, ed. 5. Boston, Little, Brown

Hochman JS, Gersh BJ, 1998: Acute myocardial infarction: Complications. In Topol EJ (ed): Comprehensive Cardiovascular Medicine. Philadelphia, Lippincott Williams & Wilkins

Hudak CM, Gallo BM, Morton PG, 1998a: Anatomy and physiology of the cardiovascular system. In Critical Care Nursing: A Holistic Approach, ed. 7. Philadelphia, Lippincott Williams & Wilkins

Hudak CM, Gallo BM, Morton PG, 1998b: Acute myocardial infarction. In Critical Care Nursing: A Holistic Approach, ed. 7. Philadelphia, Lippincott Williams & Wilkins

ISIS-2 (Second International Study of Infarct Survival) Collaborative Group, 1988: Randomised trial of intravenous streptokinase, oral aspirin, both, or neither among 17,187 cases of suspected acute myocardial infarction: ISIS-2. Lancet 1:349

Johnson RG, Sirois C, Thurer RL, et al., 1997: Predictors of CABG within one year of successful PTCA: a retrospective, case-control study. Ann Thorac Surg 64:3

Jue NH, Cunningham SL, 1998: Stages of exercise behavior change at two time periods following coronary artery bypass surgery. Prog Cardiovasc Nurs 13:23

Kessler KM, 1991: Cardiac arrhythmias following myocardial infarction. In Hurst JW (ed): Current Therapy in Cardiovascular Disease, ed. 3. Philadelphia, BC Decker

King SB, 1996: Indications for nonsurgical coronary revascularization. In Baue AE, Geha AS, Hammond GL, et al. (eds): Glenn's Thoracic and Cardiovascular Surgery, ed. 6. Stamford, CT, Appleton & Lange

Kirklin JW, Barratt-Boyes BG, 1993a: Stenotic arteriosclerotic coronary artery disease. In Cardiac Surgery, ed. 2. New York, Churchill Livingstone

Kirklin JW, Barratt-Boyes BG, 1993b: Left ventricular aneurysm. In Cardiac Surgery, ed. 2. New York, Churchill Livingstone

Kirklin JW, Barratt-Boyes BG, 1993c: Mitral incompetence from ischemic heart disease. In Cardiac Surgery, ed. 2. New York, Churchill Livingstone

Kirklin JW, Barratt-Boyes BG, 1993d: Postinfarction ventricular septal defect. In Cardiac Surgery, ed. 2. New York, Churchill Livingstone

Komeda M, Fremes SE, David TE, 1990: Surgical repair of postinfarction ventricular septal defect. Circulation 82(Suppl IV):IV-243

Kutcher MA, 1991: Angina pectoris: Stable. In Hurst JW (ed): Current Therapy in Cardiovascular Disease, ed. 3. Philadelphia, BC Decker

LaRosa JC, 1998: Lipid lowering. In LaRosa JC (ed): Medical Management of Atherosclerosis. New York, Marcel Dekker

Lee KF, Wechsler AS, 1996: Cardiogenic shock secondary to myocardial infarction. Baue AE, Geha AS, Hammond GL, et al. (eds): Glenn's Thoracic and Cardiovascular Surgery, ed. 6. Stamford, CT, Appleton & Lange

Levy D, Wilson PW, 1998: Atherosclerotic cardiovascular disease: An epidemiologic perspective. In Topol EJ (ed): Comprehensive Cardiovascular Medicine. Philadelphia, Lippincott Williams & Wilkins

Lincoff AM, Topol EJ, 1997: Interventional catheterization techniques. In Braunwald E (ed): Heart Disease: A Textbook of Cardiovascular Medicine, ed. 5. Philadelphia, WB Saunders

Loop FD, 1998: Coronary artery bypass surgery. In Topol EJ (ed): Comprehensive Cardiovascular Medicine. Philadelphia, Lippincott Williams & Wilkins

Luke RG, 1997: Evaluation of the patient with hypertension. In Alpert JS (ed): Cardiology for the Primary Care Physician, ed. 2. Philadelphia, Current Medicine

Madsen JC, Daggett WM Jr, 1997: Postinfarction ventricular septal defect and free wall rupture. In Edmunds LH Jr (ed): Cardiac Surgery in the Adult. New York, McGraw-Hill.

Madsen JC, Dagget WM Jr, 1996: Postinfarction ventricular septal rupture. In Baue AE, Geha AS, Hammond GL, et al. (eds): Glenn's Thoracic and Cardiovascular Surgery, ed. 6. Stamford, CT, Appleton & Lange

Mehta JL, Saldeen TG, Rand K, 1998: Interactive role of infection, inflammation and traditional risk factors in atherosclerosis and coronary artery disease. J Am Coll Cardiol 31:1217

Nixon JV, 1997: The aging heart. In Alpert JS (ed): Cardiology for the Primary Care Physician, ed. 2. Philadelphia, Current Medicine

Ornish D, Scherwitz LW, Billings JH, et al., 1998: Intensive lifestyle changes for reversal of coronary heart disease. JAMA 280:2001

Paraskos JA, 1997: Evaluation of the patient with chest pain. In Alpert JS (ed): Cardiology for the Primary Care Physician, ed. 2. Philadelphia, Current Medicine

Passen EL, Schaer GL, 1991: Acute myocardial infarction. In Parrillo JE (ed): Current Therapy in Critical Care Medicine, ed. 2. Philadelphia, BC Decker

Peberdy MA, Ornato JP, 1992: Coronary artery disease in women. Heart Dis Stroke 1:315

Pitt B, 1998: Adjunctive nonlipid-lowering strategies for the therapy of atherosclerosis. In LaRosa JC (ed): Medical Management of Atherosclerosis. New York, Marcel Dekker

Rackley CE, Schlant RC, 1994: Prevention of coronary artery disease. In Schlant RC, Alexander RW, et al. (eds): The Heart, ed. 8. New York, McGraw-Hill

Rapaport E, Gheorghiade M, 1996: Pharmacologic therapies after myocardial infarction. Am J Med 101:4A61S

Roberts R, Morris D, Pratt CM, Alexander RW, 1994: Pathophysiology, recognition and treatment of acute myocardial infarction and its complications. In Schlant RC, Alexander RW, et al. (eds): The Heart, ed. 8. New York, McGraw-Hill

Roberts R, Pratt CM, 1991: Medical treatment of coronary artery disease. In Roberts R (ed): Coronary Heart Disease and Risk Factors. Mount Kisco, NY, Futura

Roberts WC, 1980: Morphologic features of certain myocardial complications. In Moran JM, Michaelis LL (eds): Surgery for the Complications of Myocardial Infarction. New York, Grune & Stratton

Rosen CJ, 1997: The heart and endocrine diseases. In Alpert JS (ed): Cardiology for the Primary Care Physician, ed. 2. Philadelphia, Current Medicine

Rosengart TK, Isom OW, 1998: Ventricular septal defect. In Kaiser LR, Kron IL, Spray TL (eds): Mastery of Cardiothoracic Surgery. Philadelphia, Lippincott Williams & Wilkins

Ross R, 1997: The pathogenesis of atherosclerosis. In Braunwald E (ed): Heart Disease: A Textbook of Cardiovascular Medicine, ed. 5. Philadelphia, WB Saunders

Schoen FJ, 1997: Pathologic considerations in the surgery of adult heart disease. In Edmunds LH Jr (ed): Cardiac Surgery in the Adult. New York, McGraw-Hill

Schroeder JS, 1997: Unstable angina and non-Q-wave myocardial infarction. In Alpert JS (ed): Cardiology for the Primary Care Physician, ed. 2. Philadelphia, Current Medicine

Schwarz ER, Hammerman H, Kloner RA, 1997: Q-wave myocardial infarction. In Alpert JS (ed): Cardiology for the Primary Care Physician, ed. 2. Philadelphia, Current Medicine

Simandl S, Cohn PF, 1997: Chronic ischemic heart disease. In Alpert JS (ed): Cardiology for the Primary Care Physician, ed. 2. Philadelphia, Current Medicine

Smith HC, Gersh BJ, 1997: Indications for revascularization. In Edmunds LH Jr (ed): Cardiac Surgery in the Adult. New York, McGraw-Hill

Spencer FA, Goldberg RJ, Becker RC, et al., 1998: Seasonal distribution of acute myocardial infarction in the Second National Registry of Myocardial Infarction. J Am Coll Cardiol 31:1226

Spencer FC, Galloway AC, Colvin SB, 1995: Bypass grafting for coronary artery disease. In Sabiston DC, Spencer FC (eds): Surgery of the Chest, ed. 6. Philadelphia, WB Saunders

Stone NJ, 1997: Approach to the patient with hyperlipidemia. In Alpert JS (ed): Cardiology for the Primary Care Physician, ed. 2. Philadelphia, Current Medicine

Stone NJ, Green D, 1980: Sustaining factors in atherosclerosis. In Moran JM, Michaelis LL (eds): Surgery for the Complications of Myocardial Infarction. New York, Grune & Stratton

Stratton JR, Resnick AD, 1987: Increased embolic risk in patients with left ventricular thrombi. Circulation 75:5

Taylor AE, Johnson DC, Kazemi H, 1992: Environmental tobacco smoke and cardiovascular disease. Circulation 86:699

Theroux P, 1991: Management of unstable angina. In Roberts R (ed): Coronary Heart Disease and Risk Factors. Mount Kisco, NY, Futura

Tiefenbrunn AJ, Chandra NC, French WJ, et al., 1998: Clinical experience with primary percutaneous transluminal coronary angioplasty compared with alteplase (recombinant tissue-type plasminogen activator) in patients with acute myocardial infarction. J Am Coll Cardiol 31:1240

Topol EJ, Van de Werf FJ, 1998: Acute myocardial infarction: Early diagnosis and management. In Topol EJ (ed): Comprehensive Cardiovascular Medicine. Philadelphia, Lippincott Williams & Wilkins

Vogel RA, 1998: Prevention of atherosclerosis in clinical practice. In LaRosa JC (ed): Medical Management of Atherosclerosis. New York, Marcel Dekker

Vokonas PS, Kannel WB, 1997: Risk factors for and prevention of atherosclerotic cardiovascular disease. In Alpert JS (ed): Cardiology for the Primary Care Physician, ed. 2. Philadelphia, Current Medicine

Weintraub WS, Stein B, Kosinski A, et al., 1998: Outcome of coronary bypass surgery versus coronary angioplasty in diabetic patients with multivessel coronary artery disease. J Am Coll Cardiol 31:10

White HD, Van de Werf FJ, 1998: Thrombolysis for acute myocardial infarction. Circulation 16:1632

Willerson JT, 1996: Myocardial revascularization without thoracotomy. In Edmunds LH Jr (ed): Cardiac Surgery in the Adult. New York, McGraw-Hill

Wynne J, Braunwald E, 1997: The cardiomyopathies and myocarditides. In Braunwald E (ed): Heart Disease: A Textbook of Cardiovascular Medicine, ed. 5. Philadelphia, WB Saunders

2

Valvular Heart Disease

V*alvular heart disease* (VHD) is a significant health problem in the United States, although it is far less common than coronary artery disease. It is characterized by impaired function of one or more of the four cardiac valves. Either or both of two functional abnormalities may be present: stenosis (impeded forward flow through an opened valve) or regurgitation (backward leaking of blood through a closed valve). When both stenosis and regurgitation are present in the same valve, one process usually predominates (Schoen, 1997).

Valvular heart disease affects the left-sided valves (mitral and aortic) more commonly than those on the right (tricuspid and pulmonic). Mitral valve disease is most prevalent. Tricuspid valve disease usually occurs secondary to left-sided valvular lesions. Pulmonic valve disease is rare in adults. In some patients, more than one valve is diseased. For example, end-stage mitral regurgitation may cause right ventricular enlargement that leads to annular dilatation and regurgitation of the tricuspid valve.

▶ Etiologies

A variety of etiologies can lead to VHD, including myxomatous degeneration, congenital malformation, infective endocarditis, rheumatic heart disease, and other acquired disorders. In most cases, pathologic changes in valvular endothelium occur gradually and the heart compensates for progressively worsening valve function for many years. Less commonly, etiologic factors, such as myocardial infarction or infective endocarditis, cause acute valvular dysfunction and precipitous hemodynamic instability.

Mitral Valve Prolapse and Myxomatous Degeneration

Mitral valve prolapse (MVP) is the systolic billowing of one or both mitral leaflets into the left atrium with or without mitral regurgitation (Bonow et al., 1998). Also known as Barlow's syndrome, it is the most commonly diagnosed valvular deformity in the United States, occurring in 6% to 10% of young women and in 4% of young men (American Heart Association, 1998). The cause of MVP is likely congenital, due to defective fibroelastic connective tissue in the leaflets, chordae tendineae, and annulus (Fann et al., 1997). Although usually a benign condition, MVP comprises a continuum of degrees of valvular abnormality. In its most common form, it is not associated with valvular regurgitation or any significant clinical sequelae. It is detected only by the presence of an auscultatory ejection click and its characteristic echocardiographic features. Only 5% to 10% of people with MVP experience progression of mitral regurgitation, and most remain asymptomatic (Fann et al., 1997).

Despite the benignity of MVP in most people, myxomatous valvular degeneration occurs in others and is an important cause of VHD. Myxomatous degeneration is the leading cause of mitral regurgitation requiring surgical intervention in the United States (Gillinov et al., 1998). Affected patients have severely myxomatous and redundant valve leaflets that prolapse into the left atrium during systole. These patients are likely to have clinically significant mitral regurgitation, which may be chronic or which may increase acutely if a chordal structure tears. Also, because the anterior leaflet of the mitral valve and the aortic annulus have a fibrous continuity, patients with advanced myxomatous changes of the mitral valve often have annuloaortic ectasia (ie, enlargement of the aortic annulus) (David, 1998).

Congenital Malformation

Except for MVP, which is likely a congenital abnormality, the most common congenital valve malformation is a bicuspid aortic valve (Fig. 2-1). Normally, the aortic valve is tricuspid, composed of three leaflets or cusps. If one or two of the valve commissures is absent, the valve is bicuspid or unicuspid, respectively. Bicuspid aortic valves are estimated to occur in 2% of the general population (Perloff, 1998). The abnormality is most common in men and may be accompanied by other congenital cardiac defects. A bicuspid aortic valve is predisposed to calcification and is susceptible to infective endocarditis (Nugent et al., 1994). During childhood, the abnormal valve frequently produces no hemodynamic dysfunction. As the person ages, however, progressive sclerosis, thickening, and calcification may cause the valve to become increasingly stenotic. A bicuspid aortic valve also may become regurgitant owing to progressive fibrosis and calcification of the leaflets or because of leaflet distortion (Glower, 1995).

Congenital pulmonic valve stenosis also can occur. The valve usually appears dome shaped during systole with a central opening and fused commissures. Hemodynamically significant pulmonic stenosis almost always is corrected during childhood and thus is rare in adults. Congenital mitral valve malformation is rare. Marfan's syndrome, a heritable connective tissue disorder, can produce myxomatous valvular degeneration and can be

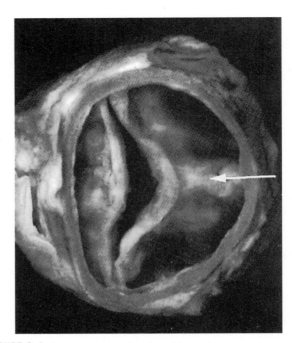

FIGURE 2-1. Bicuspid aortic valve viewed from above; note the raphe or seam (*arrow*) fusing the right and left coronary leaflets. The valve is also thickened and stenotic. (Hurst JW, Nugent EW, Anderson RH, Wilcox BR, 1988: Congenital heart disease. In Hurst JW, Anderson RH, Becker AE, Wilcox BR [eds]: Atlas of the Heart, p. 3.39. London, Times Mirror International)

associated with aortic, mitral, or tricuspid valve regurgitation. Marfan's syndrome is discussed in more detail in Chapter 3, Disorders of the Thoracic Aorta.

Infective Endocarditis

Infective endocarditis is localized infection of one or more of the cardiac valves. It occurs when organisms (usually bacteria, but occasionally fungi) enter the bloodstream and invade cardiac valvular endothelial tissue. Although the term *subacute bacterial endocarditis* traditionally was used to describe this condition, *infective endocarditis* has been adopted more recently because the condition is usually acute and the invading pathogen may not be bacterial.

Bacteria or other organisms can enter the bloodstream from the mouth, gastrointestinal tract, skin, or contaminated needles used for venipuncture. Bacteremia may occur spontaneously, may complicate a focal infection, or may result from surgical or dental instrumentation involving mucosal surfaces or contaminated tissues (Dajani et al., 1997). The frequency of bacteremia is highest with dental and oral procedures, intermediate with procedures involving the genitourinary tract, and lowest with gastrointestinal diagnostic procedures (Bonow et al., 1998). Ordinary dental procedures in susceptible people are one of the most common sources of infection. However, in many cases the precipitating cause of the bacteremia is never identified.

In 55% to 75% of cases, native valve endocarditis occurs in patients with a valve or valves already damaged by another disease, such as MVP, rheumatic endocarditis, congenital malformation, or degenerative heart disease (Karchmer, 1997). Normal cardiac valves, however, also are susceptible when exposed to particularly virulent organisms (eg, *Staphylococcus aureus*), when the person is immunocompromised, or when there is repetitive blood contamination from intravenous drug abuse. Native valve endocarditis in patients who are not intravenous drug abusers usually is caused by streptococci or *S. aureus;* in intravenous drug abusers, *S. aureus* is the predominant causative organism, but *Pseudomonas aeruginosa,* other gram-negative bacilli, and *Candida* species are other important causes (Karchmer, 1997).

The infective process causes erosion of leaflet tissue and deposition of fibrin, leukocytes, and platelets on the leaflet, forming particulate matter known as a *vegetation* (Fig. 2-2). Leaflet perforation may occur, or, in the case of mitral or tricuspid valve endocarditis, chordae tendineae may be destroyed. The degree of valvular damage depends on the pathogenicity of the infecting organism, the duration of infection, and the timeliness of appropriate antibiotic therapy (Larbalestier et al., 1992). Especially with the most virulent organisms, such as *S. aureus,* infection often extends beyond endocardial tissue of the valve leaflets to form intramyocardial abscesses. In aortic valve endocarditis, the infective process may involve the adjacent aortic root, resulting in periannular abscess or intracardiac fistula formation.

Rheumatic Heart Disease

Chronic *rheumatic valvular disease* is the result of an inflammatory process caused by acute rheumatic fever. Rheumatic fever or rheumatic heart disease affects an estimated 1.8 million Americans (American Heart Associ-

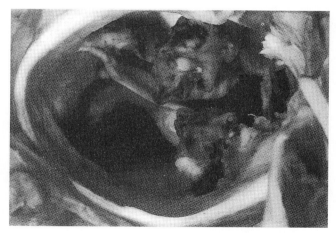

FIGURE 2-2. Infective endocarditis of this aortic valve has caused extensive destruction of leaflet tissue with resultant acute aortic regurgitation. (Hurst JW, Rackley CE, Becker AE, Wilcox BR, 1988: Valvar heart disease. In Hurst JW, Anderson RH, Becker AE, Wilcox BR [eds]: Atlas of the Heart, p. 4.18. London, Times Mirror International)

ation, 1998). The incidence has decreased substantially in the United States owing to widespread, effective prophylaxis against rheumatic fever in children. In developing countries, however, which contain two thirds of the world's population, rheumatic fever is responsible for almost half of cardiovascular deaths in all age groups and is the leading cause of death in the first five decades of life (Kaplan, 1994). In these countries, a rapid and progressive form of valvular disease may follow rheumatic fever in children and young adults (John et al., 1990).

Acute rheumatic fever occurs primarily in children between 5 and 15 years of age (Kaplan, 1994). The exact mechanism for its development is not clear, but the primary etiologic factor is known to be a group A streptococcal infection of the pharynx, more commonly known as *strep throat.* The syndrome is insidious, producing generalized malaise, low-grade fevers, and arthralgias. Diagnosis is based on a constellation of clinical and laboratory findings. Patients with a presumed diagnosis of acute rheumatic fever are given penicillin or another appropriate antibiotic to treat the group A streptococcal infection. After the clinical presentation has fully evolved, treatment also includes aspirin to treat arthritic symptoms and, in patients with carditis, corticosteroids (Kaplan, 1994). People who have had an episode of rheumatic fever are at high risk for recurrent episodes, and those who have had carditis are prone to similar episodes with subsequent attacks (Bonow et al., 1998).

Rheumatic endocarditis occurs when endothelial tissue, usually that comprising the cardiac valves, becomes inflamed. Rheumatic valvulitis initially produces edema, lymphocytic infiltration, and neovascularization of leaflets (Glower, 1995). With each subsequent bout of acute rheumatic fever, damage is compounded. Chronic rheumatic valvulitis produces at least three distinct pathologic changes in valvular structures: (1) fusion of the valve leaflets at the commissures; (2) fibrosis of leaflets with subsequent stiffening, contraction, and calcification; and (3) in the atrioventricular valves, fusion and shortening of chordae tendineae (Spencer et al., 1995) (Fig. 2-3). Although the interval is variable, in the United States it usually takes two decades or more after acute rheumatic fever for clinically significant rheumatic valve disease to develop. A growing number of American patients, and especially women, acquire symptoms after 50 years of age. In the tropics, however, and particularly in underdeveloped areas, the disease advances more rapidly and severe valvular disease may be present in adolescence (Braunwald, 1997). The mitral valve is affected most often, in isolation or with associated aortic or tricuspid valve involvement. Rheumatic endocarditis of only the aortic or tricuspid valve is uncommon.

Other Acquired Diseases

Acquired aortic valvular stenosis (aortic valve sclerosis) is the most common valvular abnormality in elderly people. It occurs secondary to degenerative calcification and fibrosis of the aortic valve (Fig. 2-4). As the number of

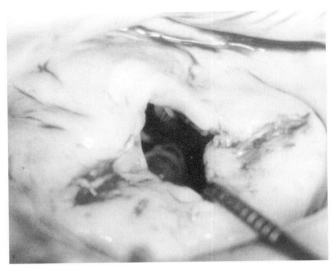

FIGURE 2-3. Resected mitral valve demonstrating leaflet thickening and commissural fusion due to rheumatic endocarditis. (Alpert JS, Sabik J, Cosgrove DM, 1998: Mitral valve disease. In Topol EJ [ed]: Comprehensive Cardiovascular Medicine. p. 541. Philadelphia, Lippincott Williams & Wilkins)

elderly people increases, severe aortic stenosis in persons in the eighth or ninth decade of life has become more common. When degenerative calcification is superimposed on a congenitally bicuspid aortic valve, clinically significant aortic stenosis develops earlier, usually in the sixth or seventh decade (Schoen, 1997).

Ischemic heart disease can produce dysfunction or rupture of the mitral valve's supportive apparatus (chordae tendineae or papillary muscles) or annular dilatation.

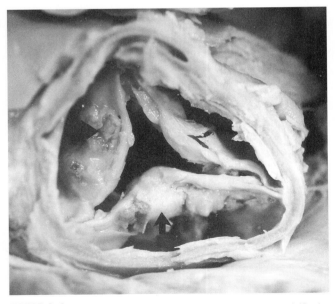

FIGURE 2-4. Senile calcific aortic stenosis. There are heavy calcific deposits at the depths of the sinuses (*arrows*) and no commissural fusion is present. (Friesinger GC, Gravanis MB, 1993: Aging and the cardiovascular system: Implications in health and disease. In Gravanis MB [ed]: Cardiovascular Disorders: Pathogenesis and Pathology. p. 305. St. Louis, Mosby)

Diseases of the ascending aorta often lead to aortic regurgitation. For example, aortic dissection that extends in a retrograde fashion to the aortic valve annulus produces valvular incompetence. An ascending aortic aneurysm also can cause aortic regurgitation by dilating and distorting the valve annulus. Rarely, damage to cardiac valves occurs secondary to blunt or penetrating chest trauma.

► Mitral Valve Disease

The mitral valve is a complex structure comprising leaflets, chordae tendineae, papillary muscles, and annulus. Abnormalities of any of these structures can produce functional problems. Mitral valve disease most often is caused by MVP, coronary artery disease, or rheumatic fever. Causes of mitral valve disease are listed in Table 2-1.

Mitral Stenosis

Mitral stenosis is narrowing of the mitral valve orifice that impedes blood flow into the left ventricle during diastole. A stenotic valve may represent one or more pathologic changes in valve structure, including (1) calcification, thickening, or scarring of leaflets; (2) fusion of commissures; and (3) fusion or shortening of chordae tendineae. Mitral stenosis in adults usually is caused by rheumatic endocarditis. Approximately 50% of patients

TABLE 2-1

Etiologies of Mitral Valve Disease

MITRAL STENOSIS
Rheumatic heart disease
Atrial myxoma
Vegetation
Annular calcification
Congenital deformity

MITRAL REGURGITATION
Mitral valve prolapse and myxomatous degeneration
Rheumatic heart disease
Coronary artery disease
    Papillary muscle dysfunction or rupture
    Annular dilatation
Infective endocarditis
Cardiomyopathies
    Dilated
    Hypertrophic
Connective tissue disorders
Congenital deformity
Systemic lupus erythematosus
Trauma
Anorectic drugs

with symptomatic mitral stenosis can provide a history of rheumatic fever, usually occurring approximately 20 years before presentation (Frankel et al., 1998). Two thirds of patients with rheumatic mitral stenosis are women (Smith & Willis, 1997). Rare causes of mitral stenosis include congenital deformity of the valve, atrial myxoma, thrombus, vegetations, and calcification of the mitral annulus and leaflets (Gaasch et al., 1994).

Severity of valvular stenosis is described in two ways. First, an estimated valve area may be calculated. The orifice of the open mitral valve normally measures 4 to 6 cm^2. A valve opening less than 2.5 cm^2 is moderately stenotic; in severe stenosis, the valve area may measure less than 1 cm^2. Second, pressures in the chambers retrograde and antegrade to the valve may be measured. In contrast to the normal similarity of left atrial and ventricular pressures during ventricular diastole, a stenotic mitral valve produces an abnormal pressure gradient between the two chambers.

As left atrial pressure rises to compensate for mitral valve narrowing, a mean transvalvular pressure gradient of 10 to 15 mm Hg may occur at rest; the left atrial pressure and gradient rise substantially with exercise (Fann et al., 1997). Because there are no valves between the left atrium and pulmonary vasculature, the elevated atrial pressure is transmitted into the pulmonary veins and capillaries. If the left atrium is poorly compliant (ie, it does not distend in response to increased left atrial pressure), more of the pressure is transmitted to the pulmonary vascular bed and mitral stenosis is not well tolerated. More commonly, chronically elevated left atrial pressure produces left atrial enlargement (dilatation and hypertrophy). This compensatory mechanism allows the pulmonary circulation to tolerate better the increased left atrial pressure.

Chronically increased left atrial pressure eventually produces damaging changes in left atrial muscle, pulmonary vasculature, lungs, and right ventricle. Atrial muscle architecture disintegrates, leading to intractable atrial fibrillation with a resultant reduction in cardiac output and increased left atrial pressure (Kirklin & Barratt-Boyes, 1993a). Because the fibrillating atria fail to contract in an organized fashion, stasis of blood along atrial walls may lead to intra-atrial thrombosis. Systemic embolization may result, producing arterial occlusion at any of a variety of sites throughout the systemic circulation. Patients at increased risk for systemic embolism, particularly a cerebral vascular accident, include those with decreased cardiac output, left atrial enlargement, or advanced age. Occasionally, systemic embolization, especially in association with atrial fibrillation, is the first symptom of mitral stenosis (Smith & Willis, 1997). Left atrial enlargement also can produce hoarseness due to compression of the left recurrent laryngeal nerve, dysphagia due to esophageal displacement, or cough due to bronchial irritation (Goldberger, 1982).

In 10% to 20% of patients with mitral stenosis, pulmonary vascular disease and disproportionate pulmonary hypertension develop (Schlant, 1991). When pulmonary artery pressure exceeds the oncotic pressure of plasma, transudation of fluid into the pulmonary interstitial tissues occurs, and pulmonary edema may develop, depending on the transport capacity of the pulmonary lymphatic circulation (Spencer et al., 1995). To compensate for chronic fluid transudation, lymphatic channels hypertrophy and drain the flooded alveoli. Chronic pulmonary congestion also causes thickening of alveolar walls and may produce areas of pulmonary infarction or hemorrhage. The right ventricle hypertrophies in response to increased pulmonary artery pressure and eventually dilates. When the distended right ventricle can no longer compensate, the patient experiences debilitating symptoms of right-sided heart failure. Although the left ventricle is protected from chronic dilatation and failure by the stenotic mitral valve, it probably does not remain normal.

The most common symptom of mitral stenosis is shortness of breath, specifically dyspnea on exertion, paroxysmal nocturnal dyspnea, or orthopnea. Exertional dyspnea is most common and episodes of pulmonary edema may occur. The classic symptom of dyspnea on exertion occurs as the heart attempts to increase cardiac output with exercise, resulting in increased left atrial pressure and lung congestion (Spencer et al., 1995). Fatigue and muscle wasting are thought to occur secondary to the heart's impaired capacity to increase cardiac output in response to increased metabolic demand because of chronically reduced left ventricular preload. Other common symptoms of mitral stenosis include cough and palpitations. Hemoptysis also may occur as blood enters the bronchioles from engorged pulmonary vessels that have ruptured.

Fatigue and exercise intolerance typically cause patients with mitral stenosis to adopt an increasingly sedentary lifestyle. With such adaptations and appropriate medical therapy, a stenotic mitral valve usually is tolerated for many years before corrective therapy becomes necessary. Often, a pregnancy, with its associated hemodynamic alterations (ie, increased blood volume and cardiac output), precipitates functional status deterioration.

Mitral Regurgitation

Mitral regurgitation is the leakage of a portion of left ventricular stroke volume into the left atrium during ventricular systole. Functional competence of the mitral valve depends on proper, coordinated interaction of the mitral annulus and leaflets, chordae tendineae, papillary muscles, left atrium, and left ventricle (Fann et al., 1997). Dysfunction of one or more of these structures can cause valvular incompetence. Myxomatous degeneration of the valve (MVP) is the most common cause of pure mitral regurgitation in the United States. Other significant etiologies include (1) scarring and retraction of leaflets due to rheumatic heart disease, (2) ischemic damage to the subvalvular apparatus of the valve or annulus, and (3) distortion of the relationship between leaflets and subvalvular apparatus secondary to left ventricular dilatation. Anorectic drugs also have been reported to cause mitral regurgitation (Bonow et al., 1998). Although myxomatous disease of the mitral valve is more prevalent in women, mitral regurgitation occurs more often in men (David et al., 1998). Mitral regurgitation is most often chronic but can develop acutely.

Regurgitation of a portion of each stroke volume through a malfunctioning mitral valve causes increased volume and pressure in the left atrium with resultant marked chamber dilatation. The severity of valvular incompetence in combination with the degree of resistance to forward flow (afterload) determines the degree of regurgitation (LeDoux, 1995). Valvular regurgitation is categorized by echocardiographic or angiographic techniques using a four-point grading system, ranging from 1+ (mild) to 4+ (severe). In contrast to mitral stenosis, the left ventricle is not protected in the presence of mitral regurgitation. Left ventricular hypertrophy develops as the ventricle pumps more forcefully to maintain adequate forward flow. If significant regurgitation continues, left ventricular hypertrophy is followed eventually by ventricular dilatation and failure. Pulmonary congestion occurs as with mitral stenosis, and the right ventricle may eventually fail.

Symptoms develop late in the course of chronic mitral regurgitation and often are insidious (Raizner & Siegel, 1991). They include fatigue, dyspnea on exertion, orthopnea, palpitations, and paroxysmal nocturnal dyspnea. As with mitral stenosis, the heart's ability to increase cardiac output in response to increased demand is impeded. Therefore, limitation of activities is common. With severe mitral regurgitation, atrial fibrillation and systemic embolization may occur.

Mitral regurgitation sometimes develops acutely as a result of (1) papillary muscle or chordae tendineae dysfunction or rupture secondary to myocardial infarction, (2) infective endocarditis, or, rarely, (3) blunt trauma. Acute mitral regurgitation usually produces precipitous hemodynamic instability. Because the left atrium is poorly distensible, pulmonary venous pressure increases suddenly. As a result, pulmonary edema and left ventricular failure develop rapidly.

▶ Aortic Valve Disease

Aortic Stenosis

Aortic stenosis is narrowing that obstructs left ventricular outflow into the aorta during systole. In adults, aortic stenosis almost always is due to abnormalities of the valve leaflets. The two most common causes of aortic stenosis are degenerative calcification of a normal valve and calcification of a congenital bicuspid valve. Risk factors that have been identified thus far for progressive calcific degeneration of the aortic valve include smoking, high cholesterol, and hypertension. Less commonly, aortic stenosis occurs secondary to rheumatic fever. Supravalvular (narrowing of the ascending aorta) or subvalvular (left ventricular fibrous ring or tunnel) stenosis occurs rarely (Saenz et al., 1987) (Table 2-2).

TABLE 2-2

Etiologies of Aortic Valve Disease

AORTIC STENOSIS
Congenital bicuspid valve
Aortic valve sclerosis
Rheumatic heart disease
Supravalvular stenosis
Subvalvular stenosis

AORTIC REGURGITATION
Rheumatic heart disease
Infective endocarditis
Congenital bicuspid valve
Aortic dissection
Aortic aneurysm
Annuloaortic ectasia
Connective tissue disorders
   Cystic medial necrosis
   Marfan's syndrome
Trauma
Aortitis
Arthritic inflammatory diseases

The degree of orifice narrowing can vary from mild to severe and determines the compensatory responses and symptoms. The open aortic valve orifice normally measures 3.0 to 4.0 cm^2. When the orifice narrows to approximately 0.8 cm^2, significant obstruction to left ventricular outflow exists. As left ventricular pressure increases to maintain normal systemic arterial pressure, a gradient develops between systolic left ventricular and aortic pressures. A gradient greater than 50 mm Hg represents significant aortic stenosis, and gradients as high as 100 to 120 mm Hg can occur.

Over time, the left ventricular muscle mass hypertrophies to generate adequate pressure to eject blood through the stenotic valve orifice. As a result of the chronic pressure overload, the left ventricle develops concentric hypertrophy with an increased ventricular mass and ratio of wall thickness to cavity radius without appreciable dilatation; because the vasculature does not proliferate commensurate with the increased cardiac mass, the hypertrophied myocardium is usually relatively deficient in blood vessels (Schoen, 1997). Systolic function (contractility) is initially preserved by the compensatory hypertrophy, but diastolic filling (compliance) of the ventricle is impaired (Rapaport et al., 1994). Eventually, the ventricle dilates and systolic function deteriorates as well. Left-sided failure occurs as the left ventricle is forced to work increasingly harder to eject blood into the aorta. Left ventricular end-diastolic pressure rises, causing a corresponding rise in pulmonary arterial pressure, decreases in cardiac output and ejection fraction, and eventual congestive heart failure (Rapaport et al., 1994).

The heart usually compensates for a stenotic aortic valve for many years, producing no symptoms until middle or late life (Ronan, 1991). During this long latent period, morbidity and mortality are very low (Bonow et al., 1998). Once symptoms develop, however, average life expectancy is 5 years or less (Kirklin & Barratt-Boyes, 1993b). The classic symptoms of aortic stenosis are angina, dyspnea on exertion, and syncope. Angina occurs in approximately two thirds of patients with critical aortic stenosis (Braunwald, 1997). It is produced by the imbalance between oxygen demand and supply; demand is increased because of left ventricular muscle hypertrophy and supply is compromised because the stenotic valve is obstructive to left ventricular output.

The hypertrophied, poorly compliant ventricle also impairs diastolic filling of the coronary arteries. Angina caused by aortic stenosis may be attributed erroneously to coronary artery disease. In other cases, both aortic stenosis and coronary artery disease are present and the angina may be produced by either condition. Because both disease processes produce similar symptomatology, coronary angiography often is necessary to determine the correct etiology of the angina.

Effort dyspnea, orthopnea, paroxysmal nocturnal dyspnea, or frank pulmonary edema occurs in 30% to 40% of patients; these symptoms are associated with increased left ventricular end-diastolic pressure and systolic wall stress and decreased cardiac output and ejection fraction (Kirklin & Barratt-Boyes, 1993b). Syncopal episodes also may occur. The precise pathologic mechanism for syncope is not well understood but may be related to an inability to increase cardiac output in response to effort.

Ventricular arrhythmias and conduction disturbances are common in patients with aortic stenosis. Sudden cardiac death is estimated to occur in 15% to 20% of symptomatic patients and has been attributed to arrhythmias and myocardial ischemia (Rapaport et al., 1994). The risk of sudden cardiac death increases markedly when the gradient across the valve is high. Although all patients with aortic stenosis are at increased risk of sudden death, it is unusual in asymptomatic patients. Patients with severe aortic stenosis also are notoriously difficult to resuscitate if cardiac arrest occurs because ventricular tachycardia and fibrillation are easily sustained in the hypertrophic left ventricle. Because ventricular arrhythmias associated with aortic stenosis may be related to the abnormal ventricle rather than to the valve itself, the arrhythmic disorder usually is not corrected by valve replacement, and lifelong antiarrhythmic therapy may be necessary. In patients with extensive calcification of a stenotic aortic valve, complete heart block develops occasionally (Kirklin & Barratt-Boyes, 1993b).

The loss of sinus rhythm (ie, onset of atrial fibrillation) may cause rapid clinical deterioration in patients with moderate aortic stenosis. In contrast to the normal heart, in which atrial contraction contributes approximately 20% of stroke volume, atrial contraction supplies up to 40% of ventricular filling during diastole in the presence of aortic stenosis (Jamieson, 1997). Also, patients with aortic stenosis are particularly sensitive to afterload reduction or hypovolemia. Because of fixed obstruction to ventricular output and poor compliance of the ventricle, vasodilating medications, volume loss, or bleeding are poorly tolerated and may lead to catastrophic hemodynamic compromise. Therapeutic maneuvers, such as induction of general anesthesia or administration of diuretic or afterload-reducing agents, must be performed with caution.

Aortic Regurgitation

Aortic regurgitation is leakage of a portion of left ventricular stroke volume from the aorta backward into the ventricle during diastole. It may be caused by primary disease of the aortic valve leaflets, the wall of the aortic root, or both (Braunwald, 1997). Calcific aortic valve degeneration may cause aortic regurgitation because of leaflet fixation that prevents full closure of the leaflets during diastole (Glower, 1995). Chronic aortic regurgitation also may result from rheumatic endocarditis or a congenitally bicuspid aortic valve. In other cases, aortic regurgitation develops as a result of annuloaortic ectasia, or enlargement of the aortic annulus, associated with aortic diseases such as ascending aortic aneurysm, chronic aortic dissection, cystic medial necrosis, or inflammatory, bacterial, or syphilitic aortitis (see Table 2-2).

The size of the regurgitant valve orifice and the pressure gradient between the aorta and left ventricle during diastole determine the severity of aortic regurgitation. In the early stages of aortic regurgitation, ventricular hypertrophy produces an increased ventricular ejection fraction and a compensatory decrease in systemic vascular resistance occurs to facilitate forward flow. Peripheral vasodilatation and regurgitation of blood into the left ventricle result in a low diastolic arterial pressure. Systolic arterial pressure, on the other hand, is high as the ventricle works to maintain an adequate ejection fraction. Chronic volume overload of the left ventricle causes both hypertrophy of the myocardium and chamber dilatation, in which both ventricular wall thickness and radius are increased (Schoen, 1997). The combination of volume overload during both systole and diastole produces marked cardiomegaly. Eventually, left ventricular dilatation compromises effective contractility and systolic impairment develops.

Patients with mild or moderate chronic aortic regurgitation may remain asymptomatic for many years. However, as ventricular contractility becomes increasingly impaired, ejection fraction decreases and symptoms of left-sided heart failure, particularly dyspnea on exertion, develop. Angina pectoris is a presenting symptom in 25% of patients (Jamieson, 1997). It occurs secondary to subendocardial ischemia caused by decreased diastolic coronary perfusion pressure, increased diastolic ventricular pressure, left ventricular hypertrophy, and increased left ventricular workload (Glower, 1995). With severe aortic regurgitation, patients may become aware of an audible heartbeat, head bobbing, or tickling in the throat from pressure on the uvula. Severe aortic regurgitation also is associated with a number of signs that may be apparent during physical examination. These include a widened pulse pressure (high systolic and low diastolic blood pressure), bounding or "water-hammer" peripheral pulses (rapid upstroke and descent on arterial pressure tracing), and Quincke's sign (alternating paling and flushing of lightly compressed nail beds or mucous membranes) (Hillis et al., 1995).

Acute aortic regurgitation can result from acute aortic dissection involving the aortic valve annulus, infective endocarditis, or trauma (Treasure, 1991). In acute aortic regurgitation, the left ventricle has no time to undergo the compensatory changes associated with chronic aortic regurgitation. Consequently, acute left ventricular failure with pulmonary edema or cardiogenic shock is likely to occur.

► Tricuspid and Pulmonic Valve Disease

Tricuspid valve disease is uncommon and usually occurs secondary to left-sided valvular disease. When associated with rheumatic mitral or aortic valve disease, either regurgitation or stenosis may be present. Tricuspid regurgitation also can result from annular dilatation secondary to right ventricular enlargement; the precipitating cause is usually severe disease of the left-sided heart valves in association with pulmonary hypertension (Kirklin & Barratt-Boyes, 1993c). Tricuspid valve endocarditis, with resultant tricuspid regurgitation, may occur secondary to intravenous drug abuse, immunodeficiency, or indwelling vascular catheters (Crawley, 1991).

Infrequently, blunt trauma produces acute tricuspid regurgitation from injury to the tricuspid valve leaflets or its subvalvular apparatus. Unusual causes of tricuspid regurgitation are myocardial infarction, carcinoid, prolapsed leaflet, and congenital abnormalities such as atrial septal defect and Ebstein's anomaly (Rackley et al., 1994) (Fig. 2-5). Tricuspid stenosis is uncommon and results almost exclusively from rheumatic fever; unusual causes include tricuspid valve vegetations, tumor, and constrictive pericarditis (Pitts & Hillis, 1997). Tricuspid valve disease produces elevated right atrial pressure and subsequent symptoms of right-sided heart failure.

Pulmonic valve disease is rare in adults. Pulmonic stenosis almost always is congenital. The most common causes of pulmonic regurgitation are pulmonary hypertension, pulmonary artery dilatation, either idiopathic or due to a connective tissue disorder, and infective endocarditis (Braunwald, 1997).

► Diagnosis

In contrast to coronary artery disease, physical examination often reveals important clues about the nature and severity of VHD. Auscultation of heart sounds may reveal a change in quality or intensity of a murmur that represents a worsening in the patient's condition. Mitral stenosis usually is diagnosed by auscultation of a characteristic low-pitched, apical diastolic murmur. Mitral regurgitation produces a late systolic or holosystolic

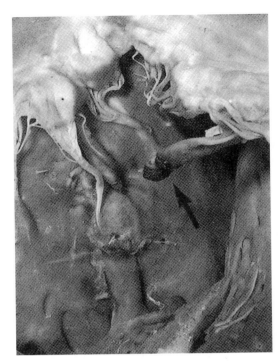

FIGURE 2-5. Resected tricuspid valve demonstrating papillary muscle rupture (*arrow*) due to myocardial infarction with resultant severe tricuspid regurgitation. (Hurst JW, Rackley CE, Becker AE, Wilcox BR, 1988: Valvar heart disease. In Hurst JW, Anderson RH, Becker AE, Wilcox BR [eds]: Atlas of the Heart. p. 4.53. London, Times Mirror International)

murmur at the apex of the heart. Aortic stenosis is associated with a systolic ejection murmur best heard in the second intercostal space to the right of the sternum with radiation into both carotid arteries (Glower, 1995). A high-pitched, decrescendo, diastolic murmur characterizes aortic regurgitation.

Another important diagnostic guide is clinical symptomatology produced by the dysfunctional valve. Assessment of the patient's ability to perform daily activities and of the presence and severity of associated symptoms aids in evaluating effectiveness of medical therapy and establishing optimal timing of surgical intervention. The classic method for categorizing severity of functional impairment in patients with VHD is the New York Heart Association (NYHA) Functional Classification System (Criteria Committee of the New York Heart Association, 1964) (Table 2-3). A four-point scale is used to rate degree of exertion with which the classic symptoms of heart disease (ie, chest pain, shortness of breath, palpitations, and fatigue) occur. The NYHA functional rating system is used widely because of its simplicity and usefulness in categorizing patients in a standardized fashion.

The echocardiogram, electrocardiogram, and chest roentgenogram are the primary diagnostic studies used for evaluation of VHD. Either transthoracic or transesophageal echocardiography is performed to provide important information about valve leaflet motion, the presence of a gradient or regurgitant flow across the

TABLE 2-3

New York Heart Association Functional Classification System

Class	Description
I	Ordinary physical activity does not cause undue fatigue, palpitation, dyspnea, or angina.
II	Ordinary physical activity causes undue fatigue, palpitation, dyspnea, or angina.
III	Less than ordinary physical activity causes undue fatigue, palpitation, dyspnea, or angina.
IV	Fatigue, palpitation, dyspnea, or angina occur at rest.

Adapted from Criteria Committee of the New York Heart Association, 1964: Physical capacity with heart disease. In Diseases of the Heart and Blood Vessels: Nomenclature and Criteria for Diagnosis, ed. 6. Boston, Little, Brown.

valve, and the presence of vegetations or thrombus. Serial electrocardiograms and chest roentgenograms are important because of the information they provide about progressive cardiac chamber hypertrophy or dilatation.

In the past, cardiac catheterization almost always was performed before surgical treatment of VHD. However, the sophisticated echocardiographic techniques now available often can provide all necessary diagnostic information. Therefore, cardiac catheterization is sometimes omitted if relevant information can be obtained with less invasive studies. However, because of the prevalence of coronary artery disease, catheterization with coronary angiography almost always is performed in middle-aged and older adults before surgical therapy to define coronary anatomy and detect coexisting coronary artery lesions that might be treated at the time of the valve operation.

Cardiac catheterization can provide the following information about valvular abnormalities and cardiac function: (1) measurement of intracardiac pressures with calculation of valve area and pressure gradient across the valve; (2) visualization of valve leaflet appearance (eg, abnormal thickening, redundant tissue, or presence of calcium) and movement; (3) assessment of regurgitant flow across a valve; and (4) estimation of ventricular contractility (ventriculogram).

▶ Treatment

The presence of any significant valvular abnormality mandates lifelong medical supervision. Treatment varies depending on the specific valvular lesion, its etiology, and its acuity. In most cases of chronic valvular disease, the patient can be managed with medical treatment for many years before valve repair or replacement is required. However, it is essential to restore adequate valve function before the heart or pulmonary vasculature is damaged irreversibly. Although patient symptomatology remains an important criterion for determining management strategy, advances in diagnostic modalities have made it possible to base recommendations for surgical intervention increasingly on objective measures of cardiovascular function.

In patients with mitral stenosis, percutaneous balloon valvotomy or surgical commissurotomy often is recommended when mitral valve area decreases to less than 1.0 to 1.5 cm², even if the patient is asymptomatic. Early mitral valve repair may allow the patient to maintain normal sinus rhythm, thus lessening the risk of embolism, and prevent progressive valve fibrosis and calcification that would necessitate replacement rather than repair of the valve (Spencer et al., 1995).

In asymptomatic patients with hemodynamically significant aortic stenosis, medical evaluation at 3- to 6-month intervals is recommended for the detection of symptoms that would prompt surgical intervention, and the patient is advised to refrain from occupations and sports that require heavy exertion (Fifer, 1997). Once symptoms occur, early surgical correction of moderate to severe aortic stenosis is essential because of the limited life expectancy with medical therapy alone. Even mild symptoms, such as exertional dyspnea, warrant prompt surgical intervention when severe aortic stenosis is present (Otto, 1998).

Management of patients with chronic mitral or aortic regurgitation varies greatly depending on severity of valvular incompetence. Asymptomatic patients with mild regurgitation may not require either pharmacologic therapy or restriction of normal activities. Moderate but asymptomatic valvular regurgitation may be treated with medications and avoidance of strenuous physical activities. In patients with severe valvular regurgitation, early operative therapy may be important to avoid irreversible ventricular damage. The current trend in the treatment of mitral regurgitation is earlier surgical intervention; patients with a NYHA II functional class may undergo surgery if signs of left ventricular dysfunction are present (Quinones, 1998). In patients with aortic regurgitation, aortic valve replacement is recommended once significant symptoms develop, or if there is reliable evidence of left ventricular contractile dysfunction at rest or extreme left ventricular dilatation (Bonow, 1998).

Acute mitral or aortic regurgitation often necessitates emergent surgical therapy to restore valve competence and correct cardiogenic shock. In patients with acute mitral regurgitation, intra-aortic balloon counterpulsation provides important preoperative cardiac support. Its use is contraindicated, however, in patients with aortic regurgitation because balloon inflations during diastole would worsen regurgitant flow.

Pharmacologic Therapy

Pharmacologic treatment of VHD is aimed at improving the heart's ability to compensate for the poorly functioning valve or valves. Digitalis is used if ventricular contractility is impaired. Diuresis and sodium restriction are important in controlling congestive heart failure. Angiotensin-converting enzyme inhibitors, such as captopril, are important for reducing afterload in mitral or aortic regurgitation. Afterload reduction enhances forward blood flow from the left ventricle, reducing regurgitant flow through the incompetent mitral or aortic valve.

Treatment of mitral valve disease often includes pharmacologic therapy for management of associated atrial fibrillation or, less commonly, atrial flutter. Medications, such as digoxin, beta-blocking agents, or calcium channel blocking agents are used to control the rapid ventricular response to these atrial arrhythmias. However, pharmacologic agents that slow the ventricular rate when the patient is in atrial flutter may result in unacceptably slow ventricular rates with atrial fibrillation. If so, a permanent pacemaker may become necessary. Patients with atrial fibrillation also require long-term anticoagulation.

Antibiotic prophylaxis before certain dental and surgical procedures is an important component of medical therapy because transient bacteremia in people with valvular dysfunction may cause infective endocarditis. Accordingly, the American Heart Association has well established recommendations to guide prophylactic antibiotic therapy (Dajani et al., 1997). At highest risk for infective endocarditis are people with prosthetic cardiac valves, including bioprostheses and homografts, and those with previous endocarditis; at moderate risk are people with acquired valvular dysfunction and those with MVP associated with regurgitation or thickened leaflets (Dajani et al., 1997). People in these high- and moderate-risk categories require appropriate antibiotic prophylaxis before dental procedures and certain procedures involving the respiratory, genitourinary, and gastrointestinal tissues (Table 2-4).

Probably the most common source of infection is bacteremia resulting from gum disease, dental abscesses, or dental procedures. Because endocarditis can occur after even minor dental procedures, antibiotic prophylaxis is recommended in susceptible patients before all dental procedures likely to cause bleeding from hard or soft tissues, periodontal surgery, scaling, and professional cleaning of teeth (Dajani et al., 1997).

TABLE 2-4

Procedures Requiring Antibiotic Prophylaxis in Patients at Risk for Endocarditis

---

Dental procedures (eg, prophylactic cleaning, extractions, periodontal procedures)
Rigid bronchoscopy
Tonsillectomy or adenoidectomy
Cystoscopy
Prostatic surgery
Biliary tract surgery

Adapted from Dajani AS, Taubert KA, Wilson W, et al., 1997: Prevention of bacterial endocarditis: Recommendations by the American Heart Association. JAMA 277:1794.

Treatment of Infective Endocarditis

The increased population of intravenous drug abusers and of immunocompromised people has made infective endocarditis a more prevalent problem. Infective endocarditis should be suspected in any febrile patient who has a valve that is known to be abnormal, who has a history of intravenous drug abuse, who has an immunodeficiency disorder or is receiving immunosuppressive therapy, or who has been septic. Because of the tricuspid valve's location on the right (venous) side of the heart, it is most likely to be infected by intravenous contaminants.

Clinical manifestations of endocarditis include fever, a changing murmur, peripheral emboli, and elevated white blood cell count. Blood cultures are obtained to detect and identify the responsible pathogen. If endocarditis is caused by a fungal agent, however, blood cultures often remain negative (Rubinstein & Lang, 1995). If blood cultures are positive or infective endocarditis is suggested by clinical findings, an echocardiogram is performed to detect vegetations or perivalvular abscesses and to evaluate valve function. Transesophageal echocardiography often is used because of its greater than 90% sensitivity in identifying vegetations in patients with infective endocarditis (Ewy, 1997). Endocarditis sometimes occurs in the absence of vegetations, and thus the diagnosis may be based on clinical findings alone.

Patients with confirmed infective endocarditis are treated with appropriate organism-specific intravenous antibiotics for 6 to 8 weeks. Streptococcal infections often can be cured with antibiotic therapy alone, sparing the native valve. S. aureus, P. aeruginosa, Serratia marcescens, or fungal infections are more virulent, often destroying valve leaflets and producing valvular incompetence (David, 1997). Valve replacement may be the only effective therapy for particularly virulent or drug-resistant endocarditis. Failure of antibiotic therapy to control endocarditis is evidenced by signs of progressive invasion of the myocardium with abscess formation, heart block, or fistulae; persistent sepsis; progressive hemodynamic instability; or repeated emboli (Ewy, 1997).

Embolization of vegetations to the brain, abdominal viscera, or extremities is a potential threat from endocarditis of the left-sided valves, and to the lungs from right-sided valves. Septic emboli are more damaging than ordinary bland emboli. Because they contain pathogenic organisms, an additional area of infection may develop at the site of the embolus. For example, a cerebral embolus may cause a brain abscess as well as a stroke. In intravenous drug abusers, recurrent embolism of septic vegetations from the tricuspid valve to the pulmonary arteries is common. The resulting pulmonary infarction can produce infection (eg, pneumonitis or lung abscess) and atelectasis of substantial portions of lung tissue with secondary pleural effusion. Prosthetic valve endocarditis (infection of valvular prostheses) is discussed in Chapter 16, Surgical Treatment of Valvular Heart Disease.

Balloon Valvotomy for Valvular Stenosis

Balloon valvotomy, also called balloon valvuloplasty, is an invasive, nonsurgical procedure performed in the cardiac catheterization laboratory. It is appropriate for selected patients with valvular stenosis. Balloon valvotomy is an important component of therapy for children and young adults who might otherwise face multiple surgical procedures and for patients who are too elderly or medically compromised to withstand an operation that includes general anesthesia, an incision in the thoracic cavity, use of cardiopulmonary bypass, and surgical manipulation of the heart. Balloon valvotomy is performed most commonly in patients with rheumatic mitral stenosis. The morphology of the mitral apparatus is the most important determinant of outcome after valvotomy; other important factors include the absence of significant mitral regurgitation or left atrial thrombus (Bruce & Nishimura, 1998).

Balloon valvotomy consists of dilatation of a cardiac valve by inflation of a balloon passed by catheter technique across the valve (Fig. 2-6). For mitral balloon valvotomy, a balloon flotation catheter is inserted into the femoral vein and passed through the inferior vena cava into the right atrium. The catheter is passed through a patent foramen ovale, if present, or a hole is punctured in the atrial septum with a needle tip passed through the catheter. Once the catheter is in the left atrium, it is advanced until one large or two smaller balloons extend across the mitral valve orifice. The balloon is then inflated repetitively to split the fused commissures of the valve. At the conclusion of the procedure, the pressure gradient between the left atrium and ventricle is measured to assess residual stenosis, and ventriculography is performed to detect new regurgitation resulting from the balloon inflations.

In patients with favorable valvular anatomy, percutaneous mitral balloon valvotomy usually produces immediate hemodynamic improvement and a long-term clinical outcome that is similar to that achieved with surgical mitral valve repair (Lincoff & Topol, 1997). Complications of mitral balloon valvotomy include cerebral embolic events, cardiac perforation, and development of mitral regurgitation severe enough to require operation (Braunwald, 1997).

Pulmonic stenosis occurs rarely in adults but also may be treated with balloon valvotomy. Results of balloon valvotomy for aortic valve stenosis in adults with calcified valves have been disappointing. In approximately

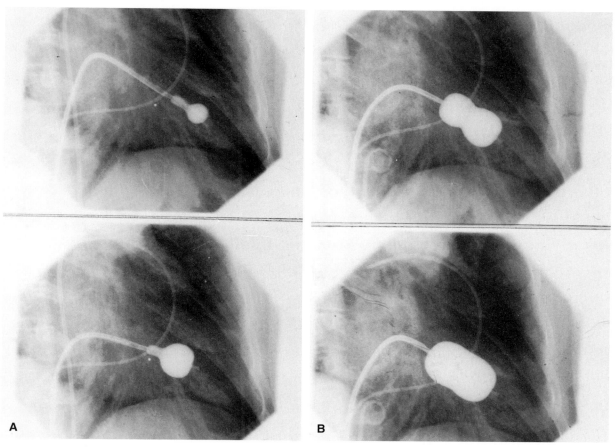

A   **B**

FIGURE 2-6. One technique (Inoue) of mitral balloon valvotomy. **(A)** Inflation of the distal portion of the balloon, which is then pulled back and anchored at the mitral valve. **(B)** Subsequent inflation of proximal and middle portions of the balloon. At full inflation, the waist of the balloon at its midportion has disappeared. (Vahanian AS, 1998: Valvuloplasty. In Topol EJ [ed]: Comprehensive Cardiovascular Medicine. p. 2509. Philadelphia, Lippincott Williams & Wilkins)

50% of adults with critical, calcified aortic stenosis who undergo balloon valvotomy, restenosis develops within 6 months (Braunwald, 1997). In addition, balloon dilatation of the aortic annulus may produce aortic dissection. Therefore, aortic balloon valvotomy usually is performed only in patients considered at prohibitive risk for surgical valve replacement.

Surgical Therapy

Surgical therapy is a major component in the treatment of moderately severe or severe VHD. Improvements in myocardial protection techniques and cardiopulmonary bypass, successful reparative techniques for preserving native valves, and better valvular prostheses have led to operative therapy being performed earlier in the course of many forms of VHD. Although valve replacement with an artificial prosthetic valve is most common, valve repair is possible for some valvular lesions. Valve repair is performed most often as the surgical treatment of choice for mitral regurgitation, particularly that due to degenerative valve disease (Gillinov, 1998). Surgical therapy is discussed in detail in Chapter 16, Surgical Treatment of Valvular Heart Disease.

REFERENCES

American Heart Association, 1998: 1999 Heart and Stroke Statistical Update. Dallas, American Heart Association

Bonow RO, 1998: Chronic aortic regurgitation: Role of medical therapy and optimal timing for surgery. Cardiol Clin 16:449

Bonow RO, Carabello B, de Leon AC, et al., 1998: American College of Cardiology/American Heart Association guidelines for the management of patients with valvular heart disease. J Am Coll Cardiol 32:1486

Braunwald E, 1997: Valvular heart disease. In Braunwald E (ed): Heart Disease: A Textbook of Cardiovascular Medicine, ed. 5. Philadelphia, WB Saunders

Bruce CJ, Nishimura RA, 1998: Clinical assessment and management of mitral stenosis. Cardiol Clin 16:375

Crawley IS, 1991: Acquired tricuspid and pulmonary valve disease. In Hurst JW (ed): Current Therapy in Cardiovascular Disease, ed. 3. Philadelphia, BC Decker

Criteria Committee of the New York Heart Association, 1964: Physical capacity with heart disease. In Diseases of the Heart and Blood Vessels: Nomenclature and Criteria for Diagnosis, ed. 6. Boston, Little, Brown

Dajani AS, Taubert KA, Wilson W, et al., 1997: Prevention of bacterial endocarditis: Recommendations by the American Heart Association. JAMA 277:1794

David TE, 1998: Annuloaortic ectasia. In Kaiser LR, Kron IL, Spray TL (eds): Mastery of Cardiothoracic Surgery. Philadelphia, Lippincott Williams & Wilkins

David TE, 1997: Complex operations of the aortic root. In Edmunds LH Jr (ed): Cardiac Surgery in the Adult. New York, McGraw-Hill

David TE, Omran A, Armstrong S, et al., 1998: Long-term results of mitral valve repair for myxomatous disease with and without chordal replacement with expanded polytetrafluoroethylene. J Thorac Cardiovasc Surg 115:1279

Ewy GA, 1997:Infectious endocarditis. In Alpert JS (ed): Cardiology for the Primary Care Physician, ed. 2. Philadelphia, Current Medicine

Fann JI, Ingels NB Jr, Miller DC, 1997: Pathophysiology of mitral valve disease and operative indications. In Edmunds LH Jr (ed): Cardiac Surgery in the Adult. New York, McGraw-Hill

Fifer MA, 1997: Aortic stenosis and regurgitation. In Alpert JS (ed): Cardiology for the Primary Care Physician, ed. 2. Philadelphia, Current Medicine

Frankel SK, Lilly LS, Bittl JA, 1998: Valvular heart disease. In Lilly LS (ed): Pathophysiology of Heart Disease, ed. 2. Baltimore, Williams & Wilkins

Gaasch WH, O'Rourke RA, Cohn LH, Rackley CE, 1994: Mitral valve disease. In Schlant RC, Alexander RW, et al. (eds): The Heart, ed. 8. New York, McGraw-Hill

Gillinov AM, Cosgrove DM, Blackstone EH, et al., 1998: Durability of mitral valve repair for degenerative disease. J Thorac Cardiovasc Surg 116:734

Goldberger E, 1982: Valvular cardiovascular syndromes. In Textbook of Clinical Cardiology. St. Louis, CV Mosby

Glower DD, 1995: Acquired aortic valve disease. In Sabiston DC Jr, Spencer FC (eds): Surgery of the Chest, ed. 6. Philadelphia, WB Saunders

Hillis LD, Lange RA, Winniford MD, Page RL, 1995: Chronic aortic regurgitation. In Manual of Clinical Problems in Cardiology, ed. 5. Boston, Little, Brown

Jamieson WR, 1997: Mechanical and bioprosthetic aortic valve replacement. In Edmunds LH Jr (ed): Cardiac Surgery in the Adult. New York, McGraw-Hill

John S, Ravikumar E, Jairaj PS, et al., 1990: Valve replacement in the young patient with rheumatic heart disease. J Thorac Cardiovasc Surg 99:631

Kaplan EL, 1994: Acute rheumatic fever. In Schlant RC, Alexander RW, et al. (eds): The Heart, ed. 8. New York, McGraw-Hill

Karchmer AW, 1997: Infective endocarditis. In Braunwald E (ed): Heart Disease: A Textbook of Cardiovascular Medicine, ed. 5. Philadelphia, WB Saunders

Kirklin JW, Barratt-Boyes BG, 1993a: Mitral valve disease with or without tricuspid valve disease. In Cardiac Surgery, ed. 2. New York, Churchill Livingstone

Kirklin JW, Barratt-Boyes BG, 1993b: Aortic valve disease. In Cardiac Surgery, ed. 2. New York, Churchill Livingstone

Kirklin JW, Barratt-Boyes BG, 1993c: Tricuspid valve disease. In Cardiac Surgery, ed. 2. New York, Churchill Livingstone

Larbalestier RI, Kinchla NM, Aranki SF, et al., 1992: Acute bacterial endocarditis. Circulation 86(Suppl II):II-68

LeDoux D, 1995: Acquired valvular heart disease. In Woods SL, Froelicher ESS, Halpenny CJ, Motzer SU (eds): Cardiac Nursing, ed. 3. Philadelphia, JB Lippincott

Lincoff AM, Topol EJ, 1997: Interventional catheterization techniques. In Braunwald E (ed): Heart Disease: A Textbook of Cardiovascular Medicine, ed. 5. Philadelphia, WB Saunders

Nugent EW, Plauth WH, Edwards JE, Williams WH, 1994: The pathology, pathophysiology, recognition, and treatment of congenital heart disease. In Schlant RC, Alexander RW, et al. (eds): The Heart, ed. 8. New York, McGraw-Hill

Otto CM, 1998: Aortic stenosis: Clinical evaluation and optimal timing of surgery. Cardiol Clin 16:353

Perloff JK, 1998: Survival patterns without cardiac surgery or interventional catheterization: A narrowing base. In Perloff JK, Child JS (eds): Congenital Heart Disease in Adults, ed. 2. Philadelphia, WB Saunders

Pitts WR, Hillis LD, 1997: Tricuspid and pulmonic valve disease. In Alpert JS (ed): Cardiology for the Primary Care Physician, ed. 2. Philadelphia, Current Medicine

Quinones MA, 1998: Management of mitral regurgitation. Cardiol Clin 16:421

Rackley CE, Wallace RB, Edwards JE, Katz NM, 1994: Tricuspid and pulmonary valve disease. In Schlant RC, Alexander RW, et al. (eds): The Heart, ed. 8. New York, McGraw-Hill

Raizner AE, Siegel CO, 1991: Mitral regurgitation. In Hurst JW (ed): Current Therapy in Cardiovascular Disease, ed. 3. Philadelphia, BC Decker

Rapaport E, Rackley CE, Cohn LH, 1994: Aortic valve disease. In Schlant RC, Alexander RW, et al. (eds): The Heart, ed. 8. New York, McGraw-Hill

Ronan JA Jr, 1991: Aortic stenosis in adults. In Hurst JW (ed): Current Therapy in Cardiovascular Disease, ed. 3. Philadelphia, BC Decker

Rubinstein E, Lang R, 1995: Fungal endocarditis. Eur Heart J 16(Suppl B):84

Saenz A, Hopkins CB, Humphries JO, 1987: Valvular heart disease. In Chung EK (ed): Quick Reference to Cardiovascular Diseases, ed. 3. Baltimore, Williams & Wilkins

Schlant RC, 1991: Mitral stenosis. In Hurst JW (ed): Current Therapy in Cardiovascular Disease, ed. 3. Philadelphia, BC Decker

Schoen FJ, 1997: Pathologic considerations in the surgery of adult heart disease. In Edmunds LH Jr (ed): Cardiac Surgery in the Adult. New York, McGraw-Hill

Smith SC Jr, Willis PW IV, 1997: Mitral stenosis and regurgitation. In Alpert JS (ed): Cardiology for the Primary Care Physician, ed. 2. Philadelphia, Current Medicine

Spencer FC, Galloway AC, Colvin SB, 1995: Acquired disease of the mitral valve. In Sabiston DC Jr, Spencer FC (eds): Surgery of the Chest, ed. 6. Philadelphia, WB Saunders

Treasure CB, 1991: Aortic regurgitation. In Hurst JW (ed): Current Therapy in Cardiovascular Disease, ed. 3. Philadelphia, BC Decker

3

Disorders of the Thoracic Aorta

The thoracic aorta is subject to three major types of pathologic conditions. An *aneurysm* is the localized enlargement of a segment of aorta, *dissection* is longitudinal separation of the three layers of aortic wall, and *transection* is traumatic disruption of aortic wall. Although these terms sometimes mistakenly are used synonymously, they represent three distinct entities. Sometimes, however, one type of lesion leads to a second (eg, acute transection causing chronic aneurysm) or two types coexist (eg, dissection and aneurysm).

▶ Etiologies of Aortic Pathologic Conditions

Pathologic conditions of the aorta can result from various diseases, iatrogenic injury, trauma, or congenital anomalies. Atherosclerosis is the most common disease affecting the thoracic aorta. Atherosclerosis initially affects the intimal layer of arterial wall, but advanced lesions penetrate the underlying media, producing scarring and atrophy (Lindsay et al., 1994). Hypertension frequently is present and may accelerate the degenerative process. The ulcerated atherosclerotic plaques that characterize aortic atherosclerosis can (1) release atheroemboli; (2) become covered with mural thrombus that may dislodge to yield peripheral thromboemboli; or (3) impinge on the media with resultant dilatation, aneurysm formation, or rupture (Schoen, 1997). Atherosclerosis is discussed in more detail in Chapter 1, Coronary Artery Disease.

Aortic disease also can result from degeneration of the medial (middle) layer of the aortic wall. A certain degree of elastic fiber fragmentation and loss of smooth muscle cell nuclei in the aortic media is an almost universal consequence of aging, resulting in the common de-

velopment of aortic tortuosity and ectasia (Lindsay et al., 1994). Such changes usually are not clinically significant. Severe medial degeneration, known as *cystic medial necrosis*, occurs in some people. It can lead to aneurysm, dissection, or both as a result of loss of elastic fibers and medial weakening. Although the entire aorta is susceptible, medial degeneration is most severe at the aortic root. Therefore, the ascending aorta and aortic valve are most likely to be affected.

The cause of cystic medial necrosis is unknown. It commonly is associated with Marfan's syndrome, a heritable connective tissue disorder that primarily affects the skeletal, ocular, and cardiovascular systems (Pyeritz, 1979). Marfan's syndrome is estimated to occur in 4 to 6 people per 100,000, although the incidence in China is considerably higher, where it is reported to be 17 people per 100,000 (Svensson & Crawford, 1997a). Persons with Marfan's syndrome often have a distinctive general appearance, with long extremities, an arm span that exceeds the height, a longer lower segment (pubis to foot) than upper segment (head to pubis), and arachnodactyly (abnormally long and slender fingers and toes) (Perloff & Braunwald, 1997) (Figs. 3-1 and 3-2). Other physical stigmata of Marfan's syndrome include bilateral lens displacement, chest wall deformities, kyphosis, hyperextensibility of the joints, high-arched palate, and sparse muscle mass.

Cardiovascular complications are a prevalent problem in Marfan's syndrome and are responsible for a shortened life expectancy. A number of studies based on echocardiographic findings have documented cardiovascular abnormalities in as many as 95% of people with Marfan's syndrome (Geva et al., 1987). All portions of the aorta may be affected, as well as the aortic valve. Mitral or tricuspid valve regurgitation also may occur, caused by the same myxomatous changes that affect the

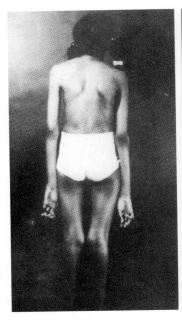
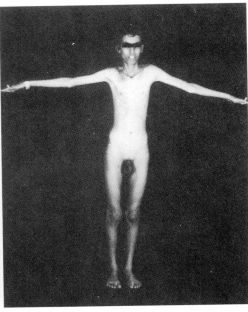

FIGURE 3-1. Typical stigmata of Marfan's syndrome; note long extremities and digits, tall stature, and scoliosis. (Pyeritz RE, 1997: Genetics and cardiovascular disease. In Braunwald E [ed]: Heart Disease: A Textbook of Cardiovascular Medicine, ed. 5, p. 1670. Philadelphia, WB Saunders)

aorta and aortic valve, or by ventricular dilatation that occurs secondary to aortic regurgitation. The most common cardiovascular features are dilatation of the sinuses of Valsalva and mitral valve prolapse; associated clinical problems of aortic regurgitation, aortic dissection, and mitral regurgitation, if untreated, account for most of the early mortality (Pyeritz, 1997). The average age at death in people with Marfan's syndrome is approximately 32 years (Downing & Kouchoukos, 1997). Only 50% of men and women with the syndrome reach 40 and 50 years of age, respectively (Murdoch et al., 1972).

Cystic medial necrosis is found in virtually all cases of Marfan's syndrome (Isselbacher et al., 1997). However, the converse is not true because cystic medial necrosis sometimes occurs in people with no physical stigmata of Marfan's syndrome. It is unclear whether cystic medial necrosis of the aorta identical to that seen

in Marfan's syndrome, but in people without skeletal or ocular manifestations of Marfan's syndrome, represents a forme fruste (atypical or incomplete form) of the syndrome or a separate disease.

Various forms of aortitis (inflammation of the aorta) also may cause aortic disease, particularly aneurysm. Granulomatous aortitis is a rare condition in which aortic tissue has the microscopic appearance of infectious changes but no bacterial organisms are present (Kirklin & Barratt-Boyes, 1993a). It typically occurs in older people, particularly women (Isselbacher et al., 1997). Aortitis also has been demonstrated in a sizable minority of people with autoimmune disorders, such as ankylosing spondylitis and Reiter's syndrome (Lindsay et al., 1994).

Takayasu's arteritis is an unusual inflammatory arterial disease that produces stenosis or aneurysm in the aorta or its major branches and in the pulmonary and

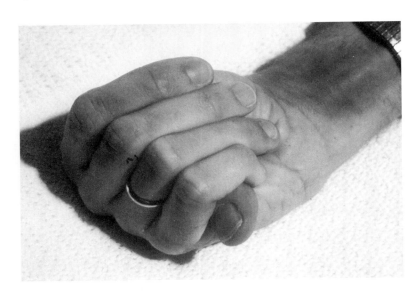

FIGURE 3-2. Arachnodactyly in a person with Marfan's syndrome. Note the thumb extends beyond the fifth digit with the hand clenched in a fist. (Spittell PC, 1998: Diseases of the aorta. In Topol EJ [ed]: Comprehensive Cardiovascular Medicine. p. 3047. Philadelphia, Lippincott Williams & Wilkins)

coronary arteries. All three layers of the arterial wall are affected, and the arteritis may be diffuse or segmental. The disease is characterized by an early stage of active inflammation with progression to a later sclerotic stage with intimal hyperplasia, medial degeneration, and adventitial fibrosis (Isselbacher et al., 1997). The etiology of Takayasu's disease is unknown, although a genetic predisposition and an autoimmune process are thought to play a role (Lindsay et al., 1994). Women younger than 30 years of age, and especially Asian women, are affected most commonly (Isselbacher et al., 1997; Peyton & Isom, 1995).

Bacterial aortitis occurs when bacteria invade the aortic wall. Aortic endothelium normally is quite resistant to bacterial invasion; bacterial aortitis almost always occurs in a previously diseased or injured segment of aorta (Lindsay et al., 1994). Bacterial infection also can develop in vascular prosthetic grafts placed during operations on the thoracic aorta. Syphilitic aortitis is a late complication of syphilis. It has become rare since the widespread availability of antibiotic therapy to treat primary syphilis. Nevertheless, syphilitic aortitis can occur, typically many years after the primary infection. The ascending thoracic aorta is affected most often and the sinuses of Valsalva sometimes are involved; occasionally the aortic arch or abdominal aorta is affected (Svensson & Crawford, 1997b).

Congenital anomalies of the aorta include coarctation and anomalies of the aortic arch. Occasionally, aortic disease results from iatrogenic injury or from trauma. Iatrogenic aortic injury, occurring as a complication of cardiac operations or operations on the aorta itself, or femoral artery cannulation, can lead to aneurysm formation or dissection (Table 3-1). Severe blunt chest trauma, especially that associated with rapid horizontal or vertical deceleration, can cause aortic transection.

TABLE 3-1

Procedures Associated With Iatrogenic Aortic Injury

CARDIAC OPERATIONS
Aortic cannulation
Saphenous vein–aorta anastomoses
Cross-clamping
Aortotomy

AORTIC OPERATIONS
Aortic–prosthetic graft anastomoses
Aortotomy
Aortic cannulation

CARDIAC CATHETERIZATION, INTRA-AORTIC BALLOON COUNTERPULSATION, CARDIOPULMONARY BYPASS
Femoral artery cannulation
Retrograde arterial perfusion

▶ Types of Aortic Pathologic Conditions

Annuloaortic Ectasia

The term *annuloaortic ectasia* is used to denote marked dilatation of the sinuses of Valsalva and the aortic valve annulus (Kouchoukos, 1996). The sinuses of Valsalva are the three pouch-like areas of aortic wall that originate at the aortic valve annulus and extend just beyond the coronary artery ostia (DeBakey & McCollum, 1987). Annuloaortic ectasia often is associated with Marfan's syndrome; forme fruste of Marfan's syndrome; aortic dissection; aortitis; and other disorders that cause weakness of the aortic wall (David, 1998). Aortic regurgitation, aneurysmal dilatation, or aortic dissection may occur in the presence of annuloaortic ectasia.

Thoracic Aortic Aneurysm

Any condition that weakens aortic wall integrity can produce localized dilatation of the aorta, with eventual aneurysm formation. *Thoracic aortic aneurysms* are much less common than aneurysms of the abdominal aorta, and their incidence has not increased markedly, as has that of abdominal aortic aneurysms (Isselbacher et al., 1997). Most thoracic aneurysms are true aneurysms. A true aneurysm is one in which all layers of the aortic wall remain intact. In a false aneurysm, there is partial or complete disruption of the aortic wall and aortic blood is contained only by the adventitial layer and periaortic fibrous tissue (Cohn, 1995). Abnormalities of the aorta that are sometimes confused with aortic aneurysm include aortic enlargement secondary to aortic regurgitation and poststenotic dilatation in patients with aortic stenosis.

Aneurysms are described according to shape and location. A fusiform aneurysm is characterized by circumferential dilatation, whereas a saccular aneurysm is a balloon-like dilatation on one side of the aorta (Fig. 3-3). Most etiologic conditions produce diffuse, fusiform aneurysmal dilation, although infection (ie, mycotic aneurysm) often produces a saccular aneurysm (Coselli, 1997). The lumen of both fusiform and saccular aneurysms virtually always contains laminated thrombus (Lindsay et al., 1994). Thoracic aneurysms are categorized by location as ascending (between aortic valve annulus and origin of innominate artery), transverse arch (between origins of innominate and left subclavian arteries), or descending (distal to origin of left subclavian artery). An aneurysm of the descending thoracic aorta that extends below the diaphragm is termed thoracoabdominal.

Of all thoracic aortic aneurysms, the ascending aorta is affected in approximately 50% of cases, the arch in 10%, and the descending aorta in 40% (Fann & Miller, 1996). The anatomic distinction is significant because etiology, natural history, and therapy differ depending on the thoracic aortic segment involved (Isselbacher et al., 1997). Aneurysms of the aortic arch usually are a

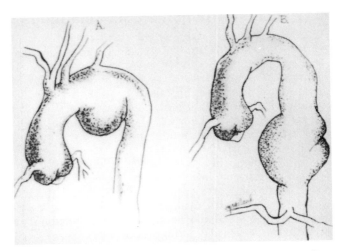

FIGURE 3-3. Thoracic aneurysms are categorized by shape as sacciform **(A)** or fusiform **(B)**. (Weiland AP, Walker WE, 1986: Thoracic aneurysms. Critical Care Quarterly 9(3):21; Aspen)

manifestation of more diffuse aortic disease that involves either the ascending or descending aorta, or both (Griepp & Ergin, 1997). Sometimes, multiple discrete aneurysms are present or the entire thoracic aorta is aneurysmal. Rarely, an aneurysm occurs in one of the sinuses of Valsalva.

The most common etiology of thoracic and thoracoabdominal aneurysms is atherosclerosis (Kirklin & Barratt-Boyes, 1993a). Atherosclerotic aortic disease usually affects people older than 50 years of age and often coexists with coronary or peripheral arterial manifestations of the disease. Although atherosclerosis usually is more severe in the abdominal aorta, aneurysms of atherosclerotic origin sometimes develop in the thoracic aorta. They are more common in the ascending than the descending thoracic aorta, and least common in the aortic arch (Cohn, 1995). Atherosclerotic aneurysms are most often fusiform.

Aortic aneurysm also is common in people with Marfan's syndrome or cystic medial necrosis. Such aneurysms commonly begin at the aortic valve in the area of the sinuses of Valsalva and extend to the origin of the innominate artery. Aortic regurgitation frequently is present owing to annuloaortic ectasia and the resulting loss of valve leaflet coaptation (Kouchoukos, 1996). Other processes that affect the aortic wall, such as aortitis, also can cause thoracic aneurysms. Granulomatous aortitis is a common cause of diffuse aneurysmal disease, sometimes involving the entire thoracic segment or even the entire aorta. Syphilis once was a common cause of very large saccular aneurysms in the ascending aorta or aortic arch, but syphilitic aneurysms are now rare as a result of aggressive antibiotic treatment of syphilis in its early stage (Isselbacher et al., 1997; Pairolero et al., 1976). An aneurysm that develops secondary to syphilis is called a *luetic aneurysm*.

A mycotic aneurysm is one that is caused by infective aortitis. Mycotic aneurysms can result from (1) septic embolism to a normal or atherosclerotic aorta; (2) contigu-

ous spread from recent abscesses, infected lymph nodes, or empyema; and (3) sepsis due to trauma, intravenous injections, or a previous surgical procedure (Cohn, 1995). For unexplained reasons, mycotic aneurysms tend to occur along the lesser curvature of the transverse aortic arch or in the upper abdominal aorta immediately posterior to the origin of the visceral vessels (Coselli, 1997). Sepsis, distal embolization, and a significant threat of aortic rupture are characteristic of mycotic aneurysms (Akins, 1989).

Another cause of aneurysm formation is persistence of a false lumen after acute aortic dissection. The thin outer wall of the false lumen has a tendency to weaken gradually; as wall stress increases, an aneurysm may develop and enlarge (Kirklin & Barratt-Boyes, 1993a). An unusual cause of thoracic aneurysm formation is aortic transection due to trauma (Finkelmeier et al., 1982). If rupture resulting from aortic transection is contained by adventitia, the lesion may evolve into a chronic false aneurysm. Chronic traumatic aneurysm classically occurs at the thoracic isthmus (near the origin of the left subclavian artery), but may arise from tears in other locations as well. Depending on the circumferential extent of the initial aortic laceration, chronic traumatic aneurysms may be fusiform or saccular (Bavaria & Edmunds, 1997). Occasionally, an aneurysm develops in the thoracic aorta that is caused by iatrogenic aortic injury that occurred during previous cardiac or aortic surgery.

Aneurysms sometimes develop secondary to aortic stenosis or coarctation because of poststenotic dilatation. The change in velocity of blood flow through an area of stenosis increases lateral pressure on the aortic wall just beyond the stenotic area, producing a jet lesion with eventual aneurysm formation. Congenital aneurysms can occur near the ligamentum arteriosum or in the sinuses of Valsalva. Etiologies of thoracic aneurysm are listed in Table 3-2.

TABLE 3-2

Etiologies of Thoracic Aortic Aneurysm

Atherosclerosis
Cystic medial necrosis
Marfan's syndrome
Annuloaortic ectasia
Aortitis
   Granulomatous
   Syphilis (luetic)
Infection (mycotic)
Aortic transection
Iatrogenic injury
Poststenotic dilatation
Chronic aortic dissection with persisting false lumen
Congenital anomalies
   Sinus of Valsalva
   Ductus (ligamentum arteriosum)

Thoracic aortic aneurysm often is diagnosed when its appearance is noted on a chest roentgenogram. Aneurysms of the descending thoracic aorta, in particular, are likely to be detected before development of any symptoms because of a chest roentgenogram obtained for another reason. Aortography remains the diagnostic gold standard for clearly defining aneurysm location and its relationship to arteries branching from the aorta, whether the branches are stenosed or occluded, and the quality of the aorta beyond the aneurysm (Bayfield & Kron, 1998). Computed tomography (CT) of the chest with contrast infusion sometimes is performed as well. If the aortic valve is involved in the aneurysmal process, echocardiography and coronary angiography usually are performed.

The most significant feature of thoracic aortic aneurysm is the known propensity for aortic rupture. Studies have suggested that mortality from aortic aneurysm approaches 75% at 5 years, with one third to one half of deaths due to rupture (Lindsay et al., 1994). Likelihood of aortic rupture is directly related to aneurysm size and the development of symptoms. The law of Laplace states that as the size of a sphere increases, the wall tension of that sphere increases; thus, larger aneurysms are more prone to rupture than smaller ones (Cohn, 1995). Aortic rupture may occur precipitously as the initial manifestation, causing exsanguination into the mediastinum, pleural space, esophagus, or tracheobronchial tree (Lindsay et al., 1994). Occasionally, aortic rupture occurs without exsanguination because bleeding is contained by periaortic, pericardial, or pleural tissue. Patients with contained rupture usually experience severe chest pain and have roentgenographic evidence of a widened mediastinum or pleural effusion. Precipitous disruption of a contained rupture with rapid exsanguination can occur at any time. Rarely, a contained rupture remains intact, forming a false aneurysm.

Thoracic aneurysms often expand over time. Aneurysm expansion is worrisome because it increases the likelihood of aortic rupture. Depending on its location, an aneurysm can produce a variety of symptoms as it enlarges because of encroachment on surrounding structures (Table 3-3). Symptomatic patients have a much poorer prognosis than do those without symptoms, primarily because the onset of symptoms is frequently a harbinger of aortic rupture (Isselbacher et al., 1997). Between 25% to 33% of patients with ascending aortic aneurysms have chest pain as a presenting symptom (Downing & Kouchoukos, 1997). If the aortic root is aneurysmal, distortion of the aortic valve annulus may lead to aortic regurgitation and symptoms of congestive heart failure. Aortic regurgitation also may produce angina because low diastolic blood pressure impairs coronary artery filling and ventricular dilatation increases myocardial oxygen demand. Arch aneurysms may be associated with dyspnea, stridor, hoarseness, hemoptysis, cough, or chest pain (Coselli, 1996). Uncommonly, an arch aneurysm causes neck vein distention from venous compression (Spittell, 1998) (Fig. 3-4). Although as many as 50% of patients with descending tho-

TABLE 3-3

Signs and Symptoms of Thoracic Aortic Aneurysm Enlargement

Sign or Symptom	Due to Compression of
Superior vena cava syndrome	Superior vena cava
Chest wall pain	Ribs
Back pain	Vertebrae, spinal nerves
Hoarseness	Recurrent laryngeal nerve
Left hemidiaphragm elevation	Phrenic nerve
Dysphagia	Esophagus
Wheezing, cough, stridor, dyspnea	Trachea or bronchus

racic aortic aneurysms are asymptomatic at the time of diagnosis, back or chest pain, usually localized to the area of the aneurysm, is the most common symptom (Fann & Miller, 1996).

The only treatment for thoracic aortic aneurysm is operative repair. The decision to proceed with surgical resection of the aneurysm is based primarily on two factors: (1) any symptoms or radiographic evidence of enlargement, and (2) aortic diameter size. Operative repair is recommended for any symptomatic aneurysm, any aneurysm that exceeds twice the transverse diameter of an adjacent normal-caliber aortic segment, or any aneurysm that is 6 cm in diameter or larger (Duke et al., 1998). Larger aneurysms not only are more prone to rupture, they appear to have a more rapid growth rate than small aneurysms (Isselbacher et al., 1997). In people with Marfan's syndrome, operative repair often is

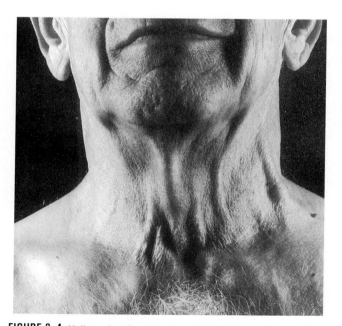

FIGURE 3-4. Unilateral neck vein distention (left internal jugular vein) in a patient with an aortic arch aneurysm. (Spittell PC, 1998: Diseases of the aorta. In Topol EJ [ed]: Comprehensive Cardiovascular Medicine. p. 3039. Philadelphia, Lippincott Williams & Wilkins)

recommended when an aneurysm reaches 5.0 to 5.5 cm because of the friable quality of aortic tissue associated with cystic medial necrosis. Normal diameter of the ascending aorta is 2.5 to 3.0 cm.

The nature of the aortic repair is determined primarily by location and extent of the aneurysm. The diseased segment of aorta usually is replaced with a prosthetic tubular graft. Blood flow to arterial branches supplied by the diseased segment must be preserved. Arteries are reimplanted into the side of the tubular graft. In the case of the great vessels, an island of aortic tissue containing the arch vessel origins is attached to an opening in the graft, or a human cadaver allograft may be used to replace the arch segment. If the aortic valve is regurgitant, valve resuspension or valve replacement to restore competency may be necessary. Operative repair of the thoracic aorta is discussed in greater detail in Chapter 17, Surgery on the Thoracic Aorta.

Aortic Dissection

Aortic dissection is the most common catastrophic condition involving the aorta, occurring almost twice as frequently as rupture of the abdominal aorta (Ergin & Griepp, 1996). The disorder is estimated to occur in approximately 5 to 10 people per million population (Wheat, 1987). Those at highest risk are men, African Americans, and people between 50 and 70 years of age. Acute aortic dissection has a grim prognosis. Without treatment, more than 25% of patients die within 24 hours, more than 50% within 1 week, and more than 75% within 1 month; fewer than 10% of patients survive 1 year (Isselbacher et al., 1997).

Dissection of the aortic wall occurs as an acute event secondary to a disruption in the intima. Two factors promote development of an intimal tear: (1) repeated motion of the ascending and proximal descending aorta secondary to the force of cardiac contractions; and (2) intraluminal hydrodynamic force of the pulse wave propagated by each cardiac contraction, particularly in the ascending aorta and exaggerated in the presence of systemic hypertension (Wheat, 1987). Approximately two thirds of dissections involve the ascending aorta (Lindsay et al., 1994). By far the two most frequent sites of aortic dissection origin (ie, intimal disruption) are the ascending aorta, within 5 cm of the aortic valve, and just distal to the left subclavian artery near the ligamentum arteriosum (Isselbacher et al., 1997).

When intimal disruption occurs, blood from the true lumen of the aorta dissects the abnormal medial layer, forming a false lumen between the intima and adventitia. Systemic blood pressure in the aorta causes blood to track retrograde, antegrade, or in both directions, separating intimal and adventitial layers for a variable length of the aorta. Progression of the dissection is enhanced by continued hypertension, anticoagulation, or an elevated dP/dt (ie, the force of left ventricular ejection). Multiple reentry points may be present where blood in the false lumen ruptures the intima to reenter the true lumen. Al-

ternatively, the dissection may stop at a point where further dissection is precluded by atherosclerotic changes in the aortic wall. The term *dissecting aneurysm* frequently is used to label this disorder. However, the word *aneurysm* is a misnomer because the pathologic abnormality really is a dissecting hematoma and not an aneurysm. The two conditions sometimes coexist.

Although the etiology of aortic dissection is not well defined, a number of factors are thought to play a role in its occurrence (Table 3-4). Of these factors, arterial hypertension remains most consistent (Ergin & Griepp, 1996). Seventy-five to 90% of patients with aortic dissection are hypertensive at the time of presentation or have a history of hypertension (Stone & Borst, 1997; Wheat, 1987). Although hypertension has not been definitively linked to initiation of aortic dissection, it is the major factor in promoting progression of dissection (Ergin & Griepp, 1996).

Cystic medial necrosis is present in approximately 20% of patients with acute aortic dissection (Kirklin & Barratt-Boyes, 1993b). In affected people, cohesiveness of inner (intimal) and outer (adventitial) wall layers is diminished. Medial degeneration most is often related to a connective tissue disorder, such as Marfan's syndrome. Even in patients without physical stigmata of Marfan's syndrome, cystic medial degeneration often is detected on pathologic examination of the aortic tissue. Other disorders that affect aortic wall integrity, such as aortitis and Ehlers-Danlos syndrome, a congenital connective tissue disorder, also are causative factors.

Additional factors associated with increased risk for aortic dissection, particularly in young people, are pregnancy, a congenitally deformed aortic valve, and coarctation. Of aortic dissections in young women, 50% occur during pregnancy, mostly during the third trimester and in patients with congenital malformation of the aorta or connective tissue disorders (Ergin & Griepp, 1996; Isselbacher et al., 1997). A congenitally bicuspid or unicuspid aortic valve is another well recognized risk factor for dissection of the proximal aorta (Spittell, 1997). Coarctation of the aortic isthmus also predisposes the aorta to dissection, particularly in older patients (Stone & Borst, 1997). Rarely, iatrogenic aortic

TABLE 3-4
Etiologic Factors in Aortic Dissection

Cystic medial necrosis
Marfan's syndrome
Aortitis
Ehlers-Danlos syndrome
Coarctation of the aorta
Bicuspid aortic valve
Pregnancy
Hypertension
Iatrogenic arterial injury
Blunt chest trauma

dissection occurs secondary to femoral artery or aortic cannulation for cardiopulmonary bypass, intra-aortic balloon catheter insertion, or aortic cross-clamping during cardiovascular operations.

Aortic dissections are categorized according to location and extent of aortic involvement. Anatomic categorization of aortic dissection is important because therapy is distinctly different. Two classification systems are used commonly. The Stanford classification system categorizes aortic dissection according to ascending aortic involvement, regardless of the origin of intimal disruption (Fig. 3-5). Type A dissection involves the ascending aorta. The dissection may be confined only to the ascending aorta or extend beyond the aortic arch to involve the descending aorta as well. Type B dissection involves only the descending aorta, distal to the left subclavian artery.

The DeBakey classification system also remains in common use: type I dissection extends from the ascending aorta to beyond the left subclavian artery; type II is limited to the ascending aorta, proximal to the left subclavian artery; and type III involves only the descending aorta, distal to the left subclavian artery (DeBakey & McCollum, 1987) (Fig. 3-6). DeBakey types I and II are combined in the Stanford system as type A, and DeBakey type III is the same as Stanford type B. Aortic dissections are further classified as acute or chronic. Because most of the mortality from dissection occurs within 2 weeks of onset, a dissection recognized during this period is considered acute, whereas one recognized more than 2 weeks after onset is chronic (Spittell, 1997).

Acute dissection is a catastrophic event that can produce several life-threatening consequences. Sudden death can occur when (1) rupture causes tamponade or exsan-

guination, or (2) proximal extension of the dissection causes occlusion of the coronary ostia or severe acute aortic regurgitation. Rupture of the dissected aorta, with hemorrhage into the pericardium, mediastinum, pleural space, or abdomen, is the most common cause of death. Although rupture can occur anywhere along the length of aorta, proximal dissections most commonly rupture into the pericardium and distal dissections into the left pleural space (Eagle et al., 1989). Free rupture is invariably fatal owing to rapid exsanguination. Bleeding into the pericardial sac or mediastinum may cause cardiac tamponade. In some instances, the rupture is temporarily contained by periaortic fibrous, pericardial, or pleural tissue.

Type A (ie, ascending) aortic dissection frequently extends retrograde to involve the aortic valve. Acute aortic regurgitation can occur as a result of annular dilatation, altered geometry of the aortic root, or leaflet or annular tear (Fann et al., 1991). Unlike chronic aortic regurgitation, in which the left ventricle over time develops compensatory adaptations to the regurgitated stroke volume, acute aortic regurgitation produces severe congestive heart failure, pulmonary edema, or frank cardiogenic shock.

The coronary ostia, particularly that of the right coronary artery, may become involved in the dissection, leading to inferior wall myocardial ischemia or infarction. Aortic dissection also can occlude any of the other aortic branches, causing acute ischemia to organs supplied by affected branches. Thirty to 50% of patients have signs or symptoms of acute peripheral arterial occlusion as a consequence of extrinsic compression of the arterial true lumen by the false lumen (Fann et al., 1989). Stroke, paraplegia, or peripheral neuropathy can result from compromised blood flow to the brain, spinal cord, or peripheral nerves, respectively. These neurologic manifestations occur in 6% to 19% of patients with aortic dissection (Isselbacher et al., 1997). Renal failure, bowel infarction, or limb ischemia also may develop as supplying arteries become occluded by the dissection.

The most prevalent symptom associated with aortic dissection is the sudden onset of excruciating chest or back (interscapular) pain, often described as tearing, shearing, or "knife-like." Frequently, pain migrates from its origin to other sites, usually following the path of the dissection as it extends through the aorta (Isselbacher et al., 1997). Acute aortic dissection and myocardial infarction are sometimes difficult to differentiate, and both conditions should be considered during the evaluation of any patient with severe chest pain. In such cases, the diagnosis of aortic dissection must be excluded before administering thrombolytic therapy for treatment of MI. Occasionally, aortic dissection is not accompanied by any pain or the pain waxes and wanes or dissipates after a short duration.

Shock may be present because of (1) loss of blood volume from the false channel into periaortic tissues and spaces, (2) acute aortic regurgitation, or (3) rupture into the pericardium with cardiac tamponade (Kirklin & Barratt-Boyes, 1993b). Other possible manifestations include abdominal pain, extremity weakness, hematuria,

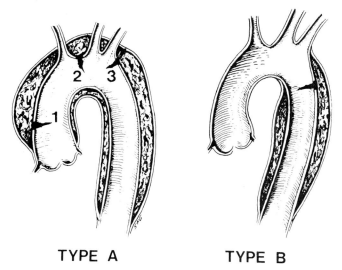

TYPE A   **TYPE B**

FIGURE 3-5. Stanford classification of aortic dissection. The primary intimal disruption in type A dissections can be in the ascending aorta (1), transverse arch (2), or descending aorta (3). (Wheat MW Jr, 1987: Acute dissection of the aorta. In McGoon DC [ed]: Cardiac Surgery, ed. 2, p. 250. Philadelphia, FA Davis)

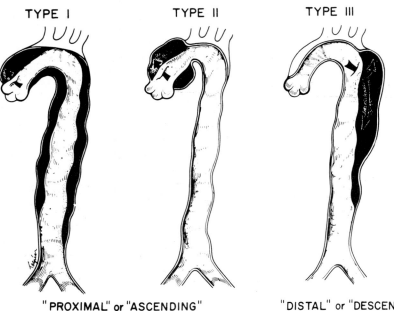

FIGURE 3-6. DeBakey classification of aortic dissection. (Eagle KA, Doroghazi RM, DeSanctis RW, Austen WG, 1989: Aortic dissection. In Eagle KA, Haber E, DeSanctis RW, Austen WG [eds]: The Practice of Cardiology, ed. 2, p. 1371. Boston, Little, Brown)

hemiparesis, hemiplegia, paraplegia, syncope, and speech or visual disturbances.

Physical examination may reveal unequal pulses or blood pressure in the extremities, a diminishing hematocrit, and a new diastolic murmur of aortic regurgitation. The occurrence of aortic dissection often is associated with a dramatic sympathetic response, which causes an exacerbation or persistence of marked hypertension (Gardner, 1998). Thus, hypertension may be present despite a general appearance of shock. Neurologic signs and symptoms as well as blood flow to one or several extremities can wax and wane as pressure in the dissecting hematoma (false lumen) increases or decreases (Wheat, 1987).

The diagnosis is suggested by the clinical presentation in combination with a chest roentgenogram that reveals widening of the mediastinum. Mediastinal width is difficult to interpret, however, because prior chest roentgenograms may be unavailable or may have been taken using a posteroanterior projection. A chest film taken for evaluation of acute dissection is almost always done at the bedside and, therefore, is performed using an anteroposterior projection. The mediastinum, by virtue of the anteroposterior projection, appears somewhat wider than it does on the posteroanterior film. Also, aortic dissection does not always produce radiographic evidence of mediastinal widening. The chest roentgenogram also may demonstrate pleural effusion (usually left sided) or cardiomegaly secondary to pericardial effusion (Kirklin & Barratt-Boyes, 1993b).

Although symptoms and roentgenographic demonstration of a widened mediastinum are helpful in suggesting the presence of dissection, they should not be used to rule out the diagnosis. Either CT of the chest with contrast infusion or transesophageal echocardiography is used to confirm the diagnosis of aortic dissec-

tion, and often provides all the information needed to proceed with definitive treatment. CT scanning has relatively high, but not absolute, sensitivity and specificity, and conventional CT may not detect a rapidly moving intimal flap (Finkelmeier, 1997). Unless ultrafast scanning techniques are available, the rapidly moving, disrupted intima is not always demonstrated. Transesophageal echocardiography is highly reliable in detecting dissection and provides information about aortic valve function, but care must be taken to avoid exacerbation of hypertension with the passage of a probe into the esophagus in a conscious patient. Transthoracic echocardiography usually is not helpful in diagnosing aortic dissection. Aortography, formerly the gold standard for diagnosis of dissection, now is used selectively in patients with aortic dissection. It can provide more detailed information about the perfusion status of important branches supplied by the dissected aorta, and more effectively demonstrates the origin (intimal flap), the true and false lumens, and the distal extent of dissection.

Acute aortic dissection is associated with devastating complications and has a lethal nature, particularly if diagnosis or treatment is delayed. Consequently, the patient with acute dissection is monitored in a cardiothoracic surgical intensive care unit and a cardiothoracic surgeon oversees initial patient evaluation and management. The patient is at highest risk for death during the first hours after onset of dissection, particularly if hypertension is not corrected. Thorough, serial assessments are essential to monitor occurrence and progression of complications of the dissection. Type A aortic dissection is treated as a surgical emergency, unless irreversible complications of dissection already have occurred. Emergent surgical intervention is recommended because of a nearly 100% probability of early death with type A dissection due to aortic rupture or coronary artery occlusion (Gardner, 1998). The operative mortality rate for repair of type A dissection ranges from 5% to 20%, depending on the interval between the onset of dissection and operation (Cohn, 1995).

In contrast, the primary treatment for patients with type B (ie, descending) aortic dissection is pharmacologic therapy to control hypertension. A cardiothoracic surgeon usually directs acute management of type B dissection because urgent operative intervention may become necessary if the dissection extends or rupture occurs. Persistent pain or evidence of threatened perfusion to abdominal viscera, the spinal cord, or lower extremities indicates extension of the dissection. Repair of acute type B dissection is associated with an operative mortality rate of 10% to 20%, primarily because the operation most often is performed selectively in patients with complications of dissection (Cohn, 1995).

Surgical therapy also is recommended for both type A and type B dissections in patients with Marfan's syndrome (Isselbacher et al., 1997). Operative repair of aortic dissection is discussed in Chapter 17, Surgery on the Thoracic Aorta.

Regardless of whether surgical therapy is undertaken, immediate treatment of hypertension is the most important component of medical therapy in all patients with aortic dissection. Antihypertensive therapy is essential to prevent further dissection and must be instituted as soon as the diagnosis is suspected, even before diagnostic confirmation. Medications that are effective in reducing systolic arterial pressure and the force of left ventricular ejection (dP/dt) are used. Intravenous nitroprusside is almost always the drug of choice because of its immediate and potent antihypertensive effect. However, nitroprusside alone may cause a reflex increase in dP/dt, possibly accelerating dissection progression (Isselbacher et al., 1997). Therefore, a beta-blocking agent such as esmolol also must be used acutely to reduce dP/dt. Systolic blood pressure usually is maintained between 90 and 100 mm Hg, or at the lowest level that continues to provide adequate organ perfusion.

With either surgical or medical treatment, long-term management of hypertension is essential. An oral beta-blocking agent, such as propranolol, often is used for chronic blood pressure control. For patients who are successfully discharged after treatment of aortic dissection, there is a 75% to 82% probability of surviving 5 years (Isselbacher et al., 1997). Residual aortic and cardiovascular disease are significant causes of late death and morbidity in people with aortic dissection, regardless of the mode of treatment of the disease (Glower et al., 1990).

Rarely, acute dissection remains unrecognized. Such patients, and those who have received medical therapy only, are considered to have chronic aortic dissection. In chronic dissection, gradual aneurysmal dilatation of the false channel occurs (Ergin & Griepp, 1996). Type A chronic dissection (ie, type A dissection that was undetected during its acute phase) usually is treated with elective operative repair if any of the following develop: (1) significant aortic regurgitation, (2) aneurysm formation, or (3) progression of dissection (Cohn, 1995; Eagle et al., 1989). Elective repair of type B chronic dissection is considered in patients in whom aortic diameter exceeds 6 cm, especially in association with uncontrolled hypertension (Neya et al., 1992). The risk of operative death is 5% to 10% for repair of both type A and type B chronic aortic dissection (Cohn, 1995).

Aortic Transection

Acute transection of the aorta occurs as a consequence of severe blunt chest trauma. Motor vehicle accidents are thought to account for 80% of acute aortic transections; other causes include kicks, falls from heights, and crush injuries (Miller & Calhoon, 1998). Injury to the aorta almost always occurs in one of two sites: (1) in the descending aorta just distal to the origin of the left subclavian artery, and (2) in the aortic root just above the aortic valve. These two locations are classic sites of aortic injury because of the stress to which they are subjected. The heart and the descending aorta are relatively fixed in position by contiguous structures. However, the ascending and transverse aorta (aortic arch), from the aortic root to the ligamentum arteriosum, are not tethered. Therefore, these two junctures of fixation are likely injury points.

Transection just distal to the left subclavian artery most often is produced by rapid horizontal deceleration, such as occurs with high-speed motor vehicle accidents. Rapid vertical deceleration, such as occurs with a fall from a building or airplane, usually causes disruption of the ascending aorta, usually just above the aortic valve. Aortic disruption that occurs in this location almost always is immediately fatal, and that which occurs at the aortic isthmus usually is. Untreated survivors of acute thoracic aortic transection have a grim prognosis. Of the 10% to 20% of patients who survive initially, one half are estimated to die within 24 hours, and an additional 5% of the remaining survivors die per day; only a few untreated patients survive long enough for development of a chronic traumatic thoracic aneurysm (Miller & Calhoon, 1998). Aortic transection is described in more detail in Chapter 32, Cardiac and Thoracic Trauma.

REFERENCES

Akins CW, 1989: Nondissecting aneurysms of the thoracic aorta. In Eagle KA, Haber E, DeSanctis RW, Austin WG (eds): The Practice of Cardiology, ed. 2. Boston, Little, Brown

Bavaria JE, Edmunds LH Jr, 1997: Traumatic aortic rupture. In Edmunds LH Jr (ed): Cardiac Surgery in the Adult. New York, McGraw-Hill

Bayfield MS, Kron IL, 1998: Repair of chronic thoracic and thoracoabdominal aortic aneurysms. In Kaiser LR, Kron IL, Spray TL (eds): Mastery of Cardiothoracic Surgery. Philadelphia, Lippincott Williams & Wilkins

Cohn LH, 1995: Thoracic aortic aneurysms and aortic dissection. In Sabiston DC Jr, Spencer FC (eds): Surgery of the Chest, ed. 6. Philadelphia, WB Saunders

Coselli JS, 1997: Descending and thoracoabdominal aortic aneurysms. In Edmunds LH Jr (ed): Cardiac Surgery in the Adult. New York, McGraw-Hill

Coselli JS, 1996: Aneurysms of the transverse aortic arch. In Baue AE, Geha AS, Hammond GL, et al. (eds): Glenn's Thoracic and Cardiovascular Surgery, ed. 6. Stamford, CT, Appleton & Lange

David TE, 1998: Annuloaortic ectasia. In Kaiser LR, Kron IL, Spray TL (eds): Mastery of Cardiothoracic Surgery. Philadelphia, Lippincott Williams & Wilkins

DeBakey ME, McCollum CH, 1987: Diseases of the aorta. In Chung EK (ed): Quick Reference to Cardiovascular Diseases, ed. 3. Baltimore, Williams & Wilkins

Downing SW, Kouchoukos NT, 1997: Ascending aortic aneurysm. In Edmunds LH Jr (ed): Cardiac Surgery in the Adult. New York, McGraw-Hill

Duke MD, Miller DC, Mitchell RS, et al., 1998: The "first generation" of endovascular stent-grafts for patients with aneurysms of the descending thoracic aorta. J Thorac Cardiovasc Surg 116:689

Eagle KA, Doroghazi RM, DeSanctis RW, Austen WG, 1989: Aortic dissection. In Eagle KA, Haber E, DeSanctis RW, Austin WG (eds): The Practice of Cardiology, ed. 2. Boston, Little, Brown

Ergin MA, Griepp RB, 1996: Dissections of the aorta. In Baue AE, Geha AS, Hammond GL, et al. (eds): Glenn's Thoracic and Cardiovascular Surgery, ed. 6. Stamford, CT, Appleton & Lange

Fann JI, Glower DD, Miller DC, et al., 1991: Preservation of aortic valve in type A aortic dissection complicated by aortic regurgitation. J Thorac Cardiovasc Surg 102:62

Fann JI, Miller DC, 1996: Descending thoracic aortic aneurysms. In Baue AE, Geha AS, Hammond GL, et al. (eds): Glenn's Thoracic and Cardiovascular Surgery, ed. 6. Stamford, CT, Appleton & Lange

Fann JI, Sarris GE, Miller C, et al., 1989: Surgical management of acute aortic dissection complicated by stroke. Circulation 80(Suppl I):I-257

Finkelmeier BA, 1997: Dissection of the aorta: a clinical update. J Vasc Nurs 15:97

Finkelmeier BA, Mentzer RM, Kaiser DL, et al., 1982: Chronic traumatic aneurysm. J Thorac Cardiovasc Surg 84:257

Gardner TJ, 1998: Acute aortic dissection. In Kaiser LR, Kron IL, Spray TL (eds): Mastery of Cardiothoracic Surgery. Philadelphia, Lippincott Williams & Wilkins

Geva T, Hegesh J, Frand M, 1987: The clinical course and echocardiographic features of Marfan's syndrome in childhood. American Journal of Diseases of Children 141:1179

Glower DD, Fann JI, Speier RH, et al., 1990: Comparison of medical and surgical therapy for uncomplicated descending aortic dissection. Circulation 82(Suppl IV):IV-39

Griepp RB, Ergin MA, 1997: Aneurysms of the aortic arch. In Edmunds LH Jr (ed): Cardiac Surgery in the Adult. New York, McGraw-Hill

Isselbacher EM, Eagle KA, DeSanctis RW, 1997: Diseases of the aorta. In Braunwald E (ed): Heart Disease: A Textbook of Cardiovascular Medicine, ed. 5. Philadelphia, WB Saunders

Kirklin JW, Barratt-Boyes BG, 1993a: Chronic thoracic and thoracoabdominal aortic aneurysms. In Cardiac Surgery, ed. 2. New York, Churchill Livingstone

Kirklin JW, Barratt-Boyes BG, 1993b: Acute aortic dissection. In Cardiac Surgery, ed. 2. New York, Churchill Livingstone

Kouchoukos NT, 1996: Aneurysms of the ascending aorta. In Baue AE, Geha AS, Hammond GL, et al. (eds): Glenn's Thoracic and Cardiovascular Surgery, ed. 6., Stamford, CT, Appleton & Lange

Lindsay J Jr, DeBakey ME, Beall AC, 1994: Diagnosis and treatment of diseases of the aorta. In Schlant RC, Alexander RW et al. (eds): The Heart, ed. 8. New York, McGraw-Hill

Miller OL, Calhoon JH, 1998: Acute traumatic aortic transection. In Kaiser LR, Kron IL, Spray TL (eds): Mastery of Cardiothoracic Surgery. Philadelphia, Lippincott Williams & Wilkins

Murdoch JL, Walker BA, Halpern BL, et al., 1972: Life expectancy and causes of death in the Marfan syndrome. N Engl J Med 286:15

Neya K, Omoto R, Kyo S, et al., 1992: Outcome of Stanford type B acute aortic dissection. Circulation 86(Suppl II):II-1

Pairolero PC, Bernatz PE, 1976: Aneurysms. In Gay WA (ed): Cardiovascular Surgery (Goldsmith Practice of Surgery, rev. ed.). Philadelphia, Harper & Row

Perloff JK, Braunwald E, 1997: Physical examination of the heart and circulation. In Braunwald E (ed): Heart Disease: A Textbook of Cardiovascular Medicine, ed. 5. Philadelphia, WB Saunders

Peyton RB, Isom OW, 1995: Occlusive disease of branches of the aorta. In Sabiston DC Jr, Spencer FC (eds): Surgery of the Chest, ed. 6. Philadelphia, WB Saunders

Pyeritz RE, 1979: The Marfan syndrome: Diagnosis and management. N Engl J Med 300:772

Pyeritz RE, 1997: Genetics and cardiovascular disease. In Braunwald E (ed): Heart Disease: A Textbook of Cardiovascular Medicine, ed. 5. Philadelphia, WB Saunders

Schoen FJ, 1997: Pathologic considerations in the surgery of adult heart disease. In Edmunds LH Jr (ed): Cardiac Surgery in the Adult. New York, McGraw-Hill

Spittell PC, 1998: Diseases of the aorta. In Topol EJ (ed): Comprehensive Cardiovascular Medicine. Philadelphia, Lippincott Williams & Wilkins

Spittell PC, 1997: Aortic dissection: diagnosis and management. In Brown DL (ed): Cardiac Intensive Care. Philadelphia, WB Saunders

Stone C, Borst H, 1997: Dissecting aortic aneurysm. In Edmunds LH Jr (ed): Cardiac Surgery in the Adult. New York, McGraw-Hill

Svensson LG, Crawford ES, 1997a: Marfan syndrome and connective tissue diseases. In Cardiovascular and Vascular Disease of the Aorta. Philadelphia, WB Saunders

Svensson LG, Crawford ES, 1997b: Aortic infections. In Cardiovascular and Vascular Disease of the Aorta. Philadelphia, WB Saunders

Wheat MW, 1987: Acute dissection of the aorta. In McGoon DC (ed): Cardiac Surgery, ed. 2. Philadelphia, FA Davis

4

Cardiac Rhythm Disorders

Recurring or persistent cardiac arrhythmias represent a cardiac rhythm disorder, usually occurring secondary to underlying cardiac disease or other abnormality. An estimated 4,300,000 Americans have heart rhythm disorders (American Heart Association, 1998). *Chronic rhythm disorders* requiring long-term therapy with antiarrhythmic drugs, implantable devices, or catheter or surgical ablation are the focus of this chapter. Cardiac arrhythmias also may occur as transient events, triggered by specific precipitants, such as myocardial ischemia, proarrhythmic agents, or electrolyte imbalance. Characteristics and acute management of such transient arrhythmias are discussed in Chapter 25, Cardiac Arrhythmias.

▶ Electrical Activation of the Heart

Electrical activation of the heart normally occurs as a coordinated, progressive excitation process by means of specialized conductive tissue. Impulses originate in the sinus node, a small group of automatic cells located just beneath the epicardial surface at the junction of the superior vena cava and right atrium. Automatic cells differ from contractile cells of the myocardium in that the membrane potential does not remain constant during the final phase (phase 4) of the action potential. Instead, the hallmark of automatic cells is that the membrane permeability of the cells allows a slow inward leak of current during phase 4, leading to spontaneous depolarization (White, 1998). This property of automaticity enables the sinus node to initiate action potentials independent of any prior impulse.

Although there are automatic cells in other areas of the heart (atrioventricular [AV] node, some atrial cells, and Purkinje fibers), the sinus node has the most rapid rate of spontaneous depolarization and, under normal conditions, acts as the dominant pacemaker. Its rich innervation with postganglionic adrenergic and cholinergic nerve terminals increases and decreases the rate of spontaneous depolarization, accounting for variations in sinus heart rate (Zipes, 1997a). Whereas the sympathetic nervous system exerts a dominant effect on heart rate during times of stress, the parasympathetic nervous system is the major mediator at rest (Sabatine et al., 1998).

From its origin in the sinus node, the electrical impulse spreads in relatively concentric circles to excite muscle cells throughout both atria (Bond & Halpenny, 1995). Impulse conduction between the sinus and AV nodes does not occur at the same velocity through all parts of the atria, but instead appears to travel more rapidly by means of thick atrial muscle bundles. These muscle bundles, however, are not specialized, insulated conduction tracts comparable with the ventricular bundle branches, and their surgical transection does not block internodal conduction (Cox, 1995). Thus, the precise role that these preferential pathways play in transmitting impulses between the sinus and AV nodes remains unclear.

The impulse passes through the AV node to the ventricles after a slight delay. The AV node functions both as the means of conducting impulses to the ventricles and as the origin of the cardiac rhythm in the presence of sinus nodal dysfunction (eg, sinus arrest, sinus bradycardia, and sinus block) (Chung, 1989). Except for AV nodal and bundle of His tissue, an electrically inert barrier, the fibrous skeleton, separates the atria and ventricles. Therefore, the AV node is normally the only pathway for electrical conduction between atria and ventricles. When it is dysfunctional, the ventricles no longer receive impulses originating in the atria.

Impulses traveling through the AV node are conducted to ventricular myocardium through the bundle of His, bundle branches, and Purkinje fibers. This specialized conductive network spreads the impulse almost simultaneously to the entire right and left ventricular endocardium. Activation then spreads from the endocardium toward the epicardium, depolarizing all regions of the ventricles.

▸ Pathogenesis of Arrhythmias

Mechanisms of arrhythmogenesis can be categorized as disorders of impulse formation, disorders of impulse conduction, or a combination of both.

Abnormal Impulse Formation

The most common disorder of impulse formation is enhanced automaticity, a phenomenon in which the spontaneous depolarization rate of myocardial pacemaker cells becomes abnormally accelerated. Enhanced automaticity of sinus node cells produces sinus tachycardia. Atrial, nodal, or ventricular tachycardias may result from enhanced spontaneous depolarization of normally latent automatic cells. Clinical conditions that enhance spontaneous depolarization in automatic cells include ischemia, hypokalemia, and beta-adrenergic receptor stimulation (Ruskin & Schoenfeld, 1989).

Alternatively, impulse formation in automatic cells may become abnormally slow. If the sinus depolarization rate still surpasses that of other automatic cardiac cells, sinus bradycardia results. Pronounced slowing of the sinus depolarization rate sometimes allows a latent or ectopic pacemaker to initiate the cardiac rhythm. Because the AV node usually has the second-fastest spontaneous depolarization rate, a nodal escape rhythm typically occurs. Causes of decreased sinus node automaticity include excessive vagal stimulation, such as carotid sinus massage; medications, such as digitalis or beta-adrenergic blocking agents; and diseases, such as sick sinus syndrome or inferior wall myocardial infarction (MI) (Jacobson, 1995).

In addition to enhanced or slowed impulse formation in automatic cells, arrhythmias can arise from abnormal automaticity, that is, myocardial contractile fibers that abnormally exhibit automaticity. Atrial and ventricular myocardial cells outside the specialized conducting system normally do not have spontaneous depolarizations and thus do not initiate spontaneous impulses, even when not excited for long periods of time by propagating impulses (Waldo & Wit, 1994). Abnormal automaticity occurs when these contractile cells acquire the ability to initiate abnormal rhythms because of pathologic cellular changes caused by tissue injury (Sabatine et al., 1998).

Abnormal Impulse Conduction

Two primary disorders of impulse conduction can occur: blocked or slowed conduction and a phenomenon known as *reentry*. Blocked conduction occurs when an impulse reaches a region of the heart that is electrically unexcitable; the block may be transient or permanent, and unidirectional or bidirectional (Sabatine et al., 1998). If an area of conduction tissue is abnormal but still excitable, conduction may occur but be slower than normal. Blocked or slowed conduction may result in bradycardia, tachycardia, or no change in heart rate. For example, injury to the AV node may cause complete heart block with a ventricular escape rhythm (bradycardia). Alternatively, a tachycardia may result when slowed conduction provides the substrate for establishment of a reentry tachycardia. An example of slowed conduction that does not affect heart rate is delayed conduction through the bundle branches. Although ventricular depolarization is prolonged, as evidenced by a widened QRS complex, the heart rate usually does not change.

Reentry, or continuous circulating excitation, is the second type of abnormal impulse conduction. It is the likely mechanism for most recurrent arrhythmias in chronic heart disease (Grant & Whalley, 1998). Reentry occurs when an impulse depolarizes an area of myocardium and then reenters and depolarizes the same area again (Jacobson, 1995). Under normal conditions, an impulse originates in the sinus node, activates all cardiac cells in turn, and is extinguished when all fibers have been depolarized and are completely refractory (Zipes, 1997a). The refractory period after cellular depolarization ensures that all cells are depolarized only once by the impulse.

A reentry circuit may be established, however, when an area of unidirectional block is present in combination with slowed conduction through an alternative pathway. In the area of unidirectional block, antegrade impulse propagation is blocked and cells distal to the area are depolarized through the alternate pathway. If conduction velocity through the alternate pathway is sufficiently slow, the electrical wave front travels retrograde through the area of unidirectional block, then reenters previously depolarized cells in the alternate pathway that have recovered and are capable of reexcitation (Fig. 4-1). The impulse again travels retrograde through the area of unidirectional block and, because the wave front continues through excitable tissue, the circular excitation can continue indefinitely, producing a reentrant arrhythmia. Reentry circuits may involve anatomically large portions of myocardium or may be confined to small areas of tissue. The reentry circuit may produce either supraventricular or ventricular tachyarrhythmias, depending on its location.

▸ Classification of Arrhythmias

Bradyarrhythmias

A variety of etiologic factors can produce *bradyarrhythmias*, including degenerative changes in the conductive system, MI, cardiac operations, hypersensitive carotid sinus syndrome, and certain medications. Diagnosis of bradyarrhythmias usually is accomplished with a standard 12-lead electrocardiogram (ECG) or Holter moni-

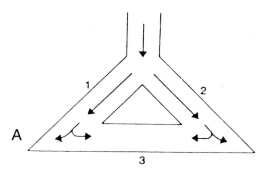
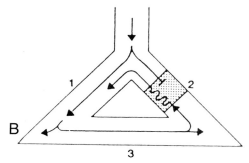

FIGURE 4-1. Schematic representation of reentry phenomenon. **(A)** Normal conduction of an impulse through cardiac muscle. **(B)** Conditions required to permit reentry. The impulse depolarizes pathway 1 normally, but antegrade conduction is blocked (*shaded area*) in pathway 2. The electrical wave front traveling through pathway 1 proceeds retrograde through the area of unidirectional block in pathway 2 and reenters myocardial cells in pathway 1 that have recovered and are capable of reexcitation. (Adapted from Rosen RM, Danilo P, 1979: The electrophysiological basis for cardiac arrhythmias. In Narula OS [ed]: Cardiac Arrhythmias: Electrophysiology, Diagnosis, and Management, p. 9. Baltimore, Williams & Wilkins)

toring. An electrophysiologic study (EPS) may be necessary in symptomatic patients in whom noninvasive studies fail to document suspected sinus nodal dysfunction or high-grade AV block in association with symptoms (Wolbrette & Naccarelli, 1998). Results of an EPS help determine arrhythmic risk and clarify the need for specific treatment.

The need for treatment of bradyarrhythmias is based primarily on (1) presence and severity of associated symptoms; (2) ventricular rate; and (3) clinical circumstances, specifically the presence and severity of organic heart disease and the direct cause of the arrhythmia (Lowe & Wharton, 1995). Bradycardia of a transient nature is treated with intravenous administration of atropine or isoproterenol, or with temporary pacing, using an external pulse generator to stimulate the myocardium through transvenous, epicardial (after cardiac surgery), or, rarely, transthoracic leads. Implantation of a permanent pacing system is required for significant symptomatic bradycardia that persists or can be expected to recur. Temporary and permanent pacing systems are discussed in Chapter 26, Temporary Pacing and Defibrillation, and Chapter 20, Permanent Pacemakers and Implantable Cardioverter Defibrillators, respectively.

Tachyarrhythmias

Tachyarrhythmias can be subdivided into supraventricular tachycardias (SVTs) and ventricular tachycardias (VTs) according to whether the site of origin is above or below the bifurcation of the bundle of His. Reentry is thought to cause most tachyarrhythmias. However, there is increasing evidence that the autonomic nervous system is also an important factor in arrhythmogenesis. Indeed, the electrophysiologic mechanism for most clinically occurring arrhythmias may be presumptive because current diagnostic methods do not provide unequivocal determination of the etiologic mechanism (Zipes, 1997a).

Supraventricular Tachyarrhythmias

Supraventricular tachyarrhythmias may be caused by a variety of mechanisms. Reentry is most common, although an automatic mechanism is presumed responsible for some forms of SVT. For example, ectopic foci in the left or right atrium can precipitate automatic atrial tachycardia (Kirklin & Barratt-Boyes, 1993). Automatic atrial tachycardias typically occur in younger patients, do not respond to vagal maneuvers, often display an incessant nature, and when incessant, can lead to dilated cardiomyopathy and congestive heart failure (Waldo & Biblo, 1998).

The various forms of reentry SVT are categorized by location of the reentrant circuit. Atrial-ventricular reentry describes a circuit within an anomalous tract of electrically active cardiac tissue extending directly from atrium to ventricle and bypassing the AV node. AV nodal reentry refers to a circuit located within the AV node or perinodal tissue, and intra-atrial reentry describes a reentrant pathway within the atrial muscle. Early data supporting a reentrant mechanism for SVT were developed in the electrophysiologic evaluation of patients with anomalous atrial-ventricular conduction, as occurs in patients with Wolff-Parkinson-White (WPW) syndrome. The anatomic and electrophysiologic data obtained in these patients have since been applied successfully to support the existence of a reentrant mechanism in AV nodal and atrial tachycardias as well.

Atrial-ventricular reentrant tachycardia occurs in the presence of an accessory pathway that bypasses the AV node. Patients with WPW syndrome have such an anomalous pathway, called a Kent bundle, that is present at birth and which may become manifest clinically at any age. The Kent bundle consists of a band of myocardium, electrically similar to atrial tissue, that is positioned such that it abnormally connects atrial and ventricular myocardium (Sabatine et al., 1998).

The anomalous atrial-ventricular pathway usually is

categorized according to its anatomic location in the heart at the level of the AV groove (ie, left free wall, right free wall, posterior septum, or anterior septum) (Ferguson & Cox, 1996) (Fig. 4-2). The Kent bundle also may be referred to as a type A or type B pathway. Type A pathways usually are between the left atrium and ventricle, and type B pathways are between the right atrium and ventricle. Twenty percent of patients have more than one accessory pathway (Hood et al., 1991).

The following ECG features characterize WPW syndrome: a short PR interval (≤0.12 second), a prolonged QRS complex (≥0.12 second), slurring of the ascending limb of the QRS wave (delta wave), and secondary ST segment and T wave changes (Fisch, 1997) (Fig. 4-3). An EPS is necessary to confirm definitively the presence and location of the anomalous pathway.

In patients with WPW syndrome, conduction may occur intermittently or continuously through the accessory tract and in an antegrade or retrograde direction. Antegrade conduction through the accessory pathway during sinus rhythm or an atrial arrhythmia may occur before AV nodal conduction and cause ectopic early activation of the ventricles, a phenomenon known as ventricular preexcitation (Fig. 4-4). When preexcitation occurs, the protection against rapid ventricular response rates normally provided by the AV node is absent. Retrograde, or concealed, conduction through the AV node or accessory tract provides the necessary alternate pathway for atrial-ventricular reentrant tachycardias.

Although some patients with WPW syndrome have no significant tachyarrhythmias, the frequency of paroxysmal tachycardia appears to increase with age. Most common is a reciprocating SVT, which occurs in 80% of patients who have WPW and tachyarrhythmias; atrial fibrillation occurs in 15% to 30% and atrial flutter in 5% (Zipes, 1997b; Kirklin & Barratt-Boyes, 1993). Although patients with WPW rarely experience sudden cardiac death (SCD), it can occur when atrial fibrillation with conduction through the accessory pathway causes

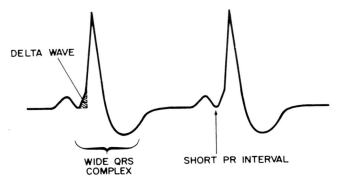

FIGURE 4-3. Characteristic electrocardiographic features during normal sinus rhythm in a patient with Wolff-Parkinson-White syndrome. (Cox JL, 1990: The surgical management of cardiac arrhythmias. In Sabiston DC Jr, Spencer FC [eds]: Surgery of the Chest, ed. 5, p. 1866. Philadelphia, WB Saunders)

a rapid ventricular rate with subsequent degeneration into ventricular fibrillation (VF) (Prystowsky, 1997a).

Atrioventricular nodal reentrant tachycardia arises from the presence of dual conduction pathways in the region of the AV node (Ferguson & Cox, 1996). These dual AV nodal conduction pathways, one slow and one fast, provide the anatomic-electrophysiologic substrate for a reentrant circuit (Cox, 1995). Most common is so-called "slow-fast" AV nodal reentry tachycardia, in which antegrade conduction of a premature atrial impulse blocks in the fast pathway, alternatively propagates antegrade

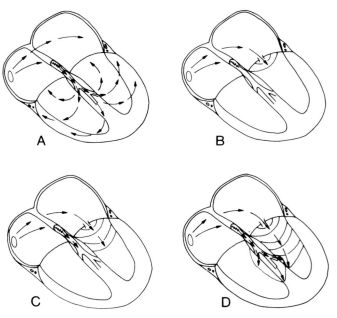

FIGURE 4-4. (A) Normal spread of electrical activation in the heart during sinus rhythm; the electrical impulse is delayed approximately 100 msec in the AV node. **(B–D)** Spread of electrical activation during sinus rhythm in Wolff-Parkinson-White syndrome with an accessory pathway in the left free wall. (Cox JL, 1990: The surgical management of cardiac arrhythmias. In Sabiston DC Jr, Spencer FC [eds]: Surgery of the Chest, ed. 5, p. 1866. Philadelphia, WB Saunders)

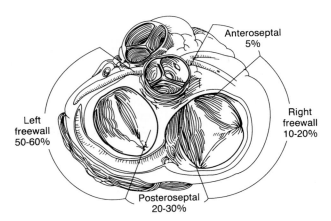

FIGURE 4-2. Distribution of accessory pathways. The most common location is the left free wall position. (Packer DL, 1998: AV node-dependent tachycardias. In Topol EJ [ed]: Comprehensive Cardiovascular Medicine. p. 1897. Philadelphia Lippincott Williams & Wilkins)

through the slow pathway, and returns retrograde through the fast pathway (Prystowsky, 1997b; Zipes, 1997a). AV nodal reentry is the most common mechanism of paroxysmal SVT, accounting for 60% to 65% of cases (Morady, 1999). It is characterized on the ECG by an abrupt onset and abrupt termination, and the absence of P waves or inverted P waves just after the QRS complexes (Hendel, 1998).

Experimental and intraoperative mapping studies suggest that atrial fibrillation and atrial flutter are *intra-atrial reentrant tachycardias*. Atrial fibrillation appears to be caused by multiple reentrant wavelets in the atrium that are maintained by inhomogeneity of tissue refractoriness in the atrial myocardium; atrial flutter most likely arises from a large reentrant circuit in the right atrial tissue (Ferguson & Cox, 1993). Atrial fibrillation is the most common sustained rhythm disorder in humans. Its prevalence increases with age, especially after the age of 60 years, and it is slightly more common in men (Prystowsky & Katz, 1998; American Heart Association, 1998).

Ventricular Tachyarrhythmias

Ventricular tachyarrhythmias arise within or distal to the bundle of His. They represent a continuum of severity that can be categorized as (1) premature ventricular complexes; (2) nonsustained VT (ie, >100 beats per minute and <30 seconds in duration); (3) sustained VT (ie, >100 beats per minute and ≥30 seconds in duration or requiring intervention to eradicate); and (4) VF. Ventricular tachyarrhythmias are a major cause of cardiac arrest and the cause of approximately 50% of cardiac-related deaths (Tchou, 1998). The most common ventricular arrhythmia requiring therapy is VT, usually due to a reentry phenomenon. Sustained VT may cause symptoms, including syncope or SCD.

Chronic ventricular rhythm disorders usually are categorized by etiology (Table 4-1). Patients who experience sustained, symptomatic VT almost always have organic

heart disease, usually coronary artery disease. Ventricular tachyarrhythmias associated with coronary artery disease almost always arise in the left ventricle or on the left ventricular side of the septum (Zipes, 1997c). These arrhythmias may be the result of either ischemia-mediated or scar-mediated electrical disorders. Ischemia-mediated tachyarrhythmias arise from tissue that is acutely or chronically ischemic secondary to obstructive lesions in the coronary arteries. Scar-mediated ventricular tachyarrhythmias are caused by changes in electrical properties of endocardial tissue that has been damaged by MI. The heterogeneity of the scar tissue provides a focus for reentrant arrhythmogenesis. Serious ventricular arrhythmias related to endocardial scar almost always are associated with major left ventricular wall motion abnormalities and often with significantly compromised left ventricular function.

Ventricular arrhythmias that occur in the absence of coronary artery disease may be associated with various other forms of organic heart disease. A congenital form of cardiomyopathy, termed *arrhythmogenic right ventricular dysplasia,* is characterized by intractable VT originating from pathologic tissue in the infundibulum, apex, or posterior basilar region of the right ventricle (Cox, 1995). Both dilated and hypertrophic forms of cardiomyopathy are associated with serious ventricular rhythm disturbances, most likely related to pathologic changes in the ventricular myocardium. Specific forms of valvular heart disease, particularly mitral valve prolapse and aortic stenosis, may be associated with ventricular tachyarrhythmias. Once present, the ventricular rhythm disorder usually is not eradicated by valve replacement.

Long QT syndrome is another etiologic mechanism for ventricular tachyarrhythmias. Long QT syndrome may occur as a hereditary disorder or as an acquired disorder due to medications, electrolyte imbalance, or hypothermia. The syndrome is characterized by abnormal ventricular repolarization, manifested primarily by prolongation of the QT interval on the ECG. QT prolongation increases susceptibility to subsequent ventricular stimulation during the vulnerable recovery period, with resultant serious ventricular arrhythmias. It sometimes is associated with torsades de pointes, a distinctive form of polymorphic VT that can degenerate into VF (Zipes, 1997b; Keating & Curran, 1998).

People with inherited long QT syndrome usually have no other physical abnormalities and typically begin to experience symptoms during young adulthood (Keating & Curran, 1998). Affected people are susceptible to arrhythmogenic syncope or SCD, commonly associated with episodes of adrenergic stimulation (eg, emotional stress or sudden loud noises).

Electrocardiographic manifestations may be present consistently or may become evident only when a person with the disorder receives certain medications, such as epinephrine, quinidine, or erythromycin. Others may be carriers of long QT syndrome without manifesting any electrocardiographic evidence of the disorder. For this reason, and because of the insidious and potentially lethal nature of the condition, it is essential that family

---

TABLE 4-1

Etiologies of Ventricular Rhythm Disorders

Coronary artery disease
  Ischemia-mediated
  Scar-mediated
Dilated cardiomyopathy
Hypertrophic cardiomyopathy
Valvular heart disease
Primary electrical disorder
Prolonged QT syndrome
Medications
Metabolic disturbances
Endocrine abnormalities
Autonomic influences

members of people diagnosed with long QT syndrome receive adequate genetic counseling and testing for presence of the causative genes.

A number of medications are known to predispose to ventricular tachyarrhythmias. In fact, pharmacologic therapy for arrhythmic disorders is limited by the tendency for many commonly used antiarrhythmic agents to have proarrhythmic properties; that is, the drug itself may cause serious ventricular arrhythmias. Ventricular arrhythmias also can develop secondary to metabolic or endocrine abnormalities. Still other ventricular arrhythmias are related to autonomic influences and occur in the setting of stress or exertion. Primary electrical disorder is a rhythm disorder that occurs in the absence of underlying structural heart disease, proarrhythmic agents, or metabolic imbalance. This entity may sometimes account for sudden, unexplained deaths that occur in presumably healthy young adults.

▶ Sudden Cardiac Death

Sudden cardiac death is defined as unexpected cardiac death without preceding symptoms or with symptoms less than 1 hour in duration (Stein & Roberts, 1994). It is the most common cause of death in adults younger than 65 years of age (Prystowsky, 1997a). Instantaneous death almost always is due to a catastrophic arrhythmia. The initial documented arrhythmia is VF in 75% of SCD victims, asystole in 20%, and electromechanical dissociation in 5% (Greene, 1990). SVT in the presence of an anomalous atrial-ventricular conduction pathway also can cause arrhythmic death. SCD due to bradycardia may occur as a result of sick sinus syndrome with sinus arrest or AV block (Chung, 1988).

An estimated 300,000 people experience SCD each year in the United States; the worldwide incidence varies largely as a function of the prevalence of coronary artery disease in different countries (Myerburg & Castellanos, 1997). At highest risk are African-American men (American Heart Association, 1998). Most SCD survivors have significant coronary artery disease. Often they have had a previous MI, congestive heart failure, or both (Hillis et al., 1995). Although a previous MI can be identified in up to 75% of patients who experience SCD, only a minority of survivors of out-of-hospital SCD have clinical evidence of a new transmural MI associated with the SCD event (Myerburg & Castellanos, 1997). Etiologic factors for SCD other than coronary artery disease are the same as those for ventricular arrhythmic disorders.

Episodes of SCD usually occur outside of hospitals during routine activities of daily living. Survival of SCD has become more common owing to widespread community awareness of cardiopulmonary resuscitation techniques and development of emergency systems that provide trained personnel capable of defibrillating victims in the field. Many SCD victims, however, do not survive the initial event. Depending on the level of community-based emergency services, only 10% to 30% of patients receiving resuscitation for out-of-hospital cardiac arrest subsequently are discharged from the hospital alive (Prystowsky, 1997a).

Those patients who do survive SCD comprise a challenging patient population requiring aggressive therapy. Unless the precipitating factor is controlled, these patients remain at increased risk for future major arrhythmic events. A number of factors have been identified that predispose to SCD recurrence. One important marker is whether the cardiac arrest occurred in association with an acute MI. Arrhythmias that occur in association with an acute MI are likely the result of electrophysiologic and biochemical abnormalities in the infarcted muscle. When the acute phase of the MI is over, the risk for arrhythmia recurrence decreases in most patients. Patients who experience an arrhythmogenic cardiac arrest without associated acute MI are more likely to have recurrent SCD. Although the 1-year mortality rate is only 2% after SCD associated with acute MI, it is 22% for those who have SCD without an associated MI (Prystowsky, 1997a).

In SCD survivors with coronary artery disease and history of a prior MI, a number of risk factors for subsequent arrhythmic events have been identified. One useful predictor is left ventricular dysfunction, as demonstrated by a left ventricular ejection fraction that is less than 40% or by left ventricular wall motion abnormalities. Other predictors of increased risk for SCD after MI include the presence of nonsustained VT, occurrence of syncope, presence of late potentials on a signal-averaged ECG (SAE), and inducible, sustained VT during EPS (Tchou, 1998).

▶ Diagnosis

Electrophysiologic study is the definitive diagnostic modality for defining arrhythmic disorders and guiding therapy. It allows assessment of individual portions of the cardiac electrical system, including evaluation of spontaneous function, responses to stresses, and vulnerability to induced tachycardias (Fisher, 1998). EPS provides a sophisticated method of analyzing cardiac electrical activation and defining abnormalities of impulse formation and conduction. Guidelines on indications for EPS have been developed jointly by the American College of Cardiology, American Heart Association, and North American Society for Pacing and Electrophysiology (Zipes et al., 1995). Types of information that can be obtained during EPS are displayed in Table 4-2.

The EPS procedure, which is performed in a laboratory setting, consists of placing intracardiac catheters with the aid of fluoroscopy in various locations in the heart. These catheters are used for two purposes: (1) recording intracardiac action potentials, and (2) programmed electrical stimulation (PES). PES consists of using pacing stimuli to induce and terminate clinical arrhythmias and to identify abnormal activation sequences, thus localizing reentrant pathways. During PES, repetitive electrical stimuli are delivered at specific points in the cardiac cycle to provoke an arrhythmia that

TABLE 4-2

Purposes of Electrophysiologic Study

Recording intracardiac electrograms
    Assessment of sinus node function
    Definition of atrioventricular nodal function (site of block)
    Mapping of cardiac activation during arrhythmias
Programmed electrical stimulation
    Initiation of arrhythmias
    Determination of inducibility and sustainability
    Determination of arrhythmia mechanism (reentrant vs. autonomic)
    Termination of arrhythmia
Evaluation of antiarrhythmic medication or intervention effectiveness
Assessment of sensing and response by antiarrhythmic device

has occurred clinically. Extra stimuli can be delivered at progressively shorter intervals until tissue refractoriness occurs. PES defines the origin and nature of the arrhythmia and reveals prognostic information about the likelihood of arrhythmia recurrence. Therapy then can be more specifically directed at a particular arrhythmia, thus enhancing its efficacy. PES also is performed during ablative or surgical procedures to eradicate arrhythmogenic tissue.

Clinically occurring arrhythmias provoked by PES are referred to as *inducible*. In general, inducible arrhythmias are thought to reflect a reentrant mechanism. A clinically occurring arrhythmia caused by an autonomic mechanism is more likely to be noninducible during PES (ie, it cannot be provoked) (Cox, 1995). An important characteristic of an induced arrhythmia is sustainability. Sustained arrhythmias during PES are defined as those of at least 30 seconds' duration or requiring intervention for hemodynamically compromising symptoms.

Inducibility and sustainability have important prognostic implications. For example, inducible, sustained VT correlates with a high probability of clinical arrhythmia recurrence. Similarly, inability to induce VT suggests a decreased risk of arrhythmia recurrence and, in selected patients, antiarrhythmic therapy may not be indicated. Finally, if arrhythmia provocation is reproducible, serial PES may be performed to evaluate efficacy of antiarrhythmic therapy. The effectiveness of a particular medication in preventing laboratory provocation of a clinically occurring tachyarrhythmia correlates in most cases with prognosis for clinical arrhythmia recurrence.

In SVT due to an accessory pathway (ie, WPW syndrome), the type and location of pathway can be identified by the sequence of electrical activation through the heart after the clinical arrhythmia has been induced. The reentry circuit may be either orthodromic (ie, antegrade conduction over the AV node and retrograde conduction over the anomalous pathway) or, less commonly, antidromic (ie, antegrade conduction through the anomalous pathway and retrograde conduction through the AV node) (Wellens, 1998). Tracking the pathway of electrical activation helps localize the anomalous path-

way. Similar techniques are used to track the electrical activation sequence in other reentrant tachycardias.

Electrophysiologic testing has greatly enhanced understanding of a variety of rhythm disorders and provides valuable descriptive and prognostic information about cardiac rhythm disorders in individual patients. However, caution must be used in interpretation of findings. PES is not uniformly helpful in its predictive information; the ability of PES to predict arrhythmic outcome is variable based on the clinical situation. Therefore, particular consideration must be given to the clinical arrhythmia and the type and extent of underlying cardiac disease.

For example, inducible monomorphic VT (uniform QRS morphology) often is due to endocardial scar from a remote MI and typically is reproducible. In contrast, the induction of nonsustained, monomorphic VT or polymorphic VT (frequent changes in QRS morphology or axis) is less specific and of less clinical significance, particularly in patients with limited underlying structural heart disease. PES also is less predictive for patients with cardiomyopathic heart disease and in those with greater left ventricular dysfunction. The use of PES to evaluate drug efficacy in patients with inducible arrhythmias is limited by the fact that noninducibility is achieved in only a small percentage of patients who undergo subsequent PES while receiving antiarrhythmic drug therapy. Also, because the arrhythmia substrate changes over time, it is difficult to predict long-term efficacy of an antiarrhythmic medication based on a single episode of noninducibility at a given point in time.

The *signal-averaged electrocardiogram* (SAE) provides another noninvasive diagnostic study for evaluation of ventricular arrhythmias. An SAE is a high-gain electrocardiogram that attempts to detect low-voltage propagation through scarred areas of the myocardium extending beyond the QRS complex (Tchou, 1998). Thus, an SAE magnifies QRS complexes and characterizes them by voltage and duration criteria. Patients with an abnormal SAE (prolonged QRS complex duration of predominantly low-voltage activity) may have an increased incidence of symptomatic ventricular tachyarrhythmias. Interpretation of SAEs in patients with a paced cardiac rhythm or complete bundle branch block is limited.

Before development of EPS, arrhythmia analysis and the plan of therapy were based primarily on the standard ECG, Holter monitoring, and exercise stress testing. Today, these diagnostic modalities provide valuable adjunctive information to supplement EPS. They are described in more detail in Chapter 8, Diagnostic Evaluation of Cardiac Disease.

▶ Treatment

Supraventricular tachyarrhythmias most often necessitate treatment because the arrhythmic episodes produce bothersome or disabling symptoms or because episodes increase in frequency, duration, or severity of associated symptoms over time. Uncommonly, treatment is necessary to prevent SCD, such as might occur in a person with an accessory atrial-ventricular pathway and SVT. Antiarrhythmic therapy almost always is necessary for patients with ventricular tachyarrhythmias and underlying structural heart disease. In the absence of structural heart disease, patients with nonsustained or asymptomatic VT are thought to be at low arrhythmic risk; specific antiarrhythmic therapy is not indicated.

Treatment of chronic cardiac rhythm disorders begins with elimination of any correctable etiologic factors, such as proarrhythmic medications. If the arrhythmia is attributed to active myocardial ischemia, coronary artery bypass grafting, percutaneous coronary intervention, or antianginal medications may be indicated. In the absence of correctable precipitants, there are several forms of antiarrhythmic therapy: (1) antiarrhythmic drugs, (2) catheter ablation of arrhythmogenic foci or anomalous conduction pathways, (3) antitachycardia devices, and, rarely, (4) surgical excision or ablation. Often a combination of therapies is required for effective treatment of the cardiac rhythm disorder.

Antiarrhythmic Medications

Antiarrhythmic medications once were the mainstay of therapy for patients with chronic heart rhythm disorders. The development of curative catheter ablative techniques and sophisticated antitachycardia devices has dramatically increased the use of interventional modalities and shifted drug therapy to a more adjunctive role. In addition, significant problems are associated with chronic antiarrhythmic drug therapy. First, all available antiarrhythmic drugs have significant adverse effects and may not be tolerated as chronic therapy. Second, some antiarrhythmic drugs produce significant myocardial depression and may be contraindicated in patients with organic heart disease, who often have poor left ventricular function. Also, many antiarrhythmic agents have proarrhythmic properties. Finally, serious arrhythmia recurrences develop in a significant number of patients despite all available antiarrhythmic agents.

The use of chronic drug therapy for supraventricular tachyarrhythmias has lessened considerably because of the evolution of curative catheter ablation techniques for many forms of SVT and the problems associated with drug therapy. Antiarrhythmic medications may be selected as the initial mode of therapy, but many patients receiving chronic drug therapy eventually experience break-through arrhythmias despite the medication or are unable to tolerate an effective agent's adverse effects. Antiarrhythmic drug therapy is further limited in women of child-bearing years because many of the drugs are contraindicated during pregnancy.

The use of antiarrhythmic drug therapy as the primary treatment modality for patients with ventricular tachyarrhythmias also has waned. The proven efficacy of antitachycardia devices in reducing arrhythmic deaths, in combination with previously discussed problems associated with antiarrhythmic medications, has caused drug therapy to be relegated to an adjunctive role for life-threatening ventricular arrhythmias.

A variety of medications are available for antiarrhythmic therapy. Medications unlikely to be proarrhythmic and with a good side effect profile are used most often. Antiarrhythmic medications are classified into four categories or classes, according to their mechanism of action: I, membrane-stabilizing agents; II, beta-adrenergic blocking agents; III, agents that prolong repolarization; and IV, calcium channel antagonist agents.

Class II beta-blocking agents (eg, propranolol) or sotalol (a class III agent with beta-blocking properties) often are chosen for treatment of supraventricular tachyarrhythmias. Class III agents that prolong repolarization (eg, amiodarone or sotalol) are used most commonly for life-threatening ventricular arrhythmias. Amiodarone is considered in general the most effective antiarrhythmic agent in treatment of patients with ventricular rhythm disorders who have survived SCD. However, the efficacy of this potent agent must be weighed carefully against the arrhythmic risk. Amiodarone has many potentially serious side effects, including pulmonary, hepatic, neuromuscular, and thyroid toxicity. Ongoing medical supervision is essential in patients receiving the drug.

Catheter and Surgical Ablation

Difficulties with antiarrhythmic drug therapy have led to development of ablative therapy to eradicate arrhythmogenic tissue. Ablative therapy consists of catheter or, uncommonly, open heart surgical techniques for disruption of a reentrant pathway. It is indicated for patients with either SVT or VT to prevent frequent, disabling, or life-threatening arrhythmic episodes.

Radiofrequency catheter ablation, performed in the electrophysiology laboratory, has largely replaced antiarrhythmic drug therapy and surgical therapy for the treatment of several types of tachyarrhythmias. The therapeutic ablative procedure typically is performed in combination with the diagnostic EPS. After identifying the endocardial site of earliest activation during the arrhythmia, radiofrequency energy is delivered through a transvenous, intracardiac electrode catheter positioned in the area of the reentrant pathway (Fig. 4-5). Radiofrequency ablation produces localized thermal destruction of arrhythmogenic cardiac tissue. Lesions created by radiofrequency energy are small; typical ablation catheters create lesions approximately 5 to 6 mm in diameter and 2 to 3 mm deep (Morady, 1999). Because the area of tissue charge is localized, the technique is associated with few complications. The risk of associated complications ranges from 1.8% to 4% and includes events such as complete heart block, MI, valvular injury, stroke, and death (Haines, 1998).

Radiofrequency catheter ablation most commonly is used to interrupt reentrant pathways responsible for supraventricular tachyarrhythmias, typically AV nodal reentrant pathways or anomalous atrial-ventricular connections associated with WPW syndrome (Fig. 4-6). Suc-

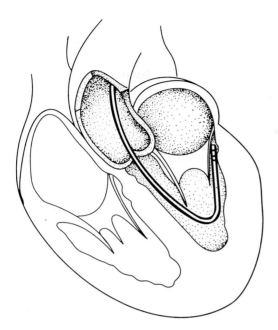

FIGURE 4-5. Retrograde catheterization of the left ventricle for radiofrequency ablation of left free wall accessory pathway. Catheter tip is positioned near mitral valve annulus in region of identified reentrant pathway. (Scheinman MM, 1991: Catheter ablation: Present role and projected impact on health care for patients with cardiac arrhythmias. Circulation 83:1492; Reproduced with permission. © 1991, American Heart Association)

cessful arrhythmia eradication is achieved in 95% to 98% of patients. Atrial flutter also may be treated with catheter ablation, with an acute success rate of 90% or greater and a late recurrence rate of 10% to 20% (Haines, 1998). In patients with atrial fibrillation, complete AV nodal eradication may be performed in combination with implantation of a single-chamber (those with chronic atrial fibrillation) or dual-chamber (those with paroxysmal atrial fibrillation) pacemaker (Kay et al., 1998). Techniques for delivering radiofrequency current to the left or right atrium to ablate atrial fibrillation are under investigation.

Ventricular tachyarrhythmias also are sometimes treated with radiofrequency ablation. Catheter ablation is most effective for reentrant VT in patients with nonischemic cardiomyopathy and for monomorphic VT in patients with otherwise structurally normal hearts (Tchou, 1998). In patients with VT due to coronary artery disease, radiofrequency ablation usually is used as an adjunct to other therapies. The most common indication in this group of patients is VT refractory to drug therapy that results in frequent discharges from an implantable cardioverter-defibrillator (ICD), is too slow to be detected by an ICD, or that is incessant (Morady, 1999).

Occasionally, surgical ablation is used in the treatment of supraventricular or ventricular tachyarrhythmias to eradicate arrhythmogenic tissue or interrupt reentrant circuits. Direct surgical excision and cryoablation are ab-

lative techniques performed during cardiac operations. Cryoablation is the direct application of an extremely cold (−60°C) probe to arrhythmogenic cardiac tissue to destroy it. It is used as an adjunctive ablative therapy along with surgical excision. With the successful evolution of catheter techniques for arrhythmia ablation, the indications for surgical ablation have become rare.

Supraventricular tachyarrhythmias may be treated surgically with mapping-directed division or cryoablation of reentrant pathways. Except for selected pathways that can be divided on the epicardial surface, most must be interrupted on the endocardial surface and therefore require atriotomy (incision into the atrium) and cardiopulmonary bypass. Radiofrequency ablation has replaced direct surgical ablation in all but the occasional patient in whom catheter ablation fails or who is having cardiac surgery for another reason (Zipes, 1997c).

Uncommonly, intra-atrial reentry arrhythmias are treated with surgical therapy. The *Cox maze procedure,* used primarily to eradicate atrial fibrillation, consists of multiple atrial incisions made to direct sinus impulses through a surgically created path or "maze" to reach the AV node (Prystowsky & Katz, 1998). Indications for the Cox maze procedure include (1) atrial fibrillation or atrial flutter associated with a failure of medical therapy (either symptomatic intolerance despite pharmacologic rate control or inability to achieve pharmacologic rate control); (2) patient intolerance of antiarrhythmic medications; or (3) the occurrence of at least one previous thromboembolic episode attributable to the atrial arrhythmia (Sundt & Cox, 1998). The Cox maze procedure is very effective in eliminating atrial fibrillation. Nearly 100% of patients maintain sinus rhythm more than 3 months after the procedure, although 30% to 40% of patients require a pacemaker because of chronotropic incompetence of the sinus node (Zipes, 1997c).

Occasionally, patients with symptomatic, drug-resistant ventricular tachyarrhythmias undergo surgical ventriculotomy and mapping-directed excision of endocardial scar. *Endocardial resection* is performed using cardiopulmonary bypass and intraoperative mapping of the left ventricular endocardium during induced VT to identify the arrhythmogenic tissue, which is then surgically excised (Cleveland & Harken, 1998). Because ventriculotomy further damages an already compromised ventricle, the procedure is used selectively, typically in patients with a discrete anterior aneurysm, fairly good ventricular function, and frequent, monomorphic VT. Surgical resection is not possible in patients with ventricular arrhythmias due to diffuse myopathic heart disease, as opposed to discrete areas of endocardial scarring. Endocardial resection may carry a prohibitive operative risk in patients with severe left ventricular dysfunction and congestive heart failure.

Antitachycardia Devices

An *implantable cardioverter-defibrillator* (ICD) is the most appropriate form of therapy for most patients with serious ventricular tachyarrhythmias. It is the most ef-

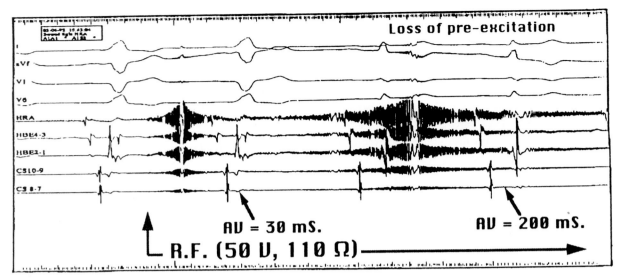

FIGURE 4-6. Loss of preexcitation during radiofrequency ablation in a patient with Wolff-Parkinson-White syndrome. Electrocardiographic tracings from top to bottom include surface leads (I, aVf, V_1, and V_6), and electrograms recorded from high right atrium (HRA), the region of the His bundle (HBE4-3, HBE2-1), and the coronary sinus (CS10-9, CS8-7). First arrow on left represents application of radiofrequency energy; second and third arrows demonstrate lengthening of AV interval with loss of preexcitation. (Finkelmeier BA, 1994: Ablative therapy in the treatment of tachyarrhythmias. Critical Care Nursing Clinics of North America 6:106)

fective modality for preventing arrhythmic death in patients with poor ventricular function and sustained or nonsustained ventricular tachyarrhythmias. ICDs initially were approved to prevent SCD in patients with prior MI, poor left ventricular function, and sustained, inducible VT or VF. Indications for ICD implantation more recently have been expanded based on the improved survival outcomes demonstrated in the Multicenter Automatic Defibrillator Implantation Trial (MADIT) (Gregoratos et al., 1998; Mushlin et al. 1998) (Table 4-3).

Implantable cardioverter-defibrillators sense tachyarrhythmias and in response deliver one or more shocks to defibrillate the heart and restore an intrinsic cardiac rhythm. Devices are available that offer comprehensive pacing therapy (antibradycardia and antitachycardia modalities) as well as both low- and high-energy defibrillating shocks. Selection of the specific device to be implanted is based on a careful evaluation of the patient's current and potential need for both pacing and defibrillation therapies. Planning for potential pacing needs at the time of ICD implantation eliminates the need for separate pacemaker and defibrillating devices and the inherent problematic interactions between two separate devices.

For example, an ICD with dual-chamber, antibradycardia pacing capabilities may be selected for patients susceptible to bradycardia-mediated ventricular tachyarrhythmias or to allow higher dosages of antiarrhythmic medications that would otherwise induce unacceptable bradycardia. In addition to its therapeutic use for dual-chamber pacing, an atrial electrode can be used diagnostically to record atrial electrograms that better de-

fine the origin of tachyarrhythmic events. Antitachycardia pacing allows for the painless termination of many episodes of sustained monomorphic VT, whereas defibrillation shocks are used for more rapid or polymorphic VT or VF (Pinski & Chen, 1998).

Defibrillator implantation almost always can be performed transvenously and, in contrast to endocardial resection, does not necessitate a major thoracic operation

---

TABLE 4-3

Class I Indications for Implantable Cardioverter-Defibrillator Therapy*

- Cardiac arrest due to VF or VT, where VF or VT is not due to a transient or reversible cause
- Spontaneous sustained VT
- Syncope of undetermined origin with clinically relevant, hemodynamically significant sustained VT or VF induced at EPS when drug therapy is ineffective, not tolerated, or not preferred
- Nonsustained VT with coronary artery disease, prior myocardial infarction, left ventricular dysfunction, and inducible VF or sustained VT at EPS that is not suppressible by a Class I antiarrhythmic drug

EPS, electrophysiologic study; VF, ventricular fibrillation; VT, ventricular tachycardia.

*Class I indications are conditions for which there is evidence and/or general agreement that a given procedure or treatment is beneficial, useful, and effective.

Adapted from Gregoratos G, Cheitlin MD, Conill A, et al., 1998: ACC/AHA guidelines for implantation of cardiac pacemakers and antiarrhythmia devices: A report of the American College of Cardiology/American Heart Association Task Force on Practice Guidelines. J Am Coll Cardiol 31:1175.

with cardiopulmonary bypass and ventriculotomy. The mortality rate associated with ICD implantation is less than 1%, although complications, such as lead failure, infection, spurious shocks for supraventricular tachyarrhythmias, and psychological morbidity, do occur (Pinski & Chen, 1998). An ICD does nothing to prevent an arrhythmia from occurring; rather, it provides conversion of the arrhythmia when it occurs. Therefore, in patients requiring frequent discharges for arrhythmic episodes, it is used in combination with antiarrhythmic medications or, rarely, with endocardial resection. Availability of defibrillating devices as an additional therapeutic modality has reduced greatly the indications for surgical endocardial resection. Surgical ablation therapies and ICDs are described in more detail in Chapters 18, Surgical Treatment of Cardiac Rhythm Disorders and 20, Permanent Pacemakers and Implantable Cardioverter-Defibrillators, respectively.

REFERENCES

American Heart Association, 1998: 1999 Heart and stroke statistical update. Dallas, American Heart Association

Bond EF, Halpenny CJ, 1995: Physiology of the heart. In Woods SL, Froelicher ES, Halpenny CJ, Motzer SU (eds): Cardiac Nursing, ed. 3. Philadelphia, JB Lippincott

Chung EK, 1988: Sudden cardiac death. In Manual of Acute Cardiac Disorders. Boston, Butterworths

Chung EK, 1989: Some aspects of the anatomy, electrophysiology, and hemodynamics of the heart. In Principles of Cardiac Arrhythmias, ed. 4. Baltimore, Williams & Wilkins

Cleveland JC, Harken AH, 1998: Rational strategies in the surgical therapy of malignant ventricular tachyarrhythmias. In Kaiser LR, Kron IL, Spray TL (eds): Mastery of Cardiothoracic Surgery. Philadelphia, Lippincott Williams & Wilkins

Cox JL, 1995: The surgical management of cardiac arrhythmias. In Sabiston DC Jr, Spencer FC (eds): Surgery of the Chest, ed. 6. Philadelphia, WB Saunders

Ferguson TB, Cox JL, 1996: Surgery for supraventricular arrhythmias. In Baue AE, Geha AS, Hammond GL, et al. (eds): Glenn's Thoracic and Cardiovascular Surgery, ed. 6. Stamford, CT, Appleton & Lange

Ferguson TB, Cox JL, 1993: Surgical treatment of cardiac arrhythmias. Heart Disease and Stroke 2:37

Fisch C, 1997: Electrocardiography. In Braunwald E (ed): Heart Disease: A Textbook of Cardiovascular Medicine, ed. 5. Philadelphia, WB Saunders

Fisher JD, 1998: Electrophysiologic testing. In Topol EJ (ed): Comprehensive Cardiovascular Medicine. Philadelphia, Lippincott Williams & Wilkins

Grant AO, Whalley DW, 1998: Mechanisms of cardiac arrhythmias. In Topol EJ (ed): Comprehensive Cardiovascular Medicine. Philadelphia, Lippincott Williams & Wilkins

Gregoratos G, Cheitlin MD, Conill A, et al., 1998: ACC/AHA guidelines for implantation of cardiac pacemakers and antiarrhythmia devices: A report of the American College of Cardiology/American Heart Association Task Force on Practice Guidelines. J Am Coll Cardiol 31:1175

Greene HL, 1990: Sudden arrhythmic cardiac death—mechanisms, resuscitation, and classification: The Seattle perspective. Am J Cardiol 65:4B

Haines DE, 1998: Catheter ablation therapy for arrhythmias. In Topol EJ (ed): Comprehensive Cardiovascular Medicine. Philadelphia, Lippincott Williams & Wilkins

Hendel RC, 1997. Interpreting noninvasive cardiac tests. In

Alpert JS (ed): Cardiology for the Primary Care Physician, ed. 2. Philadelphia, Current Medicine

Hillis LD, Lange RA, Winniford MD, Page RL, 1995: Ventricular tachycardia and ventricular fibrillation. In Manual of Clinical Problems in Cardiology, ed. 5. Boston, Little, Brown

Hood MA, Smith WM, Robinson C, et al., 1991: Operations for Wolff-Parkinson-White syndrome. J Thorac Cardiovasc Surg 101:998

Jacobson C, 1995: Arrhythmias and conduction disturbances. In Woods SL, Froelicher ES, Halpenny CJ, Motzer SU (eds): Cardiac Nursing, ed. 3. Philadelphia, JB Lippincott

Kay GN, Ellenbogen KA, Giudici M, et al., 1998: The Ablate and Pace Trial: A prospective study of catheter ablation of the AV conduction system and permanent pacemaker implantation for the treatment of atrial fibrillation. Journal of Interventional Cardiac Electrophysiology 2:121

Keating MT, Curran ME, 1998: Molecular genetics. In Topol EJ (ed): Comprehensive Cardiac Care. Philadelphia, Lippincott Williams & Wilkins

Kirklin JW, Barratt-Boyes BG, 1993: Tachycardia. In Cardiac Surgery, ed. 2. New York, Churchill Livingstone

Lowe JE, Wharton M, 1995: Cardiac pacemakers and implantable cardioverter-defibrillators. In Sabiston DC Jr, Spencer FC (eds): Surgery of the Chest, ed. 6. Philadelphia, WB Saunders

Morady F, 1999: Radio-frequency ablation as treatment for cardiac arrhythmias. N Engl J Med 340:534

Mushlin AI, Hall WJ, Zwanziger J, et al., 1998: The cost effectiveness of Automatic Implantable Cardiac Defibrillators: Results from MADIT. Circulation 97:2129

Myerburg RJ, Castellanos A, 1997: Cardiac arrest and sudden cardiac death. In Braunwald E (ed): Heart Disease: A Textbook of Cardiovascular Medicine, ed. 5. Philadelphia, WB Saunders

Pinski SL, Chen PS, 1998: Implantable cardioverter-defibrillators. In Topol EJ (ed): Comprehensive Cardiovascular Medicine. Philadelphia, Lippincott Williams & Wilkins

Prystowsky EN, 1997a: Evaluation of the patient resuscitated from cardiac arrest. In Alpert JS (ed): Cardiology for the Primary Care Physician, ed. 2. Philadelphia, Current Medicine

Prystowsky EN, 1997b: Atrioventricular node reentry: Physiology and radiofrequency ablation. Pacing Clin Electrophysiol 20:552

Prystowsky EN, Katz A, 1998: Atrial fibrillation. In Topol EJ (ed): Comprehensive Cardiovascular Medicine. Philadelphia, Lippincott Williams & Wilkins

Ruskin JN, Schoenfeld MH, 1989: Mechanisms of ventricular arrhythmias. In Eagle KA, Haber E, DeSanctis RW, Austin WG (eds): The Practice of Cardiology, ed. 2. Boston, Little, Brown

Sabatine MS, Antman EM, Ganz LI, et al., 1998: Mechanisms of cardiac arrhythmias. In Lilly LS (ed): Pathophysiology of Heart Disease, ed. 2. Baltimore, Williams & Wilkins

Stein B, Roberts R, 1994: Syncope, presyncope, palpitations, and sudden death. In Schlant RC, Alexander RW (eds): The Heart, ed. 8. New York, McGraw-Hill

Sundt TM, Cox JL, 1998: Maze III procedure for atrial fibrillation. In Kaiser LR, Kron IL, Spray TL (eds): Mastery of Cardiothoracic Surgery. Philadelphia, Lippincott Williams & Wilkins

Tchou PJ, 1998: Ventricular tachycardia. In Topol EJ (ed): Comprehensive Cardiovascular Medicine. Philadelphia, Lippincott Williams & Wilkins

Waldo AL, Biblo LA, 1998: AV nodal-independent supraventricular tachycardias. In Topol EJ (ed): Comprehensive Cardiovascular Medicine. Philadelphia, Lippincott Williams & Wilkins

Waldo AL, Wit AL, 1994: Mechanisms of cardiac arrhythmias and conduction disturbances. In Schlant RC, Alexander RW (eds): The Heart, ed. 8. New York, McGraw-Hill

Wellens HJ, 1998: The electrocardiographic diagnosis of arrhythmias. In Topol EJ (ed): Comprehensive Cardiovascular Medicine. Philadelphia, Lippincott Williams & Wilkins

White J, 1998: Disorders of cardiac rhythm and conduction. In Porth CM (ed): Pathophysiology: Concepts of Altered Health States, ed. 5. Philadelphia, Lippincott Williams & Wilkins

Wolbrette DL, Naccarelli GV, 1998: Bradycardias. In Topol EJ (ed): Comprehensive Cardiovascular Medicine. Philadelphia, Lippincott Williams & Wilkins

Zipes DP, 1997a: Genesis of cardiac arrhythmias: Electrophysiological considerations. In Braunwald E (ed): Heart Disease: A Textbook of Cardiovascular Medicine, ed. 5. Philadelphia, WB Saunders

Zipes DP, 1997b: Specific arrhythmias: Diagnosis and treatment. In Braunwald E (ed): Heart Disease: A Textbook of Cardiovascular Medicine, ed. 5. Philadelphia, WB Saunders

Zipes DP, 1997c: Management of cardiac arrhythmias: Pharmacological, electrical, and surgical techniques. In Braunwald E (ed): Heart Disease: A Textbook of Cardiovascular Medicine, ed. 5. Philadelphia, WB Saunders

Zipes DP, DiMarco JP, Gillette PC, et al., 1995. Guidelines for clinical intracardiac electrophysiological and catheter ablation procedures. J Am Coll Cardiol 26:555

5

Cardiomyopathies

The term *cardiomyopathy* is used to describe any of a group of primary disorders of the heart muscle. Although several causative agents and systemic syndromes are known to produce myocardial dysfunction, a specific etiology is not identified in most cases. Therefore, pathophysiology, instead of etiology, usually is used to categorize cardiomyopathy into three major forms: (1) dilated, (2) hypertrophic, and (3) restrictive. Because of the differing anatomic and functional characteristics, each produces different hemodynamic consequences and requires different types of therapy.

Dilated cardiomyopathy is characterized by ventricular dilatation with impaired systolic function, hypertrophic cardiomyopathy by an abnormally thickened ventricle with abnormal diastolic relaxation, and restrictive cardiomyopathy by impaired diastolic relaxation due to a myocardium stiffened by fibrosis or infiltration, with systolic function that usually is preserved (Grayzel et al., 1998). Ventricular failure that occurs not as a primary disorder of the heart muscle, but rather secondary to another condition, such as myocardial infarction (so-called "ischemic cardiomyopathy"), systemic arterial hypertension, or valvular heart disease is not a true cardiomyopathy and thus is not included in the discussion in this chapter.

▶ Dilated Cardiomyopathy

Dilated cardiomyopathy (DCM), formerly known as *congestive cardiomyopathy,* is the most commonly occurring form of heart muscle disorder in the United States. It accounts for 87% of all cases of cardiomyopathy (American Heart Association, 1998). DCM is characterized by dilatation and impaired systolic function of one or both ventricles (Fig. 5-1). Marked enlargement of all four cardiac chambers is typical and chamber dilatation is out of proportion to any hypertrophy (Grayzel et al., 1998).

The cause or causes of DCM remain unclear. Research interest has focused on three possible etiologic mechanisms of damage: viral myocarditis and other cytotoxic insults, genetic factors, and immunologic abnormalities. Clinical conditions known to be associated with DCM include alcohol and cocaine abuse, human immunodeficiency virus infection, metabolic abnormalities, and the cardiotoxicity of anticancer drugs (Wynne & Braunwald, 1997). In a great many cases, no specific etiologic factor is identified and the condition is termed *idiopathic DCM.*

Myocarditis is a well recognized cause of DCM. Usually due to viral infection, it also can occur due to infection by fungal, parasitic, rickettsial, or spirochetal organisms (Goldman, 1997). Acute viral myocarditis most often is caused by coxsackievirus group B or echovirus infection and usually affects young, previously healthy people (Grayzel et al., 1998). A spectrum of clinical manifestations may occur, including (1) a completely asymptomatic response; (2) myalgia, rhinorrhea, fatigue, and fever; (3) symptoms that mimic myocardial infarction; or (4) severe congestive heart failure or life-threatening arrhythmias (Goldman, 1997). An insidious and benign course is most common but, for unexplained reasons, serious cardiovascular complications develop in some patients. Viral myocarditis is particularly difficult to diagnose because of the highly variable clinical presentation and the infrequency with which the presence of viral organisms can be detected histologically. As a result, it frequently remains undiagnosed until chronic cardiac dysfunction and congestive heart failure develop (Grady & Costanzo-Nordin, 1989).

Dilated cardiomyopathy also can result from heavy ingestion of alcoholic beverages over a prolonged period. A history of chronic alcoholism can be elicited in approximately 20% of patients with DCM (Schoen, 1997). The relationship between alcohol abuse and DCM is well documented, but the causative mechanism remains unclear. DCM related to alcohol abuse develops

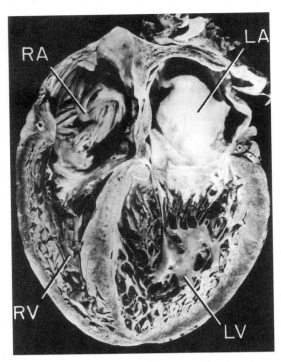

FIGURE 5-1. Autopsy specimen demonstrating dilated cardiomyopathy. Note all four cardiac chambers are dilated, particularly the left ventricle (LV). The ventricular walls are hypertrophied, but not disproportionately to the degree of chamber dilation. RA, right atrium; LA, left atrium; RV, right ventricle. (Johnson RA, Fifer MA, Palacios IF, 1989: Dilated and restrictive cardiomyopathies. In Eagle KA, Haber E, DeSanctis RW, Austen WG [eds]: The Practice of Cardiology, ed. 2, p. 896. Boston, Little, Brown)

most often in middle-aged people who have consumed large amounts of alcohol for more than 10 years (Hillis et al., 1995a). *Alcoholic cardiomyopathy* differs from other forms of DCM in that ceasing alcohol consumption early in the course of the disease may halt progression or even reverse left ventricular contractile dysfunction (Wynne & Braunwald, 1997). For this reason, it is one of the few potentially reversible causes of DCM. With continued alcohol abuse, however, myocardial damage becomes irreversible, leading to a progressively downward course despite drinking patterns.

Pregnancy also may precipitate DCM. *Peripartum cardiomyopathy* in the United States is most common in women with twin pregnancies, and in those who are multiparous, older than 30 years of age, or African American (Elkayam, 1997). It is characterized by the development of congestive heart failure during the final month of pregnancy or in the months after delivery and may recur with subsequent pregnancies (Burlew et al., 1997). Factors leading to peripartum DCM are not well understood.

Patients with DCM may remain asymptomatic for a period. Congestive heart failure is the major clinical manifestation. Exertional dyspnea, generalized weakness, and fatigue typically develop gradually over weeks or months (Bush & Healy, 1987). Both systemic and pulmonary embolism can occur as a result of thrombus as-

sociated with atrial fibrillation, poorly contractile ventricles, or peripheral venous stasis. As left ventricular dysfunction progresses, complex ventricular arrhythmias often develop, placing the patient at increased risk for sudden cardiac death (Gilbert & Bristow, 1994).

The natural history of patients with DCM is variable, but development of symptoms usually is followed by a downward course. Only 50% of patients diagnosed with DCM survive 5 years, and only 25% are alive 10 years after diagnosis (American Heart Association, 1998). Indicators of a poor prognosis include age at onset greater than 55 years, New York Heart Association (NYHA) class IV functional status, marked cardiomegaly detected by radiograph and echocardiogram, ejection fraction less than 20%, cardiac index less than 2 L/min/m², left ventricular end-diastolic pressure greater than 20 mm Hg, and symptomatic ventricular tachycardia (Gay, 1995). Death in patients with DCM frequently is due to ventricular tachycardia or fibrillation (Grayzel et al., 1998).

In some cases, a treatable cause of DCM is identified. However, in most cases, there is no curative therapy. Medical treatment is aimed at palliating symptoms of progressive heart failure by controlling salt and water retention, reducing the workload on the heart, and improving contractility (Gilbert & Bristow, 1994). Angiotensin-converting enzyme inhibitors (eg, enalapril) and beta-blocking agents (eg, carvedilol and bisoprolol) also are major components of pharmacologic therapy and have proven effective in improving functional status and prolonging survival (CIBIS-II Investigators and Committees, 1999; Wynne & Braunwald, 1997). Typically, loop diuretics and digoxin also are prescribed. Intravenous infusions of dobutamine or milrinone may be used for patients with heart failure refractory to conventional oral medications (Smith et al., 1997). Patients with symptomatic ventricular arrhythmias require electrophysiologic evaluation and may need antiarrhythmic therapy or an implantable cardioverter-defibrillator. Anticoagulation is recommended to reduce the risk of thromboembolism.

Cardiac transplantation is recommended for patients with DCM who remain severely symptomatic (ie, NYHA class III or IV functional status) despite optimal pharmacologic therapy and who are suitable candidates for the procedure. A ventricular assist device may be necessary to support ventricular function during the often lengthy waiting period for a donor organ. If heart transplantation is accomplished successfully, survival prognosis is increased substantially. Availability of transplantation, however, is limited by the scarcity of donor hearts. Many patients with DCM do not meet eligibility criteria for transplantation or die while waiting for a donor organ. The use of ventricular assist devices as an alternative to transplantation is under investigation. Ventricular assist devices and cardiac transplantation are discussed in detail in Chapter 30, Circulatory Assist Devices, and Chapter 31, Heart, Lung, and Heart-Lung Transplantation, respectively.

Dynamic cardiomyoplasty is an alternative form of surgical therapy that is being performed for patients with DCM in selected centers (Moreira et al., 1991). The procedure consists of wrapping the heart with skeletal muscle. A cardiomyostimulator (device used to deliver electrical impulses), implanted and attached to the muscle wrap by stimulating and sensing leads, is used to stimulate the skeletal muscle to contract in synchrony with ventricular contractions. The procedure, which remains investigational in the United States, is best suited to patients with heart failure that is controlled with medical therapy but is causing cardiac enlargement, worsening symptoms, or deteriorating left ventricular function (Magovern & Magovern, 1998).

Dynamic cardiomyoplasty is discussed further in Chapter 21, Surgical Treatment of Other Cardiovascular Disorders.

► Hypertrophic Cardiomyopathy

Hypertrophic cardiomyopathy (HCM) is a genetically transmitted form of cardiomyopathy characterized by impaired diastolic ventricular function and hypertrophy of ventricular muscle mass (Fig. 5-2). HCM formerly has been called *idiopathic hypertrophic subaortic stenosis* (IHSS), *hypertrophic obstructive cardiomyopathy*, and *asymmetric septal hypertrophy* (Nishimura et al., 1991). The pathophysiology of HCM is not well understood, but the process involves fibrosis of myofibrils, leading to

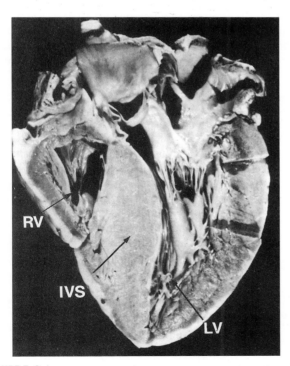

FIGURE 5-2. Autopsy specimen demonstrating hypertrophic cardiomyopathy. Ventricular walls are disproportionately thickened relative to the ventricle chambers; note massively thickened interventricular septum (IVS). RV, right ventricle; LV, left ventricle. (Johnson RA, Fifer MA, Palacios IF, 1989: Dilated and restrictive cardiomyopathies. In Eagle KA, Haber E, DeSanctis RW, Austen WG [eds]: The Practice of Cardiology, ed. 2, p. 896. Boston, Little, Brown)

impaired ventricular relaxation. Ventricular cavity size is small or normal, and systolic function is usually hyperdynamic (Bush & Healy, 1987). Ventricular hypertrophy may occur in an asymmetric or concentric fashion. Most common is asymmetric hypertrophy of the ventricular septum, which occurs in approximately 90% of cases (Grayzel et al., 1998). Increased septal thickness and abnormal anterior displacement of the mitral valve produce anatomic narrowing of the left ventricular outflow tract; mitral regurgitation also may be present owing to increased leaflet area, abnormal papillary muscle insertion, or systolic anterior motion of the anterior valve leaflets (Glower, 1995).

In contrast to valvular aortic stenosis, left ventricular obstruction associated with HCM is dynamic; that is, it changes with varying hemodynamic conditions. Therefore, the intensity of the systolic murmur produced by outflow obstruction varies directly with increases or decreases in the pressure gradient between the left ventricle and aorta. Maneuvers that decrease left ventricular preload and cavity size increase the pressure gradient and murmur intensity; conversely, those that increase preload and cavity size decrease the gradient and murmur intensity. For example, the murmur is increased with the Valsalva maneuver and during standing from a squatting position; it is decreased by maneuvers such as squatting from a standing position, passive leg elevation, and hand grip (Wynne & Braunwald, 1997). The most important study for diagnostic evaluation of HCM is Doppler echocardiography.

Hypertrophic cardiomyopathy occurs more commonly in men. It can be manifested at any age from early infancy to the sixth or seventh decade, but most commonly becomes evident in the second or third decade (Kirklin & Barratt-Boyes, 1993a). The most frequently occurring symptoms are (1) dyspnea, present in up to 90% of patients with HCM; (2) angina, occurring in 70% to 80%; and (3) syncope, in approximately 20% (Nishimura et al., 1991). Symptoms commonly are associated with exertion when ventricular contractility and oxygen demands are increased.

One of the most distressing aspects of HCM is a propensity for sudden death. Sudden death occurs in 2% to 3% of adults with hypertrophic cardiomyopathy per year and is particularly likely in young men with familial hypertrophic cardiomyopathy or with a family history of sudden death (Schoen, 1997). Almost half of the sudden deaths in patients with HCM occur during or just after strenuous physical activity (Wynne & Braunwald, 1997). Sudden death may occur in previously asymptomatic patients, in people who were unaware they had HCM, and in patients with an otherwise stable course (Wynne & Braunwald, 1997). Data demonstrate that 36% of young athletes who die suddenly have probable or definite HCM (American Heart Association, 1998). Although pathogenesis of sudden cardiac death in patients with HCM is not clearly defined, it may be related to a primary electrical disorder, abnormality of conductive tissue, or hypotension secondary to left ventricular outflow tract obstruction.

Pharmacologic therapy for HCM is directed toward (1) reducing left ventricular outflow tract obstruction by decreasing contractility, and (2) improving diastolic relaxation. Both beta-adrenergic blocking and calcium channel antagonistic medications may be useful in reducing symptoms because of their negative inotropic effects. Beta-blocking agents also enhance diastolic filling by increasing ventricular compliance and lowering heart rate (Bush & Healy, 1987). More recently, dual-chamber pacing has been added to the treatment strategy for HCM. Data from multiple centers worldwide have demonstrated effectiveness of dual-chamber pacing in reducing left ventricular outflow obstruction and associated mitral regurgitation, reducing drug-refractory symptoms, and improving exercise performance (Fananapazir & McAreavey, 1998).

Antibiotic prophylaxis against infective endocarditis is recommended because of the increased risk of endocardial infection due to turbulent blood flow through the narrowed left ventricular outflow tract and associated mitral regurgitation (Grayzel et al., 1998). Patients with HCM are advised to avoid strenuous exercise because of the risk of sudden death. Antiarrhythmic medications may be administered to patients with evidence of ventricular arrhythmias. Inotropic medications, such as digoxin, are contraindicated in patients with HCM because they increase contractility and thereby increase the degree of outflow tract obstruction.

Surgical treatment of HCM is reserved for patients who have severe symptoms or who are considered at high risk for sudden cardiac death (Schonbeck et al., 1998). The most common reparative procedure is a septal myectomy, or resection of a portion of the hypertrophied ventricular septum. Mitral valve replacement may be necessary in some cases. Surgical therapy is described in detail in Chapter 21, Surgical Treatment of Other Cardiovascular Disorders.

► Restrictive Cardiomyopathy

Restrictive cardiomyopathy is the least common form of primary myocardial dysfunction. It is more common in Africa, the tropics, and subtropics than in North America and Europe (Goldman & Fisher, 1997). Restrictive cardiomyopathy is characterized by diffuse ventricular hypertrophy and impaired diastolic function with loss of compliance (Kirklin & Barratt-Boyes 1993b). It may occur as a primary myocardial disorder, or secondary to a generalized disease or infiltration of the myocardium with an abnormal substance. Causative disorders include (1) amyloidosis, a disorder of unknown etiology in which eosinophilic fibrous protein is deposited in the myocardium and other tissue; (2) sarcoidosis, a multisystem granulomatous disorder of unknown etiology; (3) hemochromatosis, characterized by excessive deposition of iron in body tissues, including the myocardium; and (4) glycogen deposition in the myocardium (Goldman & Fisher, 1997; Hillis et al., 1995b). Restrictive cardiomy-

opathy also may occur secondary to mediastinal irradiation or a collagen-vascular disorder, such as scleroderma. Endomyocardial fibroelastosis is a form of restrictive cardiomyopathy in which the pathologic process occurs in the endocardium (Kirklin & Barratt-Boyes, 1993b). In some instances, etiology is unknown.

The restrictive process in the myocardium or endocardium produces abnormal rigidity of the ventricular chambers. The resultant inability of the myocardium to relax during diastole impedes ventricular filling and results in decreased cardiac output. Both ventricles are likely to be affected by the process and presenting symptoms may include either right or left heart failure. Exercise intolerance commonly is present in patients because the reflex tachycardia that occurs to increase cardiac output further compromises ventricular filling (Wynne & Braunwald, 1997). The clinical manifestations of restrictive cardiomyopathy frequently are difficult to distinguish from those caused by constrictive pericarditis. Endomyocardial biopsy is used to differentiate the two conditions definitively.

The biventricular failure that results from restrictive cardiomyopathy is difficult to treat with conventional medical therapy. Because of the systemic nature of the underlying disease process and the potential for disease recurrence in a transplanted heart, these patients usually are not considered candidates for cardiac transplantation. Treatment is directed toward relief of the symptoms caused by restricted diastolic filling and subsequent passive right- and left-sided congestion (Goldman & Fisher, 1997). A progressive downhill course is typical, and most patients die within 1 or 2 years of diagnosis.

REFERENCES

American Heart Association, 1998: 1999 Heart and Stroke Statistical Update. Dallas, American Heart Association

Burlew BS, Horn HR, Sullivan JM, 1997: Pregnancy and the heart. In Alpert JS (ed): Cardiology for the Primary Care Physician, ed. 2. Philadelphia, Current Medicine

Bush DE, Healy BP, 1987: Cardiomyopathies. In Chung EK (ed): Quick Reference to Cardiovascular Diseases, ed. 3. Baltimore, Williams & Wilkins

CIBIS-II Investigators and Committees, 1999: The Cardiac Insufficiency Bisoprolol Study II (CIBIS-II): A randomised trial. Lancet 353:9

Elkayam U, 1997: Pregnancy and cardiovascular disease. In Braunwald E (ed): Heart Disease: A Textbook of Cardiovascular Medicine, ed. 5. Philadelphia, WB Saunders

Fananapazir L, McAreavey D, 1998: Therapeutic options in patients with obstructive hypertrophic cardiomyopathy and severe drug-refractory symptoms. J Am Coll Cardiol 31:259

Gay WA, 1995: Cardiac transplantation. In Sabiston DC Jr, Spencer FC (eds): Surgery of the Chest, ed. 6. Philadelphia, WB Saunders

Gilbert EM, Bristow MR, 1994: Idiopathic dilated cardiomyopathy. In Schlant RC, Alexander RW, et al. (eds): The Heart, ed. 8. New York, McGraw-Hill

Glower DD, 1995: Acquired aortic valve disease. In Sabiston DC Jr, Spencer FC (eds): Surgery of the Chest, ed. 6. Philadelphia, WB Saunders

Goldman ME, 1997. Infectious myocarditis. In Alpert JS (ed): Cardiology for the Primary Care Physician, ed. 2. Philadelphia, Current Medicine

Goldman ME, Fisher EA, 1997: Restrictive cardiomyopathy. In Alpert JS (ed): Cardiology for the Primary Care Physician, ed. 2. Philadelphia, Current Medicine

Grady KL, Costanzo-Nordin MR, 1989: Myocarditis: Review of a clinical enigma. Heart Lung 18:4

Grayzel D, Dec GW, Lilly LS, 1998: The cardiomyopathies. In Lilly LS (ed): Pathophysiology of Heart Disease, ed. 2. Baltimore, Williams & Wilkins

Hillis LD, Lange RA, Winniford MD, Page RL, 1995a: Dilated cardiomyopathy. In Manual of Clinical Problems in Cardiology, ed. 5. Boston, Little, Brown

Hillis LD, Lange RA, Winniford MD, Page RL, 1995b: Restrictive cardiomyopathy. In Manual of Clinical Problems in Cardiology, ed. 5. Boston, Little, Brown

Kirklin JW, Barratt-Boyes BG, 1993a: Hypertrophic obstructive cardiomyopathy. In Cardiac Surgery, ed. 2. New York, Churchill Livingstone

Kirklin JW, Barratt-Boyes BG, 1993b: Primary cardiomyopathy and cardiac transplantation. In Cardiac Surgery, ed. 2. New York, Churchill Livingstone

Magovern JA, Magovern GJ, 1998: Cardiomyoplasty. In Kaiser LR, Kron IL, Spray TL (eds): Mastery of Cardiothoracic Surgery. Philadelphia, Lippincott Williams & Wilkins

Moreira LF, Stolf NA, Jatene AD, 1991: Benefits of cardiomyoplasty for dilated cardiomyopathy. Semin Thorac Cardiovasc Surg 3:140

Nishimura RA, Giuliani ER, Tajik AJ, Brandenburg RO, 1991: Hypertrophic cardiomyopathy. In Giuliani ER, Fuster V, Gersh BJ, et al. (eds): Cardiology Fundamentals and Practice, ed. 2. St. Louis, Mosby–Year Book

Schoen FJ, 1997: Pathologic considerations in the surgery of adult heart disease. In Edmunds LH Jr (ed): Cardiac Surgery in the Adult. New York, McGraw-Hill

Schonbeck MH, Brunner-La Rocca HP, Vogt PR, et al., 1998: Long-term follow-up in hypertrophic obstructive cardiomyopathy after septal myectomy. Ann Thorac Surg 65:1207

Smith TW, Kelly RA, Stevenson LW, et al., 1997: Management of heart failure. In Braunwald E (ed): Heart Disease: A Textbook of Cardiovascular Medicine, ed. 5. Philadelphia, WB Saunders

Wynne J, Braunwald E, 1997: The cardiomyopathies and myocarditides. In Braunwald E (ed): Heart Disease: A Textbook of Cardiovascular Medicine, ed. 5. Philadelphia, WB Saunders

Congenital Heart Disease in Adults

Approximately 32,000 infants are born each year with one or more congenital heart defects, and an estimated 1 million people with *congenital heart disease* (CHD) are currently alive in the United States (American Heart Association, 1998). A combination of genetic predisposition and environmental factors is thought to cause congenital cardiac anomalies. Some defects, such as those that occur with Down's syndrome, are primarily genetic; others are caused by exposure to environmental teratogens (agents that produce developmental malformations) during a critical period of fetal development (Nugent et al., 1994). Innovations in surgical techniques over the past several decades have made possible correction of most congenital cardiac defects. As a result, most people with CHD undergo surgical correction during infancy or early childhood. Between 1986 and 1996, death rates in the United States among people with CHD declined 25% and the actual number of deaths declined 14% (American Heart Association, 1998).

Adults with CHD may be grouped into one of three categories. Most common in a cardiac surgical setting are those who require surgical correction of an isolated defect that was undiagnosed or asymptomatic during childhood. The diagnosis in such patients frequently is made when, as an adult, the person first receives a physical examination, chest roentgenogram, or electrocardiogram. In other cases, the defect is detected when a period of increased hemodynamic demands, such as occurs with pregnancy, provokes the development of symptoms. With some defects, such as bicuspid aortic valve or mitral valve prolapse, the diagnosis is known, but harmful sequelae of the lesion appear only after several decades, precipitated by degenerative tissue changes or endocarditic infection. Whereas ventricular septal defect (VSD) is the most common congenital lesion in the pediatric population, atrial septal defect (ASD) and aortic stenosis secondary to a bicuspid aortic valve are most common in adults (Henning & Grenvik, 1989).

The second group of adults with CHD are those who have already undergone surgical correction. Because many congenital heart defects are repaired during infancy or childhood, the number of adults with repaired lesions is increasing steadily. Although lifelong medical supervision for management of postoperative sequelae is necessary, treatment in a cardiac surgical setting is required only rarely. However, a small number of patients with previously repaired defects require further surgical therapy during adulthood. Revision of prosthetic conduits and replacement of prosthetic valves or homografts are the most common reasons for reoperation.

The third group of adults with CHD are those with lesions for which no corrective surgery is available. Survival to adulthood is rare in these patients. Of those who do reach adulthood, some may have undergone a palliative procedure during childhood. Rarely, a subsequent palliative operation is performed.

▶ Classification of Defects

Nearly 100 types of anatomic congenital deformities of the heart exist; most are rare or represent combinations of isolated lesions (Nolan, 1974). The anatomic and physiologic abnormalities are extensive, complex, and beyond the scope of this chapter. Adults with CHD represent only a small segment of the population of affected people. Similarly, with rare exceptions, untreated defects in adults consist of only a handful of the most common and least complex isolated cardiac deformities. Only those congenital heart lesions that are present most commonly in adults are included in this chapter. For an in-depth discussion of the multitude of cardiovascular deformities that constitute CHD, the reader is referred to a textbook of pediatric cardiology.

The common congenital anatomic deformities of the heart may be classified into four categories, according to the type of physiologic abnormality. Individual defects in each category differ in anatomic location but are similar in the resulting pathophysiologic effects (Table 6-1). The categories are (1) abnormal communication between systemic and pulmonary circulations, producing a left-to-right shunt; (2) valvular or vascular obstruction, with or without a right-to-left shunt; (3) transposition of great vessels or cardiac chambers; and (4) venous anomalies (Nolan, 1974). Almost all untreated defects in adults that require surgical intervention are in the first two categories.

▶ Defects With Left-to-Right Shunts

Atrial septal defect, VSD, and patent ductus arteriosus (PDA) are the most common defects associated with left-to-right shunts. In each, an abnormal communication allows shunting of blood from the left side of the heart with its high systemic resistance to the right side with its low pulmonary vascular resistance. The three defects differ primarily in the anatomic level of systemic-pulmonary communication. The opening is between the atria with ASD, between the ventricles with VSD, and between the great vessels (aorta and pulmonary artery) with PDA.

The predominant hemodynamic effect of each of these lesions is left-to-right shunting of blood. The resultant increased blood flow through the pulmonary vasculature produces congestive heart failure and pulmonary hypertension that may evolve to pulmonary vascular obstruction, that is, an irreversible increase in pulmonary vascular resistance. Patients with chronically increased pulmonary vascular pressure may be

TABLE 6-1
Classification System for Common Forms of Congenital Heart Disease

I. LEFT-TO-RIGHT SHUNT
(Abnormal communication between systemic and pulmonic circuits)

Defect	Level of Communication
Atrial septal defect	Atria
Ventricular septal defect	Ventricles
Patent ductus arteriosus	Great vessels (aorta to pulmonary artery)

II. VALVULAR OR VASCULAR OBSTRUCTION
(With or without abnormal communication proximal to obstruction)

Defect	Level of Obstruction	Level of Communication
Aortic stenosis	Aortic valve	None
Pulmonic stenosis	Pulmonic valve	None
Coarctation	Aorta	None
Tetralogy of Fallot	Right ventricular outflow tract	Ventricle

III. TRANSPOSITION OF GREAT VESSELS OR CARDIAC CHAMBERS
Transposition of great vessels

IV. VENOUS ANOMALIES
Total or partial anomalous pulmonary venous connection

From Nolan SP, 1974: Congenital heart disease: Indications for and timing of operation. Paediatrician 3:144.

comfortable at rest but experience such symptoms as tachypnea, dyspnea, cough, fatigue, and orthopnea with exercise (McNamara, 1989). Often, the person does not recognize such exercise intolerance as abnormal because it always has been present.

Eventually, right-sided pressure may increase substantially, decreasing the shunt and causing a diminution in intensity of the heart murmur associated with the defect. This indicates worsening, not improvement, of the patient's condition. If pulmonary hypertension remains uncorrected, pulmonary artery pressure eventually exceeds systemic arterial pressure and the shunt direction reverses to right to left. This condition, known as Eisenmenger's syndrome, is discussed later in the chapter.

Atrial Septal Defect

Atrial septal defects comprise 30% to 40% of CHD in adults (Marelli & Moodie, 1998). ASDs are classified by their location in the interatrial septum (Fig. 6-1). Most common is ostium secundum, or fossa ovalis ASD, located in the middle portion of the atrial septum. Secundum-type defects occur in 10% to 15% of all patients with CHD and are twice as common in women as in men (Galloway et al., 1995).

Less common are sinus venosus ASDs, located at the junction of the superior vena cava. Sinus venosus ASDs

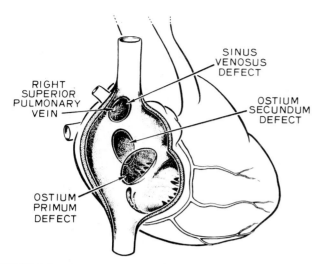

FIGURE 6-1. Location of the most common types of atrial septal defect. (Watson SP, Watson DC Jr, 1982: Anatomy, physiology, and hemodynamics of congenital heart disease. In Ream AK, Fogdall RP [eds]: Acute Cardiovascular Management: Anesthesia and Intensive Care, p. 584. Philadelphia, JB Lippincott)

often are associated with partial anomalous pulmonary venous connection (PAPVC), a structural abnormality in which the anomalous location of one or both right pulmonary veins causes part or all of the venous (oxygenated) blood from the right lung to empty through the septal defect into the right instead of the left atrium. Rarely, the left pulmonary veins drain anomalously (Liberthson, 1989a). PAPVC occasionally occurs without an ASD and, like an ASD, produces left-to-right shunting of blood. Ostium primum ASDs are located at the base of the septum. They also are referred to as *endocardial cushion* or *incomplete atrioventricular canal defects*. Ostium primum defects often are associated with defects in the mitral or tricuspid valve. If the entire septum fails to develop, a common or single atrium is said to exist.

The pressure gradient between the left and right atria is minimal and is not responsible for left-to-right shunting. Instead, the size of the defect and the compliance of the left and right ventricles during diastole determine the direction and amount of blood flow across an ASD (Kopf & Laks, 1996). Most shunting occurs during ventricular diastole when the atria are emptying blood into the ventricles. Because the thin-walled right ventricle is more compliant, blood shunts across the defect from left to right. Increased blood flow through the right ventricle and pulmonary vasculature causes right atrial enlargement, right ventricular hypertrophy and enlargement, and pulmonary hypertension. The degree of shunting is described using a ratio that compares the amount of pulmonary blood flow in relation to systemic blood flow ($Q_P : Q_S$). For example, with a 2 : 1 shunt, cardiac output from the right ventricle into the pulmonary artery is twice that of the left ventricle into the aorta.

In most instances, an ASD is diagnosed during childhood when a systolic ejection murmur, caused by increased flow across the pulmonic valve, is auscultated.

Fixed splitting of the second heart sound also is common. Increased blood flow across the pulmonic valve delays its closing, causing the two components of the second heart sound (aortic and pulmonic valve closure) to be heard separately throughout the respiratory cycle. The term *fixed splitting* is used to describe this finding. Increased blood flow through the pulmonary artery may produce a palpable thrill over the pulmonic valve area.

An abnormal electrocardiogram or chest roentgenogram also may lead to diagnosis of ASD. Electrocardiographic signs associated with ASD include incomplete right bundle branch block, right axis deviation, and right ventricular hypertrophy. The chest roentgenogram may demonstrate increased pulmonary vascular markings as well as enlargement of the pulmonary artery and right atrium and ventricle. Echocardiography is used to confirm the diagnosis and define the pulmonary venous drainage.

Although many children appear asymptomatic, careful study reveals easy fatigability and dyspnea with limited endurance in as many as 50% to 60% of patients, particularly those with large shunts (Kopf & Laks, 1996). Children with ASDs also may be shorter and of slighter stature than their peers (Kirklin & Barratt-Boyes, 1993a). Occasionally, an asymptomatic ASD is not detected until adulthood. An ASD in an adult may become apparent when a condition common to older adults, such as hypertension or ischemic heart disease, decreases left ventricular compliance and thereby increases left-to-right shunting (Henning & Grenvik, 1989). Conversely, if right ventricular compliance is acutely decreased (eg, due to right ventricular myocardial infarction) or pulmonary vascular resistance increases (eg, due to pulmonary embolism), transient right-to-left shunting with resultant arterial desaturation may occur.

The likelihood of harmful consequences of an ASD, including atrial arrhythmias, pulmonary vascular obstruction, and right ventricular failure, increases with age. Typically, an unrepaired ASD causes a gradual decrease in exercise capacity as the person enters his or her teens and 20s, with a progressive decline in exercise tolerance over the next 10 to 20 years coincident with deterioration in right ventricular function (Mainwaring & Lamberti, 1998). Although atrial arrhythmias are uncommon in children with ASDs, atrial fibrillation or flutter commonly develops in older adults with unrepaired defects, augmenting the left-to-right shunt and precipitating right ventricular failure (Perloff, 1998).

Pulmonary embolism and paradoxical systemic embolism are fairly common in older patients with ASDs (Liberthson, 1989a). Paradoxical embolization is the migration of venous thrombus or air into the arterial circulation through an anomalous intracardiac communication. Although flow across an ASD is predominantly left to right, some degree of right-to-left shunting across the defect occurs as well, allowing thrombus or air from the right atrium to enter the left side of the heart. Not infrequently, the initial symptom of ASD in an adult is a cerebral vascular accident caused by paradoxical embolism. Women who become pregnant with unrepaired ASDs have a 20% to 30% incidence of fetal mortality and a 2% risk of maternal mortality (Mainwaring & Lamberti, 1998). ASD is not associated with an increased risk of infective endocarditis.

Surgical repair of an ASD is recommended regardless of age in patients with significant shunts ($Q_P : Q_S > 1.5 : 1$). The primary indication for operative repair is the unpredictable development of irreversibly elevated pulmonary vascular resistance. Pulmonary vascular disease eventually develops in approximately 15% to 20% of children with an ASD (Laks et al., 1997). In affected people, increased pulmonary vascular resistance and decreased right ventricular compliance cause blood to shunt from right to left, producing cyanosis (Kopf & Laks, 1996). When this occurs, operative repair is no longer possible because obliterating the right-to-left shunt in a patient with severely elevated pulmonary vascular resistance would lead to right ventricular overload and failure. Although some patients survive to old age with unrepaired ASDs, average life expectancy for people with a shunt greater than 1.5 : 1 is approximately 45 years (Mainwaring & Lamberti, 1998). Death in persons with unrepaired defects usually occurs as a consequence of pulmonary hypertension or heart failure.

Ventricular Septal Defect

Ventricular septal defect is one of the most common congenital defects, accounting for 20% to 30% of all congenital cardiac malformations (Knott-Craig, 1998). De-
spite the prevalence of this form of CHD, unrepaired congenital VSDs are quite uncommon in adults. An estimated 40% of VSDs close spontaneously during infancy, and 60% close by 5 years of age (Warnes et al., 1991a). Although large defects rarely close, those associated with significant shunts produce symptoms of congestive heart failure in early life that lead to operative repair during childhood. VSDs in adults are likely to be small defects resulting from partial spontaneous closure of a larger defect or from residual leakage of a previously repaired VSD (Laks et al., 1997).

Defects in the ventricular septum are categorized according to location. There are three primary components of the septum: (1) the inlet septum, extending from the tricuspid annulus to the valve's distal attachments; (2) the muscular, or trabecular, septum that extends from the inlet septum to the apex and upward to the outlet septum; and (3) the outlet, or infundibular, septum that extends from the muscular septum to the pulmonic valve (Fig. 6-2). The membranous septum is sometimes categorized separately as a fourth component of the septum; composed of fibrous tissue, it is located beneath the atrioventricular valves and between the inlet and outlet septum. Defects in the membranous component of the septum are the most common, accounting for more than 80% of VSDs (Tchervenkov & Shum-Tim, 1996). Often, a VSD occurs in association with another congenital cardiac defect.

The degree of shunting through an isolated VSD is determined by the size of the defect and the degree of pul-

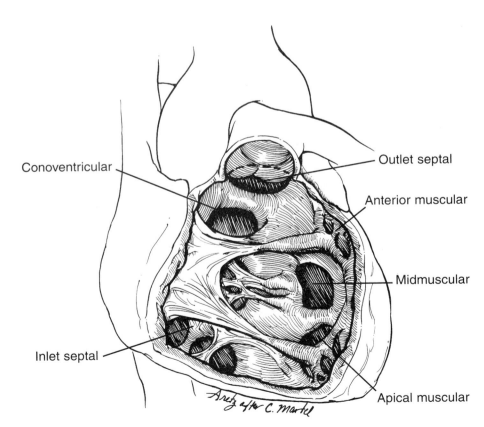

Conoventricular

Outlet septal

Anterior muscular

Midmuscular

Inlet septal

Apical muscular

FIGURE 6-2. The right ventricular free wall has been resected to show the various types of ventricular septal defects; muscular defects may be midmuscular, anterior, or apical; conoventricular = perimembranous. (Knott-Craig CJ, 1998: Ventricular septal defects. In Kaiser LR, Kron IL, Spray TL [eds]: Mastery of Cardiothoracic Surgery, p. 688. Philadelphia, Lippincott Williams & Wilkins)

monary vascular resistance (Perloff, 1998). In small to moderate-sized defects, the pressure gradient between the left and right ventricles results in shunting of blood from left to right with increased blood flow into the pulmonary vasculature. In large defects, systolic pressures in the ventricles, aorta, and pulmonary artery are essentially the same. The relative resistances of the aortic and pulmonary vasculature therefore determine the degree and direction of shunting (Nugent et al., 1994). VSDs are associated with a harsh, holosystolic murmur, enlargement of the left atrium and left and right ventricles, and dilatation of the pulmonary artery (DeAngelis, 1991).

An unrepaired VSD with significant left-to-right shunting ($Q_P : Q_S > 1.8 : 1$) eventually leads to progressive congestive heart failure and, sometimes, irreversible pulmonary vascular obstruction and resultant right-to-left shunting. Severe pulmonary vascular disease develops in approximately 50% of patients with large defects by the third decade of life, with eventual death from complications of Eisenmenger's syndrome (Laks et al., 1997). Table 6-2 categorizes VSDs by hemodynamic severity. Operative repair is recommended for defects with a $Q_P : Q_S$ ratio greater than 1.5 : 1 as long as the calculated pulmonary vascular resistance is less than 6 units/m² (Laks et al., 1997).

Patent Ductus Arteriosus

The ductus arteriosus is a vascular connection between the descending thoracic aorta and the pulmonary artery (Fig. 6-3). A normal vessel in fetal circulation, the ductus routes blood flow from the pulmonary artery into the distal aorta, bypassing the lungs. At or shortly after birth, the walls of the ductus, which contain smooth muscle fibers in the medial layer, actively contract to obliterate the lumen (Hallman et al., 1987). The residual fibrous, connective tissue is known as the *ligamentum arteriosum*. If the fetal ductus arteriosus fails to close, a *patent ductus arteriosus* remains. Hypoxemia is thought to contribute to failure of the ductus to close. Premature infants and those born at high altitude have a higher incidence of the defect (Hillis et al., 1995a). PDA occurs twice as often in girls, is particularly common when the mother contracts rubella during the first trimester of pregnancy, and may occur in siblings (Kirklin & Barratt-

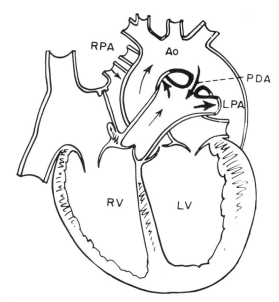

FIGURE 6-3. Patent ductus arteriosus (PDA). Ao, aorta; LPA, left pulmonary artery; LV, left ventricle; RPA, right pulmonary artery; RV, right ventricle. (Edwards BS, Edwards JE, 1987: Classification. In Roberts WC [ed]: Adult Congenital Heart Disease, p. 19. Philadelphia, FA Davis)

Boyes, 1993b). It often coexists with other congenital cardiac defects.

Shortly after birth, systemic vascular resistance rises and pulmonary vascular resistance falls. As soon as this occurs, a PDA allows shunting of blood from the aorta to the pulmonary artery (left to right), opposite the direction of blood flow through the ductus during fetal life. This shunting of blood continues through both systole and diastole, producing a characteristic continuous murmur often described as a "machinery" murmur. Because of the easily recognized murmur, most PDAs are detected, definitively diagnosed with echocardiography, and repaired during infancy or early childhood.

The size of the ductal lumen and the resistance in the pulmonary vasculature determine the degree of left-to-right shunting (Canobbio, 1995). The degree of shunting in turn determines the presence and severity of symptoms. If only a small shunt exists, the patient is likely to remain asymptomatic. However, if a large shunt is present, exertional dyspnea may result from the left ventric-

TABLE 6-2

Hemodynamic Severity of Ventricular Septal Defect

Defect	Size	Ventricular Pressures	$Q_P : Q_S$	Pulmonary Pressure
Small	0.5 cm²	Not equal	<1.75 : 1	<1/2 systemic
Moderate	0.5–1.0 cm²	Not equal	3 : 1	1/2 systemic
Large	>1.0 cm²	Equal	>3 : 1	Systemic

$Q_P : Q_S$, ratio of pulmonary to systemic blood flow.
From Liberthson RR, 1989: Ventricular septal defect. In Congenital Heart Disease. Boston, Little, Brown.

ular failure and pulmonary hypertension that develop secondary to volume overload of the left ventricle and pulmonary vasculature. Congestive heart failure, irreversible pulmonary vascular obstruction, and infective endocarditis all can occur as a consequence of the PDA. A PDA also may become markedly dilated and aneurysmal; degenerative changes in the ductal tissue occur with aging and rarely lead to aortic dissection or rupture (Liberthson, 1989b). Natural history data reveal a dramatically shortened life span for people with PDAs. The mortality rate associated with an unrepaired PDA is 1% per year in early adulthood and increases to 2% to 4% by midlife (Laks et al., 1997). Average age at death is only 40 years (Henning & Grenvik, 1989). Consequently, surgical repair of PDA is recommended regardless of whether the defect is associated with symptoms. Operative repair is not performed if prolonged pulmonary hypertension has caused reversal of the shunt or if the patient is dependent on the PDA to compensate for other inoperable cardiac defects (Hillis et al., 1995a).

▶ Defects With Outflow Obstruction

Aortic stenosis, pulmonic stenosis, and coarctation of the aorta are obstructive lesions in which no abnormal communication between cardiac chambers is present. The primary consequence of obstructive lesions is heart failure resulting from the increased work of pumping blood across an obstructed pathway. Tetralogy of Fallot (TOF), rarely seen in adults, is an example of a congenital heart defect that has an obstructive component (pulmonic stenosis) with a communication proximal to the obstruction (VSD) that allows right-to-left shunting of blood.

Aortic Stenosis

Congenital *aortic stenosis* includes lesions obstructive to left ventricular outflow that are valvular, subvalvular, or supravalvular. Subvalvular stenosis occurs in two forms: (1) type 1 (discrete), caused by a diaphragm-like membrane beneath the aortic valve; and (2) type 2 (diffuse), a more extensive combination of outflow tract and valvular abnormalities that rarely permits survival beyond infancy (Liberthson, 1989c). Supravalvular stenosis is rare. Stenosis of the valve itself is most common. Congenital aortic stenosis most often occurs because the valve is bicuspid instead of tricuspid. The incidence of bicuspid aortic valve in the general population is estimated at 2% and a bicuspid aortic valve accounts for 98% of congenital aortic valve malformations (Perloff, 1998). Rarely, only one cusp is present, and the valve is said to be unicuspid. A bicuspid aortic valve often is not recognized in childhood because it does not produce stenosis. However, the valve can become increasingly stenotic with aging due to fibrosis, calcification, or endocarditic infection. Congenital aortic stenosis is more common in boys.

The primary hemodynamic consequence of aortic stenosis is fixed obstruction to left ventricular outflow. As a result, left ventricular pressure increases, leading to left ventricular hypertension, secondary concentric hypertrophy, and heart failure. Once symptoms develop, average life expectancy without surgical treatment is 5 years or less (Kirklin & Barratt-Boyes, 1993c). Classic symptoms of aortic stenosis include angina, dyspnea on exertion, and syncope. When severe obstruction is present, sudden cardiac death may occur. In addition, a congenitally abnormal valve is more susceptible to bacterial infection. Recurrent bouts of endocarditis may occur, further impairing valve function. Significant aortic stenosis is treated with valvotomy in children and with valve replacement in adults. Repair or replacement of the valve is recommended for symptomatic patients and for those with valvular stenosis and a valve area of less than 0.6 cm² or a transvalvular gradient of 80 mm Hg or greater (Marelli & Moodie, 1998). Aortic stenosis and aortic valve replacement are discussed in more detail elsewhere in the text.

Coarctation of the Aorta

Coarctation of the aorta, in its most common form, is a segmental narrowing of the aortic lumen, created by a discrete fibrous infolding of the aortic wall near the origin of the left subclavian artery, opposite the ligamentum arteriosum (Liberthson, 1989d) (Fig. 6-4). Aortic coarctation often occurs in association with other cardiac defects that impact on physiology of the defect and presenting symptomatology (Ungerleider, 1998). Isolated

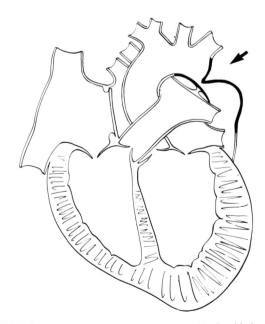

FIGURE 6-4. Coarctation of the aorta represented by focal indentation in the superior aspect of the aorta (*arrow*), which causes the aortic lumen to be eccentric and narrow. (Edwards BS, Edwards JE, 1987: Classification. In Roberts WC [ed]: Adult Congenital Heart Disease, p. 10. Philadelphia, FA Davis)

coarctation is more than twice as common in boys (Kirklin & Barratt-Boyes, 1993d). Infants with coarctation may develop severe left heart failure with poor distal perfusion because of obstruction to left ventricular and distal aortic blood flow (Ungerleider, 1998).

In asymptomatic people, coarctation occasionally remains undiagnosed until adulthood. In such cases, the lesion often is detected during a routine physical examination of peripheral pulses and blood pressure. Coarctation produces arterial hypertension above the narrowing and a gradient between blood pressure in the upper and lower extremities. A difference in quality of upper and lower extremity pulses, the presence of severe hypertension in a child or young adult, and a gradient between upper and lower extremity blood pressure measurements are highly suggestive of coarctation. Auscultation reveals a systolic murmur, best heard over the back between the left scapula and spine (Pickering, 1997). A suprasternal notch thrill, fourth heart sound, and a bruit over the left posterior thorax also are common.

The chest roentgenogram in a person with coarctation often demonstrates erosion or notching along the inferior posterior rib edges, representing collateral arteries that have developed over time to enhance blood supply to the aorta distal to the coarctation. These prominent collateral blood vessels also may produce visible or palpable pulsations in the scapular region. Collateral blood vessels, which increase with the duration and severity of aortic obstruction, arise mainly from branches of the subclavian, intercostal, scapular, and internal thoracic arteries (Liberthson, 1989d).

In contrast to other obstructive lesions, such as aortic stenosis, severity of obstruction is not accurately reflected by a pressure gradient across the coarcted segment because of the well-developed collateral blood vessels in adults that supply the distal aorta beyond the area of obstruction. Instead, severity of obstruction is measured by the degree of aortic narrowing and anatomic and physiologic consequences, such as hypertension and left ventricular failure.

In patients without significant symptoms during infancy, symptoms of coarctation may not occur until after 20 to 30 years of age (Perloff, 1997). Symptoms and complications almost always are present by 40 years of age. Systemic hypertension is the predominant clinical manifestation of coarctation. Occurring in 90% of those affected, it is primarily systolic with a wide pulse pressure (Liberthson, 1989e). The abnormally high blood pressure above the coarctation may produce symptoms of hypertension, including headache, epistaxis, dizziness, and palpitations (Hillis et al., 1995b). Stroke from intracranial hemorrhage may occur. In addition to hypertension, left ventricular hypertrophy almost always is present. Heart failure occurs in two thirds of patients (Liberthson, 1989e). The aorta may become aneurysmal, intercostal arteries may develop aneurysmal dilatation and rupture, and aortic dissection or rupture can occur (Laks et al., 1997). Coarctation also imposes an increased risk of infective endocarditis.

Adults with uncorrected coarctation often have precocious coronary atherosclerosis (Liberthson, 1989d). Also, because blood flow to the distal aorta is diminished, poorly developed lower extremities, renal insufficiency, and, occasionally, claudication may be present. Aortic valve disease also may develop during adulthood. The frequently associated bicuspid aortic valve may become calcified and stenotic. In addition, aortic regurgitation may result from the association of systemic hypertension and the abnormal valve (Fuster et al., 1991). Pregnancy in a woman with unrepaired coarctation may be associated with a number of complications, including aortic dissection, hypertension, congestive heart failure, angina, infective endocarditis in the mother, or CHD in the fetus (Elkayam, 1997). For this reason, coarctation usually is repaired before anticipated pregnancy.

Operative repair of coarctation is the treatment of choice and has been performed since 1945. Natural history studies before that time revealed markedly reduced life expectancy in patients with unrepaired coarctation. More than three fourths of patients with uncorrected coarctation die by 50 years of age, usually from congestive heart failure, aortic rupture, intracranial hemorrhage, or infective endocarditis (Perloff, 1998; Maron, 1982). The objectives of operative repair include reducing or preventing worsening of hypertension and lessening the risk of endocarditis or aneurysm formation at the coarctation site.

Despite surgical correction of coarctation, long-term medical supervision is essential. Coexisting cardiovascular disease is prevalent and many patients have persistent hypertension after surgical repair. The older the child or adult at the time of repair, the less likely is hypertension to be corrected by surgical treatment. Accordingly, most people who have undergone coarctation repair in adulthood require lifelong antihypertensive therapy with angiotensin-converting enzyme inhibiting, beta-adrenergic blocking, or calcium channel antagonist medications. Recurrent coarctation occurs in 5% to 20% of patients, depending on age at the time of repair, the extent of the lesion, the reparative technique, and the length of the follow-up period (Ungerleider, 1998).

Pulmonic Stenosis

Pulmonic valve stenosis is reported to account for 8% to 10% of all congenital heart anomalies (Laks & Plunkett, 1998). The valvular abnormality usually consists of a dome-shaped valve with a central opening and fused commissures (Warnes et al., 1991b). Uncorrected pulmonic stenosis in adults is rare and when present usually is not severe enough to produce symptoms. Severity of obstruction sometimes increases with aging, however, and symptoms become more prevalent. The defect is suggested by a systolic ejection murmur in the pulmonic area and evidence of right ventricular hypertrophy.

Moderate to severe pulmonic stenosis produces hypertrophy of the right ventricular infundibulum, which in turn can lead to right-sided heart failure, tricuspid regurgitation, and mild cyanosis due to right-to-left shunting across a patent foramen ovale in the presence of elevated right atrial pressure (Henning & Grenvik, 1989). Right ventricular failure, usually after the fourth decade of life, is the most common cause of death, and patients with moderate to severe pulmonic stenosis are at increased risk for infective endocarditis (Perloff, 1998).

Intervention for pulmonic stenosis is recommended in patients with a transvalvular gradient of 50 mm Hg or greater (Marelli & Moodie, 1998). Pulmonic stenosis is most often corrected with balloon valvotomy or, less commonly, with surgical valvuloplasty. Replacement of the pulmonic valve usually is not necessary because the small degree of pulmonic regurgitation that may develop secondary to reparative interventions is usually well tolerated. Because operative repair has been performed in children for many years, postoperative adults are more commonly encountered than are adults with unrepaired pulmonic stenosis. Further surgical intervention is almost never required.

Tetralogy of Fallot

Tetralogy of Fallot represents 10% of all CHD and is the most common form of cyanotic CHD (Perryman & Jaquiss, 1998). The occurrence of unrepaired TOF in adults is quite rare because survival into adulthood without correction is unlikely and because corrective surgery has been possible for years. In patients with unrepaired TOF of all degrees of severity, only 11% survive to 20 years of age and only 3% to 40 years (Perloff, 1998). Before the development of corrective surgery, children died secondary to hypoxia, brain abscess, cerebral vascular accident, or infective endocarditis (Nolan, 1974).

The defect TOF derives its name from its four classic components: (1) VSD, (2) aorta that overrides the VSD and communicates with both the right and left ventricles, (3) right ventricular hypertrophy, and (4) pulmonic stenosis (Fig. 6-5). The primary manifestations of TOF are cyanosis and hypoxia. Correction of TOF includes closure of the VSD and widening of the right ventricular outflow tract to relieve pulmonic stenosis. If the patient has a previously placed palliative shunt, it is closed at the time of definitive repair.

▸ Complications of Congenital Heart Disease

Congenital heart defects are associated with a number of potential complications, including infective endocarditis, pulmonary hypertension, paradoxical embolism, arterial desaturation, and aneurysm formation.

Infective Endocarditis

Almost all congenital heart defects subject the person to an increased risk of *infective endocarditis.* The cardiac or vascular abnormality provides a potential site for de-

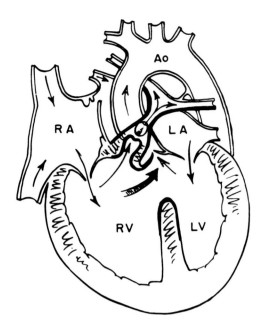

FIGURE 6-5. Classic tetralogy of Fallot. Ao, aorta; LA, left atrium; LV, left ventricle; RA, right atrium; RV, right ventricle. (Edwards BS, Edwards JE, 1987: Classification. In Roberts WC [ed]: Adult Congenital Heart Disease, p. 24. Philadelphia, FA Davis)

position of pathogenic organisms and development of infection. Factors that place a person at greatest risk are listed in Table 6-3. Adults with congenital lesions are thought to be more susceptible to infective endocarditis than are children, probably because of two factors: (1) a longer period has elapsed for development of degenerative changes on valves, septal walls, or vessels; and (2) chronic gum disease and dental abscesses (a frequent source of bacteremia) are more prevalent in adults (McNamara, 1989). Unrepaired congenital defects that are associated with a moderate or high risk of infective endocarditis include bicuspid aortic valves (functionally normal, stenotic, or regurgitant), coarctation, pulmonic valve stenosis, VSD, PDA, and TOF (Child et al., 1998).

TABLE 6-3

Conditions Associated With Increased Risk for Endocarditis

HIGH-RISK CATEGORY

Prosthetic heart valves
Previous infective endocarditis
Complex cyanotic congenital heart disease
Surgically constructed systemic pulmonary shunts or conduits

MODERATE-RISK CATEGORY

Unrepaired patent ductus arteriosus, ventricular septal defect, atrial septal defect, coarctation, bicuspid aortic valve

---

From Dajani AS, Taubert KA, Wilson W, et al., 1997: Prevention of bacterial endocarditis: Recommendations by the American Heart Association. JAMA 277:1794.

Surgical correction of a congenital defect usually substantially lowers, but does not eradicate, the potential risk for endocarditis. Important exceptions (ie, patients who continue at high risk) are patients in whom prosthetic valves have been implanted and those with surgically constructed systemic pulmonary shunts or conduits (Dajani et al., 1997). Prosthetic material other than cardiac valves is of lesser concern after the early postoperative period because the material becomes covered with intimal cells or fibrous tissue. Complications of infective endocarditis include valvular destruction with resultant heart failure and septic embolization. Embolization into the pulmonic, as well as systemic, circulation can occur with a left-to-right intracardiac shunt. Patients at increased risk for infective endocarditis should receive appropriate antibiotic prophylaxis before certain types of dental procedures and instrumentation or surgery involving the respiratory, genitourinary, or gastrointestinal tissues (Dajani et al., 1997).

Eisenmenger's Syndrome

A complication of defects that produce left-to-right shunting and chronic volume overload of the pulmonary vasculature is irreversible pulmonary vascular obstruction. Pulmonary vascular resistance becomes irreversibly elevated because of prolonged hypertension and resultant changes in the pulmonary arterioles. Severe pulmonary vascular obstruction leads to a condition known as *Eisenmenger's syndrome*, defined as a communication between the pulmonic and systemic circulations and associated obliterative pulmonary vascular disease that is severe enough to cause right-to-left shunting of blood through the defect (Hillis et al., 1995c). The resultant right-to-left shunt allows desaturated blood to enter the systemic circulation, producing arterial desaturation. Although Eisenmenger's syndrome is classically associated with unrepaired VSD, it can result from uncorrected left-to-right shunting at the atrial (ASD) or aortic (PDA) level as well.

Once Eisenmenger's syndrome has developed, surgical correction of the cardiac anomaly is no longer possible. Closure of the defect eliminates the right-to-left shunt, which has been providing compensatory decompression of the right ventricle. Profound right-sided heart failure would then result because of the irreversibly elevated right ventricular afterload (pulmonary vascular resistance). Eisenmenger's syndrome may be associated with chest pain resembling angina, exertional syncope, hemoptysis, cerebral thrombosis secondary to polycythemia, or cerebral abscess; death usually occurs by the third decade (Warnes et al., 1991a). Patients with Eisenmenger's syndrome typically succumb to arrhythmias, heart failure, embolism, or abscess.

Paradoxical Embolism

Paradoxical embolism, defined earlier, is more common with right-to-left shunts but can occur in the presence of defects in which shunting of blood is predominantly left to right, particularly ASD. During periods of increased right atrial pressure, such as occurs with a Valsalva maneuver, right-to-left shunting increases and venous thrombus can travel into the systemic circulation. Because air or thrombus from intravenous catheters also can travel into the arterial circulation through an ASD, particular attention must be given to handling of intravenous catheters so that no air or thrombus is introduced from the catheter into the right side of the heart.

Paradoxical embolism occasionally occurs across a patent foramen ovale, a tiny opening located in the midportion of the atrial septum. Patent foramen ovale exists normally in approximately 20% of people and is not considered a form of ASD. In conditions that acutely increase right atrial pressure, such as right ventricular myocardial infarction or pulmonary embolism, right-to-left shunting through the patent foramen ovale can occur, causing arterial desaturation or paradoxical embolism.

Arterial Desaturation

Arterial desaturation in adults with CHD is uncommon and should become increasingly so because of the aggressive approach to surgical correction of defects in infants and children. It occurs with lesions that allow a right-to-left shunt primarily or with those in which a left-to-right shunt has reversed because of chronically elevated pulmonary vascular resistance. Desaturated blood enters the systemic circulation, producing decreased arterial saturation that can lead to hypoxemia, cyanosis, polycythemia, and clubbing. Increased blood viscosity secondary to polycythemia predisposes the person to cerebral vascular accidents and spontaneous hemorrhage (Nolan, 1974). The presence of right-to-left shunting also provides the conditions necessary for systemic embolization of venous thrombus.

Aortic Aneurysm

Conditions with abnormal blood flow through the aorta (turbulent flow or jetting of blood) are sometimes associated with aortic aneurysm formation. Coarctation, PDA, and aortic stenosis are examples of congenital defects associated with aortic aneurysm formation. Bacterial infection of an abnormal segment of aortic wall can lead to formation of a mycotic aneurysm (ie, aneurysm caused by infective aortitis) with possible aortic rupture (Lindsay et al., 1994).

Complications Associated With Pregnancy

Congenital heart disease can produce significant complications during pregnancy. Support of a growing fetus causes major hemodynamic alterations in the mother. Cardiac decompensation, usually in the form of congestive heart failure, may occur as physiologic demands on

TABLE 6-4

Risk Associated With Pregnancy and Congenital Heart Disease

LOW RISK

Isolated pulmonic stenosis
Functionally normal bicuspid aortic valve
Repaired without residual:
  Atrial septal defect
  Ventricular septal defect
  Patent ductus arteriosus
  Tetralogy of Fallot (NYHA functional class I)

INTERMEDIATE RISK

Aortic valve disease
Unrepaired:
  Perimembranous ventricular septal defect
  Coarctation

HIGH RISK

Cyanotic congenital heart disease
Increased pulmonary vascular resistance
Heart failure (NYHA functional class III or IV)

NYHA, New York Heart Association.
From Canobbio MM, 1995: Congenital heart disease. In Woods SL, Froelicher ES, Halpenny CJ, Motzer SU (eds): Cardiac Nursing, ed. 3. Philadelphia, JB Lippincott

the heart increase. Depending on the nature of the underlying defect and severity of symptoms, abortion of the fetus or surgical repair of the cardiac defect in the mother may become necessary to save the life of the mother, the infant, or both. Table 6-4 displays the risk associated with pregnancy in the presence of various forms of CHD. Cardiac disease and pregnancy are discussed further in Chapter 7, Other Cardiovascular Disorders.

REFERENCES

American Heart Association, 1998: 1999 Heart and Stroke Statistical Update. Dallas, American Heart Association

Canobbio MM, 1995: Congenital heart disease. In Woods SL, Froelicher ES, Halpenny CJ, Motzer SU (eds): Cardiac Nursing, ed. 3. Philadelphia, JB Lippincott

Child JS, Perloff JK, Kubak B, 1998: Infective endocarditis. In Perloff JK, Child JS (eds): Congenital Heart Disease in Adults, ed. 2. Philadelphia, WB Saunders

Dajani AS, Taubert KA, Wilson W, et al., 1997: Prevention of bacterial endocarditis: Recommendations by the American Heart Association. JAMA 277:1794

DeAngelis R, 1991: The cardiovascular system. In Alspach JG (ed): Core Curriculum for Critical Care Nursing, ed. 4. Philadelphia, WB Saunders

Elkayam U, 1997: Pregnancy and cardiovascular disease. In Braunwald E (ed): Heart Disease: A Textbook of Cardiovascular Medicine, ed. 5. Philadelphia, WB Saunders

Fuster V, Warnes CA, McGoon DC, 1991: Congenital heart disease in adolescents and adults: Coarctation of the aorta. In Giuliani ER, Fuster V, Gersh BJ, et al. (eds): Cardiology: Fundamentals and Practice, ed. 2. St. Louis, Mosby–Year Book

Galloway AC, Colvin SB, Spencer FC, 1995: Atrial septal defects, atrioventricular canal defects, and total anomalous pulmonary venous return. In Sabiston DC Jr, Spencer FC (eds): Surgery of the Chest, ed. 6. Philadelphia, WB Saunders

Hallman GL, Cooley DA, Gutgesell HP, 1987: Patent ductus arteriosus. In Surgical Treatment of Congenital Heart Disease, ed. 3. Philadelphia, Lea & Febiger

Henning RJ, Grenvik A, 1989: Congenital heart disease in the adult. In Henning RJ, Grenvik A (eds). Critical Care Cardiology. New York, Churchill Livingstone

Hillis LD, Lange RA, Winniford MD, Page RL, 1995a: Patent ductus arteriosus. In Manual of Clinical Problems in Cardiology, ed. 5. Boston, Little, Brown

Hillis LD, Lange RA, Winniford MD, Page RL, 1995b: Coarctation of the aorta. In Manual of Clinical Problems in Cardiology, ed. 5. Boston, Little, Brown

Hillis LD, Lange RA, Winniford MD, Page RL, 1995c: Eisenmenger syndrome. In Manual of Clinical Problems in Cardiology, ed. 5. Boston, Little, Brown

Kirklin JW, Barratt-Boyes BG, 1993a: Atrial septal defect and partial anomalous pulmonary venous connection. In Cardiac Surgery, ed. 2. New York, Churchill Livingstone

Kirklin JW, Barratt-Boyes BG, 1993b: Patent ductus arteriosus. In Cardiac Surgery, ed. 2. New York, Churchill Livingstone

Kirklin JW, Barratt-Boyes BG, 1993c: Aortic valve disease. In Cardiac Surgery, ed. 2. New York, Churchill Livingstone

Kirklin JW, Barratt-Boyes BG, 1993d: Coarctation of the aorta and interrupted aortic arch. In Cardiac Surgery, ed. 2. New York, Churchill Livingstone

Knott-Craig CJ, 1998: Ventricular septal defects. In Kaiser LR, Kron IL, Spray TL (eds): Mastery of Cardiothoracic Surgery. Philadelphia, Lippincott Williams & Wilkins

Kopf GS, Laks H, 1996: Atrial septal defects and cor triatriatum. In Baue AE, Geha AS, Hammond GL, et al. (eds): Glenn's Thoracic and Cardiovascular Surgery, ed. 6. Stamford, CT, Appleton & Lange

Laks H, Marelli D, Drinkwater DC, 1997: Surgery for adults with congenital heart disease. In Edmunds LH Jr (ed): Cardiac Surgery in the Adult. New York, McGraw-Hill

Laks H, Plunkett MD, 1998: Pulmonary stenosis and pulmonary atresia with intact septum. In Kaiser LR, Kron IL, Spray TL (eds): Mastery of Cardiothoracic Surgery. Philadelphia, Lippincott Williams & Wilkins

Liberthson RR, 1989a: Atrial septal defect. In Congenital Heart Disease: Diagnosis and Management in Children and Adults. Boston, Little, Brown

Liberthson RR, 1989b: Patient ductus arteriosus. In Congenital Heart Disease: Diagnosis and Management in Children and Adults. Boston, Little, Brown

Liberthson RR, 1989c: Congenital aortic stenosis. In Congenital Heart Disease: Diagnosis and Management in Children and Adults. Boston, Little, Brown

Liberthson RR, 1989d: Congenital heart disease in the child, adolescent and adult. In Eagle KA, Haber E, DeSanctis RW, Austin WG (eds): The Practice of Cardiology, ed. 2. Boston, Little, Brown

Liberthson RR, 1989e: Coarctation of the aorta. In Congenital Heart Disease: Diagnosis and Management in Children and Adults. Boston, Little, Brown

Lindsay J, DeBakey ME, Beall AC, 1994: Diagnosis and treatment of diseases of the aorta. In Schlant RC, Alexander RW, et al. (eds): The Heart, ed. 8. New York, McGraw-Hill

Mainwaring RD, Lamberti JJ, 1998: Atrial septal defects. In Kaiser LR, Kron IL, Spray TL (eds): Mastery of Cardiothoracic Surgery. Philadelphia, Lippincott Williams & Wilkins

Marelli AJ, Moodie DS, 1998: Adult congenital heart disease. In Topol EJ (ed): Comprehensive Cardiovascular Medicine. Philadelphia, Lippincott Williams & Wilkins

Maron BJ, 1982: Coarctation of the aorta in the adult. In Roberts WC (ed): Congenital Heart Disease in Adults, Philadelphia, FA Davis

McNamara DG, 1989: The adult with congenital heart disease. Curr Probl Cardiol 14:1

Nolan SP, 1974: Congenital heart disease: Indications for and timing of operation. Paediatrician 3:144

Nugent EW, Plauth WH Jr, Edwards JE, Williams WH, 1994: The pathology, pathophysiology, recognition, and treatment of congenital heart disease. In Schlant RC, Alexander RW, et al. (eds): The Heart, ed. 8. New York, McGraw-Hill

Perryman RA, Jaquiss RD, 1998: Tetralogy of Fallot. In Kaiser LR, Kron IL, Spray TL (eds): Mastery of Cardiothoracic Surgery. Philadelphia, Lippincott Williams & Wilkins

Perloff JK, 1998: Survival patterns without cardiac surgery or interventional catheterization: A narrowing base. In Perloff JK, Child JS (eds): Congenital Heart Disease in Adults, ed. 2. Philadelphia, WB Saunders

Perloff JK, 1997: Congenital heart disease in adults. In Braun-wald E (ed): Heart Disease: A Textbook of Cardiovascular Medicine, ed. 5. Philadelphia, WB Saunders

Pickering TG, 1997: Secondary hypertension. In Alpert JS (ed): Cardiology for the Primary Care Physician, ed. 2. Philadelphia, Current Medicine

Tchervenkov CI, Shum-Tim D, 1996: Ventricular septal defect. In Baue AE, Geha AS, Hammond GL, et al. (eds): Glenn's Thoracic and Cardiovascular Surgery, ed. 6. Stamford, CT, Appleton & Lange

Ungerleider RM, 1998: Coarctation of the aorta. In Kaiser LR, Kron IL, Spray TL (eds): Mastery of Cardiothoracic Surgery. Philadelphia, Lippincott Williams & Wilkins

Warnes CA, Fuster V, Driscoll DJ, McGoon DC, 1991a: Congenital heart disease in adolescents and adults: Ventricular septal defect. In Giuliani ER, Fuster V, Gersh BJ, et al. (eds): Cardiology: Fundamentals and Practice, ed. 2. St. Louis, Mosby–Year Book

Warnes CA, Fuster V, McGoon DC, 1991b: Congenital heart disease in adolescents and adults: Pulmonary stenosis with intact ventricular septum. In Giuliani ER, Fuster V, Gersh BJ, et al. (eds): Cardiology: Fundamentals and Practice, ed. 2. St. Louis, Mosby–Year Book

7

Other Cardiovascular Disorders

► Cardiac Neoplasms

Types of Tumors

Most *cardiac neoplasms* represent secondary tumors, or metastatic disease, most often associated with lung or breast cancer, melanoma, leukemia, or lymphoma. In fact, 10% to 20% of patients who die of disseminated cancer have cardiac metastases to the pericardium and epicardium (Hall & Anderson, 1997). Tumors can metastasize to the heart through hematogenous or lymphocytic routes or extend directly from surrounding intrathoracic structures (Schaff et al., 1991). Whereas primary neoplasms usually involve the myocardium and interior of the cardiac cavities, metastatic neoplasms to the heart most commonly involve the pericardium, and pericardial effusion and constriction are the most common manifestations (Roberts, 1998).

Primary neoplasms occasionally occur. Approximately 70% to 75% are benign (Hall & Anderson, 1997; Kirklin & Barratt-Boyes, 1993). Most common is myxoma, which accounts for half of all benign primary cardiac tumors in adults (Van Trigt & Sabiston, 1995). Other examples of benign cardiac tumors are lipoma and papillary fibroelastoma. Nearly all primary malignant cardiac tumors are a form of sarcoma; most common are angiosarcoma and rhabdomyosarcoma (Hall & Anderson, 1997; Hall et al., 1994). Sarcomas tend to metastasize widely and as many as 80% of patients have systemic metastases at the time of diagnosis (Spotnitz & Blow, 1998). The prognosis for patients with cardiac sarcomas is poor. A list of benign and malignant primary cardiac tumors is provided in Table 7-1.

Whether benign or malignant, cardiac tumors can produce lethal complications, including arrhythmias, cardiac tamponade, pericardial constriction, valvular ob-

struction, or embolism (Fallon & Dec, 1989). Prognosis varies greatly, depending on the nature and location of the tumor. Malignant cardiac tumors are invariably fatal unless surgical resection is possible. Unfortunately, operative removal of malignant tumors usually is precluded by extensive tumor infiltration into the myocardium, local invasion of adjacent structures, or distant metastases. The remainder of the discussion in this chapter is limited to myxoma, the most frequently occurring cardiac tumor in adults. For information on other cardiac tumors, the reader is referred to a textbook of cardiology.

Myxoma

A *myxoma* is a soft, gelatinous, mucoid mass that is usually grayish-white with areas of hemorrhage or thrombosis (Hall et al., 1994). The average size of the tumor is approximately 5 cm in diameter, but growth to 15 cm and larger can occur (Hall and Anderson, 1997). Myxomas arise from the endocardium and extend into a cardiac chamber, most commonly the left atrium (Fig. 7-1). They also are found sometimes in the right atrium alone, in both atria, or in the right or left ventricle. Atrial myxomas typically are attached by a pedunculated stalk to the interatrial septum near the fossa ovalis.

Although myxomas occur in people of all ages, the incidence is greatest in the third to sixth decades of life, and there is a slight predominance in women (Van Trigt & Sabiston, 1995; Schaff et al., 1991). Two forms of myxoma occur—the more common sporadic myxoma and a familial form that predominantly affects young men, less commonly arises in the left atrium, and is associated with a higher rate of recurrence (Acker & Gardner, 1996).

Myxomas typically are associated with three types of symptoms: (1) obstructive, (2) embolic, and (3) consti-

TABLE 7-1

Most Common Primary Neoplasms of the Heart and Pericardium

Benign Neoplasms	Malignant Neoplasms
Myxoma	Angiosarcoma
Lipoma	Rhabdomyosarcoma
Fibroelastoma	Fibrosarcoma
Rhabdomyoma	Mesothelioma
Fibroma	Malignant lymphoma

tutional (Van Trigt & Sabiston, 1995). Obstructive symptoms occur when the tumor occludes or interferes with blood flow through the heart. During diastole, left or right atrial myxomas can occlude or prolapse through the mitral or tricuspid valve, respectively, creating transient obstruction to blood flow between the atrium and ventricle. As a result, patients often experience clinical manifestations of valvular stenosis. Manifestations of left atrial myxoma often mimic those of mitral stenosis except that there is no antecedent history of rheumatic fever and symptoms progress more rapidly (Acker & Gardner, 1996). Right atrial myxomas cause symptoms of right heart failure. Because of mobility of the tumor mass within the cardiac chamber, episodes of dyspnea, hypotension, or syncope may occur intermittently or with positional changes. Catastrophic complications, such as sudden cardiac death or acute cardiac failure, also may be caused by tumor occlusion of outflow from a cardiac chamber.

Embolic complications occur because portions of the tumor itself or thrombus that has formed on the tumor

can embolize. Systemic emboli occur in 30% to 45% of patients with left atrial myxoma (Kirklin & Barratt-Boyes, 1993). Consequently, it is not unusual for the presenting symptom of myxoma to be stroke, sudden loss of vision, acute limb ischemia, or myocardial infarction (Table 7-2). Approximately 50% of emboli affect the brain, often producing major, irreversible neurologic deficits (Acker & Gardner, 1996). Peripheral emboli occasionally lead to a diagnosis of myxoma when embolic material removed from a peripheral artery is identified on pathologic examination as myxomatous tissue.

Constitutional manifestations are those simulating a systemic illness, such as weight loss, fatigue, fever, and arthralgias. Systemic symptoms have been reported in as many as 90% of patients with cardiac myxomas (Schaff et al., 1991). These symptom complexes may be related to tumor embolization with resultant myalgias and arthralgias and an elevated immunoglobulin response; more important, such symptom complexes tend to resolve after surgical resection of the myxoma (Hall & Anderson, 1997).

Echocardiography is the primary diagnostic study used to confirm the presence of myxoma. The diagnosis can be confirmed with transthoracic echocardiography, but transesophageal echocardiography provides the best information about tumor size, location, mobility, and attachment (Hall & Anderson, 1997). Improvements in echocardiography have greatly aided in diagnosis of myxoma and of cardiac tumors in general. Previously, diagnosis was difficult because of the transitory nature of symptoms and the absence of other objective signs of organic heart disease. It was not unusual for patients with myxomas to be treated as if symptoms were entirely psychosomatic because the diagnosis of myxoma was not suspected and other cardiac disease could not be found.

Cardiac catheterization usually is not performed in patients with suspected myxomas because of the potential for catastrophic, systemic embolization of tumor fragments that might be broken off by an intracardiac catheter. However, patients at risk for coronary artery disease may undergo coronary angiography before surgical treatment to detect the presence of significant coronary artery lesions.

Treatment of myxoma is surgical resection. Although myxomas are almost invariably benign, operative resection is necessary to eliminate the intracavitary lesion. Surgical resection of myxoma is highly successful in pro-

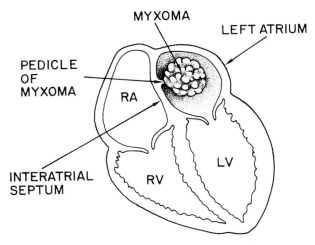

FIGURE 7-1. Most common location of cardiac myxoma is in the left atrium, attached to a broad-based pedicle arising from the interatrial septum. LV, left ventricle; RA, right atrium; RV, right ventricle. (Spotnitz WD, Blow O, 1998: Cardiac tumors. In Kaiser LR, Kron IL, Spray TL [eds]: Mastery of Cardiothoracic Surgery. p. 567, Philadelphia, Lippincott Williams & Wilkins)

TABLE 7-2

Embolic Complications of Myxoma

Site of Embolization	Clinical Manifestation
Cerebral artery	Cerebral vascular accident
Retinal artery	Sudden loss of vision
Femoral artery	Lower extremity ischemia
Coronary artery	Myocardial infarction

viding total cure. However, all myxomatous tissue must be removed to prevent tumor recurrence, particularly in those with a familial form of myxoma. The risk of a second myxoma developing after complete resection of a sporadic, nonfamilial myxoma ranges from 0% to 5%; recurrent myxomas may be benign or may become progressively more malignant with each recurrence (Acker & Gardner, 1996).

▶ Pericardial Disease

The pericardium, a sac that snugly encircles the heart, has two components: (1) parietal, with a fibrous outer coat tethered to the sternum, great vessels, and diaphragm and an inner serosal layer; and (2) visceral, comprising the epicardium and overlying serosal membrane (Shabetai, 1994) (Fig. 7-2). A small space between the visceral and parietal layers, containing 10 to 15 mL of clear, plasmalike fluid, is termed the *pericardial space.*

The pericardium is thought to perform the following functions: (1) limiting acute cardiac distention and valvular incompetence secondary to high filling pressures, (2) limiting cardiac displacement, (3) protecting the heart from inflammation of nearby tissues, and (4) reducing friction associated with cardiac movement (Brandenburg et al., 1991). Normal cardiac function, however, can occur when the pericardium is absent from birth or surgically removed. Although the pericardium can become diseased by a variety of etiologic

processes, pericardial disease usually is manifest as inflammatory pericarditis, constrictive pericarditis, or pericardial effusion.

Inflammatory Pericarditis

Inflammatory pericarditis is a syndrome involving inflammation of the parietal and visceral pericardia. It can result from any of a variety of causes, but most often is idiopathic or due to viral or bacterial infection, uremia, acute myocardial infarction, tuberculosis, pericardiotomy, tumor, or trauma (Lorell, 1997) (Table 7-3). Histopathologic manifestations of pericarditis usually include hyperemia, increased microvascularity, polymorphonuclear leukocyte accumulation, and fibrin deposition; adhesions can form between the layers of the pericardium and between pericardium and adjacent structures, such as pleura and mediastinum (Klein & Scalia, 1998).

Pericarditis is associated with chest pain, low-grade fevers, a pericardial friction rub, malaise, and characteristic electrocardiographic findings. Typically, chest pain associated with pericarditis is precordial and is aggravated by inspiration, coughing, and recumbency; patients characteristically assume a position of sitting and leaning forward to lessen the discomfort (Vaitkus et al., 1997). Pericardial or pleural effusion may be present. Acute nonmicrobial pericarditis is treated with antiinflammatory medications such as aspirin, indomethacin, or ibuprofen, and by correcting the underlying

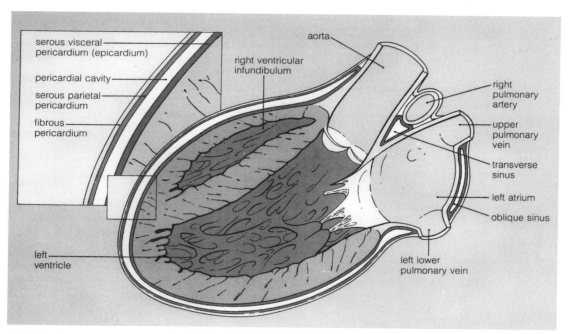

FIGURE 7-2. Diagram of the long axis of the heart demonstrates the arrangement of the pericardium. The outer (parietal) sack is firmly attached to the great arteries and veins at the base. The heart itself invaginates a second sack, the visceral pericardium. The pericardial cavity is located between the parietal and the visceral pericardium. (Anderson RH, Wilcox BR, Becker AE, 1988: Anatomy of the normal heart. In Hurst JW, Anderson RH, Becker AE, Wilcox BR [eds]: Atlas of the Heart, p. 1.2. London, Times Mirror International)

TABLE 7-3

Etiologies of Pericarditis

Idiopathic
Viral infection (coxsackievirus, mumps virus)
Bacterial infection (tuberculosis, *Pneumococcus*)
Fungal infection (histoplasmosis, coccidioidomycosis)
Other infections (toxoplasmosis, amebiasis)
Myocardial infarction (Dressler's syndrome)
Uremia
Neoplasm (lung cancer, breast cancer)
Mediastinal irradiation
Autoimmune disorders (acute rheumatic fever, scleroderma)
Other inflammatory disorders (sarcoidosis, amyloidosis)
Medications (hydralazine, procainamide)
Trauma (hemopericardium, surgical pericardiotomy)
Aortic dissection

Adapted from Lorrel BH, 1997: Pericardial diseases. In Braunwald E (ed): Heart Disease: A Textbook of Cardiovascular Medicine, ed. 5. Philadelphia, WB Saunders.

cause, if known. Some people experience recurring bouts of acute pericarditis, which may require treatment with corticosteroids.

Postpericardiotomy syndrome is pericardial inflammation precipitated by pericardiotomy (surgical incision of the pericardium). It is estimated to occur in 10% to 30% of patients who undergo cardiac operations (Landolfo & Smith, 1995). The syndrome, which typically appears in the first or second week after a cardiac operation, may last 3 to 5 weeks and is usually self-limited (Edmunds, 1996). The cause of postpericardiotomy syndrome is unknown, but clinical manifestations are similar to pericarditis from other etiologies. Symptoms are usually mild and respond to a regimen of anti-inflammatory medications or a single intravenous dose of corticosteroids. Rarely, postpericardiotomy syndrome may lead to significant pericardial or pleural effusion or even cardiac tamponade.

Pericarditis occurs in 7% to 23% of patients after acute myocardial infarction, and the risk for its development is proportional to the size of the infarction (Vaitkus et al., 1997). Dressler's syndrome is a more pronounced form of pericarditis that sometimes develops in patients weeks or months after myocardial infarction. Dressler's syndrome accompanies 1% to 3% of myocardial infarctions and is characterized by fever, chest pain, evidence of polyserositis, and a tendency to recur (Roberts et al., 1994).

Constrictive Pericarditis

Constrictive pericarditis is the end result of chronic pericardial inflammation (Fig. 7-3). The pericardium loses its elasticity, becoming thickened, fibrotic, and adherent to the heart. The pathologic process commonly extends into the myocardium, causing decreased myocardial contractility, but the major abnormality is impairment of diastolic filling of the ventricles (Harken et al., 1996). Symptoms are basically those of systemic venous congestion: peripheral edema, ascites, and liver enlargement. Vague abdominal symptoms such as postprandial fullness, dyspepsia, flatulence, and anorexia sometimes are present (Lorell, 1997). The mainstay of medical therapy is diuresis. If symptoms persist, surgical removal of the pericardium (pericardiectomy) may become necessary.

Pericardial Effusion

Pericardial effusion is abnormal accumulation of fluid (serous or purulent fluid, blood, or chyle) in the pericardial space. Abnormal fluid accumulation can occur owing to conditions that cause increased capillary permeability, increased capillary hydrostatic pressure, decreased plasma oncotic pressure, or obstruction of pericardial lymphatic drainage (Roberts & Lilly, 1998). An unusual problem, it is most often associated with tumor, infection, postpericardiotomy syndrome, or pericarditis.

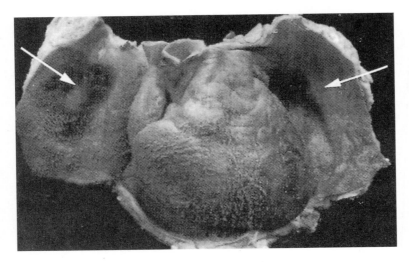

FIGURE 7-3. Resected heart demonstrating fibrinous pericarditis that is most likely of viral origin. *Arrows* point to thickened parietal surfaces of opened pericardium. (Hurst JW, Shabetai R, Becker AE, Wilcox BR, 1988: Pericardial disease. In Hurst JW, Anderson RH, Becker AE, Wilcox BR [eds]: Atlas of the Heart, p. 7.3. London, Times Mirror International)

The presence of pericardial effusion usually is detected when the patient experiences shortness of breath or hypotension. The development of increased intrapericardial pressure and consequent severity of symptoms are determined by the volume of the effusion, the rapidity with which the fluid accumulates, and the physical characteristics of the pericardium (Lorell, 1997). In the case of chronic pericardial effusion, gradual accumulation of fluid enlarges the pericardial space with little hemodynamic effect.

Rapid fluid accumulation, on the other hand, is not well tolerated hemodynamically. Two hundred to 250 mL of fluid is likely to produce cardiac tamponade, a condition in which diastolic filling of cardiac chambers is impeded by external compression. Cardiac tamponade, like constrictive pericarditis, produces equalization of intracardiac (right and left atrial and right and left ventricular end-diastolic) pressures, increased central venous pressure, and decreased cardiac output. Heart rate increases to compensate for the diminished stroke volume. Because of the similar clinical manifestations, it sometimes is difficult to differentiate between constrictive pericarditis and pericardial effusion.

Signs of pericardial effusion include distant heart sounds, distention of neck veins, hypotension, enlargement of the cardiac silhouette on chest roentgenogram, decreased QRS voltage on the electrocardiogram, and pulsus paradoxus. Pulsus paradoxus is defined as a greater than 12 to 15 mm Hg reduction in systolic arterial pressure during inspiration, compared with that measured by sphygmomanometry during expiration (Chatterjee, 1998). As cuff pressure of the sphygmomanometer is slowly decreased, the systolic pressure during expiration is noted and compared with the systolic pressure noted during inspiration.

Pulsus paradoxus is not a paradoxical phenomenon, as the term suggests, but rather an exaggeration of a normal physiologic phenomenon. Normally, systolic arterial pressure is slightly lower during spontaneous inspiration because of the decrease in left ventricular filling and ejection that occurs as intrathoracic pressure declines (Harken et al., 1996). With cardiac tamponade, the physiologic reduction in left ventricular filling and resultant stroke volume during inspiration is more pronounced, causing an exaggerated decrease in arterial pressure. Diagnosis of pericardial effusion is confirmed by echocardiographic demonstration of fluid in the pericardial sac.

Pericardiocentesis may be indicated for relief of cardiac tamponade or for cytologic examination of the fluid if the etiology of a pericardial effusion is unknown. It is performed by a physician in an intensive care setting or in a laboratory in which fluoroscopic and electrocardiographic monitoring equipment is available. Typically, a subxiphoid approach is used. Using local anesthesia, a needle is inserted between the xiphoid process and left costal margin and directed upward toward the left shoulder; aspiration is performed as the needle is advanced slowly (Roberts & Kaiser, 1998). Care must be taken to aspirate the pericardial fluid without entering one of the cardiac chambers inadvertently. Particularly in the case of a bloody effusion, it can be difficult to differentiate pericardial fluid from intracardiac blood. The pericardial catheter often is connected to a closed drainage system and left in place for 12 to 24 hours. Recurrent pericardial effusion may necessitate surgical drainage.

► Pulmonary Embolism

Pulmonary embolism is the migration of thrombotic material from another location to the pulmonary vasculature with subsequent arterial occlusion. It occurs most often as a consequence of deep venous thrombosis originating in the veins of the proximal lower extremities (Tapson, 1998). Pulmonary embolism is estimated to lead to 200,000 deaths each year in the United States, most often in people not treated because the condition remains undiagnosed (Alpert & Dalen, 1994). Autopsy studies have documented repeatedly the high frequency with which pulmonary embolism is unsuspected before death and the actual incidence of the condition in the United States may be as high as 600,000 cases per year (Tapson, 1998). Pulmonary embolism is particularly common in hospitalized elderly patients and accounts for 5% to 10% of all deaths in American hospitals (Palevsky & Edmunds, 1997). Although most often treated with medical therapy (ie, systemic anticoagulation or thrombolytic therapy), surgical treatment may be necessary for massive acute or chronic pulmonary embolism.

Massive Acute Embolism

Massive acute pulmonary embolism is defined as that which causes hemodynamic instability. It is characterized in general by thrombosis affecting at least half of the pulmonary arterial system and the presence of clot bilaterally, although it may occur with smaller occlusions in patients with preexisting cardiac or pulmonary disease (Goldhaber, 1997; Palevsky & Edmunds, 1996). Extremely large amounts of thrombus may form a saddle embolus, which is a thrombus that lodges in the main pulmonary artery and extends into both the right and left pulmonary arteries (Fig. 7-4). Massive pulmonary embolism produces acute cor pulmonale, or right-sided heart failure secondary to the abrupt rise in pulmonary vascular resistance caused by thrombotic occlusion of blood flow. When 60% to 75% of the pulmonary circulation is obstructed, the increased pulmonary vascular resistance and compensatory elevation of right ventricular pressure lead to dilatation and failure of the right ventricle (Alpert & Dalen, 1994).

Clinical manifestations of massive pulmonary embolism include acute dyspnea, tachypnea, tachycardia, hypotension, low cardiac output, severe hypoxemia, syncope, and cardiac arrest (Palevsky & Edmunds, 1997). The diagnosis should be considered in the event of an unexplained clinical deterioration or cardiac arrest, particularly in a young adult with risk factors for pulmonary em-

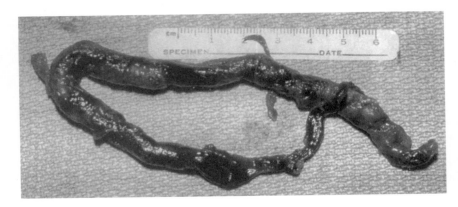

FIGURE 7-4. Giant saddle embolus removed from a 19-year-old woman with cardiovascular collapse due to acute pulmonary embolism. (Hartz RS, 1997: Reply to the editor. Ann Thorac Surg 64:883. Reprinted with permission from the Society of Thoracic Surgeons)

bolism such as smoking, oral contraceptives, or clotting abnormalities. However, clinical differentiation from catastrophic states related to conditions such as myocardial infarction or aortic dissection is difficult and proven erroneous by subsequent diagnostic studies in many patients (Palevsky & Edmunds, 1997).

Pulmonary angiography is the definitive diagnostic study for pulmonary embolism. It defines pulmonary vascular anatomy and identifies location and extent of thrombus. In all but the most extreme cases, acute pulmonary embolism is treated with heparin or thrombolytic therapy. However, patients with documented, centrally located thrombus and persistent hypotension despite maximal medical therapy may undergo emergent pulmonary embolectomy. If the patient is in cardiogenic shock or has sustained cardiac arrest, portable cardiopulmonary bypass may be necessary to provide hemodynamic support during emergent transport to the operating room for surgical evacuation. The mortality rate for patients undergoing pulmonary embolectomy for massive acute pulmonary embolism is 30% to 50% because patients who undergo the procedure are almost always in profound shock (Alpert & Dalen, 1994). In patients who experience recurring pulmonary emboli despite anticoagulation, inferior venal caval interruption also may be necessary.

Chronic Embolism

Except in the case of massive pulmonary embolism, pulmonary emboli usually resolve spontaneously as a result of intrinsic mechanisms of fibrinolysis. With appropriate anticoagulant therapy, perfusion defects usually are resolved within several weeks with no long-term sequelae. Occasionally, however, inadequate lysis or recurring emboli may lead to chronic pulmonary embolism or accumulation of thrombotic material in the pulmonary arterial system. Although more often due to lack of adequate anticoagulation, chronic pulmonary embolism sometimes occurs despite therapeutic anticoagulation.

Defective fibrinolysis begins a cycle of incomplete lysis of emboli, partial recanalization within the pulmonary vasculature, organization, and proximal thrombotic extension (Sebastian & Sabiston, 1995). The re-

sultant chronic obstruction to blood flow through the pulmonary arteries eventually leads to pulmonary hypertension, symptoms of progressive respiratory insufficiency, hypoxemia, and right ventricular failure (Sebastian & Sabiston, 1995). Although no signs or symptoms are specific to chronic thromboembolism, the most common symptom is exertional dyspnea associated with pulmonary hypertension (Palevsky & Edmunds, 1997). Recurring episodes of thrombophlebitis, hemoptysis, and chest pain also may occur (Sebastian & Sabiston, 1995).

The natural history of chronic thromboembolic pulmonary hypertension is progressive right heart failure and death for nearly all patients (Palevsky & Edmunds, 1997). In carefully selected patients, surgical thromboendarterectomy of the pulmonary arteries may be beneficial. The best candidates for surgical thromboendarterectomy are those with severe respiratory insufficiency, hypoxemia, pulmonary hypertension with proximal pulmonary artery occlusion and adequate bronchial collateral circulation, and minimally impaired right ventricular function (Sebastian & Sabiston, 1995). Diffuse involvement of small distal branches and severe right ventricular failure are relative contraindications to thromboendarterectomy.

► Cardiac Disease and Pregnancy

Rheumatic heart disease, usually mitral stenosis, accounts for approximately 50% of cardiac disorders in pregnant women; congenital disease is believed to comprise an additional 30% to 50% (Noller & Hill, 1991). Diseased cardiac valves or unrepaired congenital heart defects, such as atrial septal defect or coarctation, may be undetected or associated with no symptoms until the added physiologic demands of a pregnancy are imposed. Pregnancy in a woman with cardiac disease presents a number of complex and difficult issues. In addition to the survival of the mother, the health and integrity of the fetus must be considered.

Pregnancy produces major hemodynamic alterations. Blood volume increases 50% above baseline and resting cardiac output increases 40% to 50% (Burlew et al., 1997). As the woman's heart and lungs take on the added burden of supporting fetal life, cardiac decompensation may occur. Decompensation is most likely during the second or third trimester as demands of the growing fetus increasingly strain the mother's cardiovascular system. During labor and delivery, cardiac output increases further owing to the anxiety, pain, and increased venous return to the heart associated with uterine contractions (Canobbio, 1987).

Symptoms of congestive heart failure during pregnancy are the most common manifestation of underlying cardiac disease. If medical therapy is unsuccessful in controlling heart failure, surgical correction of the cardiac problem may become necessary. Recurrent congestive heart failure suggests that a woman will be unable to sustain a full-term pregnancy. In addition, as demands of the fetus increase, the mother's life may be jeopardized increasingly.

In women with aortic disease, aortic dissection or rupture of an aortic aneurysm is more likely to occur during pregnancy. One half of aortic dissections in women younger than 40 years of age occur during pregnancy, usually in the last trimester or during labor; contributing factors include hypercirculation during late gestation, hypertension, and loosened connective tissue secondary to hormonal changes (Stone & Borst, 1997). Pregnant women with unrepaired coarctation are at risk for hypertension, congestive heart failure, angina, infective endocarditis, or congenital heart defects in the fetus (Elkayam, 1997).

In women who require valve replacement before a possible future pregnancy, careful consideration must be given to choice of valvular prosthesis. Pregnant women with bioprosthetic valves have a 35% incidence of accelerated valvular deterioration, presumably because of changes in calcium metabolism during pregnancy (Laks et al., 1997). Mechanical valvular prostheses provide durability but systemic anticoagulation is essential and management is complex. Both warfarin and heparin have serious potential adverse effects, and insufficient data are available about their safety and efficacy during pregnancy.

Warfarin crosses the placental barrier and has the potential to cause both bleeding in the fetus and embryopathy, resulting in fetal hemorrhage, wastage, or malformation (Ginsberg & Hirsh, 1998; Badduke et al., 1991). Heparin does not cross the placental barrier and has no effect on the fetus, but its efficacy in preventing thromboembolic complications in pregnant women with mechanical cardiac valves is not well established (Ginsberg & Hirsh, 1998). Also, long-term administration of heparin can cause osteoporosis in the mother or, less commonly, development of heparin-associated antibodies resulting in thrombosis and thrombocytopenia (Baughman, 1998).

Definitive recommendations for anticoagulation during pregnancy are lacking. One recommended management strategy is administration of warfarin throughout most of the pregnancy, except during two critical periods: (1) the first 12 weeks of gestation (the period of highest risk for fetal embryopathy), and (2) the last 2 weeks of the pregnancy (to avoid delivery of an anticoagulated fetus with resultant perinatal bleeding) (Ginsberg & Hirsh, 1998; Baughman, 1998). Alternatively, therapeutic anticoagulation with subcutaneous heparin is maintained throughout gestation. Regardless of the particular regimen chosen, anticoagulation must be managed judiciously with close monitoring of therapeutic effect.

Medical or surgical interventions during pregnancy to improve or correct a cardiac problem can have profound implications for viability of the fetus. The decision to perform an operation requiring general anesthesia and cardiopulmonary bypass with systemic anticoagulation is difficult because risk to the fetus is high. Depending on severity of the mother's illness and the stage of pregnancy, abortion may be recommended. This is a difficult decision that requires input from the patient, obstetrician, and cardiologist.

REFERENCES

Acker MA, Gardner TJ, 1996: Cardiac tumors. In Baue AE, Geha AS, Hammond GL, et al. (eds): Glenn's Thoracic and Cardiovascular Surgery, ed. 6. Stamford, CT, Appleton & Lange

Alpert JS, Dalen JE, 1994: Pulmonary embolism. In Schlant RC, Alexander RW (eds): The Heart, ed. 8. New York, McGraw-Hill

Badduke BR, Jamieson WR, Miyagishima RT, et al., 1991: Pregnancy and childbearing in a population with biologic valvular prostheses. J Thorac Cardiovasc Surg 102:179

Baughman KL, 1998: The heart and pregnancy. In Topol EJ (ed): Comprehensive Cardiovascular Medicine. Philadelphia, Lippincott Williams & Wilkins

Brandenburg RO, Click RL, McGoon DC, 1991: The pericardium. In Giuliani ER, Fuster V, Gersh BJ, et al. (eds): Cardiology Fundamentals and Practice. St. Louis, Mosby–Year Book

Burlew BS, Horn HR, Sullivan JM, 1997: Pregnancy and the heart. In Alpert JS (ed): Cardiology for the Primary Care Physician, ed. 2. Philadelphia, Current Medicine

Canobbio MM, 1987: Pregnancy in women with congenital heart disease. Prog Cardiovasc Nurs 2:61

Chatterjee K, 1998: Physical examination. In Topol EJ (ed): Comprehensive Cardiovascular Medicine. Philadelphia, Lippincott Williams & Wilkins

Edmunds LH, 1996: Cardiopulmonary bypass for open heart surgery. In Baue AE, Geha AS, Hammond GL, et al. (eds): Glenn's Thoracic and Cardiovascular Surgery, ed. 6. Stamford, CT, Appleton & Lange

Elkayam U, 1997: Pregnancy and cardiovascular disease. In Braunwald E (ed): Heart Disease: A Textbook of Cardiovascular Medicine, ed. 5. Philadelphia, WB Saunders

Fallon JT, Dec GW, 1989: Cardiac tumors. In Eagle KA, Haber E, DeSanctis RW, Austin WG (eds): The Practice of Cardiology, ed. 2. Boston, Little, Brown

Ginsberg JS, Hirsh J, 1998: Use of antithrombotics during pregnancy. Chest 114:524S

Goldhaber SZ, 1997: Pulmonary embolism. In Braunwald E (ed): Heart Disease: A Textbook of Cardiovascular Medicine, ed. 5. Philadelphia, WB Saunders

Hall RA, Anderson RP, 1997: Cardiac neoplasms. In Edmunds LH Jr (ed): Cardiac Surgery in the Adult. New York, McGraw-Hill

Hall RJ, Cooley DA, McAllister HA, Frazier OH, 1994: Neoplastic heart disease. In Schlant RC, Alexander RW (eds): The Heart, ed. 8. New York, McGraw-Hill

Harken AH, Hall AW, Hammond GL, 1996: The pericardium. In Baue AE, Geha AS, Hammond GL, et al. (eds): Glenn's

Thoracic and Cardiovascular Surgery, ed. 6. Stamford, CT, Appleton & Lange

Kirklin JW, Barratt-Boyes BG, 1993: Cardiac tumor. In Cardiac Surgery, ed. 2. New York, Churchill Livingstone

Klein AL, Scalia GM, 1998: Diseases of the pericardium, restrictive cardiomyopathy and diastolic dysfunction. In Topol EJ (ed): Comprehensive Cardiovascular Medicine. Philadelphia, Lippincott Williams & Wilkins

Laks H, Marelli D, Drinkwater DC, 1997: Surgery for adults with congenital heart disease. In Edmunds LH Jr (ed): Cardiac Surgery in the Adult. New York, McGraw-Hill

Landolfo K, Smith PK, 1995: Postoperative care in cardiac surgery. In Sabiston DC Jr, Spencer FC (eds): Surgery of the Chest, ed. 6. Philadelphia, WB Saunders

Lorell BH, 1997: Pericardial diseases. In Braunwald E (ed): Heart Disease: A Textbook of Cardiovascular Medicine, ed. 5. Philadelphia, WB Saunders

Noller KL, Hill LM, 1991: Cardiac disease associated with pregnancy and its management. In Giuliani ER, Fuster V, Gersh BJ, et al. (eds): Cardiology Fundamentals and Practice. St. Louis, Mosby–Year Book

Palevsky HI, Edmunds LH Jr, 1997: Pulmonary thromboembolism. In Edmunds LH Jr (ed): Cardiac Surgery in the Adult. New York, McGraw-Hill

Roberts JR, Kaiser LR, 1998: Pericardial procedures. In Kaiser LR, Kron IL, Spray TL (eds): Mastery of Cardiothoracic Surgery. Philadelphia, Lippincott Williams & Wilkins

Roberts R, Morris DC, Pratt CM, Alexander RW, 1994: Pathophysiology, recognition, and treatment of myocardial infarction and its complications. In Schlant RC, Alexander RW (eds): The Heart, ed. 8. New York, McGraw-Hill

Roberts TG, Lilly LS, 1998: Diseases of the pericardium. In Lilly LS (ed): Pathophysiology of Heart Disease, ed. 2. Baltimore, Williams & Wilkins

Roberts WC, 1998: Cardiac neoplasms. In Topol EJ (ed): Comprehensive Cardiovascular Medicine. Philadelphia, Lippincott Williams & Wilkins

Schaff HV, Piehler JM, Lie JT, Giuliani ER, 1991: Tumors of the heart. In Giuliani ER, Fuster V, Gersh BJ, et al. (eds): Cardiology Fundamentals and Practice. ed 2. St. Louis, Mosby–Year Book

Sebastian MW, Sabiston DC Jr, 1995: Chronic pulmonary embolism. In Sabiston DC Jr, Spencer FC (eds): Surgery of the Chest, ed. 6. Philadelphia, WB Saunders

Shabetai R, 1994: Diseases of the pericardium. In Schlant RC, Alexander RW (eds): The Heart, ed. 8. New York, McGraw-Hill

Spotnitz WD, Blow O, 1998: Cardiac tumors. In Kaiser LR, Kron IL, Spray TL (eds): Mastery of Cardiothoracic Surgery. Philadelphia, Lippincott Williams & Wilkins

Stone C, Borst H, 1997: Dissecting aortic aneurysm. In Edmunds LH Jr (ed): Cardiac Surgery in the Adult. New York, McGraw-Hill

Tapson VF, 1998: Venous thromboembolism. In Topol EJ (ed): Comprehensive Cardiovascular Disease. Philadelphia, Lippincott Williams & Wilkins

Vaitkus PT, LeWinter MM, Alpert JS, 1997: Pericardial disease. In Alpert JS (ed): Cardiology for the Primary Care Physician, ed. 2. Philadelphia, Current Medicine

Van Trigt P, Sabiston DC Jr, 1995: Tumors of the heart. In Sabiston DC Jr, Spencer FC (eds): Surgery of the Chest, ed. 6. Philadelphia, WB Saunders

PREOPERATIVE EVALUATION AND PREPARATION

8

Diagnostic Evaluation of Cardiac Disease

For many years, the principal study used in diagnosis of cardiac disease was the electrocardiogram (ECG). Although electrocardiographic analysis of the heart reveals important clues about myocardial disease, the ECG is limited in the information it provides. The development of sophisticated echocardiographic, radionuclide imaging, cardiac catheterization, and electrophysiologic techniques has greatly enhanced the accurate diagnosis of cardiac diseases. A number of diagnostic modalities, both noninvasive and invasive, are available. Those studies performed most commonly in patients who undergo cardiac surgical procedures are described in this chapter.

▶ Noninvasive Studies

Electrocardiogram

The *electrocardiogram,* a graphic recording of cardiac electrical activity, is the most frequently used diagnostic study for patients with known or suspected cardiac disease. It documents cardiac rate and rhythm, provides information about impulse conduction and electrical axis of the heart, and reveals the presence of various pathologic conditions, such as myocardial ischemia or infarction, ventricular hypertrophy, or bundle branch block. The standard, or 12-lead, ECG records electrical cardiac activity from 12 different perspectives; 6 limb leads measure forces on the vertical plane, and 6 precordial (chest) leads measure forces on the horizontal plane. Because many forms of cardiac disease produce electrocardiographic abnormalities, ECGs are obtained as part of the routine preoperative evaluation of almost all adults undergoing operations that require general anesthesia.

The ECG is often an independent marker of cardiac disease, occasionally is the only indicator of a pathologic process, and sometimes provides a guide to therapy (Fisch, 1997). In patients with coronary artery disease, the ECG may reveal the presence of either myocardial ischemia or infarction. Moreover, the leads in which abnormalities are present provide information about the specific coronary artery or arteries that are obstructed. Manifestations of myocardial ischemia include ST segment elevation, horizontal or downsloping ST segment depression, symmetric T wave inversion, normalization of a previously abnormal T wave (also called pseudonormalization), or QT prolongation (Hendel, 1997). Transmyocardial infarction typically produces Q waves in leads reflective of affected myocardium and reciprocal positive forces in opposite leads. Persistent ST segment elevation may indicate presence of a ventricular aneurysm.

In patients with valvular or congenital heart disease, the development of ventricular damage may be detected by abnormalities in leads overlying the affected ventricle. Increased QRS amplitude is seen with right or left ventricular enlargement, and ST segment or T wave changes may indicate ventricular strain. Atrial enlargement may be detected by changes in amplitude, width, and configuration of the P wave. The width and morphology of the QRS complex in specific leads identify the appearance and progression of right or left bundle branch block. The ECG also may demonstrate changes produced by various medications, or by electrolyte or metabolic abnormalities. For example, a number of medications can produce hazardous prolongation of the QT interval, and hyperkalemia affects the configuration of all components of depolarization and repolarization. Hypothermia may cause bradycardia, flattening of P waves, and prolongation of the QRS complex and PR and QT intervals (Sgarbossa & Wagner, 1998). Interpretation of ECGs is described in further detail in Chapter 24,

Twelve-Lead Electrocardiography and Atrial Electrograms.

The *signal-averaged ECG* is a special type of ECG used to evaluate likelihood of future arrhythmic events in patients with clinical risk factors for ventricular tachyarrhythmias. It is a high-gain ECG that attempts to detect low-voltage propagation extending beyond the QRS complex (Tchou, 1998). These low-amplitude, high-frequency signals, known as late potentials, represent late depolarization and slowed conduction through scarred areas of ventricular myocardium. Late potentials are not visible on a standard ECG.

To obtain a signal-averaged ECG, surface electrodes are used to record cardiac electrical activity, which is digitized, amplified, and averaged to eliminate virtually all artifactual noise (Hillis et al., 1995). The resultant signal-averaged ECG characterizes QRS complexes by voltage and duration criteria. The presence of late potentials may indicate an increased risk for symptomatic ventricular tachyarrhythmias. Interpretation of signal-averaged ECGs in patients with a paced cardiac rhythm or complete bundle branch block is limited.

Ambulatory Electrocardiographic Monitoring

Ambulatory monitoring, also referred to as *Holter monitoring*, is an extended recording of the cardiac rhythm over time, usually 24 hours. The recording device is contained in a portable, compact unit that the patient carries using a shoulder harness or belt. Commonly, two leads, reflecting the anterior and inferior ventricular walls, are recorded continuously through four or five electrodes placed on the patient's anterior chest wall (Hudak et al., 1998). The device continuously records the ECG while the patient performs normal daily activities. The patient is asked to keep a diary of these activities, as well as medications taken and the presence of any symptoms. In addition, most Holter monitors have an "event" button that can be pushed to mark the tape whenever symptoms occur (Hudak et al., 1998).

The recording is evaluated by computer and reviewed by a cardiologist, who characterizes heart rate and rhythm over the period of monitoring, correlating changes or abnormalities with patient activities as documented in the accompanying diary. The number and character of supraventricular and ventricular arrhythmias are quantitated, as well as changes in heart rate or ST segments. Ambulatory monitor recordings typically are obtained to identify and quantitate arrhythmias in patients with known or suspected arrhythmic disorders and to identify rhythm abnormalities in those with suggestive symptoms (eg, syncope). In patients with life-threatening arrhythmic disorders, ambulatory monitoring is used as an adjunct to electrophysiologic studies. Ambulatory monitoring also may be useful in patients with symptomatic myocardial ischemia to detect episodes of silent ischemia (ie, electrocardiographic evidence of ischemia not accompanied by clinical symptoms) that would otherwise go unrecognized (Gersh et al., 1997).

Exercise Electrocardiography

Exercise electrocardiography, or exercise stress testing (EST), is the observation, measurement, and recording of physiologic and psychological responses to a known amount of physical work (Berra & Froelicher, 1995). The study consists of monitoring the ECG, blood pressure, and heart rate while the patient walks on a treadmill or rides a bicycle ergometer and is subjected to progressively increasing, graded levels of work. The purpose of EST is to observe electrocardiographic and hemodynamic changes that occur during a dynamic state. Abnormal responses include (1) decrease or no change in systolic blood pressure; (2) excessive increase or decrease in heart rate; (3) depression of ST segments on the ECG; (4) serious arrhythmias; and (5) symptoms such as angina, dyspnea, or unusual fatigue.

Exercise stress testing remains the most widely used method for assessing the presence and severity of coronary artery disease (Okin, 1998). Because physical exertion increases myocardial oxygen consumption and because myocardial ischemia produces typical electrocardiographic manifestations, EST often provokes and defines underlying myocardial ischemia in a controlled setting (Fig. 8-1). The procedure is used both to screen people at risk and, in patients with known coronary artery disease, to assess functional capacity, severity of exercise-induced ischemia, and effectiveness of various forms of antianginal therapy. After myocardial infarction or coronary artery revascularization, EST frequently is performed to assess a patient's physical capabilities under monitored conditions. EST also may be used to assess heart rate response to exercise or to detect exercise-induced arrhythmias. Common indications for EST are displayed in Table 8-1.

In the United States, EST is performed most commonly using a treadmill and one of a number of established exercise protocols. Typically these protocols include a multistage test in which the treadmill speed and grade are increased gradually at regular intervals. The specific protocol selected should be consistent with a patient's physical capacity and the purpose of the test (Chaitman, 1997). The Bruce protocol is performed widely to diagnose and assess functional significance of obstructive lesions in the coronary arterial circulation. A modified protocol with less strenuous work levels is used for older patients and for those with limited exercise tolerance.

Because EST can precipitate severe ischemia or arrhythmias, the procedure is performed under supervision of a physician and with accessible emergency drugs and equipment. The test is terminated when the patient has signs or symptoms of myocardial ischemia, or other symptoms, such as fatigue or dyspnea (Hudak et al., 1998). In the absence of symptoms or signs that warrant termination, the study is continued until the patient achieves his or her age-predicted target heart rate (Okin, 1998).

A positive EST usually is defined as 1 mm or more of horizontal or downsloping ST segment depression or 1.5 mm or more of upsloping ST segment depression 0.08 second after the J point of the QRS complex (Hendel, 1997). Severity of coronary artery obstructive lesions can

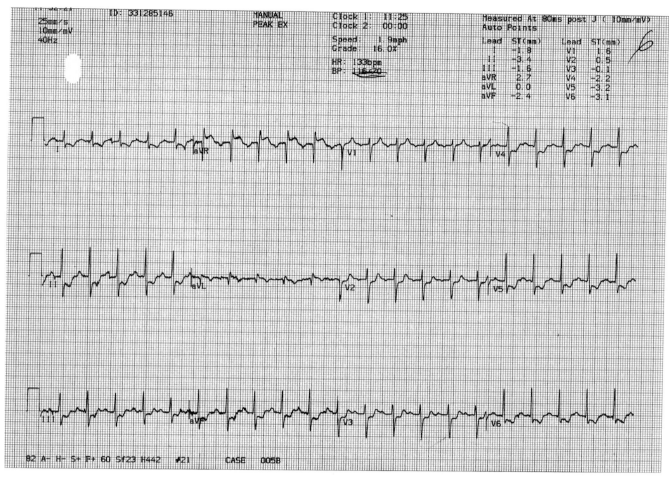

FIGURE 8-1. Twelve-lead ECG obtained at peak exercise during treadmill test in patient with a history of angina. After exercising approximately 11.5 minutes, the patient experienced chest discomfort with 2- to 3-mm downsloping ST segment depression in inferior (II, aVF) and lateral (V_4, V_5, V_6) leads consistent with myocardial ischemia. (Courtesy of James Rosenthal, MD)

be estimated by the magnitude of ST depression, level of exercise when it occurs, and persistence of ischemic changes in the recovery period (Sutherland, 1991). Severe or multivessel coronary artery disease is suggested by a marked reduction (<6 minutes) in exercise capacity, a decrease in blood pressure during exercise, or severe or prolonged symptoms or ECG changes (Hendel, 1997).

TABLE 8-1

Common Indications for Exercise Stress Testing

Screen high-risk individuals for coronary artery disease
Document exercise-induced ischemia in individuals with symptoms suggestive of coronary artery disease
Evaluate functional capacity after myocardial infarction or coronary artery revascularization
Document exercise-induced arrhythmias or determine heart rate response to exercise

Exercise electrocardiography is less reliable as a screening test for coronary artery disease in women because the prognostic value of exercise-induced ST segment depression is less in women than in men (Chaitman, 1997). Also, because EST is less definitive than cardiac catheterization, it is not always performed before cardiac catheterization in patients with signs and symptoms suggestive of significant coronary artery obstruction. In patients with unstable angina or with suspected left main or other severe coronary artery lesions, EST usually is not performed because it may produce precipitous myocardial ischemia or infarction.

Echocardiography

Echocardiography is a diagnostic modality that uses ultrasound, or sound waves of frequencies higher than the human ear can detect, to scan the heart. A transducer, which contains one or more crystals with piezoelectric (ie, ability to convert electricity into vibration and vice versa) properties, is used to transmit pulses of ultrasonic energy into the heart. Echoes reflected back from the heart are converted into electrical impulses that provide images of cardiac structures or blood flow through the heart.

Echocardiography provides a great deal of information, is rapidly available at the bedside, and is essentially risk free (Elefteriades et al., 1996). It is particularly useful in diagnosing valvular dysfunction, congenital defects, or defects caused by trauma or myocardial infarction. Cardiac chamber size, contractility, and abnormalities of the myocardium, such as calcification, hypertrophy, wall motion abnormalities, or ventricular aneurysm, also can be assessed. Finally, fluid collection (pericardial effusion) and abnormal masses, such as myxoma, vegetation, or thrombus, often are diagnosed definitively with echocardiography (Table 8-2 and Fig. 8-2).

One of several types of echocardiography may be used, depending on the type of information needed. In M-mode echocardiography, a transducer placed on the anterior chest provides a transthoracic, one-dimensional view of cardiac structures throughout the cardiac cycle. M-mode echocardiography provides rapid assessment of valvular motion and chamber wall thickness (Hudak et al., 1998). In a two-dimensional (2-D) echocardiogram, the ultrasonic beam moves in a sector, interrogating a pie-shaped slice of the heart (Feigenbaum, 1997). The device used to record the 2-D echocardiogram is a video camera, which records the two dimensions of the pie-shaped plane and movement over time (Hudak et al., 1998). In patients with coronary artery disease, 2-D exercise, or stress, echocardiography sometimes is performed to detect wall motion abnormalities that develop in ischemic myocardium with exercise or the administration of a pharmacologic stress agent (eg, dobutamine). More recently, three-dimensional echocardiographic reconstruction has become available in

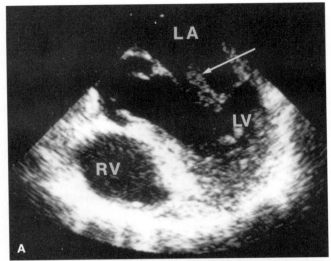
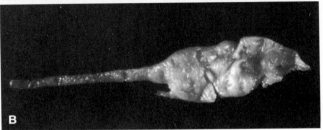

FIGURE 8-2. (A) Transesophageal echocardiogram showing a vegetation (*arrow*) on anterior leaflet of the mitral valve. LA, left atrium; RV, right ventricle; LV, left ventricle. **(B)** Gross appearance of the resected vegetation. (Courtesy of David McPherson, MD)

TABLE 8-2

Information Provided by Echocardiography

- Cardiac valves
  - ○ Characteristics, motion, and competency
  - ○ Quantification of gradient, valve area, regurgitant flow
- Ventricular wall and interventricular septum
  - ○ Systolic and diastolic ventricular dimensions and volumes
  - ○ Myocardial thickness and segmental wall motion
  - ○ Ejection fraction
- Structural abnormalities
  - ○ Intracardiac shunts (eg, atrial septal defect)
  - ○ Intracavitary lesions (eg, myxoma, vegetations, thrombus)
- Pericardium
  - ○ Effusion or constriction

---

selected centers, providing further enhanced imaging of intracardiac structures.

The Doppler echocardiogram consists of recorded sound waves reflected from moving red blood cells. Doppler echocardiography has become the principal ultrasonic technique for obtaining hemodynamic data. It provides information about blood flow through cardiac chambers, across cardiac valves, and into the great vessels. Doppler echocardiography has the highest sensitivity of all diagnostic techniques in detection of valvular regurgitation; the degree of regurgitation can be evaluated at least in a semiquantitative fashion (Flachskampf & Breithardt, 1998). Sophisticated technology now makes it possible to transform blood flow signals into a display of different colors, providing a more graphic representation known as color Doppler flow mapping.

In most cases, echocardiograms are obtained using a transthoracic approach; that is, the transducer is positioned on the anterior chest wall. However, 2-D and Doppler echocardiograms also can be obtained with a transesophageal approach. *Transesophageal echocardiography* uses an ultrasound transducer on a probe that is passed into the esophagus, usually with conscious sedation of the patient or during cardiac operations (Fig. 8-3). The transesophageal approach places the transducer close to the left atrium, eliminating the chest wall interference

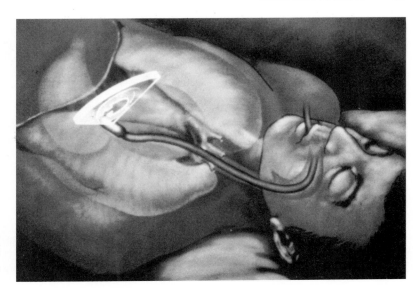

FIGURE 8-3. Transesophageal echocardiography is performed using an ultrasound transducer on a probe passed into the esophagus. (Courtesy of Hewlett-Packard, Andover, MA)

and intrathoracic attenuation that occur with a conventional transthoracic approach (Matsuzaki et al., 1990). As a result, images are clearer and more accurate than those obtained with transthoracic echocardiography.

Transesophageal echocardiography is particularly useful in diagnosing acute aortic dissection. It has become one of the primary diagnostic modalities for this condition because of its high reliability and the ease and rapidity with which it can be performed at the bedside. Transesophageal echocardiography also is advantageous in a number of other clinical situations in which a transthoracic approach is unlikely to provide adequate images (Table 8-3).

Intraoperative transesophageal echocardiography is particularly useful during cardiac operations because echocardiographic images can be obtained while the chest is open. Typical uses of intraoperative transesophageal echocardiography include (1) examination of the heart to detect intracardiac air during operations that necessitate opening the ascending aorta or a cardiac chamber, and (2) assessing competency of reconstructed cardiac valves before concluding the operation. Transesophageal echocardiography has a small but definite incidence of complications. Death, esophageal perforation, serious arrhythmias, congestive heart failure, or laryngospasm occur in less than 0.3% of patients (Griffin, 1998).

TABLE 8-3

Indications for Transesophageal Echocardiography

Obese patients
Patients with chronic obstructive pulmonary disease
Intraoperative studies
Inadequate information from transthoracic study
Patients with suspected aortic dissection
Detailed valvular anatomic assessment in infective endocarditis

Radionuclide Imaging

Radionuclide imaging (scintigraphy) is a diagnostic technique that detects pathologic cardiac conditions by tracking a small quantity of radioactive tracer injected into the bloodstream. Radionuclides are unstable atoms that emit radioactivity (gamma rays) as they spontaneously convert into a more stable configuration (Hall, 1995). As gamma rays are emitted, a gamma-scintillation camera records the presence of the radionuclides, or tracers. Current Food and Drug Administration–approved tracers include thallium-201 (Tl-201), technetium 99m (Tc-99m) sestamibi, Tc-99m teboroxime, and Tc-99m tetrofosmin (Iskandrian & Verani, 1998). The most commonly used imaging techniques are radionuclide myocardial perfusion imaging and radionuclide angiography.

Radionuclide myocardial perfusion imaging is used to evaluate regional myocardial perfusion and viability in patients with coronary artery disease. Because it demonstrates differential blood flow distribution through the left ventricular myocardium, myocardial perfusion imaging detects regional perfusion deficits that represent areas of ischemic or infarcted cardiac muscle. Myocardial perfusion imaging can be performed using planar images, acquired in three primary views, or single-photon emission computed tomography (SPECT) imaging, which collects a series of planar projections acquired as a camera rotates in an arc around the patient (Hendel, 1997) (Fig. 8-4).

The most common form of radionuclide perfusion imaging consists of injecting radioactive tracers into the bloodstream that become concentrated in perfused myocardium in a ratio proportional to coronary blood flow to the area. Thus, perfusion defects (areas of decreased uptake) appear in regions with diminished coronary blood flow or that are infarcted. Radionuclide imaging to assess myocardial perfusion is performed using Tl-201 or Tc-99m, and is performed at rest and with exercise stress or pharmacologic vasodilatation (Skorton et al., 1997).

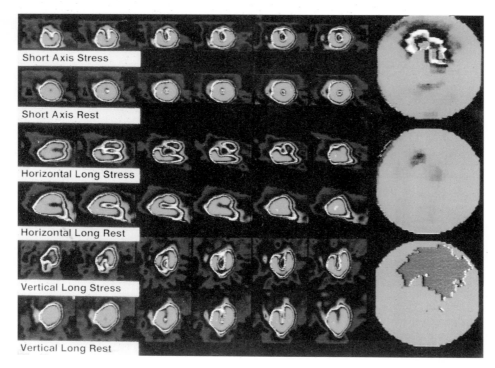

FIGURE 8-4. Single-photon emission computed tomographic images in this patient demonstrate a high-grade left anterior descending artery stenosis in its middle portion. A reversible defect involving the anterior wall, septum, and apex is depicted in the upper rows of each pair. The polar maps on the right display the tracer activity during stress (*upper panel*) and redistribution (*middle panel*). The *lower panel* localizes the defect to the left anterior descending vascular territory (Iskandrian AE, Verani MS, 1998: Nuclear imaging techniques. In Topol EJ [ed]: Comprehensive Cardiovascular Medicine, p. 1511. Philadelphia, Lippincott Williams & Wilkins)

Rest imaging may demonstrate perfusion abnormalities in patients with previous myocardial infarction or high-grade stenoses. However, because most functionally significant coronary stenoses are associated with normal resting myocardial blood flow and thus normal resting perfusion images, it is necessary to obtain images during stress to demonstrate these stenoses (Iskandrian & Verani, 1998). A reversible perfusion defect is an area of decreased tracer uptake during exercise compared with rest, and a fixed perfusion defect is an area of decreased uptake that is present on both exercise and rest scans (Hudak et al., 1998).

Exercise perfusion scanning is particularly helpful in patients in whom conventional exercise electrocardiography may be inconclusive, such as women and those with baseline ST segment abnormalities. The greater the functional severity of coronary artery disease, the more abnormal exercise myocardial perfusion images are likely to be (Wackers et al., 1997). In patients unable to achieve adequate exercise levels, intravenous dipyridamole may be administered to simulate the heart's response to exercise (ie, dilate nonstenotic coronary arteries). This type of study is termed *dipyridamole thallium scanning.*

Less commonly, myocardial perfusion imaging is performed during acute coronary syndromes to detect acute myocardial infarction, measure infarct size, assess efficacy of thrombolytic therapy or primary percutaneous coronary intervention, and assess muscle viability (Iskandrian & Verani, 1998).

The second type of radionuclide imaging, radionuclide angiography, is performed using one of two techniques: (1) first-pass radionuclide imaging samples a few cardiac cycles at the time of radionuclide injection, and (2) gated equilibrium radionuclide imaging analyzes several hundred cardiac cycles (Chaitman & Miller, 1996). Both first-pass and gated equilibrium studies may be performed at rest or in combination with exercise, obtaining measurements of left ventricular ejection fraction at each stage of exercise (Hendel, 1997).

Radionuclide angiography is used to assess ventricular size and volume and evaluate right and left ventricular ejection fraction (ie, the proportion of ventricular volume ejected with each ventricular contraction). A normally functioning ventricle ejects 50% to 60% of its blood volume; a 30% to 50% ejection fraction represents a moderately impaired ventricle; and an ejection fraction that is below 30% represents severe ventricular impairment. This type of radionuclide imaging can also detect the presence of a ventricular wall motion abnormality, which is a segment of ventricular wall that contracts poorly or paradoxically compared with other segments. Wall motion abnormalities almost always represent ventricular damage caused by myocardial infarction and are often associated with congestive heart failure and chronic arrhythmic disorders.

Positron emission tomography (PET) is another imaging technique used infrequently in patients with coronary artery disease. PET scanning uses biologically active radiopharmaceuticals to distinguish dysfunctional but viable myocardium from infarcted tissue. PET scanning in combination with perfusion tracers provides accurate diagnosis and localization of coronary artery disease, but limited availability and high cost of the scanning equipment hinders widespread clinical use (Schwaiger & Ziegler, 1998).

► Invasive Studies

Invasive diagnostic studies involve the introduction of catheters into the left or right side of the heart from peripheral arteries or veins, respectively. Invasive studies used for the diagnosis of cardiac disease include cardiac catheterization, electrophysiologic studies, and endomyocardial biopsy.

Cardiac Catheterization

Cardiac catheterization is a procedure in which catheters are placed in the heart and used to measure intracardiac pressures and oxygen saturation and to obtain fluoroscopic angiograms. Angiography is the injection of radiographic contrast material into cardiac chambers, coronary arteries, or great vessels. A full cardiac catheterization includes angiography as well as intracardiac pressure and oxygen saturation measurements from both the right and left chambers. A great deal of valuable information about the heart can be obtained during cardiac catheterization, including (1) definition of coronary anatomy; (2) estimation of ventricular wall motion and ejection fraction; (3) measurement of intracardiac pressures and hemodynamic parameters; (4) evaluation of cardiac valve function; and (5) diagnosis of structural cardiac abnormalities, such as ventricular septal defect, ventricular aneurysm, or intracavitary mass.

Left-sided heart catheterization usually includes coronary angiography and left ventriculography. Coronary angiography is the most common form of cardiac catheterization procedure. It is performed in patients with suspected coronary artery disease, typically in those who have angina that has accelerated in frequency or severity or that recurs despite pharmacologic therapy or after myocardial infarction. Coronary angiography is performed by means of percutaneous cannulation of the femoral artery or, less commonly, cannulation of the brachial artery using a cutdown approach. The brachial artery typically is used when femoral artery cannulation is rendered difficult because of extensive peripheral arterial disease, marked obesity, systemic arterial hypertension, bleeding diatheses, or disorders that markedly augment arterial pulse pressure (eg, aortic regurgitation) (Lange & Hillis, 1998).

In either case, the catheter is guided, using fluoroscopy, in a retrograde fashion through the aorta until its tip is in the ascending aorta near the coronary artery ostia. Radiographic contrast material then is injected selectively into the ostia of the right and left coronary arteries and fluoroscopy is used to visualize the arterial structures. Only a small portion of the coronary circulation is visualized (ie, major epicardial branches and their second-, third-, and perhaps fourth-order branches); the myriad small intramyocardial branches are not visualized because of their small size, cardiac motion, and limited resolution of cine imaging systems (Bittl & Levin, 1997). Cineangiograms (motion pictures) of each of the coronary arteries are obtained in at least two projections: right anterior oblique and left anterior oblique. Views from other angles also may be obtained to ensure adequate visualization of the proximal and distal portion of each vessel and to demonstrate better specific coronary artery lesions (Newton, 1995) (Fig. 8-5).

Coronary artery anatomy usually is described in terms of whether the right, left, or neither coronary artery is dominant. The term *dominance* is used to denote which artery supplies the posterior diaphragmatic interventricular septum and diaphragmatic surface of the left ventricle (Bond & Halpenny, 1995). Most common is right dominant coronary circulation, in which the posterior descending artery arises from the right coronary artery; in left dominant coronary circulation, the posterior descending artery is a branch of the left cir-

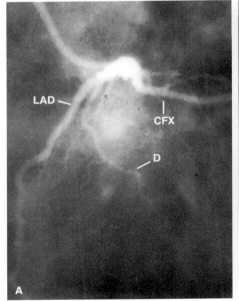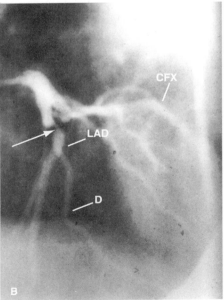

FIGURE 8-5. Two projections of the same left coronary arterial system obtained during coronary angiography. **(A)** In the left anterior oblique projection, no significant narrowings are demonstrated. **(B)** Cranially angled left anterior oblique projection demonstrates a tight stenosis in the left anterior descending (LAD) artery (*arrow*). D, diagonal branch of LAD; CFX, circumflex coronary artery. (Courtesy of Sheridan Meyers, MD)

cumflex artery (Kirklin & Barratt-Boyes, 1993). From a physiologic standpoint, the term *dominance* is somewhat misleading. Despite the fact that most people have right dominant coronary circulation, the left coronary artery in most human hearts is of wider caliber and perfuses the largest proportion of myocardium (Bond & Halpenny, 1995).

Visualization of the major coronary arteries and their branches demonstrates vessel size, areas of narrowing or irregularity, and quality of the distal portion of the vessel. Severity of stenotic lesions can be quantitated by comparing the reduction in luminal diameter with that in a normal segment of the same artery. The percentage of luminal diameter reduction usually is categorized as (1) less than 50%, (2) 50% to 75%, (3) 75% to 99%, or (4) total occlusion. Lesions that reduce luminal diameter more than 50% are considered significant because they represent a 75% reduction in cross-sectional area of the artery and can decrease blood flow reserves during exercise (Remetz & Hennecken, 1996). Because contrast material clears faster with higher flow rates, a subjective evaluation of the adequacy of perfusion can be based on how quickly an artery fills with and clears contrast (Newton, 1995).

Ventriculography (ie, opacification of a ventricular chamber using contrast material) is performed routinely in association with coronary angiography. Left ventriculography is accomplished by injecting contrast material through a catheter that has been advanced in retrograde fashion from the proximal aorta across the aortic valve into the left ventricle. A ventriculogram provides subjective demonstration of effectiveness of global and segmental ventricular contractility. Wall motion abnormalities, such as areas of akinesis (lack of motion), hypokinesis (diminished motion), or dyskinesis (abnormal motion), are identified during this portion of the study. In addition, left ventriculography is used to calculate left ventricular volumes and ejection fraction and to assess the presence and severity of mitral valve regurgitation (Lange & Hillis, 1998). In hemodynamically unstable patients, a ventriculogram is more hazardous because of the adverse effects of contrast material on a poorly functioning ventricle. In these patients, the ventriculogram may be omitted.

Aortic root aortography (injection of contrast into the ascending aorta) may be performed with coronary angiography if aortic insufficiency is suspected. Angiography of the internal thoracic (mammary) arteries occasionally is performed in preoperative patients if there is a question about the quality of the vessels.

Right-sided heart catheterization is performed through the cephalic or femoral vein with fluoroscopically guided, retrograde advancement of the catheter into the right side of the heart. Catheterization of the right side of the heart is performed for the following reasons: (1) measurement of right atrial, right ventricular, and pulmonary artery pressures, cardiac output, and oxygen saturation; (2) visualization of the right atrium, right ventricle, tricuspid and pulmonic valves, or pulmonary arterial circulation; and (3) access to the left atrium through transseptal cannulation.

Transseptal catheterization is performed by passing an intracardiac catheter from the right to left atrium. Techniques vary, but in general a combination catheter–needle is passed through the fossa ovalis in the atrial septum and the catheter then is advanced from the left atrium to the left ventricle, where left ventricular pressures and angiograms are obtained (Bashore et al., 1995). A transseptal approach to the left side of the heart most often is performed in patients in whom it is ill advised or not possible to advance a catheter through the aortic valve, such as those with an aortic valve prosthesis or severe aortic stenosis. A transseptal approach also is used for therapeutic balloon valvotomy of the mitral valve.

Improvements in catheterization techniques, contrast material, and catheters have made cardiac catheterization quite safe and have expanded indications for the procedure. More than 1.7 million cardiac catheterizations are performed annually in the United States (American Heart Association, 1998). Almost all adults who undergo cardiac operations have a cardiac catheterization before surgery. The most common reason for performing catheterization of the heart is to evaluate the presence and severity of coronary artery atherosclerosis. For patients undergoing coronary artery revascularization, preoperative definition of the coronary anatomy is essential. Because of the prevalence of coronary artery disease in this country, coronary angiography also is important to detect coronary stenoses in high-risk patients who require other types of operative procedures. As a result, greater numbers of both critically ill as well as ambulatory patients at risk for coronary artery disease are undergoing cardiac catheterization (Bashore et al., 1995).

Patients with valvular abnormalities or structural defects of the heart may undergo heart catheterization to determine intracardiac pressures, detect abnormal communications, and assess function of the cardiac valves. However, the sophisticated echocardiographic and nuclear imaging techniques that are available often provide sufficient diagnostic information. In young patients at low risk for coronary artery disease, cardiac catheterization often is unnecessary. Cardiac catheterization is performed for an increasing variety of therapeutic purposes, such as percutaneous coronary intervention and mitral balloon valvotomy. Therapeutic catheterization procedures are discussed elsewhere in the text.

Although cardiac catheterization is an invasive procedure, it is associated with minimal morbidity when performed by experienced angiographers. Mortality risk associated with the procedure ranges from 0.14% to 0.175% (Davidson et al., 1997). Patients at highest risk in the adult population include those with significant left main coronary artery disease, poor left ventricular function, advanced age, and associated valvular disease (Bashore et al., 1995). The most common complication of cardiac catheterization is peripheral arterial injury at the site of catheter insertion. Potential clinical sequelae resulting from iatrogenic arterial injury include thromboembolism, hematoma, arterial perforation, pseudoaneurysm, and arteriovenous fistula (Finkelmeier & Finkelmeier, 1991). Vascular complications appear to occur more frequently in women and when a brachial artery approach is used (Bashore et al., 1995). Other complications of cardiac catheterization include allergic reaction to the contrast material, severe vasovagal reflex, cardiac arrest, stroke, myocardial infarction, and arrhythmias.

Electrophysiologic Studies

An *electrophysiologic study* is performed to assess systematically the electrical conduction system of the heart. The assessment includes evaluation of spontaneous function, responses to stress, and vulnerability to induced tachyarrhythmias (Fisher, 1998). Electrophysiologic study is the definitive diagnostic modality for characterizing arrhythmic disorders, stratifying risk, and directing therapy. The procedure is similar to cardiac catheterization in that intracardiac catheters are positioned with the aid of fluoroscopy. The catheters serve two purposes. First, they are used to obtain intracardiac electrical recordings that demonstrate cardiac electrical activation, allow measurement of conduction and recovery times, and define abnormalities. In this portion of the study, adequacy of sinus and atrioventricular node and His bundle function can be assessed and the mechanism and characteristics of supraventricular or ventricular rhythm disorders are clarified.

The intracardiac catheters also are used to perform programmed electrical stimulation (PES), a method of provoking cardiac arrhythmias by delivering pacing stimuli at specific intervals during the cardiac cycle. PES permits the induction and termination of malignant arrhythmias under controlled conditions. During PES, abnormal activation sequences are identified, thereby localizing reentrant pathways. The ability or inability to provoke an arrhythmia that has occurred clinically is termed *inducibility*. An induced arrhythmia that is sustained for 30 seconds or more or that requires intervention for hemodynamically compromising symptoms is termed a *sustained arrhythmia*. Inducibility and sustainability provide prognostic information about likelihood of clinical recurrence as well as evaluative information about efficacy of antiarrhythmic therapy. Use of electrophysiologic studies in guiding therapy of patients with chronic arrhythmic disorders is discussed in Chapter 4, Cardiac Rhythm Disorders.

Endomyocardial Biopsy

Endomyocardial biopsy is the acquisition of a small piece of myocardium for microscopic analysis. The biopsy is obtained using a bioptome, which is a specially designed catheter with an externally controlled pinching mechanism at its distal end (Fig. 8-6). The bioptome is inserted into the right internal jugular or femoral vein and is advanced under fluoroscopic guidance into the right ventricle. Small fragments of endomyocardium are sampled, usually from the apical half of the right side of the ventricular septum (Schoen, 1997). Endomyocardial biopsy

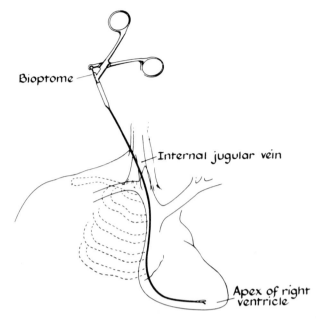

FIGURE 8-6. Bioptome is inserted through the internal jugular vein and advanced through the right atrium, across the tricuspid valve and into the right ventricle; endocardial tissue is obtained from the interventricular septum. (LeDoux D, Shinn J, 1995: Cardiac surgery. In Woods SL, Froelicher ES, Halpenny CJ, Motzer SU [eds]: Cardiac Nursing, ed. 3, p. 542. Philadelphia, JB Lippincott)

is a valuable diagnostic technique in two categories of patients: (1) those with cardiac failure of unknown etiology, and (2) those who have undergone cardiac transplantation. For adults with transplanted hearts, endomyocardial biopsy is the primary technique for detecting rejection in its early stages. Ventricular perforation, the most common complication of endomyocardial biopsy, occurs infrequently.

REFERENCES

American Heart Association, 1998: 1999 Heart and Stroke Facts, Dallas, American Heart Association

Bashore TM, Harrison JK, Davidson CJ, 1995: Cardiac catheterization, angiography, and interventional techniques in valvular and congenital heart disease. In Sabiston DC Jr, Spencer FC (eds): Surgery of the Chest, ed. 6. Philadelphia, WB Saunders

Berra KA, Froelicher ESS, 1995: Exercise testing. In Woods SL, Froelicher ESS, Halpenny CJ, Motzer SU (eds): Cardiac Nursing, ed. 3. Philadelphia, JB Lippincott

Bittl JA, Levin DC, 1997: Coronary arteriography. In Braunwald E (ed): Heart Disease: A Textbook of Cardiovascular Medicine, ed. 5. Philadelphia, WB Saunders

Bond EF, Halpenny CJ, 1995: Cardiac anatomy. In Woods SL, Froelicher ESS, Halpenny CJ, Motzer SU (eds): Cardiac Nursing, ed. 3. Philadelphia, JB Lippincott

Chaitman B, 1997: Exercise stress testing. In Braunwald E (ed): Heart Disease: A Textbook of Cardiovascular Medicine, ed. 5. Philadelphia, WB Saunders

Chaitman BR, Miller DD, 1996: Nuclear imaging in the assessment of acquired heart disease. In Baue AE, Geha AS,

Hammond GL, et al. (eds): Glenn's Cardiovascular and Thoracic Surgery, ed. 6. Stamford, CT, Appleton & Lange

Davidson CJ, Fishman RF, Bonow RO, 1997: Cardiac catheterization. In Braunwald E (ed): Heart Disease: A Textbook of Cardiovascular Medicine, ed. 5. Philadelphia, WB Saunders

Elefteriades JA, Geha AS, Cohen LS, 1996: Thoracic imaging in acute disease. In House Officer Guide to ICU Care: Fundamentals of Management of the Heart and Lungs, ed. 2. Philadelphia, Lippincott-Raven

Feigenbaum H, 1997: Echocardiography. In Braunwald E (ed): Heart Disease: A Textbook of Cardiovascular Medicine, ed. 5. Philadelphia, WB Saunders

Finkelmeier BA, Finkelmeier WR, 1991: Iatrogenic arterial injuries resulting from invasive procedures. J Vasc Nurs 9:12

Fisch C, 1997: Electrocardiography. In Braunwald E (ed): Heart Disease: A Textbook of Cardiovascular Medicine, ed. 5. Philadelphia, WB Saunders

Fisher JD, 1998: Electrophysiologic testing. In Topol EJ (ed): Comprehensive Cardiovascular Medicine. Philadelphia, Lippincott Williams & Wilkins

Flachskampf FA, Breithardt O, 1998: Doppler assessment. In Topol EJ (ed): Comprehensive Cardiovascular Medicine. Philadelphia, Lippincott Williams & Wilkins

Gersh BJ, Braunwald E, Rutherford JD, 1997: Chronic coronary artery disease. In Braunwald E (ed): Heart Disease: A Textbook of Cardiovascular Medicine, ed. 5. Philadelphia, WB Saunders

Griffin BP, 1998: Transesophageal echocardiography. In Topol EJ (ed): Comprehensive Cardiovascular Medicine. Philadelphia, Lippincott Williams & Wilkins

Hall ML, 1995: Echocardiography, radioisotope studies, magnetic resonance imaging, and phonocardiography. In Woods SL, Froelicher ESS, Halpenny CJ, Motzer SU (eds): Cardiac Nursing, ed. 3. Philadelphia, JB Lippincott

Hendel RC, 1997: Interpreting noninvasive cardiac tests. In Alpert JS (ed): Cardiology for the Primary Care Physician, ed. 2. Philadelphia, Current Medicine

Hillis LD, Lange RA, Winniford MD, Page RL, 1995: Signal-averaged electrocardiography. In Manual of Clinical Problems in Cardiology, ed. 5. Boston, Little, Brown

Hudak CM, Gallo BM, Morton PG, 1998: Patient assessment: cardiovascular system. In Critical Care Nursing: A Holistic Approach, ed. 7. Philadelphia, Lippincott Williams & Wilkins

Iskandrian AE, Verani MS, 1998: Nuclear imaging techniques. In Topol EJ (ed): Comprehensive Cardiovascular Medicine. Philadelphia, Lippincott Williams & Wilkins

Kirklin JW, Barratt-Boyes BG, 1993: Anatomy, dimensions, and terminology. In Cardiac Surgery, ed. 2. New York, Churchill Livingstone

Lange RA, Hillis LD, 1998: Cardiac catheterization and hemodynamic assessment. In Topol EJ (ed): Comprehensive Cardiovascular Medicine. Philadelphia, Lippincott Williams & Wilkins

Matsuzaki M, Toma Y, Kusukawa R, 1990: Clinical applications of transesophageal echocardiography. Circulation 82: 709

Newton KM, 1995: Cardiac catheterization. In Woods SL, Froelicher ESS, Halpenny CJ, Motzer SU (eds): Cardiac Nursing, ed. 3. Philadelphia, JB Lippincott

Okin PM, 1998: Exercise electrocardiography. In Topol EJ (ed): Comprehensive Cardiovascular Medicine. Philadelphia, Lippincott Williams & Wilkins

Remetz MS, Hennecken J, 1996: Cardiac catheterization in the evaluation of heart disease. In Baue AE, Geha AS, Hammond GL, et al. (eds): Glenn's Cardiovascular and Thoracic Surgery, ed. 6. Stamford, CT, Appleton & Lange

Schoen FJ, 1997: Pathologic considerations in surgery of adult heart disease. Edmunds LH Jr (ed): Cardiac Surgery in the Adult. New York, McGraw-Hill

Sgarbossa EB, Wagner G, 1998: Electrocardiography. In Topol EJ (ed): Comprehensive Cardiovascular Medicine. Philadelphia, Lippincott Williams & Wilkins

Skorton DJ, Brundage BH, Schelbert HR, Wolf GL, 1997: Relative merits of imaging techniques. In Braunwald E (ed): Heart Disease: A Textbook of Cardiovascular Medicine, ed. 5. Philadelphia, WB Saunders

Sutherland LJ, 1991: Patient assessment: diagnostic studies. In Kinney MR, Packa DR, Andreoli KG, Zipes DP (eds): Comprehensive Cardiac Care, ed. 7. St. Louis, Mosby–Year Book

Schwaiger M, Ziegler S, 1998: Positron emission tomography. In Topol EJ (ed): Comprehensive Cardiovascular Medicine. Philadelphia, Lippincott Williams & Wilkins

Tchou PJ, 1998: Ventricular tachycardia. In Topol EJ (ed): Comprehensive Cardiovascular Medicine. Philadelphia, Lippincott Williams & Wilkins

Wackers FJ, Soufer R, Zaret BL, 1997: Nuclear cardiology. In Braunwald E (ed): Heart Disease: A Textbook of Cardiovascular Medicine, ed. 5. Philadelphia, WB Saunders

Preoperative Management

Before any cardiac operation, the surgeon, anesthesiologist, and advanced practice nurse (1) interview and assess the patient; (2) review all diagnostic information, including laboratory, electrocardiographic, chest radiographic, and cardiac catheterization data; and (3) prepare the patient for the planned operation and postoperative regimen. Typically, this preoperative preparation is performed in an outpatient setting and the patient is admitted to the hospital on the morning of the planned operation. Same-day admission for a cardiac operation requires efficient organization of the system so that necessary evaluations can be accomplished and diagnostic studies reviewed appropriately. Because there is no inpatient observation during the night before surgery, patients need instruction to avoid ingestion of food or liquids after midnight, to take medications as directed, and to report promptly any exacerbation of symptoms that might represent myocardial ischemia or congestive heart failure. Patients with severe preoperative anxiety and coronary artery disease may require anxiolytic medication to avoid precipitous myocardial ischemia during the preoperative period.

For selected patients with special needs, preoperative hospitalization may be necessary to allow time for interventions that decrease operative risk. For example, patients with valvular heart disease and severe ventricular dysfunction may require preoperative diuresis guided by pulmonary artery pressure monitoring because of the narrow window between adequate preload and pulmonary edema. Patients with severe, long-standing cardiac disease also may have protein and calorie malnutrition requiring preoperative nutritional supplementation.

Patients who undergo coronary artery revascularization for unstable angina after acute myocardial infarction (MI) also may be hospitalized during the preoperative period. Restoring perfusion to newly infarcted muscle more than 6 hours but within 24 to 48 hours after onset of MI can cause a complex pathophysiologic process called *reperfusion injury.* Operative risk may be lessened if surgery is delayed for several days after MI, and monitoring is required during this time to detect postinfarction ischemia that might necessitate emergent operation.

▶ Patient Assessment

A primary nursing intervention in the preoperative period is a thorough assessment with documentation of significant findings. Typically, an advanced practice nurse performs the outpatient preoperative patient assessment. If a nurse practitioner has this responsibility, he or she may perform the preadmission history and physical examination as well. The preoperative nursing assessment complements the history and physical examination and provides important baseline information for comparison during the postoperative period. It also allows the nurse to establish a relationship with the patient and identify problems that will require special interventions during the hospitalization. The preoperative assessment includes information elicited from the patient, family, and medical record, as well as that obtained through physical examination. The assessment is performed in a consistent and organized manner, beginning with an overall evaluation of general status and proceeding to a more detailed evaluation of cardiovascular status (Canobbio, 1990).

Patient Interview

The preoperative interview is used to obtain baseline information about the patient's clinical history, understanding of the illness, emotional readiness for the planned procedure, and family support system (Table 9-1). Important features include (1) history of present illness (ie, the type of heart disease and associated symptoms); (2) presence of cardiac risk factors; (3) associated medical diseases, such as cerebrovascular or other peripheral arterial occlusive disease, hypertension, diabetes, peptic ulcer disease, or chronic obstructive pulmonary disease; (4) current medication regimen and any known allergies; and (5) degree of functional impairment associated with the cardiac disease. Other pertinent information includes the patient's occupation and personal habits, such as smoking, alcohol use, exercise, and diet.

Information from the clinical history may reveal factors that increase perioperative risk, such as alcohol abuse, a heavy smoking history, diabetes mellitus, or steroid dependency. It also may alter the planned perioperative therapy. For example, detection of transient ischemic attacks or amaurosis fugax may necessitate further preoperative evaluation of the carotid arteries and possible combined or staged surgical therapy. A history of gastrointestinal bleeding or peptic ulcer disease may influence the antiplatelet regimen after coronary artery revascularization or the choice of valvular prosthesis. Indications of nutritional deficiency may be ascertained, including a current weight less than 10% of ideal body weight, unintentional, significant weight loss, or inadequate daily caloric intake (<1000 calories) (Antman, 1997).

From the patient interview, the current level of symptoms is determined. Any increase in intensity or frequency of symptoms then can be identified more easily. A baseline also is established for the degree of associated functional impairment. In the presence of cardiac disease, heart function may be adequate at rest but inadequate during exertion (Braunwald, 1997). The

TABLE 9-1

Preoperative Interview: Areas of Focus

History of present illness
Presence of cardiac risk factors
Functional status
Associated medical diseases
Current medication regimen and drug allergies
Understanding of illness and planned procedure
Emotional readiness for procedure
Family support system

TABLE 9-2

Assessment of Functional Status in Patients With Heart Disease

EVALUATION OF ANGINA
Canadian Cardiovascular Society Functional Classification System

Class	Description
I	Angina occurs with strenuous or rapid or prolonged exertion at work or recreation
II	Slight limitation of ordinary activities by angina
III	Marked limitation of ordinary activities by angina
IV	Angina with any physical activity or at rest

From Campeau, 1976: Grading of angina pectoris. Circulation 54:522.

EVALUATION OF HEART FAILURE
New York Heart Association Classification System

Class	Description
I	Ordinary physical activity does not cause undue fatigue, palpitation, dyspnea, or angina
II	Ordinary physical activity causes undue fatigue, palpitation, dyspnea, or angina
III	Less than ordinary physical activity causes undue fatigue, palpitation, dyspnea, or angina
IV	Fatigue, palpitation, dyspnea, or angina occur at rest

From Criteria Committee of the New York Heart Association, 1964: Physical capacity with heart disease. In Diseases of the Heart and Blood Vessels: Nomenclature and Criteria for Diagnosis, ed. 6. Boston, Little, Brown.

Canadian Cardiovascular Classification System commonly is used in patients with coronary artery disease to describe the degree of associated disability from angina (Campeau, 1976). The New York Heart Association (NYHA) Functional Classification System (Criteria Committee of the NYHA, 1964) is more applicable for describing functional impairment due to valvular heart disease (Table 9-2).

The patient's living arrangements are addressed during the interview so that appropriate discharge planning can be initiated. An increasing number of surgical patients are elderly and have limited social and financial resources. Identification of discharge needs before hospitalization alleviates anxiety for the patient and family and makes discharge from the hospital more efficient and timely. During the preoperative interview, the nurse also evaluates the patient's understanding of the underlying illness, planned course of surgical therapy, level of anxiety, and ability to comply with the postoperative regimen. Appropriate preoperative teaching and interventions to allay anxiety can then be initiated. Preoperative education and counseling of the patient are major components of the preoperative regimen and are discussed in detail in Chapter 10, Education and Psychological Support for the Patient and Family.

Physical Assessment

The preoperative physical assessment in cardiac surgical patients is primarily a cardiovascular assessment, focusing on the heart, lungs, peripheral pulses, neck, and extremities (Table 9-3). Baseline blood pressure, temperature, and weight recordings are obtained. Heart sounds are auscultated to provide information about heart rate, rhythm, and the presence of extra sounds, murmurs, or rubs. Each of the carotid arteries is auscultated from the base of the neck to the angle of the jaw, with the patient holding his or her breath. The presence of a carotid bruit (ie, audible sound associated with turbulent flow) often represents arterial stenosis at or proximal to the site of auscultation and usually is loudest in the upper third of the neck in the area of the carotid bifurcation (Fahey, 1999). Auscultation of the lungs provides baseline data regarding respiratory rate, breath sounds, and the presence of adventitious sounds. Rales may indicate the need for preoperative diuresis. Rhonchi in a heavy smoker may warrant preoperative bronchodilator therapy and pulmonary hygiene measures.

Palpation of the abdomen may allow detection of an abdominal aortic aneurysm, except in markedly obese patients (Perloff & Braunwald, 1997). Although a pulsatile, periumbilical or upper abdominal mass is suggestive of aortic aneurysm, it may instead represent merely a tortuous abdominal aorta (Bates et al., 1995). Further diagnostic testing is necessary to confirm the diagnosis. Peripheral pulses are assessed as well as other indicators of peripheral perfusion (eg, color and temperature of extremities and capillary refill). Ankle blood pressure measurements are obtained to provide baseline information about adequacy of arterial blood flow to the lower extremities (Fig. 9-1). An ankle-brachial index may be calculated by dividing the pedal systolic pressure by the brachial systolic pressure. Systolic pressure at the ankle level normally is equal to or slightly higher than brachial systolic pressure, resulting in an ankle-brachial index of 1.0 or above (Fahey, 1999). An index of less than 0.7 is indicative of compromised blood flow to the lower extremity on that side. If the ankle-brachial index suggests compromised arterial flow in one of the extremities, the extremity with better arterial blood supply is used for harvesting saphenous vein or for insertion of an intra-aortic balloon catheter through the femoral artery.

Any abnormalities, such as jugular venous distention, ascites, or peripheral edema, are noted. The presence of varicose veins or thrombophlebitis is significant in patients who are to undergo coronary artery revascularization. These conditions, or previous vein ligation, may preclude adequate availability of saphenous vein for conduit material. For the same reason, preoperative venipuncture of saphenous veins is contraindicated in patients who are to undergo coronary artery bypass grafting to avoid damaging segments of vein that might be harvested for grafting.

Other findings of significance during the preoperative physical examination include dental infection, which increases risk of endocarditis in patients with valvular heart disease, or prior radical mastectomy, which may preclude use of an internal thoracic artery (Antman, 1997). For a more complete discussion of physical examination of the patient with cardiovascular disease, the reader is referred to a textbook of physical assessment.

Signs and Symptoms of Heart Disease

Special consideration is given during the preoperative assessment to the presence of signs and symptoms of organic heart disease. The most frequently occurring abnormalities are described in this section. Of these, recognition of acute ischemia and acute congestive heart failure are particularly important.

Most patients who undergo cardiac operations have coronary artery disease. Thus, *angina pectoris*, its cardinal manifestation, probably is the most frequently encountered symptom in preoperative cardiac surgical patients. Angina pectoris indicates transient myocardial ischemia or evolving infarction owing to an imbalance in myocardial oxygen demand and supply. Angina usually produces a sensation of substernal discomfort or pressure. However, it also may occur as an abnormal sensation in the throat, jaw, or arms (Fig. 9-2). Although angina may be manifest as a variety of somatic abnormalities, the pattern for a particular patient usually is consistent; that is, the nature of the discomfort is similar during each episode. Because of the sensory neuropathy that accompanies diabetes mellitus, diabetic patients must be evaluated carefully for the presence of silent ischemia (ie, signs of myocardial ischemia in the absence of angina) or anginal equivalent symptoms (Topol, 1998). Anginal equivalent symptoms are atypical manifestations of acute myocardial ischemia, such as shortness of breath, pulmonary edema, or ventricular tachycardia.

TABLE 9-3

Preoperative Physical Assessment: Areas of Focus

Cardiac auscultation
    Rate and rhythm
    Heart sounds
    Murmurs, clicks, rubs
Auscultation of carotid arteries
Auscultation of the lungs
Respiratory rate
    Breath sounds
    Adventitious sounds
Palpation of peripheral pulses
Blood pressure
Weight
Temperature
Examination of extremities
    Peripheral edema
    Evidence of arterial insufficiency or venous stasis
    Evidence of prior vein ligation

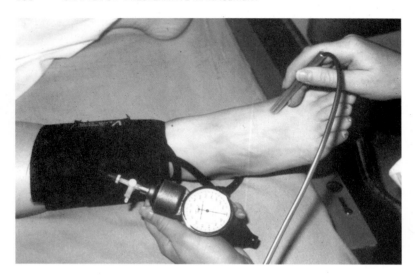

FIGURE 9-1. Measurement of ankle pressure using Doppler probe placed over the dorsalis pedis artery. (Courtesy of Victora A. Fahey, RN, MSN, CVN)

Severity of pain usually is quantified using a scale from 1 to 10, with 1 being barely noticeable pain and 10 the most severe pain. The term, "OLD CART" provides a mnemonic for characterizing features of a patient's anginal pattern: Onset, Location, Duration, Character, Aggravating Factors, Relieving Factors, and Time (how often). Typically, angina is precipitated by one of the "four Es"—exercise, emotion, eating, or exposure to cold. Because the anginal threshold is lower in the morning than at other times throughout the day, patients commonly report that activities that may cause angina in

the morning or when first undertaken do not do so later in the day (Braunwald, 1997).

Angina usually is categorized as stable or unstable. Chronic stable angina usually lasts 5 to 15 minutes and is relieved by rest or sublingual nitroglycerin. Angina is considered unstable if it (1) is new in onset or occurs at rest; (2) is accelerating (occurs more frequently or at lower workloads); (3) wakes the patient from sleep; (4) is prolonged or unresponsive to nitrates; or (5) is associated with severe nausea, weakness, dyspnea, sweating, palpitations, syncope, or pulmonary edema (Paraskos,

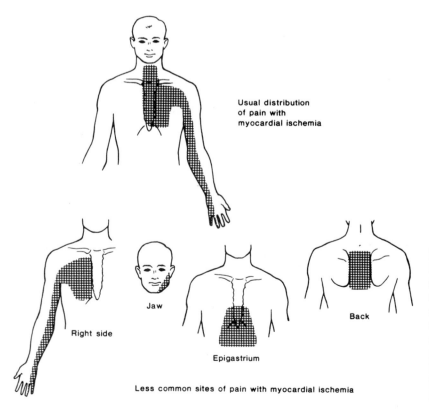

Usual distribution of pain with myocardial ischemia

Jaw

Right side

Epigastrium

Back

Less common sites of pain with myocardial ischemia

FIGURE 9-2. Pain patterns with myocardial ischemia. Most common distribution is referral to all or part of the sternal region, left side of the chest, neck, and down the ulnar side of the left forearm and hand. With severe ischemic pain, the right chest and right arm are often involved as well, although isolated involvement of these sites is rare. Less commonly involved, either alone or together with other sites, are the jaw, epigastrium, and back. (Horwitz LD, 1985: Chest pain. In Horwitz LD, Groves BM [eds]: Signs and Symptoms in Cardiology, p. 9. Philadelphia, JB Lippincott)

1997). Angina that is accelerating represents an acute coronary syndrome. It is reported promptly to the surgeon and requires increased antianginal therapy or admission to the hospital. Myocardial ischemia that is unrecognized or unrelieved can lead to death, irreversible muscle damage, or complications, such as arrhythmias or cardiogenic shock (Skov & Motzer, 1995). Acute coronary syndrome is discussed further later in the chapter.

Chest pain can occur because of other etiologies, but in preoperative patients all chest pain is assumed ischemic until proven otherwise. Probably most difficult to distinguish from angina is chest pain caused by gastroesophageal reflux. Pain due to reflux frequently occurs after eating and is relieved by antacids. Pleuritis secondary to pleural inflammation also can cause chest pain. However, unlike angina, pleuritic pain increases on inspiration when the pleura is stretched. Musculoskeletal chest pain differs from angina in that it usually is well localized and the painful area is tender to palpation. Also, in contrast to angina, musculoskeletal pain usually is provoked by movement, such as jarring, coughing, or sneezing, and is relieved by massage, heat, or manipulation. Chest pain caused by anxiety may assume any form, although it frequently occurs as a dull ache in the left inframammary hemithorax. It is persistent and often is associated with fleeting sharp pains or a sensation of anxiety or breathlessness.

Dyspnea is a second common symptom of organic heart disease. Dyspnea is a gasping sensation provoked by effort that previously did not produce an awareness of breathing. Dyspnea occurs normally with strenuous exercise in healthy, well-conditioned people and with moderate exercise in those unaccustomed to exercise; it should be regarded as abnormal only when it occurs at rest or with a level of activity not expected to produce dyspnea (Braunwald, 1997). *Paroxysmal nocturnal dyspnea, orthopnea,* and *dyspnea on exertion* are terms used to categorize the various forms of dyspnea.

Paroxysmal nocturnal dyspnea, or that which awakens the patient from sleep, most commonly represents left-sided heart failure. Orthopnea is dyspnea that necessitates elevation of the head with more than one pillow to breathe comfortably while lying down. As cardiac disease worsens, orthopnea typically increases. Dyspnea on exertion signifies that the patient breathes comfortably at rest but becomes dyspneic with activity. Dyspnea is most common in patients with valvular heart disease. It also may be present in patients with ventricular dysfunction due to prior MI. Occasionally, dyspnea occurs as an anginal equivalent; that is, as a manifestation of acute myocardial ischemia.

Less common manifestations of cardiac disease in adults include syncope, palpitations, cough, hemoptysis, hoarseness, nocturia, fatigue, cyanosis, and peripheral edema. Syncope is a loss of consciousness due to inadequate perfusion of the brain (Topol, 1998). It may occur secondary to an arrhythmia, pacemaker malfunction, aortic stenosis, hypersensitive carotid sinus syndrome, or a vasovagal response. Cardiac syncope is usually of rapid onset without aura and not associated with convulsive movements, urinary incontinence, or a postictal confusional state (Braunwald, 1997).

Palpitations are an unpleasant awareness of the heartbeat while at rest or during basal activities. Patients usually describe the sensation as heavy or rapid beating, fluttering, pounding, or skipping a beat. It is important to determine if the palpitating sensation represents simply an awareness of a forceful heartbeat or if it is produced by an arrhythmia. Palpitations are a relatively nonspecific symptom and not a reliable indicator of any particular cardiac arrhythmia; in a minority of patients, however, they may be associated with functional incapacity, severe hemodynamic sequelae, or an increased risk for sudden cardiac death (Spratt et al., 1997).

Cardiac arrhythmias are common in patients with organic heart disease. Many patients have chronic premature ventricular contractions, and often no treatment is necessary. However, documentation of their presence in the preoperative period provides useful information to formulate an appropriate response to postoperative arrhythmias. Preoperative ventricular tachycardia may represent acute myocardial ischemia or an underlying chronic rhythm disorder that requires electrophysiologic evaluation. Atrial fibrillation is another frequently occurring arrhythmia, particularly in patients with mitral valve disease. Because chronic atrial fibrillation usually necessitates anticoagulation, its presence is an important factor in determining the type of prosthesis selected for cardiac valve replacement.

Cough associated with cardiac disease usually is nonproductive and occurs at night when the patient is lying down. A dry, irritating cough with dyspnea when in the supine position usually indicates pulmonary venous congestion (Chatterjee, 1998). It also may occur because of compression of the tracheobronchial tree by an enlarged left atrium or a thoracic aortic aneurysm. Hemoptysis associated with heart disease is most likely in patients with mitral stenosis. It results from elevated pulmonary vascular pressure with resultant bleeding into alveoli. Hoarseness is unusual but may be present owing to pressure on the recurrent laryngeal nerve from an enlarged left atrium or a thoracic aortic aneurysm.

Nocturia is defined as the passage of abnormally large amounts of urine at night; it may represent early congestive heart failure. Fatigue is a difficult symptom to evaluate because it is entirely subjective. Although rarely the first or only symptom of organic heart disease, it is helpful in evaluating the degree of functional impairment imposed by cardiac disease. It may indicate low cardiac output or result from excessive diuresis or the use of beta-adrenergic blocking drugs (Topol, 1998). Cyanosis is a bluish discoloration of the skin and mucous membranes resulting from an increased quantity of reduced hemoglobin or of abnormal hemoglobin pigments in the blood perfusing these areas (Braunwald, 1997). Cyanosis, observed rarely in adults, represents chronic hypoxemia and may occur in patients with severe pulmonary disease or in those with unrepaired, cyanotic congenital heart defects. Localized peripheral cyanosis may occur due to low cardiac output or arterial occlusive disease.

Dependent edema, involving the inferior extremities, occurs as a consequence of systemic venous hypertension associated with right-sided heart failure (Chatterjee, 1998). It is unusual, except in patients with severe tricuspid valve disease or mitral stenosis. In ambulatory patients, dependent edema develops bilaterally in the lower extremities. It is symmetric, usually preceded by a 7- to 10-pound weight gain, and may progress to involve the thighs, genitalia, and abdominal wall (Braunwald, 1997). In bedridden patients, edema is likely to develop in the sacral area or back. Other signs indicative of right-sided heart failure include liver enlargement, ascites, and neck vein distention. Gastrointestinal symptoms, including nausea, anorexia, bloating, or early satiety, commonly are present because of increased intra-abdominal pressure.

► Preparatory Interventions

Diagnostic Studies

Diagnostic studies performed routinely during the preoperative period include a complete blood cell count with differential, hemostasis studies (prothrombin time, partial thromboplastin time, and platelet count), blood chemistry survey, urinalysis, electrocardiogram, and chest roentgenogram. These baseline studies are important to detect any abnormalities that may increase risk of the operation or necessitate further preoperative evaluation. Abnormalities that may alter the timing or plan of therapy include such conditions as urinary tract infection, bleeding disorder, or a pulmonary lesion.

Many patients, especially those with coronary artery disease, have associated peripheral arterial occlusive disease. A noninvasive carotid ultrasound study is obtained if the patient has a carotid bruit or a history of a transient ischemic attack or cerebral vascular accident. A Doppler arterial blood flow study of the lower extremities may be obtained in patients with claudication or evidence of limb ischemia. Venous duplex scanning (vein mapping) may be performed in selected patients undergoing coronary artery revascularization to assess the quality of venous conduit for grafting. In patients with severe pulmonary disease, a preoperative arterial blood gas on room air may be obtained to establish a baseline. Pulmonary function testing may provide additional useful information to assess operative risk in selected patients with severe pulmonary dysfunction.

Before cardiac valve replacement, patients usually undergo a dental evaluation with dental roentgenograms (Fig. 9-3). Because dental infection is a common source of bacterial endocarditis, infected teeth are extracted and oral abscesses drained before implantation of a valvular prosthesis. In patients with valvular dysfunction, appropriate antibiotic prophylaxis according to American Heart Association guidelines is administered before any dental procedures likely to cause bleeding from hard or soft tissues, periodontal surgery, scaling, or professional cleaning of teeth (Dajani et al., 1997).

Sometimes, cardiac surgery is delayed because of diagnostic studies. For example, consideration is given to nephrotoxic effects of angiographic contrast material used during cardiac catheterization. Evidence of renal insufficiency (eg, elevated blood urea nitrogen and creatinine values) after angiography usually leads to postponement of the operation until renal function improves. Occasionally, a patient becomes febrile before a planned operation. A temperature greater than 38.5°C (101.3°F) is suggestive of infection and an elective operation is post-

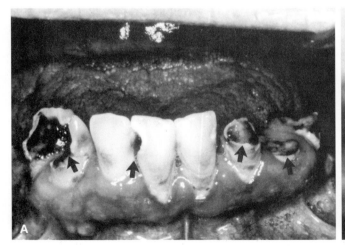
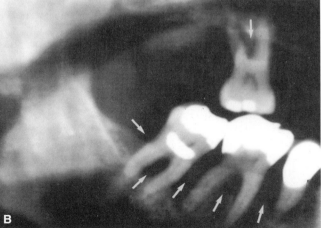

FIGURE 9-3. (A) The preoperative oral examination may reveal significant dental decay. In this patient, severe dental caries (*arrows*) and associated abscesses necessitated multiple dental extractions before cardiac valve replacement. **(B)** Although the gingival area surrounding these teeth appeared clinically healthy, the radiograph illustrates significant bone loss (radiolucent areas) around and in between the roots of the molars (*arrows*), consistent with chronic periodontal disease. (Courtesy of William Friedrich, DDS)

poned because of increased risk of wound contamination from a preexisting infection. Similarly, an operation is delayed if the screening urinalysis reveals a urinary tract infection. If an unsuspected malignancy is diagnosed, the cardiac operation may be postponed or canceled, depending on the urgency of the cardiac problem and the nature and extent of the malignancy.

Medications

Most medications are continued during the preoperative period, particularly those used for control of hypertension, angina, or arrhythmias. Withdrawal of antihypertensive medications can lead to rebound hypertension or intraoperative blood pressure lability. Acute discontinuation of beta-adrenergic blocking agents can result in a hypersympathetic state, precipitating myocardial ischemia or infarction, or arrhythmias (Mathew & Barash, 1996; Sethna et al., 1990). However, if the patient is receiving large doses or a long-acting form of beta-blocking medication, the surgeon may elect to taper the dosage or substitute a short-acting beta-blocking medication to avoid potential intraoperative myocardial depression. In patients receiving the calcium channel antagonists diltiazem or verapamil, the preoperative dose may need to be reduced to avoid postoperative bradycardia and a low cardiac-output syndrome, particularly in patients who are also receiving beta-blocking agents or amiodarone, or who are elderly (Antman, 1997).

Medications that affect hemostasis also are discontinued. Warfarin sodium (Coumadin) is usually withheld for 3 to 5 days before a planned operation so that the prothrombin time gradually decreases toward a normal level. Depending on the indication for warfarin, it may be necessary to administer heparin intravenously or enoxaparin sodium (Lovenox) subcutaneously during this period to prevent serious thrombotic or thromboembolic complications. Because of its short half-life, heparin usually is continued until the morning of the operation or, if the patient has unstable angina, until transport to the operating room.

Most patients who undergo coronary artery revascularization are receiving aspirin. Aspirin is a primary component in treatment of coronary artery disease because of its demonstrated effectiveness in reducing MI and mortality in patients with unstable angina or MI (Hillis et al., 1995; Gay, 1990). Because aspirin irreversibly inhibits platelet function, aspirin ingestion within 1 week before surgery is associated with increased perioperative bleeding that may necessitate blood transfusions or surgical reexploration. When possible, aspirin or any aspirin-containing compound is usually discontinued a full week before an elective cardiac operation. Aspirin administration is resumed in the early postoperative period in patients who receive coronary artery bypass grafts. Other antiplatelet medications, such as ticlopidine hydrochloride (Ticlid), are discontinued before surgery as well.

Oral hypoglycemic agents usually are withheld from diabetic patients on the day of surgery. In insulin-dependent patients, the insulin dosage is adjusted because food and fluids are withheld for 8 to 12 hours before operation. For example, one half the usual dose of long-acting insulin may be prescribed on the evening before surgery and supplemented with regular insulin on the morning of surgery. It is preferable to err on the side of a blood sugar that is higher than desired. Frequent blood glucose determinations are obtained during surgery, and regular insulin is administered as needed. Patients who have been taking a protamine-based insulin (eg, isophane [NPH] or protamine zinc insulin [PZI]) may have an increased risk for a sensitivity reaction to intraoperative protamine given to reverse the effects of heparin at the termination of cardiopulmonary bypass (Sather-Levine, 1990). In patients receiving preoperative steroids, intravenous steroids are administered during and after surgery until oral steroid therapy is resumed. Abrupt cessation of corticosteroids in patients who have been on chronic steroid therapy can lead to acute adrenal insufficiency (Gotch, 1991).

Patients who undergo cardiac operations almost always receive antibiotic prophylaxis immediately before operation. Although the rate of wound infection is relatively low, the consequences of sternal wound infection are significant (Waddell & Rotstein, 1994). Wound contamination is most likely during the operation itself. Potential sources of pathogenic microorganisms include a preexisting infection in the patient's body, the patient's skin, and operating room personnel and equipment. Infection of the sternal wound is particularly ominous because of the significant morbidity associated with sternal dehiscence, mediastinitis, and osteomyelitis of the sternum. The preoperative dose of antibiotics is given intravenously in the operating room as soon as an intravenous catheter is placed.

Staphylococcus aureus and *Staphylococcus epidermidis* are the most frequently encountered causative pathogens for infection of clean wounds; enteric gram-negative rods are less common (Doebbeling et al., 1990). Although numerous clinical trials have compared a variety of antimicrobial agents, no one antibiotic has emerged as the optimal choice for prophylaxis (Miedzinski et al., 1990). Cephalosporins (eg, cefazolin sodium or cefamandole nafate) often are chosen for prophylaxis because of demonstrated effectiveness against staphylococcal, streptococcal, and the most frequently encountered gram-negative organisms (van der Starre et al., 1988). In penicillin-allergic patients, an alternative antibiotic, such as vancomycin, must be selected. Vancomycin also may be used as a prophylactic agent in patients at higher risk for perioperative endocarditis, such as those undergoing implantation of a valvular prosthesis.

Blood Preparation

Blood preparation for cardiac operations is complex because of the risk of transmitting hepatitis B, hepatitis C (non-A, non-B hepatitis), or acquired immunodeficiency syndrome through allogeneic blood transfusions. Despite testing of donor blood for these agents, transmission of infection occurs in a small number of patients. The risk of transmitting infectious agents through blood product transfusion varies depending on the number of donors per recipient and the prevalence of undetected, contaminated blood in the tested blood supply (Kolins & Kolins, 1990). In addition to infection, allogeneic blood transfusions also may cause allergic reactions and sensitization to blood products (Scott et al., 1990).

If it is possible to schedule the operation several weeks in advance and if the patient's medical condition permits, autologous donation may be performed. One or 2 units of blood is donated by the patient, stored, and used as necessary during the perioperative period. Three to 4 weeks usually are necessary for recovery from anemia after collection of 400 mL of autologous whole blood, and approximately 2 months is necessary after collection of 800 mL (Watanabe et al., 1991). Iron supplementation usually is prescribed to enhance red blood cell replenishment. Recombinant human erythropoietin also may be administered. Erythropoietin, a hematopoietic hormone, is the primary regulator of erythropoiesis, or the formation of red blood cells (Levine et al., 1991).

Autologous donation is more hazardous in the presence of coronary artery disease because removal of red blood cells impairs oxygen-carrying capacity and therefore can worsen myocardial ischemia. Also, coronary artery revascularization procedures often are performed in patients who have recently experienced MI, who have just undergone cardiac catheterization, who require another operative procedure after coronary bypass grafting, or who require surgery urgently. Autologous donation is contraindicated in these situations.

Alternatively, family and friends with compatible blood types may donate blood to be used specifically for the patient. In general, several days are needed for processing these so-called "directed donations." Although patients often prefer directed blood donations, it is not clear that they are safer than other exogenous blood stores because it may be difficult for family and friends, under pressure to help the patient, to be candid about possible past exposure to hepatitis or human immunodeficiency virus infection.

Because of the limited supply and associated infectious risks of allogeneic blood, blood products are transfused judiciously. Improved mechanisms for hemostasis and blood conservation in the operating room and intensive care unit have reduced the rate of transfusion in patients who undergo elective, primary cardiac operations. However, even in patients at low risk for blood transfusion, excessive bleeding may occur and necessitate transfusion. Appropriate preoperative testing of potential recipient and donor blood and close coordination with the local blood bank are important so that adequate, type-specific blood is available as needed.

Typing of recipient blood and screening for the presence of antibodies usually are sufficient in low-risk patients to ensure adequate availability of blood for intraoperative transfusion. The type and screen must be performed within a prescribed period of time before the operation (eg, within 3 days). It is desirable to perform the type and screen during the outpatient preoperative diagnostic evaluation, before the actual day of operation, because of the possibility of detecting antibodies that could delay performance of an operation planned for the same day. Patients who have received transfusions, who have had pregnancies, or who are undergoing reoperations are at increased risk to have antibodies that require cross-matched blood.

In patients at moderate to high risk for intraoperative transfusion, specific units of donor blood (usually 2 to 4 units) are cross-matched and held in reserve for potential intraoperative use. In addition, fresh-frozen plasma and platelets should be readily available for all cardiac operations. Patients at higher risk for bleeding and allogeneic blood transfusion include those who (1) undergo redo or combined procedures (eg, valve replacement and coronary bypass grafting), (2) undergo aortic resection or a Ross procedure, (3) have preoperative anemia or abnormal bleeding studies, or (4) weigh less than 60 kg.

Preoperative Regimen

A preoperative shower or bath with an antibacterial soap is prescribed routinely to reduce the potential for wound infection. The most effective regimen for diminishing staphylococcal skin flora is showering both the evening before and the morning of the planned operation (Kaiser et al., 1988). The patient is instructed to shower at home, thoroughly cleansing the axillae, groin, and legs. No lotions or powder should be applied to areas in which incisions will be made. Shaving of the chest, groin, and legs is performed when the patient arrives in the operating room. A preoperative enema is not necessary because the abdominal cavity is not opened during cardiac operations and because patients return to a regular diet and ambulation within several days. In patients with unstable angina, a preoperative enema is contraindicated because it may precipitate myocardial ischemia.

A sleeping medication may be prescribed the night before the operation to help allay anxiety and to ensure that the patient is able to sleep comfortably. Sleeping medications are avoided in patients who are elderly or frail, or who have underlying dementia. A sedative medication is administered before transporting the patient to the operating room. In patients with ischemic heart disease, supplemental oxygen through nasal prongs may be initiated when preoperative sedation is given to minimize the possibility of hypoxemia (Mathew & Barash, 1996). Preoperative sedation facilitates patient cooperation in the operating room when invasive catheters are placed. It also suppresses physiologic stress responses so that baseline hemodynamic parameters may be measured accurately. The type and dosage usually are prescribed by the anesthesiologist based on patient age, type of cardiac disease, level of anxiety, and associated medical problems, specifically pulmonary disease. Morphine commonly is used. Scopolamine may be given adjunctively to provide perioperative amnesia and enhance the central nervous system effects of morphine (Mathew & Barash, 1996).

Accurate timing of sedative administration is important so that the patient arrives in the operating room with minimal apprehension, yet is hemodynamically stable and alert enough to cooperate with preparatory interventions (Lake, 1985). In unstable patients, preoperative sedation is withheld until the patient arrives in the operating room and is under direct observation. Unstable patients are transported to the operating room by medical and nursing personnel with appropriate monitoring and resuscitative equipment.

▶ Management of High-Risk Patients

Acute Coronary Syndrome

It is essential to identify those patients who have special needs for closer observation or intervention during the preoperative period. For example, particular attention must be given to patients with coronary artery disease who experience an accelerating anginal pattern or who have angina at rest. An increase in intensity or frequency of angina represents an acute coronary syndrome, in which portions of ventricular myocardium are ischemic but not yet damaged irreversibly. One of three conditions may be present: (1) unstable angina; (2) evolving MI (ie, prolonged ischemia over 4 to 6 hours during which muscle necrosis spreads from the subendocardium through the ventricular myocardium); or (3) a completed MI with unstable postinfarction angina.

Patients with an *acute coronary syndrome* are moved to a closely monitored setting, cardiologic consultation is obtained, and appropriate interventions are initiated to limit ischemia. Intravenous nitroglycerin is administered by continuous infusion if oral medications fail to eradicate anginal pain while the patient is at rest. Arterial blood pressure monitoring is performed to allow continuous observation of the drug's effect on systolic blood pressure. A continuous intravenous heparin infusion usually is initiated and continued until the patient is transported to the operating room. Heparin prevents extension of intracoronary thrombus, which is presumed to be present in most patients with unstable angina (Roberts & Pratt, 1991). Intra-aortic balloon counterpulsation may be instituted to augment coronary artery perfusion and decrease myocardial work. Aspirin and other antiplatelet agents (eg, ticlopidine or abciximab [ReoPro]), are discontinued. Alternatively, a decision may be made to proceed immediately with surgical revascularization.

Occasionally, ventricular tachycardia or pulmonary edema occurs as a manifestation of acute coronary syndrome. Patients with these symptoms usually are operated on urgently. Intravenous lidocaine or other antiarrhythmic medication is administered to suppress ventricular arrhythmias until the heart is revascularized. In patients with pulmonary edema, a pulmonary artery catheter may be placed to better assess intravascular preload and afterload and guide diuretic and vasodilating therapy, respectively. Preoperative intubation and mechanical ventilation also may become necessary to support the patient.

Because accelerating angina or angina that occurs at rest may represent MI, it is important that it is detected promptly and reported to the cardiac surgeon. Electrocardiograms taken during episodes of chest pain and serial measurement of isoenzyme levels help determine whether acute MI has occurred. If evolving MI is detected within 4 to 6 hours of onset, the patient may undergo emergent surgery. Prompt revascularization may limit infarct size because the evolution of necrosis and resulting infarct size are influenced by alterations in myocardial oxygen supply and demand during the first several hours after the onset of blood flow occlusion (Roberts et al., 1994).

An operation performed more than 6 hours but within 24 to 48 hours of MI onset carries an increased risk of operative death. Restoring perfusion to recently infarcted muscle can cause a complex pathophysiologic cellular process, termed *reperfusion injury*, which produces significant ventricular dysfunction. If enzymatic or electrocardiographic evidence of MI is present, the operation typically is delayed for several days. Urgent revascularization may become necessary if post-infarction angina persists despite pharmacologic antianginal therapy and balloon counterpulsation, or if counterpulsation is contraindicated. Operative risk is considerably higher in these patients.

Ventricular Dysfunction

Patients with significant acute or chronic *ventricular dysfunction* also require special management in the preoperative period. Acute ventricular dysfunction (ie, cardiogenic shock) can occur in preoperative patients with acute valvular dysfunction, postinfarction ventricular septal defect, aortic dissection, or infective endocarditis. Although left ventricular failure is more common, isolated right ventricular failure is sometimes present, such as in patients with acute tricuspid regurgitation secondary to infective endocarditis. Often it is impossible to correct cardiogenic shock with medical therapy alone, and emergent surgical therapy may be essential.

Severe chronic ventricular dysfunction occurs most often in patients with long-standing hypertension or mitral or aortic valve disease, and in those with prior left ventricular MI. Although these disorders initially affect left ventricular function, producing left-sided heart failure, manifestations of right-sided heart failure eventually develop as well (Braunwald et al., 1997) (Fig. 9-4). Patients with long-standing, severe ventricular dysfunction usually can be identified by their physical appearance, which is one of marked weight loss, malnutrition, and cachexia (Perloff & Braunwald, 1997). *Cardiac cachexia* describes the appearance of a person who is emaciated, often with anasarca (generalized body edema in nearly

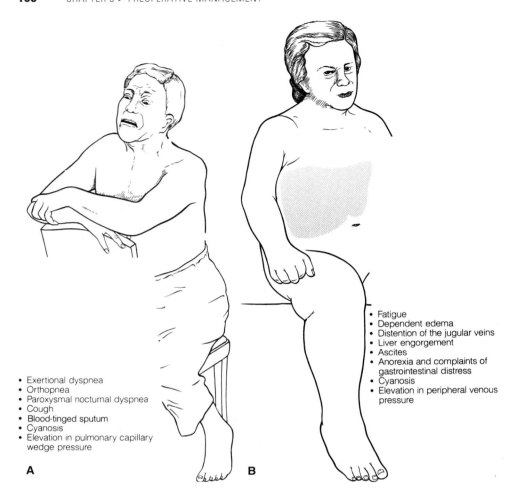

- Exertional dyspnea
- Orthopnea
- Paroxysmal nocturnal dyspnea
- Cough
- Blood-tinged sputum
- Cyanosis
- Elevation in pulmonary capillary wedge pressure

A

- Fatigue
- Dependent edema
- Distention of the jugular veins
- Liver engorgement
- Ascites
- Anorexia and complaints of gastrointestinal distress
- Cyanosis
- Elevation in peripheral venous pressure

B

FIGURE 9-4. Manifestations of left-sided **(A)** and right-sided **(B)** heart failure. (Urban N, Porth CM, 1998: Heart failure and circulatory shock. In Porth CM [ed]: Pathophysiology: Concepts of Altered Health States, ed. 5, pp. 433, 435. Philadelphia, Lippincott Williams & Wilkins)

all regions of the body), ascites, and jaundice secondary to prolonged passive congestion of the liver (Kennedy, 1988). Specific entities that can exacerbate preexisting heart failure include infection, arrhythmias, pulmonary embolus, excessive intake of alcohol, and thyroid disease (Smith et al., 1997).

The presence of congestive heart failure at the time of admission may necessitate postponement of the operation to improve cardiac function and thereby lessen operative risk. Because of the narrow window between maintaining adequate preload and precipitating congestive heart failure in such patients, closely titrated pharmacologic therapy is necessary. A pulmonary artery catheter may be placed to guide therapy. Diuresis and fluid and salt restriction are primary components of treatment. Intravenous inotropic and afterload reduction (vasodilating) agents may be necessary to treat congestive heart failure refractory to oral pharmacologic therapy. Intra-aortic balloon counterpulsation may be instituted to augment afterload reduction.

Recognition of the precarious hemodynamic status in this group of patients is essential. Although independence in self-care activities and intermittent ambulation are important in most preoperative patients to maintain strength and avoid complications of immobility, such activities in patients with severely compromised ventricu-

lar function can have lethal consequences. These patients legitimately need assistance with daily care and may not be able to ambulate safely. If a preoperative patient is unable to perform daily activities independently or is unable to ambulate, the physician is consulted regarding advisability of increasing the patient's level of activity during the preoperative period.

Infective Endocarditis

Another group of preoperative patients who require close observation are those with *infective endocarditis*. Eighty to 90% of patients with infective endocarditis of native cardiac valves are effectively treated medically with an extensive course of organism-specific antimicrobial therapy (Hendren et al., 1992). However, depending on the virility of the organism and extent of valvular damage, emergent surgical therapy sometimes becomes necessary.

Patients with infective endocarditis often are gravely ill with hemodynamic instability and multisystem organ failure (Larbalestier et al., 1992). Close observation is essential to detect findings that indicate a deterioration in the patient's condition, including (1) a new or changed heart murmur; (2) manifestations of congestive heart failure; (3) evidence of systemic (left-sided valvular endocarditis) or pulmonary (right-sided valvular endocarditis) embolism; (4) persistent fever despite antibiotic therapy; and (5) the development of complete heart block representing intramyocardial extension of the infection. Indications for proceeding urgently with surgical therapy include acute valvular regurgitation secondary to leaflet or chordae tendineae destruction, persistent sepsis despite organism-specific antimicrobial therapy, recurrent embolization from the infected valve, or evidence of intramyocardial abscess.

Severe Aortic Stenosis

Patients with severe *aortic stenosis* also require close preoperative monitoring. Patients with aortic stenosis are especially sensitive to afterload reduction or hypovolemia because of fixed obstruction to ventricular output and poor compliance of the ventricle. Therapeutic maneuvers, such as induction of general anesthesia or administration of diuretic or afterload-reducing agents, must be performed with caution. Volume loss and bleeding are poorly tolerated and may lead to catastrophic hemodynamic compromise. The patient with severe aortic stenosis who suffers cardiac arrest can seldom be successfully resuscitated because ventricular tachycardia or fibrillation is easily sustained in the hypertrophied left ventricle. In addition, the onset of atrial fibrillation may cause rapid clinical deterioration in patients with moderate or severe aortic stenosis because atrial contraction supplies up to 40% of ventricular filling during diastole in the presence of a stenotic aortic valve (Jamieson, 1997). Urgent operation may be necessary in patients with severe aortic stenosis and unstable angina because administration of nitroglycerin may cause precipitous hemodynamic instability.

REFERENCES

Antman EM, 1997: Medical management of the patient undergoing cardiac surgery. In Braunwald E (ed): Heart Disease: A Textbook of Cardiovascular Medicine, ed. 5. Philadelphia, WB Saunders

Bates B, Bickley LS, Hoekelman RA, 1995: The abdomen. In A Guide to Physical Examination and History Taking, ed. 6. Philadelphia, JB Lippincott

Braunwald E, 1997: The history. In Braunwald E (ed): Heart Disease: A Textbook of Cardiovascular Medicine, ed. 5. Philadelphia, WB Saunders

Braunwald E, Colucci WS, Grossman W, 1997: Clinical aspects of heart failure: High-output failure; pulmonary edema. In Braunwald E (ed): Heart Disease: A Textbook of Cardiovascular Medicine, ed. 5. Philadelphia, WB Saunders

Campeau L, 1976: Grading of angina pectoris. Circulation 54:522

Canobbio MM, 1990: Assessment. In Cardiovascular Disorders (Mosby's Clinical Nursing Series). St. Louis, CV Mosby

Chatterjee K, 1998: Physical examination. In Topol EJ (ed): Comprehensive Cardiovascular Medicine. Philadelphia, Lippincott Williams & Wilkins

Criteria Committee of the New York Heart Association, 1964: Physical capacity with heart disease. In Diseases of the Heart and Blood Vessels: Nomenclature and Criteria for Diagnosis, ed. 6. Boston, Little, Brown

Dajani AS, Taubert KA, Wilson W, et al., 1997: Prevention of bacterial endocarditis: Recommendations by the American Heart Association. JAMA 277:1794

Doebbeling BN, Pfaller MA, Kuhns KR, et al., 1990: Cardiovascular surgery prophylaxis. J Thorac Cardiovasc Surg 99:981

Fahey VA, 1999: Clinical assessment of the vascular system. In Fahey VA (ed): Vascular Nursing, ed. 3. Philadelphia, WB Saunders

Gay WA Jr, 1990: Aspirin, blood loss and transfusion. Ann Thorac Surg 50:345

Gotch PM, 1991: The endocrine system. In Alspach JG (ed): Core Curriculum for Critical Care Nursing, ed. 4. Philadelphia, WB Saunders

Hendren WG, Morris AS, Rosenkranz ER, et al., 1992: Mitral valve repair for bacterial endocarditis. J Thorac Cardiovasc Surg 103:124

Hillis LD, Lange RA, Winniford MD, Page RL, 1995: Anticoagulants and antiplatelet agents. In Manual of Clinical Problems in Cardiology, ed. 5. Boston, Little, Brown

Jamieson WR, 1997: Mechanical and bioprosthetic aortic valve replacement. In Edmunds LH Jr (ed): Cardiac Surgery in the Adult. New York, McGraw-Hill

Kaiser AB, Kernodle DS, Barg NL, Petracek MR, 1988: Influence of preoperative showers on staphylococcal skin colonization: A comparative trial of antiseptic skin cleansers. Ann Thorac Surg 45:35

Kennedy G, 1988: Clinical cardiac assessment. In Kern LS (ed): Cardiac Critical Care Nursing. Rockville, MD, Aspen

Kolins J, Kolins MD, 1990: Informed consent, risk, and blood transfusion. J Thorac Cardiovasc Surg 100:88

Lake CL, 1985: Preoperative evaluation and preparation of cardiac surgical patients. In Cardiovascular Anesthesia. New York, Springer-Verlag

Larbalestier RI, Kinchla NM, Aranki SF, et al., 1992: Acute bacterial endocarditis. Circulation 86 (Suppl II):II-68

Levine EA, Rosen AL, Sehgal LR, et al., 1991: Erythropoietin deficiency after coronary artery bypass procedures. Ann Thorac Surg 51:764

Mathew JP, Barash PG, 1996: Anesthesia for cardiac surgery. In Baue AE, Geha AS, Hammond GL, et al. (eds): Glenn's Thoracic and Cardiovascular Surgery, ed. 6. Stamford, CT, Appleton & Lange

Miedzinski LJ, Callaghan JC, Fanning EA, et al., 1990: Antimicrobial prophylaxis for open heart operations. Ann Thorac Surg 50:800

Paraskos JA, 1997: Evaluation of the patient with chest pain. In Alpert JS (ed): Cardiology for the Primary Care Physician, ed. 2. Philadelphia, Current Medicine

Perloff JK, Braunwald E, 1997: Physical examination of the heart and circulation. In Braunwald E (ed): Heart Disease: A Textbook of Cardiovascular Medicine, ed. 5. Philadelphia, WB Saunders

Roberts R, Morris D, Pratt CM, Alexander RW, 1994: Pathophysiology, recognition and treatment of acute myocardial infarction and its complications. In Schlant RC, Alexander RW, et al. (eds): The Heart, ed. 8. New York, McGraw-Hill

Roberts R, Pratt CM, 1991: Medical treatment of coronary artery disease. In Roberts R (ed): Coronary Heart Disease and Risk Factors. Mount Kisco, NY, Futura

Sather-Levine B, 1990: Perioperative agents. In Underhill SL, Woods SL, Froelicher ES, Halpenny CJ (eds): Cardiovascular Medications for Cardiac Nursing. Philadelphia, JB Lippincott

Scott WJ, Kessler R, Wernly JA, 1990: Blood conservation in cardiac surgery. Ann Thorac Surg 50:843

Sethna DH, Moffitt EA, Hackner EL, 1990: Anesthetic techniques for cardiac surgery. In Gray RJ, Matloff JM (eds): Medical Management of the Cardiac Surgical Patient. Baltimore, Williams & Wilkins

Skov P, Motzer SU, 1995: History taking and physical examination. In Woods SL, Froelicher ES, Halpenny CJ, Motzer SU (eds): Cardiac Nursing, ed. 3. Philadelphia, JB Lippincott

Smith TW, Kelly RA, Stevenson LW, et al., 1997: Management of heart failure. In Braunwald E (ed): Heart Disease: A Textbook of Cardiovascular Medicine, ed. 5. Philadelphia, WB Saunders

Spratt KA, Fiengo MN, Michelson EL, 1997: Evaluation of the patient with palpitations and non-life-threatening cardiac arrhythmias. In Alpert JS (ed): Cardiology for the Primary Care Physician, ed. 2. Philadelphia, Current Medicine

Topol EJ, 1998: The history. In Topol EJ (ed): Comprehensive Cardiovascular Medicine. Philadelphia, Lippincott Williams & Wilkins

van der Starre PJ, Trienekens PH, Harinck-de Weerd JE, et al., 1988: Comparative study between two prophylactic antibiotic regimens of cefamandole during coronary artery bypass surgery. Ann Thorac Surg 45:24

Waddell TK, Rotstein OD, 1994: Antimicrobial prophylaxis in surgery. CMAJ 151:925

Watanabe Y, Fuse K, Konighi T, et al., 1991: Autologous blood transfusion with recombinant human erythropoietin in heart operations. Ann Thorac Surg 51:767

Education and Psychological Support for the Patient and Family

Cardiothoracic surgical nurses play a major role in preparing patients and families for operations. In facilities where cardiac surgery is performed routinely, preoperative instruction and psychological support are an integral component of nursing care. Ideally, nurses who will provide care in the postoperative period perform preoperative teaching and counseling. The designated nurse can assess the patient before surgery, plan for any special postoperative or discharge needs, and communicate information to other nursing staff. In addition, the nurse conveys to the patient the knowledge and skill of those who will be providing postoperative care and establishes a relationship with the patient and family before surgery.

Preparation of the patient for surgery is commonly referred to as *preoperative teaching,* but the focus is actually as much on providing psychological support to the patient and family as on educational needs. Because most patients undergoing elective operations are admitted to the hospital on the morning of the planned operation, preoperative preparation usually is performed in an outpatient setting. Patients recovering from acute myocardial infarction or who have just undergone catheterization may receive preoperative instruction while in the hospital.

▶ Preoperative Education

Patient education is known to have many positive effects on patients with life-threatening illnesses, including increased knowledge retention, improved pain management, decreased length of hospitalization, and improved patient adherence to the medical regimen (Barr, 1989). The provision of concrete objective information also is effective in reducing emotional negative responses during threatening procedures. Describing the experience from the patient's point of view in unambiguous, concrete, and objective terms facilitates coping by decreasing the differences between expectations and actual experience and by increasing the patient's understanding of the experience (Clark, 1997).

Preoperative education is one type of patient education in which the patient is instructed regarding a planned operative procedure and the projected postoperative course. Just as the surgeon discusses with each patient the objectives of an operation and its potential benefits and risks, the nurse describes to the patient and family the planned perioperative events and what will be expected of the patient during the postoperative period. Preoperative education differs from other forms of patient education in that it is necessary to provide in a short time span a body of specific information that is relevant only to the period of hospitalization. In addition, the instruction must be accomplished during a time when patients are facing a major operation.

Patients usually are very apprehensive during the preoperative period. Although motivation for learning is high because of the life-threatening nature of cardiac surgery, learning capacity often is inversely diminished by anxiety. Fear, anxiety, uncertainty, loss of control, and decreased self-esteem are common in patients confronted with the need for hospitalization and surgery (Breemhaar et al., 1996). These factors can greatly impede the patient's capacity for concentration and learning. Also, patients undergoing cardiac operations often are elderly. Older patients may have neurologic or physiologic impairments that interfere with their ability to learn, and they may be less able to adapt to new and distressing stimuli.

Preoperative teaching usually is performed before the hospital admission, typically when the patient comes to the hospital for preoperative diagnostic studies. In patients hospitalized during the preoperative period, teaching typically is performed the day before the planned operation. The need to perform teaching in an outpatient setting or during an acute illness necessitates a preoperative teaching program with realistic guidelines and standard content, teaching materials, and methods of documentation. Such a program ensures that every patient receives adequate preparation for surgery and that the nurses' interventions and patients' responses are communicated appropriately. Evaluation and continued improvement of the preoperative preparation program can be achieved by soliciting feedback from postoperative patients and their families about their own recent experiences.

Before initiating preoperative teaching, the nurse reviews the patient's cardiac history, presence of risk factors, associated medical problems, planned surgical procedure, and operative risk as assessed by the surgeon. This is followed by an assessment of the patient's current level of understanding, capacity and motivation for learning new information, and emotional status. A continuum of emotional responses is represented in preoperative cardiac surgical patients. Some patients, such as those undergoing elective valve replacement, have known and planned for the operation for months. On the other end of the spectrum are patients operated on urgently, such as those with unstable angina. The latter group of patients may have had no knowledge of a heart problem before the present hospitalization. In this situation, the patient must, within a matter of hours, adjust not only to the presence of a life-threatening health problem but also to the need for a major operation.

Barriers to learning are identified and the teaching plan is formulated with these limitations in mind (Table 10-1). Principles of adult education are taken into consideration. Guiding assumptions for preoperative teaching of adults include (1) adults want to be active participants in the learning process, (2) past experiences have an impact on learning, (3) major life events stimulate a desire to learn, and (4) information that is immediately applicable is of most interest (Gessner, 1989). The nurse also must evaluate the family's norms and beliefs so that what is taught is congruent with the patient and family's health beliefs and experience (Hudak et al., 1998). Chachkes and Christ (1996) recommend several strategies to achieve a culturally sensitive approach to patient education, including (1) becoming aware of one's own cultural values and beliefs and their influence, (2) developing and maintaining an attitude of respect for the broad range of cultural differences, and (3) seeking con-

TABLE 10-1
Potential Barriers to Learning in Cardiac Patients
Severity of illness
Advanced age
Anxiety
Depression
Separation from loved ones
Time constraints on teaching
Cultural differences
Language or literacy constraints

tinuous education about predominant cultures treated in the institution.

Despite variability in learning needs, emotional responses, and cultural norms, most patients are focused principally on implications of the operation itself. Also, because teaching time is limited, content should be relevant to the patient's current problem (ie, the need for information about the perioperative course). Usually, a generalized description of the projected course is given to the patient, including the preoperative regimen, various units in which the patient will stay, the number of days in each unit, and what the patient's condition will be like during each phase. Interventions that require active participation from the patient, such as coughing and deep breathing exercises, are highlighted. Information commonly included in preoperative teaching is discussed in the next section (Table 10-2).

Content

Components of the preoperative regimen that may be discussed with the patient include evaluations by members of the surgical team; preoperative diagnostic stud-

TABLE 10-2
Scope of Information for Preoperative Teaching
Basic anatomy and pathologic condition
Description of operative procedure
Common diagnostic and preoperative studies
Description of perioperative course
Assistive catheters and tubes
Visiting procedures
Pulmonary hygiene
Progression of activity
Appetite, emotional responses, physical stamina
Pain and pain control
Information about valve prostheses or pacemakers
Available resources
Support personnel
Insurance or financial concerns
Community services after discharge

ies; antibacterial showers; preoperative sedation; withholding of food and drink after midnight; and shaving of the chest, groin, and legs. Patients are informed that they will spend the first 24 postoperative hours in an intensive care unit and the remainder of the hospitalization (3 to 4 days) on a cardiothoracic surgical unit. Basic information about monitoring and supportive catheters and devices is given. The patient usually does not need a detailed description of all the various invasive catheters and tubes. By the time the patient is alert enough to examine the attached devices, most will have been removed. In addition, catheters and tubes are placed in the operating room, so the patient will have no memory of their insertion, and once in place, they usually are not uncomfortable or bothersome.

Typically it is best to discuss specifically the need for intubation and assisted ventilation. Although most patients are extubated on the day of the operation, awareness of the endotracheal tube often is discomforting for the patient during the early postoperative hours. The tube is not painful, but the patient is unable to talk or take fluids by mouth. In addition, the sensation of assisted mechanical ventilation may be frightening. For these reasons, it is reassuring to explain to the patient in advance that a nurse will be readily available during the period of intubation to interpret and assist with basic needs. It also is helpful to prepare the patient for the presence of a urinary drainage catheter. Often patients are unaware that urine drains freely from the bladder while a catheter is in place. Particularly in men, the catheter may cause a sensation of needing to urinate.

A frequent concern of patients is separation from family during the operation and early postoperative period. Usually the family may visit during the immediate preoperative hours and accompany the patient during transfer to the operating room. It is helpful to inform the patient and family that family members will be able to stay in a comfortable area near the operating room and that the surgeon will discuss the operation with them as soon as it is completed. In addition, many cardiothoracic surgical services have advanced practice nurses who act as liaisons to facilitate communication with the family during the operation and the postoperative period. Family members usually wish to visit patients as soon as possible after the operation, and this can be arranged in most cases. Often patients are quite concerned about being able to have dentures, glasses, or a hairpiece in place as soon as possible. Although these requests may seem minor, they can take on unusual significance for some patients, and accommodating the patient's wishes provides a great deal of comfort.

The patient also is instructed about the anticipated progression of recovery during the postoperative period (eg, initiation of bathroom privileges and resumption of a regular diet). Particular attention is given to preparing the patient to participate with pulmonary hygiene measures and progressive ambulation. Incentive spirometry or other assistive device for prevention of atelectasis is demonstrated and the patient is given an opportunity to practice using the device. Expectations for getting out of bed and progressive ambulation in the corridors should be communicated to the patient. Patients who understand the rationale will be better prepared to cooperate actively with deep breathing and coughing exercises as well as early and progressive ambulation.

Excessive fatigue, depression, insomnia, and anorexia are almost universal complaints after a cardiac operation, and it is beneficial for the patient to understand that these may occur during the recovery process. Patients may be reassured that these are expected, transient problems that should diminish gradually and resolve. Often patients fear the pain that accompanies cardiac surgery. Although pain tolerance varies greatly among individuals, patients may be reassured that postoperative pain usually is not significant after sternotomy and that adequate analgesic agents will be available.

Beyond the provision of essential information, the nurse is guided by assessment of the patient's readiness to learn and emotional status. Patients usually ask questions that reveal what information will be most useful to them. In most instances, patients request information that will lessen anxiety about the loss of control and uncertain outcome associated with a major operation. Attempts to educate patients about the underlying disease process, risk factor modification, or chronic medical therapies usually are best deferred until after the operation. However, reference material should be available for patients who do want to learn more about the underlying disease during the preoperative period. The need to individualize content to individual learning needs cannot be overemphasized. Providing content that exceeds the patient's ability or desire to learn may cause the patient to become confused or increasingly anxious.

Teaching Strategies

Preoperative teaching is more efficacious if a person's learning style can be matched with an appropriate teaching technique (Lindsay et al., 1991). The phenomenon of widespread Internet availability with abundant, unfiltered health information has added a new dimension to the provision of effective patient education. Given a suitably designed interface, most patients consider information access using a computer acceptable and may find it preferable to obtain information in this way (Bental et al., 1999). Many patients have independently obtained information from Internet web sites about their illness or an impending operation before the preoperative teaching session. Nurses can play a key role in ensuring that computer-based information is used effectively to enhance patient education by directing patients to Internet web sites with reliable information and by clarifying information that patients have derived already from Internet sources.

In some facilities, group teaching sessions are performed. Although this provides patients with a forum to share concerns and support one another, it has the distinct disadvantage that individual needs for information and support are sometimes compromised by the needs of other group members. If group teaching is used, it should not replace an individualized session during the preoperative period in which a nurse devotes full attention to providing counseling to each patient and family.

A written brochure is an excellent supplement to preoperative teaching and is used in most facilities. Studies demonstrate that patients remember only 29% to 72% of information provided to them, and that the more information presented, the lower the recall rate (Houts et al., 1998). Use of a teaching booklet enhances consistency of information and provides a reference for both the patient and family. If a booklet specific to the institution is developed, lay terminology should be used and information should be presented in a supportive fashion. During preparation of a teaching booklet, the level of literacy in the patient population must be considered. A lack of reading skills, most prevalent in minority populations and in those with lower per capita income, may limit the ability of patients to access and use critical information (TenHave et al., 1997). Content is evaluated to ensure that the reading level is appropriate for most people who will be receiving it. Language barriers also must be considered for those patients whose first language is other than that in which material is presented.

Computers can provide invaluable assistance in producing patient education materials for specific subsets of patients. A major advantage of computer-generated teaching resources is that it is possible to adapt material to particular needs of individuals and organizations; material is not fixed but can be selected and presented differently depending on particular needs (Bental et al., 1999). Alternatively, a commercially prepared patient teaching booklet for cardiac surgical patients may be used.

Audiovisual aids, such as instructional videotapes, also may be helpful. Retention of learned material is enhanced when more than one sense is involved in the learning process (Oka et al., 1995). Audiovisual aids provide a creative supplement to preoperative teaching and, like written materials, enhance consistency of information presented to the patient. Opportunities for informal teaching, incorporated in performance of routine preoperative nursing interventions, allow repetition of important information. In addition, interventions and their rationale are explained as they are performed. A tour of the postoperative nursing unit is helpful for some patients.

► Psychological Support

Almost all patients experience some fear and anxiety when facing a cardiac operation. Sources of anxiety for preoperative patients include physical discomfort, socioeconomic problems, a feeling of helplessness, fear of disability, uncertainty of the outcome, separation from family, and the possibility of death (Rocey, 1990). Anxiety may be manifested by a variety of psychophysiologic symptoms, such as increased tension, increased helplessness, decreased self-assurance, sympathetic stimulation, and focusing on the perceived object of fear (Carty, 1991).

Although the provision of factual information is effective in reducing anxiety, preoperative teaching is neither the only nor the most important method of supporting patients before surgery. In fact, the need for psychological support far outweighs the need for information in many patients. One study of patients scheduled for cardiac catheterization demonstrated that once patients had been given adequate information to allow informed consent for the procedure, the presence of a caring person who interacted socially was as effective as repetition of information in reducing anxiety (Peterson, 1991).

Interventions to provide psychological support include allowing verbalization of concerns and providing reassurance about the commitment of the nurses and physicians to the patient's well-being. Scheduling one nurse to work consistently with the patient allows more thorough assessment, planning, and coordination of care, and provides the setting for development of rapport between the nurse and patient (Oka et al., 1995). In addition to the patient's primary nurse, other resources also play an important role. An advanced practice nurse who works with the patient and family throughout the hospitalization can assist staff nurses in assessing the patient's need for psychological support and also may have more flexibility in scheduling consistent time to spend with the patient and family.

Presumably, people who can mobilize strong supportive resources from within their social relationships are better able to withstand negative effects of stresses on their health (Porth, 1998). Social support is thought to help buffer the person from potentially pathogenic effects of stress by preventing the immediate appraisal of stress after an event, or by facilitating reappraisal or inhibiting an emotionally linked physiologic response after an event is perceived as stressful (Emery & Becker, 1998).

Family members almost always are a patient's greatest source of support and, as much as possible, should be included in preoperative teaching. If they have received the same information as the patient, they can better reinforce teaching with the patient, who may be too ill or anxious to retain information presented during the preoperative teaching session. Also, with shortened hospital stays, families are taking on increased responsibilities in caring for patients at home; they need appropriate information to carry out these responsibilities (Houts et al., 1998).

Patients who have undergone similar operative procedures also can provide support to the preoperative patient. Often, a visit from a convalescing patient is reassuring. In some facilities, people who have previously undergone heart surgery are permitted to visit preoperative patients and provide supportive information.

Occasionally, preoperative patients are nearly incapacitated by anxiety. Severe anxiety during the preoperative period warrants close observation and special nursing interventions. It is often these severely anxious patients in whom disorientation or frank psychosis develops after surgery. Severe anxiety may be manifested either overtly or in a more insidious fashion. If the patient is able to acknowledge the fear and anxiety, it is easier for the nurse to intervene by talking with the patient, allowing verbalization of concerns, and providing reassurance. An anxiolytic medication, such as diazepam, may be administered, particularly in patients with ischemic heart disease.

Occasionally, patients are both severely anxious and unable to acknowledge the anxiety. The resulting manifestation may be hostile, demanding, or controlling behaviors. The patient tends to alienate staff by these behaviors, which may reduce the amount of emotional support that is given when in fact more is needed. Another manifestation may be inordinate concern by the patient regarding one aspect of the perioperative care. In attempting to establish a sense of control, the patient may magnify its importance out of proportion. For example, the patient may threaten to leave if not given a private room or insist that medical or nursing students not be allowed to participate in the care.

Most often, it is the nurse at the bedside who deals with the brunt of these behaviors. Effective methods of providing support to severely anxious patients include (1) listening to the patient's concerns and requests; (2) making special accommodations if they are reasonable and do not compromise the ability of the team to care for the patient safely; (3) providing a rationale when special accommodations are not possible; and (4) throughout all interactions, maintaining an air of confidence in the team's ability to provide safe care, and an attitude of concern for making the situation as comfortable as possible for the patient. If the patient's need for support is beyond what the cardiac surgical team realistically can provide, psychiatric consultation is obtained.

REFERENCES

Barr WJ, 1989: Teaching patients with life-threatening illnesses. Nurs Clin North Am 24:639

Bental DS, Cawsey A, Jones R, 1999: Patient information systems that tailor to the individual. Patient Education and Counseling 36:171

Breemhaar B, van den Borne HW, Mullen PD, 1996: Inadequacies of surgical patient education. Patient Education and Counseling 28:31

Carty JL, 1991: Psychosocial aspects. In Alspach JG (ed): Core Curriculum for Critical Care Nursing, ed. 4. Philadelphia, WB Saunders

Chachkes E, Christ G, 1996: Cross cultural issues in patient education. Patient Education and Counseling 27:13

Clark CR, 1997: Creating information messages for reducing patient distress during health care procedures. Patient Education and Counseling 30:247

Emery CF, Becker NL, 1998: Psychosocial issues and the heart. In Topol EJ (ed): Comprehensive Cardiovascular Medicine. Philadelphia, Lippincott Williams & Wilkins

Gessner BA, 1989: Adult education. Nurs Clin North Am 24:589

Houts PS, Bachrach R, Witmer JT, et al., 1998: Using pictographs to enhance recall of spoken medical instructions. Patient Education and Counseling 35:83

Hudak CM, Gallo BM, Morton PG, 1998: Patient and family education in a changing health care environment. In Critical Care Nursing: A Holistic Approach, ed. 7. Philadelphia, Lippincott Williams & Wilkins

Lindsay C, Jennrich JA, Biemolt M, 1991: Programmed instruction booklet for cardiac rehabilitation teaching. Heart Lung 20:648

Oka RK, Burke LE, Froelicher ESS, 1995: Emotional responses and inpatient education. In Woods SL, Froelicher ES, Halpenny CJ, Motzer SU (eds): Cardiac Nursing, ed. 3. Philadelphia, JB Lippincott

Peterson M, 1991: Patient anxiety before cardiac catheterization: An intervention study. Heart Lung 20:643

Porth CM, 1998: Stress and adaptation. In Porth CM (ed): Pathophysiology: Concepts of Altered Health States, ed. 5. Philadelphia, Lippincott Williams & Wilkins

Rocey DL, 1990: Preparation of the patient and family. In Gray RJ, Matloff JM (eds): Medical Management of the Cardiac Surgical Patient. Baltimore, Williams & Wilkins

TenHave TR, Van Horn B, Kumanyika S, et al., 1997: Literacy assessment in a cardiovascular nutrition education setting. Patient Education and Counseling 31:139

INTRAOPERATIVE CONSIDERATIONS

11

Intraoperative Patient Management

Intraoperative care of the cardiac surgical patient is performed collaboratively by the cardiothoracic surgeon, cardiac anesthesiologist, perfusionist, and operating room nursing staff. Each team member, under the direction of the surgeon, assumes responsibility for specialized components of patient care and monitoring during the intraoperative period. Established patient care protocols, clear and concise communication, and a thorough understanding of the planned procedure are essential to safe conduct of the operation. Although all team members participate in intraoperative patient care, the anesthesiologist has primary responsibility for ensuring the patient's hemodynamic stability while the surgeon performs the operation.

► Preoperative Evaluation and Preparation

Anesthetic management begins with a thorough preoperative evaluation. Because most patients are admitted to the hospital on the morning of an elective cardiac operation, the preoperative evaluation typically is performed during an outpatient visit 1 or 2 days before the planned operation. Assessment of cardiovascular and pulmonary status and a review of the current medication regimen are of particular importance in the clinical history. The preoperative physical examination focuses on the heart, lungs, peripheral pulses, extremities, and abdomen. The patient also is examined to detect any potential difficulties with intubation or vascular cannulation.

Baseline vital signs are noted. The chest roentgenogram and electrocardiogram are reviewed along with information obtained from available diagnostic studies, such as cardiac catheterization and echocardiography. Pertinent preoperative laboratory studies include serum electrolytes,

blood urea nitrogen, and creatinine; complete blood cell count; blood glucose level; liver enzyme analysis; coagulation studies; and urinalysis. Correctable abnormalities that might increase morbidity, such as congestive heart failure or infection, are identified and treated before the operation. The anesthesiologist often categorizes the patient's severity of illness using the American Society of Anesthesiologists' (ASA) Physical Status Classification (Table 11-1). Accuracy of the ASA Classification system is controversial; although some research has indicated that it is useful in predicting perioperative mortality, other studies have indicated that it is not predictive (Mangano, 1999).

The anesthetic approach is formulated based on the specific type of cardiac disease, the estimated complexity of the operative procedure and the patient's functional status. Patient age and associated cardiovascular problems, such as hypertension, congestive heart failure, or cerebral vascular disease, are taken into consideration. Coexisting medical diseases, such as chronic obstructive pulmonary disease, renal insufficiency, or diabetes mellitus, also influence the planned anesthetic management. In unstable patients, such as those with acute myocardial ischemia, cardiogenic shock, or severe aortic stenosis, special anesthetic techniques are planned to avoid precipitous perioperative complications.

Unless the patient requires preoperative hospitalization (eg, for unstable angina, acute myocardial infarction, or congestive heart failure), he or she is not hospitalized until the morning of the operation. Thus, the patient is not under observation during the night before the operation and must be instructed to withhold food or liquids after midnight, to take medications as directed, and to contact the managing physician for any exacerbation of symptoms that might represent myocardial ischemia or congestive heart failure. Withholding oral intake for 6 to 8 hours before an elective operation

TABLE 11-1

American Society of Anesthesiologists' Physical Status Classification

Class I	A normally healthy patient
Class II	A patient with mild systemic disease
Class III	A patient with severe systemic disease that is not incapacitating
Class IV	A patient with an incapacitating systemic disease that is a constant threat to life
Class V	A moribund patient who is not expected to survive for 24 hours with or without operation

"E" added to the classification number signifies an emergency operation.
From Owens WD, Felts JA, Spitznagel EL, 1978: ASA physical status classifications: A study of consistency of ratings. Anesthesiology 49:239.

is recommended to reduce the potential for aspiration during and after anesthesia induction.

Most medications, particularly antianginal and antiarrhythmic agents, are continued during the preoperative period to avoid precipitous myocardial ischemia or arrhythmias. Patients with severe preoperative anxiety and coronary artery disease may require the addition of an anxiolytic medication to avoid precipitous myocardial ischemia during the preoperative period at home. Aspirin often is discontinued the week preceding a planned cardiac operation. Aspirin impairs platelet function and increases the likelihood of excessive perioperative bleeding. In patients receiving intravenous heparin, the heparin typically is continued until the morning of the operation or, if the patient has unstable angina, until transport to the operating room.

In diabetic patients, oral hypoglycemic agents are withheld on the morning of the operation. In insulin-dependent patients, a reduced dose of insulin is prescribed and blood glucose levels are measured during the operation on a frequent basis. Patients who have been receiving steroids are at risk for development of acute adrenal insufficiency and circulatory shock when exogenous glucocorticoids are withheld because of suppressed adrenal function that is insufficient to meet the stress of a surgical procedure (Murray & Torres, 1999). Therefore, patients who have been on chronic steroid therapy are given parenteral steroids before the operation and during the postoperative period until an oral diet is resumed. Preoperative evaluation and preparation of the cardiac surgical patient are described in greater detail in Chapter 9, Preoperative Management. Psychological preparation of the patient is an integral component of preoperative patient preparation and is discussed in Chapter 10, Education and Psychological Support for the Patient and Family.

Preoperative medication usually is administered before the patient leaves the nursing unit to suppress anxiety and induce sedation. Preoperative sedation facilitates patient cooperation during the preparatory period in the operating room when invasive procedures must be accomplished. In addition, it suppresses physiologic stress

responses so that baseline hemodynamic parameters may be measured accurately. The anesthesiologist prescribes the specific agents and dosage for a given patient based on a number of factors, including age, level of anxiety, type of cardiac disease, and associated medical conditions, particularly pulmonary disease.

A commonly used premedication combination is oral diazepam, with intramuscular morphine and scopolamine; diazepam is anxiolytic, and morphine and scopolamine provide analgesia and amnesia, respectively (Kaplan & Wynands, 1999). Accurate timing of administration is important so that the patient has minimal apprehension yet remains hemodynamically stable and alert enough to cooperate with preliminary intraoperative preparations. In unstable patients, preoperative medication is omitted to avoid hemodynamic alterations during patient transfer. Instead, sedatives are given in the operating room under direct observation of the anesthesiologist. Unstable patients are transported to the operating room by medical and nursing personnel with appropriate ventilatory, monitoring, and resuscitation equipment.

► Intraoperative Preparation and Monitoring

An operating room nurse greets the patient on arrival and assumes responsibility for nursing management until the patient is transferred to the postoperative unit. Prophylactic antibiotics almost always are prescribed for prevention of perioperative wound infection and are administered intravenously on the patient's arrival in the operating room. The patient is positioned, using padding as required to prevent pressure necrosis and to optimize exposure for the planned operation. For most cardiac operations, a median sternotomy approach is used. The patient is positioned supine, with the sternum parallel to the floor. A padded roll is placed between the patient's shoulders with arms lying on either side to prevent brachial plexus injury (Nolan & Zacour, 1998). An antimicrobial solution is used to cleanse the neck, chest, abdomen, both groins, and both legs (if saphenous vein harvesting is planned), and sterile drapes are applied in appropriate fashion.

During cardiac operations, any evidence of cardiac, respiratory, neurologic, or renal dysfunction must be detected and treated promptly to prevent irreversible organ damage. Accordingly, a multitude of catheters and devices are used to monitor the function of all major organ systems. As soon as the patient arrives, electrocardiographic, noninvasive blood pressure, and pulse oximetry monitoring are initiated to allow rapid identification of ischemic changes, arrhythmias, hypotension, or hypoxemia.

Ongoing electrocardiographic monitoring is performed using leads that allow adequate assessment of ST segment changes, particularly in the anterolateral (lead V_5) and inferior (lead II) myocardial wall. An esophageal lead may be used in selected patients to detect right ventricular and posterior wall ischemia and to detect P waves indicative of atrial activity during cardioplegia administration. ST segment elevation, which may be indicative of myocardial ischemia, can occur at any time before or after cardiopulmonary bypass but is most likely after removal of the aortic cross-clamp during myocardial reperfusion (London & Kaplan, 1999). Arrhythmias are most likely during insertion of the pulmonary artery catheter, intubation, surgical manipulation of the heart, reperfusion after release of the aortic cross-clamp, and episodes of myocardial ischemia (Friedman & Sethna, 1990).

Arterial, pulmonary artery, and central venous pressure monitoring are instituted before cardiac operations that involve extracorporeal circulation. Because the patient is vulnerable to myocardial ischemia or low cardiac output during anesthesia induction, these catheters usually are inserted after sedation but before induction. Myocardial ischemia is most likely in patients with coronary artery disease but also can occur in patients with valvular or congenital heart disease. Hypovolemia secondary to diuretic therapy or angiographic dye (eg, administered during a recent cardiac catheterization) may require fluid infusion before or during anesthesia induction.

An indwelling arterial cannula is placed for arterial pressure monitoring and intermittent arterial oxygen tension measurements. The radial artery almost always is used for this purpose after ulnar artery patency is confirmed with the Allen test. During the period of cardiopulmonary bypass, arterial blood gases are monitored continuously using a sensor in the arterial tubing of the bypass circuit distal to the oxygenator. A pulmonary artery catheter is inserted through the jugular or subclavian vein to allow continuous monitoring of intracardiac pressures (pulmonary artery and right atrial pressures). Cardiac output and mixed venous oxygen measurements also are obtained using the pulmonary artery catheter. Pulmonary artery diastolic pressure is used to guide perioperative fluid management. Right atrial pressures provide information about right ventricular function. For patients undergoing complex operations or with specific clinical requirements, pulmonary artery catheters are available that provide additional monitoring and therapeutic capabilities, including continuous measurement of mixed venous oxygen saturation, continuous cardiac output measurement, measurement of right ventricular volumes and ejection fraction, and temporary cardiac pacing (Lichtenthal, 1998; Headley, 1998).

A separate triple-lumen central venous catheter may be inserted to provide ports for continuous infusion of medications. A large-bore peripheral intravenous catheter is placed for administering fluids and blood products. If the need for intra-aortic balloon counterpulsation is anticipated, a femoral artery catheter or sheath may be placed to make percutaneous balloon catheter insertion easier. All invasive catheters and monitoring devices are secured to prevent inadvertent disconnection during the operation.

A urinary drainage catheter is placed to monitor adequacy of urine output in the anesthetized patient. Core body temperature is monitored using a blood (pulmonary artery catheter), urethral (urinary catheter), or esophageal thermistor. Nasopharyngeal, tympanic, or rectal temperature often is monitored as well. In some institutions, a myocardial probe is placed in the ventricular myocardium to monitor myocardial temperature directly during the period of aortic cross-clamping.

Ongoing temperature monitoring is essential during cardiac operations to evaluate the status of patient cooling and rewarming, monitor the degree of myocardial protection, and detect the presence of malignant hyperthermia. Anesthetized patients are poikilothermic—that is, body temperature is controlled by the environment rather than by intrinsic regulation by the hypothalamus. Redistribution of body heat and heat loss to the environment result in mild hypothermia before cardiopulmonary bypass (Leslie & Sessler, 1998). In addition to hypothermia due to passive heat loss, hypothermia is induced deliberately during the period of aortic cross-clamping to protect the myocardium and decrease systemic oxygen consumption (Savino & Cheung, 1997). Rewarming is performed before discontinuing cardiopulmonary bypass. Rewarming that occurs too rapidly can produce cerebral hyperthermia and postoperative cognitive dysfunction (Yao et al., 1998).

Capnometry, the monitoring of airway carbon dioxide (CO_2) partial pressure, is used routinely to allow rapid detection of disorders of ventilation, CO_2 production, or CO_2 transport that may occur because of esophageal intubation, apnea, disconnection of the breathing circuit, extubation of the trachea, or airway obstruction (Savino & Cheung, 1997). Intraoperative echocardiography, using transesophageal or epicardial transducers, may be used and provides important information regarding intraoperative myocardial performance, valve function, regional myocardial function, anatomic shunting, intrachamber air, and effectiveness of venting (Reves et al., 1995).

Electroencephalography sometimes is performed during cardiac operations to monitor intraoperative cerebral function and to detect evidence of acute (and potentially reversible) brain injury or ischemia. It also may be used to provide information about the functional state of the brain in specific clinical situations, such as when a deep hypothermic circulatory arrest technique is used or when barbiturates or other agents are administered to slow cerebral metabolism (Sebel, 1998). Although neurologic complications are one of the most significant causes of morbidity after cardiac operations, neurologic monitoring during routine cardiac operations has not been demonstrated directly to reduce the incidence of neurologic damage (Levy, 1999). Postoperative neurologic deficits occasionally occur despite the use of available intraoperative neurologic monitoring techniques.

▶ General Anesthesia

General anesthesia is a state of profound central nervous system depression during which there is a complete loss of sensation, consciousness, pain perception, and memory (Abrams, 1998a). The objectives of anesthetic man-

TABLE 11-2

Categories of Anesthetic Agents

Inhalation Agents	Narcotic Agents	Sedative-Hypnotic Agents	Muscle-Relaxing Agents
Desflurane	Alfentanil	Diazepam	Atracurium
Enflurane	Fentanyl	Etomidate	Metocurine
Halothane	Morphine	Ketamine	Pancuronium
Isoflurane	Remifentanil	Midazolam	Succinylcholine
Sevoflurane	Sufentanil	Propofol	Vecuronium
		Thiopental sodium	

agement are to achieve and maintain unconsciousness, amnesia, analgesia, muscle relaxation, and attenuation of stress responses without producing hemodynamic instability or myocardial ischemia. Because no single anesthetic agent produces all of the desired effects, multiple drugs are administered to achieve general anesthesia (Table 11-2). Each anesthetic drug has a unique spectrum of actions; careful titration of drug doses and combining drugs minimizes or counteracts the deleterious effects of individual agents (Hensley et al., 1991).

Anesthetic Agents

Two major categories of anesthetic agents commonly are used for cardiac operations: volatile anesthetics (ie, inhalation agents) and narcotics. The primary difference between inhalation and narcotic agents is that inhalation agents more effectively provide amnesia and analgesia but also cause significant myocardial depression and vasodilatation when used in concentrations sufficient to block sympathetic responses to noxious stimuli (Warner & Warner, 1989) (Table 11-3). Although they produce different perioperative hemodynamic effects, inhalational and narcotic agents are comparable with respect to incidence of postoperative myocardial infarction and death (Slogoff & Keats, 1989).

Inhalation agents are volatile liquids administered with oxygen, nitrous oxide, or air in various concentrations that the patient inspires through a face mask or endotracheal tube. The agents are absorbed from the pulmonary alveoli into the bloodstream. Inhalation agents, such as isoflurane, enflurane, and halothane, are similar in that they rapidly induce anesthesia, allow early emergence, and act as potent myocardial depressants and peripheral vasodilators. They tend to disrupt autoregulation of blood flow in a dose-dependent manner, rendering blood flow more linearly dependent on mean arterial blood pressure instead of remaining constant over a range of perfusion pressures (Savino & Cheung, 1997).

In patients with myocardial ischemia, the negative inotropic effect provided by inhalation agents is beneficial in reducing myocardial oxygen consumption; however, they may exacerbate heart failure in patients with poor left ventricular function (Hensley et al., 1991). The bronchodilating effects of inhalation agents make them useful in patients with obstructive or bronchospastic pulmonary disease (Schneider, 1989). Although inhalation agents have analgesic actions, the associated myocardial depression and vasodilatation may limit their use in doses large enough to provide adequate analgesia. Therefore, narcotics or sedatives are used as supplements to provide adequate anesthesia (ie, blocking of pain perception and physiologic responses to noxious stimuli) and amnesia. Even in the unconscious patient who is unaware of pain, it is important to prevent sympathetic responses, such as tachycardia and hypertension (Hensley et al., 1991).

Narcotics or *opioids* comprise the second major category. Narcotic agents are given intravenously directly into the bloodstream. They rapidly produce profound analgesia and attenuation of sympathetically mediated cardiovascular responses to pain without significant direct effects on myocardial contractility or vasomotor tone (Savino & Cheung, 1997). Most narcotic actions are dose dependent: the larger the dose, the greater is the level of analgesia, respiratory depression, and anesthesia (Warner & Warner, 1989). The synthetic narcotics (eg, fentanyl, sufentanil, alfentanil, and remifentanil) are used most often. Morphine is used less commonly because it produces prolonged postoperative respiratory depression and because vasodilatation and decreased peripheral resistance increase perioperative fluid requirements (Kaplan & Wynands, 1999). Morphine also is less effective in suppressing patient awareness and recall of

TABLE 11-3

Primary Characteristics of Inhalation and Narcotic Agents

INHALATION AGENTS

Dose-dependent myocardial depression
Vasodilatation
Rapid induction
Early emergence

NARCOTIC AGENTS

Potent anesthesia and analgesia
Minimal hemodynamic effects
Slow emergence

intraoperative events and may fail to attenuate cardio-vascular responses to stress (Mathew & Barash, 1996).

A *high-dose narcotic technique* sometimes is used in cardiac operations. With a high-dose technique, narcotic agents are used both to induce and to maintain the anesthetized state. However, none of the opioids provides true anesthesia despite very large doses and high serum concentrations; hypertension and tachycardia can occur in response to surgical stimuli (Kaplan & Wynands, 1999). Also, opioids do not provide hypnosis or amnesia reliably. Recall of intraoperative events, especially conversations, can occur. The period of highest risk for incomplete amnesia is during rewarming before termination of cardiopulmonary bypass; the anesthetic effect of hypothermia is removed, inhalational agents are discontinued, and intravenous agents have been diluted by the perfusate (circulating blood volume in cardiopulmonary bypass circuit) (Hensley et al., 1991). Therefore, when high doses of opioids are used, supplementation with hypnotic or inhalation agents is required to provide complete anesthesia (Kaplan & Wynands, 1999; Reves et al., 1995).

Anesthetic management has been influenced greatly by the trend toward early postoperative extubation and rapid recovery protocols. The respiratory depression associated with a high-dose narcotic technique and the resultant need for prolonged postoperative ventilation make its use impractical for routine cardiac operations because it precludes same-day extubation and rapid progression of postoperative recovery. Modifications that facilitate extubation in less than 8 hours after cardiac surgery include lower doses of opioids supplemented by other agents and the use of propofol infusion or intermittent midazolam to provide postoperative sedation (Kaplan & Wynands, 1999).

A *balanced technique* (ie, a combination of inhalation and narcotic agents) is used most often. Balanced anesthesia using multiple agents allows lower doses of individual agents to be used, thus reducing unwanted adverse effects. A balanced anesthetic technique involving the continuous administration of volatile (eg, isoflurane) or intravenous (eg, propofol) anesthetic agents before, during, and after cardiopulmonary bypass does not increase the risk of perioperative complications and is associated with a low incidence of intraoperative patient awareness (Dowd et al., 1998).

Other categories of agents are important adjuncts for anesthetic management of cardiac surgical patients. Sedative-hypnotics, including barbiturates, benzodiazepines, etomidate, propofol, and ketamine, are a broad class of anesthetic drugs used for preoperative sedation, producing immediate loss of consciousness during intravenous induction of general anesthesia, supplementing the actions of the inhaled anesthetics, and providing sedation in the immediate postoperative period (Savino & Cheung, 1997). Barbiturates (eg, thiopental) produce hypnosis and amnesia, but not analgesia, and are used commonly to induce the anesthetized state. Benzodiazepines (eg, diazepam, lorazepam, and midazolam) have hypnotic, amnesic, anxiolytic, and anticonvulsant effects (Abrams, 1998b).

Neuromuscular blocking agents (ie, muscle relaxants) are used to facilitate endotracheal intubation, provide intercostal muscle paralysis that makes sternal retraction less traumatic, prevent muscle movement during light levels of anesthesia, eliminate diaphragmatic movement, and allow controlled mechanical ventilation (Stanley, 1989). Muscle relaxants are chosen based on the desired speed of onset, duration of action, route of elimination, spectrum of cardiovascular side effects, and cost (Savino & Cheung, 1997). Succinylcholine is a muscle relaxant with a rapid onset and short duration of action; its use is limited primarily to providing neuromuscular blockade for induction and intubation. Vecuronium (intermediate acting), metocurine (long acting), and pancuronium (long acting) are muscle relaxants with longer durations of action that may be used as adjuncts to general anesthesia. Muscle relaxants do not provide analgesia, sedation, or amnesia; therefore, muscle paralysis should not be performed without sedation or general anesthesia (Reves et al., 1995).

Stages of Anesthesia

General anesthesia consists of three phases: (1) induction, (2) maintenance, and (3) emergence. Induction is the transition period from the awake to the anesthetized state. The maintenance period continues until near completion of the procedure. Emergence describes the phase when anesthetic agents are discontinued and the patient is allowed to return to the conscious state.

Before induction, the patient is preoxygenated because hypoxemia and hypercarbia from premedications or intravenous sedatives can lead to hypertension and tachycardia (Friedman & Sethna, 1990). Induction is performed after monitoring is established and just before intubation. It is accomplished using either hypnotics (ie, pharmacologic agents that produce sleep) or narcotics (eg, fentanyl). Thiopental, an ultra–short-acting barbiturate, is used commonly. Other induction agents include droperidol, ketamine, diazepam, and midazolam (Kirklin & Barratt-Boyes, 1993).

Intubation is carried out as soon as the induction agents are administered. A muscle relaxant is used to facilitate intubation by causing temporary paralysis of the jaw, diaphragm, and other skeletal muscles (Hoffer, 1991). Stressful intubation can produce release of catecholamines with resultant hypertension, tachycardia, and increased systemic vascular resistance, all of which affect myocardial blood flow adversely. Additional anesthetic agents may be necessary to attenuate these responses. Topical anesthetics or vasodilating agents may be used as well (Hensley et al., 1991). Fiberoptic bronchoscopy occasionally is necessary to facilitate intubation.

Special induction techniques are necessary to gain rapid control of the airway in patients with increased risk of aspiration. Patients more likely to aspirate during induction and intubation include (1) those with recent oral intake who undergo emergent operation, (2) those with gastroesophageal reflux, (3) diabetic patients with gastroparesis, and (4) those with other conditions associated with delayed gastric emptying. After intubation, mechanical ventilation is instituted. Oxygenation and ventilation are monitored throughout the operation. Airway management can be complicated at any point in the perioperative period by airway obstruction, aspiration of gastric contents, laryngeal or tracheal injury, or cardiovascular stimulation during airway manipulation (Hensley et al., 1991). During the period of extracorporeal circulation, ventilation of the lungs is discontinued.

Throughout the operative procedure, general anesthesia is maintained at an adequate level to ensure unconsciousness, analgesia, muscle relaxation, and attenuated stress responses. The anesthesiologist uses knowledge of the hemodynamic effects of each agent and its interactions with other drugs to anticipate and correct hemodynamic changes throughout the procedure (Warner & Warner, 1989). Administration of anesthetic agents, fluids, and vasoactive medications is titrated according to heart rate, arterial and pulmonary artery pressures, and cardiac output. Increases in blood pressure or heart rate and patient movement may indicate an inadequate depth of anesthesia. During cardiopulmonary bypass, inhalational agents must be administered through the cardiopulmonary bypass circuit because the lungs are not ventilated. Intravenous agents can be given directly into the patient's bloodstream.

Maintenance of anesthesia is designed to prevent myocardial ischemia and dysfunction and to treat them if they do occur (Wynands & O'Connor, 1989). Careful regulation of blood pressure is essential. Hypotension decreases subendocardial blood supply; hypertension, on the other hand, increases afterload and left ventricular oxygen demand. Intraoperative hypotension is treated with decreased amounts of anesthetic agents, volume replacement if preload is low, and inotropic agents. Nitroglycerin or sodium nitroprusside infusions are used commonly to control hypertension.

Consideration is given throughout the operation to the type of underlying cardiac disease. For example, coronary artery disease and ventricular hypertrophy both cause resting vasodilatation and significantly reduce the capacity of subendocardial vessels to dilate and regulate blood flow proportionate to changing oxygen needs (Buckberg & Allen, 1996). The left ventricular subendocardium is at greatest risk because compression of intramyocardial blood vessels prevents blood flow during systole. In addition, many patients who undergo coronary artery revascularization have been receiving beta-blocking or calcium channel antagonist agents. Beta-adrenergic blockers depress myocardial contractility and lower heart rate; some calcium channel antagonists produce vasodilatation in addition to depressing contractility. These drugs, in combination with volatile anesthetic agents, can produce significant myocardial depression, hypotension, bradycardia, and heart block.

Bradycardia can lower cardiac output, which is the product of stroke volume times heart rate. In patients with aortic regurgitation, bradycardia increases regurgitant flow (Buckberg & Allen, 1996). Tachycardia is particularly detrimental in patients with coronary artery disease; it further impairs coronary artery blood flow by shortening diastole when coronary artery filling occurs. Tachycardia also is poorly tolerated in patients with aortic stenosis because it further shortens diastolic filling time, which is reduced already because ejection through the narrowed valve orifice prolongs systole (Buckberg & Allen, 1996). Aortic stenosis poses other special concerns for the anesthesiologist. Vasodilating medications, volume loss, or bleeding are poorly tolerated because of fixed obstruction to ventricular output and decreased ventricular compliance, and may lead to catastrophic hemodynamic compromise.

▶ Transfer to the Intensive Care Unit

As the operation is concluded, the anesthesiologist informs nursing staff in the postoperative intensive care unit (ICU) of the patient's condition, prescribed ventilator settings, and any currently infusing intravenous medications. The transfer is postponed if the patient is hemodynamically unstable. Therapeutic manipulations are instituted in the operating room, and the patient is managed there until hemodynamic stability is achieved.

The patient is transported to the ICU using portable equipment for monitoring cardiac rhythm and arterial pressure. Ventilation is provided manually using a self-inflating bag and 100% oxygen. Vigilant observation and attention to detail are necessary during the transport period. Patient emergence from anesthesia or physiologic changes that occur with moving the patient from the operating table to the bed may cause precipitous hemodynamic instability. Potential problems during transport include sudden hypotension due to fluid shifts that occur as the patient is moved, acute hypertension due to sympathetic stimulation, and extubation or undesirable reflex responses caused by traction on the endotracheal tube (Hendren & Higgins, 1991). In addition, intravenous infusions of medications may be interrupted or the dosage changed as intravenous tubing is manipulated and equipment exchanged. Momentary lapses in monitoring may occur unless protocols are well established and carefully observed during the transfer process.

The anesthesiologist accompanies the patient to the ICU and remains until all monitoring equipment and intravenous infusions are safely reestablished and the patient's hemodynamic stability is confirmed. During this period, a summary of pertinent information is given to the ICU nurse regarding the patient's intraoperative course and current rates of fluid and medication infusion. The patient is allowed to emerge gradually from the anesthetized state. Propofol or midazolam commonly is used to prevent premature wakefulness, which may lead to undesirable hypertension, tachycardia, and resistance to mechanical ventilation. Sedation is maintained until chest tube drainage is at an acceptable level and the patient is fully rewarmed, hemodynamically stable, and ready for weaning from mechanical ventilation (Coyle, 1991).

Residual anesthetic effects can have a major influence on the cardiovascular, respiratory, and central nervous systems and must be taken into account during the early postoperative hours (Wong, 1991). If opioid-induced narcosis resolves before neuromuscular blocking agents have been eliminated or metabolized, the patient may awaken but remain paralyzed. Aggressive pharmacologic intervention with nitrates, alpha- and beta-blocking agents, and calcium channel antagonist medications may be necessary to suppress autonomic stress responses (Hendren & Higgins, 1991). In a patient who is slow to awaken, naloxone, a narcotic antagonist, may be necessary to eliminate residual narcosis. However, naloxone is not used in most circumstances because the release of catecholamines, the exacerbation of the stress response, and the resultant hypertension and tachycardia may cause myocardial ischemia with resultant hemodynamic instability and low cardiac output (Reves et al., 1995).

REFERENCES

Abrams AC, 1998a: Anesthetics. In Clinical Drug Therapy, ed. 5. Philadelphia, Lippincott Williams & Wilkins

Abrams AC, 1998b: Antianxiety and sedative-hypnotic drugs. In Clinical Drug Therapy, ed. 5. Philadelphia, Lippincott Williams & Wilkins

Buckberg GD, Allen BS, 1996: Myocardial protection during adult cardiac operations. In Baue AE, Geha AS, Hammond GL, et al. (eds): Glenn's Thoracic and Cardiovascular Surgery, ed. 6. Stamford, CT, Appleton & Lange

Coyle JP, 1991: Sedation, pain relief, and neuromuscular blockade in the postoperative cardiac surgical patient. Semin Thorac Cardiovasc Surg 3:81

Dowd NP, Cheng DC, Karski JM, et al., 1998: Intraoperative awareness in fast-track cardiac anesthesia. Anesthesiology 89:1068

Friedman AS, Sethna DH, 1990: Hemodynamic manipulation of the patient during anesthesia. In Gray RJ, Matloff JM (eds): Medical Management of the Cardiac Surgical Patient. Baltimore, Williams & Wilkins

Headley JM, 1998: Invasive hemodynamic monitoring: Applying advanced technologies. Critical Care Nursing Quarterly 21:73

Hendren WG, Higgins TL, 1991: Immediate postoperative care of the cardiac surgical patient. Semin Thorac Cardiovasc Surg 3:3

Hensley FA, Larach DR, Martin DE, 1991: Intraoperative anesthetic complications and their management. In Waldhausen JA, Orringer MB (eds): Complications in Cardiothoracic Surgery. St. Louis, Mosby–Year Book

Hoffer JL, 1991: Anesthesia. In Meeker MH, Rothrock JC (eds): Alexander's Care of the Patient in Surgery, ed. 9. St. Louis, Mosby–Year Book

Kaplan JA, Wynands JE, 1999: Anesthesia for myocardial revascularization. In Kaplan JA (ed): Cardiac Anesthesia, ed. 4. Philadelphia, WB Saunders

Kirklin JW, Barratt-Boyes BG, 1993: Anesthesia for cardiovascular surgery. In Cardiac Surgery, ed. 2. New York, Churchill Livingstone

Leslie K, Sessler DL, 1998: The implications of hypothermia for early tracheal extubation following cardiac surgery. J Cardiothorac Vasc Anesth 12(Suppl 2):30

Levy WJ, 1999: Central nervous system monitoring. In Kaplan JA (ed): Cardiac Anesthesia, ed. 4. Philadelphia, WB Saunders

Lichtenthal PR, 1998: Swan-Ganz catheter reference section. In Quick Guide to Cardiopulmonary Care. Irvine, CA, Baxter Healthcare Corporation

London MJ, Kaplan JA, 1999: Advances in electrocardiographic monitoring. In Kaplan JA (ed): Cardiac Anesthesia, ed. 4. Philadelphia, WB Saunders

Mangano DT, 1999: Preoperative assessment of cardiac risk. In Kaplan JA (ed): Cardiac Anesthesia, ed. 4. Philadelphia, WB Saunders

Mathew JP, Barash PG, 1996: Anesthesia for cardiac surgery. In Baue AE, Geha AS, Hammond GL, et al. (eds): Glenn's Thoracic and Cardiovascular Surgery, ed. 6. Stamford, CT, Appleton & Lange

Murray MJ, Torres NE, 1999: Critical care medicine for the cardiac patient. In Kaplan JA (ed): Cardiac Anesthesia, ed. 4. Philadelphia, WB Saunders

Nolan SP, Zacour R, 1998: Cardiopulmonary bypass. In Kaiser LR, Kron IL, Spray TL (eds): Mastery of Cardiothoracic Surgery. Philadelphia, Lippincott Williams & Wilkins

Reves JG, Greeley WJ, Grichnik K, 1995: Anesthesia and supportive care for cardiothoracic surgery. In Sabiston DC Jr, Spencer FC (eds): Surgery of the Chest, ed. 6. Philadelphia, WB Saunders

Savino JS, Cheung AT, 1997: Cardiac anesthesia. In Edmunds HL Jr (ed): Cardiac Surgery in the Adult. New York, McGraw-Hill

Schneider RC, 1989: Anesthesia for cardiac surgery. In Grillo HC, Austen WG, Wilkins EW Jr, et al. (eds): Current Therapy in Cardiothoracic Surgery. Toronto, Canada, BC Decker

Sebel PS, 1998: Central nervous system monitoring during open heart surgery: An update. J Cardiothorac Vasc Anesth 12(Suppl 1):3

Slogoff S, Keats AS, 1989: Randomized trial of primary anesthetic agents on outcome of coronary artery bypass operations. Anesthesia 70:179

Stanley TH, 1989: Opiates and cardiovascular anesthesia. In Estafanous FG (ed): Anesthesia and the Heart Patient. Boston, Butterworths

Warner MA, Warner ME, 1989: Anesthetic agents for cardiac surgery. In Tarhan S (ed): Cardiovascular Anesthesia and Postoperative Care, ed. 2. Chicago, Year Book

Wong CA, 1991: Physiologic responses to anesthesia. In Shekleton ME, Litwack K (eds): Critical Care Nursing of the Surgical Patient. Philadelphia, WB Saunders

Wynands JE, O'Connor JP, 1989: Anesthesia for coronary artery surgery. In Estafanous F (ed): Anesthesia and the Heart Patient. Boston, Butterworths

Yao FS, Barbut D, Deon EJ, et al., 1998: Cerebral hyperthermia during cardiopulmonary bypass rewarming in patients undergoing cardiac surgery. Anesthesiology 89:A238

Cardiopulmonary Bypass

*C*ardiopulmonary bypass (CPB) describes a system used temporarily to perform the functions of the heart (circulation of blood) and lungs (gas exchange) during operative procedures on the heart or great vessels. Development of CPB was due largely to pioneering research by Dr. John Gibbon, whose research efforts culminated in performance of the first cardiac operation using CPB in 1953 and heralded the beginning of the modern era of cardiac surgery (Mangano et al., 1999; Blanche et al., 1990). For the first time, prolonged interruption of normal circulation became possible, providing a decompressed, noncontracting heart and a bloodless field within which the surgeon could work.

Cardiopulmonary bypass is called *extracorporeal circulation* because blood is diverted from the vascular system and circulated through a circuit of plastic tubing outside the body. Because this tubing circuit transverses the skin barrier, extracorporeal perfusion systems are designed for temporary application (Edmunds, 1997). Venous cannulae are used to drain blood from the right side of the heart into the CPB circuit. As blood is pumped through the circuit, it is oxygenated, filtered, cooled or warmed, and returned by means of an arterial cannula to the systemic circulation. In this fashion, body tissues, particularly those of the brain and other vital organs, are perfused and remain viable despite temporary cessation of heart and lung function. CPB may be either total (essentially all venous blood is diverted into the extracorporeal circuit) or partial (some

venous blood returns to the heart and is ejected into the aorta). In most cardiac operations, total CPB is used and a cross-clamp is applied to the ascending aorta, excluding the coronary arteries from the extracorporeal circuit. Cardioplegic solution is infused separately into the coronary circulation to induce and maintain cardiac arrest. Any cardiac operation that involves use of CPB is correctly termed an *open heart* operation regardless of whether a cardiac chamber is opened during the procedure.

Extracorporeal circulation sometimes is used in situations other than during cardiac or great vessel surgery. Temporary circulatory support may be used to treat postoperative cardiogenic shock or as a bridge to emergent cardiac surgery in patients with sudden, profound ventricular failure. Extracorporeal membrane oxygenation is a form of CPB sometimes used to treat severe respiratory failure in infants and children. Temporary circulatory support of the heart outside the operating room is discussed in Chapter 30, Circulatory Assist Devices.

▶ Components of Cardiopulmonary Bypass

The following components comprise the CPB system: (1) venous and arterial cannulae; (2) oxygenator, reservoir, and heat exchanger; (3) arterial pump; (4) left ventricular vent; and (5) cardiotomy suction catheter (Fig. 12-1).

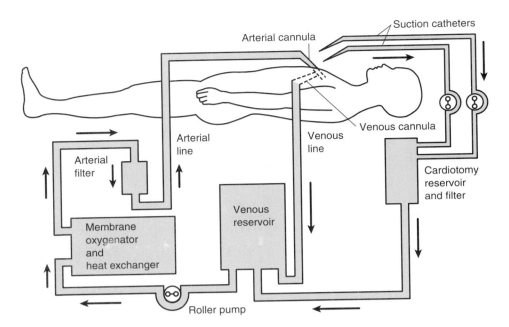

FIGURE 12-1. Diagram of a typical cardiopulmonary bypass system with a membrane oxygenator.

Venous and Arterial Cannulae

Cannulae used for CPB are designed to minimize turbulence and stagnation of blood, thus reducing hemolysis and thrombus formation (Stammers, 1999). The various cannulae necessary for CPB are inserted by small incisions through surrounding purse-string sutures that help secure the cannula to the vessel wall and prevent bleeding around the cannula. One or two large-bore cannulae are placed to divert venous blood into the CPB circuit. Most commonly, venous blood is drained through a single two-stage (ie, with two drainage ports) cannula that is inserted through a small incision in the right atrial appendage (Fig. 12-2). Single right atrial cannulation is suitable for most cardiac operations, despite the fact that a small amount of venous blood continues to enter the right atrium through the coronary sinus and thebesian veins.

Alternatively, two venous cannulae may be positioned in the superior and inferior venae cavae to divert venous return totally from the heart. Separate cannulation of the superior and inferior venae cavae is necessary during operations that require working within the right atrium or right ventricle (Edmunds, 1997). A third technique for diverting venous return into the CPB circuit is cannulation of the femoral vein with retrograde advancement of the cannula into the inferior vena cava or right atrium.

In most cases, oxygenated blood is returned to the systemic circulation by means of a cannula inserted into the ascending aorta, just proximal to the origin of the innominate artery (Fig. 12-3). The ascending aorta is used most commonly because (1) it is easily accessible through the median sternotomy incision; (2) it eliminates the need for groin dissection and femoral artery repair; and (3) it reduces the potential for arterial dissection, which is more likely with retrograde perfusion through the femoral artery (Behrendt & Austen, 1985). Potential complications of ascending aortic cannulation include intimal

damage leading to aortic dissection, disruption and embolization of intimal plaque into cerebral vessels, and inappropriate placement of the cannula tip in the innominate artery (Blanche et al., 1990).

The femoral artery may be cannulated instead of the aorta. Femoral artery cannulation provides distinct advantages in selected situations. First, cannulation of the femoral artery may be preferable in reoperations because it can be performed before opening the chest. In patients who have had one or more previous operations through a median sternotomy, internal scarring from prior procedures may result in adherence of the anterior surface of the heart to the posterior table of the sternum. Laceration of the right ventricle or aorta can occur as the sternum is divided. Without the ability to initiate extracorporeal circulation promptly in this situation, exsanguination and death can occur within minutes. Previously constructed bypass grafts, particularly an internal thoracic artery graft positioned on the anterior surface of the heart, also may be injured, causing precipitous myocardial ischemia. If femoral artery and vein cannulae have been placed already, CPB and myocardial protection measures can be initiated rapidly while the surgeon repairs the injured structure or revascularizes the myocardium. Similarly, in unstable or high-risk patients who might experience hemodynamic deterioration with induction of anesthesia, CPB can be rapidly instituted by means of femoral vessel cannulation before the median sternotomy has been performed.

Use of the femoral artery for cannulation is necessary during operative repair of the ascending aorta or aortic arch. Femoral arterial cannulation also may be preferable when the ascending aorta is heavily calcified. In such patients, embolization of calcium or atheromatous material into the cerebral circulation can occur during manipulation and cannulation of diseased tissue in the ascending aorta. In patients who have undergone previous coronary

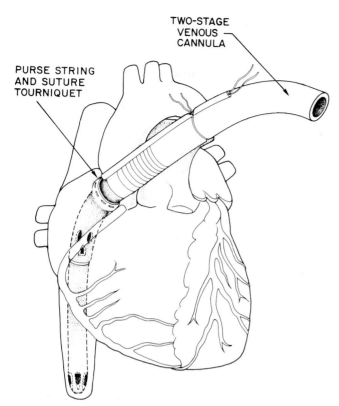

FIGURE 12-2. Single venous cannulation. The "two-stage" construction of the cannula places drainage ports in the right atrium and the inferior vena cava. (Nolan SP, Zacour R, 1998: Cardiopulmonary bypass. In Kaiser LR, Kron IL, Spray TL [eds]: Mastery of Cardiothoracic Surgery, p. 282. Philadelphia, Lippincott Williams & Wilkins)

bypass surgery with multiple saphenous vein anastomoses to the proximal aorta, femoral cannulation may be selected because there is no remaining area to insert the arterial cannula without disrupting existing vein graft anastomoses. Femoral cannulation for both arterial and venous access is used during so-called "port access" minimally invasive cardiac procedures (Reardon et al., 1997). The femoral artery and vein also are cannulated when a lateral thoracotomy incision is used for cardiac operations because the ascending aorta and right atrium are not accessible through the thoracotomy exposure.

Ascending aorta and femoral artery cannulation are similar with respect to adequacy of organ perfusion. With availability of percutaneous cannulae developed for portable CPB systems, a cutdown technique may not be needed for femoral vessel cannulation; percutaneous cannulae can be inserted quickly and used with a standard CPB system (Hartz et al., 1990). The primary complication associated with femoral artery cannulation is aortic dissection, which may not be recognized until retrograde perfusion is initiated and irreversible damage has occurred. As a result, the complication often is fatal. Femoral artery cannulation also can cause limb ischemia. Aortic dissection and limb ischemia are most likely in patients with atherosclerotic peripheral arterial occlusive disease.

Cannulae for cardioplegia delivery also must be placed if cardioplegic solution is to be administered during the course of the operation. Almost all cardiac operations are performed using cardioplegia and a period of aortic cross-clamping during CPB for myocardial protection. Cardioplegia is achieved by infusing the coronary arteries with a high potassium solution to induce and maintain cardiac arrest. Antegrade cardioplegia delivery necessitates cannulation of the ascending aorta, proximal to the cannula used for returning blood from the CPB circuit. Cross-clamping the aorta between the aortic and cardioplegic cannulae allows separation of the coronary circulation from the CPB circuit. Often, cardioplegia is delivered using both antegrade and retrograde delivery techniques. If retrograde cardioplegia administration is to be performed, a cannula is inserted through the right atrium into the coronary sinus. Methods of myocardial protection are discussed in more detail in Chapter 13, Myocardial Protection.

Oxygenator, Heat Exchanger, and Reservoir

The *oxygenator* is the device that oxygenates blood and facilitates carbon dioxide exchange. A membrane oxygenator is used most commonly. It consists of a semi-

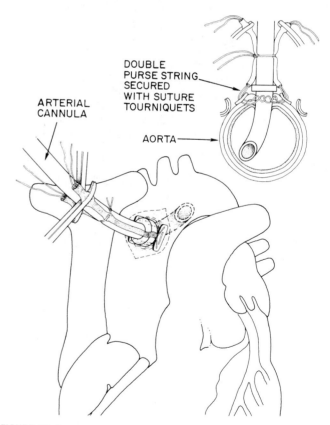

FIGURE 12-3. Placement of arterial cannula in ascending aorta; cannula position is secured with double purse-string sutures and suture tourniquets. (Nolan SP, Zacour R, 1998: Cardiopulmonary bypass. In Kaiser LR, Kron IL, Spray TL [eds]: Mastery of Cardiothoracic Surgery, p. 280. Philadelphia, Lippincott Williams & Wilkins)

permeable membrane through which oxygen and carbon dioxide diffuse. A *heat exchanger,* usually incorporated in the oxygenator, is used to adjust precisely the temperature of the blood and thereby protect the patient during the period of extracorporeal circulation. Cooling is used to minimize ischemia during the period of aortic cross-clamping and cardiac arrest; warming is used to restore normal body temperature after periods of hypothermia and to avoid hypothermia that would otherwise occur as blood circulates outside the body through the CPB circuit. The heat exchanger cools or warms by exposing the blood-filled tubing to water at a selected temperature. An ideal heat exchanger offers minimal resistance to blood flow, is without defects that would allow mixing of blood and water, requires a low priming volume, and is disposable (Stammers, 1999).

Blood flowing into the venous cannula enters a *venous reservoir* contained in the CPB circuit that collects and holds 500 to 3000 mL of blood. Its purpose is to reserve a volume of blood in the extracorporeal circuit, to allow escape of air from the blood, and to allow the rate of blood return to the patient to be manipulated somewhat independently of the patient's venous return. The reservoir contains an entry port through which blood products, crystalloids, and medications can be added to the perfusate (ie, the circulating blood volume). Blood collected in the venous reservoir is pumped through the oxygenator and added to the perfusate as additional circulating volume is needed.

Arterial Pump

A primary component of the CPB system is the *arterial pump,* which propels oxygenated blood into the patient's arterial circulation. Arterial flow during CPB can be either nonpulsatile or pulsatile. Nonpulsatile roller or centrifugal pumps usually are used (Fig. 12-4). Both are relatively simple to operate, inexpensive, and reliable (Edmunds, 1997; Blanche et al., 1990). A roller pump propels blood by external compression of the tubing and produces continuous flow. A centrifugal pump is a disposable unit that propels blood by a whirling, circular motion. It conducts fluid movement by the addition of kinetic energy to a fluid or cone in a constrained housing (Stammers, 1999). Centrifugal pumps are thought to produce less hemolysis because blood elements are not subjected to compression by a roller. In addition, air in the tubing is less likely to be propelled into the patient's arterial circulation. Instead, the centrifugal force of the pump collects minute quantities of air, which is lighter than blood, near the center of the pump.

One of two operational methods may be used to achieve pulsatile arterial blood flow: (1) a roller head that accelerates during the systolic phase and decelerates during the diastolic phase, or (2) an alternating occlusion system that uses an intermittent occlusive phase (Stammers, 1999). The superiority of pulsatile versus nonpulsatile flow has been debated since the development of CPB and remains controversial. Despite a large volume of literature comparing the physiology of nonpulsatile versus pulsatile flow, substantive clinical benefits of pulsatile flow have yet to be demonstrated (Mangano et al., 1999). Pulsatile flow is intuitively more attractive because it more closely simulates physiologic blood flow, but it actually could be more damaging to blood elements. At this time, pulsatile pumps are used rarely.

Arterial line filters are incorporated into the CPB circuit to trap particulate matter or air that inadvertently enters the circuit before blood is returned to the patient's circulation. The CPB circuit also has safety devices that detect air bubbles, low flow, and low oxygen delivery.

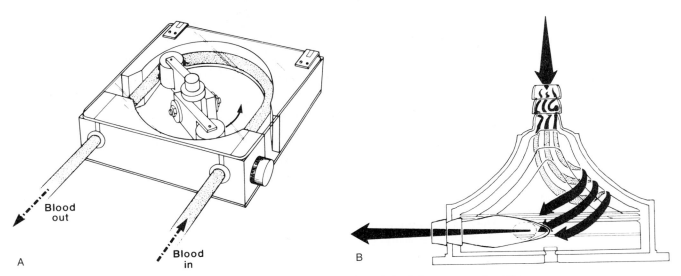

FIGURE 12-4. Types of arterial pumps. **(A)** Roller pump. (Milan JD, 1983: Blood transfusion in heart surgery. Surg Clin North Am 63:1130) **(B)** Centrifugal pump. (Kern FH, Giesser WG, Farrell DM, 1993: Extracorporeal circulation and circulatory assist devices in the pediatric patient. In Lake CL [ed]: Pediatric Cardiac Anesthesia, ed. 2, p. 154. Norwalk, CT, Appleton & Lange)

Left Ventricular Vent

Some cardiac operations necessitate placement of a vent in the left ventricle (Fig. 12-5). The purpose of a *left ventricular vent* is to prevent distention of the ventricle when it is not ejecting blood; that is, when the aorta is cross-clamped or when the ventricles are fibrillating. For most operations, a Y-catheter is placed in the aortic root, with one limb used for venting the left ventricle and the other for administration of cardioplegic solution. Alternatively, a catheter may be inserted into the superior pulmonary vein and directed through the left atrium and across the mitral valve into the left ventricle. Yet another option for left ventricular venting is insertion of the catheter through the left atrial wall and into the ventricle. These techniques avoid the injurious consequences of direct insertion through the ventricular muscle. In cases in which left ventricular decompression is more important, some surgeons prefer inserting the vent through the apex of the left ventricle.

The necessity of venting the left ventricle during all cardiac operations is controversial, and some surgeons use left ventricular vents only selectively. However, if ventricular distention occurs during a procedure in which a vent has not been placed or is not functioning properly, vent insertion or correction of the problem must be performed

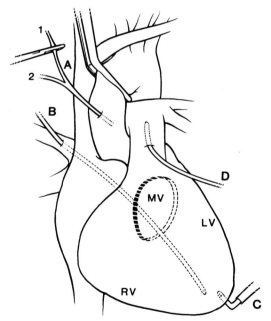

FIGURE 12-5. Alternative sites for venting the left ventricle (LV). **(A)** Aortic root cannula; one limb (1) is connected to the cardioplegia administration system and the other (2) to suction for venting the left ventricle. **(B)** Cannula is inserted at junction of right superior pulmonary vein and left atrium and advanced through left atrium and mitral valve (MV) into the left ventricle. **(C)** Cannula is inserted directly into apex of the left ventricle. **(D)** Cannula is inserted into the pulmonary artery. RV, right ventricle. (Hessel EA, 1993: Cardiopulmonary bypass circuitry and cannulation techniques. In Gravlee GP, Davis RF, Utley JR [eds]: Cardiopulmonary Bypass: Principles and Practice, p. 78. Baltimore, Williams & Wilkins)

rapidly. Distention of the left ventricle, even for a limited period, can have serious consequences. Left ventricular distention significantly reduces myocardial contractility, may reduce coronary blood flow, and sometimes produces acute lung damage from increased pulmonary venous pressure (Edmunds, 1997).

Cardiotomy Suction

The *cardiotomy suction catheter* is a specially designed catheter used to aspirate blood from the operative field. During bypass, while the blood is heparinized, a cardiotomy suction catheter is placed in the opened heart or mediastinum. Aspirated blood is directed through suction tubing into the extracorporeal circuit. Because the suctioned blood contains air and particulate matter, it is directed into a cardiotomy reservoir, where it is filtered and defoamed before being added to the extracorporeal blood volume to be oxygenated, cooled, and returned to the arterial circulation (Fig. 12-6). Vented blood from the left ventricle, pulmonary artery, or aortic root also is returned to the extracorporeal circuit through the cardiotomy reservoir (Stammers, 1999).

▶ Extracorporeal Circulation

Cardiopulmonary bypass is a highly sophisticated life support system. Its operation is directed and monitored by a certified perfusionist, who regulates the device, monitors all hemodynamic and metabolic parameters, and corrects any functional problems that occur. Because the CPB system provides total cardiopulmonary support for the patient, there is a potential for catastrophic complications should a system malfunction occur.

Initiation

A bolus of heparin, typically 300 U/kg, is injected into the right atrium in preparation for cannulation and CPB. Systemic anticoagulation is mandatory throughout the period of extracorporeal circulation while the blood is circulated outside the body and exposed to nonbiologic surfaces. Heparin combines with antithrombin III to inactivate several clotting factors (IX, X, XI, XII) and thrombin so thrombus formation is prevented (Abrams, 1998).

The CPB tubing is filled or "primed" with approximately 2 L of a crystalloid solution, similar in electrolyte composition to plasma. Albumin may be added to the priming solution to maintain colloidal osmotic pressure and reduce extravasation into the interstitial space (ie, "third spacing"). Fluid is circulated through the system for several minutes to filter air and particulate matter and to ensure proper functioning. Great care is taken to remove all air from the arterial side of the circuit to prevent delivering an air embolus into the systemic circulation. This preparatory phase usually requires 30 to 40

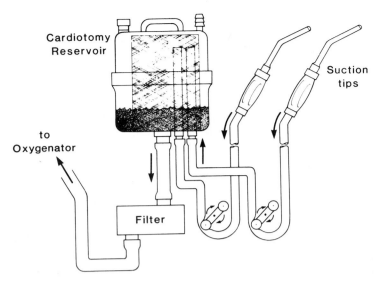

Cardiotomy
Reservoir

Suction
tips

to
Oxygenator

Filter

FIGURE 12-6. Cardiotomy aspiration system. (Milan JD, 1983: Blood transfusion in heart surgery. Surg Clin North Am 63:1130)

minutes, although it can be done more quickly if emergent initiation of CPB is necessary.

After the surgeon has inserted the cannulae, they are connected to the tubing of the CPB circuit in a manner that ensures evacuation of all air from the circulating perfusate. To begin extracorporeal circulation, the perfusionist releases the arterial line clamp and slowly transfuses the patient with volume; as soon as it is apparent that arterial flow is unobstructed, the venous clamp is released, diverting the patient's venous blood into the CPB circuit (Nolan and Zacour, 1998). The right side of the heart becomes decompressed and the rate of arterial return is gradually increased until total bypass is achieved.

As the patient's blood circulates through the CPB circuit, it is intentionally cooled before being returned to the patient to lower body temperature, and thus lower tissue metabolism and oxygen demand. Adjusting perfusate temperature to induce hypothermia, termed *core cooling,* enhances myocardial protection, minimizes ischemic damage to organs, and allows specific target organs to tolerate markedly reduced flow rates or transient interruption of circulation. Hypothermia also sustains intracellular reservoirs of high-energy phosphates essential for cellular integrity, and preserves high intracellular pH and electrochemical neutrality (Nolan & Zacour, 1998). Core cooling must be performed slowly to cool body tissues efficiently without regional temperature differences. *Moderate hypothermia* (eg, 28°C to 32°C) is used for most cardiac operations. When an adequate degree of hypothermia has been achieved, a cross-clamp is applied to the aorta and chilled cardioplegic solution is administered to provide further regional cooling of the myocardium. Typically, bladder and nasopharyngeal temperatures are monitored throughout the period of extracorporeal circulation.

As the patient's blood circulates through the extracorporeal circuit it mixes with the priming solution, producing *hemodilution,* or lowering of the hematocrit, usually to approximately 25%. Although the ideal degree of hemodilution is not established, a general guide-

line is that the hematocrit as a percentage should not exceed the desired level of hypothermia in degrees Celsius (Nolan & Zacour, 1998). Hemodilution is well tolerated during hypothermia because tissue oxygen demands are reduced. A lower hematocrit is in fact advantageous in that it lowers blood viscosity (which increases during hypothermia), thereby facilitating blood flow to the microcirculation of peripheral tissues (Whitman, 1987). In addition, hemodilution reduces the need for exogenous blood, decreases trauma to blood cells and blood proteins, and increases urine flow and excretion of sodium, potassium, and creatinine (Edmunds, 1996). Hemodilution does, however, reduce oncotic pressure, resulting in interstitial edema (Nolan & Zacour, 1998; Edmunds, 1996).

Some complex cardiovascular operations require decreasing the flow rate during CPB to very low levels or completely interrupting circulation to the brain for a period. For example, operations on the aortic arch necessitate interruption of circulation through the ascending aorta for an extended period. Profound or deep hypothermia is used in these situations and the technique is termed *deep hypothermic circulatory arrest.* Cooling is achieved by perfusion and augmented with a hypothermia blanket beneath the patient and ice packing around the head (Edmunds, 1997). In contrast to the moderate hypothermia used in most cardiac operations, the body is systemically cooled to approximately 18°C and CPB circulation is stopped. With the body cooled to this extreme degree, perfusion can be interrupted for as much as 60 minutes while the aortic reconstruction is performed. Deep hypothermia is the only available method for safely extending the duration of the brain's tolerance to ischemia. However, prolonged hypothermia below 15°C is avoided because it may damage brain tissue. To improve cerebral protection during the period of deep hypothermic circulatory arrest, many surgeons use retrograde cerebral perfusion. Using a separate roller pump, low-flow retrograde blood flow to the cerebral circulation is maintained through the superior vena cava (Rao &

Weisel, 1997). Blood exits the head vessels through the opened aortic arch and is then returned to the CPB circuit through the cardiotomy suction catheter.

Maintenance

During CPB, the perfusionist controls systemic blood flow based on arterial and central venous pressures to provide adequate oxygenation of the microcirculation. While the heart is inactive, the flow rate is adjusted to deliver 4 to 5 L/min, or a cardiac index equivalent to 2.2 to 2.5 L/min/m². Lower flow rates may be used while the patient is hypothermic. Selection of perfusion pressure during CPB is designed to balance the need for a bloodless field with ensuring adequate oxygenation (Mangano et al., 1999). A low flow rate and perfusion pressure during CPB decrease noncoronary collateral flow, which facilitates a drier operative field and prevents rewarming of the heart (Utley, 1989). Although the ideal flow rate remains a source of debate, a flow rate less than 1.6 L/min/m² during normothermia is associated with acidosis with increased lactic acid production, low oxygen consumption, and other features of cardiogenic shock (McGiffin & Kirklin, 1995). Excessive flow rates, on the other hand, may produce more trauma to blood elements and higher gradients across the arterial cannula (Kirklin & Barratt-Boyes, 1993).

During CPB, the arterial pressure is a mean, nonpulsatile pressure unless an artificial method is used to provide pulsatile flow; this mean pressure should be viewed as an index of the relationship between blood flow, volume, and arteriolar resistance, and not as a measure of perfusion adequacy (Nolan & Zacour, 1998). The ideal range for mean arterial pressure is not known. Typically, mean arterial pressure during normothermic CPB is maintained between 50 and 70 mm Hg (Edmunds, 1996).

Volume, in the form of blood, other colloid, or crystalloid solution, may be added to the reservoir to increase the flow rate, particularly when there is a major bleeding problem. Flow may be decreased by reserving volume in the reservoir. Vasoconstricting or vasodilating drugs may be added to the circulating blood volume to adjust systemic vascular resistance. If an intra-aortic balloon catheter is in place, a standby mode usually is used during CPB. Because the patient is systemically anticoagulated, thrombus formation along the catheter does not occur. If a nonpulsatile pump is being used, some surgeons prefer to maintain counterpulsation during CPB in the belief that it might provide a pulsatile quality to the blood flow.

Central venous and pulmonary artery pressures are maintained at or near 0 mm Hg to minimize interstitial fluid accumulation in the lungs and peripheral tissue. There appears to be no physiologic advantage to keeping central venous pressure above 0 mm Hg during CPB (Kirklin & Barratt-Boyes, 1993). In addition to interstitial fluid accumulation, increased venous pressure reduces circulating volume and may necessitate additional priming volume. An adequately sized venous cannula and unimpaired venous drainage are essential to achieve low venous pressures. A left ventricular vent also may be helpful. Negative venous pressure also must be avoided because it causes collapse of the thin-walled venae cavae and limits venous return to the CPB circuit (Edmunds, 1996). For this reason, most CPB systems drain venous blood by gravity.

Because venous blood is oxygenated in the CPB system, it is not necessary to ventilate the lungs during extracorporeal circulation. When CPB is initiated, the anesthesiologist turns off the ventilator. Leaving the lungs in a deflated state during the procedure makes the operative work technically easier by avoiding encroachment of the inflated lungs on the operative field. Sustained hypoinflation of the lungs, however, is a contributing factor for the atelectasis that routinely occurs in patients after cardiac operations.

Continuous monitoring of arterial blood gases is performed using a sensor placed in the arterial tubing distal to the oxygenator. Arterial oxygen pressure usually is maintained in the range of 200 to 250 mm Hg during CPB to ensure adequate tissue perfusion without producing oxygen toxicity or bubble formation. Arterial carbon dioxide levels are maintained in the normal physiologic range with appropriate adjustments for temperature.

Serial arterial blood gas measurements are obtained to assess adequacy of oxygenation and hemoglobin concentration of the perfusate. Venous oxygen measurements also are obtained. Abnormally low venous oxygenation may indicate arterial hypoxemia or an inadequate perfusion rate; adjustment of arterial oxygenation or the arterial flow rate may be necessary to correct the problem. In addition to arterial and venous oxygen measurements, the perfusionist monitors acid–base status, potassium levels, and hematocrit. Because sensitivity to and metabolism of heparin varies among patients, activated clotting time (ACT) is measured intermittently to assess the degree of anticoagulation (Edmunds, 1996). The ACT measures heparin activity rather than heparin concentration. Although the normal baseline ACT ranges between 80 and 120 seconds, the optimal range during CPB has not been defined; a typical ACT range during CPB is 400 to 600 seconds (Nolan and Zacour, 1998). Periodic boluses of heparin are administered as necessary to maintain ACT in the desired range.

Blood shed from the operative field usually can be salvaged to lessen the need for transfusion of allogeneic blood. During the period of extracorporeal circulation and systemic anticoagulation, blood aspirated from the open heart or mediastinum is returned to the CPB circuit through the venous reservoir, where it is defoamed and filtered to remove tissue debris and air. Suctioning of mediastinal blood greatly reduces intraoperative blood loss. However, the suction system is a major cause of hemolysis and is very destructive of all blood elements; in addition, aspirated blood differs from the perfusate with which it will be mixed in that it contains enzymes activated by blood contact with the wound (Edmunds, 1997).

Weaning

As reparative work on the heart or great vessels is nearing completion, the blood is rewarmed by gradually increasing the perfusate temperature. Rewarming is performed slowly (0.2°C to 0.5°C per minute) to prevent decreased blood solubility with resultant bubble formation. Rewarming is continued until the nasopharyngeal temperature is 37°C and bladder temperature exceeds 36°C (Nolan & Zacour, 1998). Blood temperature is not allowed to exceed 40°C to avoid damaging blood proteins.

During rewarming, the aortic cross-clamp is removed in preparation for weaning from CPB. Catastrophic stroke or myocardial infarction can result when the aortic cross-clamp is removed if air is ejected from the left ventricle into the cerebral or coronary circulation, respectively. A number of technical maneuvers are performed by the surgeon before removing the aortic cross-clamp to prevent this complication. If the left atrium, left ventricle, or aorta has been opened during the procedure, vigorous attempts are made to ensure that all air is evacuated from inside the chambers before removing the aortic cross-clamp and allowing the heart to eject blood into the ascending aorta.

The operating table is adjusted so that the patient is in the Trendelenburg (head down) position. Venous return to the pump is reduced, allowing the right heart to fill while the surgeon gently massages the heart and the left ventricular vent continues to drain (Nolan & Zacour, 1998). Delivery of anesthetic agents is discontinued, and the lungs are ventilated with 100% oxygen and positive pressure to allow air in the pulmonary veins to escape (Behrendt & Austen, 1985; Blanche et al., 1990). The aortic cardioplegic cannula also is placed on suction to evacuate air massaged from the heart. These maneuvers are continued until the surgeon is confident that all air has been evacuated from the heart. Transesophageal echocardiography usually is used to confirm the absence of air in the left atrium or ventricle. The patient is maintained in a head-downward position as the aortic cross-clamp is removed, ensuring that any residual air will be directed into the descending aorta.

Pump reservoir volume is adjusted to ensure adequate volume if transfusion is needed. Arterial blood gases, hematocrit, potassium, and acid–base status are measured and corrected if necessary. When the operative repair is completed and the heart has warmed sufficiently to resume a spontaneous cardiac rhythm, weaning from CPB is begun. If defibrillation is necessary to initiate an organized cardiac rhythm, it is performed with internal paddles and 5 to 10 joules of current (Mangano et al., 1999). The patient is weaned by slowly reducing the flow rate through the CPB circuit. The venous cannula is gradually occluded, decreasing the volume of blood diverted to the CPB circuit and increasing the volume traveling normally through the heart (ie, partial CPB). When the heart is functioning effectively enough to sustain an adequate arterial systolic pressure (eg, 100 mm Hg), the perfusionist terminates CPB by completely occluding the venous and arterial cannulae (Nolan and Zacour, 1998).

Successful weaning requires complete washout of cardioplegic solution, sufficient rewarming, a stable cardiac rhythm, and adequate right and left ventricular function (Blanche et al., 1990). The surgeon uses monitored hemodynamic parameters and visual observation of the heart to assess cardiac rhythm and adequacy of right and left ventricular function. If ventricular function is good and myocardial damage has not occurred during the perioperative period, the heart usually resumes normal function quickly.

If ventricular function is impaired and low cardiac output ensues, CPB is reinstituted to prevent hypoxia or ventricular overdistention (Nolan and Zacour, 1998). Two or three attempts at weaning CPB may be necessary. Various combinations of cardiotonic and vasodilating medications may be administered. Commonly used inotropic agents include dopamine, dobutamine, and epinephrine. Vasodilating agents, such as nitroglycerin or nitroprusside, may be administered for afterload reduction. Occasionally, lidocaine or another antiarrhythmic medication is required to treat ventricular ectopy. Temporary pacing may be used to increase heart rate, maintain the atrial contribution to cardiac output, or ensure an adequate ventricular rate. In some patients, intra-aortic balloon counterpulsation is necessary to augment left ventricular function.

When the patient clearly is able to sustain an adequate arterial pressure and cardiac output without support from the CPB system, protamine sulfate is administered to reverse the heparin-induced anticoagulation. One of the cannulae (usually the venous cannula) is removed. The remaining cannula is left in place for a short time and used to infuse blood remaining in the CPB reservoir as needed. Boluses of 100 to 200 mL of blood can be infused rapidly through the remaining cannula. After the cannula is removed, residual blood in the CPB system is transferred into blood bags and may be infused in the intensive care unit if the patient requires blood volume in the early postoperative hours.

► Consequences of Cardiopulmonary Bypass

Physiologic Effects

During CPB, blood is exposed to artificial, nonendothelial surfaces of the oxygenator, filters, and tubing. Exposure to nonphysiologic surfaces is detrimental to the blood elements (ie, platelets, red blood cells, white blood cells, and plasma proteins). Blood contact with large areas of synthetic surface during extracorporeal circulation dilutes and denatures plasma proteins and activates blood cells, coagulation proteins and the fibrinolytic system, and the complement system (Schoen, 1997; Edmunds, 1997).

Blood elements are damaged further by shear stresses that occur as a result of circulation through the arterial pump, suctioning forces, and turbulent flow at cannula insertion sites. The number of platelets in circulating blood after CPB is only approximately 60% of the prebypass level, platelet survival time is reduced, and platelet function is altered (Kirklin & Barratt-Boyes, 1993). Leukocyte counts increase moderately after operation, the total number of lymphocytes as well as specific subsets of lymphocytes decrease, and monocytes and endothelial cells are activated (Edmunds, 1997). This may account for a degree of immunosuppression that has been reported to exist after CPB. The blood incorporates abnormal substances, such as fibrin, air bubbles, and tissue debris, that generate the release of a host of vasoactive substances and change vasomotor tone (McGiffin & Kirklin, 1995; Edmunds, 1997).

Complement system activation induced by extracorporeal circulation produces a systemic inflammatory response, causing the release of biologically active substances that impair coagulation and the immune system. The complement system, composed of at least 20 plasma proteins, normally acts as the body's defense against traumatic, infectious, and immunologic challenges (Mangano et al., 1999). As a result of complement activation, capillary permeability increases, plasma may be lost through the capillary membranes, and fluid accumulates in the interstitial space.

A number of other physiologic changes occur as well. Changes in temperature, acid–base balance, hemodilution, heart rate, blood volume, and vasomotor tone during CPB affect many physiologic reflexes (Edmunds, 1997). Hypothermia, hemodilution, nonpulsatile flow, and insulin, prostaglandin, and renin release during CPB are all potent stimuli for catecholamine release (Mangano et al., 1999). Epinephrine levels rise dramatically after initiation of CPB and, in some patients, norepinephrine levels rise as well. Systemic vascular resistance decreases profoundly at the onset of CPB, then progressively increases, particularly as hypothermia is induced. An increase in venous tone resulting from CPB continues for several hours after CPB is terminated (Kirklin & Barratt-Boyes, 1993). Because 70% to 80% of the patient's blood volume is contained in the venous capacitance bed, medications that adjust venous compliance may be necessary to control venous return.

Clinical Sequelae

All patients have some pathophysiologic response to CPB. The variety of metabolic, hematologic, and neurohumoral effects caused by extracorporeal circulation contributes to many of the clinical problems typically observed in the early postoperative period, such as fluid, electrolyte, and metabolic imbalances, hypertension, bleeding, and low cardiac output (Weiland & Walker, 1986). A certain degree of extravasation of fluid into interstitial tissues occurs in all patients despite maintaining low central venous pressure during CPB. Body weight increases as a result of fluid infusion necessary to replenish intravascular volume. Postoperative vasoconstriction, due to the temporary elevations in catecholamines and

other vasoactive substances, occurs commonly and may necessitate vasodilating therapy (Argenziano et al., 1998). The inflammatory response resulting from complement activation during CPB is believed to contribute to postoperative myocardial dysfunction (Lazar et al., 1998).

Complications of CPB are unusual but can occur. Nonsurgical bleeding complications associated with CPB can result from heparin use, platelet dysfunction, and fibrinolysis (Edmunds, 1997). A systemic inflammatory response characterized by profound vasodilation and hypotension may occur, particularly in patients with low ejection fractions and in those who have received preoperative angiotensin-converting enzyme inhibitors (Argenziano et al., 1998). Rarely, a severe inflammatory response to CPB, termed *postperfusion syndrome,* may occur. It is characterized by pulmonary dysfunction, renal dysfunction, bleeding diathesis, increased interstitial fluid, leukocytosis, fever, vasoconstriction, hemolysis, and increased susceptibility to infection (McGiffin & Kirklin, 1995). Patients subjected to prolonged CPB are most likely to experience postperfusion syndrome.

Administration of protamine at the conclusion of CPB occasionally causes a severe adverse reaction, characterized by profound vasodilatation and hypotension. Treatment includes rapid volume infusion and administration of vasoconstricting agents and corticosteroids. Data conflict about whether protamine reactions are more likely in diabetic patients who have formed antibodies to protamine from chronic use of a protamine-containing insulin (eg, isophane [NPH] or protamine zinc insulin [PZI]); if the risk is increased in diabetic patients, it remains small (0.6%) (Horrow, 1999). Severe protamine reactions can be fatal. Other rare complications of CPB include hematologic disorders, gastrointestinal bleeding, pancreatitis, and bowel infarction.

An unusual but catastrophic complication of CPB is air embolization. Accordingly, numerous safety features are incorporated into the CPB system to prevent infusion of air into the arterial circulation. Similarly, a number of maneuvers (eg, venting, positioning, aspiration, and lung ventilation) are performed routinely by the surgeon and anesthesiologist before discontinuing CPB. Malfunction of the CPB system occurs rarely due to tubing disconnection or rupture, air lock (entry of a large amount of air into the venous cannula), tubing obstruction, or oxygenator or pump failure.

REFERENCES

Abrams AC, 1998: Anticoagulant, antiplatelet, and thrombolytic agents. In Clinical Drug Therapy, ed. 4. Philadelphia, Lippincott Williams & Wilkins

Argenziano M, Chen JM, Choudri AF, et al., 1998: Management of vasodilatory shock after cardiac surgery: Identification of predisposing factors and use of a novel pressor agent. J Thorac Cardiovasc Surg 116:973

Behrendt DM, Austen WG, 1985: Intraoperative management. In Patient Care in Cardiac Surgery. Boston, Little, Brown

Blanche C, Matloff JM, MacKay DA, 1990: Technical aspects of cardiopulmonary bypass. In Gray RJ, Matloff JM (eds):

Medical Care of the Cardiac Surgical Patient. Baltimore, Williams & Wilkins

Edmunds LH Jr, 1997: Extracorporeal perfusion. In Edmunds LH Jr (ed): Cardiac Surgery in the Adult. New York, McGraw-Hill

Edmunds LH Jr, 1996: Cardiopulmonary bypass for open heart surgery. In Baue AE, Geha AS, Hammond GL, et al. (eds): Glenn's Thoracic and Cardiovascular Surgery, ed. 6. Stamford, CT, Appleton & Lange

Hartz RS, LoCicero J III, Sanders JH Jr, et al., 1990: Clinical experience with portable cardiopulmonary bypass. Ann Thorac Surg 50:437

Horrow J, 1999: Transfusion medicine and coagulation disorders. In Kaplan JA (ed): Cardiac Anesthesia, ed. 4. Philadelphia, WB Saunders

Kirklin JW, Barratt-Boyes BG, 1993: Hypothermia, circulatory arrest, and cardiopulmonary bypass. In Cardiac Surgery, ed. 2. New York, Churchill Livingstone

Lazar HL, Hamasaki T, Bao Y, et al., 1998: Soluble complement receptor type I limits damage during revascularization of ischemic myocardium. Ann Thorac Surg 65:973

Mangano CM, Hill L, Cartwright CR, Hindman BJ, 1999: Cardiopulmonary bypass and the anesthesiologist. In Kaplan JA (ed): Cardiac Anesthesia, ed. 4. Philadelphia, WB Saunders

McGiffin DC, Kirklin JK, 1995: Cardiopulmonary bypass for cardiac surgery. In Sabiston DC Jr, Spencer FC (eds): Surgery of the Chest, ed. 6. Philadelphia, WB Saunders

Nolan SP, Zacour R, 1998: Cardiopulmonary bypass. In Kaiser LR, Kron IL, Spray TL (eds): Mastery of Cardiothoracic Surgery. Philadelphia, Lippincott Williams & Wilkins

Rao V, Weisel RD, 1997: Intraoperative protection of organs: Hypothermia, cardioplegia, and cerebroplegia. In Edmunds LH Jr (ed): Cardiac Surgery in the Adult. New York, McGraw-Hill

Reardon MJ, Espada R, Letsou GV, et al., 1997: Editorial: Minimally invasive coronary artery surgery: A word of caution. J Thorac Cardiovasc Surg 119:419

Schoen FJ, 1997: Pathologic considerations in the surgery of adult heart disease. In Edmunds LH Jr (ed): Cardiac Surgery in the Adult. New York, McGraw-Hill

Stammers AH, 1999: Extracorporeal devices and related technologies. In Kaplan JA (ed): Cardiac Anesthesia, ed. 4. Philadelphia, WB Saunders

Utley JR, 1989: Cardiopulmonary bypass in the adult. In Grillo HC, Austen WG, Wilkins EW, et al. (eds): Current Therapy in Cardiothoracic Surgery. Toronto, Canada, BC Decker

Weiland AP, Walker WE, 1986: Physiologic principles and clinical sequelae of cardiopulmonary bypass. Heart Lung 15:34

Whitman G, 1987: Cardiac surgery. In Talkington S, Raterink G (eds): Every Nurses' Guide to Cardiovascular Care. New York, Fleshner

13

Myocardial Protection

Recognition of the relationship between intraoperative myocardial ischemia and postoperative outcome was a major advance in the development of cardiac surgery. As cardiac surgeons gained experience in the early years of using cardiopulmonary bypass (CPB), it became increasingly apparent that inadequate oxygenation of myocardial tissue during CPB results in myocardial necrosis and is the major cause of perioperative myocardial infarction and death. With this knowledge came the recognition that protection of the myocardium from ischemic injury is essential to the success of operations on the heart or great vessels.

Myocardial protection may be defined as the specific intraoperative techniques designed to protect the heart from tissue damage that would otherwise result from the ischemic state associated with extracorporeal circulation. Improved techniques to protect ischemic myocardium have had a substantial impact on lowering mortality rates associated with cardiac surgery. Because the heart can now be better protected, cardiac operations of a more complex nature have become possible, and patients with significant ventricular impairment are able to withstand cardiac surgery.

Nevertheless, perioperative myocardial damage remains the leading cause of morbidity and mortality in patients undergoing heart surgery. Combinations of gross, microscopic, or histochemical evidence of myocardial necrosis, most severe in the ventricular subendocardium, are present at autopsy in as many as 90% of patients who die during the perioperative period after cardiac operations (Buckberg & Allen, 1996). In addition, damage from global myocardial ischemia may result in myocardial stunning, a condition characterized by a variable, sometimes prolonged, period of both systolic and diastolic dysfunction without muscle necrosis (Kirklin & Barratt-Boyes, 1993). Myocardium that is stunned is not yet irreversibly damaged and responds favorably to increases in coronary blood flow and inotropic stimulation (Rao & Weisel, 1997).

The focus of this chapter is myocardial protection during CPB. However, preoperative titration of cardiac medications and fluids, careful induction of general anesthesia with proper monitoring, and vigilant control of hemodynamic parameters during the early postoperative hours also play an important role in perioperative myocardial protection and are addressed elsewhere in the text.

▶ Principles of Myocardial Protection

Under normal conditions, the amount and distribution of blood flow to the heart are regulated by changes in aortic pressure, tension in the various myocardial layers, and coronary vascular resistance (Kirklin & Barratt-Boyes, 1993). Because these protective regulatory factors are altered during CPB, the myocardium is susceptible to global ischemia. A great deal of clinical and laboratory investigation has focused on how best to protect the ischemic heart during CPB. Current techniques of myocardial protection are based on the results of these investigations and an understanding of certain physiologic principles of myocardial oxygen supply and demand.

Although the heart comprises less than 0.5% of body weight, it accounts for more than 7% of oxygen consumption (Rao & Weisel, 1997). Ischemia—that is, reduced arterial blood flow—is more damaging to myocardial tissue than hypoxia, or normal blood flow with reduced oxygen content. Both conditions result in increased anaerobic metabolism that produces hydrogen ions and lactate. However, because blood flow is compromised during ischemia, these harmful metabolites accumulate instead of being washed out as occurs with the normal flow present during hypoxia.

The left ventricular subendocardium is most vulnerable to ischemic damage. Although the right ventricle and the left ventricular subepicardium are perfused throughout the cardiac cycle, the subendocardium of the left ventricle receives oxygenated blood only during diastole.

During systole, increased myocardial tension in the well-developed left ventricular muscle mass compresses intramyocardial branches of the coronary arteries that supply the subendocardium (Kirklin & Barratt-Boyes, 1993; Buckberg, 1987). Blood flow is compromised further if the ventricle is hypertrophied or if coronary artery disease is present. Both conditions cause resting vasodilatation of subendocardial vessels and substantially reduce their capacity to regulate flow proportionate to changing oxygen needs (Buckberg & Allen, 1996). In addition, hypertrophied myocardium is relatively deficient in blood vessels, rendering it particularly susceptible to ischemic damage during cardiac operations (Schoen, 1997).

The use of hypothermia during CPB reduces metabolic activity and oxygen demand. Within limits, the lower the body temperature, the longer the ischemic time that can be endured without tissue damage. Decreased tissue temperature and cardioplegic arrest of the heart slow chemical reactions and thereby protect cardiac myocytes from progressive ischemic damage (Schoen, 1997). Hypothermia also sustains intracellular reservoirs of high-energy phosphates essential for cellular integrity and preserves high intracellular pH and electrochemical neutrality (Nolan & Zacour, 1998). Although hypothermia reduces myocardial oxygen demand, the demand is not zero even with deep hypothermia (Siwek & Daggett, 1989). Because ischemic tissue injury increases exponentially with time even with advanced methods of myocardial preservation, expeditious performance of a cardiac operation is essential (Rankin & Sabiston, 1995).

► Techniques of Myocardial Protection

Most cardiac operations are performed with cardioplegia and a period of aortic cross-clamping (Fig. 13-1). This technique provides the surgeon with a still, bloodless field within which to perform precise technical maneuvers. Application of an aortic cross-clamp isolates the coronary circulation from the blood volume circulating through the CPB circuit, but not all blood flow to the myocardium is eliminated. Noncoronary collaterals in the pericardial attachments and pulmonary vein walls continue to provide some blood flow during the period of aortic cross-clamping. Blood flow through these vessels, which are more abundant in patients with most forms of cardiac disease, produce an ischemic rather than anoxic state in the myocardium.

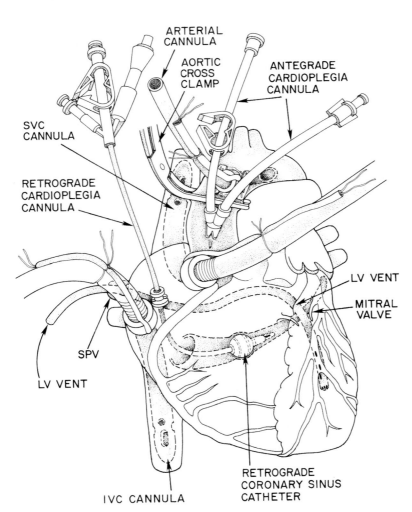

FIGURE 13-1. Completed cannulation for cardiopulmonary bypass. The superior vena cava (SVC) and inferior vena cava (IVC) have been cannulated for venous drainage and the ascending aorta has been cannulated for arterial return. A catheter for administering retrograde cardioplegia is in the coronary sinus and a catheter for antegrade cardioplegia delivery is in the ascending aorta, proximal to the aortic cross-clamp. A left ventricular (LV) vent has been inserted through the right superior pulmonary vein (SPV). (Nolan SP, Zacour R, 1998: Cardiopulmonary bypass. In Kaiser LR, Kron IL, Spray TL [eds]: Mastery of Cardiothoracic Surgery, p. 283. Philadelphia, Lippincott Williams & Wilkins)

If no cross-clamp is applied, blood flows into the coronary arteries from the CPB circuit; the heart is perfused and continues to beat. Although many cardiac operations can be performed in this fashion—that is, with an empty, perfused, and beating heart—the myocardium is more vulnerable to ischemic damage. Induction of electromechanical arrest greatly reduces myocardial energy demands and in combination with profound myocardial hypothermia increases the time that the myocardium can tolerate a globally ischemic state.

In a more recent innovation, some surgeons perform coronary artery bypass grafting without CPB, using special coronary artery retractors to perform distal anastomoses while the heart continues to beat. Data about the safety of these "off-pump" coronary artery bypass grafting operations are being evaluated, and long-term data on patency of vein grafts performed with this technique are not yet available. The following discussion focuses on the more common technique, which includes CPB and a period of ischemic cardiac arrest. The regimen used to protect the heart from global myocardial ischemia during such operations includes (1) moderate systemic hypothermia, (2) profound myocardial hypothermia, and (3) cardioplegia.

Hypothermia

A combination of three techniques is used to achieve moderate systemic and profound myocardial hypothermia: (1) systemic cooling of blood as it passes through the CPB circuit, (2) topical cooling of the heart with a cold solution or cooling jacket, and (3) infusion of the coronary arteries with chilled cardioplegic solution. In addition to active induction of systemic hypothermia, the administration of muscle relaxants, narcotics, and sedatives before surgery and of anesthetic agents during the operation inhibits the body's normal temperature-regulating mechanisms, producing a state of poikilothermia in which body temperature is environmentally controlled. Therefore, the temperature of ambient air, infused intravenous solutions, and topically applied materials contribute to maintaining a hypothermic state.

Systemic hypothermia, or core cooling of the body to 28°C to 32°C, is induced at the onset of CPB to reduce cellular metabolic demands of the myocardium and other vital organs. Before application of the aortic cross-clamp, myocardial temperature is lowered as the chilled perfusate (circulating blood volume) flows into the coronary arterial circulation. When systemic hypothermia has been achieved, the ventricles fibrillate. At this point, an occlusive clamp is applied to the aorta, proximal to the aortic cannula used for arterial return from the CPB circuit. Once the aortic cross-clamp is applied, further temperature reduction in the heart and maintenance of myocardial hypothermia are accomplished with topical bathing of the heart and infusion of cold cardioplegic solution. With these measures, myocardial temperature is lowered to approximately 10°C.

Topical (or surface) cooling of the heart minimizes re-warming between doses of cardioplegic solution. It is performed by bathing the heart continuously or intermittently with ice-cold saline or Ringer's lactate solution. Care is taken to avoid exposing the left side of the pericardium containing the phrenic nerve to the iced solution to avoid nerve injury. An isolating pad also may be placed between the heart and the left side of the pericardium for this purpose (Kirklin & Barratt-Boyes, 1993). As an alternative to bathing the heart with a cold solution, a cooling pad or "jacket" may be wrapped around the heart. Ventricular temperature and effectiveness of cooling may be measured using a thermistor probe placed in the left ventricular myocardium.

Cardioplegia

Cardioplegia is the induction and maintenance of the heart in an arrested state using a solution infused into the coronary arterial circulation. The fundamental purpose of any cardioplegic technique is protection against ischemic injury during the aortic cross-clamp period when normal antegrade coronary artery blood flow is absent (Rao & Weisel, 1997). However, the relative merits of specific ingredients of cardioplegic solutions remain controversial and optimum concentrations of various agents and additives are not standardized. Many surgeons consider hypothermia to be the most effective metabolic inhibitor and therefore the most important component of cardioplegic solution in inducing and maintaining safe arrest of the heart. Despite variations, all cardioplegic solutions are designed with the same specific objectives: safe arrest of the heart, continued energy production by the myocardium, and avoidance of ischemia (Buckberg & Allen, 1996). Usually, a standard cardioplegic solution based on the previously mentioned principles is selected for institutional use.

Major categories of cardioplegic solution include autologous blood, crystalloid, and oxygenated crystalloid solutions. Both cold blood and oxygenated crystalloid solutions provide some degree of oxygen to myocardial tissue. Myocardial metabolic processes and oxygen consumption are not entirely inhibited by hypothermia and cardiac arrest, and the presence of oxygen in the solution allows increased aerobic and decreased anaerobic metabolism (Steinberg et al., 1991). Anaerobic metabolism not only is less efficient than aerobic metabolism but its end products rapidly lead to acidosis, mitochondrial dysfunction, and myocyte necrosis (Rao & Weisel, 1997). The more efficient aerobic metabolism thus reduces the likelihood of global or regional myocardial cellular injury. Autologous *blood cardioplegia* has become the preferred type of cardioplegic solution. It is the chosen cardioplegic solution for myocardial protection in 72% of cardiac operations in the United States; crystalloid cardioplegia is used in 22% and oxygenated crystalloid in 6% (Robinson et al., 1995). Advantages of blood cardioplegia include less systemic hemodilution, the delivery of oxygen, and the provision of endogenous buffers, free radical scavengers, and proteins for controlling oncotic pressure (Loop, 1998).

Administration of cardioplegia is achieved with antegrade infusion, retrograde infusion, or a combination of both techniques. *Antegrade infusion* describes the technique of infusing cardioplegic solution through a catheter placed proximal to the aortic cross-clamp in the aortic root. With a competent aortic valve and the aorta clamped distal to the catheter, the cardioplegic solution passes directly into the coronary arteries. Aortic root pressure is measured simultaneously through a separate catheter during infusion of the cardioplegic solution.

Most often, cardiac arrest is induced and maintained with *cold cardioplegia*. Infusion of cardioplegic solution that is cold is based on the rationale that when acute ischemia is absent, a fast reduction in energy metabolism is preferable (Schlensak et al., 1996). In some situations, cardioplegia delivered at normothermic temperature, or *warm cardioplegia,* is considered preferable. Specifically, some surgeons recommend induction of cardiac arrest with warm cardioplegia in patients who come to surgery with active ischemia. An oxygenated cardioplegic solution at normothermic temperature as the initial dose to induce cardiac arrest increases myocardial oxygen uptake and is thought to provide additional benefit in patients with acute ischemia (Buckberg & Allen, 1996). Warm induction actively resuscitates the energy-depleted, ischemic heart, improving its tolerance to the subsequent interval of cold ischemia imposed for technical reasons (Elwatidy et al., 1999).

Warm cardioplegia induction usually is followed by intermittent doses of cold cardioplegia to prevent myocardial ischemia during subsequent aortic cross-clamping. An estimated 10% of cardiothoracic surgeons in the United States use warm blood cardioplegia throughout the period of aortic cross-clamping during operations for acquired heart disease (Robinson et al., 1995). Cardiac operations that use a normothermic technique necessitate near-continuous perfusion of the arrested heart with warm cardioplegic solution to prevent ischemic injury, but continuous perfusion results in an obstructed operative field and may compromise the technical quality of the operation (Rao & Weisel, 1997).

Typically, an initial dose of 1 to 1.5 L of cold cardioplegic solution is administered using an antegrade technique. The rate of administration is adjusted to maintain aortic root pressure between 80 and 100 mm Hg to ensure effective delivery of the solution and to achieve rapid diastolic arrest. Global cardiac arrest usually occurs within 30 seconds of cardioplegia infusion but may take 1 to 2 minutes in the presence of stenotic or occluded coronary arteries that impede distal distribution of the solution (Buckberg & Allen, 1996). Because blood flow from noncoronary collateral arteries washes away infused cardioplegic solution and gradually rewarms the heart, intermittent infusions of 500 to 750 mL of cardioplegic solution are administered approximately every 20 minutes during the period of aortic cross-clamping.

Because performance of a distal coronary artery graft anastomosis (vein to coronary artery) takes approximately 15 to 20 minutes for the surgeon to complete, cardioplegic solution often is administered after completion of each distal anastomosis. Cardioplegic solution can be injected directly into the proximal end of the vein graft after completion of the distal anastomosis or infused in retrograde fashion while the proximal anastomosis is being constructed. If proximal anastomoses are performed first, cardioplegic solution delivered into the aortic root after cross-clamping the aorta will flow through a graft to the myocardium it supplies as soon as the distal anastomosis is constructed. Administration of cardioplegic solution through the graft is not possible when an internal thoracic artery is used and its proximal attachment to the subclavian artery is left intact (ie, internal thoracic artery pedicle graft).

In patients with coronary artery disease, the efficacy of an antegrade cardioplegia technique is impeded by nonhomogenous distribution of coronary artery blood flow. Areas of myocardium beyond coronary stenoses are not as well cooled and display persistent electromechanical activity. Antegrade cardioplegia delivery during bypass grafting is limited by the following factors: (1) jeopardized myocardium does not receive cardioplegia until the distal anastomosis to the supplying artery is constructed; (2) muscle supplied by an artery receiving an internal thoracic artery pedicle graft is not revascularized until the end of the cross-clamp period; and (3) jeopardized muscle supplied by diseased, but not graftable, arteries is unprotected (Menasche et al., 1991). An antegrade technique for cardioplegia delivery is particularly limited in patients with diffuse distal disease and multiple totally occluded arteries. Antegrade cooling also is less effective in areas of collateral vessels and in the presence of ventricular hypertrophy (Blanche et al., 1990). Collateral blood flow, which continues despite aortic cross-clamping, is considerably warmer than the cardioplegic solution and thus interferes with the cooling provided by the chilled cardioplegic solution.

For these reasons, coronary bypass operations often are performed using *retrograde cardioplegia,* either exclusively or to supplement the initial cardioplegia dose delivered by the conventional antegrade technique into the aortic root. Most commonly, a catheter is introduced through the right atrial wall and guided by digital manipulation into the coronary sinus. With a retrograde technique, cardioplegic solution is infused through the coronary sinus and coronary veins to perfuse the myocardium in a retrograde fashion (see Fig. 13-1). The coronary venous system is an extensive and unobstructed network that provides an effective conduit to deliver cooling and cardioplegic additives throughout the thickness of the myocardium (Menasche et al., 1991). Thus, it more effectively delivers cardioplegic solution to muscle supplied by diseased coronary arteries.

Many surgeons believe a combination of antegrade and retrograde delivery of cardioplegia provides the best myocardial protection. Usually, the initial dose of cardioplegia is given using an antegrade route, with subsequent doses delivered in retrograde fashion. Proponents of retrograde coronary sinus infusion believe it provides more homogeneous distribution and better myocardial cooling distal to diseased arteries. It is particularly useful in patients with totally obstructed vessels, diffuse coronary atherosclerosis, and in reoperative procedures with atherosclerotic vein or patent internal thoracic artery grafts (Loop, 1998). Retrograde cardioplegic solution appears to be less effective in cooling the right ventricle and capillaries of the left ventricle (Rao & Weisel, 1997). Clinical studies have failed to demonstrate superiority of either the antegrade or the retrograde technique in preserving myocardial function.

Retrograde cardioplegia also is used for myocardial protection during aortic valve replacement operations in patients with aortic valvular regurgitation. In these situations, aortic root delivery of cardioplegia is ineffective because the solution would escape through the incompetent valve into the left ventricle. If aortic regurgitation is suspected before the operation, an aortic root aortogram may be obtained during the preoperative cardiac catheterization to assess valve competence. As an alternative to retrograde cardioplegia in patients with an incompetent aortic valve or during aortic valve replacement, the cardioplegic solution can be administered through small individual cannulae placed directly into the ostia of the right and left coronary arteries (Kirklin & Barratt-Boyes, 1993).

The surgeon ceases to administer cardioplegia doses when the reparative work on the heart is nearly completed. Topical myocardial cooling is discontinued, the perfusionist begins rewarming the perfusate (ie, circulating blood volume), and the aortic cross-clamp is removed. Some surgeons administer a dose of warm, substrate-enriched cardioplegia just before release of the aortic cross-clamp. The infusion of warm cardioplegia at the end of the procedure is based on the rationale that warming the myocardium in the arrested state allows for full recovery of high-energy phosphates during reperfusion (Schlensak et al., 1996). When the myocardium has warmed sufficiently to resume a spontaneous electrical rhythm, venous return to the CPB circuit is decreased gradually, allowing blood to flow through the heart normally. CPB is terminated when heart function is adequate to sustain an acceptable arterial systolic pressure.

REFERENCES

Blanche C, Matloff JM, MacKay DA, 1990: Technical aspects of cardiopulmonary bypass. In Gray RJ, Matloff JM (eds): Medical Care of the Cardiac Surgical Patient. Baltimore, Williams & Wilkins

Buckberg GD, 1987: Recent progress in myocardial protection during cardiac operations. In McGoon DC (ed): Cardiac Surgery, ed. 2. Philadelphia, FA Davis

Buckberg GD, Allen BS, 1996: Myocardial protection management during adult cardiac operations. In Baue AE, Geha AS, Hammond GL, et al. (eds): Glenn's Thoracic and Cardiovascular Surgery, ed. 6. Stamford, CT, Appleton & Lange

Elwatidy AM, Fadalah MA, Bukhari EA, et al., 1999: Antegrade crystalloid cardioplegia vs antegrade/retrograde cold and tepid blood cardioplegia in CABG. Ann Thorac Surg 68:447

Kirklin JW, Barratt-Boyes BG, 1993: Myocardial management during cardiac surgery with cardiopulmonary bypass. In Cardiac Surgery, ed. 2. New York, Churchill Livingstone

Loop FD, 1998: Coronary artery bypass surgery. In Topol EJ (ed): Comprehensive Cardiovascular Medicine. Philadelphia, Lippincott Williams & Wilkins

Menasche P, Subayi JB, Veyssie L, et al., 1991: Efficacy of coronary sinus cardioplegia in patients with complete coronary artery occlusions. Ann Thorac Surg 51:418

Nolan SP, Zacour R, 1998: Cardiopulmonary bypass. In Kaiser LR, Kron IL, Spray TL (eds): Mastery of Cardiothoracic Surgery. Philadelphia, Lippincott Williams & Wilkins

Rankin JS, Sabiston DC Jr, 1995: Physiology of coronary blood flow, myocardial function, and intraoperative myocardial protection. In Sabiston DC Jr, Spencer FC (eds): Surgery of the Chest, ed. 6. Philadelphia, WB Saunders

Rao V, Weisel RD, 1997: Intraoperative protection of organs: Hypothermia, cardioplegia, and cerebroplegia. In Edmunds LH Jr (ed): Cardiac Surgery in the Adult. New York, McGraw-Hill

Robinson LA, Schwarz GD, Goddard DB, et al., 1995: Myocardial protection for acquired heart disease surgery: Results of a national survey. Ann Thorac Surg 59:361

Schoen FJ, 1997: Pathologic considerations in the surgery of adult heart disease. In Edmunds LH Jr (ed): Cardiac Surgery in the Adult. New York, McGraw-Hill

Schlensak C, Doenst T, Beyersdorf F, 1996: Clinical experience with blood cardioplegia. Thorac Cardiovasc Surg 46:282

Siwek LG, Daggett WM, 1989: Myocardial protection. In Grillo HC, Austen WG, Wilkins EW Jr, et al. (eds): Current Therapy in Cardiothoracic Surgery. Toronto, Canada, BC Decker

Steinberg JB, Doherty NE, Munfakh NA, et al., 1991: Oxygenated cardioplegia: The metabolic and functional effects of glucose and insulin. Ann Thorac Surg 51:620

14

Preoperative Techniques

Intraoperative Techniques

Postoperative Techniques

Blood Conservation

Blood conservation may be defined as the set of techniques used to reduce perioperative bleeding, salvage shed blood, and reduce the need for allogeneic (ie, from another human donor) transfusion. It is an integral feature of cardiac operations. Perioperative bleeding is more pronounced in cardiac than in other types of surgical procedures because of the extracorporeal circulation of blood using a cardiopulmonary bypass (CPB) system. Two factors inherent to CPB increase the propensity for bleeding. First, extracorporeal circulation exposes blood to nonphysiologic surfaces and shear stresses that damage platelets and clotting factors. The resultant multiple defects in coagulation proteins, platelet dysfunction, and activation of the fibrinolytic cascade all predispose to bleeding (Bailey et al., 1997). Second, it is necessary to administer systemic anticoagulation before CPB to prevent massive thrombosis as blood is circulated through the system. Although protamine sulfate is administered at the conclusion of CPB to reverse the anticoagulated state, postoperative bleeding can be expected.

The referral of an increasingly complex population for cardiac operations has resulted in a steady increase in the number of patients who require transfusion of allogeneic blood (Jones et al., 1991). With the many less invasive forms of therapy available for treatment of heart disease, patients who undergo cardiac operations are older and have more advanced heart disease, poorer ventricular function, and more associated comorbidities. Preoperative anemia often is present and is not well tolerated postoperatively. Reoperations, associated with more intraoperative blood loss, also have become more common. Patients who require emergent coronary artery bypass grafting after failed percutaneous coronary intervention may have received the antiplatelet agent, abciximab (ReoPro), a monoclonal antibody used to promote vessel patency. Abciximab is associated with increased bleeding when administered within 12 hours of cardiac operations (Gammie et al., 1998). Other factors that increase the risk for perioperative blood transfusion include preexisting bleeding abnormalities, preoperative aspirin ingestion, intra-aortic balloon counterpulsation or thrombolytic therapy, small body size, and the performance of complex procedures.

As many as 30% to 80% of cardiac operations necessitate transfusion of allogeneic blood (Shapira et al., 1998). In addition to packed red blood cells to replace hemoglobin, administration of plasma or platelets sometimes is necessary to replace depleted clotting factors. The half-lives of the coagulation factors are variable and very short in some cases (eg, factor VI, factor VIII, and factor V); in the treatment of major coagulopathies, patients with persistent bleeding require replacement of these substances (Smith, 1998) (Table 14-1).

Appropriate transfusion of allogeneic blood products is essential. First, allogeneic blood transfusion is associated with a small but calculable risk of transmitting viral infection. Specifically, human immunodeficiency virus (HIV), human T-cell lymphotrophic virus (HTLV), hepatitis C virus, and hepatitis B virus can be transmitted through blood transfusion despite the routine testing of donor blood for these agents. The risk of transmitting viral infection by the transfusion of screened allogeneic blood is estimated to be 1 in 493,000 for HIV, 1 in 641,000 for HTLV, 1 in 103,000 for hepatitis C, and 1 in 63,000 for hepatitis B (Schreiber et al., 1996). The serious consequences of these infections have heightened efforts to avoid blood transfusion.

In addition to infection, transfusions can cause both hemolytic and nonhemolytic reactions, graft-versus-host disease, recipient alloimmunization, and hypervolemia (Stammers, 1999). An acute hemolytic transfusion reaction, the most serious type of transfusion reaction, occurs in 1 of every 3000 to 10,000 allogeneic transfusions (Hudak et al., 1998). Operative risk also is increased with excessive perioperative bleeding, particularly when transfusion of multiple allogeneic blood products or operative reexploration is necessary. Multiple transfusions can cause coagulopathies or pulmonary complications, and

TABLE 14-1

Blood Products and Coagulation Factor Concentration

Blood Product	Coagulation Factors	Fibrinogen
Fresh frozen plasma	1 U/mL	2–4 mg/mL
Platelets*	2 U/mL	4–8 mg/mL
Cryoprecipitate	5 U/mL	10 mg/mL

*Except labile factors (VIII, V).
Adapted from Smith CR, 1998: Management of bleeding complications in redo cardiac operations. Ann Thorac Surg 65(4 Suppl):S2.

TABLE 14-2

Features of Blood Conservation in Cardiac Surgery

Avoid preoperative aspirin ingestion
Autologous donation
Priming CPB circuit with crystalloid solution
Cell-saver blood processing device
Cardiotomy suction
Hemoconcentration
Adequate heparin reversal
Surgical hemostasis
Hemostatic agents
Postoperative autotransfusion
Avoidance of postoperative hypertension
Tolerance of postoperative anemia

reexploration for bleeding is an independent risk factor for mortality, renal failure, respiratory distress syndrome, sepsis, and atrial arrhythmias, especially in patients who have undergone complex procedures or reoperations (Loop, 1998). Patients who receive transfusions also have an increased risk of postoperative infection resulting from the immunosuppression associated with transfusion of allogeneic blood products (Hudak et al., 1998).

Certain patients, specifically those of the Jehovah's Witness faith, are forbidden by church law to receive transfusions of blood or blood derivatives. The Jehovah's Witnesses base their beliefs on a literal interpretation of the Bible and believe that acceptance of blood or blood products, even inadvertently, violates God's law and results in forfeiture of resurrection and eternal salvation (Grebenik et al., 1996). Jehovah's Witnesses typically accept CPB as a temporary extension of the circulation, but may consent to operation only with the understanding that they be allowed to die rather than receive allogeneic transfusion. Blood conservation techniques are essential in this group of patients if potentially life-saving operations are to be performed with an acceptable, albeit higher, operative risk.

Blood conservation in cardiac surgery also is important because allogeneic blood is a relatively scarce and expensive commodity. The supply of blood products is limited by the ongoing demand, as well as by the difficulty and expense in securing suitable donors and maintaining adequate stores of the various blood types and components. Between 12 and 14 million units of allogeneic blood products are transfused annually in the United States and cardiac surgical patients account for roughly 10% of the 3.2 million annual recipients (Kilgore & Pacifico, 1998). The techniques used before, during, and after cardiac operations to minimize allogeneic blood transfusion are described in the following sections (Table 14-2).

▶ Preoperative Techniques

Methods of blood conservation in the preoperative period include (1) avoiding aspirin, aspirin-containing products, or other antiplatelet agents (eg, ticlid); and (2) autologous blood donation. Many patients with heart disease, specifically those with coronary artery disease, take aspirin for its therapeutic antiplatelet effect. However, the impaired platelet function induced by aspirin increases perioperative bleeding. Because of its long half-life, aspirin ingestion within 7 to 10 days of surgery increases the likelihood of blood transfusion and postoperative reexploration for bleeding. Consequently, if coronary artery revascularization is planned electively, aspirin often is discontinued 1 to 2 weeks before the planned operative date, especially in patients at higher risk for bleeding. Although aspirin is withheld before surgery, it is administered routinely after coronary artery bypass grafting to promote long-term vein graft patency and, in patients without active bleeding, may be administered in the early postoperative hours by the rectal route. In the presence of significant coronary artery obstruction and unstable angina or acute myocardial infarction, it often is necessary to proceed with surgical revascularization despite recent aspirin ingestion. Also, patients hospitalized with unstable angina usually receive intravenous heparin during the preoperative period. Because of its short half-life, heparin is continued until shortly before the operation and does not significantly increase perioperative bleeding.

Preoperative *autologous donation* is collection by phlebotomy of the patient's own blood or blood components for later transfusion. This technique is used more commonly in other surgical specialties but sometimes is possible in patients undergoing cardiac operations. The cardiac surgeon determines which patients should donate blood before surgery. Autologous donation is best suited for those patients whose procedures can be scheduled several weeks or months in advance, who have a normal hemoglobin value, and who are medically stable enough to withstand a phlebotomy blood loss. Adults with valvular or congenital heart disease in whom surgery is not required urgently often are ideal candidates. A recent retrospective analysis demonstrated that patients who donated autologous blood before elective cardiac operations were less likely to require postoperative allogeneic blood transfusions than matched patients who did not donate blood before surgery (Dupuis et al., 1999).

Autologous donation is less well suited to patients with coronary artery disease. Typically, coronary artery bypass grafting operations are performed within days or weeks of obtaining angiographic evidence of significant coronary artery stenoses. The short interval before operation negates the efficacy of preoperative autologous donation. Also, decreasing the oxygen-carrying capacity of the blood by reducing hemoglobin may place patients with significant coronary artery stenoses at greater risk for acute ischemia or infarction during the preoperative period. Autologous donation is contraindicated in patients with active myocardial ischemia (ie, unstable angina) or recent myocardial infarction. Severe aortic stenosis also is a contraindication to preoperative autologous donation; reduction of intravascular volume in the presence of a fixed obstruction to ventricular output and poor ventricular compliance is tolerated poorly and may lead to catastrophic hemodynamic compromise.

In patients who undergo preoperative autologous donation, 2 units of blood may be harvested on separate occasions at least 1 week apart and several weeks before the planned operation. A period of 3 to 4 weeks usually is necessary for recovery from anemia after collection of 400 mL of autologous whole blood, and approximately 2 months is required for recovery after collection of 800 mL (Watanabe et al., 1991). Phlebotomy within 1 week of operation is counterproductive because the patient comes to surgery anemic and thus at higher risk for allogeneic transfusion. Iron supplementation usually is instituted after preoperative autologous donation to enhance red blood cell replenishment. Recombinant human erythropoietin, a hematopoietic hormone, also may be administered to stimulate bone marrow production of red blood cells. However, erythropoietin therapy is expensive and 2 to 3 weeks are required to achieve an increase in red cell volume (Loop, 1998).

▶ Intraoperative Techniques

In adults undergoing cardiac operations, intraoperative blood conservation techniques include the use of crystalloid solution to prime (ie, fill the tubing with fluid) the CPB circuit. Crystalloid priming hemodilutes the perfusate (ie, blood circulating through the CPB circuit) to a hematocrit of 25% to 30%. Blood diluted to this level still has adequate oxygen-carrying capacity, and the technique avoids the use of allogeneic blood to fill the CPB circuit. Intraoperative blood conservation also includes salvage of blood shed into the mediastinum. Although shed mediastinal blood is hemostatically abnormal due to exposure to the CPB circuit, injured tissue, air, and the collection system, salvage and retransfusion may reduce use of allogeneic blood by as much as 50% (Czer, 1990).

A *cell-saver blood processing device* often is used to salvage and process shed mediastinal blood. Because blood shed into the mediastinum during routine cardiac operations is diluted with irrigating solution and exposed to enzymes activated by blood contact with the wound, it is desirable to wash the cells and discard the diluent. The cell saver is used for this purpose before and after CPB when the patient is not anticoagulated, as well as during CPB except when bleeding is excessive. Shed blood is suctioned from the mediastinum into tubing that has an additional arm through which heparinized solution is added. Blood squeezed from blood-soaked sponges also can be returned to the cell-saver device. Once the anticoagulated blood is returned to the cell saver, the red blood cells are separated out and washed with saline or lactated Ringer's solution to remove heparin and hemolyzed red blood cells (Fig. 14-1). The red blood cells are concentrated using a centrifuge and the packed red blood cells are reserved for transfusion in the early postoperative hours. The wash, which includes the plasma constituents (with coagulation factors) and heparin, is discarded (Edmunds, 1997).

The *cardiotomy suction* in the CPB system is used to collect blood spilled from opened cardiac chambers or when substantial bleeding is present with the need for immediate volume replacement. Use of cardiotomy suction diverts shed mediastinal blood into the cardiotomy reservoir, where it is added to the perfusate for immediate return to the patient as needed. Although the cardiotomy suction system can salvage large amounts of blood that would otherwise be lost, it only filters and defoams, but does not process the blood; the aspirated blood contains enzymes and is not the same as the perfusate with which it is mixed (Edmunds, 1997). The use of cardiotomy suctioned blood also contributes to the release of proinflammatory cytokines, activation of coag-

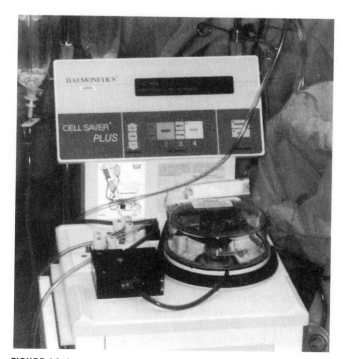

FIGURE 14-1. Haemonetics cell-saver blood processing device. (Haemonetics, Braintree, MA)

ulation, and hemolysis that occurs during and after the use of CPB (Reents et al., 1999).

In patients with preoperative renal insufficiency or excess fluid volume, *hemoconcentration* (also called hemofiltration or ultrafiltration) may be performed during CPB. Hemoconcentration removes plasma water and low–molecular-weight solutes (Edmunds, 1997). To perform hemoconcentration, shed blood is returned to the cardiotomy reservoir and then pumped through a hemofiltration device in which it is concentrated. The primary difference between hemoconcentration and a cell-saver device is that hemoconcentration effectively removes excess water while conserving and concentrating plasma components, specifically platelets and clotting factors, as well as red blood cells. The cell-saver device removes the plasma fraction with its clotting factors, salvaging only washed red blood cells. By using intraoperative blood salvaging techniques, it usually is possible to salvage 2 or 3 units of red blood cells that would otherwise be lost.

Another important component of intraoperative blood conservation is careful titration of heparin dosage during CPB and adequate reversal of systemic anticoagulation with protamine sulfate when CPB is terminated. Activated clotting time is measured to allow precise titration of the dosage of protamine to ensure adequate reversal (Elefteriades et al., 1996). Achieving surgical hemostasis also is essential to minimize blood loss and allogeneic transfusion. Hemostasis is assessed as body temperature is rewarmed and with the heart generating a normal blood pressure. The surgeon examines the mediastinum to detect sources of mechanical bleeding that require suture repair. Areas that are inspected carefully before closing the chest incision include anastomotic suture lines; cannulation sites; conduit side branches; the internal thoracic artery bed; and thymic, epicardial, sternal wire, and chest tube sites (Mahfood et al., 1991).

Hemostatic pharmacologic agents have gained widespread use as a method of blood conservation in cardiac surgery. Hemostatic agents are particularly useful to lessen diffuse bleeding in the presence of a significant coagulopathy; in patients who adamantly refuse allogeneic blood transfusion (eg, those of the Jehovah's Witness faith); and during reoperations or complex procedures, such as aortic dissection repair, heart-lung transplantation, or insertion of left ventricular assist devices. Two groups of antifibrinolytic agents are used commonly to reduce bleeding associated with cardiac operations: (1) serine protease inhibitors, most notably aprotinin; and (2) lysine analogue antifibrinolytics, either aminocaproic acid (Amicar) or tranexamic acid. Aprotinin is the most widely used agent and its efficacy and safety have been extensively evaluated. It has several possible mechanisms of action, including inhibition of the plasma enzyme systems activated by contact with the foreign surface of the CPB circuit and preservation of platelet function (Smith, 1998). Aprotinin is administered by intravenous infusion and by addition to the priming volume in the extracorporeal circuit. Intraoperative administration of aprotinin has been shown to decrease postoperative thoracic drainage volume by 43% and the requirement for red blood cell ad-

ministration by 49% (Alderman et al., 1998). Its effectiveness in reducing blood loss makes aprotinin particularly suitable for use in patients at increased risk for bleeding, such as those with known coagulopathy, those who refuse blood transfusion (eg, Jehovah's Witness faith), those undergoing reoperation, and those who have received aspirin or other antiplatelet agents in the preoperative period. Because aprotinin is a foreign protein (derived from bovine lung tissue), hypersensitivity reactions can occur. Although rare when the patient has had no prior exposure to aprotinin, they occur in 5% and 0.9% of patients who receive aprotinin within 6 months or beyond 6 months of initial use, respectively (Rich, 1998).

On the basis of direct comparisons and meta-analysis of hemostatic drugs used in cardiac surgery, aprotinin is most effective in reducing blood loss, followed in descending order by tranexamic acid and aminocaproic acid; their order with respect to cost at the most commonly recommended dose is the same (Mannucci, 1998). Although therapy with either aprotinin or the lysine analogues is associated with reduced postoperative blood loss, only aprotinin has been demonstrated consistently to reduce the transfusion of blood and blood products (Royston, 1998). However, because of its much lower cost, aminocaproic acid may provide a more cost-effective therapy when comparing bleeding-related costs associated with the use of aprotinin and aminocaproic acid (Bennett-Guerrero et al., 1997). Fibrin sealant has been used during surgery, primarily in Europe, to control small points of bleeding; products derived from pooled human fibrinogen are not yet approved by the Food and Drug Administration for use in the United States (Loop, 1998).

▶ Postoperative Techniques

Autotransfusion is performed commonly in the postoperative period as a method of blood conservation. Autotransfusion is reinfusion of shed mediastinal blood that is defibrinated by contact with the pleura and pericardium (Mahfood et al., 1991). Blood shed through the chest tubes in the initial postoperative hours is filtered and returned to the patient's venous system using a chest drainage system designed for autotransfusion and an intravenous infusion pump. The benefits of postoperative autotransfusion continue to be debated. Prospective, randomized trials have failed to show a reduction in transfusions in patients who have received autotransfusion, probably because of the very high fibrinolytic activity of the reinfused blood (Brown & Jones, 1997). Nevertheless, the practice of autotransfusion in postoperative cardiac surgery patients remains widespread. Evidence suggests that reinfusion of mediastinal and pleural drainage after coronary operation may increase cardiac enzyme levels in the patient's circulating blood, limiting the usefulness of these assays in the early postoperative period in detection of perioperative myocardial infarction (DePaulis et al., 1998).

Postoperative blood conservation also includes careful blood pressure control during the early postoperative hours to avoid hypertension. Postoperative hypertension can exacerbate bleeding or precipitate suture line disruption or loosening of a surgical clip. Even brief hypertensive episodes (eg, systolic blood pressure of 180 to 200 mm Hg) can cause a dramatic increase in chest tube output (Elefteriades et al., 1996).

Yet another method of postoperative blood conservation is tolerance of postoperative anemia. With iron supplementation, most otherwise healthy adults can tolerate a hematocrit level of 20% to 25% without untoward symptoms. In fact, many patients are extremely reluctant to receive allogeneic blood and prefer to rebuild a normal red blood cell count with time, diet, and iron supplementation. Allogeneic transfusion, in the absence of active bleeding, usually is reserved for patients with a hematocrit level less than 20%, symptomatic anemia, or advanced age. In patients with significantly impaired left ventricular function, older age, and serious comorbidities, a hematocrit level of 28% to 30% allows better perfusion pressure and hemodynamic stability (Loop, 1998).

With a comprehensive blood conservation program throughout the perioperative period, use of allogeneic blood can be substantially reduced. However, it is not possible to eliminate blood transfusions in all patients. Indeed, transfusion of allogeneic blood is an essential and sometimes life-saving form of therapy for hemorrhage and postoperative coagulopathy. These conditions are discussed in Chapter 28, Complications of Cardiac Operations.

REFERENCES

Alderman EL, Levy JH, Rich JB, et al., 1998: Analyses of coronary graft patency after aprotinin use: Results from the International Multicenter Aprotinin Graft Patency Experience (IMAGE) trial. J Thorac Cardiovasc Surg 116:716

Bailey JM, Levy JH, Hug CC, 1997: Cardiac surgical pharmacology. In Edmunds LH Jr (ed): Cardiac Surgery in Adults. New York, McGraw-Hill

Bennett-Guerrero E, Sorohan JG, Gurevich ML, et al., 1997: Cost-benefit and efficacy of aprotinin compared with epsilon-aminocaproic acid in patients having repeated cardiac operations: A randomized, blinded clinical trial. Anesthesiology 87:1373

Brown WM, Jones EL, 1997: First operation for myocardial revascularization. In Edmunds LH Jr (ed): Cardiac Surgery in the Adult. New York, McGraw-Hill

Czer LS, 1990: Mediastinal bleeding, blood conservation techniques, and transfusion practices. In Gray RJ, Matloff JM (eds): Medical Management of the Cardiac Surgical Patient. Baltimore, Williams & Wilkins

DePaulis R, Colagrande L, Seddio F, et al., 1998: Levels of troponin I and cardiac enzymes after reinfusion of shed blood in coronary operations. Ann Thorac Surg 65: 1617

Dupuis JY, Bart B, Bryson G, Robblee J, 1999: Transfusion practices among patients who did and did not predonate autologous blood before elective cardiac surgery. CMAJ 160: 997

Edmunds LH Jr, 1997: Extracorporeal perfusion. In Edmunds LH Jr (ed): Cardiac Surgery in the Adult. New York, McGraw-Hill

Elefteriades JA, Geha AS, Cohen LS, 1996: Postoperative bleeding. In House Officer Guide to ICU Care: Fundamentals of Management of the Heart and Lungs, ed. 2. Philadelphia, Lippincott-Raven

Gammie JS, Zenati M, Kormos RL, et al., 1999: Abciximab and excessive bleeding in patients undergoing emergency cardiac operations. Ann Thorac Surg 65:465

Grebenik CR, Sinclair ME, Westaby S, 1996: High risk cardiac surgery in Jehovah's Witnesses. J Cardiovasc Surg 37:511

Hudak CM, Gallo BM, Morton PG, 1998: Patient management: Cardiovascular system. In Critical Care Nursing: A Holistic Approach, ed. 7. Philadelphia, Lippincott Williams & Wilkins

Jones JW, Rawitscher RE, McLean TR, et al., 1991: Benefit from combining blood conservation measures in cardiac operations. Ann Thorac Surg 51:541

Kilgore ML, Pacifico AD, 1998: Shed mediastinal blood transfusion after cardiac operations: A cost-effectiveness analysis. Ann Thorac Surg 65:1248

Loop FD, 1998: Coronary artery bypass surgery. In Topol EJ (ed): Comprehensive Cardiovascular Medicine. Philadelphia, Lippincott Williams & Wilkins

Mahfood SS, Higgins TL, Loop FD, 1991: Management of complications related to coronary artery bypass surgery. In Waldhausen JA, Orringer MB (eds): Complications in Cardiothoracic Surgery. St. Louis, Mosby–Year Book

Mannucci PM, 1998: Hemostatic drugs. N Engl J Med 339: 245

Reents W, Babin-Ebell J, Misoph MR, et al., 1999: Influence of different autotransfusion devices on the quality of salvaged blood. Ann Thorac Surg 68:58

Rich JB, 1998: The efficacy and safety of aprotinin use in cardiac surgery. Ann Thorac Surg 66:S6

Royston D, 1998: Aprotinin versus lysine analogues: The debate continues. Ann Thorac Surg 65:S9

Schreiber GB, Busch MP, Kleinman SH, et al., 1996: The risk of transfusion-transmitted viral infections. N Engl J Med 334:1685

Shapira OM, Aldea GS, Treanor PR, et al., 1998: Reduction of allogeneic blood transfusions after open heart operations by lowering cardiopulmonary bypass prime volume. Ann Thorac Surg 65:724

Smith CR, 1998: Management of bleeding complications in redo cardiac operations. Ann Thorac Surg 65(4 Suppl):S2

Stammers AH, 1999: Extracorporeal devices and related technologies. In Kaplan JA (ed): Cardiac Anesthesia, ed. 4. Philadelphia, WB Saunders

Watanabe Y, Fuse K, Konighi T, et al., 1991: Autologous blood transfusion with recombinant human erythropoietin in heart operations. Ann Thorac Surg 51:767

CARDIOVASCULAR
OPERATIONS

15

Surgical Treatment of Coronary Artery Disease

► Coronary Artery Revascularization

Surgical revascularization of the heart has been a major component in the treatment of coronary artery disease (CAD) since the late 1960s. *Coronary artery bypass grafting* (CABG) is the principal method of surgical revascularization and continues to be one of the most common operations performed in the United States. Approximately 367,000 Americans undergo CABG annually (American Heart Association, 1998). Along with percutaneous coronary intervention (PCI), CABG is the primary interventional modality for treatment of hemodynamically significant obstructive coronary artery stenoses. As with other forms of therapy for CAD, revascularization procedures are not curative and must be accompanied by concomitant treatment of modifiable risk factors associated with disease progression. Many patients eventually are treated with more than one revascularization procedure because of disease progression, vessel restenosis, or graft failure. Thus, a significant number of patients who undergo PCI require a subsequent PCI or CABG, and a lesser number of patients who undergo CABG subsequently require PCI or repeat CABG.

In CABG operations, autologous artery and vein are used as conduits to bypass stenotic lesions in the coronary arterial circulation. Coronary atherosclerosis is a segmental disease that occurs primarily in proximal portions of the three major coronary arteries within 5 cm of their origin from the aorta; distal portions of the vessels usually are patent (Spencer et al., 1995). Bypass grafting of coronary arteries is technically feasible because the major coronary arteries course through epicardial tissue on the surface of the heart for some distance before becoming embedded deep in the myocardium. Target vessels for bypassing are identified before surgery on the coronary angiogram, a contrast study that defines coronary artery anatomy. Any of the three major coronary arteries—left anterior descending (LAD), circumflex, or right—may be grafted, as well as branches of these arteries. In patients with more diffuse CAD, CABG may be combined with coronary artery endarterectomy. Rarely, laser revascularization techniques are used.

Indications for Surgical Revascularization

Three large, randomized, prospective studies performed in the 1980s established a framework for determining the benefits of medical versus surgical treatment of CAD. Specifically, the European Cooperative Study, Coronary Artery Surgery Study (CASS), and Veterans Administration Cooperative Study provided outcome data and helped define those patients most likely to benefit from surgical therapy (European Coronary Surgery Study Group, 1982; CASS Principal Investigators, 1983; Veterans Administration Coronary Artery Bypass Cooperative Study Group, 1984). Since completion of these studies, however, treatment of CAD has continued to evolve with

149

increasingly effective antianginal medications, thrombolytic therapy, refinement of PCI, and development of intracoronary stents. As a result, indications for surgical revascularization continue to evolve as the roles of less invasive forms of treating CAD are refined. Nevertheless, the major qualitative conclusion of the early multicenter trials remains relevant to current decision making—namely, the relative benefits of CABG over medical therapy are greatest in patients with more severe ischemia, more diseased vessels, and the presence of left ventricular dysfunction (Smith & Gersh, 1996).

Whereas medical therapy achieves most of its beneficial effect through reduction in the demand side of the supply–demand coronary blood supply mismatch (eg, reducing preload, afterload, heart rate, and contractility), revascularization therapies (ie, PCI and CABG) affect the supply side of the imbalance (Smith & Gersh, 1996). Both PCI and CABG are designed to restore adequate blood flow to jeopardized myocardium to achieve one or more of three objectives: (1) control of ischemic symptoms, (2) prevention of myocardial infarction (MI), and (3) prolongation of life. Information obtained from natural history studies and clinical trials has been used to identify patients who will benefit most from these revascularization procedures. Such patients include those with significant coronary artery lesions suitable for revascularization and (1) stable angina refractory to adequate medical therapy and interfering with the patient's ability to function at an acceptable level of activity, (2) exercise-induced hypotension or ventricular arrhythmias secondary to myocardial ischemia, (3) unstable angina, or (4) evolving MI.

A great deal of judgment and consideration of relevant data affect the decision-making process about whether PCI or CABG is the most appropriate form of revascularization for a given patient because each is associated with particular benefits and risks. Patients with CAD are extremely heterogeneous in terms of clinical and angiographic severity of disease, left ventricular function, and comorbidities, such as diabetes and peripheral vascular disease (Smith & Gersh, 1996). For some patients, it remains unclear which alternative provides the best benefit–risk ratio. Ideally, in cases in which optimal therapy is controversial, the decision is made by the managing cardiologist with input from both an interventional cardiologist (who would perform PCI) and a surgeon.

Most patients with limited CAD undergo PCI as the initial revascularization procedure. Improvements in angioplasty balloon catheters, availability of intracoronary stents, and increased skill of cardiologists performing PCI have significantly expanded the use of this form of therapy. PCI is almost always the initial revascularization intervention if only one coronary artery has significant narrowing (ie, single-vessel disease). PCI offers the distinct advantage of avoiding a major thoracic operation and most patients experience substantial improvement of ischemic symptoms. Angina is decreased in 88% of patients and eliminated entirely in 76% (Lincoff & Topol, 1997).

In patients with more than one target lesion, either

PCI or CABG may be recommended, depending on the specific anatomy and status of the left ventricle. However, multivessel PCI is associated with both a greater initial risk and a higher probability of restenosis compared with single-vessel PCI (King, 1996). Other considerations also influence the choice of revascularization therapy, including age, general health status, associated cardiac disease, and associated medical problems. PCI can result in a number of complications, including acute MI and the need for emergency surgical revascularization (King, 1990). In addition, restenosis of the dilated or stented artery occurs in approximately 20% to 25% of patients. For this reason, and because of the progressive nature of CAD, many patients who initially undergo PCI eventually are treated with CABG.

The decision to recommend CABG as the initial revascularization procedure is based primarily on anatomic findings during cardiac catheterization. CABG remains the treatment of choice in several categories of patients: (1) those with triple-vessel disease with left ventricular dysfunction, (2) those with significant (>75%) left main coronary artery stenosis, and (3) those with complex lesions not well suited to balloon dilatation or with repeated restenosis after PCI.

Target Vessels

A number of characteristics of a diseased coronary artery determine its suitability for bypass grafting, including (1) degree of narrowing of the arterial lumen, (2) size of the artery distal to the stenosis, (3) presence of diffuse disease in the distal portion of the artery, and (4) viability of muscle supplied by the artery. Because lesions that produce greater than 75% narrowing of the arterial lumen significantly compromise arterial blood flow, arteries with this degree of narrowing are considered primary targets for revascularization. However, the currently recommended strategy for CABG is complete revascularization. Therefore, all arterial trunks and branches with greater than 50% narrowing usually are bypassed as well, except those of trivial size (Kirklin & Barratt-Boyes, 1993a). The native coronary artery at the site of a planned distal anastomosis should be at least 1 mm in diameter and relatively free of atherosclerotic disease. In vessels of smaller caliber, blood flow through the graft is likely to be too low to support graft patency. Arteries with diffuse narrowing throughout the length of the vessel are not suitable for bypass grafting.

A coronary artery that is totally occluded, but distally patent and perfused by collateral circulation, may be bypassed depending on viability of muscle supplied by the vessel. Most often, total occlusion of a coronary artery causes acute MI and necrosis of muscle supplied by the artery. If so, restoring blood supply to the necrotic muscle provides no benefit. However, when adequate collateral circulation to an area of muscle has prevented infarction at the time of coronary artery occlusion, it may be beneficial to bypass the artery. The ventriculogram, obtained during preoperative cardiac catheterization, provides an indication of muscle viability by demonstrating contractility of the various myocardial segments. Preoperative radionuclide scanning also is useful in determining regional muscle viability. A totally occluded artery also may be bypassed when surgical revascularization is performed during evolution of an MI (within 4 to 6 hours of onset) and muscle damage is judged to be reversible. Noninvasive techniques for determining reversibility of acute myocardial injury (ie, differentiating "stunned" from necrotic myocardium) are the focus of intense research that may revise future therapy for evolving MI.

Conduit for Bypass Grafting

Bypass grafting of the coronary arteries is performed in most patients using internal thoracic artery (ITA; also called internal mammary artery), saphenous vein, or a combination of the two.

Internal Thoracic Artery

The left and right ITAs lie on the undersurface of the anterior chest wall, on either side of the sternum. In most elective revascularization procedures, one of the ITAs, usually the left, is harvested for use in bypassing one or two stenosed coronary arteries. The ITA is the preferred conduit because its long-term patency rates have proven superior to those of saphenous veins. Use of ITA conduit significantly improves overall survival, lessens the risk of subsequent MI, and delays the need for reoperation (Kron & Bayfield, 1998). Consequently, whenever possible the ITA is selected as the conduit of choice for bypassing the LAD or other major arteries that supply large regions of myocardium (Loop, 1998).

Patency rates of 90% or greater at 10 years after operation have been demonstrated with ITA grafts, in contrast to 50% patency rates with saphenous vein grafts (Pigott & Mills, 1998). Factors thought to contribute to superior long-term patency include the following: (1) the ITA's smaller size more closely approximates coronary artery diameter; (2) flow may be less turbulent because of similarities in ITA and coronary artery geometry; (3) ITA grafts have no valves or varicosities, as do vein grafts; and (4) the ITA retains the biologic processes of an intact arterial vessel (Morris et al., 1990). The intrinsic qualities of arterial grafts make them relatively immune to the three biologic modes of graft failure affecting venous conduits: early thrombosis, subintimal fibrosis, and late atherosclerosis (Galbut et al., 1991).

For an ITA to be used for bypass grafting, it must have adequate length, be free of damage from the harvesting, and provide immediate adequate flow (Pigott & Mills, 1998). Most often, the ITA is used as a pedicle, or in situ, graft; that is, the vessel is harvested from the undersurface of the chest wall in its fat pedicle. The origin of the ITA is left intact at its connection to the subclavian artery, and the distal end is attached to the target coronary artery by constructing an end-to-side anastomosis (Fig. 15-1). After construction of an ITA pedicle

graft, oxygenated blood travels from the ascending aorta through the subclavian artery, ITA graft, and constructed distal anastomosis into the target coronary artery. Because of the anterior location of the LAD artery, a left ITA pedicle graft almost always reaches the distal portion of the vessel without tension.

Some surgeons believe the excellent patency rates associated with ITA grafts warrant elective use of both in preference to vein grafting. More commonly, bilateral ITA grafting is reserved for selected situations, such as absence of venous conduit, very young patients with accelerated atherosclerosis, and reoperation for failed vein grafts (Morris et al., 1990). Candidates for bilateral ITA grafting who lack venous conduits include patients who have undergone lower extremity amputations, previous saphenous vein ligation for varicosities, vein harvesting for coronary or peripheral arterial bypass procedures, and those who have severe and extensive varicosities. Bilateral as opposed to unilateral ITA grafting has not been proven to increase survival in patients followed up to 15 years after surgery (Brown & Jones, 1997). Bilateral ITA grafting does appear to lessen the likelihood that reoperation will be required (Lytle & Cosgrove, 1992). Data from Cosgrove and associates suggest that the superiority of using more than one arterial graft will be demonstrated primarily in younger patients in the period beyond 8 to 10 years after operation (Rankin & Morris, 1995).

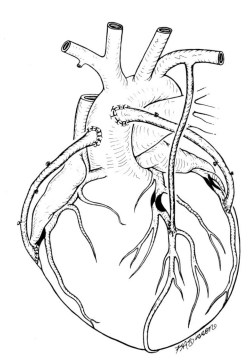

FIGURE 15-1. Typical coronary artery bypass grafting operation. In this illustration, the left internal thoracic artery has been used to construct a pedicle graft to the left anterior descending coronary artery; saphenous vein grafts have been constructed to bypass lesions in the right and circumflex coronary arteries. (Preparing for Cardiac Surgery. Division of Cardiothoracic Surgery and Department of Nursing, Northwestern Memorial Hospital)

Because of the superior patency rates offered by ITA grafts, they sometimes are used in ways that involve more complex anastomoses (eg, as a free graft, a sequential graft, or a conduit-to-conduit graft). Complex ITA grafts are more challenging technically than similar grafts using saphenous vein because the ITA is more difficult to harvest, more easily damaged, more compromised by spasm or technical error, and more difficult to anastomose owing to fragility and small size (Barner, 1998). An ITA may be used as a free graft to obtain additional graft length, when the ITA has been injured during harvesting, or to avoid placing a graft across the midline when a right ITA is used (Tashiro et al., 1998). When used as a free graft, the ITA is excised at its proximal as well as distal end. It is anastomosed proximally to the aorta in end-to-side fashion and its distal end can be used for a target coronary vessel on the side or back wall of the heart. The patency rate for ITA free grafts appears to be 5% to 8% lower than that for ITA pedicle grafts (Barner, 1998).

Using the ITA to graft vessels with less than 75% stenoses is controversial. In contrast to a vein graft, the ITA is a muscular, reactive conduit. Many surgeons believe that competitive flow through the native coronary artery (as would occur in a mildly stenosed artery) leads to low flow through the ITA graft with subsequent closure. Questions also remain regarding the influence of ITA harvesting on perioperative morbidity associated with CABG. Early reoperation for bleeding and postoperative blood loss may be somewhat increased because of the extensive intraoperative dissection with ITA harvesting. However, current blood conservation techniques and long-term superiority of ITA grafts favor routine unilateral ITA grafting despite a tendency for more bleeding.

There also is concern that diversion of a portion of the anterior chest wall blood supply may increase the incidence of sternal wound infection or dehiscence, particularly when bilateral ITA harvesting is performed in pa-tients who are obese, diabetic, or receiving chronic steroid therapy. Because the ITAs provide the major source of blood supply to the sternum, mobilization of an ITA may significantly devascularize the sternal half from which it was harvested (Ulicny & Hiratzka, 1991). Particularly susceptible to sternal infection are diabetic patients who are obese or elderly (Rankin & Morris, 1995; Spencer et al., 1995). Unfortunately, bilateral ITA grafting is particularly suited to diabetic patients because of the diffuse nature of coronary artery atherosclerosis associated with diabetes mellitus (Lytle et al., 1986).

A higher incidence of respiratory insufficiency sometimes is reported in patients undergoing ITA grafting. It may be related to phrenic nerve dysfunction during ITA harvest and usually can be avoided with proper operative technique (Rankin & Morris, 1995). Postoperative anterior chest wall discomfort or paresthesia also appears to be increased when ITA harvesting is performed. However, it is almost always transient and rarely interferes with routine postoperative recovery. A very small number of patients have persistent, pronounced discomfort or paresthesia in the chest wall overlying the area of ITA dissection.

Alternative Arterial Conduits

Bypass grafting using all arterial conduit material may be desirable in some patients, such as those who are very young or those who have demonstrated a propensity for premature failure of vein grafts (Pigott & Mills, 1998). Sources of supplemental arterial conduit, in addition to the left and right ITA, include the radial, right gastroepiploic, and the inferior epigastric artery (Fig. 15-2).

The radial artery rarely is affected by atherosclerosis and has a length and diameter suitable for bypassing the coronary arteries (Pigott & Mills, 1998). The 5-year patency rate for radial artery grafts has been demonstrated angiographically as superior to that of saphenous veins

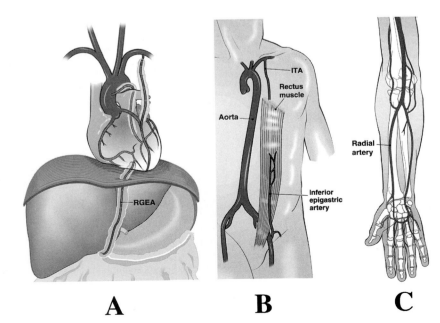

A   **B**   **C**

FIGURE 15-2. Alternative arterial conduits. **(A)** The gastroepiploic artery is mobilized from the greater curvature of the stomach, brought through the diaphragm, and usually used to graft a branch of the right coronary artery. **(B)** The inferior epigastric artery may be sewn proximally to an arterial conduit and distally to a secondary target coronary artery. **(C)** The radial artery. (Loop FD, 1998: Coronary artery bypass surgery. In Topol EJ [ed]: Comprehensive Cardiovascular Medicine, p. 2294. Philadelphia, Lippincott Williams & Wilkins)

used to graft comparable target arteries (Acar et al., 1998; Possati et al., 1998). It is regarded as the second arterial conduit of choice after both ITAs, and may be attached as an aortocoronary graft or as a "Y" graft (Loop, 1998). The gastroepiploic artery may be used as a free graft or mobilized and brought into the pericardial space as a pedicle graft. Patency rates of 92% to 97% at 8 to 10 years have been reported for gastroepiploic artery grafts (Barner, 1998). The inferior epigastric artery is used only rarely, usually to graft secondary targets such as branch vessels (Loop, 1998). Patency of inferior epigastric artery grafts is less than that of other arterial conduits (Barner, 1998).

Saphenous Vein

Most patients who undergo surgical revascularization require three or more bypass grafts, and most surgeons prefer to harvest only the left ITA in routine CABG procedures. Because the left ITA usually is used for only one distal anastomosis, the greater saphenous vein from one or both legs is harvested in almost all cases (Fig. 15-3). Saphenous vein is expendable, is of comparable size to coronary arteries, is pliable enough to allow easy suturing, and vein segments usually can be harvested as free grafts of sufficient length to bypass whichever arteries are stenosed (American College of Cardiology [ACC]/ American Heart Association [AHA] Task Force, 1991). The presence of one-way valves that occur naturally inside veins makes it necessary for the surgeon to reverse the vein segments, attaching the distal end of vein to the aorta and the proximal end to the coronary artery.

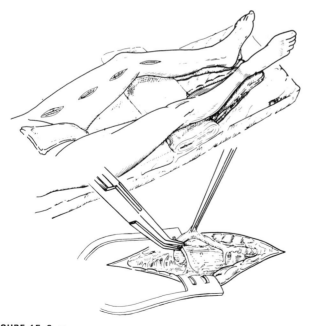

FIGURE 15-3. The greater saphenous vein is harvested from one or both legs using multiple short incisions and meticulous technique to avoid damaging the vein segments. (Loop FD, 1979: Saphenous vein bypass graft. In Cohn LH [ed]: Modern Technics in Surgery, p. 10-2. Mount Kisco, NY, Futura)

The rapidity with which the greater saphenous vein can be harvested makes it the conduit of choice in emergency situations in which the myocardium is acutely ischemic, such as failed PCI, or if the patient is hemodynamically unstable. Revascularization exclusively with saphenous vein grafts also may be preferable in very elderly patients with comorbidities. In these patients, long-term superiority of the ITA is not as important and the operation can be shortened, presumably making it safer, by using only venous conduit. Patients who receive only vein grafts have a much higher and earlier reoperation rate than patients with one or more arterial conduits (Loop, 1998).

Removal of saphenous vein from one or both legs is associated with minimal morbidity if the procedure is meticulously performed. Because there is redundant venous drainage from the legs, loss of the saphenous vein does not pose any long-term problems. Preoperative assessment of arterial blood flow to the lower extremities is important; if peripheral arterial occlusive disease is present, wound healing may be compromised. Vein is harvested from the leg with the least degree of arterial disease. Also, because lymphatic drainage from the leg is interrupted at the time of vein harvest, some degree of edema in the affected leg develops in almost all patients. The edema can be expected to resolve within weeks or, occasionally, months after the operation. In patients who are immobilized for a prolonged period after surgery, the propensity for deep venous thrombosis may be increased because of the absent vein.

Significant morphologic changes and development of atherosclerosis have been well documented in saphenous vein grafts (Grondin et al., 1979). Vein grafts undergo endothelial proliferation as soon as they are used in the arterial circulation, and diffuse intimal hyperplasia is universally present in vein grafts that have been in place more than 1 year (Loop, 1998; ACC/AHA Task Force, 1991). Saphenous vein graft occlusion occurs most frequently in the first year, at a rate of 15% to 25%; the annual rate for 2 to 7 years after grafting is 0.5% to 3% (Gall, 1997). Early postoperative vein graft failure usually is related to thrombosis from low flow, a hypercoagulable state, or technical reasons; graft failure within 2 to 3 years after surgery usually occurs secondary to intimal hyperplasia; and that occurring more than 3 years after surgery is predominantly due to atherosclerosis (Pigott & Mills, 1998).

Graft closure is more likely in vein grafts with poor distal runoff and resultant low flow (eg, grafts to coronary arteries of small caliber or arteries supplying muscle that is heavily scarred) (ACC/AHA Task Force, 1991). The intraoperative use of aprotinin also appears to affect vein graft patency adversely in patients in whom the primary target vessels for bypass grafting are less than 1.5 mm or of poor quality (Alderman et al., 1998). Strict control of postoperative serum lipids is another important factor in controlling postoperative vein graft disease, and it is possible that lipid-lowering drugs may play a role in modifying disease progression (Pigott & Mills, 1998). Data from serial postoperative angiographic studies demonstrate vein graft patency rates of

81%, 75%, and 50% at 1, 5, and more than 15 years, respectively (Loop, 1998).

Alternative Venous Conduits

If saphenous veins have been harvested previously or are of poor quality, there may be insufficient conduit material for necessary grafts. In these situations, use of alternative venous conduit may be necessary. Although all are associated with lower patency rates than greater saphenous veins, the lesser saphenous, cephalic, and basilic veins are alternative conduit sources. The lesser saphenous vein, located on the posterior aspect of the calf, is more difficult to harvest and often has many valves and branches; arm veins (cephalic or basilic) are small, thin walled, and prone to aneurysmal dilatation and graft failure (Pigott & Mills, 1998). Cryopreserved autologous saphenous vein is an alternative when the patient has inadequate sources of conduit material, although it too is associated with poor patency rates. Artificial conduits have extremely poor long-term patency rates and are used rarely.

The Operative Procedure

Operations to revascularize the heart are performed most often through a median sternotomy incision. The sternotomy incision provides excellent exposure of the heart and great vessels. An incision is made through the skin from the supraclavicular notch to the xiphoid process and electrocautery is used to dissect through the soft tissue to the anterior table of the sternum. The sternum is divided longitudinally using an oscillating saw designed for this purpose. If an ITA is to be used, the ipsilateral hemisternum is elevated with a retractor and the artery is mobilized from its intrathoracic bed on the undersurface of the anterior chest wall. Most often, the left ITA is harvested as a pedicle graft with preservation of its proximal attachment to the subclavian artery.

Great care is taken during harvest to avoid injury to the ITA or phrenic nerve, which lies medial and posterior to the artery pedicle (Jones, 1991). The distal end of the ITA graft is left intact until just before use. Typically, the graft is wrapped in a papaverine-soaked sponge after harvest is completed to eliminate any component of spasm (Cmolik & Geha, 1996). Saphenous vein for the remainder of the grafts is harvested simultaneously by a second member of the surgical team. An atraumatic technique in procuring the saphenous vein is essential. Undue traction or avulsion of small branches may damage the vein and lead to graft failure. Application of internal or external pressure causes endothelial damage, exaggerates the proliferative response, and may be a nidus for early atherosclerosis (Loop, 1998).

When ITA mobilization has been accomplished, the pericardium is opened in the midline and the pericardial edges are tied to the presternal fascia on the ipsilateral side of the incision to elevate and stabilize the cardiovascular structures (Nolan & Zacour, 1998). After administering heparin to provide systemic anticoagulation,

the right atrium and ascending aorta are cannulated. Cardiopulmonary bypass is initiated and core body temperature is cooled to approximately 28°C to 30°C. After cross-clamping the aorta, chilled cardioplegic solution is administered into the coronary circulation to produce cardiac arrest and provide additional myocardial protection. Topical iced saline may be instilled into the pericardial well surrounding the heart to provide further regional cooling. To maintain cellular viability during the period of ischemic arrest, myocardial temperature is maintained at approximately 15°C.

Typically, the vein graft anastomoses are performed first, followed by the distal ITA anastomosis. Distal vein graft anastomoses (ie, grafts to coronary arteries) are performed in the following manner. After selecting a suitable site beyond the stenosis for the distal anastomosis, the epicardium overlying the coronary artery is incised and the anterior wall of the artery is opened longitudinally. A probe is passed into the artery to measure its size and to assess proximal and distal patency (Kirklin & Barratt-Boyes, 1993a). The beveled end of the vein segment is sewn to the coronary artery with a running suture technique (Fig. 15-4). A small opening is then created in the ascending aorta (aortotomy) and the proximal end of the

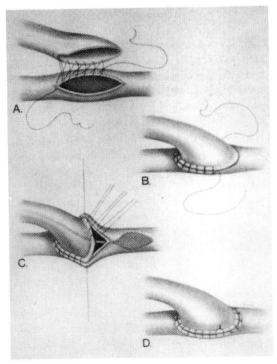

FIGURE 15-4. One technique of saphenous vein to coronary artery end-to-side anastomosis. **(A)** The anastomosis begins at the heel of the beveled end of the vein graft and **(B)** is continued for three-fourths the length of the arteriotomy on either side. **(C)** Traction is placed on both ends of the continuous suture, which opens the toe of the anastomosis, allowing excellent visualization. **(D)** Interrupted sutures are used to secure the toe of the anastomosis. (Ochsner JL, 1980: Current operative techniques for myocardial revascularization. In Moran JM, Michaelis LL [eds]. Surgery for the Complications of Myocardial Infarction, p. 152. New York, Grune & Stratton)

vein graft is sutured to the aortotomy in end-to-side fashion. The remainder of the vein graft anastomoses are performed in similar fashion.

The harvested ITA, clamped and divided at its distal end, is then prepared for grafting. Because the ITA is a reactive conduit, and vulnerable to spasm from mishandling or surgical instrumentation, many surgeons routinely instill papaverine into the distal end of the ITA to produce intraluminal dilatation and reduce the likelihood of technical anastomotic errors caused by arterial spasm (Mills, 1991). An ITA pedicle graft requires only a distal anastomosis because the native attachment of the proximal ITA to the subclavian artery is preserved. After completing the distal ITA anastomosis, the pedicle of the ITA may be tacked to the epicardial surface of the heart to prevent kinking.

Sometimes one ITA or vein graft can be used to bypass two obstructed arteries in close proximity. This type of graft is called a *tandem* or *sequential graft*. The single piece of conduit is grafted with a side-to-side anastomosis between the side of the ITA or vein and one target coronary artery and an end-to-side anastomosis between the end of the conduit and the side of the second target artery (Fig. 15-5). A *vein patch angioplasty* is an operative technique that is used occasionally during coronary artery revascularization. This technique consists of creating an arteriotomy across an identified lesion in a coronary artery and using a piece of vein to widen the arterial narrowing. Vein patch angioplasty is a useful technique for long lesions and for when an ITA pedicle graft is not long enough to reach beyond a lesion in the distal portion of an artery.

The aorta remains cross-clamped while distal graft anastomoses are performed. Because the heart gradually rewarms and collateral blood flow washes away the cardioplegic solution, repeated doses are given every 15 to 20 minutes. Cardioplegia may be administered by an antegrade or retrograde route, or a combination of both. An antegrade technique consists of infusing the solution into the coronary arteries in an antegrade direction through a small catheter in the aortic root. With antegrade delivery, however, effective distribution of the solution through significantly stenosed or occluded coronary arteries is limited. Myocardium supplied by such vessels is not as well cooled and displays persistent electromechanical activity (Buckberg, 1987). For this reason, retrograde administration of cardioplegia often is used. With retrograde delivery, the cardioplegic solution is delivered into a catheter placed through the right atrium into the coronary sinus to perfuse the myocardium in a retrograde fashion. If a combination of antegrade and retrograde administration is performed, the initial dose of cardioplegia usually is infused using an antegrade technique and subsequent doses are administered in retrograde fashion.

Coronary revascularization procedures are designed by the surgeon to minimize intraoperative myocardial injury. Because ischemic injury to myocardial tissue increases exponentially with time, the operation is planned and performed in an expedient manner. Distal anastomoses to vessels that supply muscle at most risk of ischemic injury are performed first. After construction of a distal saphenous vein graft anastomosis, cardioplegic solution can be injected directly into the proximal opening of the vein graft to cool myocardium beyond the obstructed portion of the coronary artery or cardioplegia can be administered in retrograde fashion while the proximal anastomosis is performed. Antegrade administration of cardioplegic solution through an ITA pedicle graft is not possible. A detailed description of cardiopulmonary bypass and myocardial preservation techniques is provided elsewhere in the text.

Some surgeons perform the proximal anastomoses after all distal anastomoses are completed before or after release of the aortic cross-clamp as rewarming of the patient is begun. An alternative technique is the performance of all proximal vein anastomoses (vein to aorta) before distal anastomoses. With this technique, proximal anastomoses are performed before initiating cardiopulmonary bypass, thus reducing the duration of cardiopulmonary bypass time. After both proximal and distal anastomoses of a vein graft are completed, any subsequent doses of cardioplegic solution administered into the aortic root perfuse the area of myocardium supplied by the newly constructed graft. The optimal order in which to perform distal and proximal anastomoses remains controversial, and choice of technique is determined primarily by surgeon preference.

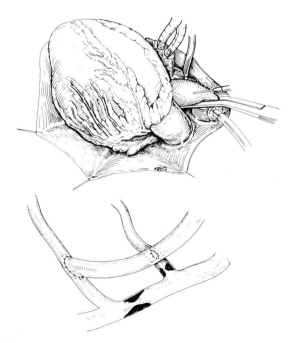

FIGURE 15-5. (*Top*) Operative exposure for sequential grafting of parallel branches of the left circumflex artery. (*Bottom*) A side-to-side anastomosis is constructed between a saphenous vein segment and the first coronary arterial branch; an end-to-side anastomosis is constructed between the distal end of the vein and the second arterial branch. (Loop FD, 1979: Saphenous vein bypass graft. In Cohn LH [ed]: Modern Technics in Surgery, p. 10-9. Mount Kisco, NY, Futura)

Warming is initiated as the bypass grafting is completed. When the myocardium has warmed sufficiently to resume a spontaneous electrical rhythm, the patient is weaned from cardiopulmonary bypass. Cannulae are removed, protamine is administered to reverse systemic heparinization, and hemostasis is achieved. A flow probe may be used to measure blood flow through each of the vein grafts. Graft flow greater than 100 mL/min is considered desirable. Measurement of graft flows provides the surgeon with valuable information about the quality of each vein graft and the likelihood of its long-term patency. If flow is less than 100 mL/min, the vein graft may be infused with a vasodilating agent, such as papaverine, to ascertain if the problem is due to vasospasm. If a technical problem is compromising graft flow, it can be corrected before concluding the operation.

Probes for measuring flow through ITA grafts are not available for clinical use. However, an estimation of graft flow is obtained after constructing the distal anastomosis and releasing the vessel clamp to allow blood flow from the graft to perfuse the myocardium. A prompt rise in myocardial temperature on release of the clamp is indicative of excellent flow. The pericardial sac usually is left open or closed loosely to avoid kinking or occluding grafts that lie on the anterior surface of the heart. The sternum is reapproximated and fastened with heavy suture material or wire, and the skin incision is closed.

Special Considerations

Minimally Invasive Coronary Artery Bypass Grafting

Recently, *minimally invasive surgical techniques* have been applied to CABG operations. The term *minimally invasive* connotes an operation performed using an incision that is smaller than a conventional incision and, sometimes, without cardiopulmonary bypass. The goals of minimally invasive CABG procedures are to reduce operative trauma, speed patient recovery, allow faster return to normal activity, and reduce costs compared with conventional CABG techniques (Society of Thoracic Surgeons/ American Association for Thoracic Surgery Ad Hoc Committee on New Technology Assessment, 1998). Minimally invasive CABG operations can be divided into two categories: (1) beating heart CABG (ie, operations performed on a beating heart without cardiopulmonary bypass); and (2) port-access CABG, performed with cardiopulmonary bypass using femoral access for arterial and venous cannulation (Reardon et al., 1997).

The first category, minimally invasive direct coronary artery bypass (MIDCAB), typically is performed through a small right or left anterior thoracotomy incision. Through this incision, the LAD and, less commonly, the right coronary artery may be grafted. Special instruments and techniques have been developed to compensate for disadvantages associated with performing the operation with limited exposure and a beating heart.

These include video-assisted thoracoscopy to facilitate visualization and dissection of the ITA, mechanical stabilizers to immobilize partially the coronary artery and reduce motion of the beating heart, and ischemic preconditioning of the myocardium and intraluminal occluders that allow distal coronary perfusion to provide a dry field for anastomosis construction (Loop, 1998).

The second category of minimally invasive CABG is performed through small "port" incisions but using cardiopulmonary bypass and cardioplegic arrest. Because the ascending aorta is not accessible for external application of a cross-clamp as in conventional cardiac operations, an aortic endovascular occluder catheter is advanced through the femoral artery into the ascending aorta. A balloon at the end of the catheter is inflated to occlude the aortic lumen and cardioplegic solution is administered into the aortic root through a port distal to the balloon or in retrograde fashion through the coronary sinus.

Minimally invasive techniques are still evolving. They are most appropriate in selected clinical situations, specifically in patients with isolated coronary artery lesions that are not amenable to PCI but are located in arteries that can be accessed adequately through a small incision. Minimally invasive techniques are used most commonly to graft isolated LAD lesions as an alternative to PCI in patients at higher risk for conventional CABG operation (Hannan & Kron, 1998; Mariani et al., 1997). Long-term data are not yet available comparing minimally invasive and conventional CABG in terms of graft patency and freedom from adverse events. Some concerns associated with the minimally invasive CABG approach are (1) the accuracy and patency of graft anastomoses, (2) incomplete revascularization of inaccessible but diseased arteries, and (3) potential morbidity and costs associated with port-access CABG (eg, multiple port sites, limited thoracotomy, groin dissection, and femorofemoral bypass) (Reardon et al., 1997).

Emergency Operation

Emergency CABG is performed to revascularize portions of myocardium that are thought to be in imminent danger of irreversible damage. It may be a primary intervention or may follow less invasive interventions (PCI or thrombolytic therapy). The most common reasons for emergency CABG are (1) ischemia that is uncontrolled by medical therapy (ie, unstable angina), (2) evolving MI, and (3) complications of PCI.

Unstable angina, or ischemic symptoms refractory to control with medical therapy, may be categorized as preinfarction or postinfarction depending on whether there is electrocardiographic or enzymatic evidence of acute MI. The most common manifestation of preinfarction angina is chest pain accompanied by characteristic electrocardiographic changes. Uncommonly, ventricular tachycardia or pulmonary edema occurs as a manifestation of acute ischemia. If symptoms cannot be controlled with intensive medical therapy (eg, nitroglycerin, heparin, beta-blocking agents, and intra-aortic balloon counterpulsation), CABG may be undertaken emergently to preserve myocardium that is presumed to be reversibly injured.

Ischemia also may be present in the early period after MI. Approximately 40% to 50% of patients with non–Q-wave MI and 15% of patients with Q-wave MI have early postinfarction angina with or without ECG changes (Franco & Hammond, 1996). Postinfarction angina indicates that there is muscle in which blood supply is jeopardized but damage remains reversible. Such patients, if treated medically, have a substantial risk of another infarction that may lead to progressive left ventricular dysfunction or death (Hochberg et al., 1984).

Surgical intervention in the immediate period after completed transmural MI is avoided if possible. Revascularization performed more than 4 to 6 hours but less than 48 hours after MI is associated with significantly increased operative mortality owing to hemorrhagic reperfusion injury. Consequently, pharmacologic therapy and intra-aortic balloon counterpulsation are the mainstays of initial treatment for postinfarction ischemia. However, if postinfarction angina is not relieved by these measures, emergent surgical therapy may become necessary. The greatest decrease in relative risk for operative mortality and perioperative MI occurs within 48 hours after transmural MI; there is little to be gained by delaying surgery beyond this time (Loop, 1998).

The second category of patients who receive emergency CABG are those with evolving MI, defined as a period of 4 to 6 hours from MI onset during which muscle damage may be reversible. The availability of thrombolytic therapy and PCI as effective methods of reestablishing blood flow through the infarct artery (artery responsible for the MI) has dramatically lessened the need for emergency surgical revascularization as an initial form of therapy. More often, CABG for evolving MI is performed as an alternative therapy when PCI or thrombolytic therapy is contraindicated or fails to reopen the infarct vessel. Surgical therapy is best suited for patients in whom coronary angiography has been performed already or can be performed within 1 to 2 hours after onset of the infarct.

The third category of emergent CABG, that required because of failed PCI, is necessary in 3% to 4% of patients who undergo PCI (Franco & Hammond, 1996). PCI can cause acute MI as a result of acute coronary artery occlusion, dissection of a coronary artery, or embolization of thrombus or atherosclerotic debris into the distal portion of a coronary artery. Each of these complications compromises antegrade flow through the artery. Chest pain, electrocardiographic manifestations of ischemia or infarction, and hemodynamic instability may result.

Surgical revascularization under emergency conditions differs in character from procedures planned and performed electively. When active ischemia is present, the primary goal is prompt restoration of blood flow to the jeopardized portion of myocardium. The vessel supplying ischemic myocardium is grafted first so that it can be perfused with cardioplegic solution while other vessels are grafted. Use of the ITA, with its long-term superior-

ity in patency, often must be abandoned in the interest of restoring flow quickly by use of a saphenous vein graft. Additional time is necessary to harvest an ITA before cardiopulmonary bypass, and thus more time elapses before ischemic muscle can be protected and revascularized. Particularly in a young patient, it is disappointing when revascularization is done emergently and only saphenous vein grafts, with lower patency rates, must be used.

Operative mortality of emergency CABG is not always higher than that of elective procedures. However, it increases profoundly, approaching 100%, if the patient is in cardiogenic shock or if cardiac arrest has occurred and the operation is initiated during cardiopulmonary resuscitation or after institution of emergency femorofemoral cardiopulmonary bypass. Patients who undergo operation after MI or with unstable angina also may be at greater risk for myocardial stunning, a period of reversible myocardial dysfunction that follows reperfusion of ischemic myocardium (Rao & Weisel, 1997). If thrombolytic therapy has been administered in the immediate preoperative period, bleeding associated with emergent CABG may be greater. The risk usually is not prohibitive unless large doses of thrombolytic agents have been used.

Patients with severe narrowing of the left main coronary artery do not necessarily require emergency operation. However, patients with significant left main stenosis usually are operated on urgently because of the tremendous amount of muscle at jeopardy. Patients in whom occlusion of the left main coronary artery develops invariably die from the ensuing global MI. For the same reason, the risk associated with PCI of a significant left main coronary artery stenosis usually is considered prohibitive. Once significant left main coronary artery disease is demonstrated, the patient is observed in a monitored setting and surgery typically is performed within 24 hours.

Reoperation

Because surgical revascularization is not curative, some patients require reoperation for disease progression or graft closure. Cosgrove and associates (1986) documented a reoperation rate of 11% at 10 years in a retrospective analysis of 8000 patients. Young age at initial operation was the most important predictor for reoperation, and the incidence of reoperation was twice as high in patients with only vein grafts compared with those who received ITA grafts (Cosgrove et al., 1986). Reoperation also is more likely in individuals who are unable to modify risk factors for disease progression, such as smoking and hypercholesterolemia (Kron & Bayfield, 1998). Reoperations are thought to represent up to 15% of CABG procedures (Cmolik & Geha, 1996).

Reentry into the chest during reoperation must be performed cautiously because of the presence of fibrous tissue from the previous operation. This internal scar tissue causes adhesion of contiguous mediastinal structures and a blurring of tissue planes between them. Grafts placed on the anterior surface of the heart and the heart muscle itself (right ventricle) become adherent to the posterior table of the sternum. Division of the sternum can be complicated by inadvertent laceration of one of the grafts, particularly an ITA pedicle graft, or by entry into the right ventricular chamber. Acute MI due to graft injury or massive hemorrhage due to right ventricular laceration can ensue. The presence of a patent left ITA graft is particularly concerning during sternal reentry because preservation of graft integrity is vital to continued perfusion of the myocardium during the period before cardiopulmonary bypass is instituted (Kron & Bayfield, 1998). In high-risk reoperations, the femoral artery and vein often are cannulated before opening the chest so that cardiopulmonary bypass can be instituted immediately if necessary. The blurring of tissue planes caused by internal adhesions also makes dissection during reoperations more tedious and prolonged. As a result, blood loss and the need for transfusion can be expected to be greater.

At the time of a reoperative procedure, the surgeon must determine if any revision of original bypass grafts is indicated. An occluded graft is not necessarily revascularized if there is good collateral circulation to the muscle it supplies or if the muscle is necrotic. The surgeon also must determine whether to replace patent vein grafts that have been in place for a number of years. A judgment must be made as to whether it is more prudent to leave a viable but old graft alone or replace it with a new graft that may or may not be as good as the original graft. Leaving original vein grafts in place risks embolization of atherosclerotic debris at the time of reoperation and premature graft stenosis or occlusion after reoperation; replacement of all vein grafts lengthens the reoperation and may use all available bypass conduits (Lytle, 1997). Another consideration in determining whether to revise vein grafts is the degree of difficulty in freeing the heart from adhesions to surrounding tissues. Regrafting coronary arteries is particularly difficult if target vessels are on the lateral or posterior surface of the heart. Patent ITA grafts are almost never revised.

As coronary revascularization has evolved, the interval between operations is increasing. As a result, patients undergoing reoperation usually are approximately 10 years older than at the first operation and have an increased prevalence of diabetes, more diffuse atherosclerosis, significantly more left main coronary artery disease, an ejection fraction that has diminished from the time of the first operation, and both vein graft stenosis and progression of native vessel disease (Gall, 1997; Loop, 1995). Reoperation is associated with a higher risk than a first operation, and risk increases substantially with a second or third reoperation. Compared with a primary operation, risk of death during repeat CABG is three to four times greater; perioperative MI, eight times greater; and stroke, more than two times greater (Cmolik & Geha, 1996). Factors associated with higher operative mortality at reoperation include emergency surgery, poor left ventricular function, older age, and female sex (Loop, 1998). Long-term survival and freedom from angina are diminished after reoperative compared with primary coronary revascularization (Gall, 1997).

Diffuse Coronary Artery Disease

Sometimes, diffuse disease of one or more coronary arteries precludes complete revascularization of all areas of viable myocardium. Incomplete revascularization adversely affects relief from symptoms, freedom from repeat operation, and survival (Johnson et al., 1989). In such patients, *coronary endarterectomy* of diffusely diseased arteries is thought to be beneficial. Coronary endarterectomy consists of removing atheromatous material from the lumen of an artery that is diffusely diseased (Fig. 15-6). It is always accompanied by bypass grafting of the vessel.

Most common is endarterectomy of the right coronary artery. Left coronary artery endarterectomy can be performed but is associated with significantly increased operative risk (Cmolik & Geha, 1996). The primary complication of endarterectomy is perioperative MI due to thrombosis of the vessel, residual obstruction, or dissection of the artery wall. Although endarterectomy is safer with current methods of myocardial protection and techniques that allow complete removal of the atherosclerotic core, the rate of associated perioperative MI is higher and vein graft patency in endarterectomized arteries is lower (Loop, 1998).

Associated Atherosclerosis

Atherosclerosis affects arteries throughout the body, and many patients with CAD also have atherosclerotic lesions elsewhere. It is not unusual for a patient who undergoes CABG to have significant carotid artery disease, aortic atheromata, an aortic aneurysm, or occlusive lesions in the arteries supplying the lower extremities. Between 3% and 12% of patients undergoing CABG are estimated to have hemodynamically significant (>70% narrowing) carotid artery stenosis (Jones & Hodakowski, 1996). In patients with combined, significant coronary and carotid artery disease, the sequence and timing of procedures remain somewhat controversial (Johnsson et al., 1991). The underlying question is whether there is greater risk for MI during carotid endarterectomy or stroke during coronary revascularization. In general, the sequence of operations is determined by the most unstable system, either neurologic or cardiac (Jones & Hodakowski, 1996).

In patients with both neurologic symptoms related to carotid artery stenosis and precarious coronary stenoses that jeopardize a significant area of myocardium, the two revascularization procedures may be performed concomitantly (Loop, 1998). The most common method for a combined procedure is to perform the carotid endarterectomy just before coronary artery revascularization. Preparations are made so that cardiopulmonary bypass can be instituted within moments should myocardial ischemia become evident. The carotid endarterectomy is performed with careful hemodynamic monitoring, either before sternotomy, or after sternotomy but before initiating cardiopulmonary bypass. As soon as the carotid endarterectomy is completed, the patient is placed on car-

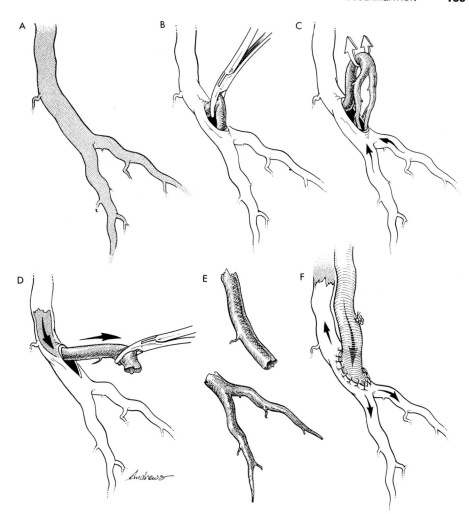

FIGURE 15-6. Technique for endarterectomy of right coronary artery (RCA). **(A)** An occluded RCA is considered for endarterectomy. **(B)** An arteriotomy is performed just above the crux and the atheromatous core is brought out through the incision. **(C)** The distal vessels are cleared individually of plaque. **(D)** The proximal portion is removed by gentle traction until it breaks free. **(E)** The atheromatous specimen after extraction from the artery. **(F)** A saphenous vein graft is anastomosed to the RCA to bypass atheromatous material in the proximal portion of the vessel. (Cooley DA, 1984: Revascularization of the ischemic myocardium. In Techniques in Cardiac Surgery, ed. 2, p. 232. Philadelphia, WB Saunders)

diopulmonary bypass and the cardiac portion of the procedure is undertaken.

Less commonly, the carotid endarterectomy is performed with the patient on cardiopulmonary bypass. Those who favor endarterectomy before bypass believe the changes in perfusion pressure associated with initiation of bypass may increase the risk of stroke. Those favoring endarterectomy during bypass believe the controlled perfusion pressure, hypothermia, and hemodilution present during cardiopulmonary bypass provide better protection against cerebral ischemia (Jones & Hodakowski, 1996; Newman & Hicks, 1988).

In patients requiring surgical treatment for both CAD and an abdominal aortic aneurysm, the coronary artery revascularization usually is performed first. MI as a complication of aneurysm repair is considered a more likely risk than aneurysm rupture complicating CABG. However, rupture of an unrepaired aortic aneurysm is a potential risk during the perioperative period. CABG is almost always performed before peripheral arterial bypass procedures.

Patients who undergo coronary artery revascularization sometimes have a significant degree of atheromatous disease in the ascending aorta. Calcification, atheromatous deposits, or ulcerated lesions in the ascending aorta are worrisome because they increase the risk of intraoperative stroke due to embolism. They also limit available sites for clamping, cannulation, and anastomosis of vein grafts to the aorta. Moderate to severe aortic atherosclerosis is more likely in patients who have associated atherosclerosis in the carotid arteries or abdominal aorta. In such patients, a preoperative chest roentgenogram, computed tomographic scan of the chest, or intraoperative transesophageal echocardiogram may detect aortic wall irregularity, calcification, or atheromata (abnormal fatty deposits).

In the presence of severe ascending aortic calcification or atherosclerosis, special care is taken during the operation to reduce the possibility of cerebral embolism from debris in the ascending aorta. Gross inspection of the outside of the aorta does not reveal the degree of atheromatous disease, which may vary among severe "porcelain" calcification; ragged, diffuse, solid atheromatous material; and yellow, semiliquid "toothpaste-like" material within the aortic wall (Mehta & Pae, 1997). The surgeon uses various techniques to decrease manipulation, clamping, or cannulation of the ascending aorta. Alternative sites for placement of the aortic cannula include the axillary artery, the femoral artery, or the aortic arch (Cmolik & Geha, 1996) (Fig. 15-7). Special operative techniques include replacing the diseased segment of aorta with a graft or performance of distal anastomoses without application of an aortic cross-clamp (Rao & Weisel, 1997). If no cross-clamp is placed on the aorta during performance of distal anastomoses, the heart is maintained in a state of hypothermic fibrillatory arrest and a left ventricular vent is placed to decompress the ventricle.

Some surgeons advocate using one or both ITAs as the sole inflow conduit in patients with atheromatous disease in the ascending aorta. An ITA pedicle graft avoids the need for a proximal ITA-to-aorta anastomosis and proximal saphenous vein graft anastomoses are constructed in end-to-side fashion to the proximal portion of the ITA graft (Peigh et al., 1991). Alternatively, the proximal end of saphenous vein grafts can be sewn to the innominate or subclavian artery. If saphenous vein grafts are anastomosed to the aorta, soft, noncalcified sites on the undersurface of the transverse arch or distal ascending aorta may be selected.

Revascularization in Young and in Elderly Adults

Patients younger than 40 years of age who require surgical revascularization appear to have a premature and more rampant form of coronary artery atherosclerosis. Both long-term survival and freedom from symptoms are decreased in these patients compared with older patients with similar disease at the time of surgical revascularization (Lytle et al., 1984). Subsequent revascularization procedures are likely to be necessary. Coronary bypass grafting in patients younger than 40 years of age often is performed using only arterial conduits because of the long-term patency superiority compared with vein grafts. Strict postoperative lipid modification therapy and diabetic management when indicated are essential (Loop, 1998).

Increased longevity in the United States and the epidemic and progressive nature of CAD have resulted in greater numbers of septuagenarians and octogenarians undergoing CABG. The mean age for patients undergoing CABG is 66 years; nearly 30% of patients are older than 70 years of age and 10% are older than 80 years of age (Loop, 1998). Most older patients who undergo CABG have an acceptable operative risk and achieve symptomatic improvement (Busch et al., 1999). Although CABG can be performed safely in elderly patients, postoperative hospitalization is significantly longer and associated costs are greater (Loop, 1998; Salomon et al., 1991). Revascularization in very elderly patients differs in that complete revascularization and long-term benefits of ITA grafting are less important than reducing operative time.

Results of Coronary Artery Bypass Grafting

By the mid 1980s, improvements in myocardial preservation and other intraoperative techniques had reduced *operative mortality* associated with CABG to less than 1%. However, the profile of patients undergoing CABG has changed, largely as a result of advances in pharmacologic and catheterization therapies, and because of increased longevity of the population. The demographic characteristics of patients undergoing CABG reflect these factors: surgical patients are older and more likely to have triple-vessel disease, left ventricular dysfunction, and comorbidities. Patients seldom have single-vessel disease, and reoperations are more common.

As a result, most centers, particularly those with higher-risk patients, are observing higher (2% to 4%) operative mortality rates associated with CABG. Risk factors associated with increased operative mortality include advanced age, emergent surgery, elevated serum creatinine, left main coronary artery disease, female sex, anemia, and moderate to severe left ventricular dysfunction (Loop, 1998). The risk of operative death also varies considerably with the patient's clinical circumstances at the time of operation. For example, the mortality rate is only 1% for patients with stable angina, 3% for those

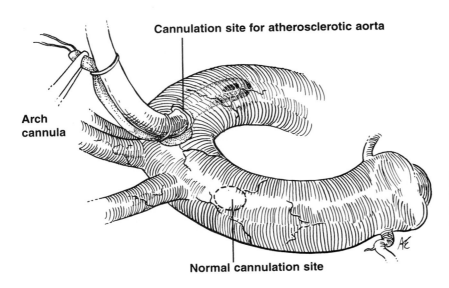

Cannulation site for atherosclerotic aorta

Arch cannula

Normal cannulation site

FIGURE 15-7. Alternative aortic cannulation site in an atherosclerotic aorta. The aortic cannula has been placed in a soft area of the aortic arch. (Ribakove GH, Galloway AC, Colvin SB, 1998: The atherosclerotic aorta. In Kaiser LR, Kron IL, Spray TL [eds]: Mastery of Cardiothoracic Surgery, p. 403. Philadelphia, Lippincott Williams & Wilkins)

with unstable angina, 5% for those with postinfarction angina or failed PCI, and 30% for those with cardiogenic shock (Franco & Hammond, 1996).

Several predictive risk models have been developed that pool multicenter data from several hundred thousand patients. These risk models are used to predict operative risk based on patient characteristics and assess institutional outcomes. Major databases for analyzing risk-adjusted operative outcome data include the Society for Thoracic Surgeons' National Cardiac Data Base and databases developed by the Department of Veterans' Affairs and the Northern New England Cardiovascular Disease Study Group (Clark et al., 1994; Grover et al., 1994; Nugent & Schults, 1994).

Perioperative complications occur in approximately 15% of patients undergoing CABG (Hammermeister et al., 1990). Common factors associated with an increased mortality or morbidity risk are displayed in Table 15-1. The most common early complications of CABG are postoperative bleeding and transient low cardiac output syndrome.

Approximately 5% of patients have significant postoperative bleeding that necessitates operative reexploration within the first 24 hours. Usually, bleeding is diffuse and represents impaired clotting. Postoperative coagulopathy is more likely with cardiac than with other types of operations because of the use of cardiopulmonary bypass. Extracorporeal circulation of blood damages platelets and other clotting factors. Also, the patient must be systemically anticoagulated during cardiopulmonary bypass. Bleeding related to a technical problem, such as a disrupted clip or suture, is unusual but also can occur, particularly if the patient is hypertensive in the early postoperative hours. Because some bleeding is inevitable, chest drainage tubes are placed in the thorax. Blood conservation techniques, such as a cell-saver system and autotransfusion, are important to lessen the need for transfusion of allogeneic blood and are discussed in Chapter 14, Blood Conservation.

Low cardiac output syndrome may represent peri-operative MI or transient depression of ventricular function secondary to effects of cardiopulmonary bypass and hypothermia. Low cardiac output syndrome usually is treated by intravenous infusion of inotropic and vasodilating medications. Occasionally, intra-aortic balloon counterpulsation is necessary. Rarely, frank cardiogenic shock refractory to pharmacologic and counterpulsation therapy occurs. In such cases, mechanical support of the heart with a circulatory assist device may become necessary. Other complications of CABG, including early graft closure, arrhythmias, cerebral vascular accident, wound infection, and respiratory failure, are described in Chapter 28, Complications of Cardiac Operations.

Long-term follow-up studies reveal that most patients do quite well after CABG, with freedom from myocardial ischemia for many years (Table 15-2). However, although CABG is quite effective in revascularizing the myocardium, it does not cure atherosclerosis. Consequently, symptoms of myocardial ischemia eventually return in most patients and often lead to the patient's death. Return of angina is the most common postoperative ischemic event. Early return of angina usually is due to graft closure or incomplete revascularization (ACC/AHA Task Force, 1991). After the first postoperative year, a 5% or greater rate of angina may accrue annually, almost always due to graft closure, progressive atherosclerosis in ungrafted arteries, or development of lesions beyond distal graft sites (Loop, 1995). At 10 years after coronary artery revascularization, 40% to 50% of patients can be expected to experience angina recurrence (Gall, 1997).

Most surgeons prescribe chronic antiplatelet therapy to augment vein graft patency. Aspirin in general is regarded as the most effective agent for this purpose (Goldman et al., 1990). Low- or regular-dose aspirin therapy may prevent platelet thrombi, the release of platelet mediators, and consequent platelet aggregation in vein grafts (Loop, 1998). It minimizes the risk of early graft closure and may decrease the extent of intimal hyperplasia (Franco & Hammond, 1996).

TABLE 15-1

Factors Associated With Increased Operative Mortality and Morbidity in Patients Undergoing Coronary Artery Bypass Grafting

Ejection fraction < 30%
Age > 70 years
Elevated serum creatinine
Left ventricular end-diastolic pressure > 25 mm Hg
Female sex
Failed percutaneous coronary intervention
Associated mitral valve disease
Previous cardiac procedure
Emergent operation
Associated peripheral arterial occlusive disease

TABLE 15-2

Long-Term Results of Coronary Artery Bypass Grafting

Outcome	Percent at		
	5 Years	*10 Years*	*15 Years*
Freedom from			
Death	92	81	57
Angina	85–90	60	
Myocardial infarction	96		64
Sudden cardiac death		97	

Spencer FC, Galloway AC, Colvin SB, 1995: Bypass grafting for coronary artery disease. In Sabiston DC Jr, Spencer FC (eds): Surgery of the Chest, ed. 6. Philadelphia, WB Saunders; Kirklin JW, Barratt-Boyes BG, 1993: Stenotic arteriosclerotic coronary artery disease. In Cardiac Surgery. ed. 2. New York, Churchill Livingstone

▶ Transmyocardial Laser Revascularization

Some patients with severe CAD are not candidates for conventional forms of coronary artery revascularization because they have diffusely diseased or small distal coronary arteries. *Transmyocardial laser revascularization* (TMR) is an alternative form of surgical revascularization. It is appropriate for patients with diffuse, end-stage CAD who have disabling symptoms of myocardial ischemia and who are not candidates for conventional forms of revascularization (Horvath et al., 1996).

Transmyocardial laser revascularization is performed through a small left anterior thoracotomy incision and does not require the use of cardiopulmonary bypass. The operative technique consists of using a carbon dioxide or other type of laser to create channels in the myocardium that allow direct perfusion of ischemic myocardium with left ventricular blood. The target area of ischemic myocardium is exposed and the laser is used to create 20 to 30 small channels, extending from the epicardium through the myocardium and into the left ventricle.

The precise mechanisms by which TMR is effective are not yet well defined. There is some investigational evidence that the laser channels may remain patent, allowing left ventricular blood to perfuse the myocardium directly. The delivery of laser energy also is thought to cause angiogenesis, or the formation of new collateral blood vessels. Effectiveness of TMR in relieving angina also may be related to denervation of the myocardium. TMR is associated with a 9% operative mortality risk, significant improvement in angina class, a decrease in perfusion defects, and a decrease in subsequent hospital admissions for angina (Horvath et al., 1997).

▶ Surgery for Complications of Myocardial Infarction

Myocardial infarction can produce several mechanical complications that may require surgical intervention. These include ventricular aneurysm, acute mitral regurgitation, and ventricular free wall or septal rupture.

Ventricular Aneurysm

In 10% to 15% of patients with acute transmural MI, a true *left ventricular aneurysm* develops (Grosso & Harken, 1995). A true ventricular aneurysm is a discrete area of necrosed, thinned myocardium that is noncontractile or that contracts paradoxically from other ventricular segments. The most common location is in the anterolateral wall of the left ventricle near the apex (Kirklin & Barratt-Boyes, 1993b). Approximately 3% to 4% of ventricular aneurysms occur posteriorly between the papillary muscles (Loop, 1998).

The classic symptoms associated with ventricular aneurysm are congestive heart failure, angina, systemic embolization, and arrhythmias. Most common is congestive heart failure. Necrotic muscle and fibrous tissue that comprise the aneurysm move paradoxically, "stealing" left ventricular stroke volume and decreasing cardiac output (Grosso & Harken, 1995). The impaired ventricular function also can produce angina. The increased ventricular cavity size increases wall tension, which can result in higher oxygen consumption in the remaining normal myocardium and decreased oxygen supply during diastole (Fiore & Jatene, 1996).

Frequently, the endocardial surface of an aneurysm contains thrombus that accumulates secondary to the endothelial injury that accompanies MI. This so-called *mural thrombus* can embolize from the left ventricle into the systemic circulation and cause stroke, MI, or mesenteric or limb ischemia. Finally, scar tissue on the endocardial surface of the aneurysmal segment may provide an arrhythmogenic focus. The differing electrophysiologic properties of conduction and refractoriness in the fibrous tissue, necrotic muscle, and viable myocardium that constitute the aneurysm and its adjacent border predispose to reentrant arrhythmias (Grosso & Harken, 1995).

The mere presence of a ventricular aneurysm does not necessitate surgical therapy. In most cases, operative repair is undertaken in patients who have symptoms associated with the aneurysm that are refractory to medical management. Even in the absence of symptoms, however, large anteroseptal aneurysms can subject the ventricle to chronic volume overload, leading to left ventricular dilatation and global dysfunction. Thus, surgical treatment also is recommended in asymptomatic patients who demonstrate signs of ventricular deterioration, such as an increase in end-systolic basilar diameter, a decrease in ventricular ejection fraction, worsening mitral regurgitation, or progressive aneurysm enlargement (Cox, 1997a).

Aneurysmectomy is performed through a median sternotomy incision and using cardiopulmonary bypass. It is technically easier if it can be performed at least 6 weeks after acute MI because the myocardial tissue is less friable than immediately after the event. One of several techniques may be used for surgical repair. A linear ventricular aneurysmectomy consists of resecting the fibrotic, aneurysmal muscle. When the heart is decompressed during extracorporeal circulation and cross-clamping of the aorta, the aneurysmal zone collapses while the remaining viable left ventricular myocardium remains firm (Gross & Harken, 1995). After making a linear incision in the aneurysm, the fibrotic tissue is excised, leaving a rim of fibrous tissue. Thrombus is evacuated from the ventricle, and the cavity is irrigated. The edges of the defect are reapproximated and closed by direct suture technique using large strips of prosthetic material to buttress the reconstruction (Fig. 15-8). Small aneurysms that do not contain mural thrombus sometimes may be repaired by plicating (ie, folding) and suturing the fibrotic tissue without opening the ventricular cavity (Glower & Lowe, 1997).

In the mid-1980s, two additional operative techniques for anteroseptal ventricular aneurysm repair were

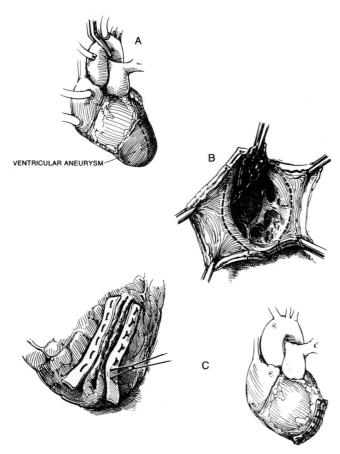

FIGURE 15-8. One technique of left ventricular aneurysm repair. **(A)** Operation is performed through a median sternotomy incision, using cardiopulmonary bypass and cardioplegic arrest. The heart is elevated from the pericardial sac and the center of the collapsed aneurysm wall is identified. **(B)** The central portion of the aneurysm is incised and any intramural clot is carefully removed. The lateral walls of the aneurysm are excised. **(C)** The edges of the defect are approximated and sutured using Teflon felt strips to reinforce the closure. (Waldhausen JA, Pierce WS, 1985: Repair of ventricular aneurysms and ventricular septal defects after myocardial infarction. In Johnson's Surgery of the Chest, ed. 5, p. 485. Chicago, Year Book)

developed separately by Jatene in Brazil and Dor in France to correct the septal portion of the aneurysm and better restore ventricular geometry in the nonaneurysmal portion of the ventricle (Cox, 1997b). Ventricular aneurysmectomy with a geometric reconstruction technique includes using a circular patch sewn to the fibrous rim of the defect to close the aneurysm. Ventricular aneurysm repair using either the Jatene or Dor technique is considered preferable to standard linear aneurysm resection in patients with large anteroseptal aneurysms.

Optimal myocardial protection during ventricular aneurysm repair is essential, as is minimal manipulation of the myocardium to prevent embolism of mural thrombus. Ventricular aneurysm resection is associated with a mortality rate of 3% to 7%; symptomatic improvement almost always is achieved and the actuarial survival rate is 80% at 5 years, with most late deaths occurring due to heart failure (Cox, 1997a). Factors that adversely affect long-term survival after ventricular aneurysm resection include left main coronary artery disease and poor left ventricular function (Gay, 1997).

Resection of a ventricular aneurysm sometimes is performed concomitantly with coronary artery revascularization. In patients with associated ventricular rhythm disorders, aneurysm resection alone does not ensure arrhythmia eradication. Concomitant intraoperative mapping and endocardial resection may be performed to treat the arrhythmic disorder. Surgical treatment of ventricular arrhythmias is discussed in Chapter 18, Surgical Treatment of Cardiac Rhythm Disorders.

Acute Mitral Regurgitation

Acute mitral regurgitation may develop secondary to MI by one of several pathophysiologic mechanisms, including papillary muscle dysfunction, papillary muscle rupture, or annular dilatation. Pulmonary edema or cardiogenic shock often accompanies acute mitral regurgitation because, in contrast to chronic mitral regurgitation, compensatory mechanisms to protect the heart have not developed. A vasodilating agent, such as nitroprusside, usually is administered to reduce afterload and facilitate forward flow. Intra-aortic balloon counterpulsation often is instituted, and emergent therapy to restore mitral valve competence may be necessary.

Ischemic papillary muscle dysfunction sometimes is reversed successfully by revascularization of ischemic muscle with thrombolytic therapy, PCI, or CABG. If a papillary muscle has ruptured or if myocardial necrosis at the base of the papillary muscles has produced annular dilatation, surgical reconstruction or replacement of the mitral valve is required. Mitral valve repair and replacement are discussed in Chapter 16, Surgical Treatment of Valvular Heart Disease.

Ventricular Rupture

Rupture of the ventricular myocardium occurs when necrotic tissue becomes too weakened to withstand intraventricular pressure. Depending on location of the MI, rupture may occur in the papillary muscles, or in the septum or free wall of the ventricle. Although the incidence is hard to assess, rupture of acutely infarcted tissue is thought to account for approximately 15% of deaths from acute MI (Antman & Braunwald, 1997).

Rupture of the free wall of infarcted ventricle occurs in as many as 10% of patients who die in the hospital of acute MI (Antman & Braunwald, 1997). Ventricular free wall rupture usually is fatal, but if detected before the patient's death is treated with emergent surgical intervention to restore ventricular wall integrity. Sometimes, ventricular rupture is small and is contained by pericardium. If sufficient pericardial inflammation and adhesions are present to localize and contain the rupture, death from pericardial tamponade is evaded and the contained rupture creates a *pseudoaneurysm* (Cooley & Walker, 1980). A pseudoaneurysm or false aneurysm differs from a true ventricular aneurysm in that its wall consists of fibrous pericardium only. Pseudoaneurysms have a great propensity to rupture (Madsen & Daggett, 1997). In addition to precipitous rupture, a pseudoaneurysm can produce the same clinical consequences as a true ventricular aneurysm. Pseudoaneurysms almost always are repaired surgically.

Resection of a true aneurysm or pseudoaneurysm in the early period after MI is technically difficult because of the fragility of tissue in the area of infarction. Also, in the case of pseudoaneurysm, the pericardium may be acting to contain the rupture. The surgeon may cannulate the aorta and right atrium through the intact pericardium so that cardiopulmonary bypass can be initiated before opening the pericardium. One technique of surgical repair is closure of the ventricular defect with horizontal mattress sutures, buttressed with Teflon strips; the closure and surrounding infarcted myocardium are then covered with a Teflon patch sutured to healthy epicardium (Madsen & Daggett, 1997).

Rupture of the interventricular septum is estimated to occur in approximately 2% of patients with acute MI (Antman & Braunwald, 1997). Although less common than free wall rupture, the condition more commonly is diagnosed before the patient's death. Ventricular septal rupture usually occurs after complete occlusion of a coronary artery and extensive transmural infarction in patients with less diffuse CAD, and thus less well-developed collateral circulation (Madsen & Daggett, 1996). Septal rupture produces a ventricular septal defect (VSD). In most cases, acute VSD occurs in the anterior or apical portion of the septum, caused by a transmural infarction in the distribution of the LAD artery. VSDs due to inferior infarction occur in the basal portion of the septum (Antman & Braunwald, 1997).

Like acute mitral regurgitation, an acute VSD after MI produces a new holosystolic murmur in association with congestive heart failure or cardiogenic shock. The differential diagnosis between acute VSD and acute mitral regurgitation is difficult from clinical criteria alone; Doppler echocardiography or right-sided heart catheterization is performed to differentiate the two conditions. When a VSD with a hemodynamically significant shunt is present, prognosis for survival is dismal unless surgical repair is performed. The defect allows shunting of blood from left to right, resulting in acute congestive heart failure in a left ventricle already damaged by acute MI. Death results from progressive cardiogenic shock and secondary organ failure. Without surgical repair, approximately 25% of patients with acute VSD die within 24 hours, 50% die within the first week, and only 20% of patients with unrepaired defects survive more than 4 weeks (Madsen & Daggett, 1997; Kirklin & Barratt-Boyes, 1993c).

Intra-aortic balloon counterpulsation usually is necessary to support the patient until operative intervention can be performed. Counterpulsation decreases afterload, thereby promoting forward flow from the left ventricle

and reducing left-to-right shunting. Inotropic and diuretic medications commonly are administered as well. Vasodilating agents are used to aid in afterload reduction if hemodynamically tolerated by the patient. Surgical closure of an acute VSD is performed emergently in hemodynamically unstable patients.

Timing of operative repair in hemodynamically stable patients is controversial. Operative repair of the defect is made technically easier if performed several weeks after the infarct when the defect edges have become fibrotic, making the tissue firmer and easier to secure with sutures. In the early period after infarction, the tissue is quite friable. Suturing is difficult and disruption of the repair is more likely. In addition, the risk of myocardial dysfunction is greater if the operation is performed early after acute MI.

Conversely, if surgical repair of the defect is delayed, precipitous, irreversible hemodynamic deterioration can occur at any time. Accordingly, many surgeons believe the risk of death to the patient during a waiting period of several weeks warrants immediate repair of a postinfarction VSD once it has been diagnosed. Although survival is usually better in those patients for whom surgical repair is delayed, patients who remain hemodynamically stable for several weeks are not comparable with those who require early operation because of cardiogenic shock. Because patients in stable condition are estimated to constitute 5% or less of the total population of patients with postinfarction VSD, most patients require prompt surgical treatment (Madsen & Daggett, 1996).

The decision about whether to perform preoperative cardiac catheterization in unstable patients with acute VSD also is controversial. If coronary angiography is performed, the surgeon will know the nature and severity of underlying CAD. Significant lesions can be bypassed concomitantly with surgical repair of the VSD. On the other hand, catheterization imposes additional risk in the presence of cardiogenic shock and delays operative repair of the immediate problem that is producing hemodynamic instability. Because balloon counterpulsation frequently produces a transient reversal of hemodynamic deterioration, it may provide a period of stability in which to perform coronary angiography before operation (Madsen & Daggett, 1997).

Operative repair of an acute VSD is performed through a median sternotomy incision and ventriculotomy through the infarcted portion of muscle (Fig. 15-9). Necrotic septal muscle is excised, and a prosthetic patch often is placed to close the defect. Defects in the posterior septum are more difficult to expose and repair than those in the anterior or apical portion of the septum (Kirklin & Barratt-Boyes, 1993c). Concomitant coronary artery revascularization may be performed, depending on the presence of suitable target vessels and hemodynamic stability. Although short-term survival is not different, significantly improved long-term survival has been demonstrated in patients who undergo coronary revascularization with VSD repair compared with patients with CAD of similar extent and no bypass grafting at the time of VSD repair (Madsen & Daggett, 1996). Concomitant mitral valve replacement is

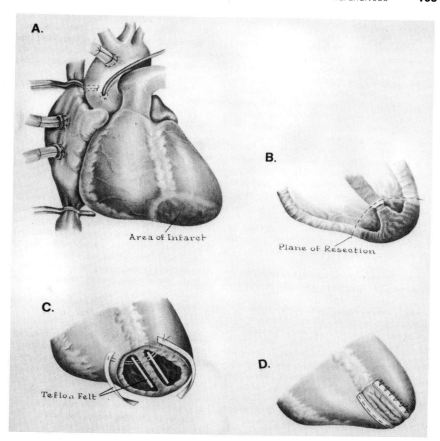

FIGURE 15-9. One technique of acute VSD repair. **(A)** Apical myocardial infarction has resulted in rupture of the ventricular septum. **(B)** The infarcted muscle is excised, including the area of the septum containing the defect and adjacent areas of right and left ventricular myocardium. **(C)** Prosthetic material is used to reinforce the closure as sutures are placed through viable myocardium surrounding the area of resection. **(D)** The apex is securely closed. (Kouchoukos NT, 1979: Infarction ventricular septal defect. In Cohn LH [ed]: Modern Technics in Surgery, p. 9-4. Mount Kisco, NY, Futura)

sometimes necessary to correct significant mitral regurgitation associated with acute VSD, particularly in patients with posterior MIs (Kirklin & Barratt-Boyes, 1993c).

REFERENCES

Acar C, Ramsheyi A, Pagny JY, et al., 1998: The radial artery for coronary artery bypass grafting: Clinical and angiographic results at five years. J Thorac Cardiovasc Surg 116:981

Alderman EL, Levy JH, Rich JB, et al., 1998: Analyses of coronary graft patency after aprotinin use: Results from the international multicenter aprotinin graft patency experience (IMAGE) trial. J Thorac Cardiovasc Surg 116:716

American Heart Association, 1998: 1999 Heart and Stroke Statistical Update. Dallas, American Heart Association

American College of Cardiology/American Heart Association Task Force on Assessment of Diagnostic and Therapeutic Cardiovascular Procedures, 1991: ACC/AHA guidelines and indications for coronary artery bypass graft surgery. Circulation 83:1125

Antman EM, Braunwald E, 1997: Acute myocardial infarction. In Braunwald E (ed): Heart Disease: A Textbook of Cardiovascular Medicine, ed. 5. Philadelphia, WB Saunders

Barner HB, 1998: Arterial grafting: Techniques and conduits. Ann Thorac Surg 66:S2

Brown WM, Jones EL, 1997: First operation for myocardial revascularization. In Edmunds LH Jr (ed): Cardiac Surgery in the Adult. New York, McGraw-Hill

Buckberg GD, 1987: Recent progress in myocardial protection during cardiac operations. In McGoon DC (ed): Cardiac Surgery, ed. 2. Philadelphia, FA Davis

Busch T, Friedrich M, Sirbu H, et al., 1999: Coronary artery bypass procedures in septuagenarians are justified: Short and long term results. J Cardiovasc Surg 40:83

CASS Principal Investigators and Their Associates, 1983: Coronary Artery Surgery Study (CASS): A randomized trial of coronary artery bypass surgery: Survival data. Circulation 68:939

Clark RE, Edwards FH, Schwartz M, 1994: Profile of preoperative characteristics of patients having CABG over the past decade. Ann Thorac Surg 58:1863

Cmolik BL, Geha AS, 1996: Coronary operations and reoperations: Techniques and conduits. In Baue AE, Geha AS, Hammond GL, et al. (eds): Glenn's Thoracic and Cardiovascular Surgery, ed. 6. Stamford, CT, Appleton & Lange

Cooley DA, Walker WE, 1980: Surgical treatment of postinfarction ventricular aneurysm: Evolution of technique and results in 1533 patients. In Moran JM, Michaelis LL (eds): Surgery for the Complications of Myocardial Infarction. New York, Grune & Stratton

Cosgrove DM, Loop FD, Lytle BW, et al., 1986: Predictors of reoperation after myocardial revascularization. J Thorac Cardiovasc Surg 92:811

Cox JL, 1997a: Left ventricular aneurysms: Pathophysiologic observations and standard resection. Semin Thorac Cardiovasc Surg 9:113

Cox JL, 1997b: Surgical management of left ventricular aneurysms: A clarification of the similarities and differences between the Jatene and Dor techniques. Semin Thorac Cardiovasc Surg 9:131

European Coronary Surgery Study Group, 1982: Long-term results of prospective randomised study of coronary artery bypass surgery in stable angina pectoris. Lancet 2:1173

Fiore AC, Jatene AD, 1996: Surgical treatment of left ventricular aneurysm. In Baue AE, Geha AS, Hammond GL, et al. (eds): Glenn's Thoracic and Cardiovascular Surgery, ed. 6. Stamford, CT, Appleton & Lange

Franco KL, Hammond GL, 1996: Surgical indications for coronary revascularization. In Baue AE, Geha AS, Hammond GL, et al. (eds): Glenn's Thoracic and Cardiovascular Surgery, ed. 6. Stamford, CT, Appleton & Lange

Galbut DL, Traad EA, Dorman MJ, et al., 1991: Bilateral internal mammary artery grafts in reoperative and primary coronary bypass surgery. Ann Thorac Surg 52:20

Gall SA Jr, 1997: Reoperative coronary surgery. In Sabiston DC Jr (ed): Textbook of Surgery: The Biological Basis of Modern Surgical Practice, ed. 15. Philadelphia, WB Saunders

Gay WA Jr, 1997: Ventricular aneurysm. In Sabiston DC Jr (ed): Textbook of Surgery: The Biological Basis of Modern Surgical Practice, ed. 15. Philadelphia, WB Saunders

Glower DD, Lowe JE, 1997: Left ventricular aneurysm. In Edmunds LH Jr (ed): Cardiac Surgery in the Adult. New York, McGraw-Hill

Goldman S, Copeland J, Moritz T, et al., 1990: Internal mammary artery and saphenous vein graft patency. Circulation 82(Suppl IV):IV–237

Grondin CM, Lesperance J, Solymoss BC, et al., 1979: Atherosclerotic changes in coronary grafts six years after operation. J Thorac Cardiovasc Surg 77:24

Grosso MA, Harken AH, 1995: Left ventricular aneurysm. In Sabiston DC Jr, Spencer FC (eds): Surgery of the Chest, ed. 6. Philadelphia, WB Saunders

Grover FL, Johnson RR, Shroyer LW, et al., 1994: The Veterans Affairs continuous improvement in cardiac surgery study. Ann Thorac Surg 58:1845

Hammermeister KE, Burchfiel C, Johnson R, Grover F, 1990: Identification of patients at greatest risk for developing major complications at cardiac surgery. Circulation 82 (Suppl IV):IV–380

Hannan RL, Kron IL, 1998: Minimally invasive coronary artery bypass grafting. In Kaiser LR, Kron IL, Spray TL (eds): Mastery of Cardiothoracic Surgery. Philadelphia, Lippincott Williams & Wilkins

Hochberg MS, Parsonnet V, Gielchinsky I, et al., 1984: Timing of coronary revascularization after acute myocardial infarction. J Thorac Cardiovasc Surg 88:914

Horvath KA, Mannting F, Cummings N, et al., 1996: Transmyocardial laser revascularization: Operative techniques and clinical results at two years. J Thorac Cardiovasc Surg 111:1047

Horvath KA, Cohn LH, Cooley DA, et al., 1997: Transmyocardial laser revascularization: results of a multicenter trial with transmyocardial laser revascularization used as sole therapy for end-stage coronary artery disease. J Thorac Cardiovasc Surg 113:645

Johnson WD, Brenowitz JB, Saedi SF, Kayser KL, 1989: Diffuse coronary artery disease. In Grillo HC, Austen WG, Wilkins EW, et al. (eds): Current Therapy in Cardiothoracic Surgery. Toronto, Canada, BC Decker

Johnsson P, Algotsson L, Ryding E, et al., 1991: Cardiopulmonary perfusion and cerebral blood flow in bilateral carotid disease. Ann Thorac Surg 51:579

Jones EL, 1991: Preparation of the internal mammary artery for coronary bypass surgery. J Cardiac Surg 6:326

Jones EL, Hodakowski GT, 1996: Combined coronary and carotid artery disease. In Baue AE, Geha AS, Hammond GL, et al. (eds): Glenn's Thoracic and Cardiovascular Surgery, ed. 6. Stamford, CT, Appleton & Lange

King SB, 1996: Indications for nonsurgical coronary revascularization. In Baue AE, Geha AS, Hammond GL, et al. (eds): Glenn's Thoracic and Cardiovascular Surgery, ed. 6. Stamford, CT, Appleton & Lange

King SB, 1990: Prediction of acute closure in percutaneous transluminal coronary angioplasty. Circulation 81(Suppl IV):IV–5

Kirklin JW, Barratt-Boyes BG, 1993a: Stenotic arteriosclerotic coronary artery disease. In Cardiac Surgery, ed. 2. New York, Churchill Livingstone

Kirklin JW, Barratt-Boyes BG, 1993b: Left ventricular aneurysm. In Cardiac Surgery, ed. 2. New York, Churchill Livingstone

Kirklin JW, Barratt-Boyes BG, 1993c: Postinfarction ventricular septal defect. In Cardiac Surgery, ed. 2. New York, Churchill Livingstone

Kron IL, Bayfield MS, 1998: Coronary artery bypass: Reoperation. In Kaiser LR, Kron IL, Spray TL (eds): Mastery of Cardiothoracic Surgery. Philadelphia, Lippincott Williams & Wilkins

Lincoff AM, Topol EJ, 1997: Interventional catheterization techniques. In Braunwald E (ed): Heart Disease: A Textbook of Cardiovascular Medicine, ed. 5. Philadelphia, WB Saunders

Loop FD, 1998: Coronary artery bypass surgery. In Topol EJ (ed): Comprehensive Cardiovascular Medicine. Philadelphia, Lippincott Williams & Wilkins

Loop FD, 1995: Repeat coronary artery bypass grafting for myocardial ischemia. In Sabiston DC Jr, Spencer FC (eds): Surgery of the Chest, ed. 6. Philadelphia, WB Saunders

Lytle BW, 1997: Coronary reoperations. In Edmunds LH Jr (ed): Cardiac Surgery in the Adult. New York, McGraw-Hill

Lytle BW, Cosgrove DM, 1992: Graft patency and revascularization strategies. Curr Probl Surg 24:769

Lytle BW, Cosgrove DM, Loop FD, et al., 1986: Perioperative risk of bilateral internal mammary artery grafting: Analysis of 500 cases from 1971 to 1984. Circulation 74 (Suppl III):III–37

Lytle BW, Kramer JR, Golding LR, et al., 1984: Young adults with coronary atherosclerosis: 10 year results of surgical myocardial revascularization. J Am Coll Cardiol 4:445

Madsen JC, Daggett WM Jr, 1997: Postinfarction ventricular septal defect and free wall rupture. In Edmunds LH Jr (ed): Cardiac Surgery in the Adult. New York, McGraw-Hill

Madsen JC, Daggett WM Jr, 1996: Postinfarction ventricular septal rupture. In Baue AE, Geha AS, Hammond GL, et al. (eds): Glenn's Thoracic and Cardiovascular Surgery, ed. 6. Stamford, CT, Appleton & Lange

Mariani MA, Boonstra PW, Grandjean JG, et al., 1997: Minimally invasive coronary artery bypass grafting versus coronary angioplasty for isolated type C stenosis of the left anterior descending artery. J Thorac Cardiovasc Surg 114:434

Mehta SM, Pae WE Jr, 1997: Complications of cardiac surgery. In Edmunds LH Jr (ed): Cardiac Surgery in the Adult. New York, McGraw-Hill

Mills NL, 1991: Preparation of the internal mammary artery graft with intraluminal papaverine. J Cardiac Surg 6:318

Morris JJ, Smith R, Glower DD, et al., 1990: Clinical evaluation of single versus multiple mammary artery bypass. Circulation 82(Suppl IV):IV–214

Newman DC, Hicks RG, 1988: Combined carotid and coronary artery surgery: A review of the literature. Ann Thorac Surg 45:574

Nolan SP, Zacour R, 1998: Cardiopulmonary bypass. In Kaiser LR, Kron IL, Spray TL (eds): Mastery of Cardiothoracic Surgery. Philadelphia, Lippincott Williams & Wilkins

Nugent WC, Schults WC, 1994: Playing by the numbers: How collecting outcomes data changed my life. Ann Thorac Surg 58:1866

Peigh PS, Disesa VJ, Collins JJ, Cohn LH, 1991: Coronary bypass grafting with totally calcified or acutely dissected ascending aorta. Ann Thorac Surg 51:102

Pigott JD, Mills NL, 1998. Venous versus arterial conduits. In Kaiser LR, Kron IL, Spray TL (eds): Mastery of Cardiothoracic Surgery. Philadelphia, Lippincott Williams & Wilkins

Possati G, Gaudino M, Alessandrini F, et al., 1998: Midterm clinical and angiographic results of radial arteries used for myocardial revascularization. J Thorac Cardiovasc Surg 116:1015

Rankin JS, Morris JJ, 1995: Utilization of autologous arterial grafts for coronary artery bypass. In Sabiston DC Jr, Spencer FC (eds): Surgery of the Chest, ed. 6. Philadelphia, WB Saunders

Rao V, Weisel RD, 1997: Intraoperative protection of organs: Hypothermia, cardioplegia, and cerebroplegia. In Edmunds LH Jr (ed): Cardiac Surgery in the Adult. New York, McGraw-Hill

Reardon MJ, Espada R, Letsou GV, et al., 1997: Editorial: minimally invasive coronary artery surgery: A word of caution. J Thorac Cardiovasc Surg 119:419

Salomon NW, Page US, Bigelow JC, et al., 1991: Coronary artery bypass grafting in elderly patients. J Thorac Cardiovasc Surg 101:209

Smith HC, Gersh BJ, 1997: Indications for revascularization. In Edmunds LH Jr (ed): Cardiac Surgery in the Adult. New York, McGraw-Hill

Society of Thoracic Surgeons/American Association for Thoracic Surgery Ad Hoc Committee on New Technology Assessment, 1998: Policy statement: Minimally invasive coronary artery bypass surgery. J Thorac Cardiovasc Surg 116:887

Spencer FC, Galloway AC, Colvin SB, 1995: Bypass grafting for coronary artery disease. In Sabiston DC, Spencer FC (eds): Surgery of the Chest, ed. 6. Philadelphia, WB Saunders

Tashiro T, Nakamura K, Sukehiro S, et al., 1998: Midterm results of free internal thoracic artery grafting for myocardial revascularization. Ann Thorac Surg 69:951

Ulicny KS Jr, Hiratzka LF, 1991: The risk factors of median sternotomy infection: A current review. J Cardiac Surg 6:338

Veterans Administration Coronary Artery Bypass Surgery Cooperative Study Group, 1984: Eleven-year survival in the Veterans Administration Randomized Trial of Coronary Bypass Surgery for Stable Angina. N Engl J Med 311:133

16

Surgical Treatment of Valvular Heart Disease

Surgical treatment of valvular heart disease (VHD) began early in the 20th century, before availability of cardiopulmonary bypass, with isolated attempts to dilate stenotic valves. The pioneering efforts of John Gibbon, Walter Lillihei, John Kirklin, and others led to development of cardiopulmonary bypass in the mid-1950s and, for the first time, the ability to perform operations successfully on intracardiac structures under direct vision (Stephenson, 1997). In the decades that followed, cardiac surgeons and scientists worked to design artificial and biologic valvular prostheses that could substitute safely for native cardiac valves and to develop operative techniques for reconstructing diseased native valves to restore adequate function.

Today, approximately 79,000 valve operations are performed in the United States each year (American Heart Association, 1998). Most patients who undergo valve repair or replacement achieve increased survival and improved quality of life. Factors that have improved operative results include (1) refined techniques for repairing valves, (2) better design of valvular prostheses, (3) improved myocardial protection during cardiopulmonary bypass, (4) earlier operative intervention, (5) more sophisticated perioperative management, and (6) more closely controlled long-term anticoagulant therapy. Still, surgical therapy remains palliative, substituting a new disease state for the old. At 15 years after valve replacement, fewer than 50% of patients remain free of valve-related morbidity (Burdon et al., 1992).

Common causes of VHD include myxomatous degeneration, aortic sclerosis, rheumatic endocarditis, infective endocarditis, and congenital anomalies. Regardless of etiology, the functional abnormality of a diseased valve is either stenosis (narrowing of the orifice when the valve is open) or regurgitation (incompetence when the valve is closed), or a combination of the two. When both stenosis and regurgitation coexist in the same valve, one process usually predominates (Schoen, 1997). Mitral valve disease is the most prevalent form of VHD, followed by aortic valve disease. The tricuspid valve occasionally is affected, usually secondary to mitral valve disease. Pulmonic valve disease is rare in adults. Operations on the mitral or aortic valve comprise most of the surgical procedures. Etiology, types of valvular lesions and their consequences, and nonsurgical therapies for VHD are discussed in detail in Chapter 2, Valvular Heart Disease.

► Indications for Surgical Therapy

In most forms of VHD, pathologic deterioration of the valve occurs gradually and the heart compensates for many years before surgical intervention becomes necessary. Optimal timing for repairing or replacing a cardiac valve depends on several factors, especially the specific valvular abnormality. With some lesions, signs and symptoms that warrant surgical intervention are well defined. With others, appropriate timing for surgical therapy is difficult to assess. It is advantageous to avoid operation and delay implantation of a prosthesis as long as possible. Conversely, it is equally important to intervene early enough to avoid irreversible damage to the heart muscle or pulmonary vasculature.

Surgical therapy often is prompted by evidence that valve dysfunction has begun to damage permanently one or both ventricles or the pulmonary vasculature. For example, severe mitral or aortic regurgitation or aortic stenosis eventually produces irreversible left ventricular enlargement and failure. Operative repair also may be recommended because the nature of the valvular lesion places the patient at risk for catastrophic consequences, such as sudden cardiac death from severe aortic stenosis or septic embolization from infected valvular vegetations. Indications for surgical correction of the most common valvular lesions are discussed in the following sections.

Mitral Stenosis

Mitral valve stenosis, which results predominantly from rheumatic fever, obstructs blood flow from the left atrium into the left ventricle. As a result, left atrial pressure becomes chronically elevated and the left atrium enlarges. Pulmonary arterial hypertension develops in 10% to 20% of patients (Schlant, 1991). Although the mechanism is not fully understood, it is thought to be related both to chronically elevated left atrial pressure and degenerative changes in the pulmonary arterioles. The time of onset and severity of pulmonary hypertension vary from patient to patient (Swain, 1996). In severe cases, systolic pulmonary artery pressure may be equal to or even greater than systolic arterial pressure. Right ventricular hypertrophy develops because of the elevated pulmonary vascular resistance or afterload against which the right ventricle must eject. Eventually, right-sided heart failure may occur.

Because mitral stenosis usually develops gradually as a consequence of rheumatic heart disease, patients remain without symptoms for years (Fann et al., 1997). Cardiac symptoms typically appear in the fourth or fifth decade in patients who live in industrialized nations; in developing countries, particularly tropical areas, the disease progresses more rapidly (Alpert et al., 1998). Dyspnea is the most characteristic symptom of mitral stenosis, and episodes of pulmonary edema are common. Chronic atrial fibrillation, or less commonly atrial flutter, usually develops secondary to atrial enlargement. Stasis of blood along the walls of the fibrillating atria predisposes to thrombus formation and the possibility of embolization. Systemic embolism occurs in approximately 20% of patients and is sometimes the first symptom of mitral stenosis (Fann et al., 1997). Although the left ventricle is protected against volume or pressure overload by the stenotic mitral valve, it probably does not remain normal. Characteristic symptoms of fatigue and progressive exercise intolerance may be related to the left ventricle's inability to increase cardiac output appropriately in response to increased metabolic demand.

In contrast to other valvular lesions in adults, mitral stenosis sometimes can be treated with a therapeutic catheterization technique, percutaneous transvenous balloon valvotomy, in addition to surgical valve repair or replacement. Interventional therapy for relief of mitral stenosis (either balloon valvotomy or operative repair) usually is prompted by the degree of disabling symptoms. An interventional procedure usually is recommended when the patient's New York Heart Association (NYHA) functional status deteriorates to class II or III or if symptoms of right-sided heart failure develop.

An interventional procedure also may be recommended in asymptomatic patients with hemodynamically significant mitral stenosis (cross-sectional valve area <1.5 cm^2). The rationale for early operation for hemodynamic rather than symptomatic indications is based on the typically insidious progression of mitral stenosis. Patients with hemodynamically significant mitral valve narrowing are at risk for two serious potential consequences. First, systemic embolism, particularly to the brain, can occur even if the patient is in normal sinus rhythm; second, progressive deterioration of the valve from fibrosis and calcification may preclude valve repair and necessitate valve replacement (Spencer et al., 1995).

In addition, it is preferable to correct mitral stenosis while the patient is still in normal sinus rhythm. Because atrial fibrillation reduces cardiac output and increases left atrial pressure, the arrhythmia exacerbates symptoms and accelerates the patient's downward course (Kirklin & Barratt-Boyes, 1993a). After years of atrial distention and atrial fibrillation, a return of normal sinus rhythm is unlikely, even after valvular repair or replacement.

The expected 10-year survival rate for patients with mitral stenosis receiving medical treatment is only 85% for asymptomatic patients (NYHA I), 50% for those in NYHA class II, and 20% for those in NYHA class III; no patients in NYHA class IV can be expected to survive 5 years (Fann et al., 1997). Because the stenotic mitral valve restricts blood flow into the left ventricle and thus preserves adequate left ventricular function, patients with mitral stenosis almost never have disease so far advanced that surgical treatment is not possible (Spencer et al., 1995). The increased pulmonary vascular resistance often associated with mitral stenosis is usually at least partially reversible after valve repair or replacement.

Mitral Regurgitation

Chronic *mitral regurgitation* may result from myxomatous degeneration, ischemic damage to the subvalvular apparatus, rheumatic endocarditis, or left ventricular dilatation. More recently, anorectic drugs also have been reported to cause mitral regurgitation (Bonow et al., 1998). Myxomatous degeneration (floppy mitral valve or mitral valve prolapse) has become the leading cause of mitral regurgitation in the United States, primarily as a result of the decline in rheumatic heart disease (Fann et al., 1997). Regurgitation in mitral valves damaged by myxomatous degeneration is caused by leaflet prolapse, usually of the posterior leaflet, secondary to chordal rupture or elongation (Alpert et al., 1998).

Regurgitation of blood through an incompetent mitral valve during systole causes increased volume and pressure in the left atrium with resultant left atrial enlargement. As the ventricle pumps more forcefully to maintain adequate forward flow, left ventricular hypertrophy and dilatation develop as well. Symptoms, which are similar to those of mitral stenosis, develop late in the course of mitral regurgitation. Ideally, surgical intervention to correct mitral regurgitation is performed early enough to preserve normal left ventricular function. Once the ventricle undergoes substantial dilatation, muscle function becomes permanently damaged despite correction of the valvular abnormality. Precise timing of operation to preserve normal ventricular function is difficult because the onset of irreversible muscle damage is not predictable.

Angiotensin-converting enzyme (ACE) inhibiting medications, such as captopril, are the mainstay of medical therapy for mitral regurgitation. Because ACE inhibitors reduce afterload and promote forward flow from the left ventricle, they produce symptomatic improvement in patients with mitral regurgitation. However, there is concern about whether afterload reduction therapy may mask progressive ventricular injury caused by ongoing left ventricular volume overload (Fann et al., 1997). With pharmacologic afterload reduction, it is possible to have left ventricular dysfunction in the presence of normal left ventricular dimensions and minimal symptoms (Dalrymple-Hay et al., 1998). Thus, the left ventricle can undergo irreversible damage despite the lack of disabling symptoms.

Preservation of adequate left ventricular function is essential because it is the most important predictor of postoperative outcome. Compared with patients who undergo surgery before development of left ventricular dysfunction, patients with excessive left ventricular dilatation or systolic dysfunction experience a greater decrease in postoperative ejection fraction, an increased incidence of heart failure, and a higher mortality (Quinones, 1998). Consequently, mitral valve repair or replacement is recommended when echocardiographic data demonstrate early left ventricular dysfunction (an ejection fraction $\leq 50\%$) or dilatation (left ventricular end-systolic volume index ≥ 55 mL/m^2, end-diastolic dimension between 65 and 68 mm, and end-systolic dimension between 44 and 45 mm) (Alpert et al., 1998).

Aortic Regurgitation

Aortic regurgitation may be caused by rheumatic endocarditis, a bicuspid aortic valve, or conditions that dilate the valve annulus or damage valve leaflets, such as ascending aortic aneurysm, aortic dissection, or Marfan's syndrome. Aortic regurgitation subjects the left ventricle to increased volume and pressure as a portion of each stroke volume is regurgitated during diastole. Initially, the left ventricle hypertrophies and systemic vascular resistance decreases to maintain adequate forward flow. Eventually, the left ventricle dilates and loses the ability to contract effectively. Ejection fraction decreases, and symptoms of left-sided heart failure develop. Mild aortic regurgitation causes no symptoms and patients with moderate to severe aortic regurgitation may remain asymptomatic for many years (Hammond & Letsou, 1996). However, the time course between the development of left ventricular dysfunction at rest and the onset of symptoms is relatively short; two thirds of asymptomatic patients with evidence of left ventricular dysfunction experience symptoms within 2 to 3 years (Bonow, 1998). The predominant symptoms of advanced aortic regurgitation are those of pulmonary venous hypertension; namely, dyspnea, orthopnea, and paroxysmal nocturnal dyspnea. Angina is a presenting symptom in 25% of patients (Jamieson, 1997).

Because of the irreversible left ventricular damage that eventually occurs, there is a trend toward earlier valve replacement for aortic regurgitation. Surgical therapy is recommended for aortic regurgitation that produces significant symptoms. In asymptomatic patients, surgical intervention is indicated for deteriorating ventricular function, as evidenced by echocardiographic demonstration of an ejection fraction less than 55% with a diastolic ventricular diameter approaching 75 mm or an end-systolic diameter approaching 50 mm (Maier & Wechsler, 1997).

Aortic Stenosis

Aortic stenosis, defined as obstruction to left ventricular outflow, can occur at a valvular, subvalvular, or supravalvular level. In adults, it nearly always is due to a valvular abnormality, often a congenitally bicuspid valve or one that has undergone calcific degeneration. Valvular aortic stenosis in adults is characterized by calcification of the valve and a diminished valve orifice. The left ventricle hypertrophies and a significant transvalvular gradient develops to generate sufficient pressure to eject blood through the narrowed valve orifice. As a result, left ventricular damage is a prominent feature of severe aortic stenosis. Diastolic filling of the ventricle is impaired, and the ventricle eventually dilates, leading to systolic impairment and symptoms of left-sided heart failure. In addition, severe aortic stenosis is associated with an increased incidence of ventricular arrhythmias, conduction disturbances, and sudden cardiac death. Although all patients with aortic stenosis are at increased risk for sudden cardiac death, the risk is highest in symptomatic patients (Jamieson, 1997).

Characteristic symptoms of aortic stenosis, which include angina, dyspnea, and syncope, occur late in the course of the disease. Onset of symptoms is associated with a limited life expectancy unless the valvular stenosis is relieved. The 1-year survival rate for untreated patients with severe, symptomatic aortic stenosis is only 57% (Frankel et al., 1998). The definitive treatment for aortic stenosis is aortic valve replacement. It is performed when significant aortic stenosis begins to produce symptoms. Even mild symptoms, such as exertional dyspnea, warrant prompt valve replacement when severe aortic stenosis is present (Otto, 1998). Because prognosis with medical therapy is so poor, surgical intervention often is recommended even for elderly patients in the eighth and ninth decades of life. Valve replacement also may be recommended for asymptomatic patients with severe aortic stenosis, as evidenced by a valve area less than 0.8 cm^2 or a mean transvalvular gradient greater than 50 mm Hg.

Tricuspid Regurgitation

Tricuspid regurgitation can occur due to rheumatic heart disease, infective endocarditis, or right ventricular enlargement with resultant dilatation of the tricuspid valve annulus. Rheumatic tricuspid regurgitation almost always occurs in association with mitral valve disease, and usually with aortic disease as well (McGrath, 1997). A regurgitant tricuspid valve causes right ventricular enlargement and progressive symptoms of right-sided heart failure. Surgical intervention usually is undertaken when diagnostic studies suggest impending irreversible right ventricular failure. However, surgical treatment for tricuspid regurgitation is not straightforward. Although tricuspid regurgitation, like other types of valvular incompetence, tends to progress, deleterious effects of ventricular volume overload on the right side of the heart develop more slowly than on the left side (Kirklin & Barratt-Boyes, 1993b). In addition, operative morbidity and mortality rates are relatively high, indications for surgical intervention are imprecisely defined, and controversy exists about whether valve repair or replacement is preferable and which type of repair or prosthesis is optimal (Silverman & Paone, 1998; McGrath, 1990).

Acute Valvular Dysfunction

Most forms of VHD are associated with slowly progressive valvular dysfunction. In some forms, however, valve dysfunction can develop precipitously. Acute mitral regurgitation most often occurs secondary to ischemic heart disease. Dysfunction or rupture of a papillary muscle or annular dilatation associated with myocardial infarction may lead to acute valvular incompetence. In contrast to chronic mitral regurgitation, compensatory mechanisms to protect the heart have not developed. Pulmonary edema or frank cardiogenic shock occur typically as a manifestation of acute left ventricular failure. Intra-aortic balloon counterpulsation usually is necessary to support cardiac function. Papillary muscle ischemia sometimes is treated effectively with revascularization therapies (ie, thrombolytic therapy, percutaneous coronary intervention, or coronary artery bypass grafting). Papillary muscle rupture or annular dilatation usually requires emergent valve repair or replacement to restore valvular competence.

Acute aortic regurgitation also may occur, most often related to aortic dissection. Sudden volume and pressure overload of the left ventricle produces acute left ventricular failure. In contrast to cardiogenic shock from other causes, that due to acute aortic regurgitation cannot be treated with intra-aortic balloon counterpulsation because balloon inflations during diastole would increase regurgitant flow through the incompetent aortic valve. Emergent surgical intervention usually is necessary if the patient is to survive.

Acute dysfunction of any of the cardiac valves may be caused by infective endocarditis. In individuals who abuse intravenous drugs, the right-sided tricuspid valve is most commonly infected by venous contamination. Most cases of infective endocarditis in intravenous drug abusers are due to *Staphylococcus aureus, Pseudomonas aeruginosa,* other gram-negative bacilli, or *Candida* species; in persons who are not drug abusers, infective endocarditis commonly is caused by streptococci or *S. aureus* (Karchmer, 1997).

In 80% to 90% of cases, infective endocarditis of native cardiac valves can be treated effectively with an extensive course of organism-specific antibiotic therapy (Hendren et al., 1992). However, surgical therapy may be the only effective treatment in patients infected by particularly virulent microorganisms. Infective endocarditis caused by *S. aureus, P. aeruginosa, Serratia marcescens,* or fungi usually necessitates surgical treatment for cure (David, 1997; Ewy, 1997). These virulent microorganisms typically cause extensive leaflet or chordae tendineae destruction, resulting in severe ventricular failure. Survival is unlikely unless valvular competence is restored. Vegetations also may form on valvular tissue and provide a source of recurring septic emboli. Although the mere presence of a vegetation is not an indication for surgical intervention, embolization of vegetative tissue is common. Twenty to 40% of patients with infective endocarditis of left-sided cardiac valves have embolic neurologic complications (Ting et al., 1991).

Optimal timing for surgical therapy in patients with infective endocarditis is difficult to determine. Patients who require surgical treatment often are gravely ill with hemodynamic instability and multisystem organ dysfunction (Larbalestier et al., 1992). Ideally, a full course (usually 6 weeks) of antibiotic therapy is given before surgery. Sterilization of the native valve before implantation of prosthetic material substantially increases the likelihood of curing the infection, which is extremely difficult to eradicate with a valvular prosthesis in place. However, depending on the virulence of the organism, the degree of valvular destruction, and the development of vegetations, it may become necessary to perform urgent valve replacement before completion of the antibiotic course.

Indications for proceeding urgently with removal of an infected valve and implantation of a valvular prosthesis include hemodynamic instability due to acute valvular regurgitation, persistent fevers or septic shock despite appropriate antibiotic therapy, or evidence of recurrent embolization from the infected valve. Surgery also is indicated when antibiotic therapy fails to control endocarditis, as evidenced by signs of progressive invasion of the myocardium with abscess formation, heart block, or fistulae (Ewy, 1997).

If septic cerebral embolization has occurred, determining timing of operative therapy is particularly challenging. Although removal of the infected valve is desirable to avoid recurrent embolization, cardiopulmonary bypass with systemic anticoagulation in a patient with recent stroke imposes the risk of cerebral hemorrhagic infarction. The major risk factor for perioperative stroke in such patients appears to be the preoperative presence of a hemorrhagic as opposed to an ischemic cerebral infarction (Ting et al., 1991).

▶ Surgical Procedures

A variety of surgical techniques are available for repairing and replacing cardiac valves. The specific valve that is diseased and the nature of the valve disease determine whether valve repair or replacement is preferable and if a minimally invasive surgical approach is advantageous. However, other factors, such as the patient's age, clinical status, and associated medical problems also are taken into consideration. Available options for the surgical management of common valvular lesions are displayed in Table 16-1.

Minimally Invasive Surgical Techniques

Operations on the mitral and aortic valve sometimes can be performed using minimally invasive surgical techniques. When used to describe valve repair or replacement, the term *minimally invasive* connotes that the operation is performed through an incision that is smaller than the standard sternotomy incision, usually either a small right parasternal or right lateral thoracotomy or partial sternotomy incision (Fig. 16-1). Cannulation of the aorta and venae cavae for cardiopulmonary bypass is performed through the chest incision, or the common femoral artery and vein are cannulated through an incision in the groin in combination with direct cannulation of the superior vena cava. In contrast to minimally invasive coronary artery bypass grafting, which sometimes describes an operation performed without cardiopulmonary bypass, extracorporeal circulation using cardiopulmonary bypass always is necessary for valve operations because the heart or aorta must be opened to access the intracardiac structures.

The objectives of minimally invasive cardiac surgery are to reduce surgical trauma in order to decrease incisional pain, lessen morbidity, shorten hospital length of stay and recovery time, reduce costs, and achieve a more cosmetically pleasing result for the patient (Aklog et al., 1998). It is imperative, however, that the long-term quality of the operation not be compromised to achieve these short-term objectives. Minimally invasive surgery is appropriate only when an operation can be performed with safety and efficacy that is equivalent to that achieved with a full sternotomy incision and standard cardiopulmonary bypass cannulation techniques.

The incision used must provide adequate exposure of valve structures and allow the safe conduct of cardiopulmonary bypass and myocardial protection. Minimally in-

TABLE 16-1	
Surgical Therapy for Valvular Heart Disease	
Valvular Lesion	*Corrective Procedure*
Mitral stenosis*	Commissurotomy
	Mitral valve replacement
Mitral regurgitation	Valvuloplasty
	Mitral valve replacement
Aortic stenosis	Aortic valve replacement
Aortic regurgitation	Aortic valve replacement
Tricuspid regurgitation	Valvuloplasty
	Tricuspid valve replacement

*Also treated with balloon valvotomy.

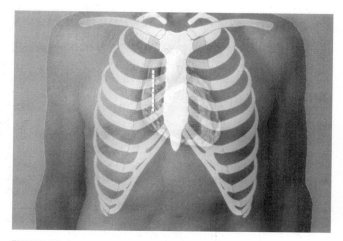

FIGURE 16-1. Minimally invasive incision for mitral valve operation. Right parasternal incision extends 8 to 10 cm, from lower border of second costal cartilage to upper border of the fifth costal cartilage. (Alpert JS, Sabik J, Cosgrove DM, 1998: Mitral valve disease. In Topol EJ [ed]: Comprehensive Cardiovascular Medicine, p. 556. Philadelphia, Lippincott Williams & Wilkins)

vasive surgical techniques may not be possible in patients who are markedly obese or in those with significant chest wall abnormalities or unusual cardiac orientation (Aklog et al., 1998). Also excluded from minimally invasive procedures are patients undergoing a Ross procedure.

Valve Repair

The repair of cardiac valves dates to the beginning of the surgical treatment of heart disease. Salvage of a native cardiac valve is attractive because all available valvular prostheses are associated with significant long-term complications. Also, valve repair usually obviates the need for chronic anticoagulation, which is necessary with all mechanical valvular prostheses. An additional advantage of reparative procedures that salvage the mitral valve is preservation of the subvalvular apparatus. The chordae tendineae anchor the anterior and posterior leaflets of the mitral valve to the papillary muscles arising from the ventricular endocardium. This supportive apparatus exerts tension during ventricular relaxation, allowing the valve to open actively during diastole. Subvalvular structures also are thought to augment ventricular contraction during systole. Thus, mitral valve repair is less compromising to left ventricular function than mitral valve replacement, if the replacement includes complete excision of the valve and removal of the subvalvular apparatus.

Reparative procedures for cardiac valves include percutaneous transvenous balloon valvotomy, commissurotomy, and surgical valvuloplasty. Balloon valvotomy (also called balloon valvuloplasty) and commissurotomy are performed to correct pure valvular stenosis. Both procedures involve splitting open fused valve commissures to widen a stenotic valve orifice and are performed most often in patients with mitral stenosis. They are appropriate only in specific situations, determined by the particular anatomy and degree of calcification of the native cardiac valve.

Balloon valvotomy of the mitral valve is best suited to patients with appropriate morphology of the valve apparatus and no significant mitral regurgitation; the procedure is contraindicated in the presence of left atrial thrombus (Bruce & Nishimura, 1998). Although balloon valvotomy spares the patient from an open heart operation, it does not allow direct visualization of the valve during the repair. It is described in more detail in Chapter 2, Valvular Heart Disease.

A *commissurotomy* is the surgical incision of valve commissures to relieve stenosis. Mitral commissurotomy has been performed for half a century and remains a mainstay in treatment of mitral stenosis throughout the world. Before development of adequate cardiopulmonary bypass, mitral commissurotomy was performed as a "closed" procedure without the aid of extracorporeal circulation. The surgeon inserted a finger through a small opening in the left atrium and, guided only by palpation of the valve, blindly fractured the valve commissures with a finger or with an instrument inserted through the left ventricle.

Mitral commissurotomy now is performed as an "open" procedure during which the surgeon can directly inspect valvular disease. Sixty to 80% of stenotic mitral valves can be repaired successfully with available techniques (Alpert et al., 1998). After initiating cardiopulmonary bypass and cardioplegic arrest, the left atrium is opened and the valve is repaired under direct visualization. When performed as an open procedure, the results are quite predictable and operative risk is low.

Surgical repair of mitral stenosis sometimes includes more than simple division of the commissures. In complex cases, the procedure is more appropriately called a surgical valvuloplasty. In addition to the commissurotomy itself, it may be necessary for the surgeon to free scarred chordae tendineae, split papillary muscles, or implant a supportive prosthetic ring in the valve annulus if commissural regurgitation results from commissurotomy. When rheumatic disease has damaged the valve leaflets, fibrous material is excised to restore leaflet pliability; if calcification is present, it may be necessary to débride the leaflet and patch it with autologous pericardium (Alpert et al., 1998).

More often, *surgical valvuloplasty* describes a reparative procedure to correct mitral regurgitation. Early attempts to repair regurgitant mitral valves rarely were successful. However, Carpentier, Duran, and others have introduced techniques that result in satisfactory and predictable results. Feasibility of valve repair for mitral regurgitation depends on the underlying valvular disease. Mitral valvuloplasty is performed most often and is the procedure of choice in patients with pure mitral regurgitation secondary to myxomatous disease (David et al., 1998). Mitral regurgitation secondary to myxomatous degeneration is well suited to a reparative procedure because, in contrast to valve dysfunction owing to a rheumatic etiology, pure regurgitation often is present. The excellent surgical results and the difficulty in reliably detecting early left ventricular dysfunction have led to earlier surgical valve repair (eg, NYHA class I or II) for patients with moderate or severe mitral regurgitation due to degenerative valve disease (Dalrymple-Hay et al., 1998). With current techniques, mitral valve repair is possible in approximately 95% of patients with myxomatous valve disease (Gillinov et al., 1998).

Repair also is possible in many cases in which mitral regurgitation is due to ischemic damage, infective endocarditis, or rheumatic valvular disease. Ischemic valve damage most often involves papillary muscles that support the posterior mitral valve leaflet. Although valves damaged by infective endocarditis often require replacement, repair of the native valve, when possible, is advantageous in that it avoids placement of a prosthetic valve in the presence of active infection. In centers with extensive experience in valve repair, such as the Cleveland Clinic, mitral valve repair is performed in 76% of patients with ischemic mitral regurgitation, 59% of patients with mitral regurgitation due to infective endocarditis, and 42% of patients with rheumatic mitral regurgitation (Alpert et al., 1998).

Satisfactory valvuloplasty necessitates thorough intraoperative assessment of native valve dysfunction. The mitral valve is a complex, dynamically integrated structure, and incompetence may be due to abnormalities of the leaflets, chordae tendineae, papillary muscles, annulus, or a combination of these. Intraoperative transesophageal echocardiography is performed to quantify the degree of regurgitation and determine the precise functional anatomy. It provides highly accurate information about the mitral valve and left ventricle to assist the surgeon in planning the repair (Lawrie, 1998).

Valvular regurgitation may be due to increased leaflet motion (ie, leaflet prolapse) or restricted leaflet movement. The subvalvular structures (the chordae tendineae and papillary muscles) may be elongated or ruptured. Dilatation of the annulus also is common.

Valve reconstruction is tailored to the identified valvular abnormality. Most common is isolated posterior leaflet prolapse due to choral rupture in a myxomatous valve. The standard reparative technique for posterior leaflet prolapse is resection of a quadrangular section of the posterior leaflet and performance of an annuloplasty (tightening the annulus with placement of a supportive ring to remodel annular shape without reducing orifice size) (Fig. 16-2). Posterior leaflet quadrangular resection with annuloplasty is the technique of mitral valve repair associated with the greatest long-term durability (Gillinov et al., 1998).

Cardiothoracic surgeons have developed expertise in several other surgical techniques to restore adequate functional anatomy. For example, quadrangular resection is not possible for repair of anterior leaflet prolapse because of the anterior leaflet's attachment to the aortic valve annulus (Alpert et al., 1998). Instead, repair is achieved by relocating or shortening chordal attachments

to restore valve competency. Secondary chordae of the anterior leaflet or posterior leaflet chordae may be relocated to the area of a ruptured or elongated chordae tendineae. Alternatively, polytetrafluroethylene suture may be used to replace ruptured chordae (Chitwood, 1998). A papillary muscle elongated by ischemic damage may be folded onto itself to restore valve competency (Fig. 16-3) (Alpert et al., 1998). Mitral valves damaged by infective endocarditis sometimes can be repaired by replacing portions of the anterior leaflet with pericardium and performing leaflet resection or chordal transposition for destroyed chordae tendineae (Alpert et al., 1998). Annular dilatation associated with left ventricular enlargement is corrected with implantation of a prosthetic annuloplasty ring. Surgical repair of cardiac valves always is followed by intraoperative assessment of valve competency with transesophageal echocardiography before concluding the procedure.

Although mitral valvuloplasty can be technically more complex and necessitate longer operative time than valve replacement, successful repair of the native mitral valve is superior to valve replacement. Compared with mitral valve replacement, valvuloplasty is associated with a lower risk of operative death, thromboembolic complications, and endocarditis; better preservation of left ventricular function; and improved long-term survival (Kon, 1998). The operative mortality rate for mitral valve repair ranges from 0% to 6% (Alpert et al., 1998). The best long-term results are associated with mitral valvuloplasty in patients with myxomatous degeneration (Kon, 1998). Not all valves can be repaired. For valves requiring complex reparative procedures, limited information is available about long-term durability, and many surgeons recommend valve

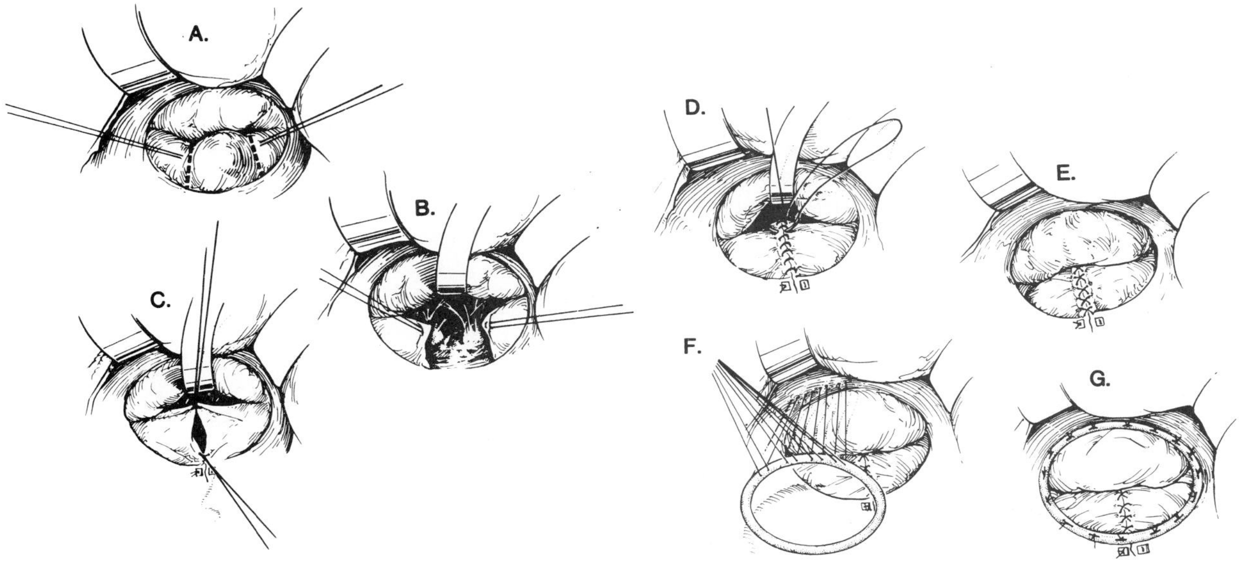

FIGURE 16-2. Initial steps in quadrilateral resection of the mitral valve posterior leaflet to correct mitral regurgitation (**A** through **C**); completion of mitral valvuloplasty with insertion of prosthetic annuloplasty ring (**D** through **G**). (Cohn LH, Disesa VJ, Couper GS, et al, 1989: Mitral valve repair for degeneration and prolapse of the mitral valve. J Thorac Cardiovasc Surg 98:988)

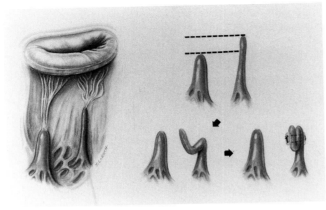

FIGURE 16-3. In this mitral valve repair, an elongated papillary muscle is folded onto itself to restore valve competence. (Alpert JS, Sabik J, Cosgrove DM, 1998: Mitral valve disease. In Topol EJ [ed]: Comprehensive Cardiovascular Medicine, p. 555. Philadelphia, Lippincott Williams & Wilkins)

replacement using a mechanical valve or tissue bioprosthesis.

Less commonly, valvuloplasty is performed on the tricuspid valve. Tricuspid regurgitation often is due to annular dilatation secondary to left-sided VHD. If untreated at the time of mitral or aortic valve replacement, regurgitation usually persists or progresses and may lead to heart or liver failure (Minale et al., 1990). Tricuspid regurgitation often can be corrected by implantation of a prosthetic ring to support the valve annulus. Because of the proximity of atrioventricular conduction tissue to the tricuspid valve annulus, heart block is a potential complication of tricuspid valve repair (Silverman & Paone, 1998).

Reparative procedures for aortic regurgitation are rare. Repair occasionally is possible in an aortic valve with an isolated perforation of one of the leaflets and no annular dilatation, calcification, or gradient indicative of aortic stenosis. In such an unusual situation, it may be possible to patch the leaflet with glutaraldehyde-treated pericardium to salvage the native valve. Pericardium is very durable and is able to withstand the systemic pressure to which the aortic valve and root are subjected. Repair of an incompetent aortic valve also is possible in some cases of regurgitation secondary to ascending aortic aneurysm or dissection. If the aortic valve itself is normal and regurgitation is caused only by annular distortion from aortic disease, it may be possible to resuspend the aortic valve, thus restoring competence.

Although many patients receive excellent palliation and never require implantation of a valvular prosthesis, all of the reparative procedures are associated with potential complications. The primary complication of valvuloplasty is breakdown of the repair, resulting in acute valvular regurgitation. The complication usually is manifest by acute onset of congestive heart failure and a new murmur. Reoperation and implantation of a valvular prosthesis is required. The risk of reoperation is low

for repaired myxomatous mitral valves but somewhat higher for repaired rheumatic valves (Lawrie, 1998).

In a small percentage of patients who undergo mitral valvuloplasty with implantation of a prosthetic ring, *systolic anterior motion (SAM)* of the anterior leaflet of the mitral valve occurs, causing obstruction of the left ventricular outflow tract (Fig. 16-4). Most often, SAM does not produce symptoms but rather is detected by intraoperative or postoperative echocardiography and the presence of a systolic murmur. More severe cases are associated with significant dynamic left ventricular outflow tract obstruction, similar to that occurring in patients with hypertrophic cardiomyopathy. Treatment of the two conditions is similar and includes administration of beta-adrenergic blocking agents and increased preload to facilitate forward flow through the left ventricular outflow tract. Beta-adrenergic receptor agonists (epinephrine or dobutamine), vasodilatation, diuresis, and cardiac glycosides are contraindicated in patients with SAM (Grossi et al., 1992). SAM usually is a self-limiting syndrome. If associated with significant symptoms that do not resolve, reoperation with implantation of a mitral valve prosthesis is performed.

Valve Replacement

Despite advances in reparative techniques, *valve replacement* is necessary in most patients who require surgical therapy for VHD. The era of cardiac valve replacement began before cardiopulmonary bypass when, in the early 1950s, Hufnagel implanted a caged-ball prosthesis in the descending thoracic aorta to treat aortic regurgitation (Stephenson, 1997). After development of cardiopulmonary bypass, successful implantation of an aortic valve prosthesis in its native anatomic position and mitral valve replacement were accomplished in 1960 by

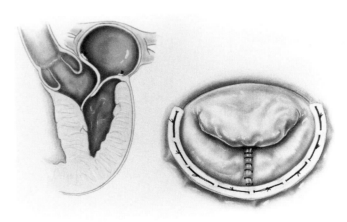

FIGURE 16-4. Diagrammatic representation of systolic anterior motion of the anterior mitral valve leaflet resulting in obstruction of the left ventricular outflow tract (*left*), after mitral valve repair with annuloplasty (*right*). (Alpert JS, Sabik J, Cosgrove DM, 1998: Mitral valve disease. In Topol EJ [ed]: Comprehensive Cardiovascular Medicine. p. 554. Philadelphia, Lippincott Williams & Wilkins)

Harken and Starr, respectively (Stephenson, 1997; Hildenberg & Austen, 1989). In the subsequent decades, thousands of valve replacement operations have been performed using a variety of mechanical and biologic tissue valves, as well as allografts.

Most valve replacement operations are performed through a median sternotomy incision, although minimally invasive approaches are possible in some patients and have gained in popularity. The aorta (aortic valve replacement), left atrium (mitral valve replacement), right atrium (tricuspid valve replacement or transeptal approach to the mitral valve), or pulmonary artery (pulmonic valve replacement) is opened and the native valve excised. An appropriately sized valvular prosthesis is selected by measuring the native annulus with a sizing instrument. A series of sutures is placed around the circumference of the native annulus and through the corresponding location on the sewing ring of the prosthesis. The valvular prosthesis is then positioned in the annulus and the sutures tied.

Mitral Valve Replacement

Mitral valve replacement usually is performed through a standard sternotomy incision or, less commonly, through a minimally invasive right parasternal or partial sternotomy incision. Cardiopulmonary bypass is achieved with cannulation of the ascending aorta for arterial return and bicaval (superior and inferior venae cavae) cannulation for venous drainage. In most cases, the operation is performed using hypothermia, aortic cross-clamping, and cardioplegic arrest of the heart. Either antegrade or a combination of antegrade and retrograde cardioplegia is used for myocardial protection.

Rarely, reoperative procedures on the mitral valve are performed through a right lateral thoracotomy incision to avoid potential injury during repeat sternotomy of cardiac structures adherent to the posterior table of the sternum. Direct access and cross-clamping of the ascending aorta is difficult when a lateral thoracotomy incision is used. Consequently, the procedure may be performed with hypothermic fibrillatory arrest (without aortic cross-clamping and cardioplegic arrest) or with cardioplegic arrest using an endovascular aortic occluding catheter inserted through the femoral artery in lieu of the external aortic cross-clamp (Alpert et al., 1998). When an endovascular aortic occluding catheter is used, a balloon on the end of the catheter is inflated to occlude the aortic lumen, and cardioplegic solution can be delivered through the catheter through a central port located beyond the inflated balloon, or using a retrograde technique through the coronary sinus.

Exposure of the mitral valve is achieved through an incision in the left atrium or, if a minimally invasive right parasternal or lateral thoracotomy incision has been used, through an incision in the right atrium and interatrial septum. The native, diseased mitral valve is débrided of calcium and any fibrous material to restore leaflet flexibility and allow insertion of an artificial valve while preserving the native leaflets and subvalvular attachments (Alpert et

al., 1998). Preservation of the subvalvular apparatus (chordae tendineae and papillary muscles) is advantageous, especially if left ventricular function is impaired. Mitral valve replacement for mitral regurgitation actually causes deterioration of left ventricular function in the early postoperative period because afterload is acutely increased when mitral valve competence is restored. Multiple studies suggest that sparing native chordal structures preserves ventricular function better than mitral valve replacement in which chordae are sacrificed (Chitwood, 1998). Preserving mitral valve chordae also decreases operative mortality rates and the incidence of left ventricular rupture, a complication described later (Alpert et al., 1998).

An appropriately sized valve is selected and implanted by placing sutures through the valve annulus and the sewing ring of the prosthesis. When preserving subvalvular structures, care must be taken in prosthesis selection and implantation technique to ensure that native leaflets or chordae tendineae do not impede proper prosthesis function. Accurate sizing of a mitral prosthesis also is imperative to achieve optimal hemodynamic performance. A prosthesis that is excessively large may compromise left ventricular contraction; one that is too small may produce an unacceptably large transvalvular gradient. When valve replacement is completed, the surgeon performs a defined series of steps and examines the heart with transesophageal echocardiography to ensure that all intracardiac air is evacuated before removing the aortic cross-clamp and allowing the heart to eject blood into the ascending aorta.

A rare but usually lethal complication of mitral valve replacement is left ventricular rupture secondary to disruption of the left atrioventricular groove. The injury is estimated to occur in approximately 1% of patients who undergo mitral valve replacement (Karlson et al., 1988). It is more likely in women and in patients with small left ventricles (Kirklin & Barratt-Boyes, 1993a). The defect typically becomes apparent within minutes after discontinuation of cardiopulmonary bypass or within hours of operation, when massive bleeding and hypotension develop in the patient. When left ventricular rupture becomes apparent, emergent surgical repair is attempted using cardiopulmonary bypass to arrest and decompress the heart and to maximize exposure. Occasionally, late ventricular rupture occurs, leading to the development of a left ventricular false aneurysm (Karlson et al., 1988).

Aortic Valve Replacement

Aortic valve replacement most often is performed through a median sternotomy incision. Because significant coronary artery disease is present in 25% to 30% of patients undergoing aortic valve replacement, especially in those with aortic stenosis, concomitant coronary artery bypass grafting often is necessary (Carabello et al., 1998). In young patients undergoing isolated aortic valve replacement, the procedure may be performed using a small right anterior thoracotomy in the second or third intercostal space; a vertical, parasternal incision over the third and fourth ribs; or a partial sternotomy incision.

Cardiopulmonary bypass is necessary and cannulation usually is achieved using the ascending aorta for arterial return and the right atrium for venous drainage. The conventional antegrade technique of administering cardioplegic solution into the aortic root for myocardial protection is not possible in the presence of significant aortic regurgitation. Instead, cardioplegic solution is delivered in a retrograde fashion using a catheter passed through the right atrium and into the coronary sinus. Although cardioplegic solution also can be delivered in antegrade fashion directly into each of the coronary artery ostia, this technique can cause coronary ostial stenosis and is avoided when possible (Carabello et al., 1998).

An incision is made in the aorta and the native valve is excised. An appropriately sized prosthesis is selected and sutured into place, and the aortotomy is closed (Fig. 16-5). Because of the small size of the aortic annular opening, it is important to select a prosthesis with the greatest effective orifice to sewing ring ratio. Special techniques may be necessary during aortic valve replacement if the aortic root is especially small or heavily calcified. In extreme cases, it may be necessary to perform an *aortoplasty*, or enlargement of the aortic root with a synthetic patch, in addition to aortic valve replacement. Annulus-enlarging procedures increase operative mortality risk, which must be weighed against the benefit of a larger valve size (Carabello et al., 1998).

Ensuring removal of all air from the aorta, left ventricle, and coronary arteries is extremely important after opening the aorta to replace the aortic valve. Air remaining in the systemic circulation can produce catastrophic embolization when cardiopulmonary bypass is discontinued and the heart is allowed to eject. Other potential problems that can complicate aortic valve replacement include (1) inadequate débridement of annular calcium resulting in perivalvular leaks, (2) vigorous débridement resulting in aortic or left ventricular perfo-

ration or interruption of conduction pathways, (3) detachment of the mitral valve anterior leaflet during aortic valve excision, (4) heart block from sutures placed in or around the bundle of His, (5) occlusion of the coronary artery ostia by the prosthesis sewing ring, and (6) lodging of detached calcium in the coronary arteries or left ventricle with subsequent embolization (Hammond & Letsou, 1996). Aortic valve replacement in combination with replacement of the ascending aorta is discussed in Chapter 17, Surgery on the Thoracic Aorta.

The Ross Procedure

The *Ross procedure* is a technique of aortic valve replacement using the patient's own pulmonic valve to replace the diseased aortic valve with implantation of an allograft (homograft) in the pulmonary position. It is an alternative surgical option for the treatment of isolated aortic valve disease in patients with a life expectancy greater than 20 years (Elkins, 1998). Because the pulmonary autograft (ie, patient's native pulmonary artery root) is anatomically identical to the aortic valve and, being autogenous, is viable, it offers the potential of superior hemodynamic performance compared with any other valve substitute (Doty, 1996). Another major advantage of the Ross procedure is that chronic anticoagulation with warfarin sodium is not required. The procedure also is well suited to patients with infective endocarditis. The pulmonary autograft is thought to provide intrinsic resistance to infection and also offers the surgeon more versatility in suturing techniques in an aortic root destroyed by infection (Jaggers et al., 1998). A disadvantage associated with the Ross procedure is that it is a more complex operation, necessitating a longer operative time and period of aortic cross-clamping than simple replacement of the aortic valve.

The Ross procedure is performed using a midline sternotomy incision and cardiopulmonary bypass with hypothermia and cardioplegic myocardial protection.

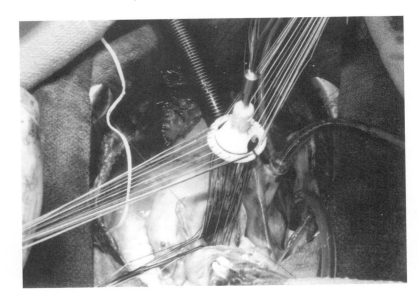

FIGURE 16-5. Implantation of a St. Jude aortic valve prosthesis. Photograph is taken from above the patient's head, looking downward into the aortic root. The native valve has been excised, and sutures have been placed around the circumference of the aortic valve annulus and the sewing ring of the prosthesis.

The patient's pulmonary artery is divided just proximal to its bifurcation and the pulmonic valve is inspected. The main pulmonary artery and pulmonic valve are then removed as a unit from the right ventricular outflow tract. Through an aortotomy incision, the aortic valve leaflets are resected and the aortic annulus is débrided of calcium. The pulmonary autograft (ie, graft that is harvested from the recipient) is sewn in place in the aortic root and the patient's coronary arteries are reimplanted into the sides of the autograft. An appropriately sized pulmonary allograft then is used to replace the pulmonic valve and proximal pulmonary artery.

In centers with surgeons experienced in performing the Ross procedure, the operative mortality rate is similar to that for mechanical aortic valve replacement (Elkins, 1998; Jaggers et al., 1998). The procedure occasionally is complicated by aortic regurgitation necessitating reoperation and aortic valve replacement. Furthermore, the procedure substitutes two valves with an unknown risk of future valve dysfunction for one abnormal valve (Carabello et al., 1998). The presence of intrinsic aortic disease (eg, Marfan's syndrome) is a contraindication to the Ross procedure because the connective tissue abnormality present in the aorta also exists in the pulmonary artery (Yun & Miller, 1997).

Multiple Valve Replacement

Multiple valve replacement is sometimes necessary. Rheumatic and, rarely, endocarditic damage of multiple valves can occur. In addition, mitral or tricuspid regurgitation due to annular dilatation may develop secondary to chronic ventricular enlargement caused by the dysfunction of another valve. When multiple prostheses are necessary, selection of the type of prostheses to be used is based partially on technical considerations of implantation. Mechanical valves are more likely to be selected because of their durability to avoid the significant risk of reoperation in these patients. Multiple valve replacement procedures require a longer duration of cardiopulmonary bypass and more dissection in the area of the conduction system. In addition, patients who require multiple valve replacement usually have more underlying ventricular dysfunction. Accordingly, double or triple valve replacement is associated with a higher operative mortality rate and a greater risk of postoperative heart block, bleeding, and low cardiac output.

Valve Replacement for Infective Endocarditis

Valve replacement for infective endocarditis includes débridement of all infected tissue and drainage of any associated abscess cavity. Usually, the surgeon bathes the endocardial surfaces with antibiotic solution before implanting the valvular prosthesis. If the prosthetic material becomes infected, it is almost impossible to sterilize and death due to intramyocardial infection follows. There is some controversy regarding the best type of valvular prosthesis to implant in patients with active endocarditis. Data suggest that allograft valves are more resistant to recurrent infection when used for aortic valve replacement in patients with active infective endocarditis (Haydock et al., 1992). Heart block is common after aortic valve replacement for infective endocarditis, especially in patients with associated abscesses in the aortic root (Carabello et al., 1998).

Valvulectomy (ie, removal of a valve without implantation of a prosthesis) is occasionally performed for infective endocarditis of the tricuspid valve (Arbulu et al., 1991). Most tricuspid endocarditis occurs in young adult drug abusers who have no underlying heart disease. Such patients usually tolerate tricuspid regurgitation that is produced by absence of the tricuspid valve. Valvulectomy avoids the necessity of placing prosthetic material in a patient in whom there is significant risk of infecting the new prosthesis. Some patients who undergo tricuspid valvulectomy experience postoperative symptoms of right-sided heart failure and eventually require implantation of a tricuspid prosthesis. However, if a new prosthesis is implanted electively after the infection has been cured, the risk of prosthetic valve endocarditis is substantially reduced. Alternatively, if the tricuspid valvular abnormality is limited to the presence of a vegetation, it may be possible to resect the vegetation from the valve leaflet and perform a reconstructive procedure, leaving a competent, native valve.

▶ Valvular Prostheses

A variety of prostheses are available for replacement of native valves (Table 16-2). Some prostheses, such as the St. Jude Medical, the CarboMedics, and the Medtronic-Hall, are mechanical, constructed of synthetic materials. Others, such as the Carpentier-Edwards or Hancock porcine, Edwards bovine pericardial, and human cadaver allograft valves, are made of biologic animal or human tissue and are called *bioprostheses*. The term *heterograft bioprosthesis* more narrowly denotes a bioprosthesis harvested from another species, whereas an *allograft bioprosthesis* is one harvested from a human cadaver.

Although the terms *allograft* and *homograft* often are used synonymously, allograft describes a human cadaver

TABLE 16-2

Selected Cardiac Valvular Prostheses

MECHANICAL
St. Jude Medical
Medtronic-Hall
CarboMedics

TISSUE
Carpentier-Edwards (porcine)
Hancock (porcine)
Allograft (human cadaver)
Carpentier-Edwards (bovine pericardial)

graft more precisely than homograft (also a graft from a donor of the same species) in that it recognizes that the graft donor and recipient are not genetically identical (O'Brien, 1996). In the Ross procedure, described earlier, two homografts are used: the patient's own pulmonary root is used as an autograft (tissue transplanted from one part of the body to another) to replace the aortic root, and a pulmonary allograft is used to replace the patient's native pulmonary root. Because allografts and autografts have functional characteristics that are different from those of either mechanical valves or animal tissue bioprostheses, they are discussed separately.

The most important characteristics of any of the valvular prostheses are (1) minimal impedance to forward flow when open and no regurgitation when closed, (2) nonthrombogenicity, and (3) durability. No available prosthesis achieves all of these objectives. Each has features that make it more or less suited for a given clinical situation. Therefore, the decision about the specific prosthesis to implant in an individual patient is based on a number of factors, including patient age, associated medical problems, underlying cardiac disease, lifestyle, and aptitude for compliance with an anticoagulant regimen.

Mechanical Prostheses

Mechanical valves account for approximately 60% of prostheses implanted in patients in the United States and worldwide (Akins, 1991). Mechanical prostheses have one of three basic design types: (1) bileaflet, (2) monoleaflet (tilting disc), or (3) caged ball. Commonly implanted mechanical prostheses include the St. Jude Medical, the CarboMedics, and the Medtronic-Hall prostheses. All of these valves have either a bileaflet or monoleaflet design with Pyrolite™ carbon leaflets and titanium or Pyrolite carbon housings (Jamieson, 1997). They all are readily available in all sizes; usually yield excellent hemodynamic function, even in smaller sizes; and are easily implanted in most situations (Carabello et al., 1998). All mechanical prostheses have a certain amount of intravalvular regurgitation, generated by closure flow backwash and by mechanisms designed to prevent deposition of thrombogenic material (Garcia, 1998). Mechanical valves also all cause some degree of subclinical hemolysis as a result of flow abnormalities particular to each valve design (Cohn & Lipson, 1996).

The St. Jude Medical valve is the most commonly implanted valvular prosthesis. More than 625,000 St. Jude valves have been implanted worldwide (Emery et al., 1996). Available since 1977, the St. Jude valve has a bileaflet design (Fig. 16-6). Bileaflet valves have a wide opening angle, thin leaflets, and a large cross-section that causes minimal disturbance to flow when the valve is open; however, they also have a larger regurgitation fraction (Cohn & Lipson, 1996). The CarboMedics valve, introduced in 1986, is a second-generation bileaflet mechanical valve. Early and midterm follow-up data suggest valve performance comparable with that of the St. Jude

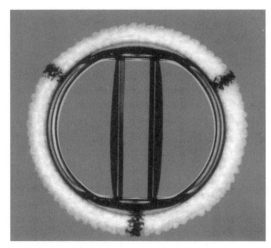

FIGURE 16-6. St. Jude® Master Series aortic valve prosthesis. (Used with permission of St. Jude Medical, Inc, St. Paul, MN)

prosthesis (Copeland, 1996). The Medtronic-Hall valve is a tilting disc prosthesis that also has excellent durability and hemodynamic performance (Akins, 1996).

The Starr-Edwards valve is a mechanical prosthesis with a caged-ball design (ie, a cage attached to the sewing ring that houses a Silastic ball). The ball moves from a closed position, occluding the ring, to an open position in the outer end of the cage (Garcia, 1998). Various models have been in use since 1961 and have displayed excellent durability. Caged-ball valves are implanted less commonly than bileaflet and tilting disc prostheses. They produce more turbulent flow because of central obstruction by the ball itself and, when used in the mitral position, the valve may partially obstruct the ventricular outflow tract because of its high profile (Cohn & Lipson, 1996).

In general, mechanical valves are associated with better hemodynamic function than porcine bioprostheses and similar function to pericardial prostheses (Carabello et al., 1998). The predominant concern with any of the mechanical prostheses is thromboembolism. Thrombogenicity remains the most serious complication of mechanical valves despite three decades of improvements in materials, design, and manufacture (Jamieson, 1997). Two factors predispose to thrombosis when a large foreign surface is in contact with the bloodstream: (1) turbulence, shearing forces, stagnation, and eddy currents trigger the release of biochemical factors that evoke clotting; and (2) valve materials themselves may precipitate thrombosis (Hildenberg & Austen, 1989).

Because of the potential for thromboembolism, long-term anticoagulation with warfarin sodium is recommended in patients with any of the available mechanical prostheses. Anticoagulation with intravenous heparin is necessary if oral anticoagulation must be withheld, such as before a planned operation or if the patient is unable to take oral medications. If gastrointestinal bleeding or another contraindication to chronic anticoagulation develops in a patient with a mechanical prosthesis, elective replacement of the prosthesis may become necessary.

Bioprostheses

Bioprosthetic heart valves are made from animal or human tissue that has been processed to make it biologically inert. Most common are glutaraldehyde-preserved heterograft bioprostheses, including porcine valves, constructed from aortic valves of pigs, and bovine pericardial valves, from the pericardial tissue of cows. Less commonly used are cryopreserved homografts from human cadavers. Biologic tissue valves are attractive because of their lower propensity for thromboembolic complications compared with mechanical prostheses, obviating the need for anticoagulation in most cases.

Heterograft Bioprostheses

Porcine valves have been used extensively since the early 1970s. The two most widely implanted porcine valves are the Hancock and the Carpentier-Edwards bioprostheses; clinical investigations directly comparing the two bioprostheses have shown no significant differences in long-term performance (Fann & Miller, 1996). Porcine bioprostheses are available in all sizes and are easily implanted. They have hemodynamic characteristics comparable with those of mechanical prostheses except in small sizes; in the smallest sizes, porcine valves may provide significant obstruction to forward flow because of the large sewing ring.

Porcine valves often are implanted in patients in whom it is desirable to avoid chronic anticoagulation (eg, elderly people in sinus rhythm and those with a medical contraindication to anticoagulation). The low rate of serious thromboembolism and virtual lack of valve thrombosis eliminate the necessity of long-term anticoagulation with its associated risk of related hemorrhagic complications (Jamieson et al., 1990). Thromboembolism can occur with bioprostheses, however, particularly in patients with mitral prostheses, atrial fibrillation, and low cardiac output (Cohn & Lipson, 1996). Anticoagulation is recommended in these patients.

The major drawback to porcine valves is the well-documented incidence of valve failure secondary to structural degeneration. Primary valve degeneration necessitating reoperation can be expected at 10 years in 20% to 40% of patients with mitral bioprostheses, although it occurs rarely in porcine valves implanted in patients older than 70 years of age (Alpert et al., 1998). The more rapid deterioration of mitral bioprostheses may be due to higher ventricular systolic pressures against the closed mitral bioprosthesis cusps compared with the lower diastolic pressures resisted by the closed aortic bioprosthesis leaflets (Cohn & Reul, 1997). Structural valve deterioration of mitral bioprostheses also appears to be accelerated in women, although the responsible mechanism has not been identified (Burdon et al., 1992). Patients who require dialysis experience accelerated structural valve deterioration as well. Hemodynamically significant structural tissue valve deterioration occurs at 10 years in 15% to 20% of porcine bioprostheses implanted in the aortic position (Carabello et al., 1998). Aside from the durability prob-

lem, porcine valves are rarely a cause of mortality, thromboembolism, or permanent morbidity.

Bovine pericardial bioprostheses are being used increasingly as an alternative to porcine valves (Fig. 16-7). Tissue valves manufactured from glutaraldehyde-preserved bovine pericardium are available in all sizes, are easily implanted, and have lesser gradients and better hemodynamic function than porcine valves in small sizes (Carabello et al., 1998). Like porcine bioprostheses, the risk of thromboembolism is low and chronic anticoagulation is unnecessary. Pericardial tissue valves appear to be more durable than porcine bioprostheses. Although they also are subject to eventual degeneration, pericardial valves implanted in the aortic position are associated with only a 4% to 9% incidence of structural valve deterioration at 10 years (Carabello et al., 1998). Advances in tissue–valve preservation are expected to increase the durability of bioprostheses further (Garcia, 1998).

More recently, stentless porcine and pericardial valves have been introduced. Because these bioprostheses have no sewing ring or stent, they provide less obstruction and thus better hemodynamic performance than standard bioprostheses. It also is hoped that the design of stentless valves will lessen tissue wear, thus improving durability (Middlemost et al., 1999). Long-term data are not yet available for stentless porcine and pericardial valves.

Allograft Bioprostheses

Aortic and pulmonary allografts are obtained from organ donors in whom the heart is unsuitable for transplantation but the cardiac valves are satisfactory. The aortic or pulmonic valve is harvested with a portion of the surrounding aorta or pulmonary artery, respectively, and cryopreserved (ie, ultrafrozen using liquid nitrogen) for long-term storage (Fig. 16-8). In some centers, in particular in the United Kingdom, allografts also are harvested from transplant recipient hearts at the time of transplantation (Lund et al., 1999). When the time from

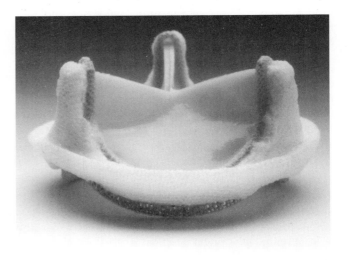

FIGURE 16-7. Baxter bovine pericardial bioprosthesis. (Courtesy of Baxter Healthcare Corporation, Cardiovascular Group, Irvine, CA)

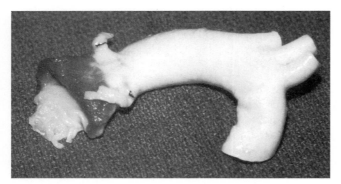

FIGURE 16-8. An aortic allograft before implantation. Most aortic allografts are implanted with only a few centimeters of the ascending aorta, excluding the great vessels. In this photograph, the great vessels are still attached. (Carabello BA, Stewart WJ, Crawford FA, 1998: Aortic valve disease. In Topol EJ [ed]: Comprehensive Cardiovascular Medicine, p. 571. Philadelphia, Lippincott Williams & Wilkins)

donor death to implantation is short, allografts harvested from transplant recipient hearts or brain-dead organ donors sometimes are implanted without cryopreservation and are termed *viable* allografts. The donor allograft is matched to a recipient by size. Although early allograft aortic valves were sewn in place using a free-hand technique, nearly all are now inserted along with the proximal aortic root from the donor, and the patient's coronary arteries are reimplanted into the wall of the allograft (Carabello et al., 1998).

Allograft aortic valves most commonly are used for valve replacement in children but also are considered the prosthesis of choice for aortic valve replacement in adults in some centers (Kirklin & Barratt-Boyes, 1993c). Aortic valve replacement using an allograft is more complex because the tissue is entirely biologic without a stiff stent or sewing ring and because precise sizing is limited by the frequent lack of availability of all sizes (Carabello et al., 1998). Pulmonary allografts are used for replacement of the pulmonic valve and pulmonary root in patients who undergo Ross procedures, as described earlier.

Allografts, like other bioprostheses, have a low incidence of thromboembolism, negating the need for chronic anticoagulant therapy. Aortic allografts and pulmonary autografts are the only tissue valves with hemodynamic performance comparable with that of native valves (Garcia, 1998). They also are associated with a very low incidence of infective endocarditis. Although allografts are more durable than other biologic valvular prostheses, they have limited durability compared with mechanical prostheses. Limited long-term data are available and there is considerable variation in the reported incidence of structural deterioration, but progressive degeneration of allograft tissue does occur and is accentuated in younger people (Carabello et al., 1998). Freedom from primary tissue failure is 62% and 18% at 10 and 20 years, respectively; long-term results are improved by avoiding older donors (Lund et al., 1999).

Prosthesis Selection

The most important determination in valve selection is whether to implant a mechanical valve, a bioprosthetic valve, or an allograft (Table 16-3). Mechanical valves are more durable and often provide better hemodynamic performance, but are more thrombogenic and necessitate chronic anticoagulation. Porcine and pericardial bioprostheses do not necessitate chronic anticoagulant therapy and are easily implanted, but are likely to degenerate, necessitating subsequent reoperation. Allografts are nonthrombogenic and, like mechanical valves, offer hemodynamic performance that is superior to that of other bioprostheses. Like porcine and pericardial bioprostheses, they are less durable than mechanical valves.

Comparison of mechanical and bioprosthetic valves at 10 years reveals that in the long term, the risk of primary valve failure in bioprostheses is counterbalanced by the risk of anticoagulant-related hemorrhage and perivalvular regurgitation in mechanical valves; survival and overall freedom from valve-related complications at 10 years are similar whether a bioprosthetic or mechanical valve is implanted (Wernly & Crawford, 1998; Hammermeister et al., 1991a, 1991b).

Older patients (>65 years) have a greater risk of valve-related complications with mechanical prostheses, whereas younger patients (<40 years) are at greater risk with bioprostheses (Jamieson, 1993). Consequently, mechanical valves usually are selected for patients younger than 70 years of age who have no contraindication to anticoagulation or who are already receiving anticoagulation therapy for another reason, such as atrial fibrillation (Alpert et al., 1998). Bioprostheses are best suited for use in the aortic position in elderly patients because chronic anticoagulation is not necessary and the prosthesis is

TABLE 16-3

Rationale for Prosthesis Selection

PATIENTS LIKELY TO RECEIVE MECHANICAL PROSTHESES
Children
Young adults (except child-bearing women)
Patients with renal failure
Patients with high reoperative risk
Patients with another indication for anticoagulation (eg, atrial fibrillation)
Patients requiring aortic root replacement

PATIENTS LIKELY TO RECEIVE TISSUE PROSTHESES
Elderly patients in whom long-term durability is less important
Persons in whom chronic anticoagulation is ill advised:
  History of major bleeding episode
  Demonstrated noncompliance with medical therapy (eg, drug or alcohol abuse)
  Lifestyle with high risk for trauma
  Advanced age (potential for dosage error or fall)
Patients at increased risk for thromboembolism

likely to remain durable for the remainder of the patient's natural life span. They seldom are implanted in patients younger than 60 years of age, in those who have experienced degeneration of a previous bioprosthesis, or in those who require anticoagulation for another reason. Allografts are most likely to be used for aortic valve replacement in young patients with an active lifestyle who wish to avoid chronic anticoagulation.

In young women in whom future pregnancy might occur, valve selection is especially complex. During pregnancy, maternal complications occur more frequently with bioprostheses, but the complications that occur with mechanical prostheses tend to be more severe; perinatal outcome does not appear to differ between mothers with bioprostheses and mechanical prostheses (Suri et al., 1999). Mechanical valves necessitate anticoagulation therapy during pregnancy, which can be hazardous. Warfarin crosses the placental barrier and may cause fetal bleeding, fetal wastage, or embryopathy; heparin does not cross the placental barrier, but may be less effective in preventing thromboembolic events and can be associated with osteoporosis or heparin-induced thrombocytopenia in the mother (Ginsberg & Hirsh, 1998; Badduke et al., 1991).

Bioprosthetic valves appear to be associated with accelerated valvular deterioration during pregnancy, presumably due to changes in calcium metabolism that occur in pregnant women (Laks et al., 1997). On the other hand, thromboembolic complications, often with long-term sequelae, are much more likely within 5 years in young women with mechanical compared with bioprosthetic valves (North et al., 1999).

▶ Postoperative Considerations

Anticoagulant Therapy

All available mechanical prostheses necessitate rigorous, lifelong anticoagulation. Anticoagulant therapy also may be recommended for the first 3 months after implantation of bioprosthetic valves in the mitral position (Stein et al., 1998). Because of the lack of standardization of tissue thromboplastin used as the reagent in prothrombin time assays and the resultant variability between laboratories in prothrombin time results, the international normalized ratio (INR) has become the standard method for reporting results of prothrombin time testing. It is a value calculated from the prothrombin time assay result, taking into account the sensitivity of the reagent used to perform the prothrombin time assay (Vanscoy & Krause, 1991).

Recommended INR values vary according to the type of prosthesis, valve position, and clinical factors. The INR must be maintained at a level sufficient to prevent thromboembolism while minimizing the risk of anticoagulant-related hemorrhage. Recommended anticoagulation levels for common types of prostheses are displayed in Table 16-4. In patients with mechanical prostheses, low doses of aspirin may be prescribed in combination with warfarin.

TABLE 16-4

Recommended Anticoagulation Levels

Prosthesis Type	Position	Recommended INR
Bileaflet mechanical	Aortic	2.0–3.0 (sinus rhythm)
		2.5–3.2 (atrial fibrillation)
Bileaflet mechanical	Mitral	2.5–3.5
Tilting disc mechanical	Mitral or aortic	2.5–3.5
Bioprostheses	Mitral	2.0–2.3 (first 3 months only)

Adapted from Stein PD, Alpert JS, Dalen JE, et al., 1998: Antithrombotic therapy in patients with mechanical and bioprosthetic heart valves. Chest 114(5 Suppl): 602S.

A low rate of both thromboembolic and bleeding complications has been demonstrated with the use of 100 mg aspirin per day in combination with anticoagulation that prolongs the INR to a range of 2.0 to 3.5 in patients with mechanical valves (Stein et al., 1998).

Administration of warfarin sodium usually is begun on the second postoperative day. Anticoagulation is not needed earlier because the use of cardiopulmonary bypass impairs coagulation during the early postoperative period. Serial prothrombin time measurements are performed and used to adjust the dosage of warfarin. It usually takes several days to establish the dose of warfarin necessary to achieve and maintain therapeutic anticoagulation in a particular patient. Warfarin is a very potent and potentially dangerous medication. Anticoagulant-related hemorrhage is a potential risk, particularly in patients who are elderly, are malnourished, or have chronic liver dysfunction secondary to VHD. The most serious form of anticoagulant-related bleeding is intracerebral hemorrhage, although gastrointestinal bleeding or profuse bleeding with trauma also can occur. Patient education is of great importance. Both the patient and family are instructed about implications of anticoagulant therapy. A plan for serial prothrombin time testing and for physician monitoring of results is essential. Conditions such as pregnancy, required surgical procedures, trauma, or development of gastric ulcers may occur subsequent to valve implantation and may greatly complicate anticoagulant therapy.

Results of Valve Replacement

Operative mortality rates with valve replacement range from 5% to 10% in most centers. However, the risk to an individual patient is quite variable depending on the specific type of operation, etiology of valvular disease, status of ventricular function, and need for concomitant procedures. Risk of operative death may be as low as 3% for a patient who undergoes elective aortic valve replacement for aortic stenosis or as high as 50% for a patient requiring emergent mitral valve replacement for acute, ischemic mitral regurgitation. Many patients who require mitral valve repair or replacement have associated coronary artery disease and significantly impaired left ventricular function. Mortality in this patient group is significant and successful results depend strongly on appropriate patient selection and the surgeon's intraoperative judgment about whether to repair or replace the diseased mitral valve. Operative mortality does not appear to be influenced by the type of prosthesis implanted.

Unless irreversible ventricular dysfunction or pulmonary hypertension has developed before surgical intervention, most patients who undergo valve replacement can expect a significant improvement in functional capacity. Dyspnea caused by a dysfunctional valve often is diminished significantly, even during the first postoperative week. However, underlying ventricular dysfunction usually is present and postoperative recovery is slower than that seen in cardiac surgical patients with normal ventricular function. Typically, it takes months or even as much as a year to achieve full improvement from valve replacement. The 5-year survival rate both for patients undergoing mitral valve replacement and for those undergoing aortic valve replacement ranges from 80% to 85% (Alpert et al., 1998; Carabello et al., 1998).

Valve-Related Morbidity

The potential for morbidity or mortality from a valvular prosthesis remains as long as the valve is in place. The major types of morbidity associated with the presence of a prosthetic cardiac valve are valve failure, thromboembolism, anticoagulant-related hemorrhage, and endocarditis. Valve failure is suggested by auscultation of a change in heart sounds and is documented by transthoracic or transesophageal echocardiography. It may be caused by (1) periprosthetic leak, (2) mechanical dysfunction (mechanical prosthesis), or (3) leaflet degeneration or calcification (bioprosthesis).

A periprosthetic leak is regurgitation of blood around the valve due to an inadequate seal between the sewing ring and the host tissue (Cohn & Lipson, 1996). It occurs unusually, most often in patients with mechanical as opposed to bioprosthetic valves. A periprosthetic leak in the early postoperative period almost always is due to suture disruption or a technical problem with placement of the prosthesis. It is most likely in those patients in whom annular tissue is friable secondary to endocarditis or myocardial infarction.

Primary valve failure is defined as dysfunction of the prosthesis itself. Primary failure of a mechanical valve can occur due to improper or failed motion of one of the valve components. Although mechanical valve failure is rare, it usually produces acute hemodynamic instability. An occasional cause of mechanical valve failure is pannus or thrombus formation on the valve. Pannus is a fibrinous coating that occasionally develops on the surfaces of a mechanical or bioprosthetic valve (Fig. 16-9). Valve thrombosis is more likely if anticoagulation is discontinued or inadequate, but occurs rarely even with therapeutic anticoagulation (Fig. 16-10). Thrombus formation or pannus ingrowth may cause acute heart failure or may occur as a slowly progressive

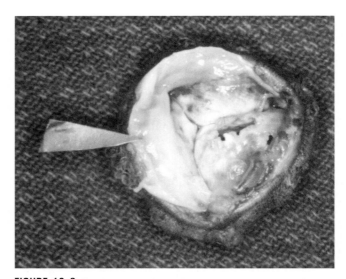

FIGURE 16-9. Porcine aortic bioprosthesis explanted 13 years after implantation; marker illustrates extensive pannus formation along valve sewing ring. (Courtesy of David J. Mehlman, MD)

disorder with protean (ie, diverse) symptomatology (Ambrose & Greenberg, 1997). Valve thrombosis has been treated successfully with thrombolytic therapy, although there is a significant associated incidence of thromboembolism, bleeding, and stroke with this form of therapy (Carabello et al., 1998). Depending on the amount and type of thrombus or fibrinous material on the valve, it may be necessary to débride the prosthesis surgically or explant the prosthesis and implant a new one.

In bioprosthetic valves, primary valve failure consists of leaflet degeneration or calcification (Fig. 16-11). In most cases, valve degeneration occurs gradually, owing

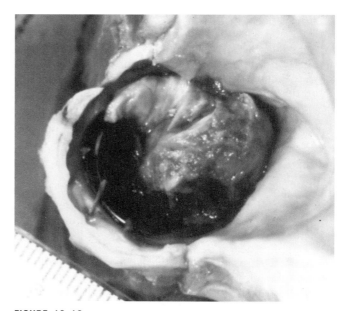

FIGURE 16-10. Autopsy specimen reveals massive thrombus covering aortic surface of mechanical aortic valve prosthesis in patient with inadequate anticoagulation. (Courtesy of David J. Mehlman, MD)

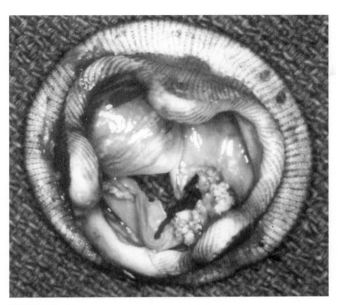

FIGURE 16-11. Explanted mitral valve bioprosthesis demonstrates leaflet degeneration and calcification. (Courtesy of David J. Mehlman, MD)

to leaflet calcification and fibrosis. Occasionally, acute leaflet rupture causes precipitous valve failure. Primary valve failure of both porcine and pericardial tissue valves occurs more rapidly in children and young adults and in patients with renal failure. Structural deterioration also occurs more frequently in mitral than in aortic bioprostheses (Jamieson et al., 1990). In patients who have undergone Ross procedures, pulmonary autograft insufficiency sometimes develops, requiring reoperation (Elkins, 1998).

Thromboembolism is another potential complication of valve replacement. No synthetic or modified biologic surface is as thromboresistant as the normal, unperturbed endothelium (Schoen, 1997). The incidence of thromboembolism has decreased because of improvements in anticoagulant therapy and because available mechanical prostheses are less thrombogenic than earlier models (Altman et al., 1991). Nevertheless, thromboembolism remains a major complication of prosthetic cardiac valves. Thromboembolic events can occur with any type of prosthesis but are more often associated with mechanical valves. The risk of thromboembolism in patients with porcine and pericardial valves is low, even without chronic anticoagulation; aortic allografts and pulmonary autografts have a negligible incidence of thromboembolism and no valve thrombosis, making anticoagulation unnecessary (Carabello et al., 1998).

Even with systemic anticoagulation, thromboembolic events occur in patients with mechanical prostheses at rates ranging between 1% and 4% per year (Alpert et al., 1998; Carabello et al., 1998). Rates of thromboembolic complications vary among the various mechanical valves, and regimens for anticoagulation are based on the thrombogenicity of the specific prosthesis. Risk of thromboembolism is lower after aortic valve replacement and great-

est after multiple valve replacement. Embolization most often occurs to the cerebral circulation, resulting in a cerebral vascular accident or transient ischemic attack, but also can occur to the peripheral circulation, resulting in ischemia or infarction of tissue distal to the embolus.

Implantation of a valvular prosthesis also imposes a higher risk of infective endocarditis. Lifelong prophylaxis against prosthetic valve endocarditis is extremely important. The American Heart Association has well-established guidelines for antibiotic prophylaxis before certain surgical procedures or instrumentation, particularly dental work (Dajani et al., 1997). The frequency of bacteremia is highest with dental and oral procedures, intermediate with procedures involving the genitourinary tract, and lowest with gastrointestinal diagnostic procedures (Bonow et al., 1998). In the early postoperative period after valve replacement, antibiotic prophylaxis is especially important before procedures such as reinsertion of a urinary catheter.

Prosthetic valve endocarditis develops in 1% to 4% of valve recipients during the first postoperative year and in approximately 1% of recipients annually thereafter (Sexton & Bashore, 1998). In industrialized countries, prosthetic endocarditis accounts for approximately 15% of the cases of infective endocarditis (Garcia, 1998). The complication occurs when transient bacteremia leads to seeding of the prosthetic material with pathogenic organisms. Infections occurring within 1 to 2 months after valve implantation most likely result from intraoperative contamination or early wound infection, whereas late infections usually occur by a hematogenous route initiated by bacteremia (Schoen, 1997). Staphylococcal infections predominate in early prosthetic endocarditis, whereas there are equal percentages of streptococcal and staphylococcal infections in late-occurring prosthetic endocarditis (Ambrose & Greenberg, 1997). With mechanical and bioprosthetic valves, prosthetic endocarditis is most common in the first 6 weeks after operation (Haydock et al., 1992). Comparison between mechanical and bioprosthetic valves at 10 years reveals no difference in the incidence of endocarditis (Hammermeister et al., 1991a). Infection is unusual in allografts and pulmonary autografts.

Prosthetic endocarditis is a potentially life-threatening complication, particularly if it occurs during the early postoperative months. At best, it necessitates prolonged hospitalization and treatment with organism-specific intravenous antibiotics for at least 6 weeks. It also may lead to urgent reoperation for removal of the infected prosthesis and reimplantation of another. The severity of the infection and type of therapy differ depending on the specific pathogenic organism. Streptococcal infections are less virulent than those due to staphylococci. Fungal infections are extremely difficult to eradicate with antimicrobial therapy and often require emergent valve replacement. Treatment of prosthetic endocarditis is complicated by the presence of artificial material, which is difficult to sterilize. Septic embolization and intramyocardial abscesses are common sequelae of prosthetic endocarditis that is not checked by antibiotic therapy or removal of the infected prosthesis (Fig. 16-12). Prosthetic

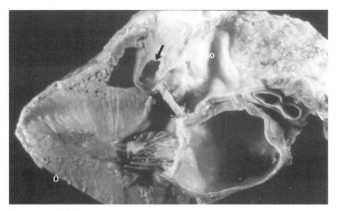

FIGURE 16-12. Autopsy specimen from patient who died of prosthetic valve endocarditis reveals intramyocardial abscess in perivalvular tissue adjacent to prosthetic aortic valve (*arrow*). (Courtesy of David J. Mehlman, MD)

valve endocarditis has an associated mortality rate of up to 65% (Haydock et al., 1992).

In patients who require valve replacement for endocarditis related to drug abuse, drug addiction is the primary disease and should be addressed while the patient is hospitalized in a controlled environment (Finkelmeier et al., 1989). As many as 49% of patients with endocarditis due to drug addiction may return to use of drugs after being cured of endocarditis (Arbulu et al., 1991). Aggressive efforts are made to enroll the patient in a drug rehabilitation program directly from the acute hospital setting. If a valvular prosthesis becomes infected through continued intravenous drug use, the prognosis for survival is dismal (Fig. 16-13).

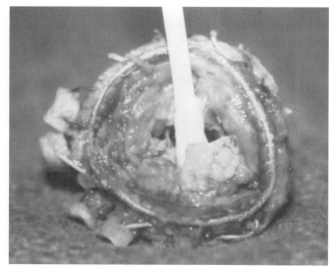

FIGURE 16-13. Porcine aortic bioprosthesis explanted at autopsy from patient who continued intravenous drug abuse after valve replacement for infective endocarditis. Note presence of extensive vegetations covering valve leaflets. (Courtesy of David J. Mehlman, MD)

REFERENCES

Akins CW, 1991: Mechanical cardiac valvular prostheses. Ann Thorac Surg 52:161

Akins CW, 1996: Medtronic-Hall prosthetic aortic valve. Semin Thorac Cardiovasc Surg 8:242

Aklog L, Adams DH, Couper GS, et al., 1998: Techniques and results of direct-access minimally invasive mitral valve surgery: A paradigm for the future. J Thorac Cardiovasc Surg 116:705

Alpert JS, Sabik J, Cosgrove DM, 1998: Mitral valve disease. In Topol EJ (ed): Comprehensive Cardiovascular Medicine. Philadelphia, Lippincott Williams & Wilkins

Altman R, Rouvier J, Gurfinkel E, et al., 1991: Comparison of two levels of anticoagulant therapy in patients with substitute heart valves. J Thorac Cardiovasc Surg 101:427

American Heart Association, 1998: 1999 Heart and Stroke Facts. Dallas, American Heart Association

Ambrose J, Greenberg BH, 1997: Acute presentations of valvular heart disease. In Brown DC (ed): Cardiac Intensive Care. Philadelphia, WB Saunders

Arbulu A, Holmes RJ, Asfaw I, 1991: Tricuspid valvulectomy without replacement. J Thorac Cardiovasc Surg 102:917

Badduke BR, Jamieson WR, Miyagishima RT, et al., 1991: Pregnancy and childbearing in a population with biologic valvular prostheses. J Thorac Cardiac Surg 102:179

Bonow RO, 1998: Chronic aortic regurgitation: Role of medical therapy and optimal timing for surgery. Cardiol Clin 16:449

Bonow RO, Carabello B, de Leon AC, et al., 1998: American College of Cardiology/American Heart Association guidelines for the management of patients with valvular heart disease. J Am Coll Cardiol 32:1486

Bruce CJ, Nishimura RA, 1998: Clinical assessment and management of mitral stenosis. Cardiol Clin 16:375

Burdon TA, Miller DC, Oyer PE, et al., 1992: Durability of porcine valves at fifteen years in a representative North American patient population. J Thorac Cardiovasc Surg 103:238

Carabello BA, Stewart WJ, Crawford FA, 1998: Aortic valve disease. In Topol EJ (ed): Comprehensive Cardiovascular Medicine. Philadelphia, Lippincott Williams & Wilkins

Chitwood WR Jr, 1998: Mitral valve repair: Ischemic. In Kaiser LR, Kron IL, Spray TL (eds): Mastery of Cardiothoracic Surgery. Philadelphia, Lippincott Williams & Wilkins

Cohn LH, Lipson W, 1996: Selection and complications of cardiac valvular prostheses. In Baue AE, Geha AS, Hammond GL, et al. (eds): Glenn's Thoracic and Cardiovascular Surgery, ed. 6. Stamford, CT, Appleton & Lange

Cohn LH, Reul RM, 1997: Mechanical and bioprosthetic mitral valve replacement. In Edmunds LH Jr (ed): Cardiac Surgery in the Adult. New York, McGraw-Hill

Copeland JG, 1996: The CarboMedics prosthetic heart valve: A second generation bileaflet prosthesis. Semin Thorac Cardiovasc Surg 8:237

Dajani AS, Taubert KA, Wilson W, et al., 1997: Prevention of bacterial endocarditis: Recommendations by the American Heart Association. JAMA 277:1794

Dalrymple-Hay MJ, Bryant M, Jones RA, 1998: Degenerative mitral regurgitation: When should we operate? Ann Thorac Surg 66:1579

David TE, 1997: Complex operations of the aortic root. In Edmunds LH Jr (ed): Cardiac Surgery in the Adult. New York, McGraw-Hill

David TE, Omran A, Armstrong S, et al., 1998: Long-term results of mitral valve repair for myxomatous disease with and without chordal replacement with expanded polytetrafluoroethylene. J Thorac Cardiovasc Surg 115:1279

Doty DB, 1996: Aortic valve replacement with homograft and autograft. Semin Thorac Cardiovasc Surg 8:249

Elkins RC, 1998: Aortic valve: Ross procedure. In Kaiser LR, Kron IL, Spray TL (eds): Mastery of Cardiothoracic Surgery. Philadelphia, Lippincott Williams & Wilkins

Emery RW, Arom KV, Nicoloff DM, 1996: Utilization of the St. Jude Medical prosthesis in the aortic position. Semin Thorac Cardiovasc Surg 8:231

Ewy GA, 1997: Infectious endocarditis. In Alpert JS (ed): Cardiology for the Primary Care Physician, ed. 2. Philadelphia, Current Medicine

Fann JI, Ingels NB Jr, Miller DC, 1997: Pathophysiology of mitral valve disease and operative indications. In Edmunds LH Jr (ed): Cardiac Surgery in the Adult. New York, McGraw-Hill

Fann JI, Miller DC, 1996: Porcine valves: Hancock and Carpentier-Edwards aortic prostheses. Semin Thorac Cardiovasc Surg 8:259

Finkelmeier BA, Hartz RS, Fisher E, Michaelis LL, 1989: Implications of prosthetic valve implantation: An eight year follow-up of patients with porcine bioprostheses. Heart Lung 18:565

Frankel SK, Lilly LS, Bittl JA, 1998: Valvular heart disease. In Lilly LS (ed): Pathophysiology of Heart Disease, ed. 2. Baltimore, Williams & Wilkins

Garcia MJ, 1998: Prosthetic valve disease. In Topol EJ (ed): Comprehensive Cardiovascular Medicine. Philadelphia, Lippincott Williams & Wilkins

Gillinov AM, Cosgrove DM, Blackstone EH, et al., 1998: Durability of mitral valve repair for degenerative disease. J Thorac Cardiovasc Surg 116:734

Ginsberg JS, Hirsh J, 1998: Use of antithrombotics during pregnancy. Chest 114:524S

Grossi EA, Galloway AC, Parish MA, et al., 1992: Experience with twenty-eight cases of systolic anterior motion after mitral valve reconstruction by the Carpentier technique. J Thorac Cardiovasc Surg 103:466

Hammermeister KE, Sethi GK, Oprian C, et al., 1991a: Comparison of occurrence of bleeding, systemic embolism, endocarditis, valve thrombosis and reoperation between patients randomized between a mechanical prosthesis and a bioprosthesis: Results from the VA randomized trial. J Am Coll Cardiol 17:362A

Hammermeister KE, Sethi GK, Oprian C, et al., 1991b: Comparison of outcome an average of 10 years after valve replacement with a mechanical versus a bioprosthetic valve: Results of the VA randomized trial. J Am Coll Cardiol 17:41A

Hammond GL, Letsou GV, 1996: Aortic valve disease and hypertrophic myopathies. In Baue AE, Geha AS, Hammond GL, et al. (eds): Glenn's Thoracic and Cardiovascular Surgery, ed. 6. Stamford, CT, Appleton & Lange

Haydock D, Barratt-Boyes B, Macedo T, et al., 1992: Aortic valve replacement for active endocarditis in 108 patients. J Thorac Cardiovasc Surg 103:130

Hendren WG, Morris AS, Rosenkranz ER, et al., 1992: Mitral valve repair for bacterial endocarditis. J Thorac Cardiovasc Surg 103:124

Hildenberg AD, Austen WG, 1989: Heart valve substitutes. In Eagle KA, Haber E, DeSanctis RW, Austen WG (eds): The Practice of Cardiology, ed. 2. Boston, Little, Brown

Jaggers J, Harrison JK, Bashore TM, et al., 1998: The Ross procedure: Shorter hospital stay, decreased morbidity, and cost effective. Ann Thorac Surg 65:1553

Jamieson WR, 1997: Mechanical and bioprosthetic aortic valve replacement. In Edmunds LH Jr (ed): Cardiac Surgery in the Adult. New York, McGraw-Hill

Jamieson WR, 1993: Modern cardiac valve devices—bioprostheses and mechanical prostheses: State of the art. J Cardiac Surg 8:89

Jamieson WR, Allen P, Miyagishima RT, et al., 1990: The Carpentier-Edwards standard porcine bioprosthesis. J Thorac Cardiovasc Surg 99:543

Karchmer AW, 1997: Infective endocarditis. In Braunwald E (ed): Heart Disease: A Textbook of Cardiovascular Medicine, ed. 5. Philadelphia, WB Saunders

Karlson KJ, Ashraf MM, Berger RL, 1988: Rupture of left ventricle following mitral valve replacement. Ann Thorac Surg 6:590

Kirklin JW, Barratt-Boyes BG, 1993a: Mitral valve disease with or without tricuspid valve disease. In Cardiac Surgery, ed. 2. New York, Churchill Livingstone

Kirklin JW, Barratt-Boyes BG, 1993b: Tricuspid valve disease. In Cardiac Surgery, ed. 2. New York, Churchill Livingstone

Kirklin JW, Barratt-Boyes BG, 1993c: Aortic valve disease. In Cardiac Surgery, ed. 2. New York, Churchill Livingstone

Kon ND, 1998: Mitral valve repair: Myxomatous/rheumatic. In Kaiser LR, Kron IL, Spray TL (eds): Mastery of Cardiothoracic Surgery. Philadelphia, Lippincott Williams & Wilkins

Laks H, Marelli D, Drinkwater DC, 1997: Surgery for adults with congenital heart disease. In Edmunds LH Jr (ed): Cardiac Surgery in the Adult. New York, McGraw-Hill

Larbalestier RI, Kinchla NM, Aranki SF, et al., 1992: Acute bacterial endocarditis. Circulation 86 (Suppl II):II-68

Lawrie GM, 1998: Mitral valve repair versus replacement: Current recommendations and long-term results. Cardiol Clin 16:437

Lund O, Chandrasekaran V, Grocott-Mason R, et al., 1999: Primary aortic valve replacement with allografts over twenty-five years: Valve-related and procedure-related determinants of outcome. J Thorac Cardiovasc Surg 117:77

Maier GW, Wechsler AS, 1997: Pathophysiology of aortic valve disease. In Edmunds LH Jr (ed): Cardiac Surgery in the Adult. New York, McGraw-Hill

McGrath LB, 1997: Tricuspid valve disease. In Edmunds LH Jr (ed): Cardiac Surgery in the Adult. New York, McGraw-Hill

McGrath LB, Gonzalez-Lavin L, Bailey BM, et al., 1990: Tricuspid valve operations in 530 patients. J Thorac Cardiovasc Surg 99:124

Middlemost SJ, Sussman M, Patel A, Manga P, 1999: The stentless quadrileaflet bovine pericardial mitral valve. J Heart Valve Dis 8:174

Minale C, Lambertz H, Nikol S, et al., 1990: Selective annuloplasty of the tricuspid valve. J Thorac Cardiovasc Surg 99:846

North RA, Sadler L, Stewart AW, et al., 1999: Long-term survival and valve-related complications in young women with cardiac valve replacements. Circulation 99:2669

O'Brien MF, 1996: Homografts and autografts. In Baue AE, Geha AS, Hammond GL, et al. (eds): Glenn's Thoracic and Cardiovascular Surgery, ed. 6. Stamford, CT, Appleton & Lange

Otto CM, 1998: Aortic stenosis: Clinical evaluation and optimal timing of surgery. Cardiol Clin 16:353

Quinones MA, 1998: Management of mitral regurgitation. Cardiol Clin 16:421

Schlant RC, 1991: Mitral stenosis. In Hurst JW (ed): Current Therapy in Cardiovascular Disease, ed. 3. Philadelphia, BC Decker

Schoen FJ, 1997: Pathologic considerations in the surgery of adult heart disease. In Edmunds LH Jr (ed): Cardiac Surgery in the Adult. New York, McGraw-Hill

Sexton DJ, Bashore TM, 1998: Infective endocarditis. In Topol EJ (ed): Comprehensive Cardiovascular Medicine. Philadelphia, Lippincott Williams & Wilkins

Silverman NA, Paone G, 1998: Tricuspid valve. In Kaiser LR, Kron IL, Spray TL (eds): Mastery of Cardiothoracic Surgery. Philadelphia, Lippincott Williams & Wilkins

Spencer FC, Galloway AC, Colvin SB, 1995: Acquired disease of the mitral valve. In Sabiston DC Jr, Spencer FC (eds): Surgery of the Chest, ed. 6. Philadelphia, WB Saunders

Stein PD, Alpert JS, Dalen JE, et al., 1998: Antithrombotic therapy in patients with mechanical and bioprosthetic heart valves. Chest 114(5 Suppl):602S

Stephenson LW, 1997: History of cardiac surgery. In Edmunds LH Jr (ed): Cardiac Surgery in the Adult. New York, McGraw-Hill

Suri V, Sawhney H, Vasishta K, et al., 1999: Pregnancy following cardiac valve replacement surgery. Int J Gynecol Obstet 64:239

Swain JA, 1996: Acquired disease of the mitral valve. In Baue AE, Geha AS, Hammond GL, et al. (eds): Glenn's Thoracic and Cardiovascular Surgery, ed. 6. Stamford, CT, Appleton & Lange

Ting W, Silverman N, Levitsky S, 1991: Valve replacement in patients with endocarditis and cerebral septic emboli. Ann Thorac Surg 51:18

Vanscoy GJ, Krause JR, 1991: Warfarin and the international normalized ratio: Reducing interlaboratory effects. Ann Pharmacother 25:1190

Wernly JA, Crawford MH, 1998: Choosing a prosthetic heart valve. Cardiol Clin 16:491

Yun KL, Miller DC, 1997: Ascending aortic aneurysm and aortic valve disease: What is the most optimal surgical technique? Semin Thorac Cardiovasc Surg 9:233

17

Surgery on the Thoracic Aorta

The most common pathologic processes necessitating surgery on the thoracic aorta are aneurysm and dissection. Although these conditions can coexist, they are distinct entities. A third pathologic process, transection, is much less common and is discussed in Chapter 32, Cardiac and Thoracic Trauma. Repair of congenital aortic abnormalities, such as coarctation and patent ductus arteriosus, is discussed in Chapter 19, Surgical Treatment of Congenital Heart Disease in Adults.

▶ Thoracic Aortic Aneurysm

Thoracic aortic aneurysm, or localized, transmural thinning and dilatation of the aortic wall, is a relatively uncommon but life-threatening condition. Thoracic aneurysms most commonly are atherosclerotic in origin but also can develop secondary to other conditions, including Marfan's syndrome, cystic medial necrosis, aortitis, trauma, chronic dissection, or infection. A true aneurysm is one in which blood is contained by aortic wall composed of the three normal layers (intima, media, and adventitia). A false aneurysm is one in which disruption of the aortic wall has occurred and blood is contained only by the adventitial layer and periaortic fibrous tissue (Cohn, 1995).

Aneurysms are described according to shape and location. A fusiform aneurysm widens the aorta circumferentially, and a saccular aneurysm distorts only one side of the aortic wall. Diffuse, fusiform aneurysms are most common, although mycotic aneurysms (ie, aneurysms resulting from aortic infection) often are saccular (Coselli, 1997). Because aneurysmal dilatation usually is localized, thoracic aneurysms typically are categorized by anatomic location. Ascending aneurysms are those occurring between the aortic valve and innominate artery origin; transverse arch aneurysms occur between the innominate and left subclavian artery origins; descending thoracic aneurysms originate distal to the left subclavian artery but above the diaphragm; and thoracoabdominal aneurysms involve both descending thoracic and abdominal aortic segments. Thoracoabdominal aneurysms are further categorized using the Crawford classification system to describe their location and extent (Coselli, 1997) (Fig. 17-1).

Aneurysms in the ascending aorta account for 50% of all thoracic aortic aneurysms (Fann & Miller, 1996). Most ascending aortic aneurysms are associated with cystic degeneration of the medial layer; other etiologies include atherosclerosis, chronic aortic dissection, aortitis, pyogenic infection, trauma, and false aneurysms from previous surgical procedures (Kouchoukos, 1996). Aneurysms of the descending thoracic aorta comprise 40% of thoracic aneurysms, and approximately 90% of these develop secondary to atherosclerosis; only 10% of thoracic aneurysms involve the aortic arch (Fann & Miller, 1996). Uncommonly, aneurysms occur in multiple segments, or the entire thoracic aorta is aneurysmal.

The most threatening consequence of an aortic aneurysm is spontaneous aortic rupture with almost certain death. Thoracic aneurysm is fatal in 75% of patients within 5 years of diagnosis, and one third to one half of deaths are due to rupture (Lindsay et al., 1994). Although the natural history is complex, size is known to be an important predictor for the risk of aortic aneurysm rupture (Isselbacher et al., 1997). Increased diameter of the aortic wall increases wall tension at constant arterial pressure (Laplace's law), making rupture more likely in larger aneurysms (Spittell, 1998).

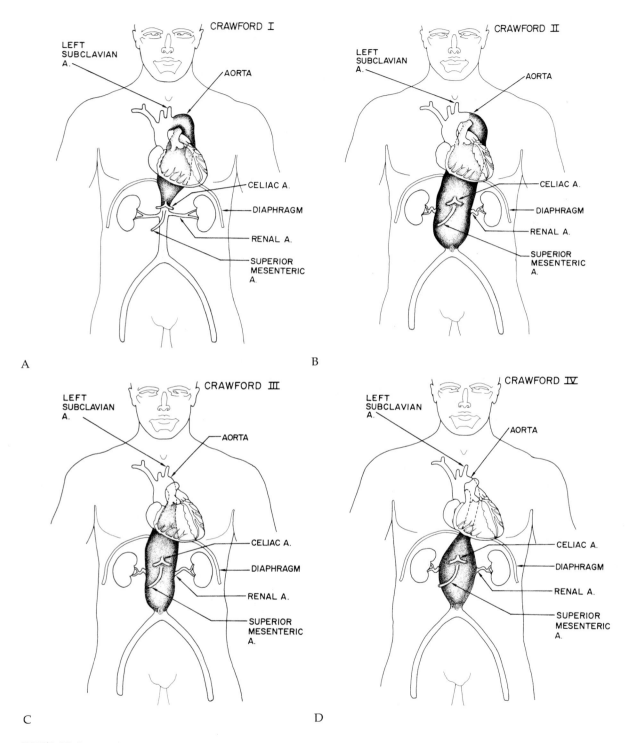

FIGURE 17-1. Crawford classification of thoracoabdominal aneurysms. **(A)** Type I, most of the descending thoracic aorta from left subclavian artery to renal arteries; **(B)** type II, left subclavian artery to the infrarenal abdominal aorta; **(C)** type III, distal half or less of the descending thoracic aorta and substantial segments of the abdominal aorta; **(D)** type IV, upper abdominal aorta and all or none of the infrarenal aorta. (Bayfield MS, Kron IL, 1998: Repair of chronic thoracic and thoracoabdominal aortic aneurysms. In Kaiser LR, Kron IL, Spray TL [eds]: Mastery of Cardiothoracic Surgery, p. 489. Philadelphia, Lippincott Williams & Wilkins)

Most thoracic aortic aneurysms are detected before the development of symptoms, during a radiologic examination performed for another reason. However, as the aneurysm expands, disabling symptoms can occur as the enlarging aortic segment encroaches on surrounding structures. Patients with ascending aortic aneurysms often have chest pain as an initial symptom (Downing & Kouchoukos, 1997). Ascending aortic aneurysms also can distort the aortic valve annulus, leading to annuloaortic ectasia (dilatation of the sinuses of Valsalva and aortic valve annulus) and progressive symptoms of aortic regurgitation. Arch aneurysms may be associated with dyspnea, stridor, hoarseness, hemoptysis, cough, or chest pain (Coselli, 1996). Back or chest pain, usually localized to the area of the aneurysm, is the most common symptom of a descending thoracic aneurysm (Fann & Miller, 1996). Rarely, aortic aneurysms produce physical signs, such as neck vein distention from venous compression (Spittell, 1998).

Indications for Operation

A thoracic aortic aneurysm is a life-threatening condition for which surgical therapy is the only treatment. Resection of a thoracic aneurysm formerly was associated with considerable mortality. More recently, technical advances have lowered the risk associated with operations on the aorta. As a result, indications for surgical repair of thoracic aortic aneurysms have expanded.

The decision to proceed with surgical aneurysm resection is based primarily on the presence of associated symptoms and aortic diameter size. These factors are significant because the onset of symptoms is frequently a harbinger of aortic rupture, and larger aneurysms are not only more prone to rupture but also appear to have a more rapid growth rate than small aneurysms (Isselbacher et al., 1997). Consequently, operative repair is recommended for any symptomatic aneurysm, any aneurysm that exceeds twice the transverse diameter of an adjacent normal-caliber aortic segment, or any aneurysm that is 6 cm in diameter or larger (Duke et al., 1998).

In patients with Marfan's syndrome, operative intervention frequently is recommended for aneurysms that are 5.0 to 5.5 cm in diameter regardless of symptomatology. The extensive cystic medial necrosis frequently present in patients with Marfan's syndrome predisposes to degenerative changes in the aortic wall and makes aneurysm rupture or expansion more likely. Operative repair also is considered for saccular or significantly asymmetric aneurysms and for false aneurysms because these features may increase the likelihood of rupture (Griepp & Ergin, 1997).

Aortography is performed before operative therapy to assess the size and extent of the aneurysm and its relation to branch vessels arising from the aorta. Coronary angiography is performed before aneurysm repair in patients who are in high-risk categories for coronary artery atherosclerosis. If the ascending aorta is involved in the aneurysmal process, preoperative coronary angiography is essential to define the origin of the coronary arteries as they arise from the ascending aorta. Preoperative knowledge of coronary artery anatomy is crucial to the surgeon's ability to plan and perform a successful operation. Abnormalities such as coronary artery lesions, anomalous origin of the coronary artery ostia, or obstruction of the ostia by the aneurysm may be revealed.

Occasionally, aortography demonstrates diffuse aneurysmal disease in multiple segments of the aorta. Aneurysmal disease that involves the ascending aorta, arch, and descending aorta usually is approached with staged operations, unless extensive arch involvement makes staging technically difficult, or symptoms related to more than one diseased segment are present (Rokkas & Kouchoukos, 1999). The order of repair is based on size and associated symptoms or on cardiac complications of the aneurysms (Crawford, 1989).

Operative repair of an aortic aneurysm usually can be performed electively unless there is evidence of rapid expansion or impending rupture. Although aortic rupture usually is fatal, patients with contained rupture may survive long enough to be considered for emergent operative therapy. A *contained rupture* is one in which the adventitia, or outer layer of aortic wall, is disrupted but periaortic, pericardial, or pleural tissue contains the blood and prevents rapid exsanguination and death. Severe chest pain and radiographic evidence of mediastinal widening or pleural effusion suggest contained rupture. *Leaking aneurysm* and *impending rupture* are other terms commonly used to describe this condition. Urgent operative therapy also is undertaken for mycotic, or infected, aneurysms because of their propensity for rupture despite antimicrobial therapy (Crawford, 1989).

Operative Techniques

Surgical repair of aortic aneurysm consists of resecting the aneurysmal segment and replacing it with a prosthetic graft. Most commonly used for replacement of diseased aortic segments is a textile double-velour graft impregnated with collagen (Hemashield; Boston Scientific/Vascular, Natick, MA) (Fig. 17-2). Cryopreserved arterial allografts (aortic segments harvested from human cadavers) may be used for surgical treatment of mycotic aneurysms and infected aortic prosthetic grafts (Vogt et al., 1998). Allografts are thought to offer more resistance to infection than prosthetic grafts.

Operative technique is planned according to aneurysm location and underlying aortic disease. Most often, an interposition technique is used in which the aneurysmal tissue is excised and replaced with a prosthetic tube graft interposed between the two aortic remnants. Alternatively, native aorta is not resected but instead is wrapped around the graft. This so-called "inclusion technique" is thought to assist in hemostasis and may assist in protecting the prosthesis from infection. Use of the interposition technique has increased because newer prosthetic grafts are more impervious to bleeding through graft interstices,

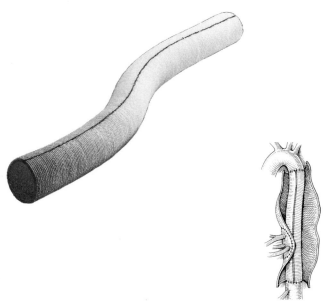

FIGURE 17-2. (Top left) Hemashield woven double velour graft used for operative repair of the thoracic aorta. **(Bottom right)** Graft used for replacement of thoracoabdominal aortic segment. (Courtesy of Boston Scientific/Vascular, Natick, MA)

lessening associated bleeding complications. In addition, the inclusion technique can be complicated by the collection of fluid between the graft and native aorta. Occasionally, local excision of saccular aneurysms, without aortic occlusion or graft placement, is possible (Akins, 1989).

Ascending Aneurysm

A median sternotomy incision is used and cardiopulmonary bypass (CPB) is necessary for repair of *ascending aortic aneurysms*. After achieving adequate exposure of the heart and ascending aorta, heparin is administered and cannulae for CPB are placed. The distal portion of the ascending aorta or the transverse arch may be used for arterial cannulation unless the aneurysm extends to the innominate artery or occurs secondary to chronic dissection. In these cases, the femoral artery is cannulated for arterial return. The right atrium is used for venous cannulation and the coronary sinus is cannulated through the right atrium for retrograde administration of cardioplegic solution. To provide ventricular decompression during the repair, a catheter is positioned in the left ventricle, often in retrograde fashion through the superior pulmonary vein.

Cardiopulmonary bypass is instituted and perfusate temperature is adjusted to induce hypothermia. When the patient's body temperature is sufficiently cooled, a cross-clamp is applied to the aorta, proximal to the arterial return cannula. Cardioplegic solution is administered into the coronary arteries (usually retrograde through the coronary sinus) to protect the myocardium from ischemic damage during the repair. Additional myocardial cooling

is achieved by irrigating the pericardial well with cold Ringer's lactate solution or with use of a cooling jacket (Downing & Kouchoukos, 1997). The diseased aortic segment is opened and a prosthetic tube graft is sewn in place. The native aorta may be reapproximated anteriorly around the tube graft.

After proximal and distal anastomoses are completed, the surgeon performs several measures to evacuate air remaining in the heart or aortic root to avoid catastrophic air embolism when blood flow is reestablished. Transesophageal echocardiography typically is performed to ascertain the absence of air before the left ventricular vent and aortic cross-clamp are removed. Suture lines are inspected carefully to ensure hemostasis before closing the incision.

If the aneurysm has caused annular dilatation of the aortic valve (annuloaortic ectasia), the valvular abnormality is addressed concomitantly, with resuspension of the valve annulus if valve leaflets are normal, or with aortic valve replacement. In patients with ascending aortic aneurysms and coexisting aortic valve disease but no intrinsic aortic root disease (eg, Marfan's syndrome or aortitis), separate aortic valve replacement and aortic graft implantation may be performed.

Prophylactic replacement of the aortic valve is recommended in patients with Marfan's syndrome because of the known propensity for myxomatous valve degeneration that may lead to aortic regurgitation in the future. In patients with Marfan's syndrome, cystic medial necrosis, or granulomatous or syphilitic aortitis, adjacent but nondiseased areas of aorta are resected to avoid future aneurysmal dilatation secondary to the underlying disease process. The entire aortic root usually is replaced in these cases to avoid possible degeneration of native aortic tissue left in place between a separately implanted tube graft and aortic valve prosthesis. Most often, a commercially available composite graft (ie, a prosthetic tube graft containing a mechanical aortic valve prosthesis) is used for this purpose (Fig. 17-3).

Less commonly used techniques for composite replacement of the aortic root include implantation of an aortic allograft or a Ross procedure. The Ross procedure consists of translocation of the patient's pulmonary artery root to the aortic position and replacement of the native pulmonary artery with a pulmonary allograft. The presence of intrinsic aortic disease (eg, Marfan's syndrome) is a contraindication to the Ross procedure because the connective tissue abnormality present in the aorta also exists in the pulmonary artery (Yun & Miller, 1997). The Ross procedure is described in more detail in Chapter 16, Surgical Treatment of Valvular Heart Disease.

When a commercial composite valve graft, allograft, or pulmonary autograft (native pulmonary artery) is implanted in the aortic position, the entire aortic root is resected, including tissue from which the coronary arteries originate. Therefore, surgical reconstruction must include reestablishment of blood flow from the aorta into the coronary arterial circulation. One of three methods may be used to accomplish this. In the first method, the Bentall procedure, the right and left coronary ostia are re-

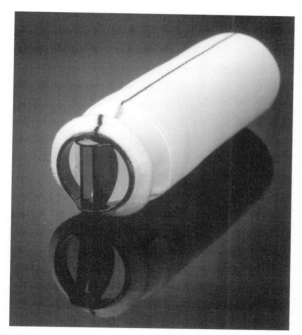

FIGURE 17-3. St. Jude Medical® Aortic Valved Graft. (Used with permission of St. Jude Medical, Inc, St. Paul, MN)

moved from the aortic wall along with a surrounding cuff of aortic tissue; the two coronary ostia are then reimplanted into the aortic graft, allograft, or pulmonary autograft (Fig. 17-4). It is imperative that the coronary ostia are reimplanted without tension on the anastomosis to prevent intraoperative bleeding or late false aneurysm (David, 1998).

Coronary artery reimplantation is not well suited for all cases. Sometimes, the coronary ostia lie so close to the

aortic root that it is impossible to reimplant them in the graft without applying undue tension to the anastomotic site. In the case of aortic dissection, surrounding aortic tissue may be friable or disrupted. A second method of restoring aorta to coronary artery continuity is the Cabrol procedure (Fig. 17-5). A prosthetic graft, comparable in size to the diameter of the coronary artery ostia, is sewn in end-to-end fashion, with one end to the right and the other end to the left coronary artery ostium, and the graft laid over the anterior surface of the composite graft. An opening is made in the posterior surface of the small graft and in the anterior surface of the aortic graft. A side-to-side anastomosis is then fashioned between the two openings. A third method of reestablishing blood flow to coronary arteries is by attaching saphenous vein grafts from the aortic graft to the native coronary arteries in the same manner as would be done during coronary artery bypass grafting.

Arch Aneurysm

Aneurysms of the aortic arch are less common than in other aortic segments, but they present a formidable challenge for the thoracic surgeon. They are likely to involve the origins of the brachiocephalic vessels (ie, the innominate, left carotid, and left subclavian arteries). Special intraoperative techniques are needed to protect the brain and heart during the repair and to reconstruct the aorta to restore circulation to the head and upper extremities (Coselli, 1996). A major advancement in reducing operative mortality associated with aortic arch replacement was the introduction by Griepp and colleagues of the technique of profound hypothermia and circulatory arrest (Griepp et al., 1975). This method of ischemia protection allows cessation of blood flow (ie, circulatory arrest) for up to 60 minutes while the aortic

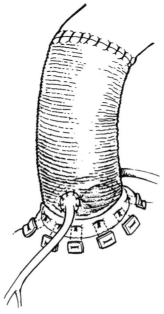

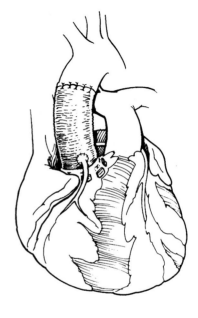

FIGURE 17-4. Replacement of the aortic valve and ascending aorta with a composite aortic graft. The right and left coronary arteries have been detached, with 4 to 5 mm of arterial wall around their orifices, and reimplanted into the anterior and posterior walls of the graft. (David TE, 1998: Annuloaortic ectasia. In Kaiser LR, Kron IL, Spray TL [eds]: Mastery of Cardiothoracic Surgery, p. 457. Philadelphia, Lippincott Williams & Wilkins)

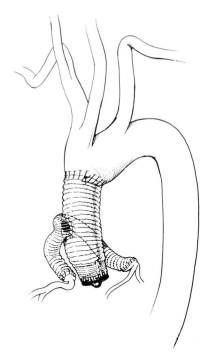

FIGURE 17-5. Composite graft with Cabrol technique of restoring aorta–coronary artery continuity. The two ends of the smaller-diameter graft are sewn in end-to-end fashion to the aorta surrounding the right and left coronary artery ostia; a side-to-side anastomosis is created between the smaller graft and the composite graft. (Coselli JS, Crawford ES, 1993: Composite aortic valve replacement and graft replacement of the ascending aorta plus coronary artery reimplantation: How I do it. Semin Thorac Cardiovasc Surg 5:61)

arch is reconstructed. Techniques for preserving circulation during aortic operations are described in more detail later in the chapter.

As with ascending aortic repair, a median sternotomy incision and CPB are used. The right atrium and femoral artery are cannulated for venous drainage and arterial return, respectively. The aortic repair is performed with deep hypothermia and circulation totally arrested or at very low flows. The repair is performed with the head in the extreme down position to allow for pooling of blood and to prevent air embolization (Coselli, 1996). Reparative techniques are variable because aneurysms of the transverse arch vary widely in size and extent (Kirklin & Barratt-Boyes, 1993a). One technique of arch reconstruction includes implanting a prosthetic tubular graft and suturing an island of aortic tissue containing the origins of the arch vessels to an opening in its superior surface (Fig. 17-6). An inclusion technique may be used to facilitate hemostasis because bleeding due to coagulopathies may develop during rewarming from deep hypothermia. Antifibrinolytic agents, such epsilon-aminocaproic acid (Amicar), typically are administered. After repair of the aortic arch, great care must be taken to evacuate all air and debris from the aortic lumen before reestablishing flow to the brain (Akins, 1989).

Descending Aneurysm

Descending thoracic aneurysms are repaired through a left posterolateral thoracotomy incision. The operation may be performed with or without CPB. A double-lumen endotracheal tube is used to provide single-lung ventilation. The right lung is ventilated while the left lung is maintained in a deflated state to provide adequate exposure of the aorta and prevent retraction injury of the lung (Crawford, 1989). Blood flow through the descending thoracic aorta is interrupted by the application of cross-clamps above and below the aortic segment to be repaired. Cross-clamping of the proximal descending aorta has two significant hemodynamic consequences. First, the application and release of a cross-clamp on the proximal aorta causes precipitous changes in left ventricular afterload. Second, diminished perfusion to organs distal to the aortic clamp can cause ischemic damage to the spinal cord, kidneys, liver, or intestines (Laschinger et al., 1987; Qayumi et al., 1992). Prevention of harmful associated effects is essential. An aortic shunt or a form of CPB may be used to reduce afterload during cross-clamping and perfuse organs distal to the clamp. These techniques are described later in the chapter. The standard repair technique for a descending thoracic aneurysm is graft interposition.

Thoracoabdominal Aneurysm

The repair of *thoracoabdominal aneurysms* can be quite complex because aortic branches to abdominal viscera are involved. Particularly large intercostal arteries identified during dissection and some or all of the visceral arteries may need to be reimplanted (Bayfield & Kron, 1998) (Fig. 17-7). As with repair of descending thoracic aneurysms, techniques to attenuate the sudden changes in left ventricular afterload and to ensure adequate perfusion of the spine and kidneys are necessary during the period of aortic cross-clamping required for thoracoabdominal aneurysm repair. Because the incision required for adequate exposure of a thoracoabdominal aneurysm (lateral chest wall, extending down the middle of the abdomen) is extensive, it is likely to compromise patient mobility and pulmonary function in the early postoperative period (Fig. 17-8).

Results of Aneurysm Resection

Mortality rates associated with thoracic aneurysm resection vary according to aneurysm location and underlying aortic disease. Cohn (1995) summarizes the risk of operative mortality as follows: ascending, 5% to 10%; arch, 10% to 20%; descending, 5% to 15%; and thoracoabdominal, 5% to 10%. Variance in results between surgical centers remains significant. Common causes of death after thoracic aortic aneurysm resection include bleeding and cardiac dysfunction. Elderly patients, those with extensive or symptomatic aneurysms, and those with underlying cardiac, renal, or pulmonary disease are at higher risk for operative death or complications.

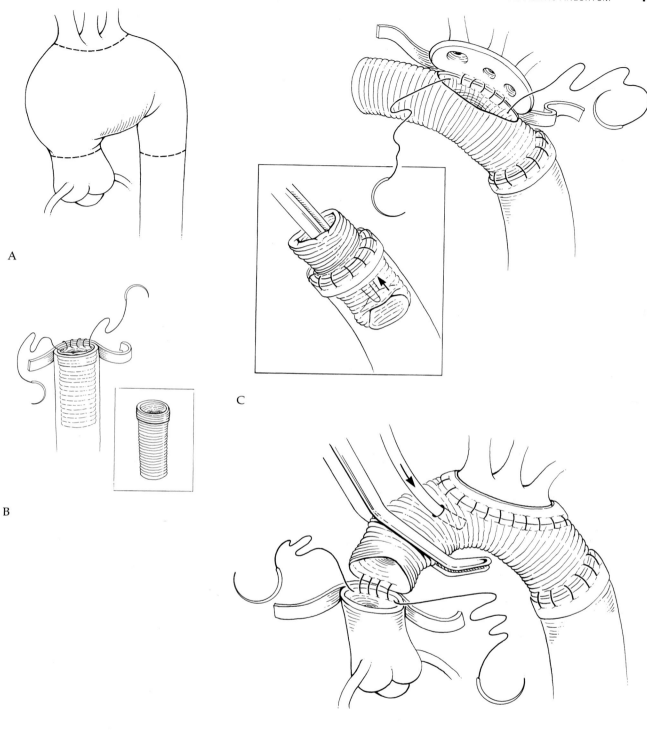

FIGURE 17-6. Operative technique for resection of aortic arch aneurysm. **(A)** Using deep hypothermic circulatory arrest, the aortic arch aneurysm is resected, as indicated by dashed lines, leaving an "island" of aortic tissue containing the origin of the arch branches. **(B)** A collagen-impregnated woven (Hemashield) graft is invaginated into itself (*inset*), creating a cuff at one end, the graft is placed inside lumen of the descending aorta, and the distal anastomosis is performed. **(C)** The graft is withdrawn from the descending aorta (*inset*); the island of arch tissue is sewn to an opening in the superior aspect of the graft. **(D)** The graft is de-aired, clamped, and cannulated so that cerebral and distal perfusion, as well as core warming, can be resumed while the proximal anastomosis is completed. (Lansman SL, Griepp RB, 1998: Resection of aortic arch aneurysms using hypothermic circulatory arrest. In Kaiser LR, Kron IL, Spray TL [eds]: Mastery of Cardiothoracic Surgery, p. 474. Philadelphia, Lippincott Williams & Wilkins)

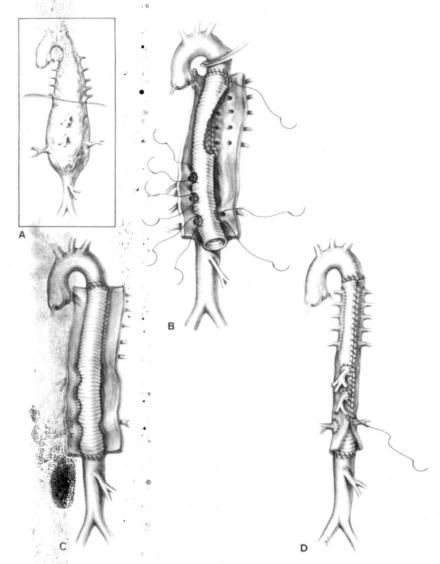

FIGURE 17-7. (A) Thoracoabdominal aortic aneurysm. **(B)** One method of surgical management. After clamping the aorta, the aneurysm is opened longitudinally. The proximal end of a prosthetic tube graft is sutured in end-to-end fashion to normal aorta. The graft is placed inside the aneurysm and side-holes are created to correspond to the ostia of the visceral, intercostal, and lumbar arteries branching from the aneurysmal portion of the aorta. Graft openings are sutured circumferentially around the corresponding vessel ostia. **(C)** The distal end of the graft is anastomosed in end-to-end fashion to the distal aorta. **(D)** After all anastomoses are completed, the wall of the aneurysm is sutured around the graft. (Robicsek F, 1984: Aneurysms of the thoracic aorta. In Haimovici H [ed]: Haimovici's Vascular Surgery: Principles and Techniques, ed. 2, p. 672. Stamford, CT. Reproduced with permission of the McGraw-Hill Companies)

▶ Aortic Dissection

Aortic dissection is the longitudinal separation of the aortic wall layers. The initiating pathologic event, disruption of the intima, or innermost layer, provides an entry point for blood from the true aortic lumen to dissect the medial layer, creating a false lumen or second channel for blood flow. Systemic blood pressure in the aorta causes blood entering the false channel to be propelled retrograde, antegrade, or in both directions, separating intimal and adventitial layers for a variable distance along the length of the aorta.

Hypertension is present in 70% to 90% of patients with aortic dissection, particularly that occurring in the distal aorta (Cohn, 1995; Ergin & Griepp, 1996). Cystic medial necrosis is present in approximately 20% of patients (Kirklin & Barratt-Boyes, 1993b). It is frequently related to a connective tissue disorder such as Marfan's syndrome or, less commonly, Ehlers-Danlos syndrome. Other etiologic factors for aortic dissection include preg-

nancy, congenital bicuspid aortic valve, and coarctation (Wheat, 1987; Wolfe & Moran, 1981). Iatrogenic aortic dissection can occur secondary to catheterization, instrumentation, or surgical procedures involving the aorta.

Aortic dissection is considered acute if it is recognized within 2 weeks of its onset because most of the associated mortality occurs during this interval (Spittell, 1997). Dissection detected or treated more than 2 weeks after its presumed occurrence is considered chronic. The Stanford classification system is used to categorize aortic dissection according to location. Type A dissection involves the ascending aorta and may involve the descending aorta as well. Type B dissection involves only the descending aorta distal to the left subclavian artery. Distinction between type A and type B dissection is important in determining therapy. The DeBakey classification system is used alternatively; DeBakey type I and type II dissections are included in Stanford type A dissection, and a DeBakey type III dissection is equivalent to a Stanford type B dissection.

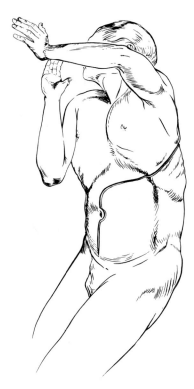

FIGURE 17-8. Thoracoabdominal incision. The patient is in the semidecubitus position. A posterolateral thoracotomy incision is begun between the T6 to T11 vertebrae, then is continued downward and anteriorly to the midline, where it is extended down the middle of the abdomen. (Ernst CB, Reddy DJ, 1989: Thoracoabdominal aortic aneurysm. In Haimovici H [ed]: Haimovici's Vascular Surgery: Principles and Techniques, ed. 3, p. 618. Stamford, CT. Reproduced with permission of the McGraw-Hill Companies)

Although dissection is the most common catastrophic illness involving the aorta, many patients do not survive long enough to receive treatment. The arterial hypertension usually associated with the condition produces progressive dissection that can occur in both retrograde and antegrade directions from the original point of intimal disruption. Without treatment, more than 25% of patients die within 24 hours, more than 50% within 1 week, and more than 75% within 1 month; fewer than 10% of patients survive 1 year (Isselbacher et al., 1997).

Three major pathologic consequences can result from aortic dissection (Eagle et al., 1989). First, retrograde dissection can disrupt the aortic valve annulus leading to acute aortic valve incompetence, with resultant left heart failure or frank cardiogenic shock. Second, rupture of intraluminal blood through the adventitia can occur anywhere along the length of the aorta. Free rupture produces rapid exsanguination; rupture into the pericardium or mediastinum causes cardiac tamponade. Third, because all body tissues receive blood from branches of the aorta, perfusion to any of the vital organs can be compromised.

Branches of the aorta may be occluded by the dissection, may stay in communication with the aorta by the false channel, or may be uninvolved (Kirklin & Barratt-Boyes, 1993b). Dissection of a coronary artery, usually the right, can cause acute myocardial infarction. Involvement of the arteries arising from the aortic arch may produce altered mental status or focal neurologic deficits (Fann et al., 1989). Compromised blood flow to the spinal cord, kidneys, intestines, or lower extremities may cause paraplegia, renal dysfunction, bowel infarction, or limb ischemia, respectively.

Patients with aortic dissection usually become acutely symptomatic, either with sudden, severe chest or back pain or with manifestations of occlusion of one of the major organs supplied by the aorta. Pain associated with dissection often migrates from its origin to other sites, generally following the path of the dissection as it extends through the aorta (Isselbacher et al., 1997). Other findings may include mediastinal widening on chest roentgenogram, hypertension despite a general appearance of shock, unequal pulses, and a diminishing hematocrit. The diagnosis is confirmed with computed tomography, transesophageal echocardiography, or aortography.

Indications for Operation

The decision to treat aortic dissection surgically is determined in large part by the location and extent of the dissection. Type A dissection (involving the ascending aorta or arch) almost always is treated with emergent surgical therapy unless the patient has already sustained irreversible major organ system damage. Without surgical intervention, type A dissection is associated with a nearly 100% probability of early death due to aortic rupture, coronary artery occlusion, or acute aortic valve regurgitation (Gardner, 1998; Fann et al., 1989).

In contrast, type B dissection (limited to the descending aorta distal to the left subclavian artery) usually is treated primarily with medical (ie, antihypertensive) therapy. Surgical and medical therapies provide equal short- and long-term survival rates in patients with uncomplicated descending (type B) aortic dissection (Schor et al., 1996; Glower et al., 1990). In addition, type B dissections more often occur in patients with preexisting atherosclerotic and hypertensive cardiovascular disease; in these patients, the pathologic process involving the aortic wall is quite different from that in patients with connective tissue disorders affecting the integrity of the aorta (Spittell, 1998). Surgical treatment sometimes becomes necessary for type B dissection because blood pressure cannot be controlled, or there is evidence of dissection progression or aortic rupture (Eagle et al., 1989). Dissection progression may be manifest by persistent pain, evidence of aortic regurgitation, or compromised blood flow to the spinal cord, abdominal viscera, or lower extremities.

Surgical therapy is recommended for either type A or type B dissection in patients with Marfan's syndrome because of the friable nature of aortic tissue in this disease and the propensity for rupture or recurrent dissection (Isselbacher et al., 1997; Eagle et al., 1989). The choice of medical or surgical therapy remains somewhat controversial for dissection that originates in the aortic arch because arch resection carries a higher operative risk. Regardless of whether surgical repair is undertaken, an integral component in treatment of all aortic dissections is aggressive pharmacologic therapy to control hypertension and prevent extension of the dissection. Antihypertensive therapy is instituted as soon as the diagnosis is suspected, even before definitive diagnostic studies are performed. Intravenous nitroprusside almost always is the agent of choice because of its immediate effect and potency; a beta-blocking agent should be administered concomitantly to prevent a reflex increase in dP/dt (ie, rate of rise of systolic arterial pressure) resulting from nitroprusside administration (Finkelmeier, 1997).

Operative Techniques

Type A Dissection

Type A aortic dissection is repaired through a median sternotomy incision. CPB, with right atrial and retrograde femoral artery cannulation, is used to maintain circulation while the ascending aorta is clamped and repaired. The proximal and distal ends of the transected ascending aorta are repaired by suturing with felt strip buttresses the intimal and adventitial layers to obliterate the false channel between the layers. After repairing both the proximal and distal aortic walls, a prosthetic tube graft is used to replace the resected segment of aorta (Fig. 17-9). Repair of type A aortic dissection includes resection of the most proximal segment of ascending aorta involved in the dissection process, thus preventing further retrograde dissection into the aortic valve annulus or pericardium.

In many cases, type A dissection is associated with some degree of aortic valvular regurgitation. Often, valve competency can be restored with resuspension of the valve commissures, reconstitution of the separated aortic wall layers (with suture buttressed with Teflon felt, or glue), and anastomosis to an appropriately sized aortic graft (Stone & Borst, 1997). Aortic valve replacement may be necessary if the degree of residual annular distortion is severe or the valve itself is abnormal (Gardner, 1998). Usually, a composite valve graft is used to replace both the aortic root and aortic valve because the underlying disease process makes future dissection or aneurysmal dilatation likely. In patients with Marfan's syndrome, replacement of the aortic root with a composite valve graft is recommended regardless of the degree of valvular damage to avoid likely myxomatous valve degeneration requiring a future operation.

The site of intimal disruption is included in aortic dissection repair if it is located in the ascending aorta. If the intimal disruption is located in the arch or descending aorta, the resection for type A aortic dissection still may be limited to repairing the ascending aorta. However, resection of the intimal tear, including tears located in the aortic arch, is believed to reduce the incidence of long-term, dissection-related complications (Ergin & Griepp, 1996). The aortic arch also is included in the operative repair in patients with (1) excessive enlargement and impending or actual rupture of the false channel in the arch, or (2) a large degenerative aneurysm in the arch (Crawford et al., 1992).

Repair of an intimal disruption in the arch requires deep hypothermic circulatory arrest so that the surgeon can remove the aortic cross-clamp, transect the distal ascending aorta or proximal arch, visualize the inner walls of the arch, and restore aortic wall integrity. Most

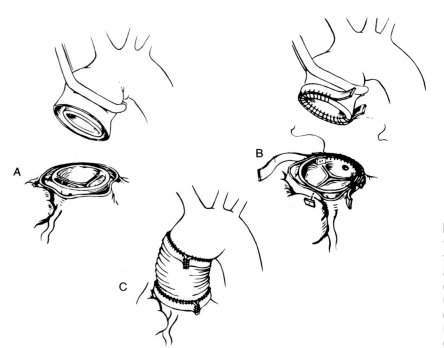

FIGURE 17-9. Surgical repair of type A aortic dissection. **(A)** Resection of the ascending aorta containing the intimal tear. **(B)** Resuspension of the aortic valve at commissures and preparation of the proximal and distal aortic walls for anastomosis of the graft. **(C)** Completed resection and graft replacement of the ascending aorta. (Ergin MA, Galla JD, Lansman S, Griepp RB, 1985: Acute dissections of the aorta: Current surgical treatment. Surg Clin North Am 65:730)

amenable to repair are limited intimal disruptions arising in the lesser curvature of the arch away from the origin of the cephalic branches (Stone & Borst, 1997). Reconstruction of the aortic arch in the face of extensive intimal disruption increases operative risk because of the technical difficulties associated with replacing the entire arch. In other cases, intimal disruption beyond the arch may not be accessible with a sternotomy exposure.

Type B Dissection

Type B dissection, that involving only the aorta distal to the left subclavian artery, is repaired through a left thoracotomy incision. With proximal and distal control, the aorta is clamped and the segment containing the intimal disruption and dilated portion of aorta is resected (Ergin & Griepp, 1996). Aortic continuity is restored with a tubular graft, obliterating the false lumen at the proximal and distal ends. If blood flow into arterial branches of the aorta has been compromised, adequate blood supply to organs supplied by the branches must be restored.

The same considerations related to occluding the descending thoracic aorta during aneurysm resection apply to dissection repair. However, the risk of spinal cord damage associated with repair of aortic dissection is higher than that for operative repair of atherosclerotic aortic aneurysms or congenital coarctation, in which collateral vessels to the spinal cord usually are well developed. Also, the false channel in type B dissection frequently involves the origins of the distal thoracic intercostal and spinal cord branches (Gardner, 1998). Repair of type B aortic dissection is associated with a 10% to 20% incidence of paraplegia.

Chronic Dissection

Surgical treatment of *chronic dissection* may become necessary because of chronic aortic regurgitation or aneurysmal dilatation of the false lumen in the distal aorta (Ergin & Griepp, 1996). Surgery for chronic proximal dissection usually is associated with a lower operative risk than for acute dissection because the procedure can be performed electively and the outer aortic wall is stronger and firmer than in acute dissection (Stone & Borst, 1997). During operative repair of chronic dissection of the distal aorta, the false channel is not obliterated because it may be the source of blood supply to aortic branches. Fenestrations are created in the prosthetic graft, and the distal end of the graft is sutured to the outer wall of the dissected aorta to direct blood flow into both the true and false aortic lumens (Ergin & Griepp, 1996).

Results of Dissection Repair

The operative mortality rate is 5% to 11% for acute type A and 6% to 16% for type B dissections (Ergin & Griepp, 1996). Residual aortic disease and coexisting cardiovascular disease are significant causes of late death and morbidity. Aneurysmal deterioration can develop late after surgical resection at fenestration or reentry sites distal to the graft replacement, and in patients with underlying connective tissue disorders, distal aneurysmal segments frequently develop owing to degenerative progression (Gardner, 1998).

▶ Preservation of Circulation During Aortic Operations

During operative procedures on the aorta, it is necessary to occlude blood flow through a segment of the aorta. Because the aorta supplies blood to all vital organs, maintenance of adequate perfusion to these organs is a particular challenge. The reduction in mortality and morbidity associated with aortic surgery largely is due to better techniques of CPB and organ preservation during the period of aortic cross-clamping. The specific techniques used depend on what segment of the thoracic aorta must be repaired.

Involvement of the aortic root or ascending aorta in the disease process necessitates use of CPB to maintain circulation while blood flow into the proximal aorta is interrupted. Depending on the type and location of the disease, arterial perfusion is accomplished with cannulation of the femoral artery, distal ascending aorta, subclavian artery, or transverse arch. Cardioplegia is administered during the period of aortic cross-clamping to protect the myocardium from ischemic injury, and a vent is inserted into the left ventricle to provide left ventricular decompression. For operations necessitating aortic root reconstruction, cardioplegic solution is delivered directly into the coronary artery ostia through balloon-tipped cannulae (David, 1998). Alternatively, a retrograde technique may be used for delivery of cardioplegic solution to the myocardium. Techniques of CPB and myocardial protection are described in more detail elsewhere in the text.

Operations on the aortic arch require attention to protection of cerebral circulation because blood flow through the carotid arteries must be interrupted. Instead of the moderate hypothermia and CPB perfusion techniques used in most cardiac operations, deep hypothermia and circulatory arrest are used. With the patient on CPB, body temperature is lowered to 18°C to 20°C. The patient's head is packed in crushed ice to provide topical cooling of the brain and to lessen rewarming during deep hypothermic circulatory arrest (Lansman & Griepp, 1998). Deep hypothermic circulatory arrest protects the brain against ischemic damage for a limited time during which cerebral blood flow is interrupted. The safe period for circulatory arrest, however, is not known precisely. An ischemic period of greater than 45 minutes is associated with an increased risk of neurologic damage, and morbidity and mortality increase significantly when the circulatory arrest period exceeds 60 minutes (Yamashita et al., 1998).

Retrograde cerebral perfusion may be used as an adjunct to hypothermic circulatory arrest in patients undergoing operative procedures on the aortic arch. With the patient in a slight Trendelenburg position, the body temperature sufficiently cooled, and the aortic arch open, the inferior vena cava cannula is clamped. A bridging circuit is used to redirect the flow of cold oxygenated blood from the CPB system through the superior vena cava cannula in retrograde fashion into the subclavian and jugular veins (Gardner, 1998). Deoxygenated blood exits the head vessels through the opened aortic arch and is returned to the CPB circuit through the cardiotomy suction catheter.

Retrograde cerebral perfusion potentially augments the cerebral protection offered by deep hypothermia and circulatory arrest by providing some cerebral blood flow and uniform cooling, thus supporting minimal cerebral metabolic needs and clearing byproducts of cerebral anaerobic metabolism (Bavaria & Pochettino, 1997). Retrograde cerebral perfusion also may facilitate the flushing of debris from aortic arch vessels (Stone & Borst, 1997). Deep hypothermic circulatory arrest, retrograde cerebral perfusion, and shorter periods of cerebral vessel occlusion have decreased the incidence of neurologic sequelae. Despite these protective measures, neurologic complications remain the predominant morbidity associated with operative procedures on the aortic arch.

Operations on the descending thoracic aorta (eg, type B aortic dissection, descending thoracic and thoracoabdominal aneurysms, and aortic transection) necessitate occlusion of the descending thoracic aorta. Proximal clamping of the aorta produces a sudden increase in afterload, and cross-clamp release precipitates sudden afterload reduction with relative hypovolemia and acute systemic hypotension (Bayfield & Kron, 1998). The abrupt rise in afterload that occurs when the clamp is applied increases cardiac work and myocardial oxygen consumption. Aortic pressure above the clamp must be carefully regulated during the period of cross-clamping to prevent left ventricular failure. Pharmacologic vasodilatation with sodium nitroprusside is used to counteract proximal hypertension. To prepare for sudden afterload reduction when the cross-clamp is released, vasodilating agents are discontinued and rapid infusion of volume is initiated (Bayfield & Kron, 1998).

One of three techniques may be used for distal perfusion and to relieve proximal hypertension: (1) a heparin-bonded shunt, (2) left-sided heart (ie, partial) bypass, or (3) CPB with femoral artery and vein cannulation (femorofemoral bypass). In the first method, a heparin-bonded shunt is placed proximal (in the aorta, left subclavian artery, or left ventricular apex) and distal (in the descending thoracic aorta or femoral artery) to the occluded aortic segment (Akins, 1989). In the second method, left atriofemoral ("left heart") bypass, blood is drained from a cannula in the left atrium, circulated through a centrifugal pump, and returned to the systemic circulation through a femoral artery cannula. Because blood still flows through the right side of the heart and pulmonary vasculature normally, an oxygenator in the circuit is not necessary. These methods have the advantage of requiring little or no anticoagulation, thus reducing the likelihood of hemorrhagic complications.

In the third method, the femoral artery and vein are cannulated and CPB is instituted for distal perfusion.

Some of the venous return to the heart is diverted through the venous cannula and circulated through the CPB circuit before being returned to the body through the femoral artery cannula to perfuse organs below the distal aortic clamp. Femorofemoral CPB necessitates higher doses of heparin than left atriofemoral bypass because the extracorporeal circuit is more complex and contains an oxygenator/heat exchanger (Bayfield & Kron, 1998). Consequently, this technique is associated with a higher incidence of bleeding complications. With either left atriofemoral or femorofemoral bypass, continued upper body perfusion by the heart must occur and the patient must be protected from excessive cooling (Gardner, 1998). Also, none of the three described techniques has eradicated the occurrence of postoperative paraplegia. Consequently, if a short cross-clamp time is anticipated, repair of the descending thoracic aorta may be performed with a "clamp and sew" technique in which the aorta is clamped and the repair is performed without a shunt or either form of CPB (Fig. 17-10).

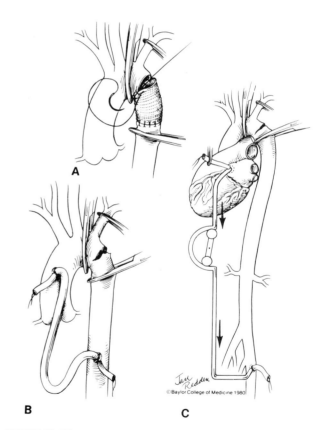

FIGURE 17-10. Several of the techniques described in the text are demonstrated in this drawing depicting repair of a traumatic transection of the descending thoracic aorta, including the "clamp and sew" technique **(A)**, a heparinized shunt placed proximal and distal to the clamped segment of aorta **(B)**, and partial (left heart) bypass with cannulation of the left atrium and femoral artery **(C)**. (Mattox KL, 1996: Thoracic trauma. In Baue AE, Geha AS, Hammond GL, et al [eds]: Glenn's Thoracic and Cardiovascular Surgery, ed. 6, p. 108. Stamford, CT. Reproduced with permission of The McGraw-Hill Companies)

► Perioperative Considerations

Patients undergoing aortic reparative operations that do not necessitate CPB are susceptible to intraoperative hypothermia. Recall that when CPB is used, the patient's body temperature may be precisely manipulated by heating or cooling the blood as it courses through the extracorporeal circuit. During operations on the descending or thoracoabdominal aorta, CPB may not be used. Anesthetized patients lose the normal intrinsic regulation of body temperature by the hypothalamus (Savino & Cheung, 1997). Instead, body temperature fluctuates with environmental temperature. Hypothermia may occur as a result of the large skin incision, cold operating room, cold, wet surgical drapes, and the administration of cold intravenous solutions (Savino & Cheung, 1997). Hypothermia can cause excessive bleeding and development of arrhythmias. In addition, it potentiates the effects of anesthetic drugs and neuromuscular blockers, increases vascular resistance, and contributes to postoperative shivering (Savino & Cheung, 1997).

An important feature of early postoperative management in patients who have undergone aortic surgery is ensuring adequate blood pressure control. Many patients with aortic aneurysm or dissection have underlying hypertension. After aortic operations, systolic arterial pressure is maintained in a low normal range (80 to 90 mm Hg) to protect the multiple anastomotic suture lines. Often, patients previously have been taking a beta-blocking medication, such as propranolol. Antihypertensive therapy is resumed when oral medications are reinstituted. Because hypertension is a predominant risk factor and one that usually can be controlled with pharmacologic therapy, it is imperative that affected patients understand the need for lifelong medical supervision with sustained control of hypertension.

The most common complications of aortic surgery are bleeding and ischemic organ injury. Procedures that include extensive replacement of the thoracic aorta may be associated with 2000 to 7000 mL of blood loss; hemorrhage may be more severe in the event of technical problems, prolonged CPB, excessive hemodilution, or coagulation defects (Kouchoukos & Wareing, 1991). Antifibrinolytic agents, such as aprotinin and aminocaproic acid, often are used to lessen perioperative coagulopathy. Operations on the ascending aorta or aortic arch may be complicated by stroke or generalized cerebral dysfunction. Brain injury is a major source of postoperative morbidity after operations with profound hypothermia and circulatory arrest and is related to the duration of circulatory arrest (Rokkas & Kouchoukos, 1999). Other potential complications of aortic root operations include low cardiac output, myocardial infarction, and heart block (David, 1998).

After operations on the descending thoracic aorta, paraplegia occurs unpredictably despite all current techniques used to predict or prevent it. The risk of paraplegia is higher in patients with acute aortic disease (eg, acute dissection or transection) and for those with more extensive disease (eg, type II thoracoabdominal aneu-

rysm). The incidence of spinal cord injury also increases when the duration of aortic cross-clamping exceeds 30 minutes, but can occur with shorter clamp times and may not occur with longer times (Miller & Calhoon, 1998).

Pathogenesis of perioperative spinal cord injury is ill defined and probably multifactorial. Major causes are thought to be (1) the duration and degree of ischemia, (2) failure to reestablish blood flow after the aortic repair, and (3) a biochemically mediated reperfusion injury caused by ischemia to the spinal cord (Stenson, 1997). Significant reduction of upper body arterial pressure during cross-clamping or hypotension after the cross-clamp is removed also can produce ischemic damage to the spinal cord (Kirklin & Barratt-Boyes, 1993a). The significant anatomic variation in spinal cord blood supply is thought to contribute to the unpredictability of postoperative paraplegia as well.

An unusual but very serious complication of surgical procedures on the thoracic aorta is infection of the vascular prosthesis. Graft infections occur in 1% to 2% of patients who undergo aortic replacement; the mortality rate for graft infection may be as high as 75% (Downing & Kouchoukos, 1997). In most instances, graft infection is thought to be due to contamination at operation (Kouchoukos & Wareing, 1991). Risk factors associated with development of vascular prosthesis infection include presence of infection elsewhere in the body, diabetes, preoperative use of steroids, and postoperative sepsis. The infection usually produces a false aneurysm at the anastomotic site (Crawford, 1989).

Continued medical supervision of patients with aortic disease is essential, especially in those with aortic dissection, cystic medial necrosis, or Marfan's syndrome. Recurrent dissection or fusiform aneurysm formation can develop in weakened areas of aortic wall (Crawford, 1989). Also, the remainder of the patient's aorta is subject to the same pathologic process that affected the resected segment of aorta. In patients with Marfan's syndrome, multiple segments or even the entire aorta eventually may be affected by aneurysm formation or dissection. Multiple operations for repair of diseased ascending aortic, aortic arch, or descending aortic segments may be necessary and may considerably extend life expectancy (Crawford, 1989).

REFERENCES

Akins CW, 1989: Nondissecting aneurysms of the thoracic aorta. In Eagle KA, Haber E, DeSanctis RW, Austin WG (eds): The Practice of Cardiology, ed. 2. Boston, Little, Brown

Bavaria JE, Pochettino A, 1997: Retrograde cerebral perfusion (RCP) in aortic arch surgery: Efficacy and possible mechanisms of brain protection. Semin Thorac Cardiovasc Surg 9:222

Bayfield MS, Kron IL, 1998: Repair of chronic thoracic and thoracoabdominal aortic aneurysms. In Kaiser LR, Kron IL, Spray TL (eds): Mastery of Cardiothoracic Surgery. Philadelphia, Lippincott Williams & Wilkins

Cohn LH, 1995: Thoracic aortic aneurysms and aortic dissection. In Sabiston DC Jr, Spencer FC (eds): Surgery of the Chest, ed. 6. Philadelphia, WB Saunders

Coselli JS, 1997: Descending and thoracoabdominal aneurysms. In Edmunds LH Jr (ed): Cardiac Surgery in the Adult. New York, McGraw-Hill

Coselli JS, 1996: Aneurysms of the transverse aortic arch. In Baue AE, Geha AS, Hammond GL, et al. (eds): Glenn's Thoracic and Cardiovascular Surgery, ed 6. Stamford, CT, Appleton & Lange

Crawford ES, 1989: Replacement of the thoracic aorta. In Grillo HC, Austen WG, Wilkins EW Jr, et al. (eds): Current Therapy in Cardiothoracic Surgery. Toronto, Canada, BC Decker

Crawford ES, Kirklin JW, Naftel DC, et al., 1992: Surgery for acute dissection of ascending aorta. J Thorac Cardiovasc Surg 104:46

David TE, 1998: Annuloaortic ectasia. In Kaiser LR, Kron IL, Spray TL (eds): Mastery of Cardiothoracic Surgery. Philadelphia, Lippincott Williams & Wilkins

Downing SW, Kouchoukos NT, 1997: Ascending aortic aneurysm. In Edmunds LH Jr (ed): Cardiac Surgery in the Adult. New York, McGraw-Hill

Duke MD, Miller DC, Mitchell RS, et al., 1998: The "first generation" of endovascular stent-grafts for patients with aneurysms of the descending thoracic aorta. J Thorac Cardiovasc Surg 116:689

Eagle KA, Doroghazi RM, DeSanctis RW, Austen WG, 1989: Aortic dissection. In Eagle KA, Haber E, DeSanctis RW, Austin WG (eds): The Practice of Cardiology, ed. 2. Boston, Little, Brown

Ergin MA, Griepp RB, 1996: Dissections of the aorta. In Baue AE, Geha AS, Hammond GL, et al. (eds): Glenn's Thoracic and Cardiovascular Surgery, ed 6. Stamford, CT, Appleton & Lange

Fann JI, Miller C, 1996: Descending thoracic aortic aneurysms. In Baue AE, Geha AS, Hammond GL, et al. (eds): Glenn's Thoracic and Cardiovascular Surgery, ed. 6. Stamford, CT, Appleton & Lange

Fann JI, Sarris GE, Miller C, et al., 1989: Surgical management of acute aortic dissection complicated by stroke. Circulation (Suppl I):I–257

Finkelmeier BA, 1997: Dissection of the aorta: A clinical update. J Vasc Nurs 15:88

Gardner TJ, 1998: Acute aortic dissection. In Kaiser LR, Kron IL, Spray TL (eds): Mastery of Cardiothoracic Surgery. Philadelphia, Lippincott Williams & Wilkins

Glower DD, Fann JI, Speier RH, et al., 1990: Comparison of medical and surgical therapy for uncomplicated descending aortic dissection. Circulation 82 (Suppl IV):IV–39

Griepp RB, Ergin MA, 1997: Aneurysms of the aortic arch. In Edmunds LH Jr (ed): Cardiac Surgery in the Adult. New York, McGraw-Hill

Griepp RB, Stinson EB, Hollingsworth JF, et al., 1975: Prosthetic replacement of the aortic arch. J Thorac Cardiovasc Surg 70:1051

Isselbacher EM, Eagle KA, DeSanctis RW, 1997: Diseases of the aorta. In Braunwald E (ed): Heart Disease: A Textbook of Cardiovascular Medicine, ed. 5. Philadelphia, WB Saunders

Kirklin JW, Barratt-Boyes BG, 1993a: Chronic thoracic and thoracoabdominal aortic aneurysm. In Cardiac Surgery, ed. 2. New York, Churchill Livingstone

Kirklin JW, Barratt-Boyes BG, 1993b: Acute aortic dissection. In Cardiac Surgery, ed. 2. New York, Churchill Livingstone

Kouchoukos NT, 1996: Aneurysms of the ascending aorta. In Baue AE, Geha AS, Hammond GL, et al. (eds): Glenn's Thoracic and Cardiovascular Surgery, ed 6. Stamford, CT, Appleton & Lange

Kouchoukos NT, Wareing TH, 1991: Management of complications of aortic surgery. In Waldhausen JA, Orringer MB (eds): Complications in Cardiothoracic Surgery. St. Louis, Mosby–Year Book

Lansman SL, Griepp RB, 1998: Resection of aortic arch aneurysms using hypothermic circulatory arrest. In Kaiser LR, Kron IL, Spray TL (eds): Mastery of Cardiothoracic Surgery. Philadelphia, Lippincott Williams & Wilkins

Laschinger JC, Izumoto H, Kouchoukos NT, 1987: Evolving concepts in prevention of spinal cord injury during operations on the descending thoracic and thoracoabdominal aorta. Ann Thorac Surg 44:667

Lindsay J Jr, DeBakey ME, Beall AC, 1994: Diagnosis and treatment of diseases of the aorta. In Schlant RC, Alexander RW, et al. (eds): The Heart, ed. 8. New York, McGraw-Hill

Miller OL, Calhoon JH, 1998: Acute traumatic aortic transection. In Kaiser LR, Kron IL, Spray TL (eds): Mastery of Cardiothoracic Surgery. Philadelphia, Lippincott Williams & Wilkins

Qayumi AK, Janusz MT, Jamieson WR, Dyster DM, 1992: Pharmacologic interventions for prevention of spinal cord injury caused by aortic cross-clamping. J Thorac Cardiovasc Surg 104:256

Rokkas CK, Kouchoukos NT, 1999: Single-stage extensive replacement of thoracic aorta: The arch-first technique. J Thorac Cardiovasc Surg 117:99

Savino JS, Cheung AT, 1997: Cardiac anesthesia. In Edmunds HL Jr (ed): Cardiac Surgery in the Adult. New York, McGraw-Hill

Schor JS, Yerlioglu E, Galla JD, et al., 1996: Selective management of acute type B dissection: Long term follow-up. Ann Thorac Surg 61:1339

Spittell PC, 1998: Diseases of the aorta. In Topol EJ (ed): Comprehensive Cardiovascular Medicine. Philadelphia, Lippincott Williams & Wilkins

Spittell PC, 1997: Aortic dissection: diagnosis and management. In Brown DL (ed): Cardiac Intensive Care. Philadelphia, WB Saunders

Stenson LG, 1997: New and future approaches for spinal cord protection. Semin Thorac Cardiovasc Surg 9:206

Stone C, Borst H, 1997: Dissecting aortic aneurysm. In Edmunds HL Jr (ed): Cardiac Surgery in the Adult. New York, McGraw-Hill

Vogt PR, Brunner-LaRocca HP, Carrel T, et al., 1998: Cryopreserved arterial allografts in the treatment of major vascular infection: A comparison with conventional surgical techniques. J Thorac Cardiovasc Surg 116:965

Wheat MW, 1987: Acute dissection of the aorta. In McGoon DC (ed): Cardiac Surgery, ed. 2. Philadelphia, FA Davis

Wolfe WG, Moran JF, 1981: Dissecting Aneurysms. In Gay WA (ed): Cardiovascular Surgery (Goldsmith Practice of Surgery, rev. ed.). Philadelphia, Harper & Row

Yamashita C, Okada M, Yoshimura T, et al., 1998: Impact of retrograde cerebral perfusion with posterolateral thoracotomy on distal arch aneurysm repair. Ann Thorac Surg 65:955

Yun KL, Miller DC, 1997: Ascending aortic aneurysm and aortic valve disease: What is the most optimal surgical technique? Semin Thorac Cardiovasc Surg 9:233

18

Surgical Treatment of Cardiac Rhythm Disorders

Cardiac arrhythmias are categorized as bradyarrhythmias or tachyarrhythmias. Persistent or recurring symptomatic bradycardia is treated primarily with permanent pacing. Pacemakers are discussed in detail in Chapter 20, Permanent Pacemakers and Implantable Cardioverter-Defibrillators. Tachyarrhythmias most commonly are treated with antiarrhythmic medications, radiofrequency ablation, or antitachycardia devices. Occasionally, surgical procedures are performed for tachyarrhythmias; these procedures are the focus of discussion in this chapter.

▶ Pathogenesis of Tachyarrhythmias

Most recurrent arrhythmias in chronic heart disease are thought to arise due to a *reentrant mechanism* (Grant & Whalley, 1998). Normally, an impulse originating in the sinus node is transmitted to all cardiac cells and is extinguished when all cells have been depolarized and are completely refractory (Zipes, 1997a). The substrate for reentry exists when there is an area of unidirectional block and slow conduction through an alternate pathway. Retrograde conduction through the region of unidirectional block can initiate a continuous, circuit-like electrical wavefront, or reentry. Reentrant tachyarrhythmias almost always occur secondary to underlying cardiac disease or abnormality. Patients who have the substrate for reentrant tachyarrhythmias are likely to experience recurrent arrhythmic episodes, which in some cases may be associated with syncope or sudden cardiac death.

Although many tachyarrhythmias result from reentry, some tachyarrhythmias are presumed to arise from an *automatic mechanism*. In other words, they occur due to enhanced spontaneous depolarization of normally latent automatic cardiac cells. Determination of arrhythmogenesis is somewhat presumptive because current diagnostic modalities cannot unequivocally define the etiologic mechanism of most clinically occurring arrhythmias (Zipes, 1997a).

▶ Treatment of Tachyarrhythmias

Treatment of supraventricular and ventricular tachyarrhythmias consists of (1) pharmacologic antiarrhythmic agents, (2) catheter ablation therapy, (3) antitachycardia devices, and (4) surgical therapy. Frequently, a combination of therapies is necessary. Supraventricular tachycardia (SVT) and some forms of ventricular tachycardia (VT) usually are treated with antiarrhythmic medications or radiofrequency catheter ablation. Ventricular tachyarrhythmias most often are treated with antiarrhythmic medications or implantable cardioverter-defibrillator (ICD) implantation.

Chronic therapy with antiarrhythmic medications is limited by several factors. All available antiarrhythmic medications have associated adverse effects that make chronic therapy unappealing, particularly in young patients. Many of the agents are proarrhythmic; that is, they can cause arrhythmias. Some significantly depress myocardial contractility. Most important, none has proven completely effective in preventing arrhythmia recurrence. Life-threatening arrhythmias can recur despite predicted success. Although antiarrhythmic medications often are the initial mode of therapy, many patients experience breakthrough arrhythmias despite chronic medication therapy or are unable to tolerate an effective agent's adverse effects. Also, many drugs are contraindicated during pregnancy, thus limiting their usefulness in women of childbearing years.

Catheter ablation and antitachycardia devices are the most rapidly expanding forms of therapy. Catheter ablation consists of using radiofrequency delivered through an intracardiac catheter to eradicate arrhythmogenic tissue. The procedure is curative and, in contrast to surgical intervention, does not necessitate general anesthesia, sternotomy, or cardiopulmonary bypass. Catheter ablation techniques are effective in eradicating reentrant pathways responsible for most forms of supraventricular tachyarrhythmias, specifically atrioventricular (AV) nodal reentrant pathways and anomalous atrial-ventricular connections associated with Wolff-Parkinson-White (WPW) syndrome.

Radiofrequency ablation of the AV node sometimes is used to treat atrial fibrillation in combination with implantation of a single-chamber (patients with chronic atrial fibrillation) or dual-chamber (patients with paroxysmal atrial fibrillation) pacemaker (Kay et al., 1998). Also, techniques for delivering radiofrequency current to the left or right atrium to ablate atrial fibrillation are under investigation. Catheter ablation also is useful for eradication of some forms of VT. It has proven most effective for reentrant VT in patients with nonischemic cardiomyopathy and for monomorphic VT in patients with otherwise structurally normal hearts (Tchou, 1998). Radiofrequency ablation is discussed further in Chapter 4, Cardiac Rhythm Disorders.

Transvenous antitachycardia devices are used commonly in the treatment of patients with ventricular tachyarrhythmias. Current ICDs have increased applicability because they are multiprogrammable in the therapies they offer and are capable of sophisticated electrocardiographic monitoring. All current devices have the ability to defibrillate, cardiovert, and provide antitachycardia and antibradycardia pacing. Indications for implantation of an antitachycardia device include (1) cardiac arrest not due to a reversible cause; (2) spontaneous sustained VT; (3) syncope of undetermined origin with clinically relevant, hemodynamically significant sustained VT or ventricular fibrillation (VF) induced at electrophysiologic study when drug therapy is ineffective, not tolerated, or not preferred; and (4) nonsustained VT with coronary artery disease, prior myocardial infarction, left ventricular dysfunction, and inducible VF or sustained VT at electrophysiologic study that is not suppressed by a class I antiarrhythmic drug (Gregoratos et al., 1998). ICDs are discussed further in Chapter 20, Permanent Pacemakers and Implantable Cardioverter-Defibrillators.

▶ Surgical Therapy

Indications for surgical treatment of tachyarrhythmias have been reduced substantially by the development of effective catheter ablation techniques and programmable transvenous pacemakers/ICD devices. Today, cardiac operations to eradicate tachyarrhythmias are per-

formed infrequently and surgeons with expertise in arrhythmia surgery are available only in a few centers.

The objective of surgical treatment is to excise, isolate, or interrupt cardiac tissue responsible for the initiation, maintenance, or propagation of the tachycardia while preserving or improving myocardial function (Zipes, 1997b). Surgical techniques developed for the treatment of tachyarrhythmias include (1) intraoperative mapping to localize reentrant pathways or arrhythmogenic foci, (2) cryoablation (ie, direct application of an extremely cold [−60°C] probe to arrhythmogenic tissue to destroy it), (3) strategically placed incisions to interrupt reentrant pathways, and (4) surgical excision of arrhythmogenic tissue.

Supraventricular Tachyarrhythmias

Reentrant SVT is categorized according to location of the reentrant pathway. Atrial-ventricular reentry signifies the presence of anomalous, electrically active tissue extending between atrium and ventricle and bypassing normal conduction through the AV node. AV nodal reentry occurs due to a reentrant pathway within the AV node or perinodal tissue. Atrial reentry tachycardia is caused by a reentrant pathway in atrial muscle. Although surgical therapies exist to eradicate several reentrant forms of SVT, they are performed only rarely because of the increasingly successful application of radiofrequency catheter ablation techniques (Guiraudon, 1996). Currently, surgical treatment for SVT is confined essentially to treatment of atrial fibrillation and for atrial-ventricular or AV nodal reentry when catheter ablation is unsuccessful.

Atrial-Ventricular Reentry Tachyarrhythmias

Atrial-ventricular reentrant tachycardia occurs in patients with WPW syndrome because of the existence of an anomalous conduction pathway. Those affected have accessory atrial-ventricular pathways, also called Kent bundles, that are present from birth and that may clinically manifest at any time. The Kent bundle consists of a band of myocardium, electrically similar to atrial tissue, that is positioned such that it abnormally connects atrial and ventricular myocardium (Sabatine et al., 1998). The anomalous atrial-ventricular pathway usually is categorized according to its anatomic location in the heart at the level of the AV groove (ie, left free wall, right free wall, posterior septum, or anterior septum) (Ferguson & Cox, 1996a) (Fig. 18-1). Most common is a left posterior free wall Kent bundle, and some patients have more than one accessory pathway.

Intermittent or continuous conduction through the accessory pathway can occur antegrade only, retrograde only, or, in some patients, in both an antegrade and retrograde fashion. Because the AV node is bypassed, paroxysmal atrial tachycardia or atrial fibrillation with a rapid ventricular response rate can occur and produce significant hemodynamic compromise. Radiofrequency catheter ablation successfully eradicates reentrant atrial-

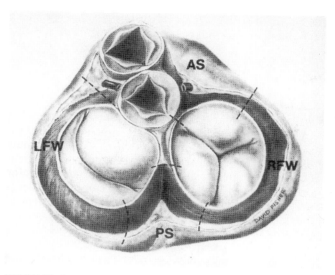

FIGURE 18-1. The heart is sectioned at the AV junction; dotted lines indicate the borders of the four anatomic regions of the coronary sulcus in which Kent bundles may be located: AS, anteroseptal space; RFW, right free wall; PS, posteroseptal space; LFW, left free wall. (Holman WL, Kirklin JK, Epstein AE, et al. 1992: Wolff-Parkinson-White syndrome. J Thorac Cardiovasc Surg 104:804)

ventricular arrhythmias associated with WPW syndrome. It has largely replaced surgical intervention except for the occasional patient in whom ablation is unsuccessful or who is having concomitant cardiac surgery for another reason (Zipes, 1997b).

Surgical division of an anomalous pathway in a patient with WPW syndrome was first performed successfully by Will Sealy in 1968 (Cobb et al., 1968). One of two surgical approaches may be used to eradicate accessory atrial-ventricular pathways. The endocardial technique is designed to divide the ventricular end of the accessory pathway and the epicardial technique is directed toward the atrial end of the pathway (Ferguson & Cox, 1997).

The endocardial technique can be used for accessory pathways in all locations. It is performed through a median sternotomy incision and using cardiopulmonary bypass with aortic and bicaval cannulation. An intraoperative mapping procedure is performed to identify the exact location of the abnormal AV connection and to determine if additional accessory pathways exist that were not identified by the preoperative electrophysiologic study (Lowe, 1997). Intraoperative mapping is important because it is more precise than preoperative programmed electrical stimulation. After the procedure, a postoperative electrophysiologic study is performed to confirm successful arrhythmia eradication.

The epicardial approach can be performed when the pathway is localized to the right or left free wall or to the posterior septal area. It does not necessitate the inducement of hypothermic, cardioplegic arrest and, for right free wall or posterior septal pathways, sometimes can be performed without cardiopulmonary bypass. Surgical division of an anomalous atrial-ventricular pathway is almost universally successful in eradicating the arrhythmia, and the operative mortality risk with either the endocardial or epicardial technique is 0% to 0.5% (Ferguson & Cox, 1997).

Atrioventricular Nodal Reentry Tachyarrhythmias

The electrophysiologic substrate for *AV nodal reentrant tachycardia* is the presence of dual AV conduction pathways, one fast and one slow, through the AV node or perinodal tissues (Ferguson & Cox, 1996a). Most common is so-called "slow-fast AV nodal reentry tachycardia" in which antegrade conduction of a premature atrial impulse blocks in the fast pathway, alternatively propagates antegrade through the slow pathway, and returns retrograde through the fast pathway (Prystowsky, 1997; Zipes, 1997a).

Although catheter ablation is the preferred interventional technique, AV nodal reentry tachycardia may be treated with surgical therapy in patients in whom catheter ablation is unsuccessful. The objective is to interrupt one of the two conduction pathways through the AV node while leaving the other conduction pathway intact (Ferguson & Cox, 1997). *Perinodal cryosurgical ablation* is performed by application of a cryoprobe to atrial tissue immediately adjacent to the AV node to ablate arrhythmogenic tissue (Cox et al., 1990) (Fig. 18-2). The cryolesions eliminate the reentrant pathway while preserving antegrade AV conduction. Heart block is a potential complication.

Atrial Reentry Tachyarrhythmias

Atrial fibrillation, an *atrial reentry tachyarrhythmia*, is the most common clinically occurring arrhythmia. It is present in 0.4% of the general population, in 10% of people older than 60 years of age, in 30% of people with idiopathic cardiomyopathy, and in approximately 60% of patients who undergo surgery for mitral valve disease (Sundt & Cox, 1998). Atrial fibrillation is thought to be caused by multiple reentrant circuits that may be simultaneously active, precluding synchronous activation of enough atrial myocardium to generate an identifiable P wave (Cox et al., 1991).

Pharmacologic therapy or electric cardioversion often fails to restore sustained sinus rhythm. Although antiarrhythmic medications may control the ventricular rate, many patients continue to experience symptoms from the arrhythmia. In addition, atrial fibrillation imposes an increased risk for cerebral vascular accident due to embolization of thrombus from the left atrium and may decrease cardiac output 10% to 40% because of loss of the atrial contribution to ventricular filling (Sundt & Cox, 1998; Repique et al., 1992).

The *Maze procedure*, developed by Cox and associates, may be performed in selected patients with paroxysmal atrial flutter/fibrillation or chronic atrial fibrillation. Indications for the procedure include arrhythmia intolerance despite the maximal amount of tolerable drug therapy or a documented cerebral thromboem-

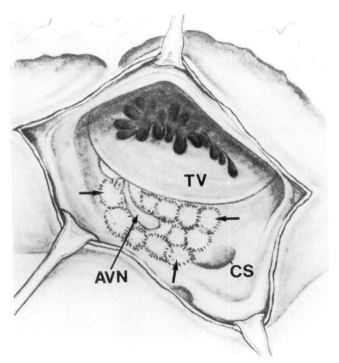

FIGURE 18-2. Cryoablation of AV nodal reentrant tachycardia. Drawing demonstrates surgical exposure through right atriotomy incision with patient's head to left. TV, tricuspid valve; CS, coronary sinus; AVN, region of AV node; short arrows point to several of the overlapping 3-mm cryolesions placed in the perinodal region of the atrial septum. (Adapted from Cox JL, Ferguson B, Lindsay BD, Cain ME, 1990: Perinodal cryosurgery for atrioventricular node reentry tachycardia in 23 patients. J Thorac Cardiovasc Surg 99:446)

bolism (Cox, 1995). It also may be performed in selected patients who require cardiac surgery for another reason, such as mitral valve repair or replacement in patients with chronic atrial fibrillation, and atrial septal defect repair in adults with a history suggestive of paroxysmal atrial fibrillation or flutter (Sundt & Cox, 1998).

First performed in 1987, the Maze procedure has been modified subsequently by Cox and associates to improve operative results. At present, the Maze III procedure represents the state-of-the-art surgical procedure for atrial fibrillation (Ferguson & Cox, 1996b). It is performed through a median sternotomy incision and using cardiopulmonary bypass with cardioplegia and a period of aortic cross-clamping. A series of carefully located atrial incisions and cryolesions prevents a critical mass of contiguous atrial tissue from sustaining atrial fibrillation and allows sinus impulses to activate the entire atrial myocardium. The procedure thus creates a "maze" of electrical propagation roots involving the entire atrial myocardium with only one side of entrance (the sinus node) and one side of exit (the AV node) (Lowe, 1997) (Fig. 18-3). The results reported by Cox and associates demonstrate successful control of atrial flutter and fibrillation in 100% of patients (93% of whom require no antiarrhythmic medications) and restoration of AV syn-

chrony in all patients (two thirds without insertion of a dual-chamber pacemaker) (Sundt & Cox, 1998).

Ventricular Tachyarrhythmias

Ventricular tachyarrhythmias most often occur in patients with coronary artery disease and significant left ventricular dysfunction. Malignant ventricular arrhythmias (ie, VT and VF) often are lethal. Approximately 400,000 Americans die each year secondary to ventricular tachyarrhythmias; sudden cardiac death accounts for more lives lost than all kinds of cancer combined (Cleveland & Harken, 1998). Patients who have experienced either cardiac arrest or an episode of VT with syncope have a 22% to 30% risk of significant arrhythmia recurrence within 1 year (Gartman et al., 1990).

In a limited number of patients, ventricular tachyarrhythmias are ischemia mediated; that is, they occur secondary to myocardial ischemia. Typically, the patient has anginal symptoms as well as the arrhythmia. For patients who experience VT during ischemia, coronary artery revascularization as a primary therapeutic approach may be recommended. It is most useful in patients with coronary artery disease resuscitated from sudden cardiac death who have no inducible arrhythmias at electrophysiologic study (Zipes, 1997b).

More often, ventricular arrhythmias are scar mediated; that is, they occur because of a reentrant pathway in the subendocardial borders of infarcted myocardium. The focus of VT commonly resides in the periphery of a prior MI (eg, at the rim of a postinfarction left ventricular aneurysm), where the border zone between scar and normal muscle manifests electrical instability (Elefteriades et al., 1996). Pharmacologic therapy for scar-mediated tachyarrhythmias is limited by the ineffectiveness and, in fact, proarrhythmic properties of most conventional antiarrhythmic medications and the frequency of intolerable side effects produced by effective agents. Conventional antiarrhythmic drug therapy successfully controls life-threatening arrhythmias in only 20% to 50% of patients (DeMaio, 1991).

In contrast to ischemia-mediated arrhythmias, coronary artery revascularization does not prevent recurrence of arrhythmias caused by the abnormal electrophysiologic properties of endocardial scar. Left ventricular aneurysmectomy as a means of eradicating arrhythmogenic scar tissue also is ineffective. Current treatment of scar-mediated tachycardia most often includes (1) implantation of an antitachycardia device (ie, an ICD), (2) antiarrhythmic medications, or (3) a combination of both therapies. However, in carefully selected patients with scar-mediated ventricular arrhythmias and a mappable morphology, surgical arrhythmia eradication may be performed. The therapies differ in that procedures to eradicate arrhythmogenic tissue are designed to eliminate arrhythmia recurrence, whereas ICDs do not prevent recurrence but rather treat the arrhythmia each time it occurs.

Surgical procedures to eradicate arrhythmogenic tissue in the ventricle began in the late 1970s with introduc-

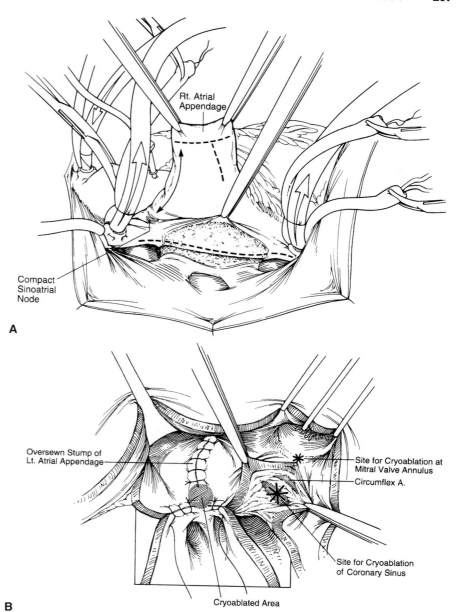

FIGURE 18-3. Intraoperative views demonstrating incisions and cryolesions used in the Maze III operation. **(A)** In this view, dashed lines represent right atrial incisions for amputating the right atrial appendage, incising the free wall laterally and opening the lateral wall of the right atrium immediately above and parallel to the septum. **(B)** This view demonstrates oversewn stump of the left atrial appendage, which has been amputated, a cryoblated area in the tissue between the incision lines, and cryoablation sites at the mitral valve annulus and coronary sinus. (Sundt TM, Cox JL, 1998: Maze III procedure for atrial fibrillation. In Kaiser LR, Kron IL, Spray TL (eds): Mastery of Cardiothoracic Surgery, pp. 532, 536. Philadelphia, Lippincott Williams & Wilkins)

tion of the encircling endocardial ventriculotomy by Guiraudon and associates and endocardial resection by Josephson and associates (Elefteriades et al., 1990). Encircling endocardial ventriculotomy is a procedure in which infarcted and bordering endocardium is excluded from electrical continuity with normal myocardium through an incision made perpendicular to the endocardial surface (Geha & Lee, 1996). The procedure is no longer in common use. Endocardial resection is the surgical excision of arrhythmogenic endocardial scar. Moran and associates refined endocardial resection, using epicardial and endocardial mapping to direct performance of an extended endocardial resection, in which not only the localized area of arrhythmogenesis but all visible fibrotic endocardium is removed (Moran et al., 1982).

Map-directed endocardial resection is the surgical procedure most commonly performed for eradication of ventricular arrhythmias. Endocardial resection is best suited to patients with a discrete anterior aneurysm, fairly good ventricular function, and frequent episodes of VT due to a mappable morphology. Before operation, coronary angiography and left ventriculography are performed to identify coronary artery lesions and evaluate left ventricular function.

The operation is performed through a median sternotomy incision. With the patient on cardiopulmonary bypass and at normothermic temperature, VT is induced and mapping is performed to identify arrhythmogenic foci. Normothermia is maintained during induction of VT because the arrhythmia often cannot be induced in a hypothermic heart (Geha & Lee, 1996). Intraoperative mapping is performed by sampling the electrogram at

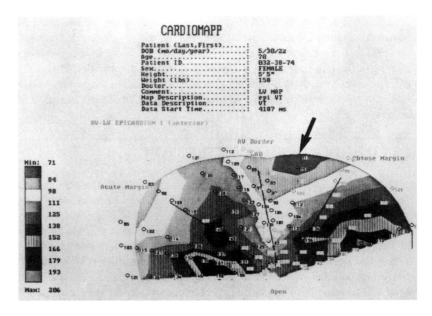

FIGURE 18-4. A computer-generated epicardial map of ventricular tachycardia. The site of earliest activation is the arrhythmogenic focus. (Elefteriades JA, Geha AS, Cohen LS, 1996: Arrhythmia surgery: Postoperative care. In House Officer Guide to ICU Care: Fundamentals of Management of the Heart and Lungs, p. 168. Philadelphia, Lippincott-Raven)

many different sites, often with computer analysis of the data; the area of earliest activation on the electrogram during VT locates the arrhythmogenic focus, which is morphologically indistinguishable by any other means (Elefteriades et al., 1996) (Fig. 18-4). When intraoperative mapping is completed, hypothermia is induced, the aorta is cross-clamped, and cardioplegia is administered. After resecting the ventricular aneurysm, and guided by the results of mapping, the surgeon resects the subendocardial tissue identified as responsible for arrhythmogenesis (Fig. 18-5). Often coronary artery bypass grafting is performed with endocardial resection.

Endocardial resection is curative if successful but carries a significant operative mortality risk, particularly in patients with impaired left ventricular function. The procedure remains useful in carefully selected situations

but is performed in only a few centers, by cardiothoracic surgeons with a special interest and expertise in arrhythmia surgery. In such patients, the risk of operative death is not prohibitive and long-term freedom from arrhythmia recurrence has been achieved.

Sometimes arrhythmogenic scar is located on the inferior wall of the left ventricle and involves portions of the papillary muscles. If the reentrant circuit is mapped to the deep septum or the base of a papillary muscle, cryoablation is recommended (Cleveland & Harken, 1998) (Fig. 18-6). Cryoablation is a useful adjunct because it destroys electrically active tissue while leaving structural elements intact (DeMaio, 1991).

Endocardial resection is unsuited to patients with VF, which, by virtue of its constant chaotic electrical activity, is not mappable (Elefteriades et al., 1996). Endocar-

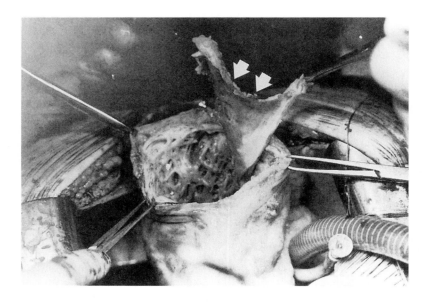

FIGURE 18-5. Intraoperative photograph demonstrating endocardial resection. The aneurysmal segment of the left ventricular wall has been resected; endocardial tissue is being removed from the left ventricular chamber (*arrows*). (Geha AS, Lee JH, 1996: Surgery for ventricular tachyarrhythmias. In Baue AE, Geha AS, Hammond GL, et al. [eds]: Glenn's Thoracic and Cardiovascular Surgery, ed. 6, p. 2170. Stamford, CT, Appleton & Lange. Reproduced with permission of the McGraw-Hill Companies)

left ventricular dysfunction with an ejection fraction less than 20%, and no discrete aneurysm.

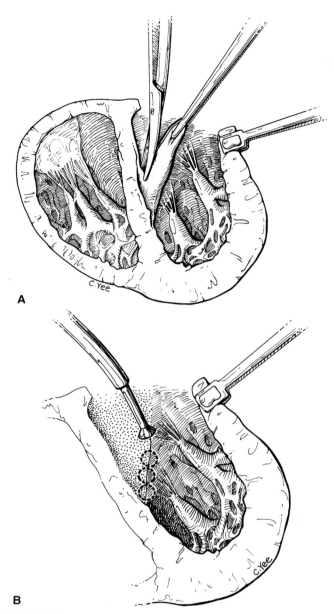

FIGURE 18-6. (A) Coronal section of the heart demonstrating excision of a thin layer of endocardial scar from the left side of the septum. **(B)** After the excision, overlapping cryolesions are applied at the perimeter of the target area to isolate potential deep septal foci of ventricular tachycardia. (Mickleborough LL, Takagi Y, Ohashi M, 1998: Left ventricular aneurysm: Linear closure. In Kaiser LR, Kron IL, Spray TL [eds]: Mastery of Cardiothoracic Surgery, p. 442. Philadelphia, Lippincott Williams & Wilkins)

dial resection also is not appropriate for patients with global left ventricular dysfunction, polymorphic VT, or extensive scar that involves the papillary muscles or mitral valve annulus. In such patients, a combination of pharmacologic antiarrhythmic therapy and ICD implantation is preferable. Cardiac transplantation may be considered in patients with noninducible VT or VF, global

REFERENCES

Cleveland JC, Harken AH, 1998: Rational strategies in the surgical therapy of malignant ventricular tachyarrhythmias. In Kaiser LR, Kron IL, Spray TL (eds): Mastery of Cardiothoracic Surgery. Philadelphia, Lippincott Williams & Wilkins

Cobb FR, Blumenschein SD, Sealy WS, et al., 1968: Successful surgical interruption of the bundle of Kent in a patient with Wolff-Parkinson-White syndrome. Circulation 38:1018

Cox JL, 1995: The surgical management of arrhythmias. In Sabiston DC Jr, Spencer FC (eds): Surgery of the Chest, ed. 6. Philadelphia, WB Saunders

Cox JL, Ferguson TB, Lindsay BD, Cain ME, 1990: Perinodal cryosurgery for atrioventricular node reentry tachycardia in 23 patients. J Thorac Cardiovasc Surg 99:440

Cox JL, Schuessler RB, Boineau JP, 1991: The surgical treatment of atrial fibrillation (I). J Thorac Cardiovasc Surg 101:402

DeMaio SJ Jr, 1991: Surgical and catheter ablative therapy of ventricular arrhythmias. In Hurst JW (ed): Current Therapy in Cardiovascular Disease, ed. 3. Philadelphia, BC Decker

Elefteriades JA, Biblo LA, Batsford WP, et al., 1990: Evolving patterns in the surgical treatment of malignant ventricular arrhythmias. Ann Thorac Surg 49:94

Elefteriades JA, Geha AS, Cohen LS, 1996: Arrhythmia surgery: Postoperative care. In House Officer Guide to ICU Care: Fundamentals of Management of the Heart and Lungs, ed. 2. Philadelphia, Lippincott-Raven

Ferguson TB, Cox JL, 1996a: Surgery for supraventricular arrhythmias. In Baue AE, Geha AS, Hammond GL, et al. (eds): Glenn's Thoracic and Cardiovascular Surgery, ed. 6. Stamford, CT, Appleton & Lange

Ferguson TB, Cox JL, 1996b: Arrhythmia surgery. Coron Artery Dis 7:36

Ferguson TB, Cox JL, 1997: Surgical treatment of arrhythmias. In Edmunds LH Jr (ed): Cardiac Surgery in the Adult. New York, McGraw-Hill

Gartman DM, Bardy GH, Allen MD, et al., 1990: Short-term morbidity and mortality of implantation of automatic implantable cardioverter defibrillator. J Thorac Cardiovasc Surg 100:353

Geha AS, Lee JH, 1996: Surgery for ventricular tachyarrhythmias. In Baue AE, Geha AS, Hammond GL, et al. (eds): Glenn's Thoracic and Cardiovascular Surgery, ed. 6. Stamford, CT, Appleton & Lange

Grant AO, Whalley DW, 1998: Mechanisms of cardiac arrhythmias. In Topol EJ (ed): Comprehensive Cardiovascular Medicine. Philadelphia, Lippincott Williams & Wilkins

Gregoratos G, Cheitlin MD, Conill A, et al., 1998: ACC/AHA guidelines for implantation of cardiac pacemakers and antiarrhythmia devices: A report of the American College of Cardiology/American Heart Association Task Force on Practice Guidelines (Committee on Pacemaker Implantation). J Am Coll Cardiol 31:1175

Guiraudon GM, Klein GJ, Yee R, Guiraudon CM, 1996: Surgery for supraventricular tachycardia. Arch Mal Coeur Vaiss 89:123

Kay GN, Ellenbogen KA, Giudici M, et al., 1998: The Ablate and Pace Trial: A prospective study of catheter ablation of the AV conduction system and permanent pacemaker implantation for the treatment of atrial fibrillation. Journal of Interventional Cardiac Electrophysiology 2:121

Lowe JE, 1997: Arrhythmia surgery: Then and now. Pacing Clin Electrophysiol 20:585

Moran JM, Kehoe RF, Loeb JM, et al., 1982: Extended endocardial resection for the treatment of ventricular tachycardia and ventricular fibrillation. Ann Thorac Surg 34:538

Prystowsky EN, 1997: Atrioventricular node reentry: Physiology and radiofrequency ablation. Pacing Clin Electrophysiol 20:552

Repique LJ, Shah SM, Marais GE, 1992: Atrial fibrillation 1992: Management strategies in flux. Chest 101:1095

Sabatine MS, Antman EM, Ganz LI, et al., 1998: Mechanisms of cardiac arrhythmias. In Lilly LS (ed): Pathophysiology of Heart Disease, ed. 2. Baltimore, Williams & Wilkins

Sundt TM, Cox JL, 1998: Maze III procedure for atrial fibrillation. In Kaiser LR, Kron IL, Spray TL (eds): Mastery of Cardiothoracic Surgery. Philadelphia, Lippincott Williams & Wilkins

Tchou PJ, 1998: Ventricular tachycardia. In Topol EJ (ed): Comprehensive Cardiovascular Medicine. Philadelphia, Lippincott Williams & Wilkins

Zipes DP, 1997a: Genesis of cardiac arrhythmias: Electrophysiological considerations. In Braunwald E (ed): Heart Disease: A Textbook of Cardiovascular Medicine, ed. 5. Philadelphia, WB Saunders

Zipes DP, 1997b: Management of cardiac arrhythmias: Pharmacological, electrical, and surgical techniques. In Braunwald E (ed): Heart Disease: A Textbook of Cardiovascular Medicine, ed. 5. Philadelphia, WB Saunders

19

Surgical Treatment of Congenital Heart Disease in Adults

Surgical treatment of *congenital heart disease* (CHD) began over 50 years ago with the repair of vascular abnormalities such as patent ductus arteriosus and coarctation of the aorta. With the development of cardiopulmonary bypass in the 1950s, it became possible to repair intracardiac defects as well. Innovative techniques were devised to correct most of the major cardiac deformities. Operative repairs to correct all but the most complex defects have been available since the early 1970s. Today, intraoperative techniques to protect organ function and sophisticated perioperative management allow most repairs to be performed safely during infancy.

Congenital heart surgery in adults is relatively uncommon, comprising only a small percentage of adult operative procedures requiring extracorporeal circulation (cardiopulmonary bypass). Untreated CHD in adults is uncommon because of increased awareness and improved noninvasive diagnostic techniques that result in detection of most defects early in life. Nevertheless, a small percentage of congenital defects do remain untreated until adulthood.

In some cases, an asymptomatic lesion is first diagnosed during a physical examination or diagnostic study in an adult. Although the defect may be asymptomatic at the time of diagnosis, natural history data about CHD reveal that many defects are associated with life-threatening complications or a shortened life expectancy. In other cases, pregnancy or aging may precipitate the onset of symptoms that warrant operative correction of the defect.

Adults with unrepaired congenital heart defects almost always have one of the most common and least complex of the many possible types of cardiac deformities. Most are isolated defects that are associated with ei-

ther (1) a left-to-right shunt, or (2) valvular or vascular obstruction. The discussion in this chapter is limited to surgical treatment of these lesions. Surgical intervention, however, is occasionally required in two other categories of adults with CHD. First, an increasing number of individuals who underwent childhood repair of a congenital lesion now have survived to adulthood. Surgical therapy is occasionally required in these patients to treat a complication of the operative repair. Second, some people with noncorrectable lesions survive to adulthood. Palliative procedures performed during childhood in such patients may require revision.

Surgical issues of concern in adults undergoing either initial operation or reoperation for a congenital cardiac defect include the presence of pulmonary vascular disease, the status of ventricular function, myocardial protection, blood salvage techniques, and the risk of endocarditis (Drinkwater et al., 1998). The spectrum of CHD is discussed in greater depth in Chapter 6, Congenital Heart Disease in Adults.

► Defects With Left-to-Right Shunts

The most common defects associated with left-to-right shunting are atrial septal defect (ASD), ventricular septal defect (VSD), and patent ductus arteriosus (PDA). In all of these defects, left-to-right shunting occurs across the defect because of the differences between systemic (left-sided) vascular resistance and pulmonic (right-sided) vascular resistance. The primary difference between the defects is the level at which shunting occurs: in ASD, the atria; VSD, the ventricles; and PDA, the aorta and pulmonary artery. The degree of shunting is quantified using a ratio that compares the amount of pulmonary blood flow with the amount of systemic blood flow (Qp:Qs) or cardiac output from the right ventricle compared with cardiac output from the left ventricle.

The primary consequence of left-to-right shunting is increased blood flow through the pulmonary vasculature. Congestive heart failure and pulmonary hypertension result and may progress to pulmonary vascular obstruction, a condition characterized by an irreversible increase in pulmonary vascular resistance. In its most severe form, pulmonary arterial pressure eventually may exceed systemic pressure, producing a reversal in direction of shunting. When right-to-left shunting secondary to increased pulmonary vascular resistance replaces left-to-right shunting, Eisenmenger's syndrome is said to exist. The development of Eisenmenger's syndrome precludes surgical correction of the defect. In the presence of irreversible pulmonary vascular obstructive disease, correcting the intracardiac defect (ie, obliterating the shunt) would produce severe right-sided heart failure.

Atrial Septal Defect

Atrial septal defects account for 30% to 40% of congenital heart defects in adults (Marelli & Moodie, 1998). Although ASDs may occur at the junction of the superior vena cava (sinus venosus ASD) or at the base of the septum (ostium primum ASD), those that remain unrepaired until adulthood almost always are ostium secundum ASDs, located in the middle of the septum in the region of the fossa ovalis. An ASD is different than a patent foramen ovale, often found incidentally during right heart catheterization, which is usually benign unless right-to-left shunting develops and allows paradoxical passage of emboli into the left atrium (Hillis et al., 1995a).

The direction and amount of blood flow across an ASD depend on the size of the defect and the compliance of the left and right ventricles during diastole (Kopf & Laks, 1996). Common diseases acquired in adulthood (eg, hypertension or ischemic heart disease) may decrease left ventricular compliance and increase left-to-right shunting. Conversely, conditions that decrease right ventricular compliance (eg, right ventricular myocardial infarction or failure) or those that increase pulmonary vascular resistance (eg, pulmonary embolism or pulmonary vascular obstructive disease) may produce significant right-to-left shunting with arterial desaturation. In addition, some right-to-left shunting occurs even when the predominant direction of shunting is left to right. As a result, venous thrombus may migrate across the septal opening and into the systemic circulation. This phenomenon, known as paradoxical embolism, is an occasional cause of cerebral vascular accidents in young adults.

Many adults with ASDs are asymptomatic, but may complain of easy fatigability and exertional dyspnea (Canobbio, 1995). Because symptoms develop gradually, they may not be recognized as abnormal. Natural history data reveal a shortened life expectancy. The average life span for those with uncorrected ASDs is 50 years, with most patients dying of progressive heart failure (Kopf & Laks, 1996). Typically, an unrepaired ASD causes a gradual decrease in exercise capacity as individuals enter their teens and twenties, with a progressive decline in exercise tolerance over the next 10 to 20 years coincident with deterioration in right ventricular function (Mainwaring & Lamberti, 1998).

Although some patients survive to old age without symptoms, most acquire progressive, disabling symptoms. Chronic congestive heart failure with fluid retention, hepatomegaly, and severe cardiac cachexia can occur in older adults (Kirklin & Barratt-Boyes, 1993a). Atrial arrhythmias, especially atrial fibrillation, also increase in frequency with aging, augmenting the left-to-right shunt and precipitating right ventricular failure (Perloff, 1998). Atrial fibrillation commonly develops by the third or fourth decade and may be present in more than 50% of patients older than 60 years of age (Laks et al., 1997; Schaff & Danielson, 1987).

Atrial septal defect closure is recommended for most patients with defects larger than 1 to 2 cm, particularly when associated with a greater than 1.5:1 left-to-right shunt (Galloway et al., 1995). Even in the absence of symptoms and in patients older than 60 years of age, operative repair is recommended to prevent the development of pulmonary hypertension and right ventricular dysfunction from chronic volume overload (Hillis et al., 1995a). The operation most often is performed through a median sternotomy incision and using cardiopulmonary bypass. Alternatively, a submammary skin incision with sternotomy or a small right anterolateral thoracotomy with femoral cardiopulmonary bypass cannulation may be used if desired for cosmetic reasons (Laks et al., 1997).

After application of a cross-clamp to the aorta and administration of cardioplegic solution, an incision is made in the right atrium to expose the interseptal defect and significant intracardiac structures. ASDs often are closed by direct suturing of the defect in children. In adults, the defect more often is patched with a piece of autogenous pericardium. Great care is taken after the repair to remove any air from the left side of the heart. The absence of air is then confirmed with transesophageal echocardiography before removing the aortic cross-clamp.

When a sinus venosus ASD is present, it often is associated with partial anomalous pulmonary venous drainage. That is, one or both right pulmonary veins empties venous (oxygenated) blood from the right lung into the right atrium instead of the left atrium. Thus, oxygenated blood enters the right side of the heart and once again circulates through the pulmonary vessels. If anomalous pulmonary veins are present, ASD repair must include baffling of the pericardial patch to redirect blood flow from anomalous veins into the left atrium (Fig. 19-1). Failure to revise anomalous drainage at the time of ASD repair results in a residual left-to-right shunt and the continued potential for right ventricular failure and pulmonary hypertension.

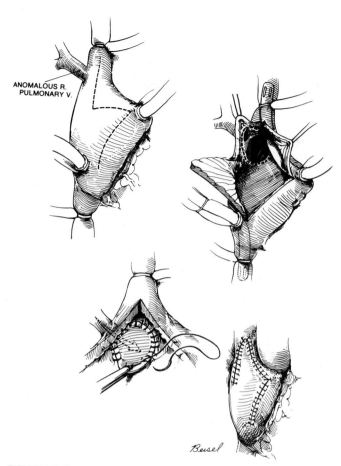

FIGURE 19-1. Repair of sinus venosus ASD with partial anomalous pulmonary venous connection. After initiating cardiopulmonary bypass, right atrium is opened (*top left*), revealing sinus venosus defect and orifice of anomalous right pulmonary vein (*top right*). Pericardial patch is placed to close defect and redirect flow from anomalous vein into the left atrium behind the patch (*lower left*). Incision in right atrial wall and superior vena cava is closed (*lower right*). (Waldhausen JA, Pierce WS, 1985: Congenital heart disease. In Johnson's Surgery of the Chest, ed. 5, p. 331. Chicago, Year Book)

Patients who undergo ASD repair are usually young, otherwise healthy adults. If pulmonary vascular resistance is normal, the operation is associated with a less than 1% mortality rate and minimal morbidity (Galloway et al., 1995). Except for temporary limitations imposed by the sternotomy, patients usually can return to previous activities within weeks of the operation.

Repair of isolated, ostium secundum ASDs before 25 years of age is followed by long-term survival similar to that of an age- and sex-matched control population; even in middle-aged and elderly patients, surgical repair of ASDs appears to improve longevity and reduce functional limitations due to heart failure (Kaplan & Perloff, 1998). In 70% of patients with preoperative arrhythmias, the abnormal rhythm persists, and in 10% to 25% of patients, new-onset atrial arrhythmias develop despite the repair (Marelli & Moodie, 1998). Sinus node dys-

function is common after repair of a sinus venosus ASD and complete heart block requiring permanent pacemaker implantation occasionally occurs after repair of an ostium primum defect (Hillis et al., 1995a).

Ventricular Septal Defect

A defect in the ventricular septum also may cause a left-to-right shunt. *Ventricular septal defects* are described according to their location in one of the four components of the septum: the membranous septum and three muscular components—the inlet septum, the apical (trabecular) septum, or the outlet (infundibular) septum. Over 80% of all congenital VSDs are categorized as perimembranous because the margins of the defect include the membranous septum or its remnant; the VSD may extend into the inlet, apical or outlet septum (Tchervenkov & Shum-Tim, 1996).

Although VSD is one of the most common congenital lesions, large VSDs in adults are infrequent. It is estimated that 40% of VSDs close spontaneously during infancy and 60% close by 5 years of age (Warnes et al., 1991). Those VSDs that remain open and associated with a significant shunt usually produce symptomatic congestive heart failure that prompts operative repair during childhood. Adults with small VSDs usually are asymptomatic, are unlikely to aquire pulmonary vascular obstructive disease, and may not require surgical repair; they do, however, have an increased risk of infective endocarditis and require antibiotic prophylaxis (Hillis et al., 1995b). In patients with large VSDs, the probability of development of pulmonary vascular disease is approximately 50% by the third decade of life, and unoperated patients eventually die of complications of Eisenmenger's syndrome (Laks et al., 1997). Infective endocarditis also is a major risk in persons with significant ventricular shunting, especially when a high-velocity jet of blood causes a traumatic lesion on the right ventricular endocardium (Hillis et al., 1995b).

Surgical repair is recommended for VSDs associated with greater than 1.5:1 left-to-right shunting to prevent progressive heart failure and irreversible pulmonary vascular obstructive disease. It is performed using a median sternotomy approach and cardiopulmonary bypass. Most defects can be repaired through an incision in the right atrium, thus avoiding the damaging effect of an incision in the ventricle (Fig. 19-2). However, a right ventriculotomy may be necessary for closure of VSDs in certain locations. A prosthetic patch almost always is used to close the defect. Pulmonary artery pressure is monitored in the early postoperative period, and acute pulmonary hypertension is treated with nitroglycerin or prostaglandin E_1 infusion, or nitric oxide inhalation (Laks et al., 1997).

Rhythm disturbances, specifically conduction abnormalities and tachyarrhythmias, sometimes occur after VSD repair. Right bundle branch block develops in 30% to 60% of patients, first-degree atrioventricular block in approximately 10%, nonsustained ventricular tachycardia in 5%, complete heart block in 1% to 3%, and, for unexplained reasons, sudden cardiac death occurs in 2%

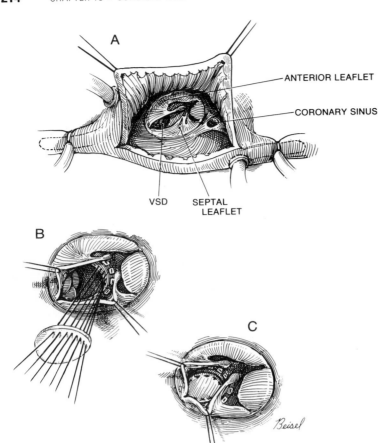

Beisel

FIGURE 19-2. Transatrial repair of a perimembranous VSD. **(A)** After establishing cardiopulmonary bypass and inserting a left ventricular vent, cardioplegia is administered and the right atrium is opened widely. The perimembranous VSD is exposed by retracting the septal leaflet of the tricuspid valve. **(B, C)** A patch is sutured into place to close the VSD. (Waldhausen JA, 1985: Congenital heart disease. In Johnson's Surgery of the Chest, ed. 5, p. 341. Chicago, Year Book)

of patients (Marelli & Moodie, 1998). Continuation of antibiotic prophylaxis against infective endocarditis is recommended after VSD closure because a small, hemodynamically insignificant, residual VSD persists in up to 25% of patients (Hillis et al., 1995b; Warnes et al., 1991). In patients with residual areas of turbulent flow, the risk of endocarditis continues despite surgical correction of a congenital heart defect (McNamara, 1989).

Adults with large VSDs and Eisenmenger's syndrome may require heart-lung transplantation or lung transplantation with VSD repair (Laks et al., 1997). These procedures are discussed in Chapter 31, Heart, Lung, and Heart-Lung Transplantation. Repair of acquired VSDs that develop secondary to myocardial infarction is discussed in Chapter 15, Surgical Treatment of Coronary Artery Disease.

Patent Ductus Arteriosus

Patent ductus arteriosus is a vascular connection between the descending thoracic aorta and the pulmonary artery. Its presence represents a failure of the fetal ductus arteriosus to close at or shortly after birth. A left-to-right shunt occurs because of the gradient between systemic pressure in the aorta and the much lower pulmonary artery pressure. The degree of shunting de-

pends on the size of the ductal lumen and the resistance in the pulmonary vascular bed (Canobbio, 1995). Typically, pulmonary blood flow is increased, producing symptoms of congestive heart failure that prompt surgical repair in infancy or childhood.

Even small PDAs without associated symptoms usually are detected during childhood because of the characteristic, continuous murmur produced by left-to-right shunting throughout the cardiac cycle. The diagnosis can be confirmed by echocardiography; cardiac catheterization is not necessary. Occasionally, a small or medium-sized PDA remains undetected until adulthood. One third of adults with unrepaired PDAs are asymptomatic; exercise intolerance and dyspnea are the most common presenting symptoms (Fisher et al., 1986). Repair is performed regardless of whether symptoms are present because PDAs are known to be associated with a shortened life expectancy. The mortality rate associated with an unrepaired PDA is 1% per year in early adulthood and increases to 2% to 4% by midlife (Laks et al., 1997). Morbidity occurs because of heart failure, pulmonary hypertension, and infective endarteritis, which usually occurs on the pulmonary side of the ductus (Marelli & Moodie, 1998). Aortic aneurysm or dissection secondary to degenerative changes in the ductal tissue also may occur.

Interventional cardiac catheterization techniques have

DEFECTS WITH OUTFLOW OBSTRUCTION **215**

been developed that allow nonsurgical closure of a ductus arteriosus. As a result, PDA closure in adults often can be performed in a cardiac catheterization laboratory using a catheter-deployed occluding device. Transcatheter occlusion is comparable with surgical repair in safety and efficacy; complications include residual shunts, usually detected only by echocardiography, in less than 8% of patients, and device embolization in 2% of patients (Marelli & Moodie, 1998).

Surgical closure of a PDA in an adult usually is performed through a small, left posterior thoracotomy incision. The ductus is clamped and divided and the two segments are closed by direct suture technique (Fig. 19-3). Operative repair of PDA in an adult may be complicated by several features that occur more often than with repair during childhood. These include (1) the frequent presence (21% to 81%) of pulmonary hypertension, (2) a tendency for the ductus to be giant in size, (3) the common occurrence of ductal calcification, and (4) the presence of prior or concurrent infective endarteritis (Fuster et al., 1991). Ductal calcification increases technical difficulty of the repair because the ductus may be torn eas-

ily when manipulated (Myers & Waldhausen, 1991). In patients with demonstrated calcification or in older patients, median sternotomy with cardiopulmonary bypass is recommended to increase the safety of the procedure (Laks et al., 1997).

Operative complications are unusual after PDA repair and the procedure in general is considered curative. However, when the operation is performed in patients with severe, chronic congestive heart failure, death may occur owing to the preexisting cardiomyopathy caused by long-standing volume overload of the left ventricle (Kirklin & Barratt-Boyes, 1993b).

▶ Defects With Outflow Obstruction

The following defects are associated with valvular or vascular obstruction: aortic stenosis, coarctation of the aorta, pulmonic stenosis, and tetralogy of Fallot (TOF). TOF differs from the other three in that, in addition to the obstructive component, right-to-left shunting of blood occurs through an associated intracardiac defect (VSD).

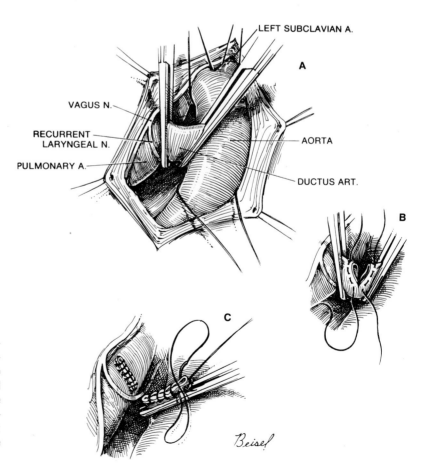

FIGURE 19-3. Surgical division of a patent ductus arteriosus (PDA). **(A)** After exposure of the PDA through a left thoracotomy incision, clamps are applied to the ductus close to the aorta and pulmonary artery. **(B)** The ductus is divided halfway through and partially sutured. **(C)** Each end of the divided ductus is closed with a running mattress suture followed by an over-and-over suture. (Waldhausen JA, 1985: Congenital heart disease. In Johnson's Surgery of the Chest, ed. 5, p. 291. Chicago, Year Book)

Aortic Stenosis

Aortic stenosis includes lesions that obstruct left ventricular outflow at the valvular, subvalvular, or supravalvular level. In adults, aortic stenosis nearly always is due to an abnormality at the valvular level. The most common type of congenitally abnormal aortic valve is one that is bicuspid rather than tricuspid. Bicuspid aortic valves are estimated to occur in 2% of the population (Perloff, 1998). Although a bicuspid aortic valve may remain functionally normal, more often fibrosis and calcification occur with aging, gradually leading to stenosis (Kaplan, 1991). In fact, approximately one half of the cases of isolated calcific aortic stenosis requiring operation in adults are caused by calcification of a bicuspid aortic valve that formerly was functionally normal (Drinkwater et al., 1998).

Congenital aortic valve stenosis usually is progressive. The obstruction to left ventricular outflow causes left ventricular hypertrophy and eventual left-sided heart failure. The mortality rate in untreated patients reaches 60% by 40 years of age, and few patients survive beyond 60 years without serious signs and symptoms (Ungerleider, 1995). A bicuspid aortic valve is also more susceptible to infective endocarditis. Classic symptoms associated with aortic stenosis include dyspnea, angina, and syncope. Ventricular arrhythmias or sudden cardiac death also may occur. The development of symptoms is ominous, signifying a downward course and the likelihood of death within the next several years.

Consequently, the presence of symptoms is an indication for repair or replacement of the stenotic valve. Surgical therapy also may be recommended in asymptomatic patients with a high transvalvular gradient because of an increased propensity for sudden cardiac death. Valve repair or replacement is recommended for symptomatic patients and for those with valvular stenosis and a valve area of less than 0.8 cm² or a mean transvalvular gradient of 50 mm Hg or greater.

Balloon valvotomy has been safely and effectively used to dilate stenotic aortic valves in children and adolescents. The repaired valve, however, has at least the same, if not a greater tendency than a functionally normal bicuspid valve to become thickened, calcified, and stenotic over time, and the patient remains at risk for infective endocarditis (Kaplan & Perloff, 1998). In adults with a stenotic, bicuspid aortic valve, calcification of the valve usually has occurred already. Balloon valvotomy is not recommended in the presence of valvular calcification because of the high incidence of restenosis and the increased likelihood of embolic complications of the procedure.

Aortic stenosis in adults is corrected by surgical replacement of the valve with a prosthesis. Through a median sternotomy incision and using cardiopulmonary bypass, aortic cross-clamping, and cardioplegic arrest, an incision is made in the ascending aorta. The stenotic, native valve is excised and a valvular prosthesis is implanted in its place. Either a mechanical valve or a bioprosthesis may be used.

Mechanical valves are preferable in young adults be-cause they are far more durable than bioprostheses. However, all of the mechanical prostheses require chronic anticoagulation with warfarin sodium. In young women who become pregnant, complex anticoagulant management is required if a mechanical valve is in place. Warfarin crosses the placental barrier and has the potential to cause both bleeding in the fetus and embryopathy (Ginsberg & Hirsh, 1998). Heparin does not cross the placental barrier, but long-term administration can cause osteoporosis in the mother or, less commonly, development of heparin-associated antibodies resulting in thrombosis and thrombocytopenia (Baughman, 1998).

Bioprostheses do not require chronic anticoagulant therapy but are very likely to necessitate reoperation when implanted in a young adult. Pregnant women with bioprosthetic valves have a 35% incidence of accelerated valvular deterioration, presumably because of changes in calcium metabolism during pregnancy (Laks et al., 1997). Other options for aortic valve replacement include the use of an allograft or performance of a Ross procedure, in which the patient's native pulmonary artery root with the pulmonic valve is translocated to the aortic position and a pulmonary allograft is implanted in its place. Aortic valve replacement and the various valvular prostheses are discussed in detail in Chapter 16, Surgical Treatment of Valvular Heart Disease.

Coarctation of the Aorta

Coarctation of the aorta in adults typically consists of a discrete narrowing of the aortic lumen, just distal to the left subclavian artery in the region of the ligamentum arteriosum. In some cases, coarctation remains undetected until adulthood. In others, coarctation repaired during childhood recurs in an adult. The incidence of recurrent coarctation ranges between 5% and 20%, depending on patient age at the time of initial repair, extent of the original coarctation, the reparative technique, and the length of follow-up (Ungerleider, 1998). Coarctation often is associated with a coexisting bicuspid aortic valve; less common coexistent anomalies include obstruction above or below the aortic valve, malformation of the mitral valve apparatus, VSD, and PDA (Marelli & Moodie, 1998).

The presence of a coarcted segment in the aorta causes a series of complex and poorly understood cardiovascular responses designed to maintain needed blood flow to organs below the stricture (Sealy, 1990). Patients have proximal hypertension and a significant gradient in arterial blood pressure between upper and lower extremities. In two thirds of patients with unrepaired coarctation, symptoms of congestive heart failure develop after 40 years of age (Hillis et al., 1995c). By 50 years of age, more than three fourths of patients with unrepaired coarctation have died (Perloff, 1998). Death can occur secondary to left ventricular hypertrophy and failure, premature coronary artery disease, aortic dissection or rupture, stroke (secondary to hypertension), or infective endarteritis.

Because of the potential complications of unrepaired coarctation, surgical correction is undertaken when the condition is diagnosed. In addition to a preoperative aortogram, cardiac catheterization often is performed because of the frequency of associated cardiac defects. Coarctation repair is performed through a left lateral thoracotomy incision. Cardiopulmonary bypass usually is not necessary. The aorta is clamped above and below the site of coarctation while the narrowed segment is removed. In infants, coarctation often is repaired with resection and extended end-to-end anastomosis (Backer et al., 1998). In older children and young adults, the coarcted segment is resected and aortic continuity usually is restored with end-to-end anastomosis of the remaining aortic segments. However, the aorta in adults is less elastic and, particularly in older adults, a prosthetic tube graft may be necessary to replace the resected area of coarctation (Fig. 19-4).

Adults with coarctation usually have well-developed

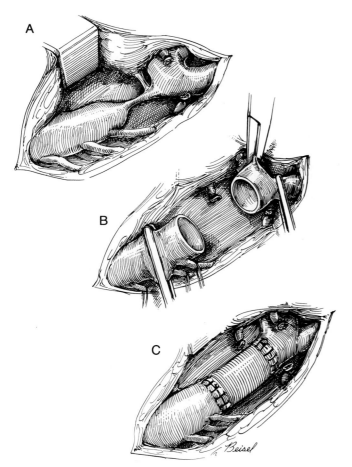

FIGURE 19-4. Surgical repair of coarctation of the aorta using a tubular graft prosthesis. **(A)** The coarctation is exposed through a left lateral thoracotomy incision. **(B)** Clamps are applied to the aorta above and below the area of coarctation and the coarcted segment is excised. **(C)** A tubular prosthetic graft is placed to bridge the defect and is sutured to the aorta in end-to-end fashion. (Waldhausen JA, 1985: Congenital heart disease. In Johnson's Surgery of the Chest, ed. 5, p. 313. Chicago, Year Book)

collateral blood vessels that bypass the narrowed segment to augment perfusion to the distal aorta. Collateral circulation through internal thoracic, scapular, and intercostal branches provides perfusion to the spinal cord during aortic cross-clamping, but the vessels are fragile; great care must be taken during the initial incision and mobilization of the aortic segment to prevent excessive bleeding from these vessels (Drinkwater et al., 1998).

Blood pressure control is of primary importance in postoperative management after coarctation repair. Hypertension occurs despite complete relief of the gradient, secondary initially to increased epinephrine and then to increased norepinephrine secretion (Myers & Waldhausen, 1991). Intravenous agents may be necessary in the early postoperative period to achieve and maintain blood pressure in a desirable range. Coarctation repair does not necessarily produce normalization of systemic blood pressure. Persistent postoperative hypertension can occur, particularly in patients who undergo operation at an older age with a longer duration of preoperative hypertension that results in baroreceptor abnormalities and compliance changes in the walls of major arteries (Perloff, 1997). Fifty percent of adults who undergo coarctation repair after 40 years of age have residual hypertension (Marelli & Moodie, 1998). Thus, many adults continue to require chronic antihypertensive therapy.

In a small percentage of patients undergoing coarctation repair, postoperative arteritis develops in arteries arising from the aorta below the coarctation (Sealy, 1990). This acute regional arteritis may produce abdominal pain, ileus, and, in severe cases, small bowel necrosis in the early postoperative period. Accordingly, a nasogastric tube is placed prophylactically at the time of operation and oral feedings are withheld for at least 24 hours until normal bowel function returns. Despite the presence of well-developed collateral arteries, coarctation repair rarely is complicated by postoperative paraplegia. Ischemic injury to the spinal cord and resultant paraplegia can occur with any operation that necessitates temporary occlusion of blood flow through the descending thoracic aorta. The risk of paraplegia is significantly higher during repair of recurrent coarctation.

Other complications of coarctation repair include restenosis, aneurysm formation, progressive enlargement of the ascending aorta, and infection of the prosthetic graft. Despite operative repair, patients may die prematurely because of associated aortic or mitral valve disease, congestive heart failure, infective endarteritis, or aortic or cerebral artery rupture (Maron, 1987). Therefore, adults with repaired coarctation require ongoing medical supervision for potential postoperative sequelae.

Pulmonic Stenosis

Congenital *pulmonic stenosis* is an unusual lesion in adults. In its most common variety, pulmonic stenosis is an isolated and uncomplicated lesion (Perloff, 1998). The valve usually appears dome shaped during systole, with a central opening and fused commissures. The functional consequences of pulmonic stenosis depend on the degree of obstruction and the adaptive response of the right ventricle. Over time, right ventricular outflow obstruction may increase because of right ventricular hypertrophy in response to the stenotic valve and because of degenerative changes, such as thickening, fibrosis, and calcification in the congenitally deformed valve; severe pulmonic stenosis eventually leads to tricuspid regurgitation and right ventricular failure (Canobbio, 1995).

An intervention to correct pulmonic stenosis is recommended in patients with peak pulmonary gradients of 50 mm Hg or more (Marelli & Moodie, 1998). In most patients, the lesion is corrected by balloon valvotomy in a cardiac catheterization laboratory. Less commonly, surgical valvotomy or, rarely, pulmonic valve replacement is performed. Surgical valve repair is performed using a median sternotomy incision, cardiopulmonary bypass, and cardioplegic arrest. Through a pulmonary arteriotomy incision, the pulmonic valve is inspected and repaired. Fused commissures and valvar adhesions to the pulmonary arterial wall are incised and a partial valvectomy may be performed to remove thickened valve tissue, dense scarring of leaflets, or dysplastic portions of the valve (Laks & Plunkett, 1998). Repair of pulmonic stenosis in adults usually yields excellent long-term results. However, patients with severe pulmonic stenosis and a right ventricle that has been subjected to chronic increased afterload are at risk for late postoperative death from right ventricular failure (Kaplan & Perloff, 1998).

Tetralogy of Fallot

Tetralogy of Fallot is a congenital malformation of the heart comprising four components: (1) VSD, (2) aorta overriding the VSD and communicating with both ventricles, (3) right ventricular outflow tract obstruction, and (4) right ventricular hypertrophy. The physiologic consequences of TOF are determined by the degree of right ventricular outflow obstruction, size of the VSD, and systemic vascular resistance (Canobbio, 1995). In most cases, the right ventricular outflow tract obstruction is significant, producing right-to-left shunting of blood through the VSD. Cyanosis is a central feature of TOF, the degree varying with the ratio of total pulmonary vascular resistance to systemic vascular resistance (Karl, 1996).

Total correction of TOF now is almost always performed during childhood. Adults with uncorrected TOF thus are encountered rarely. Often, such patients have had palliative procedures designed to increase blood flow through the pulmonary vasculature and therefore decrease the cyanosis associated with TOF. Typically, such patients have undergone either a Potts or Blalock-Taussig shunt procedure (Kaplan & Perloff, 1998). Reoperation often is required because of progressive cyanosis as the person outgrows the shunt or because of the effects of volume overload from a large systemic to pulmonary artery shunt (Laks et al., 1997).

More often, surgery in adults with TOF is performed to revise a previous corrective procedure that has become physiologically dysfunctional. Reoperation becomes necessary in approximately 5% of patients after initial corrective surgery for TOF (Warnes, 1993). Persistent or recurrent right ventricular outflow tract obstruction, significant pulmonic regurgitation, and residual or recurrent VSD are the most common abnormalities necessitating reoperation (Pacifico et al., 1990).

Rarely, corrective surgery may be performed initially during adulthood. Operative intervention usually is indicated in adults with uncorrected TOF to avoid troublesome symptoms and a shortened life expectancy. In most adults, uncorrected TOF can be definitively repaired with a low mortality rate and favorable long-term outcome (Marelli & Moodie, 1998; Laks & Pearl, 1991). Corrective repair is performed through a median sternotomy incision and using cardiopulmonary bypass. A right atriotomy or ventriculotomy is performed and the VSD is closed with a prosthetic patch. If the pulmonic valve itself is stenotic, pulmonic valvotomy may be necessary. The right ventricular outflow tract and main pulmonary artery usually require enlargement with patch augmentation. If this does not improve right ventricular outflow, a transannular patch, with sacrifice of the native pulmonic valve, is required. Adults with long-standing hypoxia and right ventricular pressure overload may not tolerate acute pulmonic valve insufficiency; for this reason, a pulmonary allograft or bioprosthetic valve may be implanted (Perryman & Jaquiss, 1998). Previously constructed palliative shunts are closed at the time of correction.

In most adults who undergo total correction of TOF, cyanosis is relieved and functional status improves (Presbitero et al., 1988). Postoperative sequelae can include residual pulmonic stenosis with elevated right ventricular pressure, some degree of pulmonic valve insufficiency, residual VSDs, and benign complete right bundle branch block (Marelli & Moodie, 1998).

REFERENCES

Backer CL, Mavroudis C, Zias EA, et al, 1998: Repair of coarctation with resection and extended end-to-end anastomosis. Ann Thorac Surg 66:1365

Baughman KL, 1998: The heart and pregnancy. In Topol EJ (ed): Comprehensive Cardiovascular Medicine. Philadelphia, Lippincott Williams & Wilkins

Canobbio MM, 1995: Congenital heart disease. In Woods SL, Froelicher ES, Halpenny CJ, Motzer SU (eds): Cardiac Nursing, ed. 3. Philadelphia, JB Lippincott

Drinkwater DC Jr, Laks H, Perloff JK, 1998: Operation and reoperation. In Perloff JK, Child JS (eds): Congenital Heart Disease in Adults, ed. 2. Philadelphia, WB Saunders

Fisher RG, Moodie DS, Sterba R, Gill CC, 1986: Patent ductus arteriosus in adults—long-term follow up: Nonsurgical versus surgical treatment. J Am Coll Cardiol 8:280

Fuster V, Driscoll DJ, McGoon DC, 1991: Congenital heart disease in adolescents and adults: Patent ductus arteriosus and other aorticopulmonary and coronary abnormal communications. In Giuliani ER, Fuster V, Gersh BJ, et al. (eds):

Cardiology: Fundamentals and Practice, ed. 2. St. Louis, Mosby–Year Book

Galloway AC, Colvin SB, Spencer FC, 1995: Atrial septal defects, atrioventricular canal defects, and total anomalous pulmonary venous return. In Spencer FC, Sabiston DC Jr (eds): Surgery of the Chest, ed. 6. Philadelphia, WB Saunders

Ginsberg JS, Hirsh J, 1998: Use of antithrombotics during pregnancy. Chest 114:524S

Hillis LD, Lange RA, Winniford MD, Page RL, 1995a: Atrial septal defect. In Manual of Clinical Problems in Cardiology, ed. 5. Boston, Little, Brown

Hillis LD, Lange RA, Winniford MD, Page RL, 1995b: Ventricular septal defect. In Manual of Clinical Problems in Cardiology, ed. 5. Boston, Little, Brown

Hillis LD, Lange RA, Winniford MD, Page RL, 1995c: Coarctation of the aorta. In Manual of Clinical Problems in Cardiology, ed. 5. Boston, Little, Brown

Kaplan S, 1991: Natural adult survival patterns. J Am Coll Cardiol 18:311

Kaplan S, Perloff JK, 1998: Survival patterns after cardiac surgery or interventional catheterization: A broadening base. In Perloff JK, Child JS (eds): Congenital Heart Disease in Adults, ed. 2. Philadelphia, WB Saunders

Karl TR, 1996: Tetralogy of Fallot. In Baue AE, Geha AS, Hammond GL, et al. (eds): Glenn's Thoracic and Cardiovascular Surgery, ed. 6. Stamford, CT, Appleton & Lange

Kirklin JW, Barratt-Boyes BG, 1993a: Atrial septal defect and partial anomalous pulmonary venous connection. In Cardiac Surgery, ed. 2. New York, Churchill Livingstone

Kirklin JW, Barratt-Boyes BG, 1993b: Patent ductus arteriosus. In Cardiac Surgery, ed. 2. New York, Churchill Livingstone

Kopf GS, Laks H, 1996: Atrial septal defects and cor triatriatum. In Baue AE, Geha AS, Hammond GL, et al. (eds): Glenn's Thoracic and Cardiovascular Surgery, ed. 6. Stamford, CT, Appleton & Lange

Laks H, Marelli D, Drinkwater DC Jr, 1997: Surgery for adults with congenital heart disease. In Edmunds LH Jr (ed): Cardiac Surgery in the Adult. New York, McGraw-Hill

Laks H, Pearl JM, 1991: The surgeon's responsibility: Operation and reoperation: The UCLA experience. J Am Coll Cardiol 18:327

Laks H, Plunkett MD, 1998: Pulmonary stenosis and pulmonary atresia with intact septum. In Kaiser LR, Kron IL, Spray TL (eds): Mastery of Cardiothoracic Surgery. Philadelphia, Lippincott Williams & Wilkins

Mainwaring RD, Lamberti JJ, 1998: Atrial septal defects. In Kaiser LR, Kron IL, Spray TL (eds): Mastery of Cardiothoracic Surgery. Philadelphia, Lippincott Williams & Wilkins

Marelli AJ, Moodie DS, 1998: Adult congenital heart disease. In Topol EJ (ed): Comprehensive Cardiovascular Medicine. Philadelphia, Lippincott Williams & Wilkins

Maron BJ, 1987: Aortic isthmic coarctation. In Roberts WC (ed): Adult Congenital Heart Disease. Philadelphia, FA Davis

McNamara DG, 1989: The adult with congenital heart disease. Curr Probl Cardiol 14:57

Myers JL, Waldhausen JA, 1991: Management of complications following repair of coarctation of the aorta, patent ductus arteriosus, interrupted aortic arch, and vascular rings. In Waldhausen JA, Orringer MB (eds): Complications in Cardiothoracic Surgery. St. Louis, Mosby–Year Book

Pacifico AD, Kirklin JK, Colvin EV, et al., 1990: Tetralogy of Fallot: Late results and reoperations. Semin Thorac Cardiovasc Surg 2:108

Perloff JK, 1998: Survival patterns without cardiac surgery or interventional catheterization: A narrowing base. In Perloff JK, Child JS (eds): Congenital Heart Disease in Adults, ed. 2. Philadelphia, WB Saunders

Perloff JK, 1997: Congenital heart disease in adults. In Braunwald E (ed): Heart Disease: A Textbook of Cardiovascular Medicine, ed. 5. Philadelphia, WB Saunders

Perryman RA, Jaquiss RD, 1998: Tetralogy of Fallot. In Kaiser LR, Kron IL, Spray TL (eds): Mastery of Cardiothoracic Surgery. Philadelphia, Lippincott Williams & Wilkins

Presbitero P, Demarie D, Aruta E, et al., 1988: Results of total correction of tetralogy of Fallot performed in adults. Ann Thorac Surg 46:297

Schaff HV, Danielson GK, 1987: Advances in the surgical management of congenital heart disease in adults. In McGoon DC (ed): Cardiac Surgery, ed. 2. Philadelphia, FA Davis

Sealy WC, 1990: Paradoxical hypertension after repair of coarctation of the aorta: A review of its causes. Ann Thorac Surg 50:323

Tchervenkov CI, Shum-Tim D, 1996: Ventricular septal defect. In Baue AE, Geha AS, Hammond GL, et al. (eds): Glenn's Thoracic and Cardiovascular Surgery, ed. 6. Stamford, CT, Appleton & Lange

Ungerleider RM, 1995: Congenital aortic stenosis. In Sabiston DC Jr, Spencer FC (eds): Surgery of the Chest, ed. 6. Philadelphia, WB Saunders

Ungerleider RM, 1998: Coarctation of the aorta. In Kaiser LR, Kron IL, Spray TL (eds): Mastery of Cardiothoracic Surgery. Philadelphia, Lippincott Williams & Wilkins

Warnes CA, 1993: Tetralogy of Fallot and pulmonary atresia/ventricular septal defect. Cardiol Clin North Am 11:643

Warnes CA, Fuster V, Driscoll DJ, McGoon DC, 1991: Congenital heart disease in adolescents and adults: Ventricular septal defect. In Giuliani ER, Fuster V, Gersh BJ, et al. (eds): Cardiology: Fundamentals and Practice, ed. 2. St. Louis, Mosby–Year Book

Permanent Pacemakers and Implantable Cardioverter-Defibrillators

Jane Kruse, RN, BSN, and
Betsy Finkelmeier, RN, MS, MM

▶ Permanent Pacemakers

Permanent pacemakers have significantly increased survival and improved quality of life for many patients with bradyarrhythmias due to cardiac conduction abnormalities or other disorders. Worldwide, approximately 400,000 pacemakers are implanted each year, and approximately 500,000 people in the United States have pacemakers currently (Barold & Zipes, 1997). Pacemakers initially were developed and remain the primary modality for maintaining an adequate ventricular heart rate in patients with life-threatening bradycardia. However, technologic advances in the 1990s have resulted in increasingly complex systems capable of pacing the heart in a more physiologic manner. As a result, pacemaker therapy has become more sophisticated, with new terminology, new indications, changing criteria for selection of a pacing system, and increasingly complex electrocardiographic manifestations (Kusumoto & Goldschlager, 1996). Standard features of current systems include permanent electrodes that can be reliably positioned in the atrium, pulse generator microcircuitry that can be reprogrammed noninvasively, and sensor systems that detect physiologic indicators of increased metabolic need. Major developments responsible for increased capabilities of permanent pacing systems include mode switching, improved rate sensor features, single-lead technology for dual-chamber sensing, and advanced monitoring features, including patient-activated arrhythmia detection.

Indications for Pacing

Decision making regarding the need for permanent pacemaker implantation can be complex and controversial. To standardize better the indications for pacemaker therapy, a joint committee of the American College of Cardiology (ACC) and American Heart Association (AHA) published guidelines in 1991 categorizing cardiac conditions for which pacemaker implantation may be considered (Dreifus et al., 1991). Updated guidelines were published by this committee in 1998 (Gregoratos et al., 1998). Class I indications are those for which there is general agreement that pacemaker implantation is beneficial, useful, and effective. Class II indications include conditions for which pacemakers are commonly implanted but for which there is not general agreement about their usefulness or efficacy. Class III indications are those conditions for which there is general agreement that pacemaker implantation is not indicated.

The most common class I indication for permanent pacing is complete heart block. Other indications include symptomatic bradycardia associated with sinus node dysfunction or second-degree heart block; acute myocardial infarction with persistent, advanced second- or third-degree heart block; recurrent syncope associated with hypersensitive carotid sinus syndrome; advanced block with atrial fibrillation or atrial flutter and a symptomatic, slow ventricular rate; and bradycardia secondary to necessary pharmacologic therapy (Gregoratos et al., 1998). In symptomatic patients, temporary pacing may be necessary until a permanent pacemaker is implanted.

Although sophisticated electrophysiologic (EP) studies are necessary in some patients, diagnosis of impulse formation or conduction abnormalities in most instances can be established with patient-activated event monitoring or ambulatory (Holter) monitoring. Provocative maneuvers, such as carotid sinus massage, may be necessary to elicit vagally induced arrhythmias. *Event monitors* are typically more helpful in diagnosis of arrhythmias because they are given to patients for a longer time, usually a minimum of 30 days. This two-lead system is worn all of the time (or at least during activity that provokes episodes) and is activated by the patient to record an electrocardiogram during symptoms. The recording is then transmitted over the phone. An *insertable loop recorder* is available to diagnose arrhythmia problems that are not determined by routine methods. This device is surgically implanted for up to 14 months. It can record a cardiac electrogram for a much longer length of time and does not require a patient to wear external leads. If an event occurs, the patient activates storage of the electrogram, which can be played back later.

Pacing System Components

All permanent pacing systems have several basic components: pulse generator, lead, and electrodes (Fig. 20-1). The *pulse generator,* which is quite compact and minimally disfiguring, is implanted under the skin in a subcutaneous pocket. It houses the power source and hybrid circuitry, which are encased in a hermetically sealed metal container that is airtight and fluid tight (Lowe & Wharton, 1995). A lithium-iodine battery is used as the power source in implanted generators. Although factors

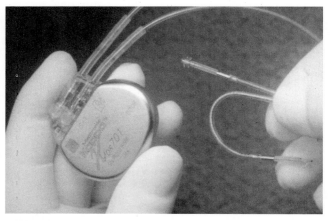

FIGURE 20-1. Dual-chamber pacemaker with bipolar atrial and ventricular leads. (Courtesy of Medtronic, Inc., Minneapolis, MN)

such as frequency of pacing, appropriate programming, and voltage requirements influence battery life, lithium-powered pulse generators usually perform for 5 to 10 years or more before replacement is required. The lithium-iodine battery has predictable characteristics that permit early warning of battery depletion; as voltage drops near the end of life, the pacing rate on magnet application declines as an indicator of the elective replacement time (Barold & Zipes, 1997).

Electronic components of a pulse generator include (1) an output circuit that transforms energy from the power source into an electrical pacing impulse, (2) a timing circuit that determines frequency of stimulation, and (3) a sensing circuit that detects intrinsic cardiac depolarization signals. Pulse generators designed for pacing both the atrium and ventricle have output, timing, and sensing circuits for both chambers as well as a separate timing circuit for the atrioventricular (AV) delay (Harthorne, 1989). In addition, many current pacemakers have circuitry that performs other functions, such as (1) allowing pacing parameters (eg, pacing rate and shape of the pacemaker pulse) to be noninvasively reprogrammed by an external computer, (2) storing and transmitting data regarding pacemaker function, and (3) automatically switching pacing modes based on detection of tachyarrhythmias. Newer devices have numerous other programmable features designed to mimic the variations inherent in normal sinus rhythm. These features vary among different brands of pacemakers.

The *pacemaker lead* is an insulated length of wire that provides a conduit for electrical energy between the pulse generator and cardiac muscle. The lead is a two-way conductor transmitting current from the generator through the lead to the myocardium (pacing) and receiving cardiac depolarization signals from the myocardium to the pulse generator (sensing). Pacing systems are categorized as single chamber or dual chamber, according to whether sensing or pacing can occur only in the atria or ventricles or in both. In a standard single-chamber pacing system, a lead is placed only in the chamber to be paced; leads in both the atrium and ventricle are required in a dual-chamber system. More recently, single-lead pacing systems have been developed to provide dual-chamber sensing and ventricular demand pacing. In these systems, an atrial sensing electrode is located in the atrial cavity on the proximal portion of the ventricular lead. This system is an alternative to dual-lead pacing systems in patients with normal sinus node function and AV block (Wiegand et al., 1999).

Leads may be placed either on the endocardial surface of a cardiac chamber (transvenous) or on the outer surface of the heart (epicardial). Nearly all pacemaker implantations are performed using transvenous leads. Transvenous leads are further categorized as passive or active. Passive leads are designed with flanges or tines near the tip that catch beneath endocardial trabeculations and hold the lead in position until growth of fibrous tissue around the lead tip permanently fixes its position. Active fixation leads are constructed with a sharpened screw at the tip that can be remotely activated and retracted (Fig. 20-2) (Lowe & Wharton, 1995). Formerly, passive leads had better sensing and pacing thresholds. More recently, steroid-eluting active leads have been shown to be effective and reliable in minimizing acute and chronic rises in pacing thresholds (Crossley et al., 1995). Active leads are less easily dislodged and may be preferable if lead fixation is difficult. In the ventricular location, active fixation leads are used when the right ventricle is smooth walled, when significant tricuspid regurgitation is present, or when a site other than the ventricular apex is desired; active leads may be used in the atrium when the right atrium is markedly dilated or the atrial appendage has been traumatized by a prior cardiac operation (Lowe & Wharton, 1995).

Epicardial leads are used rarely. Problems with epicardial leads include fatigue-related lead fractures, more traumatic fixation methods, and less satisfactory chronic pacing thresholds (Spotnitz, 1997). Also, if the pacing system becomes infected, a major operation, including sternotomy and dissection of the electrodes from the surface of the heart, may become necessary. Epicardial leads must be used in patients with prosthetic tricuspid valves to avoid positioning the lead across a valvular prosthesis. Epicardial leads also may be preferable in young children and in patients with a right-to-left shunt, subclavian vein thrombosis, or tricuspid regurgitation.

Electrodes are electrically conductive material that provide the negative (cathode) and positive (anode) terminals of the circuit. Electric current from the pulse generator travels from the cathode to the anode through the patient's tissues, which provide a conductive pathway between the two. The cathode always is located at the distal end of the lead, in contact with viable myocardium. The location of the anode distinguishes a bipolar from a unipolar system (Fig. 20-3). In a bipolar system, both electrodes are located on the lead, spaced several millimeters apart so that they both lie within the heart. A unipolar system has a single electrode (cathode) on the lead's tip; the positive electrode (anode) that is required to complete the electrical circuit is located on the casing of the pulse generator (Lowe & Wharton, 1995). Current medical opinion favors the use of bipolar leads. They are less likely to sense skeletal muscle myopotentials or other forms of electromagnetic interference and are less likely to stimulate the patient's skeletal muscles.

Pacing Objectives

The primary objectives of a permanent pacing system are to compensate for dysfunction of the intrinsic pacemaker (ie, the sinus node) or the conduction system and

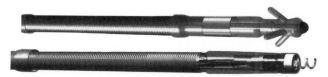

FIGURE 20-2. Transvenous bipolar tined (*top*) and bipolar active fixation (*bottom*) pacing leads. (Courtesy of Medtronic, Inc., Minneapolis, MN)

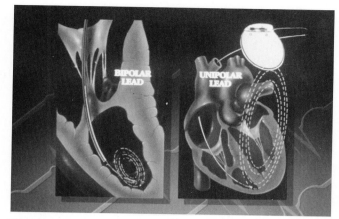

FIGURE 20-3. Bipolar and unipolar pacing systems. With a bipolar system (*left*), electric current flows from the pacemaker through the insulated lead to the negative electrode (cathode) and endocardium; electric current stimulates the heart muscle and flows back to the anode, located on a second intracardiac electrode. In a unipolar system (*right*), electric current from the pacemaker flows through the insulated lead and negative electrode (cathode) to the endocardium; electric current stimulates the heart muscle and flows back to the anode, located on the pacemaker itself. (Courtesy of Guidant Corporation, St. Paul, MN)

to simulate as closely as possible normal physiologic cardiac depolarization and conduction. Recall that repetitive, spontaneous depolarization of the sinus node and propagation of depolarization throughout atrial and ventricular tissue produce normal sinus rhythm. In this normal pattern of electrical excitation, the impulse propagation wave travels in an orderly fashion from the atria, through the AV node and bundle of His, to the ventricles, providing AV synchrony.

When a pacemaker is used to generate a cardiac rhythm, it provides one or more of three basic functions, depending on the type of system: (1) prevention of profound bradycardia, (2) preservation of AV synchrony, and (3) a mechanism for physiologic rate responsiveness or rate modulation. Either a single- (atrial or ventricular) or dual- (atrial and ventricular) chamber system is selected, depending on the type of conduction disorder and pacing objective. Expanded applications of pacing have begun to include the use of pacemakers in patients with hypertrophic cardiomyopathy (to reduce the outflow tract gradient), dilated cardiomyopathy (to improve cardiac output), and atrial fibrillation (to prevent episodes of paroxysmal atrial fibrillation). Studies are underway to define further the long-term benefits and specific applications of pacing in these patient populations (Gregoratos et al., 1998).

Prevention of bradycardia is achieved most easily and requires only a single-chamber system. If AV nodal function is normal, an electrical stimulus delivered in the atrium (ie, atrial pacing) is propagated through myocardial cells of both atria and by way of the AV node through both ventricles. In the absence of normal AV nodal function, single-chamber pacing is achieved only with direct electrical stimulation of ventricular myocardium through a ventricular pacing lead. AV synchrony—that is, an appropriately timed atrial contraction preceding each ventricular contraction—is present with atrial pacing but absent with ventricular pacing. A dual-chamber system is required to achieve AV synchrony in the presence of AV nodal dysfunction.

Atrioventricular synchrony provides significant hemodynamic benefit in patients with normal, as well as in those with impaired, ventricular function. First, atrial systole increases ventricular filling. AV synchrony increases stroke volume 5% to 15% in the normal heart, and atrial contraction is of even greater importance in the presence of left ventricular hypertrophy or heart failure (Spotnitz, 1997). Second, the atria empty more completely with AV synchrony, which decreases atrial pressure and results in increased venous return to the atria. Third, appropriately timed closing of the mitral and tricuspid valves prevents regurgitation across open valves during ventricular systole and elevated venous pressure resulting from closed valves during atrial systole. Finally, absence of AV synchrony may be associated with retrograde activation of the atria. Ventriculoatrial conduction decreases cardiac output, elevates atrial pressure, and may produce pacemaker-mediated arrhythmias or pacemaker syndrome (Hayes & Holmes, 1993). Pacemaker syndrome is a phenomenon that sometimes occurs in individuals who have single-chamber, ventricular pacemakers and fixed or intermittent normal sinus rhythm. It is discussed later in the chapter.

Atrioventricular synchrony also may be important for patients with hypersensitive carotid sinus syndrome, a disorder characterized by an extreme reflex response to carotid sinus stimulation. In affected persons, lightheadedness or syncope may result from pressure on the carotid artery in the area of the carotid sinus. A collar that is too tight or turning the head suddenly may produce recurring syncope with asystolic periods of 3 seconds or more. Two components comprise hypersensitive carotid sinus syndrome. The cardioinhibitory component results from increased parasympathetic tone and is manifest by slowing of the sinus rate or prolongation of the P-R interval and AV block. The vasodepressor component produces vasodilatation and hypotension secondary to a reduction in sympathetic activity. In patients with a primarily cardioinhibitory component of the syndrome, AV sequential pacing is very effective in relieving symptoms. Patients with a primarily vasodepressor component (vasovagal or vasodepressor syncope) require careful evaluation to determine the potential benefits of pacing therapy (Gregoratos et al., 1998).

A third function incorporated into some pacemakers is *rate modulation,* which describes a pulse generator's capacity to respond to changing physiologic demands by increasing or decreasing heart rate. Patients who require permanent pacing often are unable to generate an increased heart rate to meet physiologic demand because of the underlying arrhythmia problem or drug therapy. This condition is known as *chronotropic incompetence.* The use of rate modulation can dramatically decrease symptoms of fatigue, shortness of breath, and dizziness

that are associated with chronotropic incompetence by allowing increases in heart rate during exercise. The ability to vary heart rate according to physiologic need can provide a significant benefit in young and active people (Reynolds, 1996).

In patients with normal sinus node function, rate responsiveness is achieved with a dual-chamber pacing system capable of atrial tracking or the delivery of a ventricular pacing impulse after each sensed atrial depolarization. When the patient's sinus rate increases, the ensuing P waves trigger appropriately timed ventricular pacing impulses, resulting in a pacing rate that varies with the patient's sinus rate. In patients with sinus node dysfunction, stimuli other than atrial depolarizations must be used to adjust the ventricular pacing rate. A variety of physiologic indicators that reflect changes in metabolic need can be used to modulate changes in pacing rate (Table 20-1) (Morton, 1991). Rate modulation features typically require a period of "fine-tuning" to achieve the best fit for an individual patient. Some devices incorporate combinations of various sensors to enhance further the ability to meet individual patient needs.

Pacing Modes

Several factors are considered in selecting the particular type of pulse generator, including type of conduction abnormality, presence of supraventricular arrhythmias, and age and lifestyle of the patient. If pacing needs are likely to change over time, a dual-chamber or single-chamber rate-modulated pulse generator with multiprogrammable capability is selected (Finkelmeier, 1991). However, the technology of these devices is complex and the units are more costly. Selection of the proper pacing mode requires careful evaluation of the patient's pacing needs and sometimes is controversial (Connolly et al., 1996). The choice is based on reliable knowledge of the patient's history and current medications, as well as on the pathophysiology of the underlying cardiac illness. Table 20-2 provides basic guidelines for pacing mode selection according to type of conduction abnormality.

NBG Code

The various methods by which the pulse generator electrically stimulates the heart (paces) and responds to intrinsic cardiac activity (senses) are called the *modes* of

---

TABLE 20-1

Selected Physiologic Indicators Used in Rate-Modulated Pacing

Mechanical vibration
Minute ventilation
Respiratory rate
Central venous temperature
Q-T interval

TABLE 20-2

Recommended Pacing Modes

Diagnosis	Pacing Mode
Sinus node dysfunction	AAI-R
Atrioventricular block	DDD
Sinus node dysfunction and atrioventricular block	DDD-R or DDI-R
Chronic atrial fibrillation with atrioventricular block	VVI-R
Hypersensitive carotid sinus syndrome	DDD

pacing. A standardized coding system for describing pacing modalities was introduced by the Inter-Society Commission for Heart Disease (ICHD) Resources in 1974 (Parsonnet et al., 1974). The coding system has subsequently undergone several revisions as more sophisticated pacing modalities have been developed. The *NBG (NASPE/BPEG generic) pacemaker code* is used today and represents the most recent revision by the North American Society of Pacing and Electrophysiology (NASPE) and British Pacing and Electrophysiology Group (BPEG) (Bernstein et al., 1987).

The NBG Code is a system of classifying pulse generator function using a five-letter code (Table 20-3). The first three letters of the code describe pulse generator functions used to treat bradycardia. The first letter describes the heart chamber in which pacing can occur (eg, "A" means that the generator is capable of atrial pacing only; "V" means that ventricular pacing only is possible; and "D" signifies that pacing can occur in both chambers). Similarly, the second letter reveals the chamber(s) in which sensing of intrinsic electrical activity occurs. The third letter in the sequence designates pulse generator response to sensed cardiac events. "T" signifies that the pulse generator delivers a ventricular pacing impulse in response to sensed intrinsic atrial activity, "I" means that sensed intrinsic activity inhibits the pulse generator from delivering a pacing impulse, and "D" means that both triggered and inhibited responses are possible under various circumstances.

The fourth letter describes two functions: programmability and rate modulation. The following letters in the fourth position signify a hierarchical progression in function complexity from absence of programmability to rate modulation, with each level incorporating features of all levels below it: "O" signifies absence of programmability; "P," simple programmability (one or two programmable parameters); "M," multiple (more than two) programmable parameters; "C," communicating function (telemetry that allows interrogation of the pulse generator); and "R," rate modulation in response to physiologic parameters (Teplitz, 1991). Because current systems all include telemetry and multiprogrammable functions, the fourth letter is typically used, if needed, to signify "R" for the presence of rate modulation. The fifth letter of the code refers to antitachycardia functions. The fifth letter is often omitted in routine clinical practice. The most commonly selected pacing modes are discussed in the following sections.

Single-Chamber Modes

AAI

The *AAI pacing mode* provides atrial pacing at a fixed rate with inhibition of pacing by sensed intrinsic atrial activity. The pacing rate is programmable. AAI pacing is used in patients who have sinus node dysfunction but intact AV nodal conduction. If rate modulation is desired, AAI-R pacing may be used additionally to provide the rate-responsive feature. Second- and third-degree AV block are contraindications to AAI pacing.

VVI

The *VVI pacing mode* is identical to the AAI pacing mode except that pacing and sensing occur in the ventricle and intrinsic ventricular activity inhibits delivery of pacing impulses. Pacing occurs at a programmable, but fixed, rate. It is most appropriate for patients with (1) no significant atrial contribution to cardiac output (eg, patients with chronic atrial fibrillation), (2) no evidence of pacemaker syndrome, or (3) special circumstances in which pacing simplicity is a prime concern (eg, senility) (Dreifus et al., 1991). VVI-R signifies that the pulse gen-

TABLE 20-3

The NASPE/BPEG Generic (NBG) Pacemaker Code

I Chamber Paced	II Chamber Sensed	III Mode of Response	IV Programmable Functions	V Tachyarrhythmia Functions
O—None	O—None	O—None	O—None	O—None
A—Atrium	A—Atrium	T—Triggered	P—Simple programmable	P—Pacing
V—Ventricle	V—Ventricle	I—Inhibited	M—Multiprogrammable	S—Shock
D—Dual	D—Dual	D—Dual	C—Communicating	D—Dual
			R—Rate modulation	

NASPE, North American Society of Pacing and Electrophysiology; BPEG, British Pacing and Electrophysiology Group.
Adapted from Bernstein AD, Camm AJ, Fletcher RD, et al., 1987: The NASPE/BPEG generic pacemaker code for antibradyarrhythmia and adaptive-rate pacing and antitachyarrhythmia devices. Pacing Clin Electrophysiol 10:794.

erator also has a rate-responsive feature—that is, the pacing rate increases in response to a selected parameter indicative of increased physiologic demand, usually due to exercise. The VVI-R pacing mode provides rate modulation in patients with an atrial arrhythmia that precludes dual-chamber pacing.

Dual-Chamber Modes

DDD

The *DDD pacing mode* is the most sophisticated form of dual-chamber pacing. It provides pacing and sensing in both chambers, as well as the dual responses of triggering and inhibition. Four different cardiac rhythms can occur as a result of normal DDD function: (1) normal sinus rhythm, (2) atrial pacing, (3) AV sequential pacing, and (4) P-synchronous pacing (Hayes, 1998) (Fig. 20-4). Normal sinus rhythm at a rate greater than the programmed pacing rate inhibits both atrial and ventricular outputs. An intrinsic atrial rate less than the programmed pacing rate results in atrial pacing that produces intrinsic ventricular depolarization (atrial pacing) or is followed by appropriately timed ventricular pacing (AV sequential pacing). If the intrinsic atrial rate is greater than the pacing rate, it is sensed, inhibits the atrial output, and triggers ventricular pacing (atrial tracking), producing P-synchronous pacing. Spontaneous ventricular events are sensed and inhibit ventricular pacing. DDD pacemakers can be programmed to most other pacing modes if the patient's needs change or if malfunction of one of the leads occurs. Because of its versatility, DDD pacing has gained widespread use.

Pacemakers capable of pacing in a DDD-R mode provide AV synchrony and rate modulation for patients who have fixed sinus bradycardia and complete heart block. It is beneficial for patients who require consistent AV synchrony at rates that vary according to metabolic demands and whose sinus nodes have lost the ability to respond appropriately to such demands.

DDI

DDI pacing allows atrial sensing but not atrial tracking to occur. Intrinsic atrial activity inhibits discharge of an atrial pacing impulse, thereby avoiding competition between the pacemaker and an underlying atrial rhythm (Stephenson & Combs, 1991). Because atrial tracking is not possible with a DDI pacing mode, AV synchronous pacing occurs only at the programmed pacing rate. DDD pacemakers with automatic mode conversion temporarily reprogram to this mode when atrial activity is sensed above a programmed rate. This avoids atrial tracking during episodes of supraventricular tachycardia. Once the sensed atrial rate falls to a normal range, the pacemaker reverts to the DDD mode.

Pacemaker Implantation

Pacemaker implantation may be performed on an outpatient basis, but typically requires at least an overnight stay in the hospital. Significant preparation of the patient is required before implant, including education, informed consent, laboratory testing and chest roentgenogram, discussion of postprocedure restrictions, and evaluation of special postimplantation needs. If the patient's condition does not require immediate hospitalization, these activities may be done on an outpatient basis (Table 20-4). Anticoagulant therapy must be withheld for several days before implantation to allow prothrombin time to return to near normal. In patients with prosthetic heart valves, anticoagulation with heparin may be necessary during the period in which sodium warfarin (Coumadin) is discontinued. An individualized plan should be implemented for each patient based on the indication for anticoagulation. Patients should fast for 6 to 8 hours before implantation. Antibiotics are usually given before and after implantation to help reduce the risk of infection.

Implantation of a pacemaker using transvenous leads is performed in a catheterization laboratory or operating room using sterile technique, local anesthesia, and mild sedation. The pacing lead is inserted through the right or left subclavian or jugular vein and positioned in the cardiac chamber to be paced (right atrium or ventricle). The site of implant depends on a variety of factors and requires a detailed history from the patient. Influencing factors include previous surgery (eg, mastectomy); a history of radiation therapy, infection, dermatitis, central venous catheter, or vein occlusion; patient hobbies; and dominant hand. For example, placing a pulse generator on the right side is not desirable in a right-handed patient who hunts regularly and uses the right shoulder to brace a shotgun.

Transvenous ventricular leads are positioned in the apex of the right ventricle. Atrial leads most commonly are positioned in the right atrial appendage or on the atrial wall (Hayes et al., 1993). Leads designed for atrial

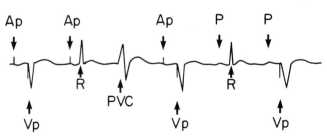

FIGURE 20-4. Simulated drawing demonstrating the possible responses with a DDD pacing mode. From left to right the tracing displays: AV sequential pacing (Ap-Vp); atrial pacing with intrinsic AV conduction resulting in inhibition of ventricular output (Ap-R); premature ventricular complex (PVC) with resetting of escape interval; AV sequential pacing (Ap-Vp); normal sinus complex (P-R), resulting in inhibition of both atrial and ventricular outputs; and sinus depolarization that fails to conduct intrinsically to ventricles, producing a triggered ventricular response (P-synchronous pacing [P-Vp]). (Finkelmeier BA, Salinger MH, 1986: Dual-chamber cardiac pacing: An overview. Critical Care Nurse 6:19)

appendage placement have a characteristic "J" shape to allow secure positioning. Fluoroscopy is used to guide lead placement in the heart. For a dual-chamber system, both leads often can be inserted in the same vein, using the same or different puncture sites. Satisfactory lead placement is confirmed by fluoroscopy and measurement of stimulation threshold, lead impedance, and cardiac signal amplitudes of the endocardial electrogram (Brinker & Midei, 1996).

The pulse generator is situated below the clavicle in a pocket created by separating pectoral muscle fascia from the overlying subcutaneous tissue (Moses et al., 1987). The pocket should be of adequate size to house the pulse generator without undue tension on overlying skin. The pocket may be irrigated with an antibiotic solution before insertion of the generator. Before closing the incision, hemostasis is achieved to prevent accumulation of blood within the pocket and resultant increased potential for infection.

Epicardial leads occasionally will have been placed prophylactically during a prior cardiac operation in patients considered at high risk for postoperative heart block. Permanent leads are easily secured through the epicardium into the atrial or ventricular myocardium while the chest is open. Alternatively, a small subxiphoid or thoracotomy incision is used for epicardial lead placement. When epicardial leads are used, the pulse generator is placed in a subcutaneous pocket in the abdominal wall.

Complications

Complications associated with permanent pacemakers are unusual but do occur. The implantation is associated with minimal morbidity. *Perforation* of the subclavian vein or right ventricle occurs rarely. It usually is detected by fluoroscopy during implantation or by the chest roentgenogram that is obtained after implantation. Venous perforation may result in hemothorax, which usually can be treated by tube thoracostomy. Right ventricular perforation can produce hemopericardium, which may require pericardiocentesis or, rarely, repair of the ventricle. Pneumothorax can occur because of lung puncture.

Pacemaker failure can occur from battery depletion, pulse generator malfunction, lead dislodgment, or lead fracture. Replacement of a pulse generator is a minor surgical procedure performed using local anesthesia. The incision overlying the generator is reopened and the indwelling generator is detached from the leads. After measuring pacing thresholds to ensure proper lead function, the leads are connected to a new pulse generator. The new generator is then inserted in the subcutaneous pocket and the incision is closed. Lead problems sometimes can be corrected by repositioning or repairing the lead. Occasionally a new lead must be placed. If a lead problem does occur, extraction of the old lead may be necessary. This may be accomplished with manual extraction techniques or with new excimer laser sheaths that deliver laser energy through the distal end of the

sheath. The laser helps release the lead from the fibrotic tissue at the lead tip without excessive force and decreases the risk of tearing tissue (Wilkoff et al., 1999).

Electromagnetic interference (EMI) is defined as any signal, biologic or nonbiologic, that falls within a frequency spectrum that may be detected by the sensing circuitry of the pacemaker and may result in rate alteration or sensing abnormalities (Hayes, 1998). EMI from common household electrical appliances is unusual with current pulse generators. For example, microwave ovens may be used freely by patients with implanted pacemakers. However, sources of major electrical or magnetic interference, such as arc welding equipment, may cause a problem with pacemaker function. Electronic sensors used for store security have been identified as possible sources of interference if the patient gets too close or leans against this equipment. Awareness of this potential problem and maintaining a safe distance help prevent inappropriate pacing (McIvor et al., 1998). Cellular phones have also been identified as sources of EMI. However, this risk can be avoided by holding the phone over the ear on the opposite side of the implant (Hayes, 1997). Muscle myopotential interference occasionally affects function of a unipolar system because the anodal electrode is located on the casing of the pulse generator and senses regional muscle activity. Although rare, it may cause disabling symptoms in some patients. It is corrected by decreasing pulse generator sensitivity or by converting to a bipolar system.

Pacemaker syndrome can occur with VVI pacing systems because of intermittent loss of AV synchrony and retrograde activation of the atrium. Pacemaker syndrome is a clinical constellation of signs and symptoms produced by adverse hemodynamic and electrophysiologic responses to ventricular pacing because of inadequate timing of atrial and ventricular contractions (Barold & Zipes, 1997). Sudden decreases in cardiac output and blood pressure occur during periods of AV asynchrony; they are thought to result from loss of the atrial contribution (ie, "atrial kick") to ventricular filling and from ventriculoatrial conduction that activates atrial stretch reflexes and leads to vagal stimulation and peripheral vasodilatation. It is estimated that some degree of pacemaker syndrome occurs in 5% to 20% of patients with VVI pacemakers (Hillis et al., 1995). The syndrome is manifest by episodes of weakness and dizziness during ventricular pacing. When the normal AV sequence of depolarization and contraction is restored by return of sinus rhythm, symptoms are relieved. Pacemaker syndrome is corrected by reprogramming or replacing the pulse generator to provide AV synchronous pacing.

Cross-talk and pacemaker-mediated tachycardia are complications unique to dual-chamber pacing systems. *Cross-talk* is inappropriate sensing of output from one lead by the other with resultant inhibition of pacing. When atrial impulses are sensed by the pacemaker as spontaneous ventricular events, ventricular pacing is inhibited and ventricular asystole may occur. Cross-talk is corrected by reprogramming the ventricular blanking period, preventing the pacemaker from sensing any ven-

TABLE 20-4

Pacemaker Placement: Low-Risk Rapid Recovery Protocol

Critical Occurence	Preprocedure	Procedure	Procedure Day Postprocedure (Hours 1 to 6)	Procedure Day Postprocedure (Hours 7 to 23)	Follow-up
Consults	• Obtain preprocedure assessments and tests • Initiate any predicted home care or special needs arrangements		Per implanting physician: • Follow-up recommendations • Wound management	Per implanting physician: • Follow-up recommendations • Wound management • Anticoagulation (if applicable) • Wound evaluation scheduled for 1 wk postimplantation	Follow-up phone call within 1 wk Incision check at 1 wk
Assessments	Preprocedure worksheet complete Preprocedure orders signed and sent to nursing unit	Documentation of periprocedural monitoring and nursing care	CCU or telemetry observation for acute change in cardiovascular, pulmonary, or neurologic status Bleeding precautions Monitor vital signs, incision, and activity	Observation for acute change in cardiovascular, pulmonary, or neurologic status Telemetry until discharge Limited activity with affected arm Monitor vital signs q 4 h	

Education	• Provide preoperative teaching for patient and family, including discussion regarding driving and activity restrictions. Provide written admission instructions		Reinforce routines, especially activity restrictions postprocedure
			Education regarding discharge instructions and follow-up
				• Reinforce teaching:
				  ○ Review new medications if applicable
				  ○ Activity restrictions
				• D/C planning to include:
				  ○ Home care and job related risks/needs	

- Provide information regarding discontinuation of warfarin and need for heparin if applicable
  - Written D/C instructions and pacemaker identification card
  - Pacemaker video watched by patient
  - Follow-up appointment scheduled
  - Transtelephonic monitor instruction
  - Transtelephonic checks every 2 wk

Tests	CBC w/differential, chemistry panel, PT/PTT/INR, urinalysis, ECG, CXR	CXR portable	12-lead ECG if needed CXR, PA and lateral
Treatments		Sling to affected arm before leaving procedure laboratory	Remove sling morning after implant
Medications	Documentation of periprocedural infusions, medications and sedation	Pain/sedation medications prn; Resume previous medications except anticoagulants	New medications as ordered; Resume warfarin if needed. No heparin
Activity		Complete bed rest with HOB ≥45°	Ambulate 6 h postimplant
Diet	NPO night before procedure	NPO	Resume diet as tolerated
Discharge			Discharge; Review patient-specific information

CBC, complete blood count; CCU, coronary care unit; CXR, chest roentgenogram; D/C, discharge; ECG, electrocardiogram; HOB, head of bed; INR, international normalized ratio; NPO, nothing by mouth; PA, posteroanterior; PT, prothrombin time; PTT, partial thromboplastin time.

Adapted from Clinical Pathway, Northwestern Memorial Hospital, Chicago, Illinois.

tricular activity immediately after delivery of an atrial pacing impulse. Cross-talk may also be avoided by activating a feature called *safety pacing,* which causes the pacemaker to deliver a ventricular stimulus when there is a sensed event on the ventricular lead immediately after an atrial stimulus has been delivered. Safety pacing can result in a shortened AV interval or may cause delivery or a pacing stimulus during intrinsic ventricular activity. These events are commonly mistaken as pacemaker malfunction (Fig. 20-5).

Pacemaker-mediated tachycardia is a rapid ventricular paced rhythm that is sustained by retrograde conduction to the atria (Fig. 20-6). Pacemaker-mediated tachycardia is possible in dual-chamber pacing systems with atrial sensing. It usually is initiated by an ectopic ventricular impulse that is conducted in retrograde fashion through intrinsic conductive tissue to the atria. The resulting P wave is sensed by the pulse generator, which responds with a triggered ventricular pacing impulse that is again conducted in retrograde fashion to the atria. A circular reentrant tachycardia is thus induced. Pacemaker-mediated tachycardia is terminated by application of a magnet over the pulse generator to disable atrial sensing and thus terminate atrial tracking. The pulse generator is then reprogrammed by increasing the postventricular atrial refractory period or eliminating atrial sensing altogether to prevent recurrence.

Pulse generator erosion through the skin occasionally occurs, particularly in elderly, cachectic patients. The skin over an edge of the generator becomes reddened and palpation reveals little or no overlying subcutaneous tissue. A new subcutaneous pocket must be created in a different location and the generator moved. If not, skin breakdown eventually occurs, allowing contamination of the device. Rarely, the suture securing the pulse generator in a fixed position becomes disrupted. If this occurs, an unknowing or disoriented patient may manipulate and rotate the pulse generator in the pocket. This so-called "Twiddler's syndrome" can produce lead dislodgment or fracture (Goldberger, 1990). Occasionally, the pulse generator migrates from the original pocket (eg, into the subcutaneous tissue of the breast in a woman). Repositioning of the generator may be necessary for comfort or cosmetic reasons.

An unusual late complication of pacemaker implantation is infection of the pacing system. Because implanted devices usually become coated with platelet-fibrin thrombus and are remote from capillary vessels, associated infections are difficult to treat with antibiotics and are resistant to host defenses (Schoen, 1997). Infection of the prosthetic material is likely to produce fistula formation and a chronic, indolent infection that continues until all prosthetic material is removed. Typically, an infected subcutaneous pocket containing the pulse generator begins to drain purulent material. The simplest corrective measure is removal of the pulse generator and as much of the leads as is possible. Although this corrects the problem for the moment, infection usually remains along the residual length of the pacing lead, and after a quiescent period, a sinus tract redevelops and begins to drain again. For this reason, many surgeons recommend removal of the entire pacing system as soon as diagnosis of infection is established.

Infection is a particularly difficult problem when epicardial leads have been secured to the ventricle and is one reason that permanent epicardial pacing systems are not used commonly. Removal of epicardial leads is a formidable task. It usually necessitates a sternotomy incision. Often the heart is densely adherent to the posterior table of the sternum because of the infection. In addition, tissue ingrowth surrounds the area where the leads are attached to the epicardium, making lead removal difficult.

Nursing Care and Follow-up

Postoperative care of the pacemaker patient includes a period of bed rest from 6 to 12 hours. Patients should be in a monitored setting to allow for early detection of pacemaker-related problems. After the initial bed rest period, patients should be encouraged to ambulate. Arm movements on the affected side may be limited, but complete restriction of arm motion is not advised because it may cause later mobility problems that outweigh the risk of lead dislodgment. Depending on the patient's typical level of activity, some restrictions may be imposed for the initial postoperative period (usually several weeks). For example, golf, tennis and other activities requiring vigorous arm movement are not advised during this period.

Before discharge from the hospital, written and verbal instructions, written descriptive information about the pacemaker, and a temporary pacemaker identification card are given to the patient. The device is registered with the manufacturer so that the patient can be notified in the event of a device recall. Comprehensive evaluation of the pacemaker is performed and adjustments to programming may be made. A chest roentgenogram is performed before discharge to document lead position and

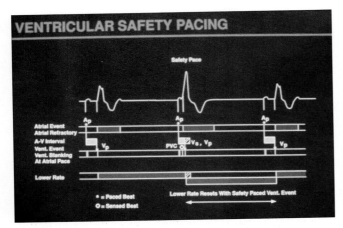

FIGURE 20-5. Example of safety pacing. Rhythm tracing demonstrates AV sequential pacing; safety pacing feature is activated during second beat due to sensing of premature ventricular contraction that occurs during cross-talk detection window. Safety pacing commonly is mistaken for ventricular undersensing. (Courtesy of Medtronic, Inc., Minneapolis, MN)

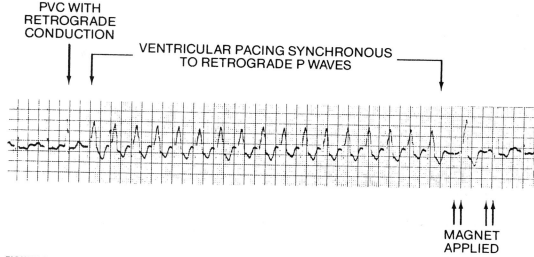

FIGURE 20-6. Pacemaker-mediated tachycardia (PMT). After two beats of P-synchronous pacing, a premature ventricular contraction (PVC) occurs and results in a retrograde P wave. The atrial channel senses the retrograde P wave and triggers ventricular pacing with subsequent retrograde conduction and ventricular pacing synchronous to the retrograde P waves. A magnet is placed over the implanted pulse generator to disable atrial sensing and terminate the PMT. (DiCola V, 1982: Modern cardiac pacing: Available pacing modes and new pacemaker "code" terminology. Intelligence Reports in Cardiac Pacing and Electrophysiology 1:1. Minneapolis, MN, Medtronic, Inc.)

to detect pneumothorax. Patients should receive clear instructions on follow-up appointments and contacts for further questions or concerns.

Intermittent evaluation of patients with implanted pacemakers is essential, particularly for those with more complex dual-chamber systems. Patients are typically given transtelephonic monitors to provide a method of frequent evaluation in the initial postoperative period. *Transtelephonic monitoring* is a technique that allows transmission of electrocardiographic tracings from the patient's home. Using electrodes placed on the patient's chest or fingertips, the cardiac rhythm tracing is converted into sound waves through a telephone mouthpiece, transmitted to a receiver at the pacemaker clinic, and converted into a printed electrocardiographic rhythm tracing (Moses et al., 1987) (Fig. 20-7). Transtelephonic recordings are supplemented with periodic visits to a physician's office or pacemaker clinic for comprehensive pacemaker interrogation and reprogramming.

Although pacemakers are highly reliable, periodic evaluation by a physician with specialized training is essential for optimal pacing. Ideally, patients receive this type of specialized surveillance through a pacemaker clinic with proper equipment (including pacemaker programming devices) and trained personnel. Continued evaluation of patients with implanted pacemakers achieves a number of important objectives: (1) assessment of pulse generator battery function, (2) optimal programming of the pacemaker, (3) detection of possible pacing system problems, and (4) maintenance of a data registry so that patients can be notified promptly in the event of a device recall.

The ability to interrogate the pacemaker is called *telemetry*. With telemetry, diagnostic data can be obtained, including pulse generator model, serial number, date of implant, number of paced and sensed beats, battery and lead impedance, and intracardiac electrograms (Finkelmeier, 1991). These diagnostic data allow assessment of intrinsic cardiac rhythm, sensing and pacing thresholds, status of AV conduction, presence of ventriculoatrial (retrograde) conduction, and status of battery life (Kleinschmidt & Stafford, 1991). Programmable parameters can be adjusted to accommodate changes in pacing needs.

Programmable pulse generators contain predetermined circuits from which one of several features or functions can be selected for variation within a specified range (Hayes, 1993). Basic parameters that are programmable include upper and lower rate limits for pacing, AV interval, pulse generator output, pacing mode, sensitivity, and refractory periods (McErlean, 1991). In rate-responsive pacemakers, settings that control the pulse generator's response to activity also are programmable. Other complex features such as mode switching, sleep modes, and data storage parameters each have a set of programmable options that vary with each device. Common reasons for reprogramming include changing the pacing mode, increasing or decreasing the pacing rate, and adjusting sensitivity. Prudent programming of the battery output settings (amplitude and pulse width) can substantially prolong battery life.

▶ Antitachycardia Devices

An *antitachycardia pacemaker* is a device capable of sensing tachycardia and delivering four or five pacing stimuli in succession at progressively shorter intervals.

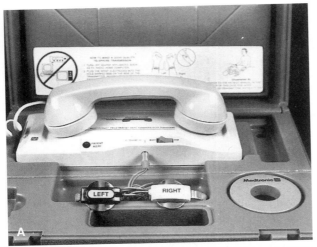

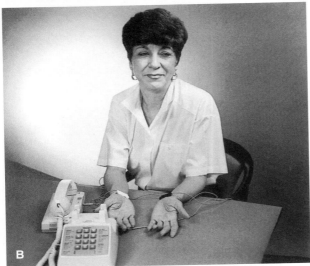

FIGURE 20-7. (A) Transtelephonic monitoring system. **(B)** Patient transmitting electrocardiogram by telephone. (Courtesy of Medtronic, Inc., Minneapolis, MN)

Antitachycardia pacemakers are activated by sensing a tachycardia of sudden onset with a stable rate (to differentiate the rhythm from atrial fibrillation). Pacing during the reentrant rhythm interrupts the tachycardia and converts it to a normal rhythm. Therapy may be delivered automatically or require activation by an external magnet. These devices are used almost exclusively to treat refractory, reentrant supraventricular tachycardia in patients in whom EP testing has demonstrated reproducible tachycardia termination by pacing without proarrhythmic effects (Rosenthal & Josephson, 1990). The effectiveness of catheter ablation for reentrant supraventricular tachycardia has made the use of antitachycardia pacing rare. It is recommended only when drug therapy is ineffective or not tolerated and ablation has been unsuccessful or refused by the patient (Barold & Zipes, 1997). Antitachycardia pacing for ventricular arrhythmias is a function incorporated into implantable

cardioverter-defibrillators and is discussed later in this chapter.

► Implantable Cardioverter-Defibrillators

The *implantable cardioverter-defibrillator* (ICD) has become widely recognized as the most effective therapy for patients with life-threatening ventricular arrhythmias. The first automatic defibrillator was implanted by Mirowski in 1980 (Mirowski et al., 1980). It was capable of delivering a single therapy for tachycardia above a single predetermined rate. Since then, remarkable changes in ICD therapy have taken place. Current devices are multiprogrammable in the therapies they offer and are capable of sophisticated electrocardiographic monitoring. State-of-the-art, dual-chamber pacemakers have been combined with ICD technology to provide the option of a single-device implant in patients who require bradycardia and tachycardia therapy (Haffajee, 1998). In 1998, over 52,000 ICDs were implanted worldwide (40,000 in the United States alone). As patients who will benefit from ICDs are identified more clearly and further technologic advances are made, the use of ICDs is expected to continue to increase.

Indications for ICD Implantation

Initial indications for ICD implantation required a patient to survive two episodes of cardiac arrest not associated with myocardial infarction (Mirowski et al., 1983). As efficacy of the ICD in prevention of sudden death was recognized in the late 1980s, implantation criteria were expanded to include any survivor of cardiac arrest (not due to a reversible cause) and any patient with recurrent ventricular tachycardia (VT) inducible at EP study and not controlled by drug therapy (Dreifus et al., 1991). At the time, ICD implant necessitated a thoracotomy. The devices were large and implanted in the abdomen. Technology rapidly improved and transvenous implantation became possible. Concurrently, research continued to demonstrate the benefits for cardiac arrest survivors. ICD implantation was shown to reduce the sudden death recurrence rate to 1% to 2% per year (Lerman & Cannom, 1998).

In response to these advances, the American College of Cardiology and the American Heart Association revised the indications for ICD implantation in 1998 (Gregoratos et al., 1998). Categories of cardiac conditions indicating ICD implant are similar to those used for pacemakers. Class I indications (evidence or general agreement that therapy is warranted) include (1) cardiac arrest not due to a reversible cause; (2) spontaneous sustained VT; (3) syncope of undetermined origin with clinically relevant, hemodynamically significant sustained VT or ventricular fibrillation (VF) induced at EP study when drug therapy is ineffective, not tolerated, or not preferred; and (4) non-sustained VT with coronary artery disease, prior myocardial infarction, left ventricular dysfunction, and inducible

VF or sustained VT at EP study that is not suppressed by a class I antiarrhythmic drug. Clinical decisions about implant in populations outside of the defined indications, such as in patients with long QT syndrome, hypertrophic cardiomyopathy, and familial history of sudden cardiac death, require careful evaluation because of the potential lethal consequences involved. Current research studies are attempting to identify patients in whom the device should be implanted as primary prevention for sudden cardiac death (Lerman & Cannom, 1998).

ICD Components

Like pacemakers, ICDs consist of a pulse generator and lead system with electrodes for sensing and pacing the heart. In addition, the ICD lead systems have shocking electrodes that deliver high-voltage energy to the heart for cardioversion or defibrillation. Because of the transition in lead systems from epicardial to transvenous beginning in 1993, patients may have either lead system in use. Before 1993, all systems necessitated a thoracotomy approach to place pace/sense leads and two defibrillating patches on the epicardial surface of the heart; some patients still have these outdated components in place. The epicardial patches used in the early implants may make external defibrillation more difficult because the outer surface of the defibrillating patch is insulated. Although the insulation properly directs energy from the ICD to the myocardium, it may inhibit delivery of energy from external defibrillators from reaching the myocardial tissue (Lerman & Deale, 1990). The presence of epicardial patches also poses a problem if coronary artery bypass grafting is needed in the future. Epicardial leads have shown a significant number of long-term complications involving lead fracture and increased impedance. Because of this, patients with epicardial lead systems require close evaluation of the lead at the time of generator replacement and yearly induction of VF to evaluate lead performance (Hammill, 1998). If the epicardial lead system malfunctions, a new transvenous system is implanted and the original epicardial system is abandoned.

Although the introduction of transvenous leads allowed ICD implantation without a thoracotomy, early devices were so large that placement of the device in the abdomen was still required. The transvenous lead incorporated shocking coils along the lead with bipolar pacing electrodes at the tip. The leads were inserted through the subclavian vein with the tip positioned in the right ventricular apex. The proximal end of the lead was then tunneled subcutaneously to an abdominal generator pocket. Depending on the size and condition of the patient's heart, the shock delivered between the two coils on the transvenous lead sometimes failed to terminate VF. If the defibrillation threshold (DFT) (ie, the lowest first-shock energy successfully terminating VF) was high, a subcutaneous lead was placed in the left chest (Fig. 20-8). The shock was then delivered between the coils on the transvenous lead and the patch, incorporating a larger portion of the myocardium.

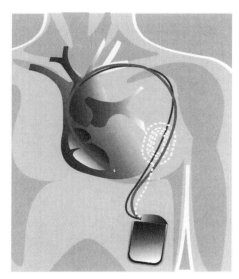

FIGURE 20-8. Transvenous ICD with abdominal placement of device; *dotted lines* indicate placement of subcutaneous patch (if necessary). (Courtesy of Medtronic, Inc., Minneapolis, MN)

Major improvements in lead technology have since occurred, resulting in ease of placement, decreased defibrillator size, and reliable long-term delivery of therapy. Although the lead design varies from one manufacturer to another, all transvenous leads used for defibrillation and pacing consist of a bipolar electrode for sensing and pacing at the distal tip of the lead and one or two shocking coils located proximally. One of the most significant changes in lead technology is the inclusion of the generator casing as part of the shocking circuit. This allows for delivery of the shock between the intracardiac coils and the generator, resulting in lower DFTs (Fig. 20-9).

A low *defibrillation threshold* is important because (1) it may increase over time owing to fibrosis at the elec-

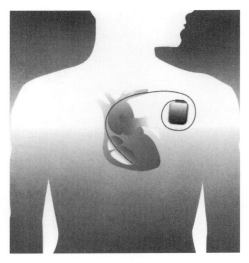

FIGURE 20-9. Transvenous ICD with pectoral device placement. (Courtesy of Medtronic, Inc., Minneapolis, MN)

trode–tissue interface, and (2) antiarrhythmic drugs that increase the DFT may be prescribed for the patient in the future. In general, the DFT must be at least 10 joules (J) lower than the maximum output of the device to allow for an adequate safety margin at the time of implant. If this margin cannot be achieved with a single lead, special leads may be added to the ICD system. The subcutaneous array and the subcutaneous patch electrode are examples of these types of leads. Both can be implanted subcutaneously in the left chest and tunneled under the skin to the generator site. Other lead advances include the ability to deliver a biphasic shock waveform and manipulate the polarity of the leads. These lead improvements have lowered the average DFT to the point that a transvenous system can provide adequate DFTs in almost 100% of patients (Kennergren, 1996). Thus, the use of subcutaneous leads has become rare.

Implantable cardioverter-defibrillator generators have also changed considerably in the 1990s. Like pacemakers, the generators contain a battery, microprocessors, and circuitry. The largest component in the generator is the capacitor, which is used to store the electrical energy as the device is charging to a programmed output. Thus, a generator with a 3- or 6-volt battery can deliver a 750-volt shock. Originally, devices were large, weighing 290 g with a volume of 160 cm³. The latest devices have been downsized to 90 g and 40 cm³ (Fig. 20-10). Part of the miniaturization has been possible because of capacitor design changes. Use of the generator's metal casing as a defibrillation surface (referred to as an *active can*) lowered DFTs and therefore the energy requirements of the device. The ability to change the polarity of the delivered energy (reversed polarity) has also decreased DFTs in patients with high thresholds (Gottlieb & Callans, 1998). Decreasing energy requirements helps make smaller generator size possible and prolongs the generator life span. Initial devices lasted up to 2 years. Projected longevity for some of the newest devices is as high as 11 years. Battery life depends on numbers of shocks delivered, types of features used, amount of pacing needed, and lead integrity. As with pacemakers,

battery life can be enhanced with appropriate programming and follow-up of the device.

The diagnostic capabilities of current ICDs vary by manufacturer, but all include electrogram storage of events that trigger therapy. These data are useful in determining the need for programming changes or adjunctive drug or ablative therapy. The devices also have the ability to document nonsustained and paced events, providing a form of ambulatory monitoring. Histograms (charts providing heart rate data) are available in ICDs with sophisticated pacemaker functions.

ICD Therapies

As ICDs became more complex, the need for nomenclature to distinguish features and functions of devices was recognized. In 1993, the NASPE/BPEG Defibrillator Code was published as an NASPE policy statement (Bernstein et al., 1993). The code is generic and patterned after the one designed for pacemakers (Table 20-5). The first letter describes the shock chamber. Thus, "A" refers to atrial defibrillation, "V" to ventricular, and "D" to dual-chamber; "O" is used if the device is turned off. The second letter indicates the location of antitachycardia pacing. The third letter provides information about the device's detection capabilities. An "E" signifies that electrogram signals alone are used to detect tachycardias. If one or more hemodynamic variables are used for tachycardia detection, an "H" is used as the third letter. The fourth letter of the code identifies the location of antibradycardia pacing without specifying the mode of pacing ("A" atrial, "V" ventricular, "D" dual-chamber, and "O" none). Manufacturers have periodically strayed from this recommended labeling, so it is possible that other letter combinations may be seen.

All currently used ICDs have the ability to defibrillate, cardiovert, and provide antitachycardia and antibradycardia pacing. Typically, defibrillation and antibradycardia pacing are the minimum functions used. The device is programmed with a defibrillation detection or "cutoff" rate above which the device begins to charge the capacitor and prepares to deliver a shock. Devices incorporate a "second-look" feature that requires verification of the tachycardia just before delivering the shock. This allows the device to abort delivery of an unnecessary shock when the patient is having nonsustained tachycardia. For patients without an indication for permanent pacing, the antibradycardia feature is programmed at a low rate (35 to 40) to provide postshock support if needed. Patients with a permanent pacing indication should receive a device capable of providing appropriate pacing modes, as discussed in the previous section.

Patients with hemodynamically tolerated VT may have the antitachycardia pacing feature activated. This allows a tiered therapy approach to treatment. A VT detection rate below the VF detection rate is programmed, creating a "VT zone." The initial therapy can be programmed to antitachycardia pacing so that the device can attempt to terminate VT without giving the patient

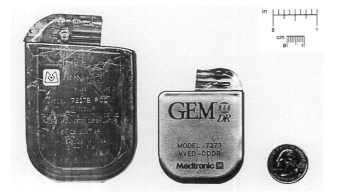

FIGURE 20-10. Comparison of early ICD (*left*) and current generation device (*right*); quarter is shown in right lower corner for size comparison. (Courtesy of Medtronic, Inc., Minneapolis, MN)

TABLE 20-5

The NASPE/BPEG Defibrillator (NBD) Code

I Shock Chamber	II Antitachycardia Pacing Chamber	III Tachycardia Detection	IV Antibradycardia Pacing Chamber
O—None	O—None	E—Electrogram	O—None
A—Atrium	A—Atrium	H—Hemodynamic	A—Atrium
V—Ventricle	V—Ventricle		V—Ventricle
D—Dual (A + V)	D—Dual (A + V)		D—Dual (A + V)

NASPE, North American Society of Pacing and Electrophysiology; BPEG, British Pacing and Electrophysiology Group.
Adapted from Bernstein AD, Camm JA, Fisher JD, et al., 1993: The NASPE/BPEG defibrillator code. Pacing Clin Electrophysiol 16:1776.

a shock. A variety of antitachycardia pacing protocols are usually available (eg, ramp, burst) and are programmable. It is helpful to test the reliability of the programmed parameters in the EP laboratory. Ideally, antitachycardia pacing terminates VT with the first attempt. Because it may accelerate the tachycardia instead of terminating it, therapies in the VT zone limit the antitachycardia pacing attempts and incorporate shocks with increasing intensity as subsequent therapy. If the ICD detects VT degenerating to VF, it switches zones and delivers the therapy programmed for VF.

Patients may require device reprogramming as frequency or types of tachycardia change. This is done noninvasively by a programmer using telemetry. Electrogram information is useful to determine the appropriateness of therapy. Interpretation of electrograms is also important in guiding changes in ICD settings or deciding to perform ablation therapy or initiate antiarrhythmic drug therapy. Stress testing may be necessary to determine the patient's maximum heart rate during exercise so that the device can be programmed to avoid shocks for sinus tachycardia (Klein & Reek, 1998).

ICD Implantation

Patients who have experienced a cardiac arrest or sustained VT are hospitalized before implantation. Other patients first learn about their need for ICD implantation after outpatient EP testing that shows inducible symptomatic VT. Regardless of the patient's presentation, there are many issues to be discussed before implantation. It is helpful to begin discussion regarding possible ICD implantation with patients before elective EP testing for suspected VT. This enables the patient to begin to consider the implications of ICD implantation and to make necessary arrangements before hospitalization. Table 20-6 provides a general plan of care for patients requiring an ICD.

Patients with an ICD may face significant lifestyle changes if they experience arrhythmias that result in loss of consciousness and they work in a setting that would increase potential injury if syncope occurred. An example is a construction worker required to work at significant heights with limited protection from a fall. It is im-

portant for the patient to realize that the arrhythmia, not the ICD, is the cause of activity restriction. Sometimes, extreme levels of EMI may exist in the workplace, prohibiting a patient with an ICD from returning to his or her job. Patients who are faced with loss of their typical work or hobbies are usually less accepting of the device.

As with pacemaker implantation, laboratory tests and a chest roentgenogram need to be obtained before implantation. Patients on anticoagulant therapy must discontinue warfarin for several days before implantation to allow the prothrombin time to return to near normal. Heparin therapy is indicated in certain circumstances (eg, prosthetic heart valve) and an individual plan should be developed accordingly. Patients are required to fast for 6 to 8 hours before implantation. Antibiotic therapy is usually given just before implantation and during the following 24 to 48 hours.

Transvenous implantation of an ICD may be done in a catheterization laboratory or operating room using sterile technique. Implantation is usually performed using local anesthesia and conscious sedation with midazolam, fentanyl, or propofol. General anesthesia or deep sedation administered by an anesthesiologist may be necessary in some circumstances. Electrocardiogram and pulse oximetry monitoring are performed throughout the procedure. In addition, external defibrillation patches are placed on the chest and monitor connections are verified before draping the patient. The transvenous lead(s) may be introduced through the cephalic or subclavian vein on the right or left side. The implantation site is determined using the same criteria discussed previously for pacemaker implantation. The generator pocket may be made in a subcutaneous or subpectoral location. For reasons that are not completely clear, when an ICD is placed in the right pectoral region, higher DFTs may be observed (Flaker et al., 1998). Occasionally, an ICD is placed in the abdomen at the patient's request for cosmetic reasons or in the case of bilateral mastectomy.

Once venous access is accomplished, the ventricular lead is positioned in the right ventricular apex under fluoroscopic guidance. Lead position is confirmed with adequate pacing threshold (<1.5 V at 0.5 milliseconds), lead impedance (300 to 1200 ohms), and R wave (≥5 mV during sinus rhythm) measurements. If dual-chamber

TABLE 20-6

Implantable Cardioverter-Defibrillator Placement: Low-Risk Rapid Recovery Protocol

Critical Occurence	Preprocedure	Procedure	Procedure Day Postprocedure (Hours 1 to 6)	Procedure Day Postprocedure (Hours 7 to 23)	Follow-up
Consults	• Obtain preprocedure assessments and tests • Initiate any predicted home care or special needs arrangements		Per implanting physician: • Follow-up recommendations • Wound management	Per implanting physician: • Follow-up recommendations • Wound management • Anticoagulation (if applicable) • Wound evaluation scheduled for 1 wk postimplant	Follow-up phone call within 1 wk Incision check at 1 wk
Assessments	Preprocedure worksheet complete Preprocedure orders signed and sent to nursing unit	Documentation of periprocedural monitoring and nursing care	CCU or telemetry observation for acute change in cardiovascular, pulmonary or neurologic status Bleeding precautions Monitor vital signs, incision and activity	Observation for acute change in cardiovascular, pulmonary, or neurologic status Telemetry until discharge Limited activity with affected arm Monitor vital signs q 4 h	

Education	• Provide preoperative teaching for patient and family including discussion regarding driving and activity restrictions. Provide written admission instructions		Reinforce routines, especially activity restrictions postprocedure
			Education regarding discharge instructions and follow-up
				• Reinforce teaching:
				  ○ Review new medications if applicable
				  ○ Activity restrictions
				  ○ D/C planning to include:	

	• Provide information regarding discontinuation of warfarin and need for heparin if applicable			○ Home care and job related risks/needs ○ Written D/C instructions and ICD identification card ○ ICD video watched by patient ○ Follow-up wound check and 1-month ICD check scheduled	
Tests	CBS w/differential, chemistry panel, PT/PTT/INR, urinalysis, ECG, CXR		CXR portable	12-lead ECG if needed CXR, PA and lateral Predischarge ICD check	ICD check with VF induction in 1–3 mo
Treatments			Sling to affected arm before leaving procedure laboratory	Remove sling morning after implant	
Medications		Documentation of periprocedural infusions, medications and sedation	Pain/sedation medications prn Resume previous medications except anticoagulants	New medications as ordered Resume warfarin if needed. No heparin	
Activity			Complete bed rest with HOB ≥45°	Ambulate 6 h postimplant	
Diet	NPO night before procedure	NPO	Resume diet as tolerated	NPO 6 hr before predischarge ICD test	
Discharge				Discharge	Review patient-specific information

CBC, complete blood count; CCU, coronary care unit; CXR, chest roentgenogram; D/C, discharge; ECG, electrocardiogram; HOB, head of bed; INR, international normalized ratio; NPO, nothing by mouth; PA, posteroanterior; PT, prothrombin time; PTT, partial thromboplastin time; VF, ventricular fibrillation.
Adapted from Clinical Pathway, Northwestern Memorial Hospital, Chicago, Illinois.

pacing is required, the atrial pacing lead is placed through the same vein and similar lead testing is documented (P wave ≥ 2 mV). Lead measurements should be stable, indicating secure lead position. Measurements must be rechecked after any lead manipulation. Once the leads have been secured to the generator, a low-energy synchronized shock is delivered during sinus rhythm to assess high-voltage lead impedance of the shocking leads, confirming the integrity of the system. This should be done before defibrillation testing.

Induction of VF is done noninvasively through a variety of techniques (burst pacing, T wave shock, programmed stimulation). Testing for reproducible termination of VF is required at implantation to ensure proper device function during a clinical arrhythmia event. One method of testing requires determination of DFTs; device output is then programmed 10 J greater than the DFT. Safety margin verification is an alternative method to DFT determination. With this method, defibrillation testing is performed two to three times at energy levels 10 to 15 J below the maximum ICD output. If testing is successful, an adequate DFT is presumed to exist and the device is programmed to maximum output. This method usually involves fewer VF inductions and shortens procedure time (Swygman et al., 1998).

Ventricular fibrillation sensing should also be assessed during implantation. If either sensing or defibrillation fails, the lead must be repositioned and retested until acceptable placement is found. In the past, device testing was done through external support devices that provided lead information and defibrillation testing without using the actual ICD. This ensured that adequate DFTs were achieved before actually using a very expensive generator. Since the introduction of technologies that have lowered DFTs, the current trend is toward device-based testing for primary implants. This method uses the implanted device for lead measurements, VF inductions, and ICD test shocks. Once acceptable measurements have been confirmed, the generator pocket is irrigated with an antibiotic solution and hemostasis is achieved. The generator is placed in the pocket and the incision is closed.

Occasionally the need for a pacemaker develops in a patient with an ICD. If the ICD leads are functioning and the generator is not approaching replacement, a separate pacemaker may be implanted. Important safeguards are followed to prevent inappropriate sensing by the ICD of pacing impulses. The ICD pulse generator detects the spike of highest amplitude as the R wave. If the pacing impulse and R wave are similar in amplitude, the ICD pulse generator may "double count" the heart rate and produce erroneous triggering of a countershock. Conversely, if VF develops in the patient, pacing impulses may be substantially taller than the fibrillatory waves and may be sensed by the ICD unit as a normal heart rate. In this case, the ICD would fail to discharge. Also, a bipolar lead system is used for the pacemaker because it produces a pacing impulse of smaller amplitude than that which occurs with a unipolar lead. The ventricular pacing lead is placed at some distance from the rate-

sensing electrodes of the ICD unit. Vigorous testing is required during implantation to verify proper function of both devices.

Complications

Serious complications during ICD implantation are rare but do exist. The implantation team must be prepared to respond to emergencies such as difficult or unattainable venous access, pneumothorax, tamponade, excessive DFTs, and refractory VF. Early postoperative complications include lead dislodgment, pocket hematoma, poor wound healing, and possible worsening of arrhythmias. Complications that may occur at a later time include infection, venous thrombosis, lead fracture, Twiddler's syndrome, and a variety of problems with device function. Incidence of complications associated with transvenous ICD implantation has been reported at rates of 2.3% to 13% (Rosenqvist et al., 1998).

Inappropriate shocks are a bothersome complication experienced by up to 25% of patients with earlier-generation ICDs (Grimm et al., 1993). Improvements in tachycardia detection (sudden onset, rate stability) will continue to decrease the incidence of spurious shocks. Information available from atrial sensing in dual-chamber pacing ICDs will also help avoid this problem.

Anxiety and depression are among the psychological complications related to ICD implantation. Patients with ICDs usually report some psychological distress. It is not clear whether the anxiety is related to the device itself or a function of living with severe underlying heart disease. Patients often have high levels of anxiety at the time of implantation that diminish over time. Younger patients and those who receive frequent, inappropriate ICD discharges have higher levels of anxiety. Early psychological intervention by a psychiatrist or clinical psychologist has been suggested for those patients identified with significant emotional distress (Conti et al., 1998). Support groups provide a less formal means of helping the patient adjust to living with an ICD. The support group offers patients a chance to meet and talk with others who have been through similar experiences. Patients and their families appreciate the reassurance that their concerns and issues are common. Support group meetings also provide an opportunity to provide new information and reinforce education for ICD patients. In general, patients are accepting of ICDs. When appropriate shocks occur, most are aware of the consequences that would have ensued had an ICD not been implanted and are appreciative of having a life-saving device.

Nursing Care and Follow-up

During the initial postoperative period, patients require bed rest for 6 to 18 hours. Patients need to be in a monitored setting so that any arrhythmia problem can quickly be addressed. Despite the presence of an ICD, standard transthoracic defibrillation is performed if sustained VT or VF occurs. External paddles are placed in the conventional position on the chest wall. Care should be taken to avoid placing the paddles directly over the ICD generator. Once the bed rest restriction has ended, patients are encouraged to ambulate. Arm movements on the affected side need to be limited, but should not be completely restricted. There is no consensus regarding postimplantation ICD testing. In some centers, patients are discharged the day of implantation. In others, a VF induction is performed in the EP laboratory the following morning before discharge. A chest roentgenogram is performed to detect pneumothorax and document proper lead placement.

Before discharge from the hospital, written and verbal instructions, written descriptive information about the ICD, and a temporary identification card are given to the patient. It is helpful to involve family members and significant others in this teaching session. Patients often have a limited capacity to absorb the tremendous amount of information they receive regarding the ICD during a short period of time. Considering that a fair amount of sedation is given during the implant and predischarge testing, written instructions for follow-up are strongly recommended. All device companies provide a general information booklet that patients should be encouraged to read. Videos are also available free of charge from device manufacturers and provide an abbreviated overview of ICD issues and commonly asked questions. The patient's demographic information is verified for correct registry with the manufacturer for device tracking purposes. It is helpful to follow up with a phone call or letter to the patient after discharge to ensure they are aware of the follow-up plan.

Common topics of concern for ICD patients are driving, concerns about EMI, and what to do if a shock occurs. Opinions vary regarding the advisability of driving. The general practice is to restrict driving for a period (1 to 6 months) in patients who have experienced a cardiac arrest or syncope related to arrhythmias. This allows time to evaluate the patient and ICD system. Most patients capable of driving before implantation are allowed to resume driving.

Sources of potential EMI are everywhere. As with pacemakers, household appliances, cellular phones, and electronic surveillance equipment do not pose any harm to the ICD or affect function as long as normal distance is maintained. The hospital setting can pose problems unique to the ICD. Patients are advised to inform any physician or health care provider (eg, dentists, physical therapists) that they have an ICD. Noise signals generated from some types of equipment used in surgical procedures (eg, electrocautery) require that the device be turned off to prevent inappropriate shocks. Once limited to the operating room, procedures using this type of equipment are now performed in many outpatient settings. People providing this type of care should be aware that if the ICD is turned off, the patient must be connected to an external defibrillator and monitored continuously until the ICD is reactivated. One test that patients with ICDs may not have is magnetic resonance imaging.

When patients receive a shock, they are instructed to call the managing physician or ICD center to report the event. Questioning the patient can help elicit clues regarding appropriateness of the shock. Patients often feel a brief period of lightheadedness, dizziness, or palpitations and are aware that an arrhythmia is occurring. Other times, the shock comes with no warning. If the patient is asymptomatic and receives one shock, he or she typically is not required to come in for immediate evaluation. However, if frequent shocks occur in a short time frame, the patient requires immediate evaluation. If the shocks are accompanied by any symptoms of myocardial ischemia or heart failure, the patient should seek immediate emergency care. Frequent shocks may also be caused by lead fracture or device malfunction; in these cases, immediate hospitalization is required as well.

Initially, patients return at 3-month intervals to a specialized clinic equipped with programmers and personnel experienced in programming ICDs. After the first year, some patients are allowed to reduce follow-up visits to every 6 months. Routine visits include an evaluation of tachyarrhythmia detections and therapies, lead measurements, pacing thresholds, and battery status. As devices become more complicated, it is increasingly important to have experienced physicians available to interpret data from the device. Determining whether a tachycardia is truly VT or a supraventricular tachycardia is not always straightforward. Decisions regarding the addition of medications or reprogramming the device may require further testing to diagnose and treat the patient adequately.

There is no standard approach to frequency of follow-up. Some of the battery tests that were performed manually in the past can be programmed to occur automatically. Some centers advise patients that they can reduce the number of visits unless they are aware of device therapy (eg, shocks). A problem with this approach is that the patient is not always aware that events have occurred (because consciousness was lost or events were terminated with antitachycardia pacing) and problems with the battery or leads do not always cause symptoms to alert the patient to the presence of a malfunction. One new feature in some devices is an alert tone emitted from the device if certain trouble criteria are met. This programmable feature can be useful in prompting patients to seek evaluation when needed.

Implantation of an ICD device does not necessarily negate the need for antiarrhythmic medications because frequent discharging of the device is not desirable or practical. Forty to 70% of patients with ICDs require chronic, concomitant antiarrhythmic medication therapy (Movsowitz & Marchlinski, 1998). Because antiarrhythmic medications can alter DFT, device function is also tested after changes in the medication regimen. Amiodarone, lidocaine, propranolol, and verapamil increase DFT, whereas sotalol decreases DFT (Barold & Zipes, 1997). Class III antiarrhythmic medications are used most commonly in patients with ICDs because they are most effective in preventing arrhythmia recurrence. In addition to affecting DFTs, class III agents may prolong VT cycle length, which may affect the ability to pace-terminate or cardiovert VT; they also have proarrhythmic potential that may affect defibrillator function (Movsowitz & Marchlinski, 1998). The interactions between ICDs and pharmacologic therapy are important considerations in long-term management of patients being treated with both modalities.

As the battery measurements show signs of energy depletion, frequency of follow-up visits is increased. Manufacturers provide guidelines for suggested replacement indicators that vary for each ICD model. When evidence of battery depletion is detected, the defibrillator is replaced. Replacement of the defibrillator battery usually can be performed as an outpatient procedure using local anesthesia. The defibrillator pocket is opened and the defibrillator is disconnected from the electrodes. Pacing and sensing thresholds of the electrodes are measured before and after being connected to a new defibrillator generator. VF is induced to assess proper function of the new device in detecting and converting the arrhythmia. The device is then anchored to the pocket with sutures to prevent twisting or migration and the incision is closed. Follow-up ICD testing with VF induction is not necessary unless a new lead has been placed. Patients have minimal restrictions as the incision heals and are then able to return to their normal activities and follow-up schedule.

REFERENCES

Barold SS, Zipes DP, 1997: Cardiac pacemakers and antiarrhythmic devices. In Braunwald E (ed): Heart Disease: A Textbook of Cardiovascular Medicine, ed. 5. Philadelphia, WB Saunders

Bernstein AD, Camm AJ, Fletcher RD, et al., 1987: The NASPE/BPEG generic pacemaker code for antibradyarrhythmia and adaptive-rate pacing and antitachyarrhythmia devices. Pacing Clin Electrophysiol 10:794

Bernstein AD, Camm JA, Fisher JD, et al., 1993: The NASPE/BPEG defibrillator code. Pacing Clin Electrophysiol 16:1776

Brinker J, Midei M, 1996: Techniques of pacemaker implantation. In Ellenbogen KA (ed): Cardiac Pacing, ed. 2. Cambridge, MA, Blackwell Science

Connolly SJ, Kerr C, Gent M, Yusuf D, 1996: Dual-chamber versus ventricular pacing: Critical appraisal of current data. Circulation 94:578

Conti JB, Sears SF, Mribal G, 1998: Psychological complications of implantable cardioverter-defibrillator therapy. Cardiac Electrophysiology Review 2:342

Crossley GH, Brinker JA, Reynolds D, et al., 1995: Steroid elution improves the stimulation threshold in an active-fixation atrial permanent pacing lead: A randomized, controlled study. Model 4068 investigators. Circulation 92:2935

Dreifus LS, Fisch C, Griffin JC, et al., 1991: Guidelines for implantation of cardiac pacemakers and antiarrhythmia devices: A report of the American College of Cardiology/American Heart Association Task Force on Assessment of Diagnostic and Therapeutic Cardiovascular Procedures. J Am Coll Cardiol 18:1

Finkelmeier NE, 1991: Pacemaker technology: An overview. AACN Clin Issues Crit Care Nurs 2:99

Flaker GC, Tummala R, Wilson J, 1998: Comparison of right-

and left-sided pectoral implantation parameters with the Jewel active can cardiodefibrillator. Pacing Clin Electrophysiol 21:447

Goldberger E, 1990: Modes of cardiac pacing. In Treatment of Cardiac Emergencies, ed. 5. St. Louis, CV Mosby

Gottlieb CD, Callans DJ, 1998: New devices: Functions and features. Cardiac Electrophysiology Review 2:272

Gregoratos G, Cheitlin MD, Conill A, et al., 1998: ACC/AHA guidelines for implantation of cardiac pacemakers and antiarrhythmia devices: A report of the American College of Cardiology/American Heart Association Task Force on Practice Guidelines (Committee on Pacemaker Implantation). J Am Coll Cardiol 31:1175

Grimm W, Flores BT, Marchlinski FE, 1993: Shock occurrence and survival in 241 patients with implantable cardioverter-defibrillator therapy. Circulation 87:1880

Haffajee CI, 1998: Comparative features, functions and longevities of implantable cardioverter-defibrillators. Cardiac Electrophysiology Review 2:263

Hammill SC, 1998: ICD lead technology: Remarkable advances during the past decade. Cardiac Electrophysiology Review 2:267

Harthorne JW, 1989: Cardiac pacing. In Grillo HC, Austen WG, Wilkins EW, et al. (eds): Current Therapy in Cardiothoracic Surgery. Toronto, Canada, BC Decker

Hayes DL, 1998: Pacemakers. In Topol EJ (ed): Comprehensive Cardiovascular Medicine. Philadelphia, Lippincott Williams & Wilkins

Hayes DL, 1997: Interference with cardiac pacemakers by cellular telephones. N Engl J Med 336:1473

Hayes DL, 1993: Programmability. In Furman S, Hayes DL, Holmes DR (eds): A Practice of Cardiac Pacing, ed. 3. Mount Kisco, NY, Futura

Hayes DL, Holmes DR, 1993: Hemodynamics of cardiac pacing. In Furman S, Hayes DL, Holmes DR (eds): A Practice of Cardiac Pacing, ed. 3. Mount Kisco, NY, Futura

Hayes DL, Holmes DR, Furman S, 1993: Permanent pacemaker implantation. In Furman S, Hayes DL, Holmes DR (eds): A Practice of Cardiac Pacing, ed. 3. Mount Kisco, NY, Futura

Hillis LD, Lange RA, Winniford MD, Page RL, 1995: Temporary and permanent pacing. In Manual of Clinical Problems in Cardiology, ed. 5. Boston, Little, Brown

Kennergren C, 1996: Impact of implant techniques on complications with current implantable cardioverter-defibrillator systems. Am J Cardiol 78(Suppl 5A):15

Klein HU, Reek S, 1998: Evaluation of the patient with frequent implantable cardioverter-defibrillator discharges. Cardiac Electrophysiology Review 2:337

Kleinschmidt KM, Stafford MJ, 1991: Dual-chamber cardiac pacemakers. J Cardiovasc Nurs 5:1

Kusumoto FM, Goldschlager N, 1996: Medical progress: Cardiac pacing. N Engl J Med 334:89

Lerman BB, Deale OC, 1990: Effect of epicardial patch electrodes on transthoracic defibrillation. Circulation 81:1409

Lerman RD, Cannom DS, 1998: Indication for implantable cardioverter-defibrillator therapy. Cardiac Electrophysiology Review 2:246

Lowe JE, Wharton JM, 1995: Cardiac pacemakers and implantable cardioverter-defibrillators. In Sabiston DC Jr, Spencer FC (eds): Surgery of the Chest, ed. 6. Philadelphia, WB Saunders

McErlean ES, 1991: Dual-chamber pacing. AACN Clin Issues Crit Care Nurs 2:126

McIvor ME, Reddinger J, Flodan E, Sheppard RC, 1998: Study of pacemaker and implantable cardioverter defibrillator triggering by electronic surveillance devices. Pacing Clin Electrophysiol 21:1847

Mirowski M, Reid PR, Mower MM, et al., 1980: Termination of malignant ventricular arrhythmias with an implanted automatic defibrillator in human beings. N Engl J Med 303:22

Mirowski M, Reid PR, Winkle RA, et al., 1983: Mortality in patients with implanted automatic defibrillators. Ann Intern Med 98:585

Morton PG, 1991: Rate-responsive cardiac pacemakers. AACN Clin Issues Crit Care Nurs 2:140

Moses HW, Taylor GJ, Schneider JA, Dove JT, 1987: Pacemaker implantation. In A Practical Guide to Cardiac Pacing, ed. 2. Boston, Little, Brown

Movsowitz C, Marchlinski FE, 1998: Interactions between implantable cardioverter-defibrillators and class III agents. Am J Cardiol 82:41-I

Parsonnet V, Furman S, Smyth NP, 1974: Implantable cardiac pacemaker status report and resource guideline. Circulation 50:A21

Reynolds DW, 1996: Hemodynamics of cardiac pacing. In Ellenbogen KA (ed): Cardiac Pacing, ed. 2. Cambridge, MA, Blackwell Science

Rosenqvist M, Beyer T, Block M, et al., 1998: Adverse events with transvenous implantable cardioverter-defibrillators: A prospective multicenter study. Circulation 98:663

Rosenthal ME, Josephson ME, 1990: Current status of anti-tachycardia devices. Circulation 82:1890

Schoen FJ, 1997: Pathologic considerations in the surgery of adult heart disease. In Edmunds LH Jr (ed): Cardiac Surgery in the Adult. New York, McGraw-Hill

Spotnitz HM, 1997: Practical considerations in pacemaker-defibrillator surgery. In Edmunds LH Jr (ed): Cardiac Surgery in the Adult. New York, McGraw-Hill

Stephenson NL, Combs W, 1991: Artificial cardiac pacemakers and implantable cardioverter defibrillators. In Kinney MR, Packa DR, Andreoli KG, Zipes DP (eds): Comprehensive Cardiac Care, ed. 7. St. Louis, Mosby–Year Book

Swygman CA, Homoud MK, Link MS, et al., 1998: Testing implantable cardioverter-defibrillator functions at implantation. Cardiac Electrophysiology Review 2:280

Teplitz L, 1991: Classification of cardiac pacemakers: The pacemaker code. J Cardiovasc Nurs 5:1

Wiegand UK, Bode F, Schneider R, et al., 1999: Atrial sensing and AV synchrony in single lead VDD pacemakers: A prospective comparison to DDD devices with bipolar atrial leads. J Cardiovasc Electrophysiol 10:513

Wilkoff BL et al., 1999: Pacemaker lead extraction with the laser sheath: Results of the pacing lead extraction with the excimer sheath (PLEXES) trial. J Am Coll Cardiol 33:1671

21

Surgical Treatment of Other Cardiovascular Disorders

► Cardiac Neoplasms

Types of Tumors

Primary cardiac neoplasms may be either benign or malignant. Approximately 75% of primary cardiac tumors are benign, and half of these are myxomas (Van Trigt & Sabiston, 1995; Kirklin & Barratt-Boyes, 1993a). Other benign tumors that occur infrequently are lipomas and papillary fibroelastomas. The most common malignant primary cardiac tumor in adults is angiosarcoma, a tumor that originates in the myocardium and invades both the cardiac chambers and pericardial space. Angiosarcomas are two to three times more common in men than in women, and most often occur on the right side of the heart (McAllister et al., 1999a).

More frequently, tumors of the heart represent metastatic spread of lung or breast cancer, melanoma, leukemia, or lymphoma. These so-called *secondary tumors* are 20 times more common than primary cardiac tumors (Hall & Anderson, 1997). Secondary cardiac tumors can metastasize to the heart through hematogenous or lymphocytic routes or extend directly from surrounding intrathoracic structures (Schaff et al., 1991). By far the most common location of metastatic cardiac neoplasms is the epicardium; epicardial tumor deposits may be multifocal, single, or extensive and essentially diffuse (Roberts, 1998).

Surgical Treatment of Tumors

Surgical treatment of intracardiac tumors became possible only after development of cardiopulmonary bypass provided a means of extracorporeal circulation. It is the recommended treatment for all cardiac tumors, even those that are benign or asymptomatic. The heart has a limited tolerance for any space-occupying lesion, and intracardiac tumors can cause lethal complications, including arrhythmias, cardiac tamponade, pericardial constriction, valvular obstruction, and embolism (Fallon & Dec, 1989; Schaff et al., 1991).

For primary malignant cardiac tumors, surgical resection is possible only occasionally. Because of their rapid growth potential, tumor removal often is precluded by extensive myocardial infiltration, local invasion of adjacent structures, or distant metastases. Because cardiac malignancies are universally fatal if not resected, prognosis for survival without surgical resection is poor. Total excision is the goal of surgical resection. However, partial excision may be necessary if the tumor involves intracardiac structures or coronary arteries (McAllister et al., 1999b).

Survival after surgical resection varies depending on the type of tumor and its location. The survival rate is 90% or greater after surgical resection for myxoma but less than 10% for primary cardiac malignancies (Van Trigt & Sabiston, 1995). Surgical treatment of metastatic malignancy to the heart is palliative and usually is confined to drainage of pericardial effusions (Hall & Anderson, 1997). The remainder of the discussion is limited to surgical resection of myxoma, by far the most common cardiac tumor treated with surgical therapy.

Surgical Resection of Myxoma

Myxomas consist of gelatinous, mucoid material and arise from the endocardial surface of one or more of the cardiac chambers. Most myxomas originate in the upper chambers of the heart. Approximately 75% arise in the left atrium, 23% in the right atrium, 2% in a ventricular cavity, and, on rare occasions, tumor is present in more than one cavity (Roberts, 1998). Typically, atrial myxomas are attached to the interatrial septum by a pedunculated stalk in the area of the fossa ovalis.

Three types of clinical manifestations are associated with myxoma: (1) symptoms related to obstruction of blood flow through the heart; (2) symptoms of systemic embolization of tumor fragments; and (3) constitutional symptoms, such as weight loss, fatigue, and fever. Symptoms may be sudden in onset, intermittent, and related to the patient's body position (Hillis et al., 1995a). Left atrial myxomas typically mimic mitral stenosis, producing dyspnea and other signs and symptoms of left-sided heart failure (Hall & Anderson, 1997).

Despite histologic benignancy, surgical removal of a myxoma always is indicated. Death or catastrophic complications may result from tumor embolization or the hemodynamic abnormalities produced by the presence of an intracardiac foreign body. Operative therapy is performed promptly after diagnosis because death from obstruction or embolism can occur precipitously. Surgical excision of myxoma is possible because the tumors are primarily intracavitary and rarely extend deeper than the endocardial layer of the heart.

A median sternotomy approach usually is used. After instituting cardiopulmonary bypass, aortic cross-clamping, and cardioplegic arrest of the heart, the appropriate cardiac chamber is opened with an incision that allows good visualization of the tumor and makes possible its removal with minimal manipulation (Fig. 21-1). For resection of atrial myxomas, one or both atria may be opened. Ventricular myxomas usually are approached through an incision in the aorta or left atrium (for left ventricular tumors) or right atrium (for right ventricular tumors) (Acker & Gardner, 1996). These approaches avoid ventricular muscle damage that would result from a ventriculotomy (ie, an incision in the ventricle).

Because myxomatous tissue is gelatinous and very friable, extreme caution is necessary to avoid embolization before and during tumor removal. The heart is handled gently during cannulation and the chamber containing the myxoma is not manipulated until the aortic cross-clamp is applied and cardioplegic arrest is achieved (Acker & Gardner, 1996). Manipulation of the tumor itself is avoided. Atrial myxomas are handled

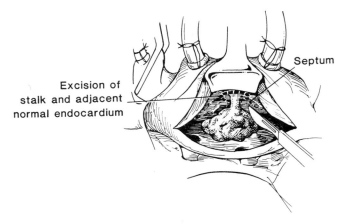

FIGURE 21-1. Left atriotomy performed after initiation of cardiopulmonary bypass reveals myxoma attached to atrial septum; myxoma stalk is excised with adjacent normal endocardium. (DiSesa VJ, Collins JJ Jr, Cohn LH, 1988: Considerations in the surgical management of left atrial myxoma. J Cardiac Surg 3:19)

only by the stalk that anchors the tumor to the interatrial septum.

All myxomatous tissue must be removed because the tumor can recur despite its benignancy (Fig. 21-2). Atrial septal tissue surrounding the tumor pedicle is excised en bloc, creating a small atrial septal defect that is repaired by direct suture technique or with an autogenous pericardial patch (Van Trigt & Sabiston, 1995). After the tumor is evacuated, the chamber is thoroughly irrigated and inspected to remove any residual tumor fragments or thrombus that might embolize when the heart is again allowed to eject blood into the systemic circulation. The cardiac valves that contacted the tumor also are inspected carefully for damage. Occasionally, valve replacement is necessary because of damage caused by prolapsing of an atrial myxoma through the valve during diastole (Roberts, 1998).

The operative mortality rate for removal of an atrial myxoma is approximately 5%, and usually is related to

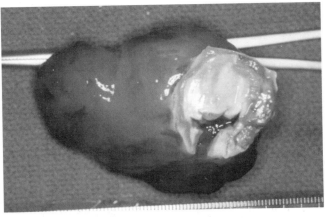

FIGURE 21-2. Left atrial myxoma has been excised with interatrial septum attachment. (Courtesy of Paul Levy MD)

advanced age and comorbid conditions (Spotnitz & Blow, 1998; Hall & Anderson, 1997). Surgical resection usually is curative. Hemodynamic improvement occurs immediately, the risk of embolism is eliminated, and most constitutional symptoms resolve completely (Schaff et al., 1991). Tumor recurrence is unusual except in patients with a familial form of myxoma. Recurring myxomatous tissue may be histologically benign or may become more malignant with each recurrence and may appear in unusual locations, such as the pulmonary artery or aorta (Acker & Gardner, 1996). Serial echocardiographic surveillance is recommended in patients with risk factors for recurrence, such as multicentric tumors, unusual tumor location, and incomplete resection (Hall & Anderson, 1997).

► Cardiomyopathies

Hypertrophic Cardiomyopathy

Hypertrophic cardiomyopathy (HCM), formerly known as *idiopathic hypertrophic subaortic stenosis,* is a primary disease of the heart muscle. HCM is characterized by inappropriate myocardial hypertrophy, usually primarily involving the interventricular septum of a nondilated left ventricle, and hyperdynamic ventricular function (Wynne & Braunwald, 1997). Deformity of the mitral valve apparatus and mitral regurgitation often are present as well. The etiology of HCM is unknown. It is thought to be genetic, often with an autosomal dominant pattern of inheritance, although sporadic cases also occur (Glower, 1995; David, 1997).

Clinical Manifestations

The primary abnormality of HCM is dynamic obstruction of the left ventricular outflow tract during systole. Two factors contribute to the obstruction: (1) septal hypertrophy, and (2) abnormal anterior displacement of the mitral valve apparatus and systolic anterior motion of the anterior mitral valve leaflet. The hypertrophied septum interferes with outflow to a varying degree depending on the contractile state of the heart and left ventricular systolic volume; anterior motion of the mitral valve anterior leaflet during systole exacerbates the obstruction (Ungerleider, 1995).

The anatomic and functional obstruction of the left ventricular outflow tract produces clinical manifestations similar to those resulting from aortic stenosis (Hammond & Letsou, 1996). Symptoms, including dyspnea, angina, syncope, and fatigue, most often occur in young adults. They commonly develop with exertion when ventricular contractility and oxygen demands are increased. The severity of symptoms usually correlates with the extent of ventricular disease and outflow obstruction (Stone et al., 1990).

Symptoms associated with HCM usually can be treated effectively with pharmacologic therapy. Beta-adrenergic blocking agents and the calcium channel antagonist, verapamil, usually are used to reduce left ventricular outflow obstruction by decreasing contractility of the hypertrophied muscle. Dual-chamber pacing has been added as a more recent treatment strategy for HCM, based on its demonstrated efficacy in reducing left ventricular outflow obstruction and associated mitral regurgitation, reducing drug-refractory symptoms, and improving exercise performance (Fananapazir & McAreavey, 1998).

One of the most distressing aspects of HCM is a propensity for sudden cardiac death, which affects even those with no or only minor symptoms of left ventricular outflow tract obstruction. Sudden death occurs in 2% to 3% of adults with HCM per year and is particularly likely in young men with familial HCM or in those with a family history of sudden death (Schoen, 1997). Despite the efficacy of beta-adrenergic blocking agents and verapamil in controlling symptoms of HCM, there is little convincing evidence that these medications reduce the incidence of serious ventricular arrhythmias or sudden death (McKenna & Elliott, 1998). In persons with high clinical or genetic risk for sudden death, antiarrhythmic medications or an implantable cardioverter-defibrillator may be necessary.

Antibiotic prophylaxis against infective endocarditis also is recommended. Patients with HCM are at increased risk of endocardial infection because of turbulent blood flow through the narrowed left ventricular outflow tract and associated mitral regurgitation (Grayzel et al., 1998).

Surgical Therapy

Surgical treatment is indicated in patients with significant left ventricular outflow tract gradients and severe symptoms or a high risk of sudden cardiac death (Schonbeck et al., 1998). The operative procedure most commonly performed for HCM is septal myectomy, also called the Morrow procedure. The operation consists of removing a wedge of the hypertrophied ventricular septum to reduce the dynamic left ventricular outflow tract obstruction; the procedure usually diminishes the degree of mitral regurgitation as well.

Myectomy is performed through a median sternotomy incision and with cardiopulmonary bypass, aortic cross-clamping, and cardioplegic arrest. Intraoperative transesophageal echocardiography is used to locate precisely the left ventricular outflow tract obstruction, guide the surgeon in planning the operative approach, and provide an assessment of operative results. Through an incision in the ascending aorta, the aortic valve leaflets are retracted and a wedge of ventricular septal myocardium is excised (Fig. 21-3). Some surgeons concomitantly plicate the anterior leaflet of the mitral valve to limit its encroachment on the outflow tract (ie, to eliminate systolic anterior motion) (Cooley, 1991). Replacement of the mitral valve may be necessary if a significant left ventricular outflow gradient or severe mitral regurgitation remains after myectomy.

The operative mortality rate of septal myectomy is less

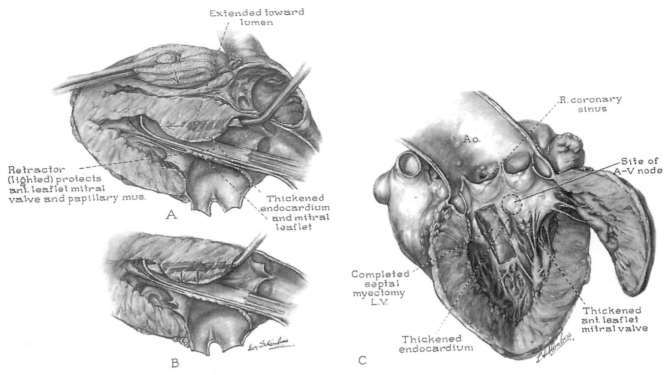

FIGURE 21-3. Myectomy. **(A, B)** A lighted ribbon retractor is passed through the aortic valve annulus to the apex; it protects the mitral valve and papillary muscles. An angled knife is used to excise a rectangular piece of the hypertrophied septum. **(C)** View of the left ventricular septum after completion of the septal myectomy. (Morrow AG, 1978: Hypertrophic subaortic stenosis: Operative methods utilized to relieve left ventricular outflow obstruction. J Thorac Cardiovasc Surg 76:425, 429)

than 5% (Lupinetti, 1998). Potential complications include left bundle branch block, complete heart block (usually due to left bundle branch block in a patient with preexisting right bundle branch block), and iatrogenic ventricular septal defect (Kirklin & Barratt-Boyes, 1993b). Mild to moderate aortic regurgitation also may occur, although it usually is not of hemodynamic significance (McKenna & Elliott, 1998; Brown et al., 1991). The long-term survival rate is 72% at 15 years after myectomy (Schonbeck et al., 1998).

Surgical correction of the dynamic outflow obstruction relieves symptoms and improves quality of life in most patients. However, the major abnormality of HCM is a myopathic process causing abnormal diastolic compliance (Nishimura et al., 1991). Diastolic dysfunction and ischemic events cannot be prevented completely by any of the therapeutic modalities, including myectomy (Schonbeck et al., 1998).

Myectomy is of limited value in patients with thin septums. In such patients, relief of outflow tract obstruction usually is incomplete and the risk of creating a ventricular septal defect is increased. Mitral valve replacement sometimes is performed alternatively as a primary surgical therapy for relief of symptoms caused by HCM. Because of potential complications inherent to valvular prostheses, valve replacement usually is reserved for patients who have (1) a thin ventricular septum, (2) signifi-

cant left ventricular outflow tract obstruction after myectomy, or (3) severe mitral regurgitation.

Dilated Cardiomyopathy

Dilated cardiomyopathy (DCM) is a primary heart muscle disease characterized by ventricular dilatation and congestive heart failure. The condition usually is progressive and often is fatal. Medical treatment is aimed at palliating symptoms of progressive heart failure by controlling salt and water retention, reducing the workload of the heart, and improving contractility (Gilbert & Bristow, 1994). Angiotensin-converting enzyme inhibitors (eg, enalapril) and beta-blocking agents (eg, carvedilol and bisoprolol) have been demonstrated to improve functional status and prolong survival (CIBIS-II Investigators and Committees, 1999; Wynne & Braunwald, 1997).

Heart failure, however, remains a lethal condition, with 5- and 10-year survival rates of 40% to 50% and 20% to 25%, respectively, from the time of diagnosis (Starling, 1998; American Heart Association, 1998; Kirklin & Barratt-Boyes, 1993c). Cardiac transplantation is recommended for patients with DCM who remain severely symptomatic (ie, New York Heart Association [NYHA] class III or class IV functional status) despite optimal pharmacologic therapy and who are suitable candidates for the procedure. However, transplantation is limited by the scarcity of donor organs and is available only to a subset of patients with DCM. Cardiac transplantation is discussed in Chapter 31, Heart, Lung, and Heart-Lung Transplantation.

Dynamic cardiomyoplasty is an evolving surgical therapy for those patients with severe heart failure who are not acceptable transplantation candidates or for whom a donor heart is not available. The operation consists of mobilizing a skeletal muscle pedicle graft and wrapping it around the ventricles. A cardiomyostimulator (burst electrical stimulator) is then used to stimulate the skeletal muscle electrically in synchrony with ventricular systole. A key principle of dynamic cardiomyoplasty is the gradual conversion of skeletal muscle from a fatigue-prone to a fatigue-resistant state with chronic electrostimulation (Starling & Young, 1998).

Positive features of cardiomyoplasty compared with other forms of ventricular support include the use of autogenous tissue and the avoidance of implanting artificial hardware. Because it is still an investigational procedure, it is reserved for patients who have a limited life expectancy with medical therapy alone. However, the beneficial effects of cardiomyoplasty do not occur immediately after the operation and candidates must therefore be stable enough to withstand a long operation, general anesthesia, and a waiting period while conditioning of the skeletal muscle graft is achieved. The best candidates for cardiomyoplasty are those with a NYHA class

III functional status, no prior cardiac surgery, a left ventricular ejection fraction greater than 20%, and preserved right ventricular function; it is not effective in patients with end-stage heart failure (NYHA class IV) who have failed all other forms of therapy (Magovern & Magovern, 1998; Frazier & Myers, 1998).

Cardiomyoplasty is performed without cardiopulmonary bypass. Two separate incisions are required for the procedure: a longitudinal incision on the lateral chest wall from the axilla to the iliac crest for harvesting the latissimus dorsi muscle graft, and a median sternotomy incision for cardiac access (Fig. 21-4). The left latissimus dorsi muscle usually is selected for grafting. It is harvested through the thoracic flank incision, preserving its intact neurovascular bundle. Muscle-stimulating electrodes are implanted in the muscle near the thoracodorsal nerve and the graft is rotated into the left hemithorax through space created by removal of the anterolateral portion of the left third rib (Magovern & Magovern, 1998). The incision is closed, the patient is repositioned, and a median sternotomy is performed.

Through the sternotomy incision, the muscle graft is wrapped around the ventricles and secured in place. An epicardial sensing electrode is placed on the anterior surface of the right ventricle. The muscle pacing and heart sensing electrodes are connected to a cardiomyostimulator device, which is then implanted in a subcutaneous pocket over the left rectus muscle in the upper abdomen. Stimulation of the muscle graft is not initiated for the first 2 postoperative weeks to allow time for the muscle

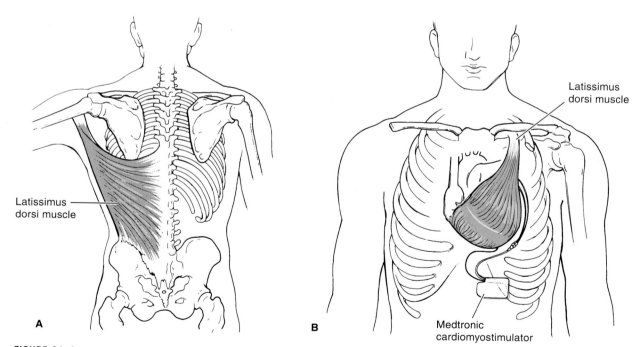

FIGURE 21-4. Two stages of cardiomyoplasty. **(A)** A left latissimus dorsi muscle graft is harvested through a longitudinal flank incision and rotated into the left chest cavity. **(B)** A median sternotomy incision is performed; the muscle graft is wrapped around the ventricles and pacing and sensing electrodes are connected to the cardiomyostimulator. (Hudak CM, Gallo BM, Morton PG, 1998: Cardiac surgery. In Critical Care Nursing: A Holistic Approach, ed. 7, p. 421. Philadelphia, Lippincott Williams & Wilkins)

to recover from the effects of mobilization and translocation (Magovern & Magovern, 1998). Electrical stimulation is then initiated using a progressive muscle-conditioning protocol.

The operative mortality rate for cardiomyoplasty ranges from 5% to 12% (Starling & Young, 1998; Frazier & Myers, 1998). Sudden cardiac death is the primary cause of postoperative death. Clinical experience with cardiomyoplasty remains limited and available long-term data demonstrate somewhat inconsistent results. The degree of benefit varies greatly among individual patients (Renlund, 1998). Also, although cardiomyoplasty improves functional capacity, cardiac function, and quality of life, the 1-year survival rate of 68% after the procedure is not better than the natural history of heart failure without surgical intervention (Magovern & Cmolik, 1996).

► Pericardial Disease

The *pericardium* is a fibroserous sac that encloses the heart. It is composed of an outer (parietal) layer and an inner (visceral) layer. The space between the parietal and visceral layers contains a small amount of clear, plasma-like fluid. The physiologic importance of the pericardium is not precisely defined. The pericardium maintains the heart in a relatively fixed position and shape within the mediastinum, limits distention and valvular incompetence at high filling pressures, and isolates the heart from inflammation in nearby tissues; however, no adverse consequences are associated with its congenital absence or surgical removal (Shabetai, 1994; Brandenburg et al., 1991).

Pericardial Pathology

A wide variety of conditions can affect the pericardium, including infection, myocardial infarction, trauma, autoimmune disorders, radiation, uremia, and malignancy. These various etiologies can produce three forms of pericardial disease: (1) inflammatory pericarditis, (2) pericardial effusion (abnormal fluid accumulation in the pericardial space), or (3) constrictive pericarditis. Often a combination of these processes occurs. Inflammatory pericarditis, in the absence of pericardial effusion or constriction, is managed with medical therapy, primarily anti-inflammatory agents or corticosteroids. Pericardial effusion and constrictive pericarditis, on the other hand, may require surgical intervention and are the focus of this discussion. It often is difficult to distinguish clinically between pericardial effusion and pericardial constriction. Echocardiography usually is used to differentiate the two conditions.

Pericardial effusion can result from malignancy, infectious processes, postpericardiotomy syndrome, or pericarditis. The development of increased intrapericardial pressure and consequent severity of symptoms are determined by the volume of the effusion, the rapidity with which the fluid accumulates, and the physical characteristics of the pericardium (Lorell, 1997). Rapid fluid accumulation, such as occurs with hemorrhage after cardiac surgery, causes cardiac tamponade and acute hemodynamic compromise. Gradual fluid accumulation, such as might occur secondary to malignancy, is more likely to produce progressive shortness of breath.

Constrictive pericarditis is characterized by marked thickening, scarring, or calcification of the pericardium (Harken et al., 1996). It is the end result of chronic pericardial inflammation that may be idiopathic or caused by one of a number of disease processes, such as infection (eg, viral, tuberculous, fungal), uremia, or myocardial infarction. Constrictive pericardial thickening compromises cardiac function by impeding diastolic ventricular filling. Clinical manifestations include ascites, peripheral edema, dyspnea, and fatigue (Hillis et al., 1995b). Vague abdominal symptoms such as postprandial fullness, dyspepsia, flatulence, and anorexia sometimes are also present (Lorell, 1997).

Surgical Procedures

Symptomatic pericardial effusion usually is treated initially with pericardiocentesis. Surgical treatment may be required for recurrent effusions or those inadequately drained by a catheter technique. Surgical drainage of the pericardium is achieved by placement of a chest tube under direct exposure. With a subxiphoid approach and a small incision in the pericardium, a chest tube is placed and connected to gravity drainage for several days. Removal of the tube can be performed at the bedside. In some cases, chest tube drainage is ineffective because the fluid is too viscous or because areas of parietal and visceral pericardium have become adherent to one another, producing loculation (ie, compartmentalization) of fluid.

In such cases, or for large, recurring pericardial effusions, it may be necessary to remove a portion of the pericardium. A *pericardial window* describes a surgical procedure that includes removal of a portion of parietal pericardium and disruption of adhesions to allow free drainage of fluid. It usually is performed through a subxiphoid incision or, less commonly, by video-assisted thoracoscopy. When performed through a subxiphoid incision, a generous disc of the anterior pericardium is excised and finger dissection is used to disrupt adhesions between the visceral and parietal pericardium (Fig. 21-5). A drain is inserted into the pericardial sac and typically remains for several postoperative days until the amount of drainage is minimal. Thoracoscopic pericardial windows may be created on either the left or right side to allow drainage of pericardial fluid into the ipsilateral pleural space, providing pleural surfaces to absorb excess fluid (Roberts & Kaiser, 1998).

Constrictive pericarditis may necessitate performance of a *radical pericardiectomy* (ie, removal of most of the pericardium) to restore adequate cardiac function. Surgical pericardiectomy is the only definitive treatment of constrictive pericarditis and should be performed before calcification and myocardial involvement progress (Klein

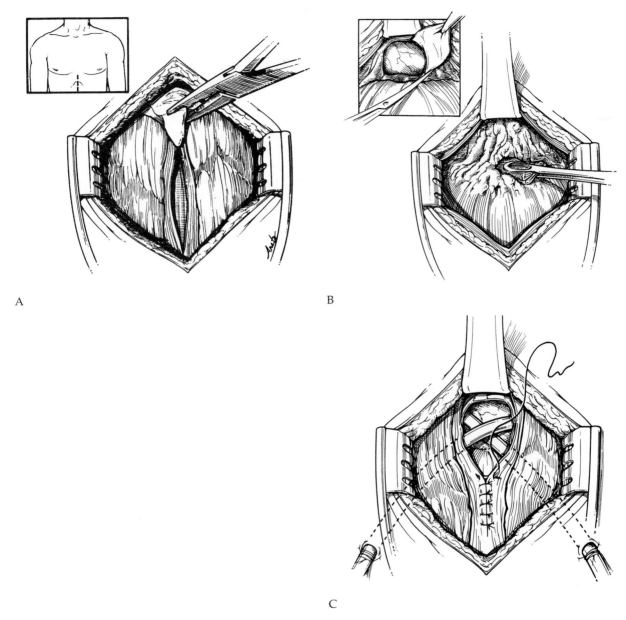

A

B

C

FIGURE 21-5. Subxiphoid pericardial window. **(A)** The subcutaneous tissue is divided with cautery and the linea alba is divided in the midline to expose the xiphoid process, which is then resected at the junction with the sternum. (*Inset*) The subxiphoid incision begins just superior to the xiphosternal junction and extends 5 to 6 cm inferior in the midline. **(B)** A sponge stick is used to sweep away preperitoneal fat while a retractor is used to elevate the sternum anteriorly. The pericardium is identified just posterior to the sternum and superior to the diaphragm. (*Inset*) A small segment of pericardium is excised and a finger is swept within the pericardium to disrupt loculations. Pericardial edges are sutured to extrapericardial tissues to keep the window open. **(C)** The pericardial space is drained with two chest tubes. (Roberts JR, Kaiser LR, 1998: Pericardial procedures. In Kaiser LR, Kron IL, Spray TL [eds]: Mastery of Cardiothoracic Surgery, p. 223. Philadelphia, Lippincott Williams & Wilkins)

& Scalia, 1998). Pericardiectomy is recommended on diagnosis of the condition because poor preoperative hemodynamic function is a major determinant of postoperative morbidity and mortality (Harken et al., 1996).

Usually, all of the anterior pericardium between the right and left phrenic nerves and sometimes pericardium beneath the left phrenic nerve is removed (Fig. 21-6). It is desirable to decorticate (remove the surface layer of pericardium) both ventricles, both atria, and both venae cavae (Harken et al., 1996). Pericardiectomy usually is performed through a median sternotomy incision. A median sternotomy approach is preferable for complete pericardiectomy of the right ventricle and venae cavae; a left thoracotomy approach better exposes the left ventricle and atrium, and allows for easy preservation of the left phrenic nerve (Roberts & Kaiser, 1998).

Cardiopulmonary bypass occasionally is used to make pericardiectomy technically easier. Extracorporeal circulation allows decompression of the heart, thereby facilitating removal of parietal pericardium from the epicardial surface. Cardiopulmonary bypass also may become necessary if manipulation of the heart induces ventricular fibrillation. Blood loss often is significant during pericardiectomy because of inflammation and adhesions, especially if the procedure is performed with cardiopulmonary bypass and systemic anticoagulation. Transfusion may be necessary.

Most patients experience significant clinical improvement if pericardiectomy is performed early after onset of constrictive pericarditis. Sometimes, symptomatic improvement occurs gradually after the operation, over several months. Results often are disappointing in patients with postirradiation constriction, probably because of underlying myocardial fibrosis (Hillis et al., 1995b). Prognosis also is worse in patients with inadequate resection, worse NYHA functional class, myocardial involvement, residual coronary artery disease, older age, chronic disease, and arrhythmias (Klein & Scalia, 1998).

► Chronic Pulmonary Embolism

Pulmonary emboli usually resolve spontaneously owing to intrinsic methods of fibrinolysis. Occasionally, however, *chronic pulmonary embolism* develops as a result of recurring emboli, inadequate lysis, or lack of adequate anticoagulant therapy. In patients with chronic pulmonary embolism, incapacitating pulmonary hypertension may eventually develop from accumulation of thrombus in major branches of the pulmonary arteries. Symptoms of progressive respiratory insufficiency and right ventricular failure typically develop. Therapy includes anticoagulation and inferior vena cava filter placement, but pulmonary thromboendarterectomy is

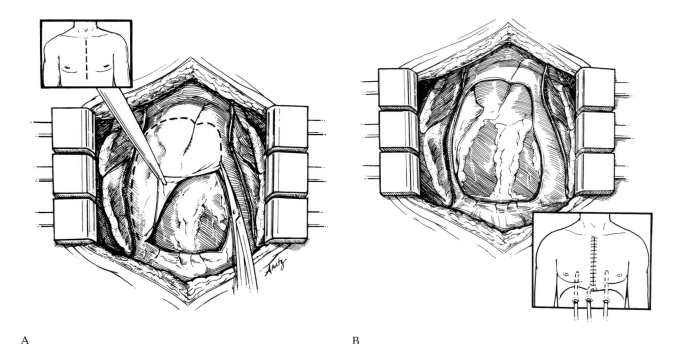

A   B

FIGURE 21-6. Pericardiectomy through a median sternotomy. **(A)** The resection usually is begun at the diaphragmatic junction and carried to both phrenic nerves and to the aorta and pulmonary artery above. (*Inset*) Typical median sternotomy incision from the sternal notch to just below the xiphoid process. **(B)** A completed resection frees the right atrium, aorta, and pulmonary artery. (*Inset*). The space is drained with chest tubes for several days. (Roberts JR, Kaiser LR, 1998: Pericardial procedures. In Kaiser LR, Kron IL, Spray TL [eds]: Mastery of Cardiothoracic Surgery, p. 227. Philadelphia, Lippincott Williams & Wilkins)

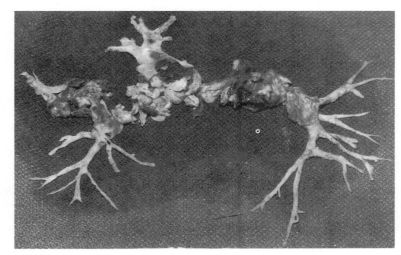

FIGURE 21-7. Endarterectomy specimen; thrombotic material has been removed from the upper, middle, and lower lobe pulmonary artery branches bilaterally. (Jamieson SW, Auger WB, Fedullo PF, et al., 1993: Experience and results with 150 pulmonary thromboendarterectomy operations over a 29-month period. J Thorac Cardiovasc Surg 106:120)

the treatment of choice for patients with pulmonary hypertension due to chronic thromboembolic disease and is the only means by which to alleviate symptoms and improve survival (Restrepo & Tapson, 1998).

Pulmonary thromboendarterectomy is a surgical procedure performed in selected centers to evacuate thrombotic material and lessen the degree of pulmonary hypertension. Appropriate candidates for surgical therapy are patients with (1) severe respiratory insufficiency and hypoxemia, (2) pulmonary hypertension with proximal pulmonary arterial occlusion and adequate bronchial collateral circulation, and (3) minimal impairment of right ventricular function (Sebastian & Sabiston, 1995). Pulmonary thromboendarterectomy is performed through a median sternotomy incision with cardiopulmonary bypass and cardioplegic arrest. Through incisions in the pulmonary arteries, endarterectomy of each of the bronchopulmonary segmental arteries and their subsegmental branches is performed (Daily et al., 1990) (Fig. 21-7).

The operative mortality rate associated with pulmonary thromboendarterectomy ranges from 6% to 20%; complications specific to the operation include reperfusion pulmonary edema, malignant pulmonary hypertension, hemorrhagic lung, and neurologic complications of deep hypothermia and cerebral ischemia (Palevsky & Edmunds, 1997). Long-term data demonstrate persistent hemodynamic, respiratory, and functional improvement, with many patients achieving a NYHA class I functional status (Jamieson, 1996). Irreversible pulmonary hypertension alternatively is treated with lung or heart-lung transplantation, discussed in Chapter 31, Heart, Lung, and Heart-Lung Transplantation.

REFERENCES

Acker MA, Gardner TJ, 1996: Cardiac tumors. In Baue AE, Geha AS, Hammond GL, et al. (eds): Glenn's Thoracic and Cardiovascular Surgery, ed. 6. Stamford, CT, Appleton & Lange

American Heart Association, 1998: 1999 Heart and Stroke Statistical Update. Dallas, American Heart Association

Brandenburg RO, Click RL, McGoon DC, 1991: The pericardium. In Giuliani ER, Fuster V, Gersh BJ, et al. (eds): Cardiology Fundamentals and Practice, ed. 2. St. Louis, Mosby–Year Book

Brown PS, Roberts CS, McIntosh CL, Clark RE, 1991: Aortic regurgitation after left ventricular myotomy and myectomy. Ann Thorac Surg 51:585

CIBIS-II Investigators and Committees, 1999: The cardiac insufficiency bisoprolol study II (CIBIS-II): A randomised trial. Lancet 353:9

Cooley DA, 1991: Surgical techniques for hypertrophic left ventricular obstructive myopathy including mitral valve plication. J Cardiac Surg 6:29

Daily PO, Dembitsky WP, Iverson S, et al., 1990: Risk factors for pulmonary thromboendarterectomy. J Thorac Cardiovasc Surg 99:670

David TE, 1997: Complex operations on the aortic root. In Edmunds LH Jr (ed): Cardiac Surgery in the Adult. New York, McGraw-Hill

Fallon JT, Dec GW, 1989: Cardiac tumors. In Eagle KA, Haber E, DeSanctis RW, Austin WG (eds): The Practice of Cardiology, ed. 2. Boston, Little, Brown

Fananapazir L, McAreavey D, 1998: Therapeutic options in patients with obstructive hypertrophic cardiomyopathy and severe drug-refractory symptoms. J Am Coll Cardiol 31:259

Frazier OH, Myers TJ, 1998: Surgical therapy for severe heart failure: Cardiomyoplasty. Curr Probl Cardiol 23:749

Gilbert EM, Bristow MR, 1994: Idiopathic dilated cardiomyopathy. In Schlant RC, Alexander RW, et al. (eds): The Heart, ed. 8. New York, McGraw-Hill

Glower DD, 1995: Acquired aortic valve disease. In Sabiston DC Jr, Spencer FC (eds): Surgery of the Chest, ed. 6. Philadelphia, WB Saunders

Grayzel D, Dec GW, Lilly LS, 1998: The cardiomyopathies. In Lilly LS (ed): Pathophysiology of Heart Disease, ed. 2. Baltimore, Williams & Wilkins

Hall RA, Anderson RP, 1997: Cardiac neoplasms. In Edmunds LH Jr (ed): Cardiac Surgery in the Adult. New York, McGraw-Hill

Hammond GL, Letsou GV, 1996: Aortic valve disease and hypertrophic cardiomyopathies. In Baue AE, Geha AS, Hammond GL, et al. (eds): Glenn's Thoracic and Cardiovascular Surgery, ed. 6. Stamford, CT, Appleton & Lange

Harken AH, Hall AW, Hammond GL, 1996: The pericardium. In Baue AE, Geha AS, Hammond GL, et al. (eds): Glenn's

Thoracic and Cardiovascular Surgery, ed. 6. Stamford, CT, Appleton & Lange

Hillis LD, Lange RA, Winniford MD, Page RL, 1995a: Primary cardiac tumors. In Manual of Clinical Problems in Cardiology, ed. 5. Boston, Little, Brown

Hillis LD, Lange RA, Winniford MD, Page RL, 1995b: Constrictive pericarditis. In Manual of Clinical Problems in Cardiology, ed. 5. Boston, Little, Brown

Jamieson SW, 1996: Pulmonary embolism. In Baue AE, Geha AS, Hammond GL, et al. (eds): Glenn's Thoracic and Cardiovascular Surgery, ed. 6. Stamford, CT, Appleton & Lange

Kirklin JW, Barratt-Boyes BG, 1993a: Cardiac tumor. In Cardiac Surgery, ed. 2. New York, Churchill Livingstone

Kirklin JW, Barratt-Boyes BG, 1993b: Hypertrophic obstructive cardiomyopathy. In Cardiac Surgery, ed. 2. New York, Churchill Livingstone

Kirklin JW, Barratt-Boyes BG, 1993c: Primary cardiomyopathy and cardiac transplantation. In Cardiac Surgery, ed. 2. New York, Churchill Livingstone

Klein AL, Scalia GM, 1998: Diseases of the pericardium, restrictive cardiomyopathy and diastolic dysfunction. In Topol EJ (ed): Comprehensive Cardiovascular Medicine. Philadelphia, Lippincott Williams & Wilkins

Lorell BH, 1997: Pericardial diseases. In Braunwald E (ed): Heart Disease: A Textbook of Cardiovascular Medicine, ed. 5. Philadelphia, WB Saunders

Lupinetti FM, 1998: Left ventricular outflow tract obstruction and aortic stenosis. In Kaiser LR, Kron IL, Spray TL (eds): Mastery of Cardiothoracic Surgery. Philadelphia, Lippincott Williams & Wilkins

Magovern JA, Cmolik BL, 1996: Cardiomyoplasty. In Kaiser LR, Kron IL, Spray TL (eds): Mastery of Cardiothoracic Surgery. Philadelphia, Lippincott-Raven

Magovern JA, Magovern GJ, 1998: Cardiomyoplasty. In Baue AE, Geha AS, Hammond GL, et al. (eds): Glenn's Thoracic and Cardiovascular Surgery, ed. 6. Stamford, CT, Appleton & Lange

McAllister HA, Hall RA, Cooley DA, 1999a: Tumors of the heart and pericardium: Primary cardiac tumors. Curr Probl Cardiol 24:63

McAllister HA, Hall RA, Cooley DA, 1999b: Tumors of the heart and pericardium: General considerations. Curr Probl Cardiol 24:63

McKenna WJ, Elliott PM, 1998: Hypertrophic cardiomyopathy. In Topol EJ (ed): Comprehensive Cardiovascular Medicine. Philadelphia, Lippincott Williams & Wilkins

Nishimura RA, Giuliani R, Tajik AJ, Brandenburg RO, 1991: Hypertrophic cardiomyopathy. In Giuliani ER, Fuster V, Gersh BJ, et al. (eds): Cardiology Fundamentals and Practice, ed. 2. St. Louis, Mosby–Year Book

Palevsky HI, Edmunds LH Jr, 1997: Pulmonary thromboem-
bolism. In Edmunds LH Jr (ed): Cardiac Surgery in the Adult. New York, McGraw-Hill

Renlund DG, 1998: Cardiac transplantation. In Topol EJ (ed): Comprehensive Cardiovascular Medicine. Philadelphia, Lippincott Williams & Wilkins

Restrepo CI, Tapson VF, 1998: Pulmonary hypertension and cor pulmonale. In Topol EJ (ed): Comprehensive Cardiovascular Medicine. Philadelphia, Lippincott Williams & Wilkins

Roberts JR, Kaiser LR, 1998: Pericardial procedures. In Kaiser LR, Kron IL, Spray TL (eds): Mastery of Cardiothoracic Surgery. Philadelphia, Lippincott Williams & Wilkins

Roberts WC, 1998: Cardiac neoplasms. In Topol EJ (ed): Comprehensive Cardiovascular Medicine. Philadelphia, Lippincott Williams & Wilkins

Schaff HV, Piehler JM, Lie JT, Giuliani ER, 1991: Tumors of the heart. In Giuliani ER, Fuster V, Gersh BJ, et al. (eds): Cardiology Fundamentals and Practice, ed. 2. St. Louis, Mosby–Year Book

Schoen FJ, 1997: Pathologic considerations in the surgery of adult heart disease. In Edmunds LH Jr (ed): Cardiac Surgery in the Adult. New York, McGraw-Hill

Schonbeck MH, Brunner-La Rocca HP, Vogt PR, et al., 1998: Long term follow-up in hypertrophic obstructive cardiomyopathy after septal myectomy. Ann Thorac Surg 65:1207

Sebastian MW, Sabiston DC Jr, 1995: Chronic pulmonary embolism. In Sabiston DC Jr, Spencer FC (eds): Surgery of the Chest, ed. 6. Philadelphia, WB Saunders

Shabetai R, 1994: Diseases of the pericardium. In Schlant RC, Alexander RW (eds): The Heart, ed. 8. New York, McGraw-Hill

Spotnitz WD, Blow O, 1998: Cardiac tumors. In Kaiser LR, Kron IL, Spray TL (eds): Mastery of Cardiothoracic Surgery. Philadelphia, Lippincott Williams & Wilkins

Starling RC, 1998: The health-care impact of heart failure. In Topol EJ (ed): Comprehensive Cardiovascular Medicine. Philadelphia, Lippincott Williams & Wilkins

Starling RC, Young JB, 1998: Surgical therapy for dilated cardiomyopathy. Cardiol Clin North Am 16:727

Stone CD, Hennein HA, McIntosh CL, et al., 1990: The results of operation in patients with hypertrophic cardiomyopathy and pulmonary hypertension. J Thorac Cardiovasc Surg 100:343

Ungerleider RM, 1995: Congenital aortic stenosis. In Sabiston DC Jr, Spencer FC (eds): Surgery of the Chest, ed. 6. Philadelphia, WB Saunders

Van Trigt P, Sabiston DC Jr, 1995: Tumors of the heart. In Sabiston DC Jr, Spencer FC (eds): Surgery of the Chest, ed. 6. Philadelphia, WB Saunders

Wynne J, Braunwald E, 1997: The cardiomyopathies and myocarditides. In Braunwald E (ed): Heart Disease: A Textbook of Cardiovascular Medicine, ed. 5. Philadelphia, WB Saunders

POSTOPERATIVE MANAGEMENT

Postoperative Patient Management

Diane Marolda, RN, MSN, ACNP, and

Betsy Finkelmeier, RN, MS, MM

Patient recovery from cardiac surgery usually follows a routine and predictable course that, when coupled with managed care incentives, makes it amenable to the development of rapid recovery programs. Many institutions throughout the United States have created clinical pathways for cardiac surgery to help reduce cost, shorten length of stay, and streamline patient care (Riegel et al., 1996; Riddle et al., 1996). Such a pathway also supports continuous quality improvement in standards of care. Results from participating institutions have been positive, indicating lower direct and indirect costs without an increase in mortality or readmission rates (Velasco et al., 1996). Typically, intensive care is necessary for the first 24 hours. An intermediate unit, if available, may be used for postoperative care on the second day. Discharge from the telemetry unit within 4 to 6 days of surgery is common. Table 22-1 demonstrates an example of a clinical pathway for the postoperative care of a patient after coronary artery bypass surgery.

▶ Intensive Care

Ideally, the postoperative intensive care unit (ICU) is located adjacent to the cardiac surgical operating rooms. In facilities where the two are geographically separate, it is desirable to keep patients in a recovery room near the operating suite for several hours. This minimizes transfer time, during which monitoring and the ability to treat problems are compromised. Also, the patient can be rapidly transferred back to the operating room should excessive bleeding or other urgent reasons for operative reexploration develop.

Transfer from the operating room to the ICU is performed after the operation is concluded and when the patient is hemodynamically stable. A self-inflating bag with 100% oxygen is used to ventilate the intubated patient during transport. Portable units with the capacity for electrocardiographic and pressure monitoring also are used. Continued visibility of the heart rhythm and arterial pressure adds a dimension of safety to the transfer process. First, attachment of monitoring equipment in the ICU can be performed in a less urgent fashion. Second, it allows prompt detection of arrhythmias, hypertension, or hypotension during transfer. Common problems that can occur during patient transport include sudden hypotension due to fluid shifts that occur as the patient is moved, acute hypertension due to sympathetic stimulation, extubation or reflex responses caused by traction on the endotracheal tube, and alteration in dosage or disconnection of intravenous medication infusions (Hendren & Higgins, 1991).

Admission and Assessment

Patient admission to the ICU is performed in a systematic manner. Priorities on patient arrival are (1) reestablishing mechanical ventilation, monitoring capabilities, and chest tube suction; (2) confirming hemodynamic stability; and (3) technology assessment (ie, identifying all catheters and pacing equipment for function and correlation). Usually, two nurses participate in the admission process so that necessary tasks can be performed quickly and any sudden problems treated promptly. The anesthesiologist or surgeon who accompanies the patient

TABLE 22-1

Clinical Pathway: Coronary Artery Bypass Surgery

Interventions	DOS: ICU	POD #1	POD #2	POD #3	POD #4
Tests	CBC/platelets, BCP ABG per protocol BG q6h if diabetic Portable CXR 12-lead ECG	CBC/platelets, BCP Glucometer q6h if diabetic Portable CXR		CBC, BCP 12-lead ECG PA/lateral CXR	
Treatments	Cardiac monitor VS per protocol Initiate weaning protocol, I&O q1h Chest tube − 20 cm suction Foley catheter	Telemetry D/C IVs, Foley, chest tubes Transfer to floor VS q4h × 24h I&O q1h, PIL Daily weight	Telemetry VS qs, daily weight Incision and pacer wire care Wean oxygen IS q1h w/a	Telemetry D/C pacer wires, then D/C telemetry 4 h later VS qs, incision care Daily weight IS q1h w/a	VS qs IS q1h w/a Incision care Daily weight
Medications	ATB × 3 doses Vasoactive gtts prn ASA suppository K & Mg prn, digoxin Volume therapy prn	D/C vasoactive gtts ECASA, MVI Digoxin, Lasix Beta blocker, Kdur IV/IM/PO analgesia	Beta blocker Digoxin ECASA, MVI IM/PO analgesia Lasix, Kdur	Beta blocker Digoxin ECASA, MVI IM/PO analgesia Lasix, Kdur	Beta blocker Digoxin ECASA, MVI IM/PO analgesia Lasix, Kdur
Diet	NPO, clear liquids 4 h after extubation	Full liquid diet AAT to cardiac diet	Cardiac diet, or as ordered	Cardiac diet, or as ordered	Cardiac diet, or as ordered
Activity	Bed rest, consult Cardiac rehab	OOB to chair Cardiac rehab	Ambulate × 2 Cardiac rehab	Ambulate × 4 Cardiac rehab	Ambulate × 6 Cardiac rehab
Education and discharge planning	Discuss plan of care with family Orient to ICU	Discuss plan of care Functional assessment Pastoral care prn	Provide cardiac rehab materials Consult HHS Consult SW prn	Discharge instructions Discharge plan finalized Prescriptions reviewed	Review discharge instructions and prescriptions Discharge home

AAT, advance as tolerated; ABG, arterial blood gases; ASA, acetylsalicylic acid; ATB, antibiotics; BCP, blood chemistry panel; BG, blood glucose; CBC, complete blood count; CXR, chest roentgenogram; D/C, discontinue; DOS, day of surgery; ECASA, enteric-coated aspirin; ECG, electrocardiogram; gtts, drips; HHS, home health service; ICU, intensive care unit; IM, intramuscular; I&O, intake and output; IS, incentive spirometry; IV, intravenous; K, potassium; Mg, magnesium; MVI, multivitamin; NPO, nothing by mouth; OOB, out of bed; PIL, peripheral heparin lock; PO, oral; POD, postoperative day; SW, social worker; VS, vital signs; w/a, while awake.

Adapted from Clinical Pathway, Northwestern Memorial Hospital, Chicago, IL.

communicates the following information to the ICU nurse: the procedure performed, the type of anesthesia used, any significant intraoperative findings or complications, whether the patient has received blood transfusions, current medication and fluid infusions, and desirable hemodynamic parameters.

A mechanical ventilator with appropriately set parameters should be in place at the bedside when the patient arrives so that mechanical ventilation can be instituted promptly. Electrocardiographic leads are connected to the bedside monitor, and arterial and pulmonary artery catheter transducers are transferred. Chest tube suction is reestablished. The arterial catheter should be assessed for patency, waveform analysis, and correlation with manual cuff pressure. All intravenous

catheters are assessed for patency and proper infusion rates. Catheters typically present include a subclavian or jugular pulmonary artery catheter, a multiple-lumen central venous catheter for administration of medications and fluid, one or two peripheral intravenous catheters, and a radial arterial catheter (Fig. 22-1). If volumetric pumps used in the operating room for infusion of intravenous medications also can be used in the ICU, no exchange of equipment is necessary. If a separate set of pumps is used, a consistent system of exchanging equipment is important so that drug infusion rates are not altered while medication solutions or infusion pumps are changed.

Temporary atrial and ventricular epicardial pacing wires are inspected and properly secured with an insulat-

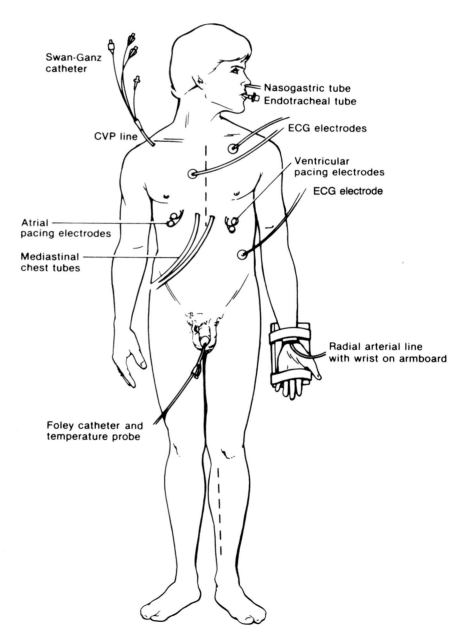

FIGURE 22-1. Typical appearance of postoperative patient; dotted lines represent median sternotomy incision and leg incision for harvesting of saphenous vein. (Hudak CM, Gallo BM, Morton PG, 1998: Cardiac surgery. In: Critical Care Nursing: A Holistic Approach, ed. 7, p. 405. Philadelphia, Lippincott Williams & Wilkins)

ing cover or are attached to an external pulse generator. Depending on the initial heart rhythm after surgery, a pacemaker set in a synchronous mode is often attached to the ventricular pacing wire. This allows the patient's intrinsic rhythm to dominate while offering protection from bradycardia or heart block that may occur during rewarming. Drainage tubes and catheters, including mediastinal and sometimes pleural chest drainage tubes, a urethral drainage catheter, and a nasogastric tube, are examined for proper functioning. If saphenous veins have been harvested, a drain may be present in the leg and is usually connected to bulb or low continuous suction.

As soon as all necessary equipment attachments are made and the admission process is completed, a thorough *patient assessment* is performed. The purpose of the assessment is to provide a summarized description of all significant findings at a particular time (Table 22-2). Information included should complement and expand on that recorded on flow sheets used for vital signs and other parameters. Baseline information observed at the time of admission to the ICU is invaluable in evaluating the patient's clinical course over time. The assessment is repeated by each new nurse assuming care of the patient (usually every 8 to 12 hours). A standardized unit protocol for documentation of the patient assessment ensures that information is consistently recorded and easily available to all nurses and physicians caring for the patient.

Often, experienced nurses can integrate performance of the assessment with nursing interventions required during the admission process. The order of patient assessment is less important than its performance in a consistent and thorough fashion so that all relevant data are included. However, certain observations are priorities and should be performed as soon as the patient arrives. These include observation of symmetric chest movement; auscultation of bilateral breath sounds; and documentation of heart rate and rhythm, blood pressure, hemodynamic parameters, chest tube output, and infusion rates of intravenous fluids. Intravenous medication infusions are reviewed for proper concentration, rate of infusion, and location and integrity of infusion site (Le Doux & Shinn, 1995). Because neurologic complications most often become apparent in the early postoperative hours, the patient's ability to move all extremities and follow simple commands is documented as soon as it is noted.

Early Postoperative Care

In most cases, the admission and early postoperative hours are routine and nursing care can be performed in an organized fashion. However, the first few hours are critical in that potentially life-threatening problems are most likely during this period. The patient, the cardiac rhythm, and the hemodynamic parameters are observed continuously, and vital signs are documented every 15 to 20 minutes to ensure prompt detection of developing complications, particularly hemorrhage, low cardiac out-

TABLE 22-2

Assessment of the Postoperative Patient

NEUROLOGIC STATUS
Level of consciousness
Reactivity of pupils
Ability to move extremities
Level of orientation
Presence of any neurologic deficits or abnormal reflex responses

CARDIOVASCULAR STATUS
Heart rate, cardiac rhythm
Arterial blood pressure (systolic, diastolic, and mean)
Pulmonary artery pressure (systolic, diastolic, and mean)
Pulmonary capillary wedge pressure, mixed venous oxygen saturation, left atrial pressure*
Central venous pressure
Cardiac output/cardiac index
Systemic vascular resistance
Heart sounds
Pacing wires, pulse generator settings
Peripheral perfusion (pulses, capillary refill, color, temperature)
Chest tube output

RESPIRATORY STATUS
Respiratory rate (ventilator and patient)
Breath sounds
Symmetry of chest movement
Current ventilator settings
Arterial blood gas or oxygen saturation
Respiratory effort

GASTROINTESTINAL STATUS
Bowel sounds
Presence and function of nasogastric tube
Presence of abdominal distention or tenderness

RENAL STATUS
Urine output
Urine color

OTHER
Adequacy of pain control and sedation
Intravenous fluids and medications
Chest x-ray and electrocardiogram
Laboratory measurements
Incisional drainage

*Measured in selected patients only.

put, or arrhythmias. Ongoing monitoring of temperature is performed using a pulmonary artery catheter equipped with a thermistor. Alternatively, rectal or tympanic temperature is checked every hour.

A portable chest roentgenogram is obtained within the first postoperative hour. The film demonstrates the position of intrathoracic tubes and catheters and provides baseline information for radiographic detection of postoperative problems. The critical care nurse is often the first to review the film and identify problems that require correction. Specifically, attention should be directed toward the following: (1) position of the endotracheal tube, (2) presence of pneumothorax or mediastinal shift, (3) pleural fluid collections, (4) size of the mediastinal silhouette, (5) correct intravascular position of pulmonary artery and central venous catheters, and (6) normal position of chest and nasogastric tubes, and sternal wires, if present (Landolfo & Smith, 1995). Atelectasis, particularly of the left lower lobe, is a common occurrence after cardiac operations because of reduced lung volume and small airway closure (Valta et al., 1992). Chest roentgenograms are discussed in further detail in Chapter 44, Postoperative Chest Roentgenogram Interpretation.

A 12-lead electrocardiogram (ECG) is obtained within several hours of the patient's arrival in the ICU. Because hypothermia can produce electrocardiographic changes that confuse interpretation, the ECG usually is deferred until the patient is normothermic and not shivering. If a temporary pacemaker is being used but the patient has an adequate underlying cardiac rhythm, pacing is discontinued while the ECG is recorded. In patients who are pacemaker dependent, the ECG usually is omitted.

Standard *hemodynamic monitoring* of the postoperative patient includes arterial blood pressure, central venous pressure, pulmonary artery pressure, cardiac output, cardiac index, and systemic vascular resistance (SVR). Mixed venous oxygen saturation also may be monitored to assist in assessing systemic perfusion, using a specialized oximetric pulmonary artery catheter. Rarely, patients undergoing valvular heart surgery have a left atrial catheter for direct measurement of left atrial pressure. Management of these catheters and principles of hemodynamic monitoring are discussed in detail in Chapter 23, Hemodynamic Monitoring.

Because adequacy of cardiovascular function is the primary concern in the early postoperative period, the most important hemodynamic indicator is cardiac output (Lee & Geha, 1996). No one parameter, however, should be considered or treated in isolation. Rather, all are evaluated in combination to determine appropriate therapeutic interventions. A thorough understanding of the interplay between the hemodynamic variables is essential. The goal is to maintain adequate systemic perfusion to protect cerebral, myocardial, and visceral function.

Measurement of arterial blood pressure, particularly mean arterial pressure, provides essential information about perfusion of the heart, brain, kidneys, and other vital organs. In addition to invasive pressure monitoring, the quality of peripheral pulses, color and temperature of the extremities, level of mentation, and adequacy of urine output are other important indicators of peripheral perfusion.

Cardiac output is measured using the pulmonary artery catheter and a thermodilution technique. To correct for differences in patient size, the measured cardiac output is divided by body surface area to obtain cardiac index. Cardiac output is determined by the interrelation of preload, afterload, cardiac rhythm (heart rate), and

myocardial contractility. It is often necessary to manipulate these individual parameters in the early postoperative hours to achieve and maintain a normal cardiac index (ie, 2.5 to 4.0 L/min/m²). However, altering preload, afterload, cardiac rhythm, and contractility affects the work done by the heart. When the heart works harder, oxygen consumption is greater. In patients with cardiac disease, clinical methods for measuring oxygen consumption and determining the optimal relationship between work and energy consumption remain unclear.

Preload is the end-diastolic volume in the ventricle and serves as an estimation of average diastolic fiber length (Landolfo & Smith, 1995). The relationship between cardiac muscle fiber length at the end of diastole and cardiac output is expressed in Starling's law, that is, within limits, cardiac output increases directly with increases in end-diastolic fiber length (Hudak et al., 1998a). As ventricular filling pressure (as measured indirectly by pulmonary artery diastolic, left atrial, or right atrial pressure) increases, cardiac output also increases until a point is reached at which further filling produces a decrease in cardiac output and congestive heart failure (Fig. 22-2). The preload that provides optimal cardiac output varies from patient to patient. Normal pulmonary artery diastolic pressure is 8 to 15 mm Hg, but in a diseased heart cardiac function is often better when it is 15 to 20 mm Hg.

The cardiac surgeon has an excellent opportunity to assess cardiac function in relation to various levels of preload while the patient is being weaned from cardiopulmonary bypass (CPB). During weaning, venous return to the extracorporeal circuit is partially occluded, allowing blood volume to enter and be ejected by the

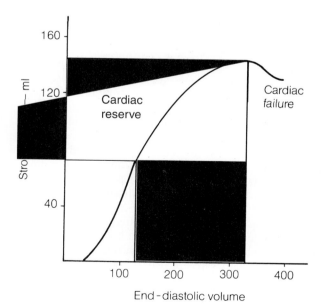

FIGURE 22-2. The Starling curve. Cardiac output increases with end-diastolic fiber length to a critical point at which further stretching precipitates heart failure. (Hudak CM, Gallo BM, Morton PG, 1998: Heart failure. In Critical Care Nursing: A Holistic Approach, ed. 7, p. 351. Philadelphia, Lippincott Williams & Wilkins)

heart. As a result, the surgeon in effect controls the patient's preload by manipulating the proportion of venous blood that is diverted through the venous cannula to that which is returned to the heart. Contractility of the ventricles can be observed directly and cardiac output measured to determine the optimal preload level. When the patient is transferred to the ICU, the surgeon communicates preload values associated with most effective cardiac function. If the patient recovers normally, cardiac function should steadily improve from the time the heart was weaned from CPB. Therefore, the required preload level would be expected not to exceed and gradually to decrease from that required by the heart at the time of weaning from CPB.

Afterload, or the impedance to left ventricular contraction, is assessed by measuring SVR. Typically, SVR is elevated in the early postoperative hours secondary to hypothermia and peripheral vasoconstriction. If left untreated, this may lead to several negative effects: (1) a decrease in stroke volume; (2) an increase in aortic wall tension, which may threaten sutures and suture lines; and (3) an increase in left ventricular metabolic demands, which may exacerbate any latent myocardial ischemia (Kirklin & Barratt-Boyes, 1993). To avert these negative effects, pharmacologic vasodilating agents may be used to decrease afterload. Eventually, as the patient's body temperature returns to normal, the SVR decreases and pharmacologic therapy can be weaned. Less commonly, pharmacologic agents are needed to increase afterload that has been abnormally decreased by anesthetic agents or an allergic reaction to protamine sulfate. The clinical indicator for right ventricular afterload is pulmonary vascular resistance. Elevated pulmonary vascular resistance is unusual except in patients with cardiac disease associated with pulmonary artery hypertension.

A third variable affecting cardiac output is *heart rate* and rhythm. Because of the importance of this factor and the prevalence of cardiac arrhythmias in the early postoperative period, continuous electrocardiographic monitoring is essential and usually is performed through the third or fourth postoperative day. An optimal cardiac rhythm provides synchronous atrial and ventricular contractions at an acceptable rate. Epicardial pacing wires routinely are placed on the right atrium and ventricle so that temporary pacing can be performed to manipulate the cardiac rhythm. The epicardial pacing wires are often left in place until the day before discharge. The wires are quite useful therapeutically, are associated with almost no morbidity, and can be detached easily before the patient's discharge from the hospital. In addition, the atrial wire can be used for diagnostic purposes.

Changes in heart rate are usually transient yet common after cardiac surgery. Several factors may account for this variation, including preoperative beta blockade, intraoperative antiarrhythmic agents, metabolic damage during cardioplegia administration, or, less commonly, ischemia or direct surgical injury to the conduction system (Ellis et al., 1980; Smith et al., 1983a, 1983b, 1983c). A heart rate that is too slow decreases cardiac output, which is the product of heart rate and stroke volume. Temporary pacing is used to increase the heart rate to 90 to 100 beats per minute, the range that usually provides the best cardiac output during the early postoperative period (Geha & Whittlesey, 1996). Atrial (if atrioventricular [AV] nodal function is normal) or AV synchronous pacing usually is selected to maintain the added ventricular filling that results from an appropriately timed atrial systole. This "atrial kick" is responsible for approximately 25% of cardiac output in the postoperative setting (Skinner et al., 1963; Finkelmeier & Salinger, 1986). If atrial fibrillation or other supraventricular arrhythmia is present, ventricular pacing must be used to increase heart rate.

Tachycardia may develop in the early postoperative hours as a manifestation of hypovolemia or sympathetic overstimulation. A rapid heart rate lowers the stroke volume by reducing the diastolic time for ventricular filling. The net effect is a decrease in cardiac output and decreased coronary perfusion. Tachyarrhythmias require correction of the precipitating cause or suppression with antiarrhythmic medication.

Myocardial contractility, or the inotropic state of the heart, describes the ability of heart muscle to shorten, develop tension, or both, independent of variations induced by altering preload or afterload (Bond & Halpenny, 1995). Myocardial contractility is enhanced, if necessary, by using inotropic pharmacologic agents. Increased inotropic performance, however, may occur at the expense of myocardial oxygen demand. Therefore, the use of inotropic agents should be considered only after optimal manipulation of heart rate, preload, and afterload has been achieved (Landolfo & Smith, 1995). There are a number of inotropic agents available, with differing associated effects on the heart and blood vessels. Most act on adrenergic receptors, and clinical experience demonstrates a synergistic effect when multiple agents are used concomitantly (Vernon et al., 1992). Ultimately, the choice of agent is individualized to the specific clinical situation. These drugs are discussed in detail in Chapter 27, Cardiovascular Medications.

Sedatives usually are administered until the patient is fully rewarmed, neuromuscular blocking agents are eliminated or metabolized, the patient is hemodynamically stable, and chest tube drainage is acceptable (Coyle, 1991). Propofol or midazolam commonly is used to prevent premature wakefulness, which may lead to undesirable hypertension, tachycardia, and resistance to mechanical ventilation. The shorter half-life of propofol, compared with midazolam, allows a shorter weaning time and subsequent earlier extubation and transfer from the ICU setting. Despite marked differences in the cost of these two agents, the overall economic profile for them is comparable (Barrientos-Vega et al., 1997; Tagliente, 1997). Occasionally, a patient awakens before neuromuscular blocking agents are eliminated or metabolized, resulting in an awake but paralyzed patient. Aggressive pharmacologic therapy with nitrates, alpha- and beta-blocking agents, or calcium channel blocking medications may be necessary to suppress the autonomic instability resulting from the patient's distress (Hendren &

Higgins, 1991). Intravenous bolus doses of morphine are administered intermittently as necessary during the first 24 hours to provide adequate analgesia.

An oral or nasal endotracheal tube remains in place during the early postoperative hours. Intubation and mechanical ventilation with a volume-cycled ventilator are necessary until the patient has awakened from anesthesia and is able to do the work of breathing independently. During the period of intubation, the patient is turned side to side every 2 hours and endotracheal suctioning is performed as needed. To prevent gastric distention, a nasogastric tube usually is placed during or immediately after surgery, and is removed at the time of extubation. Mechanical ventilation usually is performed using an intermittent mandatory ventilation (IMV) mode, which provides early patient control and allows easy weaning. Specific ventilator settings are individualized for each patient. Typical parameters are as follows: respiratory rate = 8 to 10 breaths per minute; tidal volume = 10 to 15 mL/kg; FiO_2 = 50% to 60%; positive end-expiratory pressure = 5 cm H_2O; pressure support = 5 cm H_2O; and dead space = 50 mL.

Most centers have instituted protocols for early extubation of cardiac surgical patients, usually within 1 to 6 hours after completion of surgery. Several randomized trials have demonstrated significantly reduced costs, earlier transfer from the ICU, and earlier discharge from the hospital without a significant increase in clinical complications (Silbert et al., 1998; Kollef et al., 1997). Weaning from mechanical ventilation is accomplished by limiting sedation and decreasing the IMV rate. In addition to measurement of blood gases, evaluation of weaning tolerance can be achieved with assessment of respiratory rate, minute volume, end-tidal PCO_2, and continuous pulse oximetry. Unless clinically indicated, blood gases are not repeated routinely. Most of the needed clinical data can be obtained by less expensive measurements. Table 22-3 lists the criteria for extubation. Other factors that influence timing of extubation include efficacy of rewarming, hemodynamic status of the patient, and the expected likelihood of reexploration for bleeding (Hendren & Higgins, 1991).

Humidified oxygen by means of a face mask is provided for 24 hours after extubation. A nasal cannula may be used alternatively for oxygen delivery; it usually is more comfortable for the patient, although the inspired oxygen is not as well humidified. Providing supplemental humidity is helpful in loosening pulmonary secretions so that they are more easily expectorated. Unless there is a specific respiratory problem, supplemental oxygen usually is not necessary after the first 48 hours.

Typically, two mediastinal chest tubes are placed in cardiac surgical patients for evacuation of blood. One is positioned within the pericardium and one is in the posterior mediastinum. If the pleural space has been opened, a pleural chest tube will be present as well. Protocols for routine "stripping" or "milking" of chest tubes vary from institution to institution. Some surgeons believe stripping tubes is important to maintain patency; others believe the excessive negativity created in the mediastinum by rou-

TABLE 22-3

Criteria for Extubation

pH = 7.35–7.45 or at preoperative baseline
PaO_2 >60 mm Hg on 40% FiO_2
$PaCO_2$ <45 mm Hg or at preoperative baseline
Respiratory rate <30/min
Negative inspiratory force > −20
Tidal volume >4–5 mL/kg
Vital capacity >10 mL/kg
Minute volume <10 L/min
Continuous positive airway pressure ≤5 cm
Awake and alert, able to protect airway
Hemodynamically stable
Absence of increased work of breathing, use of accessory muscles
Chest tube drainage <100 mL/h
Temperature >36°C (96.8°F), absence of shivering
Minimal secretions

Adapted from Housestaff Manual for Cardiothoracic Surgery, 1999. Northwestern University, Division of Cardiothoracic Surgery, Chicago, IL.

tine stripping causes more bleeding and might disrupt vein graft anastomoses. Regardless of whether chest tubes are stripped routinely, they are monitored closely during the early postoperative hours to ensure patency and to record hourly the amount of blood loss. Hematocrit levels are measured on admission to the unit and the following day or sooner if bleeding is excessive.

In some institutions, autotransfusion is performed routinely (Fig. 22-3). Autotransfusion is the reinfusion of shed mediastinal blood that is defibrinated by contact with the pleura and pericardium (Mahfood et al., 1991). Because average blood loss after cardiac operations is approximately 1 L, autotransfusion represents a significant method of blood conservation (Scott et al., 1990). Furthermore, the reinfusion of shed mediastinal blood has been found significantly to reduce the incidence of operative reexploration and of homologous blood transfusion (DeVarennes et al., 1996). Standardized protocols are used to guide the nurse in performing autotransfusion.

There are two equally effective methods of autotransfusion: continuous and intermittent (Sutton et al., 1993). The continuous method uses a closed chest drainage system, filter, and intravenous infusion pump. This method has several advantages over the intermittent method, including smooth maintenance of the patient's blood volume, less additional equipment, and the ability to integrate the procedure as a standard part of the postoperative care. Ultimately, the choice of autotransfusion method is determined by individual institutional practice. Autotransfusion usually is discontinued after approximately 6 hours, when active bleeding has subsided. In patients who have a postoperative coagulopathy or have received large amounts of banked blood, autotransfusion may be discontinued because the shed blood is depleted of clotting factors. Conversely, some surgeons elect to continue autotransfusion in these circumstances to conserve red blood cells.

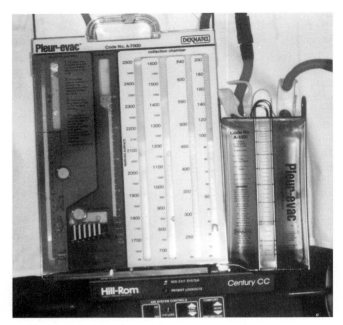

FIGURE 22-3. Example of chest drainage system with autotransfusion bag attached.

Monitoring fluid status is an important component of early postoperative care. Intake and output are recorded hourly during the first 24 hours and every 2 hours during the next 24 hours to document the amount of fluid administered compared with that lost as urine and chest tube drainage. Patients commonly gain 2 to 5 kg of fluid weight during cardiac surgical operations owing to the effects of CPB and hormonal changes associated with a major operation. Both antidiuretic hormone and aldosterone levels are elevated by surgical stress, leading to increased sodium and water retention (Behrendt & Austen, 1985).

Despite increased body weight (representing increased total body fluid), intravascular volume actually may be depleted. Fluid moves from the intravascular to the interstitial space as a result of increased capillary permeability secondary to vasoactive substances released during CPB and decreased plasma colloid osmotic pressure caused by hemodilution (Hudak et al., 1998b). Thus, the extra fluid is primarily in the interstitial tissue (ie, the "third space"). In addition, most patients experience an osmotic diuresis in the early postoperative hours. Therefore, volume repletion may be necessary to maintain an adequate preload despite increased body weight. If preload is adequate, total fluid administration is limited to 50 mL/h for the first several days. With the exception of the arterial line, intravenous fluids that contain sodium are not used so that fluid retention is not exacerbated.

After removal of the pulmonary artery and central venous catheters, weights provide the most accurate parameter for assessing fluid status. They are obtained at a consistent time each morning. The preoperative weight provides a baseline value for comparison unless the patient had some degree of heart failure before surgery or the operation was performed emergently and the patient was not weighed. Oral liquids usually are administered beginning on the first postoperative day, after the endotracheal tube has been discontinued and the patient is alert enough to protect the airway. Oral fluids are restricted until the patient returns to preoperative weight. Most patients experience a spontaneous diuresis 48 to 72 hours after surgery as fluid is mobilized into the vascular space. Although this may provide sufficient diuresis for some patients, many require the administration of diuretic agents to hasten the process.

Common Problems

Problems that arise in the early postoperative hours are often of a precipitous nature, requiring immediate interventions by the nurse at the bedside. Consequently, cardiothoracic surgical nurses require a thorough understanding of principles of cardiac physiology, the meaning and relationship of the various hemodynamic parameters, the characteristics of anesthetic agents, the consequences of CPB and rewarming, and the actions of commonly used pharmacologic agents. As previously mentioned, standardized protocols and pathways provide nurses with the flexibility to respond to typical problems. Only the more common transient postoperative problems are included in this discussion. The various postoperative complications are discussed in Chapter 28, Complications of Cardiac Operations.

Postoperative bleeding may be caused by a surgically correctable problem, such as a disrupted surgical clip or sutured anastomosis, or by a coagulopathy related to intraoperative anticoagulation, hemodilution, and the extracorporeal circulation of blood during CPB. The most important hemostatic derangement in cardiac surgical patients and a primary cause of postoperative coagulopathy is the reduction in quantity and quality of platelets after CPB (Halfman-Franey & Berg, 1991).

Adequate hemostasis is achieved before transferring a patient out of the operating room. However, bleeding that was not apparent or that was minimal during closure of the chest may increase as the patient's body temperature and blood pressure rise. Bleeding is exacerbated by postoperative hypertension that can occur secondary to elevated SVR or increasing wakefulness and agitation. Factors that increase circulating catecholamines, such as hypoxia, hypercarbia, hypothermia with shivering, and visceral distention, also may contribute to development of hypertension (Hendren & Higgins, 1991). In most situations, mean arterial pressure is maintained below 75 to 80 mm Hg during the early postoperative hours to avoid excessive bleeding. Vasodilating agents, such as nitroprusside or nitroglycerin, commonly are used to accomplish this goal. Sedation of the patient also may be necessary.

Chest tube output is monitored closely to detect sudden increases in the amount of drainage. Patients with more than ordinary amounts of bleeding are observed carefully so that reexploration and hemostasis can be achieved before hemodynamic instability develops. The decision to take a patient back to the operating room for mediastinal reexploration is influenced by the rate and amount of bleeding, the nature of the operation, and the surgeon's assessment of the likelihood of a surgically correctable etiology. A dramatic increase in the rate of bleeding is usually indicative of disruption of a clip or suture. In such cases, surgical reexploration is performed at once. Other indications for reexploration include (1) chest tube output between 300 and 500 mL/h for the first hour, (2) 200 to 300 mL/h for the second hour, and (3) greater than 100 mL/h for 6 to 8 hours (Baumgartner et al., 1997). Each clinical situation should be viewed individually, however, and aggressive correction of abnormal coagulation parameters should occur as soon as possible. A mechanical (surgically correctable) cause of bleeding is found in approximately half the patients who undergo surgical reexploration (Anderson et al., 1991).

If postoperative bleeding is excessive or if chest tubes become clotted, *cardiac tamponade* may occur. As blood accumulates in the pericardial space or mediastinum, the abnormally positive pressure in the finite space is transmitted to the ventricular cavity, eliminating the intercavitary pressure gradients responsible for normal ventricular filling during diastole (Elefteriades et al., 1996). Because the heart is unable to fill adequately, cardiac output falls. Arterial pressure initially is preserved by alpha-adrenergic–mediated peripheral vasoconstriction, but eventually decreases as a premortal event (Klein & Scalia, 1998). Other clinical manifestations of cardiac tamponade include minimal hemodynamic improvement with initiation of inotropic agents, decreased urine output, and a widened mediastinum on the chest roentgenogram.

Emergent reopening of a portion of the sternal incision may be necessary to prevent cardiac arrest. If an operating room and personnel are not immediately available, the surgeon may open the lower portion of the sternal incision in the ICU to detect and relieve possible tamponade. For this reason, wire cutters and staple removers as well as a chest-opening tray should be readily accessible. If hemodynamic compromise is due to cardiac tamponade, evacuating blood from the mediastinum allows the heart once again to fill adequately. Reopening the chest incision increases the risk of subsequent sternal wound infection, particularly if performed in the ICU and if the patient also requires sternal compressions (during closed chest massage).

A second common problem in the early postoperative period is *low cardiac output*. A low cardiac output state is said to exist when the cardiac index is less than 2.0 L/min/m². The more common causes of low cardiac output syndrome after cardiac surgery include hypovolemia, bleeding, myocardial dysfunction, cardiac tamponade, arrhythmia, and increased afterload (Kirklin & Barratt-Boyes, 1993). Clinical manifestations include cold, clammy extremities, hypotension, tachycardia, diminished peripheral pulses and capillary refill, decreased urine output, and persistent obtundation (Moreno-Cabral et al., 1988). However, classic signs of shock do not always accompany low cardiac output in the early postoperative hours because of the patient's thermal instabil-

ity, residual effects of anesthesia, and the osmotic diuresis that usually follows CPB (DiSesa, 1991). Low cardiac output may occur in the presence of adequate filling pressures and with or without obvious hypotension.

Hypovolemia or inadequate preload is a common etiology of low cardiac output because of the vasodilatation, urinary diuresis, and mediastinal bleeding that occur after cardiac operations. Accordingly, the first method of treatment is to provide sufficient preload to maximize cardiac output without overfilling the heart. In patients with normal left ventricular function, filling pressures are increased to approximately 15 mm Hg. However, if reduced ventricular compliance and diastolic dysfunction are present in the early postoperative period, a higher left ventricular end-diastolic pressure is required to achieve an adequate preload (Vander Salm & Stahl, 1997). Sustained low filling pressures despite volume replacement suggest hemorrhage.

Low cardiac output in association with elevated filling pressures indicates a problem with cardiac function. Impaired cardiac function may result from a number of etiologies, including perioperative myocardial infarction, reperfusion of ischemic or infarcted myocardium, inadequate intraoperative myocardial protection, preexisting ventricular damage, or cardiac tamponade. The primary therapy for low cardiac output due to myocardial dysfunction (except that due to tamponade) is continuous intravenous infusion of one or more inotropic pharmacologic agents. Commonly used drugs include dopamine, dobutamine, epinephrine, and milrinone. Dopamine often is selected as the initial agent of choice for low cardiac output because, in low doses, it also stimulates renal dopaminergic receptors, thereby increasing renal perfusion.

Often, a low cardiac output state is accompanied by increased afterload, as measured by SVR. Afterload reduction usually is achieved by infusing sodium nitroprusside, a vasodilating agent that directly relaxes smooth muscle in both arteriolar and venous beds, thus lowering SVR, pulmonary vascular resistance, and preload (Greco, 1990). Adequate preload levels must exist before nitroprusside is infused to avoid precipitous hypotension. Nitroglycerin may be used alternatively, or additionally. Because it vasodilates coronary and pulmonary as well as systemic vessels, it may be preferable for low cardiac output associated with coronary artery spasm, incomplete coronary artery revascularization, or increased pulmonary vascular resistance. In severe cases of low cardiac output secondary to left ventricular failure, intra-aortic balloon counterpulsation also may be used to provide mechanical afterload reduction. Prostaglandin E₁ infusion or nitric oxide inhalation may be used to produce pulmonary arterial vasodilatation in patients with postoperative right ventricular dysfunction associated with pulmonary hypertension.

Temporary pacing and antiarrhythmic agents are used as necessary to optimize cardiac rate and rhythm. Sedatives are administered to minimize sympathetic overstimulation and its deleterious effects on heart rate and SVR (Moran & Singh, 1989). Mechanical ventilation is continued so that the patient is not subjected to the work of respiration.

Occasionally, *profound hypotension* occurs precipitously in the early postoperative hours. Hypotension detected by arterial pressure monitoring should be verified by cuff measurement or palpation of the femoral artery. All medication infusions are inspected to detect possible interruption of inotropic infusion or bolus of vasodilator infusion. The chest tube drainage system is examined for a sudden increase in blood loss and chest tubes are stripped to ensure patency. In addition to bleeding, diuretic therapy or vasodilatation secondary to rewarming may cause hypovolemia (Hendren & Higgins, 1991). If filling pressures are low, a fluid bolus is administered. Infusion of dopamine or another inotropic agent is instituted or increased.

Cardiac tamponade, low cardiac output, or profound hypotension can lead to *cardiac arrest*. When cardiac arrest occurs, the endotracheal tube is disconnected from the ventilator and hand ventilation is begun, using a self-inflating bag and 100% oxygen. The heart rhythm is assessed, and ventricular pacing is instituted for bradycardia or asystole. Defibrillation is performed for ventricular tachycardia (VT) or ventricular fibrillation (VF). Although defibrillation is ineffective in converting asystole, what appears to be asystole on the oscilloscope in fact may be a fine VF that can be converted. Chest compressions (or open cardiac massage if the sternal incision has been opened) are performed, and advanced life support measures are instituted.

Hypertension commonly develops in the early postoperative hours as a consequence of patient emergence from anesthesia, endotracheal suctioning, resistance to mechanical ventilation, or pain (Whitman, 1991). It also can occur as a paroxysmal event in the absence of any of these factors. Certain types of heart disease, such as coarctation of the aorta or aortic valve disease, are particularly likely to be associated with postoperative hypertension. Although individual patients may require somewhat higher systemic arterial pressures, a mean arterial pressure of 65 to 75 mm Hg is appropriate in most patients in the early postoperative period. Higher arterial pressure increases myocardial work and oxygen consumption. Postoperative hypertension also exacerbates bleeding and may precipitate suture line disruption or loosening of a surgical clip. Careful monitoring of blood pressure and prompt intervention are important components of postoperative nursing management. Vasodilating agents, such as sodium nitroprusside or nitroglycerin, commonly are used to treat postoperative hypertension. In patients with acceptable cardiac output, beta-blocking agents, such as labetalol or esmolol, may be used (Hendren & Higgins, 1991). Sedation with morphine, midazolam, or propofol may be administered if patient agitation is contributing to hypertension.

Patients are usually mildly hypothermic during the first few postoperative hours. *Hypothermia* is actively induced during cardiac operations to reduce oxygen consumption and thereby diminish the harmful effects of myocardial ischemia. Intraoperative hypothermia is achieved by three techniques: (1) systemic cooling of the blood as it is circulated through the CPB tubing, (2) topical bathing of the heart with a chilled saline solution, and (3) perfusion of the coronary arteries with chilled cardioplegic solution. In addition, anesthetic agents inhibit the body's normal temperature-regulating mechanisms, allowing the temperature to be environmentally controlled (Phillips & Skov, 1988). Thus, a cool room, administration of room-temperature intravenous solutions, unwarmed anesthetic gases, exposure of the mediastinal viscera to room air while the incision is open, and application of cold antimicrobial solutions to the skin all play a passive role in cooling the patient (Whitman, 1991).

Rewarming is performed before terminating CPB by increasing the temperature of the circulating blood volume. However, the presence of excessive peripheral vasoconstriction allows retention of cooled blood in peripheral vessels. As these vessels gradually dilate over the next 45 to 90 minutes, they release cold blood to mix with the warmed central blood, producing a 2°C to 5°C decrease in body temperature, referred to as *afterdrop* (Whitman, 1991). The patient's body temperature gradually returns to normal with vasodilatation and restoration of patient thermoregulation (Fig. 22-4).

While the patient is hypothermic, cardiac arrhythmias are common. Hypothermia decreases myocardial conductivity and predisposes the patient to brady-arrhythmias, which may in turn lead to premature ventricular contractions (PVCs) or VT (Strong, 1991). Many patients also experience shivering in response to postoperative hypothermia. Although it is a normal compensatory mechanism to produce heat, it increases the metabolic rate, heart rate, blood pressure, carbon dioxide production, myocardial oxygen demand, and

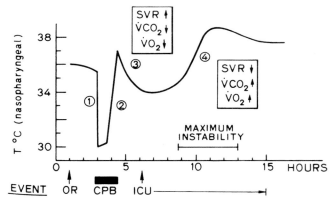

FIGURE 22-4. Nasopharyngeal temperature changes during and after cardiac surgery. (1) Hypothermia on cardiopulmonary bypass (CPB). (2) Rewarming on CPB. (3) Redistribution of heat to the periphery after CPB. (4) Rewarming after surgery. Systemic vascular resistance (SVR), CO_2 production ($\dot{V}CO_2$) and oxygen consumption ($\dot{V}O_2$) vary markedly with temperature changes. A lesser degree of fluctuation is observed in body temperature as measured by thermistors in the bladder or pulmonary artery. (Sladen RN, 1982: Management of the adult cardiac patient in the intensive care unit. In Ream AK, Fogdall RP [eds]: Acute Cardiovascular Management: Anesthesia and Intensive Care, p. 495. Philadelphia, JB Lippincott)

peripheral vasoconstriction (Whitman, 1991). Vasodilating or neuromuscular blocking agents may be administered to eliminate shivering. External measures such as warm blankets or warming devices may be used to facilitate the return to normothermia. As rewarming and vasodilatation occur in the early postoperative hours, the vascular space increases, with a resultant decrease in preload. Occasionally, rapid fluid infusion may be necessary to restore adequate intravascular volume and correct precipitous hypotension. Volume replacement may be accomplished with crystalloid, colloid, or, in actively bleeding patients, with blood component therapy.

Electrolyte imbalances may occur during the early postoperative period because of fluid shifts between the vascular space and interstitial tissues and because of manipulation of intravascular volume with intravenous fluids and diuretics. Hypokalemia is most common due to the urinary diuresis that commonly follows operations in which CPB is used. Potassium levels are measured every 4 to 8 hours and after the administration of intravenous potassium supplements. Ideally, the serum potassium level is kept between 4.0 and 5.0 mEq/L to avoid ventricular arrhythmias associated with hypokalemia.

Potassium supplementation usually is given along with diuretic therapy, unless there is a contraindication, such as renal failure. A sliding scale protocol often is used to guide potassium replacement during the early postoperative period. A central venous catheter should be used for administration of intravenous potassium because of its caustic effect on peripheral veins. A rate-regulating pump is also necessary because rapid infusion of intravenous potassium can produce cardiac asystole.

Maintaining a normal acid–base balance is essential. Fluctuations may occur in arterial pH during the early postoperative hours as a result of any of a number of physiologic factors. Most common is metabolic alkalosis, which results from extracellular volume and potassium depletion (Landolfo & Smith, 1995). It is corrected with volume and potassium repletion. Metabolic acidosis may occur as a result of low cardiac output. The diminished metabolic rate and carbon dioxide production associated with hypothermia may compensate for a moderate degree of metabolic acidosis during the first few postoperative hours (Moreno-Cabral et al., 1988). However, as rewarming occurs, metabolic acidosis may be unmasked.

Serum glucose almost always is elevated owing to the intraoperative administration of large volumes of intravenous solutions that contain glucose and the surgically induced increases in serum catecholamine and cortisol levels (Gray, 1990). Except in patients with diabetes, blood glucose gradually returns to normal levels without treatment. In diabetic patients, fluctuations in postoperative insulin requirements are common owing to hormonal responses to surgery, immobility, and anorexia. Serial measurements of blood glucose are performed to guide titration of insulin doses until the dosage requirement stabilizes.

Generalized ST segment and T wave changes are common on the postoperative ECG because of operative manipulation of the heart. However, new, localized ST segment elevation, peaked T waves, or Q waves may indicate acute myocardial ischemia or a perioperative myocardial infarction. Electrocardiographic findings are likely to precede clinical manifestations of ischemia in the sedated patient and should be communicated to the surgeon immediately. In patients who have undergone coronary artery revascularization, ischemia may represent acute graft occlusion or spasm of an internal thoracic artery (also called internal mammary artery) graft or native coronary artery. Vasodilating agents may be indicated to relieve spasm. Emergent reexploration for examination of graft patency and revision or replacement of jeopardized grafts may be necessary for acute graft closure.

Postoperative arrhythmias occur commonly after cardiac operations and necessitate familiarity with antiarrhythmic agents, competence in performing the various forms of temporary pacing and defibrillation, and easy access to emergency drugs and equipment. Regardless of the type of arrhythmia, initial nursing interventions consist of prompt assessment of the patient's hemodynamic status, ventricular rate response, and associated signs and symptoms.

Premature ventricular contractions are fairly common. A number of factors are considered in determining the seriousness of new ventricular ectopy. PVCs are of concern if (1) they occur in succession, (2) they have different morphologies (polymorphic), (3) they fall on the T wave of the previous complex, and (4) their frequency is more than 6 to 10 per minute. Treatment options include observation, overdrive pacing, and drug therapy. The most easily treatable causes should be corrected first. Because the two most likely causes are hypokalemia and hypoxemia, the appearance of ventricular ectopy should prompt measurement of serum potassium and arterial oxygen saturation. Lidocaine is the drug of choice for acute suppression of ventricular ectopy. An initial intravenous bolus is usually followed by a continuous intravenous infusion. Some patients have chronic ventricular ectopy that was well controlled before surgery with antiarrhythmic medication. Such ectopy can be expected to persist after surgery, and resumption of the antiarrhythmic agent usually is initiated in the postoperative period.

The incidence of PVCs may herald the development of VT. Several conditions may predispose the patient to development of VT, including perioperative myocardial injury due to prolonged ischemia, incomplete myocardial revascularization, graft closure, hypokalemia, acidosis, hypoxia, hypomagnesemia, use of catecholamines, and malposition of intracardiac catheters. VT usually occurs at a rate of 140 to 220 beats per minute and may be nonsustained (<30 seconds in duration) or sustained (Moore & Wilkoff, 1991) (Fig. 22-5). VT that occurs in the presence of hemodynamic stability typically is treated with an intravenous lidocaine infusion. Intravenous amiodarone, procainamide, or bretylium may be used to control VT that is refractory to lidocaine therapy.

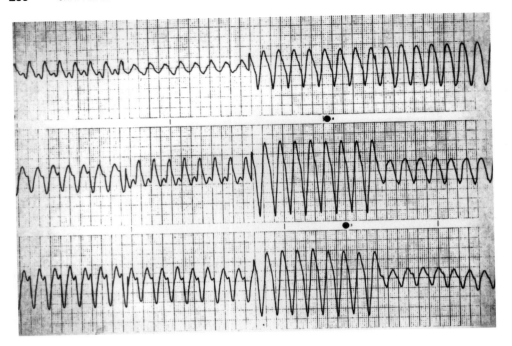

FIGURE 22-5. Ventricular tachycardia in a postoperative patient at a rate of 197 beats per minute. The ventricular origin of this tachyarrhythmia is suggested by concordance of the precordial leads, left axis deviation, and a QRS interval greater than 0.14 second. (Courtesy of Linda Hellstedt, RN, MS)

Defibrillation should be performed at once if hemodynamic compromise or VF ensues. VF causes immediate cessation of peripheral perfusion and irreversible neurologic injury within minutes (Hillis et al., 1995). Defibrillation is the single most effective resuscitative measure for improving survival (Marino, 1998). It is most likely to be successful if performed within 1 to 2 minutes of the arrhythmia's onset (Goldberger, 1990). Consequently, cardiothoracic surgical nurses are trained to defibrillate promptly a patient in whom VF or VT with profound hypotension develops. Sustained VT with hemodynamic compromise or VF also necessitates initiation of cardiopulmonary resuscitation and advanced cardiac life support protocols (Strong, 1991). Cardiopulmonary resuscitation is continued until a stable rhythm ensues.

In the past, conventional wisdom led to the assumption that chronic suppression of PVCs would improve long-term outcome. However, the Cardiac Arrhythmia Suppression Trial (CAST) and CAST II, which examined pharmacologic treatment of asymptomatic or mildly symptomatic ventricular arrhythmias after myocardial infarction, revealed that some antiarrhythmic agents increase morbidity and mortality (CAST Investigators, 1989, 1992). Thus, the decision to initiate chronic therapy for ventricular arrhythmias in postoperative patients should be made with caution, weighing the proarrhythmic risks versus benefits of arrhythmia suppression.

Although wide QRS tachycardias in postoperative cardiac surgical patients are most often of ventricular origin, aberrantly conducted supraventricular tachycardia (SVT) also can occur. Aberrant complexes are the result of supraventricular impulses that are conducted abnormally through intraventricular pathways, resulting in a wide QRS complex tachycardia that may be difficult to distinguish from VT. Differentiation of the two types of arrhythmias is important. Untreated VT can produce profound hypotension or progress to VF. Unless aberrancy is confirmed, it is safer to treat the patient as if the arrhythmia were ventricular.

Impaired AV nodal conduction occurs occasionally in patients undergoing valvular surgery and rarely in those undergoing coronary artery revascularization. Usually transient, it may be caused by ischemia, manipulation of cardiac tissue with resultant edema, digoxin toxicity, perioperative myocardial infarction, or mechanical injury to conduction tissue. Temporary pacing is instituted and medications that slow AV conduction are discontinued. Because of the ease of using pacing wires and the fact that temporary AV pacing in a demand mode is now possible, an external pulse generator usually is connected to the atrial and ventricular pacing wires if there is any reason to believe that complete heart block may develop. Pacing thresholds are assessed daily to ensure dependable pacing (Finkelmeier & O'Mara, 1984).

Complete heart block is best treated with AV synchronous (dual-chamber) pacing, which preserves the atrial contribution to cardiac output. Ventricular pacing is used in patients with atrial fibrillation because atrial capture is not possible. If pacing wires are not present, atropine or isoproterenol should be readily accessible, as well as the necessary equipment to provide for emergency pacing by means of a transvenous or transthoracic pacing system. If a patient is totally reliant on some form of pacing system, an extra pulse generator and cable are placed at the bedside or attached to another set of epicardial wires, if present, to provide backup pacing should the operational pacing system malfunction. If the underlying cardiac rhythm is asystole or profound bradycardia or if external pacing wires are not present, patients remain in an ICU or intermediate care unit for close monitoring until bradycardia is adequately treated.

Supraventricular tachycardia includes paroxysmal

SVT (arising from the atrium or AV node), atrial flutter, and atrial fibrillation. All are rapid heart rhythms in which the site of impulse formation is above the bifurcation of the bundle of His. These tachyarrhythmias decrease stroke volume, and therefore cardiac output, by 15% to 20% by compromising diastolic filling time, and thus the effective preload, as well as by decreasing myocardial contractility as a result of altered myocardial oxygen supply and demand (Lee & Geha, 1996).

Atrial flutter and atrial fibrillation are particularly common after cardiac surgical procedures, occurring in 25% to 50% of patients (Leitch et al., 1990; Lauer et al., 1989). The incidence is related to a number of risk factors, including advanced patient age, discontinuation of preoperative beta-adrenergic blocking agents, postoperative pericardial effusion, prolonged cross-clamp times with inadequate atrial protection, chronic obstructive pulmonary disease, and chronic renal disease (Creswell et al., 1993; Kirklin & Barratt-Boyes, 1993). The etiology is not well understood. The search for an effective prophylactic agent to prevent the occurrence of postoperative SVT has long been a focus of research. Multiple studies indicate that the prophylactic administration of a beta-blocking agent after cardiac surgery controls the incidence and severity of atrial arrhythmias (Ali et al., 1997; Kowey et al., 1992). Amiodarone also has been demonstrated to provide effective preoperative prophylaxis in high-risk populations (Daoud et al., 1997). Use of amiodarone is limited, however, because of its high adverse effect profile.

In most postoperative patients, SVT produces unpleasant palpitations or sensations but does not significantly affect blood pressure. However, in those with low cardiac output or underlying ventricular impairment, hemodynamic compromise can occur from loss of effective atrial contraction and the rapid ventricular rate. Diagnosis of SVT may be difficult because ectopic P waves may be indistinguishable in standard ECG leads used for monitoring. An atrial electrogram, obtained using the atrial epicardial wire, can be extremely useful. Atrial electrograms increase the amplitude of atrial activity and diminish that of other electrical components and extracardiac artifact (Finkelmeier & Salinger, 1984). Treatment of postoperative SVT may consist of oral or intravenous medications, rapid atrial pacing, or cardioversion.

Atrial fibrillation, the most common form of postoperative SVT, is usually a self-limited phenomenon and rarely requires long-term therapy. Nevertheless, it can cause an increase in morbidity and mortality in postoperative patients (Almassi et al., 1997). Often, pharmacologic control of ventricular rate is sufficient therapy and facilitates spontaneous conversion to sinus rhythm. This is usually accomplished with intravenous digitalization, followed by a maintenance regimen of oral digoxin. In addition, beta-adrenergic blocking (eg, propranolol) or calcium channel blocking (eg, verapamil) agents may be added if digoxin is inadequate for control of the ventricular rate. If atrial fibrillation persists despite these interventions, chemical cardioversion with ibutilide, procainamide, or amiodarone may be considered. Electrical cardioversion is performed immediately for SVT that produces significant hypotension. It also is considered for persistent SVT in a patient who was in normal sinus rhythm before surgery.

In patients who have atrial fibrillation for more than 48 hours before conversion to sinus rhythm, the presence of new atrial thrombus must be considered. Anticoagulation with warfarin sodium for several weeks after conversion to sinus rhythm may be recommended in patients who have had persistent atrial fibrillation. The risk of thrombus formation remains during this period because forceful atrial contractions may not resume for 2 weeks or longer. Furthermore, a newly formed thrombus may take at least 2 weeks to become firmly attached to the atrial myocardium (Prystowsky et al., 1996).

Postoperative SVT less commonly occurs in the form of atrial flutter. Type I atrial flutter is defined as atrial flutter with an atrial rate between 250 and 350 beats per minute. It typically occurs with an atrial rate of 300 beats per minute, a characteristic "sawtooth" pattern of flutter waves, 2:1 AV block, and a ventricular rate of 150 beats per minute. Type I atrial flutter often can be interrupted effectively with rapid atrial pacing using the temporary atrial epicardial pacing wires. The procedure, which is relatively painless and easy to perform, usually is combined with pharmacologic therapy to prevent arrhythmia recurrence. Type II, or atypical, atrial flutter has elements of both atrial flutter and atrial fibrillation. The atrial rate ranges from 320 to 430 beats per minute (Conover, 1996). Because the flutter waves are less uniform and vary in morphology and spacing, type II atrial flutter also is called atrial flutter-fibrillation. Type II atrial flutter is much more difficult to interrupt and rarely is responsive to pacing. The spectrum of cardiac arrhythmias is discussed in depth in Chapter 25, Cardiac Arrhythmias. Temporary pacing techniques and defibrillation are discussed in Chapter 26, Temporary Pacing and Defibrillation.

▶ Care on the Postoperative Unit

Progression of Activity

Patients who recover in routine fashion are transferred to a general cardiothoracic surgical unit with telemetry monitoring after 24 to 48 hours (Fig. 22-6). If recovery is routine, almost all invasive catheters will have been removed by this point and the patient can ambulate freely. The plan for progression of activity is based on the patient's age, baseline functional status, degree of ventricular impairment, associated medical problems, type of surgical procedure, and perioperative course. Most patients are able to walk to the bathroom on the second postoperative day and ambulate in the hallway on the following day. By the time of discharge from the hospital, most patients are ambulating independently and taking 6 to 10 walks in the corridors each day.

Certain groups of patients are much slower in recov-

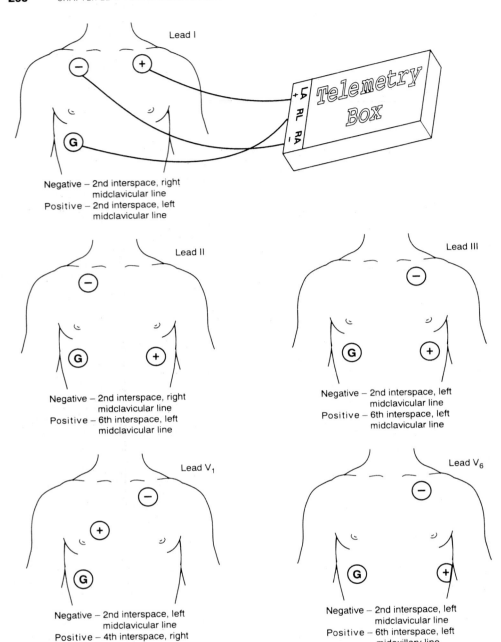

FIGURE 22-6. Telemetry monitoring; various leads may be monitored depending on electrode positions. (Huff J, Doernbach DP, White RD, 1993: Cardiac monitors. In ECG Workout, ed. 2, p. 23. Philadelphia, JB Lippincott)

ering and should not be expected to progress according to the routine regimen. Specifically, patients with the following conditions require more recovery time and assistance with ambulation: (1) end-stage valvular heart disease, (2) perioperative myocardial infarction, (3) prolonged preoperative immobility or debilitation, and (4) severe underlying ventricular dysfunction secondary to ischemic damage or cardiomyopathy. Elderly patients also progress more slowly and may require more assistance with daily activities.

Many institutions implement a cardiac rehabilitation program for patients after cardiac surgery. Such a program usually involves supervised exercise as well as education and cardiac risk reduction strategies that begin during the postoperative hospital phase and continue after discharge on an outpatient basis. The beneficial effects of cardiac rehabilitation are well documented in the literature. Specifically, in the cardiac surgery population, participation in a postoperative cardiac rehabilitation program has been shown to improve exercise tolerance, decrease blood lipid levels, reduce cigarette smoking, improve psychosocial well-being, reduce stress, and enable a quicker return to work (Wenger et al., 1995).

Pulmonary Hygiene

The provision of adequate pulmonary hygiene is one of the most important components of nursing care on the postoperative unit. Postoperative lung function and respiratory mechanics may be substantially impaired by the adverse effects of anesthetic agents, the thoracic incision and surgical manipulation, and CPB (Sivak, 1991). Routine pulmonary hygiene measures include encouraging deep breathing and coughing every hour. Diminished breath sounds, rhonchi, fever, and hypoxemia are signs of atelectasis or retained secretions and indicate the need for more aggressive interventions. Intermittent ultrasonic nebulization administered by face mask helps loosen secretions so that they may be more easily expectorated. Nasotracheal suctioning is necessary occasionally to remove secretions and allow airway expansion if the patient cannot cough effectively. Wheezing is indicative of bronchospasm and may be treated with bronchodilating agents, such as albuterol or ipratropium. Bilateral rales (crackles) suggest pulmonary edema and the need for diuresis.

Incision Care

The sternum is palpated daily for stability (Fig. 22-7). Failure of the sternal halves to heal (ie, sternal nonunion) or separation of the sternal halves (ie, sternal dehiscence) is most likely in patients who are obese, diabetic, or re-

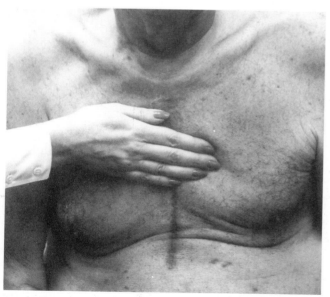

FIGURE 22-7. Sternal stability is assessed by applying firm pressure over the sternal incision while the patient turns his head from side to side or coughs.

ceiving corticosteroids, or who have had previous sternotomy, postoperative reexploration of the incision, or closed-chest massage. Female patients with large, pendulous breasts are instructed to wear a brassiere except when bathing during the first several weeks to help support the breasts and reduce tension on the sternal incision. Patients who are paraplegic, who have had lower extremity amputations, or who must use crutches require special nursing and physical therapy assistance to avoid injuring the sternal closure during the early postoperative period. Use of the upper extremities for transferring in and out of bed or for manipulating crutches or an overbed trapeze is avoided because it may lead to sternal dehiscence.

After the first 24 hours, the incision is cleaned daily with soap and water and left uncovered. Close attention is given to the appearance of the sternal incision to detect evidence of infection. Any incisional redness or drainage is reported to the surgeon. Small amounts of serous drainage may occur, usually representing necrosis of subcutaneous fat. Purulent or copious drainage is more ominous.

Leg incisions are cared for in the same manner. As ambulation is increased, lower extremity edema almost always develops owing to disruption of lymphatic channels in the leg or legs from which saphenous veins were harvested. Supportive stockings and elevation of the lower extremities when sitting are prescribed. Leg swelling may persist for several months but almost always resolves. Occasionally, a seroma, or cyst-like collection of serous fluid, develops under the skin and drains through the leg incision. If there is no evidence of incisional infection, dry dressings are the only necessary treatment until the drainage abates.

Medications

Unless contraindicated by another medical problem, aspirin therapy is initiated in all patients who undergo coronary artery revascularization. In general, aspirin is regarded as the most effective antiplatelet agent for augmenting long-term patency of vein grafts (Goldman et al., 1990). Often aspirin therapy is initiated on the operative day with administration of a rectal suppository. When an oral diet is resumed, one enteric-coated aspirin tablet a day usually is prescribed and continued indefinitely.

Postoperative anticoagulation with warfarin sodium may be necessary for patients with prosthetic heart valves, chronic atrial fibrillation, or a history of pulmonary embolism. If so, it usually is initiated on the second postoperative day, after chest drainage tubes have been removed. In most patients, anticoagulation is begun with an initial dose of 5 to 10 mg of warfarin. Daily measurement of the prothrombin time (PT) with calculation of an international normalized ratio (INR) is performed to determine subsequent doses. The INR has gained recognition in the United States as a more accurate measure of anticoagulation (Vanscoy & Krause,

1991). Calculated from the PT assay result, the INR corrects for lack of standardization in the reagent (tissue thromboplastin) used to perform the PT assay.

Usually, the PT/INR measurement is obtained in the morning and warfarin is given in the evening because the peak effect of a dose of warfarin is reached 36 to 72 hours after its administration. Serial PT/INR levels and daily warfarin doses are documented and monitored by both physicians and nurses (Table 22-4). Vigilant attention is given to determining the proper dose. Before administering warfarin, the most recent PT/INR value is considered. The INR must be maintained at a level sufficient to prevent thromboembolism while minimizing the risk of anticoagulant-related hemorrhage. Optimal INR ranges vary, depending on the reason for treatment. The INR usually is maintained at between 2.5 to 3.5 in patients with mechanical valves. Lower values (2.0 to 3.0) are acceptable for patients with atrial fibrillation or bioprosthetic cardiac valves (Hirsh et al., 1995). In patients with implanted cardiac valves, recommended INR values also may vary according to the specific prosthesis, valve position, and other clinical factors. For example, an INR between 2.0 and 2.9 may be adequate for a St. Jude Medical prosthesis in the aortic position, whereas an INR between 3.0 and 3.9 is preferable for those with Medtronic-Hall or Bjork-Shiley valves; patients with ball-and-cage prostheses or multiple mechanical prostheses may require an INR between 4.0 and 4.9 (Garcia, 1998).

Certain groups of patients require more cautious anticoagulation. These include small, elderly, or frail people; those with long-standing mitral or tricuspid valve or liver disease; and those receiving the antiarrhythmic medication amiodarone. A single dose of 10 mg in these patients may produce a significant rise in the PT/INR to dangerous levels. If this occurs, ambulation is permitted only with direct supervision to prevent potential life-threatening bleeding that could occur with a fall.

Selected patients, particularly those in whom prolonged immobilization is anticipated, may require short-term anticoagulation with intravenous heparin as prophylaxis against deep venous thrombosis and pulmonary embolism. Patients at greatest risk for postoperative deep venous thrombosis and pulmonary embolism include those requiring prolonged ventilatory or circulatory support; obese, elderly, or debilitated patients; and those who lack lower extremity muscle tone to augment venous return (paraplegic or hemiplegic patients and those with lower extremity amputations).

Specific regimens for postoperative antibiotic prophylaxis vary. Typical is a daily dose of a broad-spectrum cephalosporin (vancomycin for penicillin-allergic patients) through the first postoperative day after coronary artery revascularization. If a prosthetic cardiac valve has been implanted, some surgeons continue antibiotic prophylaxis several days longer. However, antibiotic use longer than 48 hours has not been demonstrated to be beneficial and may lead to development of resistant organisms and increased toxicity (Doebbeling et al., 1990).

Common Problems

Low-grade fevers are common during the first few postoperative days. The most common etiology is atelectasis. However, sputum, urine, and blood cultures are obtained when a temperature greater than 38.5°C (101.3°F) occurs after the first 48 hours. Wounds are examined carefully for any evidence of infection. Particularly if prosthetic material has been placed in or around the heart, the source of the fever must be promptly identified and treated.

Avoidance of postoperative infection is particularly important in patients who have undergone implantation of prosthetic material, such as a prosthetic cardiac valve, an implantable cardioverter-defibrillator, pacemaker, or vascular graft. In this group of patients, invasive catheters are discontinued as early as possible. If instrumentation such as reinsertion of a urethral catheter is performed in patients with prosthetic heart valves, prophylactic antibiotics are given according to the American Heart Association recommendations (Dajani et al., 1997).

Pain control rarely is a significant problem after cardiac operations performed through a median sternotomy. In contrast to thoracic and abdominal incisions, no muscles need be divided during sternotomy and the divided sternum is secured tightly at the completion of the operation. Although some postoperative chest discomfort is usually present, it is easily controlled with analgesic medications and usually does not interfere with patient mobility. However, because the muscles throughout the chest wall are stretched when the sternal halves are separated, pain in the back, particularly between the shoulder blades and in the neck, is typical. Also, patients who have undergone harvesting of one or both internal thoracic arteries can be expected to experience more anterior chest wall discomfort.

Oral pain medications usually are administered as necessary. Sneezing and coughing are particularly painful because they provoke forceful movement of the chest wall. A pillow may be used to brace the sternum during these times. Heat is often effective in relieving chest wall discomfort; hot showers or a heating pad may provide relief during the latter portion of the hospitalization and

TABLE 22-4

Example of Regulating Anticoagulant Therapy

Postoperative Day	Prothrombin Time	International Normalized Ratio	Warfarin (Coumadin) Dose
3	11.3	0.9	5.0 mg
4	11.3	0.9	10.0 mg
5	13.6	1.4	5.0 mg
6	18.0	2.5	2.5 mg
7	16.4	2.1	5.0 mg

the first weeks at home. A heating pad should not be applied directly over the incision.

Disorientation is a common postoperative phenomenon, particularly in elderly patients. Factors thought to contribute include general anesthesia, narcotic analgesics, sleep deprivation, severe preoperative anxiety, use of CPB, and the ICU environment. Alertness to the development of disorientation during the first few postoperative days is important to prevent patient injury. Most commonly, disoriented patients attempt to disconnect attached invasive catheters or tubes or they attempt to get out of bed. If a patient demonstrates any tendency to pull at necessary tubes or catheters, wrist restraints may be necessary. Patients who attempt to climb out of bed or ambulate without adequate assistance may require a sitter in the room, particularly at night. A restraining vest also may be used but may increase the risk of sternal wound disruption caused by the patient straining against the vest. From a legal perspective, nurses are particularly vulnerable if they fail to protect disoriented

patients adequately from injury. Other typical problems that affect patients on the postoperative unit are listed in Table 22-5.

Preparation for Discharge

Most patients are ready for discharge from the hospital by the fourth or fifth postoperative day. Discharge preparation usually is considered before hospital admission and is finalized several days before discharge. Consideration of discharge needs as early as possible allows ample time to arrange the necessary provisions for transition back to the home environment. Written and oral instructions are given to the patient and family regarding (1) medications, (2) activity, (3) restrictions, (4) diet, and (5) follow-up appointments. Most of the discharge information can be standardized for all types of cardiac surgery. Special attention should be given to those instructions that are specific to a particular patient.

TABLE 22-5

Miscellaneous Postoperative Problems

Problem	Possible Causes	Treatment
Anorexia	General anesthesia	Liberalization of dietary restrictions
	Iron supplementation	
	Pain medication	
	Decreased activity	
	Digoxin toxicity	Discontinue digoxin
Constipation	General anesthesia	Laxative therapy
	Iron supplementation	
	Pain medications	
	Decreased activity	
Diarrhea	*Clostridium difficile*	Antibiotic therapy
	Impaction	Disimpaction
	Digoxin therapy	Discontinue digoxin
	Quinidine	Discontinue quinidine
Emotional lability	Hormonal response to surgical stress	Supportive counseling
	Impaired physical stamina	
Fatigue	Effects of general anesthesia and surgical procedure	Scheduled rest periods interspersed with periods of activity
	Use of caloric intake for wound healing	
	Altered sleep patterns	
Fever	Atelectasis	Identify source and treat
	Postpericardiotomy syndrome	
	Infection	
Insomnia	Decreased activity	Progressive activity during the day
	Altered sleep patterns	Sleep medications
Pleural effusion	Harvesting internal thoracic artery	Diuresis (small to moderate and asymptomatic)
	Intraoperative regional cooling	Thoracentesis (moderate to large or symptomatic)
	Postpericardiotomy syndrome	
Postpericardiotomy syndrome	Surgical opening of pericardial sac	Nonsteroidal anti-inflammatory agents
		Steroids (if severe)
Sore throat	Endotracheal intubation	Lozenges, viscous lidocaine
Ulnar paresthesia	Nerve compression during operation	Usually none; self-limited
		Hand exercises if persistent
Weight loss	Decreased caloric intake	Ensure adequate calories to meet nutritional needs

Discharge medications vary depending on the specific operation performed and the patient's underlying cardiac disease. Most patients who undergo coronary artery revascularization procedures are discharged on antiplatelet therapy (aspirin) to enhance graft patency. A coated or buffered aspirin is often better tolerated during the early postoperative period. However, for long-term use, many patients tolerate a less expensive, generic form of aspirin. If the patient has a history of ulcer disease or gastrointestinal bleeding, aspirin therapy may be contraindicated.

Patients who have undergone valve replacement or who have other indications for chronic anticoagulation are discharged on warfarin sodium, and it is imperative that thorough instructions be given to the patient and family. Dosage errors or lack of appropriate monitoring can lead to lethal hemorrhage. Medications and activities that are contraindicated while taking warfarin are reviewed and patients may be encouraged to obtain an identification bracelet, necklace, or wallet card describing anticoagulant use. Written instructions given to the patient and included in the medical record should contain documentation that clearly states (1) current dosage regimen, (2) name of the physician who will monitor PT/INR, and (3) date and place for the next PT/INR measurement. Although warfarin is available in a variety of doses, it is practical to use either 2- or 5-mg tablets. The tablets are scored, and thus can be easily divided. Therefore, a 2-mg tablet allows 1-mg dose modification increments for patients requiring doses in the range of 1 to 5 mg. Similarly, for those patients requiring doses in the range of 2.5 to 12.5 mg, adjusting the dose in increments of 2.5 mg is possible with the 5-mg tablets.

Iron supplementation usually is prescribed for the first few months. Because infectious hazards of homologous blood transfusions have become more apparent, patients more commonly are discharged with a moderate degree of anemia. Unfortunately, iron preparations often are not well tolerated in patients who are already somewhat anorexic and constipated. If the patient cannot tolerate oral iron supplementation, it may take somewhat longer for postoperative anemia to resolve.

Oral pain medications may be prescribed for the first few weeks at home. Pain tolerance is quite variable, and many patients do not desire pain medications, even while in the hospital. Patients can be advised that chest wall discomfort will vary in intensity with level of activities, weather changes, and positioning during sleep. In patients who have undergone harvesting of one or both internal thoracic arteries, pain may be more of a problem. In a small number of these patients, chest wall pain and paresthesia may persist for several months.

Epicardial pacing wires typically are removed the day before patient discharge from the hospital, or before achieving therapeutic anticoagulation levels in patients receiving postoperative warfarin therapy. The patient always is monitored for several hours after wire removal because of the rare but potentially lethal complication of cardiac tamponade caused by atrial or ventricular laceration during wire removal. Although extremely uncommon, bleeding after pacing wire removal can cause pre-cipitous hemodynamic deterioration that is usually fatal unless detected and treated rapidly. For this reason, any evidence of hemodynamic instability after pacing wire removal should be reported to the surgeon immediately. Emergent thoracotomy may be necessary to relieve cardiac tamponade and save the patient's life.

Most patients are ambulatory and able to perform self-care activities before discharge. The specific regimen for increasing activity at home depends on a number of factors, including general functional status before the operation, underlying cardiac disease, presence of recent myocardial infarction, and the perioperative course. Fatigue is common during the first postoperative month. Because it causes patients to be less active during the day, insomnia is an almost universal complaint. The patient should spend most of the day out of bed and incorporate several periods of walking into the daily schedule. Family members are instructed to limit visitors in the early days at home because this can be quite tiring for the patient.

Discharge instructions include goals to guide progression of activity. Patients are advised to increase daily activities gradually and take rest periods according to level of fatigue. In general, patients can be expected to increase their activities during the first few days at home just by virtue of being in their own surroundings. Walking is the best form of exercise. After the first week at home, the patient should begin consciously to increase the amount of walking each day. If weather is prohibitive, shopping malls provide an excellent area of level surface for walking.

Patients with good ventricular function who undergo coronary artery revascularization are usually walking 4 to 6 miles per day within 6 weeks of the operation. The pace of walking is less important than the amount. Stair climbing may be done, although this is more tiring than walking on level ground, and most patients with stairs at home choose to limit trips up and down to the minimum necessary during the first few weeks. Sexual activity usually can be resumed within several weeks of discharge when the patient is able to ambulate several blocks or one flight of stairs without tiring excessively.

Many patients are eager to resume work. If the job is fairly sedentary and the patient can control the amount of hours worked, working on a limited basis usually can be resumed within several weeks of discharge. The patient is cautioned against taking on responsibilities that require undue physical or emotional stamina. Similarly, the patient should avoid social engagements that might prove too tiring. Heavy physical labor should not be resumed for at least 2 to 3 months. Occasionally, cardiac function is compromised to the point that job modification or change may be necessary. The managing cardiologist usually makes this determination.

There are very few activities that are specifically contraindicated during the early period at home. One of these is lifting items that weigh more than 10 pounds. Because the sternum has been surgically divided and the halves reapproximated with heavy suture or wire, it must be treated like a broken bone. Although initial healing produces sternal stability within a few weeks, it is 2 to 3 months before the bone regains its full strength. Thus, the sternum should not be subjected to undue stress by using the arms for heavy lifting. Likewise, any exercise or sport that involves vigorous upper extremity motion should be deferred for the same period. This includes golf, swimming, tennis, using a rowing machine or exercise bicycle with movable handlebars, push-ups, sit-ups, and chin-ups. In addition, common household activities that stress the sternum, such as manually raising a garage door or shoveling snow, should be avoided during this period.

Most surgeons instruct patients not to drive for at least 1 month after the operation. This prevents patients from attempting to drive when reaction times may still be somewhat slowed by the surgery and postoperative course or by pain medications. In addition, it avoids injury to the healing sternum should an accident occur and result in a forceful blow of the sternum against the steering wheel or airbag. It is acceptable for patients to ride in a car and, in most cases, travel by train or airplane.

Instructions are given about any necessary dietary modifications. Patients with coronary artery disease are instructed in low-cholesterol diets. If the patient has hypercholesterolemia, more extensive dietary counseling may be necessary, and usually is prescribed by the managing cardiologist. Modifications in salt intake often are necessary for those patients with valvular heart disease or hypertension.

The cosmetic appearance of the incisions may be a source of great concern, particularly in younger patients. The use of a subcutaneous closure technique has greatly enhanced the appearance of surgical scars. Nevertheless, all scars are somewhat disfiguring. If the patient is concerned, a strip of paper tape may be worn over the incision, except when showering, for several months. The slight pressure of the tape flattens the scar, making it less prominent. Taping the incision is not instituted until the skin edges are healed, approximately 2 weeks after the operation. If infection or skin irritation develops from the tape, its use should be discontinued. Vitamin E or aloe lotion may also be applied to help soften the scar.

The scar darkens over the first few months and then eventually fades to approximately the patient's own skin tone. Cosmetic products designed for covering discolored skin are available in major department stores for those few patients in whom the scar remains prominent after several months and is bothersome. In rare cases, keloid scar formation occurs; corticosteroid injections may be considered if the patient is distressed by the scar's appearance.

REFERENCES

Ali IM, Sanalla AA, Clark V, 1997: Beta-blocker effects on postoperative atrial fibrillation. Eur J Cardiothorac Surg 11:1154

Almassi GH, Schowalter T, Nicolosi AC, et al., 1997: Atrial fibrillation after cardiac surgery: A major morbid event? Ann Surg 226:501

Anderson DR, Stephenson LW, Edmunds LH, 1991: Management of complications of cardiopulmonary bypass: Complications of organ systems. In Waldhausen JA, Orringer MB (eds): Complications in Cardiothoracic Surgery. St. Louis, Mosby–Year Book

Barrientos-Vega R, Mar Sanchez-Soria M, Morales-Garcia C, et al., 1997: Prolonged sedation of critically ill patients with midazolam or propofol: Impact on weaning and costs. Crit Care Med 25:33

Baumgartner FJ, Robertson J, Omari B, 1997: ICU management. In Cardiothoracic Surgery. Austin, TX, Chapman & Hall

Behrendt DM, Austen WG, 1985: Complications of other organ systems. In Patient Care in Cardiac Surgery, ed. 4. Boston, Little, Brown

Bond EF, Halpenny CJ, 1995: Physiology of the heart. In Woods SL, Froelicher ES, Halpenny CJ, Motzer SU (eds): Cardiac Nursing, ed. 3. Philadelphia, JB Lippincott

CAST Investigators, 1989: Preliminary report: Effect of encainide and flecainide on mortality in a randomized trial of arrhythmia suppression after myocardial infarction. The Cardiac Arrhythmia Suppression Trial (CAST) Investigators. N Engl J Med 321:406

CAST Investigators, 1992: The effect of the antiarrhythmic agent moricizine on survival after myocardial infarction. N Engl J Med 327:227

Conover MB, 1996: Atrial flutter. In Understanding Electrocardiography, ed. 7. St. Louis, Mosby–Year Book

Coyle JP, 1991: Sedation, pain relief, and neuromuscular blockade in the postoperative cardiac surgical patient. Semin Thorac Cardiovasc Surg 3:81

Creswell LL, Schuessler RB, Rosenbloom M, Cox JL, 1993: Hazards of postoperative atrial arrhythmias. Ann Thorac Surg 56:539

Dajani AS, Taubert KA, Wilson W, et al., 1997: Prevention of bacterial endocarditis: Recommendations by the American Heart Association. JAMA 277:1794

Daoud EG, Strickberger SA, Man KC, et al., 1997: Preoperative amiodarone as prophylaxis against atrial fibrillation after heart surgery. N Engl J Med 337:1785

de Varennes B, Nguyen D, Denis F, et al., 1996: Reinfusion of mediastinal blood in CABG patients: Impact on homologous transfusions and rate of re-exploration. J Cardiac Surg 11:387

DiSesa VJ, 1991: Pharmacologic support for postoperative low cardiac output. Semin Thorac Cardiovasc Surg 3:13

Doebbeling BN, Pfaller MA, Kuhns KR, et al., 1990: Cardiovascular surgery prophylaxis. J Thorac Cardiovasc Surg 99:981

Elefteriades JA, Geha AS, Cohen LS, 1996: Chest trauma. In House Officer Guide to ICU Care: Fundamentals of Management of the Heart and Lungs, ed. 2. Philadelphia, Lippincott-Raven

Ellis RJ, Mavroudis C, Gardner C, et al., 1980: Relationship between atrioventricular arrhythmias and the concentration of K^+ ion in cardioplegic solution. J Thorac Cardiovasc Surg 80:517

Finkelmeier BA, O'Mara SR, 1984: Temporary pacing in the cardiac surgical patient. Critical Care Nurse 4:108

Finkelmeier BA, Salinger MH, 1984: The atrial electrogram: Its diagnostic use following cardiac surgery. Critical Care Nurse 4:42

Finkelmeier BA, Salinger MH, 1986: Dual-chamber cardiac pacing: An overview. Critical Care Nurse 6:12

Garcia MJ, 1998: Prosthetic valve disease. In Topol EJ (ed): Comprehensive Cardiovascular Medicine. Philadelphia, Lippincott Williams & Wilkins

Geha AS, Whittlesey D, 1996: Postoperative low cardiac output. In Baue AE, Geha AS, Hammond GL et al. (eds): Glenn's Thoracic and Cardiovascular Surgery, ed. 6. Stamford, CT, Appleton & Lange

Goldberger E, 1990: Defibrillation and cardioversion. In Treatment of Cardiac Emergencies, ed. 5. St. Louis, CV Mosby

Goldman S, Copeland J, Moritz T, et al., 1990: Internal mammary artery and saphenous vein graft patency. Circulation 82(Suppl IV):IV-237

Gray RJ, 1990: Normal convalescence. In Gray RJ, Matloff JM (eds): Medical Management of the Cardiac Surgical Patient. Baltimore, Williams & Wilkins

Greco SA, 1990: Vasoactive drugs. In Underhill SL, Woods SL, Froelicher ES, Halpenny CJ (eds): Cardiovascular Medications for Cardiac Nursing. Philadelphia, JB Lippincott

Halfman-Franey M, Berg DE, 1991: Recognition and management of bleeding following cardiac surgery. Critical Care Nursing Clinics of North America 3:675

Hendren WG, Higgins TL, 1991: Immediate postoperative care of the cardiac surgical patient. Semin Thorac Cardiovasc Surg 3:3

Hillis LD, Lange RA, Winniford MD, Page RL, 1995: Ventricular tachycardia and ventricular fibrillation. In Manual of Clinical Problems in Cardiology, ed. 5. Boston, Little, Brown

Hirsh J, Dalen JE, Deykin D, et al., 1995: Oral anticoagulants: Mechanism of action, clinical effectiveness, and optimal therapeutic range. Chest 108:231S

Hudak CM, Gallo BM, Morton PG, 1998a: Heart failure. In Critical Care Nursing: A Holistic Approach, ed. 7. Philadelphia, Lippincott Williams & Wilkins

Hudak CM, Gallo BM, Morton PG, 1998b: Cardiac surgery. In Critical Care Nursing: A Holistic Approach, ed. 7. Philadelphia, Lippincott Williams & Wilkins

Klein AL, Scalia GM, 1998: Diseases of the pericardium, restrictive cardiomyopathy and diastolic dysfunction. In Topol EJ (ed): Comprehensive Cardiovascular Medicine. Philadelphia, Lippincott Williams & Wilkins

Kirklin JW, Baratt-Boyes BG, 1993: Postoperative care. In Cardiac Surgery, ed. 2. New York, Churchill Livingstone

Kollef MH, Shapiro SD, Silver P, et al., 1997: A randomized, controlled trial of protocol-directed versus physician-directed weaning from mechanical ventilation. Crit Care Med 25:567

Kowey PR, Taylor JE, Rials SJ, Marinchak RA, 1992: Meta-analysis of the effectiveness of prophylactic drug therapy in preventing supraventricular arrhythmia early after coronary artery bypass grafting. Am J Cardiol 69:963

Landolfo K, Smith PK, 1995: Postoperative care in cardiac surgery. In Sabiston DC Jr, Spencer FC (eds): Surgery of the Chest, ed. 6. Philadelphia, WB Saunders

Lauer MS, Eagle KA, Buckley MJ, DeSanctis RW, 1989: Atrial fibrillation following coronary artery bypass surgery. Prog Cardiovasc Dis 31:369

LeDoux D, Shinn J, 1995: Cardiac surgery. In Woods SL, Froelicher ES, Halpenny CJ, Motzer SU (eds): Cardiac Nursing, ed 3. Philadelphia, JB Lippincott

Lee JH, Geha AS, 1996. Postoperative care of the cardiovascular surgical patient. In Baue AE, Geha AS, Hammond GL, et al. (eds): Glenn's Thoracic and Cardiovascular Surgery, ed. 6. Stamford, CT, Appleton & Lange

Leitch JW, Thomson D, Baird DK, Harris PJ, 1990: The importance of age as a predictor of atrial fibrillation and flutter after coronary artery bypass grafting. J Thorac Cardiovasc Surg 100:338

Mahfood SS, Higgins TL, Loop FD, 1991: Management of complications related to coronary artery bypass surgery. In Waldhausen JA, Orringer MB (eds): Complications in Cardiothoracic Surgery. St. Louis, Mosby–Year Book

Marino PL, 1998: Cardiac arrest. In The ICU Book, ed. 2. Baltimore, Williams & Wilkins

Moore SL, Wilkoff BL, 1991: Rhythm disturbances after cardiac surgery. Semin Thorac Cardiovasc Surg 3:24

Moran JM, Singh AK, 1989: Cardiogenic shock. In Grillo HC, Austen WG, Wilkins EW Jr, et al. (eds): Current Therapy in Cardiothoracic Surgery. Toronto, Canada, BC Decker

Moreno-Cabral CE, Mitchell RS, Miller DC, 1988: Perioperative care. In Manual of Postoperative Management of Adult Cardiac Surgery. Baltimore, Williams & Wilkins

Phillips R, Skov P, 1988: Rewarming and cardiac surgery: A review. Heart Lung 17:511

Prystowsky EN, Benson W, Fuster V, et al., 1996: Management of patients with atrial fibrillation: A statement for healthcare professionals from the Subcommittee on Electrocardiography and Electrophysiology, American Heart Association. Circulation 93:1262

Riddle MM, Dunstan JL, Castanis JL, 1996: A rapid recovery program for cardiac surgery patients. Am J Crit Care 5:152

Riegel B, Gates DM, Gocka I, et al., 1996: Effectiveness of a program of early hospital discharge of cardiac surgery patients. J Cardiovasc Nurs 11:63

Scott WJ, Kessler R, Wernly JA, 1990: Blood conservation in cardiac surgery. Ann Thorac Surg 50:843

Silbert BS, Santamaria JD, O'Brian JL, et al., 1998: Early extubation following coronary artery bypass surgery: A prospective randomized controlled trial. The Fast Track Care Team. Chest 113:1481

Sivak ED, 1991: Management of ventilator dependency following heart surgery. Semin Thorac Cardiovasc Surg 3:53

Skinner NS Jr, Mitchell JH, Wallace AG, Sarnoff SJ, 1963: Hemodynamic effects of altering the timing of atrial systole. Am J Physiol 205:499

Smith PK, Buhrman WC, Ferguson TB Jr, et al., 1983a: Conduction block following cardioplegia arrest: Prevention by augmented atrial hypothermia. Circulation 68(Suppl):II-41

Smith PK, Buhrman WC, Ferguson TB Jr, et al., 1983b: Relationship of atrial hypothermia and cardioplegic solution potassium concentration to postoperative conduction defects. Surg Forum 34:304

Smith PK, Buhrman WC, Levett JM, et al., 1983c: Supraventricular conduction abnormalities following cardiac operations: A complication of inadequate atrial preservation. J Thorac Cardiovasc Surg 85:105

Strong AG, 1991: Nursing management of postoperative dysrhythmias. Critical Care Clinics of North America 3:709

Sutton RG, Kratz JM, Spinale FG, Crawford FA, 1993: Comparison of three blood-processing techniques during and after cardiopulmonary bypass. Ann Thorac Surg 56:938

Tagliente TM, 1997: Pharmacoeconomics of propofol in anesthesia. Am J Health Syst Pharm 54:1953

Valta P, Takala J, Elissa T, Milic-Emili J, 1992: Effects of PEEP on respiratory mechanics after open heart surgery. Chest 102:227

Vander Salm TJ, Stahl RF, 1997: Early postoperative care. In Edmunds LH Jr (ed): Cardiac Surgery in the Adult. New York, McGraw-Hill

Vanscoy GJ, Krause JR, 1991: Warfarin and the international normalized ratio: Reducing interlaboratory effects. Ann Pharmacother 25:1190

Velasco FT, Ko W, Rosengart T, et al., 1996: Cost containment in cardiac surgery: Results with a critical pathway for coronary bypass surgery at the New York Hospital-Cornell

Medical Center. Best Practice Benchmarking Healthcare 1:21

Vernon DD, Garrett JS, Banner W Jr, Dean JM, 1992: Hemodynamic effects of dobutamine in an intact animal model. Crit Care Med 20:1322

Wenger NK, Froelicher ES, Smith LK, et al., 1995: Cardiac Rehabilitation. Clinical Practice Guideline No. 17. AHCPR Publication No. 96-0672. Rockville, MD: U.S. Department of Health and Human Services, Public Health Service, Agency for Healthcare Policy and Research and the National Heart, Lung, and Blood Institute

Whitman GR, 1991: Hypertension and hypothermia in the acute postoperative period. Critical Care Nursing Clinics of North America 3:661

23

Hemodynamic Monitoring

Hemodynamic monitoring is an essential component of caring for postoperative or critically ill cardiac surgical patients. Cardiac function in these patients often is abnormal because of underlying ventricular impairment, acute dysfunction secondary to the operative procedure and use of cardiopulmonary bypass (CPB), or a combination of the two. The word *hemodynamic* literally means "blood power." Hemodynamic monitoring thus describes the observation and recording of the forces generated within the vasculature that are associated with the movement of blood. By using invasive vascular catheters and sophisticated electronic equipment, quantitative data are obtained that can be used to detect correctable abnormalities and guide therapeutic interventions.

Hemodynamic monitoring almost always is performed using intravascular catheters, pressure transducers, and an amplifier/monitoring system. The pressure wave is transmitted from the tip of the pressure-monitoring catheter to the transducer by the fluid column in the catheter (Davidson et al., 1997). The pressure is exerted on a diaphragm in the transducer, causing the diaphragm to be displaced a small amount depending on the size of the force. Most commonly used medical transducers are "strain gauge" transducers. When the diaphragm is displaced, it causes corresponding changes in the resistance of an electronic circuit in the transducer. These resistance changes cause an electric current to vary in exactly the same proportion as the patient's pressure. The varying electric current is used as the input signal to the monitoring system that amplifies it to a readable level. Both a digital numeric value and a graphic representation of the pressure waveform usually are displayed.

Pressures commonly measured in cardiac surgical patients include arterial pressure, central venous pressure, and pulmonary artery pressure. Cardiac output also is routinely measured, and a cardiac index is derived by adjusting cardiac output for an individual patient's body surface area. Cardiac output is used to calculate systemic vascular resistance (SVR) using a simple formula known as Ohm's law (ie, flow = pressure/resistance). In selected patients with complex cardiac disease, other parameters also may be useful, such as monitoring of left atrial pressure (LAP) or mixed venous oxygen saturation (SvO_2) and calculation of pulmonary vascular resistance (PVR), stroke volume index (SVI), or stroke work index (SWI).

▶ Arterial Pressure

Arterial pressure monitoring is essential in postoperative cardiac surgical patients. It allows continuous display of systolic, diastolic, and mean arterial pressures as well as vascular access for obtaining arterial blood samples for blood gas analysis. Arterial pressure is an important indicator of systemic perfusion, particularly that to the heart, brain, kidneys, and other vital organs. Systolic blood pressure (normal range, 100 to 140 mm Hg) represents the maximal pressure with which blood is ejected from the left ventricle. Diastolic pressure (normal range, 60 to 90 mm Hg) reflects the elasticity of arterial walls and the rapidity of blood flow. Mean blood pressure (normal range, 70 to 105 mm Hg) is the average of systolic and diastolic pressure with respect to time. Because the factor of time is involved, mean blood pressure is approximately equal to the diastolic pressure plus one third of the difference between systolic and diastolic pressures (Table 23-1).

All three values (systolic, diastolic, and mean) are used to assess adequacy of systemic perfusion. The same mean blood pressure can represent a wide (high systolic, low diastolic) or narrow (low systolic, high diastolic) pulse pressure; the latter is more desirable because systolic work is less and diastolic coronary perfusion is enhanced (Daily, 1989). Also, arterial pressure alone does

Calculated Hemodynamic Indices

Index	Formula	Normal Values
MAP	DP + [(SP − DP)/3]	70–105 mm Hg
CI	CO/BSA	2.5–4.0 L/min/m^2
SVR	[(MAP − RAP)/CO] × 80	800–1200 dynes·sec·cm^{-5}
PVR	[(PAPm − PCWP)/CO] × 80	100–250 dynes·sec·cm^{-5}
SVI	[CI/Heart Rate] × 1000	35–45 mL/beat/m^2
LVSWI	SVI × (MAP − PCWP) × 0.0136	45–65 g/beat/m^2

MAP, mean arterial pressure; DP, diastolic pressure; SP, systolic pressure; CI, cardiac index; CO, cardiac output; BSA, body surface area; SVR, systemic vascular resistance; RAP, right atrial pressure; PVR, pulmonary vascular resistance; PAPm, mean pulmonary artery pressure; PCWP, pulmonary capillary wedge pressure; SVI, stroke volume index; LVSWI, left ventricular stroke work index.

not adequately reflect cardiac function. Because of the relationships expressed by Ohm's law, arterial pressure may remain in a normal range despite a low cardiac output if SVR is elevated. Consequently, arterial pressure must be evaluated in concert with cardiac output and SVR. In addition to monitored arterial pressure, noninvasive indicators of systemic perfusion include quality of peripheral pulses, color and temperature of the extremities, level of mentation, and adequacy of urine output.

The graphic representation of the arterial pressure provides additional information. The highest point is read as systolic pressure, the lowest as diastolic. The waveform changes in morphology as it moves from the aortic root to the peripheral arteries (Fig. 23-1). As the pressure wave moves toward the periphery, systolic pressure gradually increases and the systolic portion of the

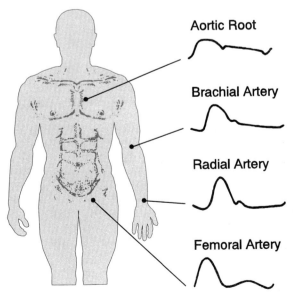

FIGURE 23-1. The arterial pulse waveform changes in morphology as it moves from the central circulation to the periphery. (Marino PL, 1998: Arterial blood pressure. In The ICU Book, ed. 2, p. 148. Baltimore, Williams & Wilkins)

waveform narrows. This effect is most pronounced in the dorsalis pedis artery, in which systolic blood pressure may be 10 to 20 mm Hg higher and diastolic blood pressure 10 to 20 mm Hg lower than in the central aorta (Reich et al., 1999). Because the increase in peak systolic pressure is offset by narrowing of the pressure wave, mean arterial pressure remains unchanged and therefore is a more accurate measure of central aortic pressure (Marino, 1998a).

The arterial pressure waveform when monitored in a peripheral artery therefore should have a sharp, rapid upstroke with a clear dicrotic notch and a definite end of diastole. An arterial pressure waveform with a slow upstroke and prolonged peak can represent partial occlusion of the catheter, aortic stenosis, or decreased stroke volume. An abrupt upstroke with a brief peak and rapid fall may be caused by anxiety, fever, anemia, vasodilatation, or aortic regurgitation. Ventricular bigeminy produces an irregular waveform rate and pulse waves of alternating amplitude.

In the early hours after cardiac operations, a mean arterial pressure in the range of 65 to 75 mm Hg is suitable for most patients. Mean pressure may be maintained at a somewhat higher level in older patients because cerebral vascular disease is more prevalent (Hendren & Higgins, 1991). A mean arterial pressure less than 60 mm Hg indicates inadequate tissue perfusion. It usually is treated with volume replacement if the patient is hypovolemic or with inotropic pharmacologic agents. Conversely, high arterial pressure in the postoperative period exacerbates bleeding and increases myocardial oxygen consumption. Pharmacologic vasodilation or sedation is used to maintain mean arterial pressure less than 90 to 100 mm Hg.

The radial artery is the first choice for arterial monitoring. It is easy to cannulate, amenable to hemostatic control, and collateral circulation to the hand usually is good. Before insertion of a radial artery catheter, an Allen test may be performed (Fig. 23-2). The Allen test is designed to assess ulnar and palmar arch blood flow during abrupt occlusion of the radial artery, although its value in predicting morbidity related to radial artery cannulation is equivocal (Savino & Cheung, 1997; Mehta & Pae, 1997).

The brachial artery is used infrequently if radial artery cannulation is not possible. It is a large vessel that is easy to catheterize and amenable to hemostatic control, but collateral blood supply to the hand is lacking. A brachial arterial catheter also limits the patient's movement of the elbow. The femoral artery sometimes is used for intraoperative monitoring but is not suitable for long-term use because insidious bleeding is more likely (particularly in obese patients), patient mobility is limited, and the catheter's location in the groin makes infection secondary to contamination likely. The dorsalis pedal artery also is used rarely. Although collateral circulation to the foot is adequate, pedal pressure does not as accurately reflect core blood pressure. Use of the dorsalis pedis artery is not recommended in diabetic patients and in those with peripheral arterial occlusive disease (Reich et al., 1999). In patients with an intra-aortic balloon catheter in place, the

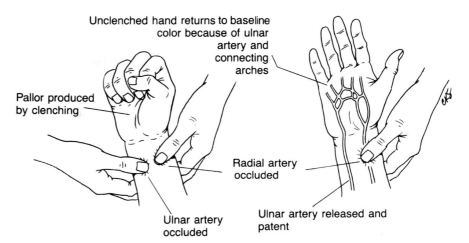

FIGURE 23-2. The Allen test. The ulnar and radial arteries are compressed while the patient clenches the hand into a fist to produce blanching. The hand is opened and compression on the ulnar artery is released. If the ulnar artery is patent, baseline color of the hand returns rapidly. (Hudak CM, Gallo BM, Morton PG, 1998: Patient assessment: Cardiovascular system. In Critical Care Nursing: A Holistic Approach, ed. 7, p. 229. Philadelphia, Lippincott Williams & Wilkins)

inner lumen of the intra-aortic catheter usually is used for monitoring arterial pressure.

▶ Intracardiac Pressures and Indices

Intracardiac pressures are measured to provide an estimation of preload which, along with afterload, heart rate, and contractility, is a major determinant of cardiac output. Preload is the end-diastolic volume in the ventricle and provides an estimation of diastolic fiber length (Landolfo & Smith, 1995). As represented by Starling's law, as end-diastolic volume increases, cardiac output also increases until a point is reached at which further filling causes a decrease in cardiac output and heart failure. Because there is no method for clinical measurement of intracardiac volumes, fluid pressure is monitored instead. Therefore, preload is defined clinically as the pressure in the ventricle just before systole, or ventricular end-diastolic pressure. Intraoperative and postoperative monitoring of left ventricular preload is essential because of wide fluctuations that can occur and the impact they have on cardiac output.

Insertion of a catheter into the left ventricle for direct measurement of left ventricular end-diastolic pressure is not feasible. Instead, diastolic pressure in the pulmonary artery or, rarely, LAP, is measured to provide an indirect method of estimating the left ventricular end-diastolic pressure (LVEDP). Similarly, right atrial pressure (RAP) provides an estimation of right ventricular end-diastolic pressure, or right ventricular preload. These indirect measurements are possible because of relationships that exist between intracardiac pressures in the normal heart. Interpretation of measured parameters requires an understanding of these relationships.

Figure 23-3 displays normal intracardiac pressures. Note that pressures in the atria are the same as diastolic pressures in the ventricles. This is because the open position of the atrioventricular (tricuspid and mitral) valves during ventricular diastole allows equilibration of atrial and ventricular pressures. Similarly, when semilunar (pulmonic and aortic) valves are open during ventricular

systole, the right and left ventricular systolic pressures in the normal heart are the same as the systolic pressures in the pulmonary artery and aorta, respectively. Finally, because there are no valves between the pulmonic and mitral valves, pulmonary artery diastolic pressure (PADP) provides a reasonable measure of LAP, which in turn approximates LVEDP.

In patients without cardiac disease, RAP also can provide an estimation of LVEDP. However, in the presence of right or left ventricular dysfunction or pulmonary vascular disease, pressure measurements obtained from the right side of the heart do not accurately reflect left-sided pressures. Patients who undergo cardiac operations typically have pathologic processes that primarily affect left ventricular function, such as coronary artery disease or valvular heart disease. The left ventricular dysfunction typically present precludes reliance on RAP monitoring to detect promptly changes in left ventricular function. In addition to preexisting dysfunction, reversible biventricular dysfunction is observed commonly in the early postoperative period because of incomplete operative correction of cardiac disease, myocardial edema, reperfusion injury, cytokine (immunoregulatory substances secreted by cells of immune system) release, and generation of nitric oxide (Bailey et al., 1997).

Pulmonary Artery Pressure

A *pulmonary artery (Swan-Ganz) catheter* usually is used in cardiac surgical patients to monitor left ventricular preload continuously. The basic pulmonary artery catheter is a triple-lumen model used to provide simultaneous recording of right atrial and pulmonary artery pressure. The catheter's proximal lumen communicates with a port positioned to lie in the right atrium, the distal lumen communicates with a port in the pulmonary artery, and the balloon inflation lumen leads to a balloon positioned just proximal to the distal port. The catheter also incorporates a thermistor several centimeters from the catheter tip in the pulmonary artery for measuring cardiac output using a thermodilution technique. Mixed

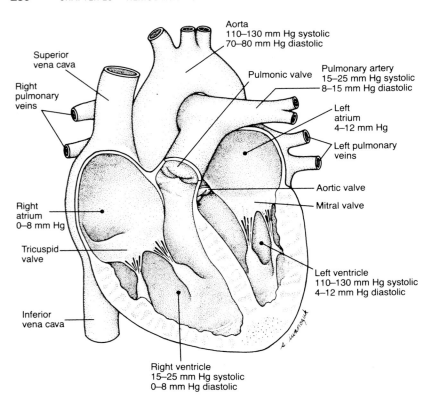

Aorta
110–130 mm Hg systolic
70–80 mm Hg diastolic

Superior
vena cava

Right
pulmonary
veins

Pulmonic valve

Pulmonary artery
15–25 mm Hg systolic
8–15 mm Hg diastolic

Left
atrium
4–12 mm Hg

Left pulmonary
veins

Aortic valve

Mitral valve

Right
atrium
0–8 mm Hg

Tricuspid
valve

Left ventricle
110–130 mm Hg systolic
4–12 mm Hg diastolic

Inferior
vena cava

Right ventricle
15–25 mm Hg systolic
0–8 mm Hg diastolic

FIGURE 23-3. A schematic representation of the heart displaying normal pressures in the cardiac chambers and great vessels. (Darovic GO, 1987: Cardiovascular anatomy and physiology. In Hemodynamic Monitoring: Invasive and Noninvasive Clinical Application, p. 38. Philadelphia, WB Saunders)

venous blood sample measurements can be obtained by sampling blood from the distal port in the pulmonary artery.

Depending on the clinical indication, a variety of catheter models are available that expand the catheter's capabilities (Fig. 23-4). Venous infusion models provide one or more additional proximal lumens in the right atrium (or right atrium and right ventricle) to allow infusion of fluid or medications without interruption of RAP monitoring; models designed for pacing incorporate pacing electrodes that allow atrial, ventricular, or atrioventricular pacing (Lichtenthal, 1998). Other models that have increased pulmonary artery catheter capabilities include (1) a rapid-response thermistor and specialized cardiac output computer to allow measurement of right ventricular volumes and ejection fraction, (2) fiberoptics and computer enhancements that provide continuous measurement of mixed venous oxygen saturation, and (3) sophisticated microprocessor algorithms that provide continuous cardiac output measurement (Headley, 1998).

A pulmonary artery catheter usually is inserted percutaneously through the subclavian or jugular vein (Fig. 23-5). Before insertion, the catheter is threaded through a sterile plastic sleeve. The balloon is then inflated to test its integrity and ensure that it extends beyond the catheter tip when inflated. The proximal and distal ports of the catheter are flushed with heparinized saline solution. A large-bore catheter (8 to 9 French), commonly referred to as an *introducer,* usually is placed in the vein initially, and the balloon-tipped, flow-directed catheter is passed

through the introducer into the vein. The external end of the distal lumen is attached to a transducer so that the pressure waveform can be used to guide catheter advancement.

Waveforms transmitted from the right atrium, right ventricle, pulmonary artery, and pulmonary artery when occluded each have characteristic features that identify location of the catheter tip (Fig. 23-6). When an RAP waveform demonstrates that the distal lumen has reached the right atrium, the balloon on the distal end of the catheter is inflated. The balloon, typically inflated with 1.5 mL of air, serves two purposes: (1) it acts as a cushion so that the catheter tip is less likely to puncture any vessels, and (2) it facilitates advancement of the catheter tip in the proper direction. Acting similarly to a sail on a boat, the inflated balloon is easily caught up in the flow of blood, hence the term *flow-directed catheter.*

The catheter is advanced across the tricuspid valve into the right ventricle and across the pulmonic valve into the pulmonary artery. Passage of the catheter through the heart is monitored by changes in the waveform tracing. When the catheter tip is advanced across the tricuspid valve and into the right ventricle, a pulsatile systolic pressure appears and the diastolic pressure is equal to RAP (Marino, 1998b). As the catheter moves through the right ventricle, transient, clinically insignificant ventricular arrhythmias almost always occur. Right bundle branch block occurs rarely.

Advancement of the catheter tip into the pulmonary artery is evidenced by an increase in the diastolic component of the pressure wave and the appearance of a dicrotic notch, representing closure of the pulmonic valve, after the systolic peak. When the balloon enters a branch of the left or right pulmonary artery, the vessel diameter narrows enough for the balloon to occlude the artery lumen, or "wedge," represented by a change in the pressure tracing from the characteristic pulmonary artery tracing to a flattened wedge tracing. The balloon is then deflated, and the sterile sleeve is extended distally and attached to the external hub of the introducer. The introducer is secured at the skin with a suture to prevent migration.

Proper positioning of the pulmonary artery catheter is assessed by a chest roentgenogram and by the shape of the pressure waveform at the catheter tip. If the catheter tip has been advanced too far, the catheter, with the balloon deflated, is withdrawn a few centimeters at a time until proper positioning is verified. While the catheter is in place, pulmonary artery systolic, diastolic, and mean pressures can be displayed continuously and pulmonary capillary wedge pressure (PCWP) may be obtained. Using measured intracardiac and arterial pressures and thermodilution cardiac output determinations, other parameters can be calculated, including SVR, PVR, SVI, and SWI (see Table 23-1).

Pulmonary artery diastolic pressure, an indirect measurement of LVEDP, is used most often to assess preload and guide clinical therapy. PADP in a normal heart is 8 to 15 mm Hg. However, patients with cardiac disease often require a PADP of 15 to 20 mm Hg to sustain an adequate cardiac output. Optimal preload varies among individual patients. During cardiac operations, the surgeon has the opportunity to assess cardiac function in relation to various levels of preload while the patient is weaned from CPB. Before terminating CPB, venous return to the extracorporeal circuit is partially occluded, allowing some volume to enter and be ejected by the heart. The degree of cannula occlusion therefore controls the patient's preload. Ventricular contractility is observed directly, and the surgeon evaluates the level of preload that provides optimal myocardial contractility.

As cardiac function improves, the level of preload necessary for adequate cardiac output and blood pressure can be expected to decrease gradually from that necessary at the termination of CPB. During the early postoperative hours, an abnormally low PADP may represent intravascular hypovolemia due to a number of physiologic sequelae of operations that necessitate CPB, including (1) active bleeding, (2) vasodilation, (3) osmotic diuresis, and (4) "third spacing" of fluid. Elevated PADP may represent transient myocardial dysfunction (ie, low cardiac output syndrome) or overzealous fluid replacement.

In most instances, PADP provides a sufficient indication of LVEDP. However, measurement of *pulmonary capillary wedge pressure* is important in selected situations. PCWP measures pressure beyond the balloon tip; that is, that transmitted from the left atrium into the pulmonary veins and capillaries (Fig. 23-7). It is obtained by inflating the balloon with a small volume (1 to 1.5 mL) of air so that the tip of the catheter is no longer exposed to pressure transmitted from the proximal pulmonary artery. Balloon inflation creates a static column of blood between the catheter tip and the left atrium (Marino,

1998c). PCWP, therefore, is a truer representation of mean LAP and LVEDP than is PADP. Conditions that increase PVR, such as cor pulmonale, pulmonary embolus, and pulmonary fibrosis, alter the correlation between PADP and PCWP, resulting in a PADP that exceeds PCWP (Becker, 1989). Thus, it may be preferable to measure PCWP intermittently in the presence of elevated PVR.

Left Atrial Pressure

Left atrial pressure is the most accurate clinical indicator of LVEDP. Monitoring of LAP is accomplished using a catheter inserted directly into the left atrium during a cardiac operation, passed through the chest wall, and connected to a pressurized fluid administration system. The LAP waveform comprises three components: (1) the a wave, representing atrial contraction; (2) the c wave, representing pressure against the closed mitral valve during ventricular systole; and (3) the v wave, representing filling of the atrium during late ventricular systole. A left atrial catheter is not used for fluid or medication administration, and zealous precautions are necessary to prevent accidental air entry into the systemic circulation.

Because of the potential catastrophic consequences of introducing air through the catheter into the systemic circulation, left atrial catheters are used only rarely. They usually are placed only when PADP or PCWP is not a reliable indicator of LAP (and indirectly of LVEDP) or when placement of a pulmonary artery catheter is not possible (eg, in patients undergoing tricuspid valve replacement).

Right Atrial Pressure

Right atrial pressure or central venous pressure monitoring is used to assess adequacy of venous return, intravascular blood volume, and right ventricular function (Schwenzer, 1990). In patients in whom right ventricular function, PVR, and the mitral valve are normal, it provides an indirect measure of left ventricular preload (Friedman & Bernstein, 1990). Continuous monitoring of RAP may be performed using the proximal port of the pulmonary artery catheter. If a pulmonary artery catheter is not in place, monitoring is accomplished using a catheter placed through the subclavian or jugular vein. Central venous pressure can be accurately measured if the catheter tip is in the right atrium or one of the large intrathoracic veins (Reich et al., 1999). In addition to pressure measurements, the catheter can be used for rapid volume infusion or continuous infusion of cardiotonic or vasoactive pharmacologic medications.

Right atrial pressure monitoring almost always is performed using a transducer rather than the formerly common water manometer method. In addition to providing a more accurate measurement of mean central venous pressure, pressures obtained with a transducer allow continuous monitoring and analysis of the actual waveform (Daily & Schroeder, 1989a). A normal right atrial waveform is similar in morphology to the left atrial waveform (Fig. 23-8).

Low RAP in conjunction with low PADP usually indicates hypovolemia or dilatation of venous capacitance vessels and the need for volume replacement. High RAP with low PADP suggests right-sided heart failure or elevated PVR. If both RAP and PADP are increased, biventricular failure may be present. Pharmacologic pulmonary artery vasodilation with nitroglycerin or isoproterenol may be instituted to decrease PVR (ie, right ventricular afterload). Occasionally, mechanical support of the right side of the heart, using a circulatory assist device, is necessary.

Calculated Indices

Cardiac output typically is measured using the triple-lumen pulmonary artery catheter and a thermodilution technique. Measurement of cardiac output using a pulmonary artery catheter and thermodilution technique is based on the assumption that cardiac output from the right and left sides of the heart are the same. A known quantity of cold solution at a known temperature is injected rapidly into the proximal port of the catheter so that it enters the right atrium. The thermistor at the distal end of the pulmonary artery catheter measures blood temperature changes as the cold bolus is ejected from the right ventricle into the pulmonary artery and past the tip of the catheter. The faster the decay of the cold bolus measured by the thermistor, the greater the cardiac output (Elefteriades et al., 1996). A computer is used to analyze the temperature changes, known as a *thermodilution curve*, and calculate cardiac output, expressed as liters per minute. Usually three measurements are obtained in succession and averaged to compensate for sampling error. Alternatively, cardiac output can be monitored continuously using a pulmonary artery catheter designed for this purpose.

Cardiac index is the measured cardiac output divided

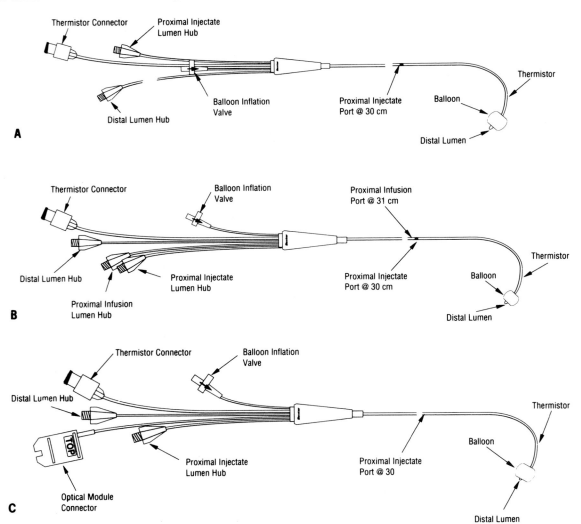

FIGURE 23-4. Various models of pulmonary artery (PA) catheters. **(A)** Standard PA catheter. **(B)** PA catheter with proximal venous infusion lumen. **(C)** Oximetry PA catheter. **(D)** Continuous cardiac output PA catheter. **(E)** Right ventricular ejection fraction oximetry PA catheter. (Courtesy of Baxter Healthcare Corporation, Edwards Critical-Care, Irvine, CA)

by the patient's body surface area to correct for body size. It is the most important hemodynamic measurement in the early period after cardiac operations (Lee & Geha, 1996). In postoperative cardiac surgical patients, a cardiac index of 1.5 to 2.2 L/min/m² represents a moderately severe reduction in cardiac output, and an index below 1.5 L/min/m² reflects severely reduced cardiac output and a high probability of death (Elefteriades et al., 1996). A low cardiac output may result from hypovolemia or transient myocardial dysfunction. It is corrected by manipulation of those factors that determine cardiac output (ie, heart rate, preload, afterload, and contractility). A high cardiac output may represent a hyperdynamic state or sepsis.

Systemic vascular resistance, or left ventricular afterload, is the impedance against which the left ventricle must eject. Although SVR cannot be directly measured, it is calculated by a formula in which the pressure difference between the proximal (mean arterial pressure) and distal (RAP) ends of the cardiovascular system is divided by the cardiac output (Daily & Schroeder, 1989b).

The result is multiplied by 80 and expressed in absolute resistance units (dyne·sec·cm⁻⁵).

Systemic vascular resistance often is elevated in the early postoperative hours secondary to peripheral vasoconstriction and hypothermia. It decreases as body temperature returns to normal, sometimes causing precipitous hypotension as it does. SVR may be lowered pharmacologically to reduce left ventricular work. Most commonly, vasodilating agents, such as sodium nitroprusside and nitroglycerin, are used. Intra-aortic balloon counterpulsation is quite effective in providing mechanical afterload reduction. Occasionally, SVR is abnormally low owing to residual effects of anesthetic agents or an allergic reaction to protamine sulfate given to reverse the effects of intraoperative systemic anticoagulation. A low SVR also may occur due to sepsis. Under these circumstances, an alpha-adrenergic agent may be administered to cause vasoconstriction and restore normal SVR.

Because right ventricular dysfunction is relatively uncommon, PVR, or right ventricular afterload, is not cal-

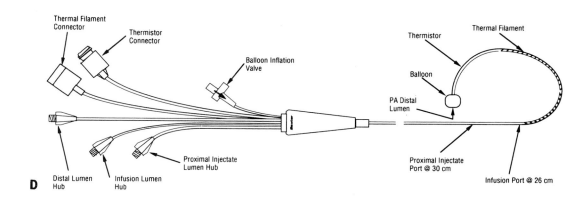

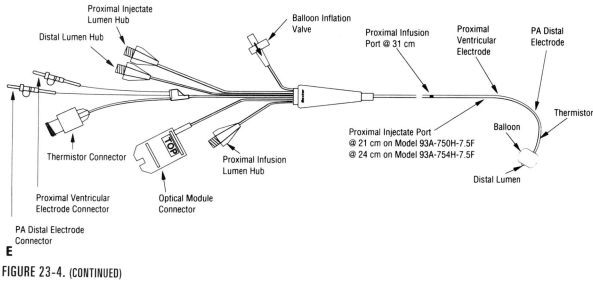

FIGURE 23-4. (CONTINUED)

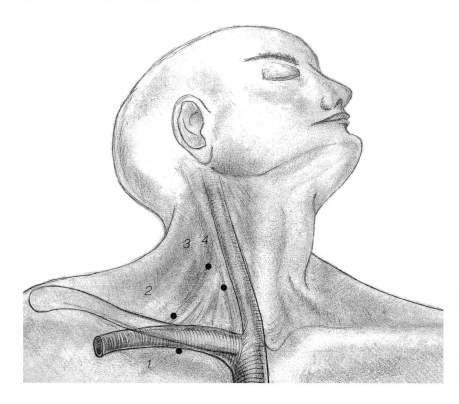

FIGURE 23-5. Diagrammatic representation of subclavian and jugular veins as they converge at the thoracic inlet. Circular markers indicate skin insertion sites for cannulation of the subclavian (1 and 2) and jugular (3 and 4) veins. (Marino PL, 1998: Vascular access. In The ICU Book, ed. 2, p. 65. Baltimore, Williams & Wilkins)

culated routinely. However, calculation of PVR is important in patients with postoperative right ventricular failure or pulmonary hypertension. It is derived in a similar manner to SVR. The pressure difference between mean pulmonary artery pressure and PCWP is divided by cardiac output, then multiplied by 80.

A *mixed venous oxygen measurement* (PvO_2) may be determined by sampling blood from the distal port of the pulmonary artery catheter while the balloon is deflated. The blood sample must be aspirated slowly and gently to avoid obtaining oxygenated blood from the pulmonary circulation. Pulmonary artery blood is used to measure

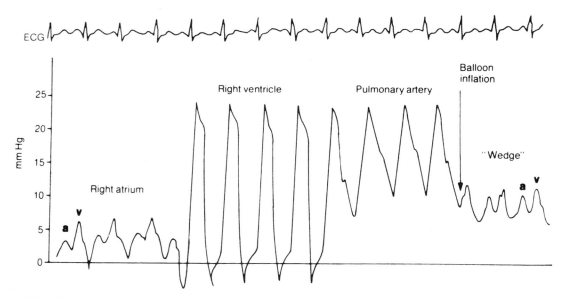

FIGURE 23-6. Characteristic waveforms transmitted from a balloon-tipped pulmonary artery catheter in the right atrium, the right ventricle, the pulmonary artery, and the occluded pulmonary artery, respectively. (Matthay MA, 1983: Invasive hemodynamic monitoring in critically ill patients. Clin Chest Med 4:234)

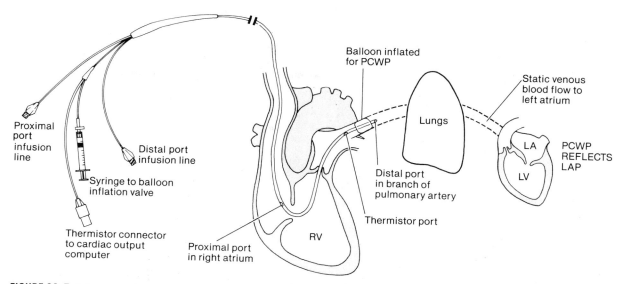

FIGURE 23-7. Pulmonary capillary wedge pressure (PCWP) is measured by momentarily inflating the balloon on the distal end of the pulmonary artery catheter. Balloon inflation creates a static column of blood between the catheter tip and left atrium, thus providing a more accurate representation of left atrial pressure (LAP). LV, left ventricle; RV, right ventricle. (Adapted from Kersten LD, 1989: Hemodynamic monitoring—respiratory applications. In Comprehensive Respiratory Nursing: A Decision Making Approach, p. 758. Philadelphia, WB Saunders)

PvO_2 because venous blood returning from various parts of the body has become mixed. In contrast, right atrial blood contains streams of highly desaturated blood entering from the coronary sinus as well as blood that is less desaturated returning from the superior and inferior venae cavae.

When arterial blood is adequately oxygenated, PvO_2 provides an indirect estimation of cardiac output and systemic perfusion. Mixed venous oxygen levels decrease as cardiac output declines and oxygen extraction increases (Mackall et al., 1996). A low PvO_2 (20 to 30 mm Hg) in the presence of a normal arterial PaO_2 indicates maximal oxygen extraction. Pulmonary artery catheters that incorporate a fiberoptic oximetry system in the catheter allow continuous monitoring of mixed venous oxygen saturation (SvO_2). Continuous monitoring of SvO_2 provides immediate feedback about effectiveness of interventions, such as adjustments in mechanical ventilation or vasoactive medication dosages, and may lessen the need for repeated arterial blood gas measurements (Gardner & Bridges, 1995). The normal range for saturation of mixed venous blood (SvO_2) is 60% to 80% and corresponds to a PvO_2 of 30 to 50 mm Hg (Elefteriades et al., 1996).

Stroke volume is the amount of blood ejected by the ventricle with each heart beat. It is derived by dividing cardiac output by heart rate. When normalized for body surface area, it is termed *stroke volume index. Stroke work index* (SWI) (ie, stroke work corrected for body surface area) reflects contractility, or the inotropic state of the myocardium, specifically the velocity of fiber shortening during systole (Daily & Schroeder, 1989c). A low SWI may indicate the need for inotropic therapy. The formula for calculating left ventricular SWI is displayed in Table 23-1.

▶ Principles of Monitoring

Hemodynamic monitoring is accomplished by attaching an appropriate intravascular catheter to an amplifier/monitor using special connecting tubing, a transducer, and a connecting cable (Fig. 23-9). The connecting tubing, also called *pressure tubing,* is noncompliant and its length is kept to a minimum to prevent distortion or reduced amplitude of transmitted fluid pressures (Hudak et al., 1998). The pressure tubing also contains stopcocks for zeroing of the transducer and aspiration of blood samples as well as a device for manually flushing the catheter. Locking connectors are used to prevent tubing disconnection, and lower-limit alarms may be adjusted to signal a decrease in pressure if disconnection occurs.

A pressurized flush solution is connected to the tubing circuit by means of a continuous, slow-flush device that delivers approximately 3 mL/h of heparinized solution and prevents backflow of blood through the catheter (Fig. 23-10). Unless contraindicated, heparin routinely is added to flush solutions to prevent thrombus formation around the catheter tip. Although the failure rate of pulmonary artery catheters does not appear to be affected by use of nonheparinized solutions, the patency rate of arterial catheters is significantly greater when a heparinized solution is used (Zevola et al., 1997). A dextrose flush solution may be used for pulmonary artery or left atrial catheters, but normal saline is used for arterial catheters because it is less injurious to the artery than dextrose.

The transducer is maintained at the level of the patient's phlebostatic axis (ie, an imaginary point that intersects the fourth intercostal space and the midaxillary line) (see Fig. 23-9). This point corresponds to the position of

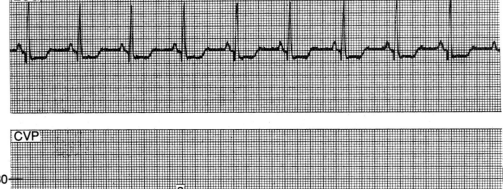
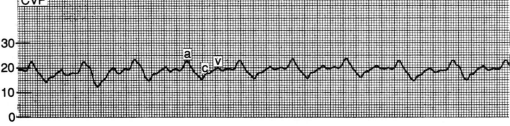

FIGURE 23-8. Right atrial waveform with a, c, and v waves present. The a wave is usually seen just after the P wave of the ECG. The c wave appears at the time of the RST junction on the ECG. The v wave is seen in the T-P interval. (Kern LS, 1993: Hemodynamic monitoring. In Boggs RL, Woolridge-King M [eds]: AACN Procedure Manual for Critical Care, ed. 3, p. 304. Philadelphia, WB Saunders)

the right and left atrium when the patient is in the supine position (Marino, 1998c). Pressure readings obtained with the transducer higher or lower than the phlebostatic reference point are falsely low or high, respectively. Zeroing of the pressure monitoring system consists of confirming that the monitor records a pressure of 0 mm Hg when the transducer is at the phlebostatic axis and is open to the atmosphere. It is performed two to three times daily and whenever there is a question about accuracy of measurements. Calibration describes the degree to which the magnitude of the output signal reflects the magnitude of the parameter being measured (Savino & Cheung, 1997). Most monitoring systems use disposable transducers and provide internal calibration. When the calibration control is activated, an electrical signal is introduced to the monitor as if calibration pressure had been applied to the transducer itself (Varon & Civetta, 1990).

Before obtaining pressure measurements, quality of the waveform is assessed and position of the transducer is verified. Accuracy of abnormal pressure measurements should be confirmed before any treatment is initiated. The term *damping* is used to describe a blunting of peaks and troughs in the displayed pressure waveform due to frictional losses in the measuring system (Savino & Cheung, 1997). Damping, or poor transmission of a pressure waveform, can occur as a result of air bubbles, blood clots, loose fittings, catheter kinking, or positioning of a catheter tip against a vessel wall (Summer & deBoisblanc, 1991). Aspiration and manual flushing may be necessary to evacuate air bubbles or thrombus from the catheter lumen. Catheter kinking may be corrected by splinting the extremity in which the catheter is inserted or by manipulating the catheter position.

Pulmonary artery pressure varies normally with respiration. In spontaneously breathing patients, pressure decreases slightly during inspiration. Conversely, it increases during inspiration in patients receiving positive-pressure mechanical ventilation. Therefore, measurements are performed consistently on or off the ventilator and at the same point in the respiratory cycle. Because inspiration causes falsely low (spontaneously breathing patient) or high (patient receiving positive-pressure ventilation) readings, filling pressures are best measured at end-expiration (ie, just before inspiration) (Elefteriades et al., 1996).

High levels of positive end-expiratory pressure (PEEP) artificially elevate pulmonary artery pressure readings because pressure is transmitted to the pulmonary artery catheter. Physiologically, PEEP lowers preload because the increased intrathoracic pressure decreases venous return to the heart. In patients receiving high levels of PEEP, disconnecting the ventilator momentarily provides a more precise measurement of filling pressures (Elefteriades et al., 1996). Pulmonary artery pressure infrequently is distorted by catheter whip artifact, caused by excessive catheter movement with right ventricular contractions. If this occurs, mean pulmonary artery pressure may provide a more accurate assessment of preload.

Inflation of the balloon when the pulmonary catheter is positioned incorrectly can cause serious complications. The balloon is always inflated slowly, while monitoring the pulmonary artery waveform for the change from a pulmonary artery pressure to a wedge pressure. If the catheter tip has migrated a short distance distally, only a small amount of air is necessary to cause wedging; inflating the balloon with the usual 1.5 mL increases the risk of pulmonary artery damage or rupture. Consequently, the balloon is inflated slowly only until a wedge tracing appears on the oscilloscope monitor, and then deflated fully after the reading is obtained (Marino, 1998b). A characteristic pulmonary artery waveform should reappear as soon as the balloon is deflated.

Sustained balloon inflation or catheter tip migration that causes pulmonary artery occlusion is detected by the presence of a PCWP waveform. It may be corrected by (1) ensuring full balloon deflation, (2) asking the patient to take deep breaths and cough, (3) repositioning the patient, or (4) withdrawing the catheter a slight distance until a pulmonary artery waveform reappears. Balloon rupture may be detected by a loss of resistance when air is injected into the balloon lumen, by an inability to pull back the syringe plunger when attempting to deflate the balloon, or by an inability to obtain a PCWP waveform. Balloon rupture does not necessitate catheter removal as long as the balloon lumen port is covered and labeled clearly to prevent subsequent attempts to inflate the balloon.

Movement of the tip of a pulmonary artery catheter into the right ventricle is evidenced by a right ventricular pressure waveform. The catheter may be advanced if a sterile sleeve was placed over the catheter before its insertion. Repositioning of an intravascular catheter should be performed only by those experienced in catheter insertion techniques. In the absence of a protective sheath, the nonsterile catheter is not advanced because it predisposes to catheter-related infection. Instead, if the patient's condition mandates continued pulmonary artery pressure measurements, the catheter is removed completely and replaced with a sterile catheter.

The insertion site of an intravascular catheter is cov-ered with an occlusive, sterile dressing, and aseptic dressing changes are performed daily. Catheter sites should not be covered with large, bulky dressings that might obscure catheter disconnection or insidious bleeding. Flush solutions and tubing are changed according to institutional standards (eg, flush solution every 24 hours, tubing every 48 hours) to minimize the risk of infection.

Intravascular monitoring catheters usually are removed 24 to 48 hours after cardiac operations. Pulmonary artery and left atrial catheters usually are removed by physicians. Before removing a pulmonary artery catheter, balloon deflation is confirmed. Because removal of left atrial catheters can cause bleeding, a chest tube often is left in place until the catheter has been removed. Removal of any catheter inserted through a central vein is performed with the patient in a supine position in the bed. The head of the bed is lowered and pressure is maintained over the insertion site as the catheter is withdrawn to prevent air embolism. Firm pressure is applied to the skin overlying the vessel puncture site for approximately five minutes. Pressure is applied for longer periods in anticoagulated patients, when removing a femoral artery catheter, or if bleeding from the puncture site does not subside.

▶ Associated Complications

Arterial pressure monitoring almost is always performed using the radial artery, and complications are rare. The most common problems associated with radial arterial cannulation are infection, embolization, and hand is-

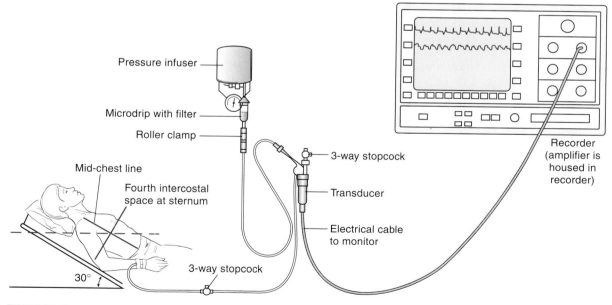

FIGURE 23-9. Diagrammatic representation of monitoring system. The arterial catheter is attached by pressure tubing to a transducer, which is connected to an amplifier/monitor that displays the waveform and systolic, diastolic, and mean pressures. A pressurized flush solution with a continuous-flush device is incorporated into the system to maintain catheter patency. (Hudak CM, Gallo BM, Morton PG, 1998: Patient assessment: Cardiovascular system. In Critical Care Nursing: A Holistic Approach, ed. 7, p. 227. Philadelphia, Lippincott Williams & Wilkins)

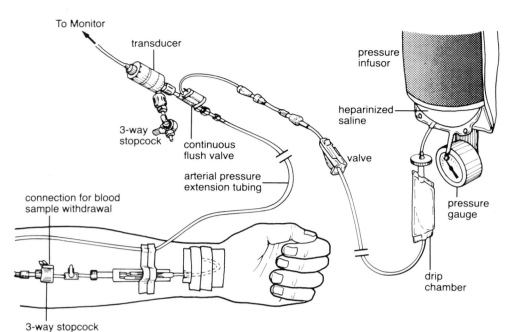

FIGURE 23-10. A pressurized flush system delivers 3 mL/h of heparinized saline through the arterial catheter. The slow infusion prevents backflow of blood into the extension tubing and thrombus formation around the catheter tip. (VanRiper J, VanRiper S, 1987: Fluid-filled monitoring systems. In Darovic GO [ed]: Hemodynamic Monitoring: Invasive and Noninvasive Clinical Application, p. 86. Philadelphia, WB Saunders)

chemia (Mehta & Pae, 1997). While the catheter is in place, the hand or limb distal to the catheter is assessed for evidence of ischemia or emboli. Loss of arterial waveform or an inability to flush the catheter suggests thrombus formation along the catheter and should prompt catheter removal unless the problem is easily corrected (Finkelmeier & Finkelmeier, 1991).

Complications associated with insertion of central venous catheters through the subclavian or jugular vein include infection, pneumothorax, hemothorax or hematoma, arterial cannulation, and vessel injury. Disconnection of an indwelling arterial or central venous catheter can result in significant blood loss if not detected promptly. Air embolism can occur with central venous catheter disconnection or if a central venous catheter is removed with the patient in an upright position. Hypovolemic, spontaneously breathing patients are most susceptible to air embolism because of low central venous pressure and cyclic negative intrathoracic pressures (Mehta & Pae, 1997).

Pulmonary artery catheters are associated with a number of potential complications. The presence of an indwelling catheter in the right ventricle may cause persistent ventricular arrhythmias that necessitate catheter removal. Serial balloon inflation can cause complications, particularly in patients with pulmonary hypertension, including pulmonary artery rupture, pulmonary infarction, and air embolism. Pulmonary artery rupture occasionally occurs even without inflating the balloon, during catheter insertion or migration. It usually causes hemoptysis, impaired oxygenation, and intrathoracic hemorrhage, and is associated with a 41% mortality rate (Mehta & Pae, 1997). Pulmonary artery catheters also can cause tricuspid or pulmonic valve damage and endocarditis (Summer & deBoisblanc, 1991).

Infection is a potential complication with any indwelling vascular catheter. Common routes of catheter-related septicemia are (1) microbe entry into the catheter lumen through break points in the system, such as stopcocks and catheter hubs; (2) migration of microbes from the skin along the subcutaneous tract created by an indwelling catheter; and (3) entrapment of microorganisms circulating in the blood into the fibrin meshwork that surrounds the intravascular segment of an indwelling catheter (Marino, 1998d). Risk factors associated with catheter-related infection include the underlying disease process, duration of catheter use (ie, >3 days), location of insertion, the number of lumens in the catheter, and insertion technique (Murray & Torres, 1999). Redness or purulent drainage at the catheter insertion site, or unexplained fever and white blood cell count elevation, are suggestive of catheter-related infection. If any of these occurs, the catheter is removed, its tip is cultured for bacteria, and, if necessary, a new catheter is inserted.

REFERENCES

Bailey JM, Levy JH, Hug CC, 1997: Cardiac surgical pharmacology. In Edmunds LH Jr (ed): Cardiac Surgery in the Adult. New York, McGraw-Hill

Becker A, 1989: Pulmonary artery catheterization: II. Interpretation of hemodynamic data. In Rippe JM (ed): Manual of Intensive Care Medicine, ed. 2. Boston, Little, Brown

Daily PO, 1989: Hemodynamic monitoring of the postoperative cardiac surgery patient. In Dailey EK, Schroeder JS (eds): Techniques in Bedside Hemodynamic Monitoring, ed. 4. St. Louis, CV Mosby

Daily EK, Schroeder JS, 1989a: Central venous and pulmonary artery pressure monitoring. In Dailey EK, Schroeder JS (eds): Techniques in Bedside Hemodynamic Monitoring, ed. 4. St. Louis, CV Mosby

Daily EK, Schroeder JS, 1989b: Intra-arterial pressure monitoring. In Dailey EK, Schroeder JS (eds): Techniques in Bedside Hemodynamic Monitoring, ed. 4. St. Louis, CV Mosby

Daily EK, Schroeder JS, 1989c: Clinical management based on hemodynamic parameters. In Dailey EK, Schroeder JS (eds): Techniques in Bedside Hemodynamic Monitoring, ed. 4. St. Louis, CV Mosby

Davidson CJ, Fishman RF, Bonow RO, 1997: Cardiac catheterization. In Braunwald E (ed): Heart Disease: A Textbook of Cardiovascular Medicine, ed. 5. Philadelphia, WB Saunders

Elefteriades JA, Geha AS, Cohen LS, 1996: Hemodynamic monitoring and the Swan-Ganz catheter. In House Officer Guide to ICU Care: Fundamentals of Management of the Heart and Lungs, ed. 2. Philadelphia, Lippincott-Raven

Finkelmeier BA, Finkelmeier WR, 1991: Iatrogenic arterial injuries resulting from invasive procedures. J Vasc Nurs 9:12

Friedman A, Bernstein H, 1990: Hemodynamic monitoring during and after cardiac surgery. In Gray RJ, Matloff JM (eds): Medical Management of the Cardiac Surgical Patient. Baltimore, Williams & Wilkins

Gardner PE, Bridges EJ, 1995: Hemodynamic monitoring. In Woods SL, Froelicher ES, Halpenny CJ, Motzer SU (eds): Cardiac Nursing, ed. 3. Philadelphia, JB Lippincott

Headley JM, 1998: Invasive hemodynamic monitoring: Applying advanced technologies. Critical Care Nursing Quarterly 21:73

Hendren WG, Higgins TL, 1991: Immediate postoperative care of the cardiac surgical patient. Semin Thorac Cardiovasc Surg 3:3

Hudak CM, Gallo BM, Morton PG, 1998: Patient assessment: Cardiovascular system. In Critical Care Nursing: A Holistic Approach, ed. 7. Philadelphia, Lippincott Williams & Wilkins

Landolfo K, Smith PK, 1995: Postoperative care in cardiac surgery. In Sabiston DC Jr, Spencer FC (eds): Surgery of the Chest, ed. 6. Philadelphia, WB Saunders

Lee JH, Geha AS, 1996: Postoperative care of the cardiovascular surgical patient. In Baue AE, Geha AS, Hammond GL, et al. (eds): Glenn's Thoracic and Cardiovascular Surgery, ed 6. Stamford, CT, Appleton & Lange

Lichtenthal PR, 1998: Swan-Ganz catheter reference section. In Quick Guide to Cardiopulmonary Care. Irvine, CA, Baxter Healthcare Corporation

Mackall JA, Buchter CM, Thames MD, 1996: Pharmacological approach to the management of the cardiac surgical patient. In Baue AE, Geha AS, Hammond GL, et al. (eds): Glenn's Thoracic and Cardiovascular Surgery, ed. 6. Stamford, CT, Appleton & Lange

Marino PL, 1998a: Arterial blood pressure. In The ICU Book, ed. 2. Baltimore, Williams & Wilkins

Marino PL, 1998b: The pulmonary artery catheter. In The ICU Book, ed. 2. Baltimore, Williams & Wilkins

Marino PL, 1998c: Central venous pressure and wedge pressure. In The ICU Book, ed. 2. Baltimore, Williams & Wilkins

Marino PL, 1998d: The indwelling vascular catheter. In The ICU Book, ed. 2. Baltimore, Williams & Wilkins

Mehta SM, Pae WE Jr, 1997: Complications of cardiac surgery. In Edmunds LH Jr (ed): Cardiac Surgery in the Adult. New York, McGraw-Hill

Murray MJ, Torres NE, 1999: Critical care medicine for the cardiac patient. In Kaplan JA (ed): Cardiac Anesthesia, ed. 4. Philadelphia, WB Saunders

Reich DL, Roskowitz DM, Kaplan JA, 1999: Hemodynamic monitoring. In Kaplan JA (ed): Cardiac Anesthesia, ed. 4. Philadelphia, WB Saunders

Savino JS, Cheung AT, 1997: Cardiac anesthesia. In Edmunds LH Jr (ed): Cardiac Surgery in the Adult. New York, McGraw-Hill

Schwenzer KJ, 1990: Venous and pulmonary pressures. In Lake CL (ed): Clinical Monitoring. Philadelphia, WB Saunders

Summer WR, deBoisblanc BP, 1991: Bedside hemodynamic monitoring. In Parrillo JE (ed): Current Therapy in Critical Care Medicine, ed. 2. Philadelphia, BC Decker

Varon AJ, Civetta JM, 1990: Hemodynamic monitoring. In Berk JL, Sampliner JE (eds): Handbook of Critical Care, ed. 3. Boston, Little, Brown

Zevola DR, Dioso J, Moggio R, 1997: Comparison of heparinized and nonheparinized solutions for maintaining patency of arterial and pulmonary artery catheters. Am J Crit Care 6:52

24

Twelve-Lead Electrocardiography and Atrial Electrograms

The *electrocardiogram* (ECG) is a graphic summary of the electrical events that make up each cardiac cycle. The six major deflections (P, Q, R, S, T, U) of the normal ECG represent the action potentials generated by depolarization and repolarization of myocardial cells. Electrical energy created by these events is detected by electrodes strategically placed on the body surface, transmitted to the electrocardiograph, amplified, and recorded in graphic form. Electrocardiographs are standardized so that both amplitude and duration of the various deflections making up the cardiac cycle can be measured. Graph paper divided in 1-mm segments is used; every fifth segment, or 5.0 mm, is designated by a darker line. Graph paper is advanced through the machine at a speed of 25 mm/sec. Thus, the space between two vertical lines (1.0 mm) represents 0.04 second and that between two darkened vertical lines (5.0 mm) represents 0.2 second. Small vertical lines or dots above the graph are spaced to mark 3-second intervals.

Voltage is similarly standardized so that 1.0 mV of electrical current produces a vertical deflection of 10 mm on the graph paper. Deflections above the baseline are considered positive, and those below the baseline are negative. If a deflection has both upward and downward components of approximately equal amplitude, it is termed *biphasic*. The isoelectric line between cardiac cycles is termed the *baseline*.

The most obvious information revealed on an ECG is cardiac rate and rhythm. Heart rate is described in beats per minute and can be quickly estimated in one of two ways. The first method is to multiply the number of

QRS complexes occurring during 6 seconds (ie, two 3-second intervals measured by the vertical lines or dots above the graph) by 10. The second method is to divide the number of seconds in 1 minute (60) by the number of seconds between two consecutive R waves (Table 24-1). Cardiac rhythm is determined using standard criteria for rhythm analysis, described in Chapter 25, Cardiac Arrhythmias.

► Electrical Components of the Cardiac Cycle

Each component of the cardiac cycle can be separately analyzed (Fig. 24-1). The morphology and duration of the various electrical components reveal important diagnostic information about conduction through the heart and the presence of cardiac disease. The first deflection of the cardiac cycle, the P wave, represents atrial depolarization. A normal P wave has a duration less than 0.12 second (3.0 mm) and voltage less than 0.2 mV (2.0 mm) (Fisch, 1997). Atrial depolarization is followed by an isoelectric line representing a physiologic conduction delay in the atrioventricular (AV) node.

The P-R interval is measured from the onset of the P wave to the initial (positive or negative) deflection of the QRS complex. It represents intra-atrial, AV nodal, and Purkinje conduction and normally lasts 0.12 to 0.20 second. Normally, the P-R interval increases with age and shortens with increasing heart rates during exercise or stress (Sgarbossa & Wagner, 1998). Atrial repolariza-

TABLE 24-1

Estimation of Heart Rate*

Number of Boxes** Between R Waves				Heart Rate
One (0.2 second)	=	60/.20	=	300
Two (0.4 second)	=	60/.40	=	150
Three (0.6 second)	=	60/.60	=	100
Four (0.8 second)	=	60/.80	=	75
Five (1.0 second)	=	60/1.0	=	60
Six (1.2 second)	=	60/1.2	=	50

*Obtained by dividing the number of seconds between two consecutive QRS complexes into the number of seconds in 1 minute.
**Large boxes separated by darkened vertical lines on electrocardiograph paper.

tion usually is not apparent on the ECG because it is obscured by manifestations of ventricular depolarization.

The QRS complex represents depolarization of ventricular tissue. The contour of the QRS complex is peaked rather than rounded because it is composed of higher-frequency signals that the P and T waves (Sgarbossa & Wagner, 1998). Duration of the QRS complex is measured from onset of the first positive or negative deflection of the QRS waveform to termination of the waveform. The point at which the QRS complex terminates is termed the J point. The normal QRS interval is 0.06 to 0.10 second. Normal voltage of the QRS complex varies depending on the lead. It should be at least 6.0 mm in V_1 and V_6, 8.0 mm in V_2 and V_5, and 10 mm in V_3 and V_4; voltage should not exceed 25 to 30 mm (Conover, 1996a). Morphology of the ventricular depolarization wave varies depending on the lead in which it is viewed. Although the term *QRS* is used to refer generically to ventricular depolarization on single-lead rhythm tracings, more precise terminology is required when multiple electrocardiographic leads are being analyzed. The standard nomenclature and definitions for the various deflections that make up ventricular depolarization are as follows:

Q wave: First negative deflection, if it is the initial event and is followed by a positive deflection

R wave: First positive deflection

S wave: First negative deflection that follows an R wave

R′ wave: Second positive deflection

S′ wave: Second negative deflection that follows an R′ wave

QS wave: Entirely negative deflection

Thus, Q and S always describe negative deflections and R always describes a positive deflection. The relative size of Q, R, and S deflections is indicated by using a lowercase or uppercase letter (Fig. 24-2).

Ventricular repolarization is represented by the ST segment and the T wave. The ST segment is the interval between termination of the QRS complex and onset of the T wave. It may be isoelectric or drift slightly above the baseline (1 mm in leads I, II, and III; as much as 2 mm in some precordial leads); it normally does not drift more than 0.5 mm below the baseline (Conover, 1996a). The T wave, representing the end of ventricular repolarization, is a gently sloping, asymmetric deflection, usually with the same polarity as the QRS complex. In some leads, a low-voltage positive deflection, the U wave, may be apparent after the T wave. Its cause and clinical significance are not well understood.

The Q-T interval defines the period from the beginning of ventricular depolarization (onset of QRS complex) to the end of ventricular repolarization (termination of T wave). It coincides with ventricular systole. Normal length of the Q-T interval varies inversely with heart rate. A general guideline is that at normal heart rates (between 60 and 100 beats per minute), the Q-T interval should be no longer than one half of the R-R interval. The Q-T interval should be measured in a lead with the most prominent T wave and with no U wave (Huff, 1997). Determination of the Q-T interval is clinically significant because abnormal prolongation is known to provide the substrate for potentially dangerous ventricular arrhythmias.

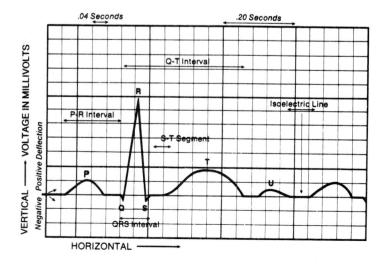

FIGURE 24-1. Electrical components of the cardiac cycle. (Hudak CM, Gallo BM, Morton PG, 1998: Patient assessment: Cardiovascular system. In *Critical Care Nursing: A Holistic Approach,* ed. 7, p. 206. Philadelphia, Lippincott Williams & Wilkins)

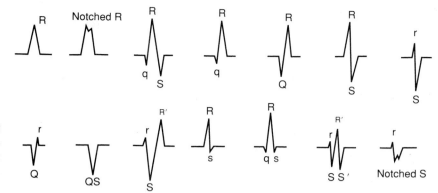

FIGURE 24-2. Diagrammatic representation of QRS variations (see text). (Huff J, 1997: Waveforms, intervals, segments, and complexes. In ECG Workout: Exercises in Arrhythmia Interpretation, ed. 3, p. 18. Philadelphia, Lippincott-Raven)

▶ Electrocardiographic Leads

An electrocardiographic lead comprises two electrodes of opposite polarity (bipolar lead), or one positive electrode and a reference point (unipolar lead) (Conover, 1996b). Each lead reflects the direction and magnitude of current flow from a particular perspective. Because the heart is three-dimensional, electrical current spreads in all directions. The more points from which this electrical energy is measured, the more accurate the depiction of conduction through atrial and ventricular muscle. The standard electrocardiograph examines electrical events of the cardiac cycle using 12 different leads. The six limb leads are called *frontal* because they provide information about left, right, superior, and inferior current flow; the six *precordial*, or horizontal plane, leads assess anterior, posterior, right, and left current flow (Conover, 1996b).

Surface electrodes are placed on each of the four limbs or representative areas on the body near the shoulders and lower abdomen; the electrical potential recorded from any one extremity should be the same no matter where on the extremity the electrode is placed (White, 1998). The right leg electrode serves only as a ground. The right arm, left arm, and left leg electrodes are used to obtain the six limb or frontal leads (I, II, III, aVR, aVL, aVF) (Fig. 24-3). The first three limb leads, I, II, and III, are bipolar. That is, each of these leads measures differences in polarity between two skin electrodes, with one acting as the negative and one as the positive pole. Lead I measures electrical polarity between the right (negative pole) and left (positive pole) arms, lead II between the right arm (negative pole) and left leg (positive pole), and lead III between the left arm (negative pole) and left leg (positive pole).

An imaginary line between the two poles of a particular lead is termed the axis of that lead. The axes of the three bipolar limb leads form Einthoven's triangle. Einthoven's law describes the relationship between the three bipolar leads: the complex in lead II is always equal to the sum of the complexes in leads I and III (Conover, 1996b). Leads aVR, aVL, and aVF are augmented unipolar leads. They measure polarity differences between the electrical center of the heart and three reference points on the body surface: the right arm, left arm, and left leg, which serve as the positive poles for aVR, aVL, and aVF, respectively. The three unipolar leads are each perpendicular to one of the three bipolar leads. They fill the wide viewing gaps resulting from the 60° angles between leads I, II, and III; the gap between leads I and II is filled by lead aVR, that between leads II and III by lead aVF, and that between leads III and I by lead aVL (Sgarbossa & Wagner, 1998).

The chest, or precordial, leads (V_1, V_2, V_3, V_4, V_5, and V_6) display electrical activity in a horizontal plane, using surface electrodes placed at six standard reference points on the chest. The precordial leads are unipolar, comparing polarity between the electrical center of the heart and six points that act as positive poles on the anterior and left lateral chest wall. Electrodes for V_1 and V_2 are placed at the fourth intercostal space, just to the right and left sides of the sternum, respectively. The V_4, V_5, and V_6 electrodes are positioned at the fifth intercostal space, on the midclavicular, anterior axillary, and midaxillary lines, respectively. The V_3 electrode is positioned equidistant between V_2 and V_4 (see Fig. 24-3). Proper placement of precordial electrodes is essential for accurate interpretation of the ECG. Deviation of as little as 1.5 to 2 cm from the standard positions can produce significant electrocardiographic abnormalities (Sgarbossa & Wagner, 1998; Hill & Goodman, 1987).

▶ Electrical Axis

The depolarization of cardiac cells produces electrical currents that flow from depolarized to polarized tissue. These currents can be represented by vectors, which have magnitude and direction. The magnitude is represented by the length of the vector arrow and the direction by the arrowhead. When analyzing a particular lead of the ECG, the axis and location of the positive pole for that lead must be considered. A positive deflection represents a depolarization wave parallel to the axis of the lead and directed toward the positive pole of the lead. Similarly, a negative deflection represents electrical activity parallel to the axis and directed away from the positive pole.

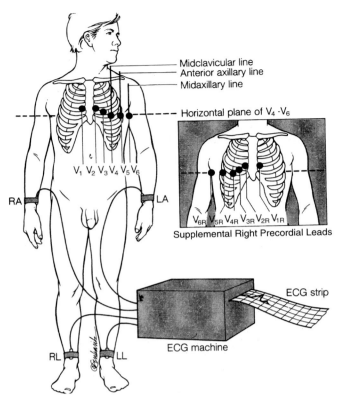

FIGURE 24-3. Placement of limb and precordial electrodes for recording 12-lead ECG. Supplemental right precordial leads may be obtained using electrodes placed across the right side of the chest, mirroring the position of standard precordial leads (inset). (Hudak CM, Gallo BM, Morton PG, 1998: Patient assessment: Cardiovascular system. In Critical Care Nursing, ed. 7, p. 189. Philadelphia, Lippincott Williams & Wilkins)

Biphasic deflections or an isoelectric line indicate electrical activity directed perpendicular to the axis of the lead. If the mean direction of current flow falls between being parallel and perpendicular to the axis of the lead, the complex is predominantly positive or negative depending on whether the bulk of electrical energy is directed toward or away from the positive pole of the lead.

Electrical axis describes the mean direction of electrical current or force through the atria (P wave axis) and ventricles (QRS axis). Although electrical current flows in a multitude of directions, cardiac depolarization basically occurs from the base to the apex of the heart and in a leftward direction. Atrial depolarization normally originates in the sinus node, located high in the right atrial myocardium, near the orifice of the superior vena cava. Accordingly, sinus node discharge depolarizes atrial cells in a right-to-left and inferior direction. Therefore, the P wave is usually upright in leads I, II, aVF, and V_3 through V_6; the P wave usually is inverted in aVR and may be inverted in V_1 and V_2 (Gilmore & Woods, 1995).

Ventricular depolarization consists of two components. The intraventricular septum is depolarized first by a branch of the left bundle. Therefore, initial electrical forces are directed from left to right. The second component is depolarization of the right and left ventricles

from the endocardial to epicardial surface. Although both ventricles are depolarized simultaneously during this phase, the thicker left ventricle is electrically dominant and the resultant electrical force is directed from the right to left side.

From a clinical perspective, the mean electrical axis of ventricular depolarization (QRS complex) is most significant. Calculated from the electrocardiographic tracings in the six frontal leads, it is a product of both the anatomic position of the heart in the chest and the manner in which the depolarization wave travels through the ventricles. To calculate the mean QRS axis, it is necessary to visualize the reference axes of the six frontal leads, with each positioned so that it intersects the electrical center of the heart, as shown in Figure 24-4. Beginning with the positive pole of lead I, each of the negative and positive poles of the six leads is labeled using numerical degrees to represent its position. Lead I is used as a starting point and is labeled 0°; positive degrees are assigned to the points moving clockwise and negative degrees to those moving counterclockwise.

Mean QRS axis may be estimated by identifying two factors: (1) the lead with a biphasic QRS complex, and (2) the lead with the R wave of tallest amplitude. Mean axis is perpendicular to the lead with the biphasic complex and at the pole with the tallest R wave. The normal adult QRS axis ranges from $-30°$ to $+110°$. Axes outside this range may represent cardiac disease. If the axis falls between $+110°$ and $+180°$, right axis deviation is present; an axis of $-30°$ to $-90°$ constitutes left axis deviation; an axis of $-90°$ to $-180°$ is considered either extreme right or extreme left axis deviation. An indetermi-

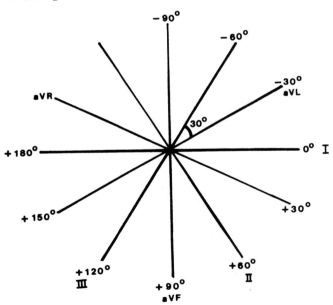

FIGURE 24-4. The hexaxial reference system divides the frontal plane into 30° intervals. All degrees in the upper hemisphere are labeled as negative degrees and all degrees in the lower hemisphere are labeled as positive degrees. (Gilmore SB, Woods SL, 1995: Electrocardiography and vectorcardiography. In Woods SL, Froelicher ES, Halpenny CJ, Motzer SU [eds]: Cardiac Nursing, ed. 3, p. 296. Philadelphia, JB Lippincott)

nate axis is present when all the QRS complexes in the frontal leads are biphasic. Electrical axis can be estimated quickly by examining the QRS complex in leads I and aVF. The axis is normal if the QRS complex is upright in both leads, shifted to the left if lead I is positive and lead aVF is negative, and toward the right if lead I is negative and aVF is positive (Hudak et al., 1998). Negative complexes in both leads I and aVF indicate extreme axis deviation (Fig. 24-5).

Right axis deviation may occur normally or as a result of pulmonary disease, right ventricular hypertrophy, lateral wall myocardial infarction, or left posterior hemiblock (Goldberger, 1990). An axis between +90° and +110° is considered borderline right axis deviation and may be due to a vertically positioned heart, particularly in a tall, thin patient. Left axis deviation may represent a normal variant, left anterior hemiblock, an inferior wall myocardial infarction, left ventricular hypertrophy, or left bundle branch block. Borderline left axis deviation (an axis between 0° and −30°) may represent a horizontally positioned heart, as would occur during pregnancy or in the presence of ascites.

The precordial leads are not used to calculate the mean electrical axis of the heart, but they provide important information about ventricular depolarization in the horizontal plane. Normally, the initial septal depolarization, which occurs from left to right, produces a small positive deflection (r wave) in the right leads (V_1, V_2) and a small negative deflection (q wave) in V_6. Septal depolarization is perpendicular to the other precordial leads. The leftward and posterior forces of left ventricular depolarization dominate the remainder of current flow through the ventricles. Thus, negative deflections (S waves) occur in leads to the right of the left ventricle and positive deflections (R waves) in those to the left. R wave progression describes the normal increase in R wave amplitude as the electrocardiographic lead is changed from V_1 through V_5 or V_6 (Fig. 24-6). The R wave is tallest in the lead that is parallel to the mean direction of electrical force.

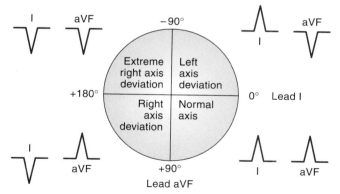

FIGURE 24-5. Rapid assessment of electrical axis based on direction of QRS complex in leads I and aVF. (Hudak CM, Gallo BM, Morton PG, 1998: Patient assessment: Cardiovascular system. In Critical Care Nursing: A Holistic Approach, ed. 7, p. 221. Philadelphia, Lippincott Williams & Wilkins)

► Electrocardiographic Abnormalities

Myocardial Ischemia and Infarction

The 12-lead ECG is one of the principal methods used to diagnose myocardial ischemia and infarction. Electrocardiographic manifestations of myocardial ischemia may include ST segment elevation, horizontal or downsloping ST segment depression, symmetric T wave inversion, pseudonormalization (normalization of a previously abnormal T wave), or Q-T prolongation (Hendel, 1997).

ST segment deviation toward the involved myocardium is the standard indicator of acute coronary artery thrombosis and threatened myocardial infarction (Sgarbossa & Wagner, 1998). A pattern of electrocardiographic changes occurs during MI evolution. The classic sequence begins with tall and peaked (hyperacute) T waves, followed by at least 1 mm of ST segment elevation in two or more contiguous leads, and then inversion of the T waves and formation of Q waves (Hendel, 1997). Abnormal Q waves appear in leads facing infarcted myocardium because necrotic tissue no longer depolarizes. Although small Q waves representing septal depolarization occur normally in a number of leads, new or large (>0.04 second in duration and >25% of R wave amplitude) Q waves are abnormal and represent myocardial infarction.

Q waves usually do not develop unless a myocardial infarction is transmural (ie, full thickness). Subendocardial, or nontransmural, myocardial infarction usually produces only ST segment elevation or depression and T wave inversion. The presence or absence of Q waves on the ECG, however, does not reliably distinguish between transmural and subendocardial infarction. Patients with transmural infarction do not always have Q waves and, conversely, Q waves are sometimes documented in patients with autopsy evidence of a subendocardial MI (Antman & Braunwald, 1997).

Changes in specific electrocardiographic leads identify the area affected by ischemia or infarction and, to some extent, the degree of damage to myocardial tissue. Most myocardial infarctions involve the left ventricle. The presence of abnormal Q waves, ST segment elevation, and T wave inversion in leads I, aVL, and V_1 through V_6 represents infarction of the anterior portion of the left ventricle (Fig. 24-7). Leads V_1 and V_2 reveal anteroseptal changes; leads V_2 through V_4, localized anterior changes; and leads V_4 through V_6, aVL, and I, anterolateral changes. Characteristic electrocardiographic changes in leads II, III, and aVF reveal inferior wall infarction.

None of the standard surface electrocardiographic leads directly reflects changes in the posterior wall. Instead, posterior infarction is indicated by reciprocal changes in leads opposite the posterior wall (ie, leads V_1 through V_3). In contrast to Q waves, inverted T waves, and ST segment elevation, reciprocal changes include tall R waves; tall, upright T waves; and ST segment depression in these right chest leads. The standard 12-lead ECG is of limited value in diagnosing infarction involving the

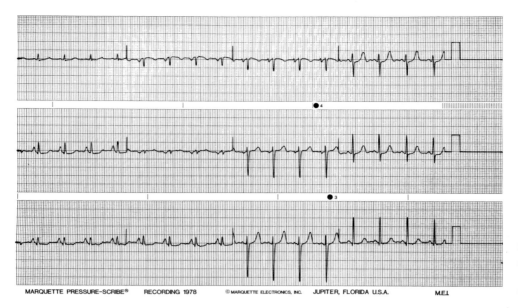

MARQUETTE PRESSURE-SCRIBE®   RECORDING 1978   © MARQUETTE ELECTRONICS, INC.   JUPITER, FLORIDA U.S.A.   M.E.I.

FIGURE 24-6. Precordial leads (V_1–V_6) in this 12-lead ECG demonstrate normal R wave progression. (Courtesy of Richard Davison, MD)

right ventricle. Right ventricular myocardial infarction, which usually occurs in association with inferior wall infarction, is best detected by recording the ECG from leads placed on the right side of the chest, in anatomic locations analogous to the conventional left-sided precordial leads (Morton, 1991).

Chamber Enlargement

Atrial enlargement or dilatation produces changes in the normal contour of the P wave (Fig. 24-8). Right atrial en-

largement causes increased P wave voltage (ie, >2.5 mm) but no increase in P wave duration. The characteristic tall, narrow P wave of right atrial enlargement (termed *P pulmonale*) is best visualized in leads II, III, and aVF.

Left atrial enlargement, on the other hand, causes a widening of the P wave because depolarization of the left atrium occurs slightly later than that of the right atrium. Left atrial enlargement is characterized by a notched P wave with a duration of 0.12 second or more (termed *P mitrale*), best observed in leads II and V_1, and a wide terminal negative deflection in lead V_1 (Sgarbossa & Wagner, 1998). The biphasic P wave in lead V_1 occurs be-

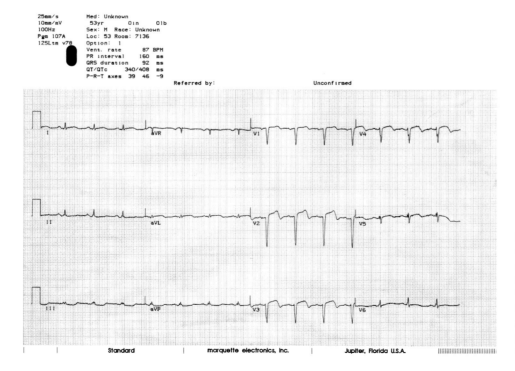

FIGURE 24-7. Twelve-lead ECG demonstrating anterolateral myocardial infarction. Diagnostic findings include Q waves in V_1 through V_2; slow R wave progression in V_3 through V_5; ST segment elevation in V_1 through V_5, I, and aVL; and reciprocal ST segment depression in leads III and aVF. (Courtesy of Richard Davison, MD)

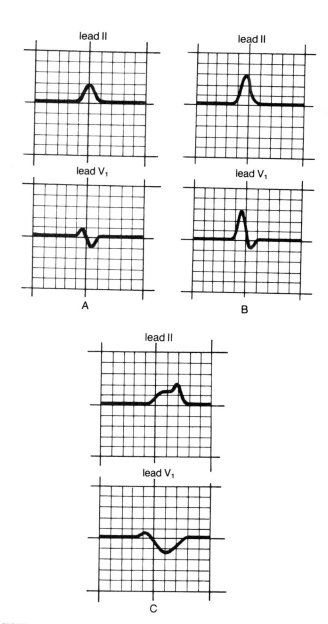

FIGURE 24-8. Right versus left atrial enlargement. **(A)** Normal P waves in leads II and V_1, **(B)** Right atrial enlargement. **(C)** Left atrial enlargement. (Hudak CM, Gallo BM, Morton PG, 1998: Patient assessment: Cardiovascular system. In Critical Care Nursing: A Holistic Approach, ed. 7, p. 223. Philadelphia, Lippincott Williams & Wilkins)

cause the lead lies opposite the posteriorly located left atrium. The initial small, positive deflection represents right atrial depolarization. It is followed by a terminal negative deflection, representing the predominant electrical activity that is directed away from V_1 and toward the enlarged left atrium.

Ventricular hypertrophy is demonstrated by increased amplitude of the QRS complex. Right ventricular hypertrophy produces large R waves in the right precordial leads (V_1, V_2) and deep S waves in the left precordial leads (V_5, V_6). The R wave progression normally apparent from right to left across the precordium is reversed (Hudak et

al., 1998). Right precordial T waves typically are inverted. Left ventricular hypertrophy produces abnormally deep S waves in V_1 or V_2 and abnormally large R waves in V_5 or V_6. ST segment and T wave changes, representing left ventricular strain, also may be evident in the left chest leads. Enlargement of both ventricles may lead to cancellation of opposite forces and result in a normal ECG; alternatively, tall R waves may develop in all precordial leads with prominent, biphasic QRS complexes in midprecordial leads (Sgarbossa & Wagner, 1998).

Bundle Branch Block

Normal intraventricular conduction occurs through specialized conduction tissue known as the bundle of His and its branches (Fig. 24-9). The bundle tissue is trifascicular, composed of a right bundle branch and a left bundle branch that bifurcates into anterior and posterior fascicles. The left bundle also gives rise to a septal branch. Abnormal width and configuration of the QRS complex reveals the presence of bundle branch block. Complete bundle branch block produces a QRS complex that is 0.12 second or greater. It does not necessarily imply total absence of conduction through the dysfunctional bundle branch, but rather that conduction is delayed long enough for the ventricles to be depolarized by the other bundle branch. Instead of being activated together, one ventricle is activated after the other and a pattern of complete bundle branch block is present on the ECG (Conover, 1996c). Bundle branch block may be fixed or may occur only with a fast (tachycardia-related) or slow (bradycardia-related) heart rate (Hillis et al., 1995).

The configurations of the widened QRS complex in V_1, a right-sided chest lead, and in V_6, a left-sided chest lead, are used to diagnose whether the right or left bundle is dysfunctional. Right bundle branch block is most common and usually is benign (Hendel, 1997). In right bundle branch block, the initial septal depolarization and left ventricular depolarization occur normally. Right ventricular depolarization occurs last, with the impulse wave traveling abnormally from the left ventricular muscle to depolarize the right ventricle. Consequently, the initial portion of the QRS is normal (rS in V_1 and qR in V_6). The terminal portion, representing right ventricular depolarization, consists of an R′ wave in V_1 and a deep, wide S wave in V_6. Therefore, right bundle branch block produces an rSR′ configuration in V_1 and a qRS configuration in V_6 (Fig. 24-10).

The most common cause of left bundle branch block is coronary artery disease (Hendel, 1997). In left bundle branch block, the depolarization of the septum and ventricles depends on the right bundle. Therefore, it occurs entirely in a right-to-left fashion. The small initial deflection representing septal depolarization is absent. Instead, V_1 displays a QS complex and V_6, a broad RR′ wave (Fig. 24-11). If incomplete bundle branch block is present, the QRS complex is typically widened to 0.11 second, although it may be narrower with incomplete right bundle branch block.

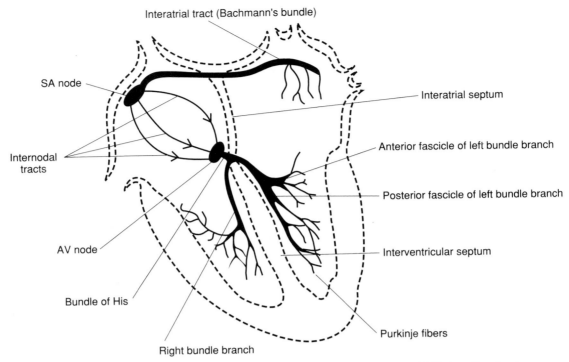

FIGURE 24-9. Electrical conduction system of the heart. (Huff J, 1997: Electrophysiology. In ECG Workout: Exercises in Arrhythmia Interpretation, ed. 3, p. 11. Philadelphia, Lippincott-Raven)

▶ Atrial Electrograms

Most often, electrical cardiac activity is assessed using electrodes on the body surface. However, because of the distance of the sensing electrodes from the heart and the small amplitude of the deflection produced by atrial depolarization, other electrical components or artifacts frequently obscure P waves (Finkelmeier & Salinger, 1984). Arrhythmia analysis may be supplemented in cardiac surgical patients with atrial electrograms obtained by recording a rhythm tracing from an atrial epicardial pac-

ing wire. Using an electrode attached directly to atrial epicardium to record intracardiac events produces amplification of atrial activity and diminution of ventricular activity. As a result, atrial activity and its relationship to ventricular activity are elucidated.

One or two pacing wires are routinely attached to the atrial epicardium during cardiac operations. The electrode end of the wire is secured to the epicardium, and the opposite end is brought out through the anterior chest wall. Two types of atrial electrograms may be obtained: (1) a bipolar electrogram in which two atrial elec-

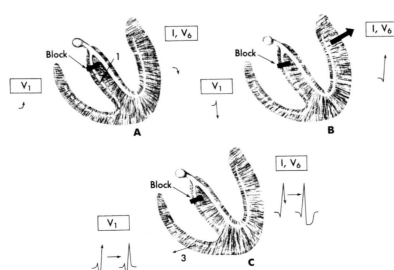

FIGURE 24-10. Schematic representation of ventricular activation in right bundle branch block (RBBB). **(A)** Initial activation of the ventricular septum (*arrow 1*) occurs normally. **(B)** Because of the RBBB, right ventricular activation is delayed and left ventricular activation occurs alone. **(C)** The right ventricle is activated after left ventricular activation, resulting in a terminal R wave in lead V_1 and a terminal S wave in leads I and V_6. (Grauer K, 1992: The QRS interval/bundle branch block. In A Practical Guide to ECG Interpretation, p. 63. St. Louis, Mosby–Year Book)

FIGURE 24-11. Schematic representation of ventricular activation in left bundle branch block (LBBB). Initial activation of the ventricular septum (*arrow 1*) occurs abnormally from right to left because of the LBBB. The electrical impulse travels by means of the intact right bundle to activate the right ventricle (2R) and spreads across the ventricular septum to activate the left ventricle (2L). Ventricular activation thus occurs primarily in a right to left direction, resulting in a QS waveform in lead V_1 and a broad RR' waveform in leads I and V_6. (Grauer K, 1992: The QRS interval/bundle branch block. In A Practical Guide to ECG Interpretation, p. 65. St. Louis, Mosby—Year Book)

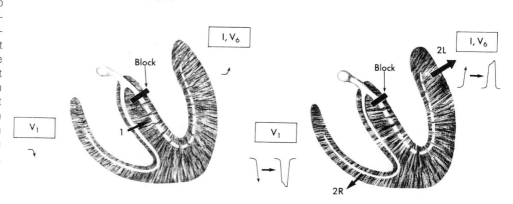

trodes are used for recording, and (2) a unipolar electrogram in which one atrial and one distant electrode are used. Bipolar atrial electrograms provide the best enhancement of atrial activity with minimal visibility of ventricular activity; unipolar atrial electrograms provide some magnification of atrial activity but also clearly demonstrate the relationship between atrial and ventricular activity (Finkelmeier & Salinger, 1984; Moore & Wilkoff, 1991) (Fig. 24-12).

An atrial electrogram is obtained easily at the bedside and should be performed any time the diagnosis of an arrhythmia is in question. If two atrial epicardial wires have been placed, both bipolar and unipolar tracings may be performed. An appropriately grounded and electrically isolated electrocardiograph is used, preferably one that can produce a simultaneous recording of a surface electrocardiographic lead.

The atrial epicardial wire is attached to the right arm electrode of the electrocardiograph. If a second epicardial wire is present, it is attached to the left arm electrode; if not, the left arm electrode is attached in the usual fashion. The right and left leg electrodes are positioned normally. If both the right and left arm electrodes are attached to atrial epicardial wires, recording a lead I tracing produces a bipolar atrial electrogram. A lead I tracing with standard electrode placement measures polarity between the right and left arm. Therefore, in this instance it measures polarity between the two atrial electrodes. When the electrocardiograph is adjusted to obtain a lead II tracing (ie, measuring polarity between right arm and left leg electrodes), it produces a unipolar electrogram (atrial and left leg electrodes).

If only the right arm electrode has been attached to an atrial wire, recording in either lead I or lead II produces a unipolar electrogram. A unipolar electrogram may be obtained alternatively by attaching all four limb electrodes in their usual positions and the atrial wire to the V electrode. Recording in the V_1 setting produces a unipolar atrial electrogram. If a telemetry monitoring system is being used, attaching the right arm electrode to an atrial wire produces an atrial electrogram. The right arm electrode of a bedside monitoring system also may be used if the equipment is electrically isolated to avoid delivery of current from the monitoring system to the heart through the pacing wire. The electrical safety of the

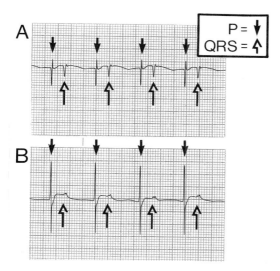

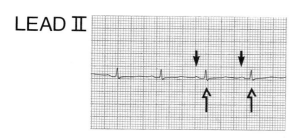

FIGURE 24-12. Normal sinus rhythm: unipolar **(A)** and bipolar **(B)** atrial electrograms are recorded simultaneously with a lead II rhythm tracing. (Finkelmeier BA, Salinger MH, 1984: The atrial electrogram: Its diagnostic use following cardiac surgery. Critical Care Nurse 4:43)

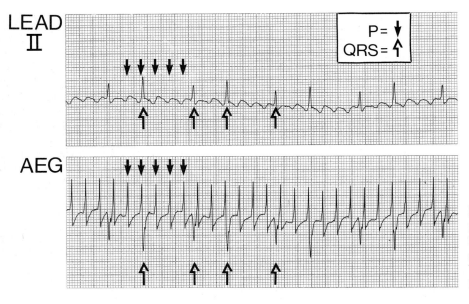

FIGURE 24-13. Atrial electrogram (AEG) recorded simultaneously with lead II rhythm tracing clearly reveals atrial flutter waves with a variable block. (Finkelmeier BA, Salinger MH, 1984: The atrial electrogram: Its diagnostic use following cardiac surgery. Critical Care Nurse 4:44)

monitoring system must be confirmed before using it to perform an atrial electrogram.

Atrial electrograms often are used when attempting to diagnose supraventricular tachycardias. During tachyarrhythmias, P wave activity frequently is obscured by the QRS complex or T wave. In addition, it is often difficult to determine if the ratio of P waves to QRS complex is more than 1:1. An atrial electrogram of atrial flutter read-

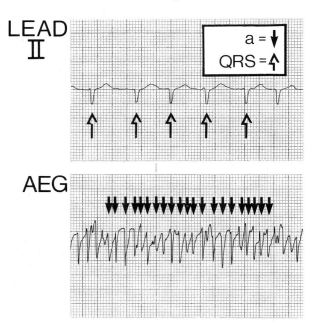

FIGURE 24-14. Atrial electrogram (AEG) recorded simultaneously with lead II rhythm tracing during atrial fibrillation reveals erratic atrial activity (a); QRS complexes are obscured in the AEG. (Finkelmeier BA, Salinger MH, 1984: The atrial electrogram: Its diagnostic use following cardiac surgery. Critical Care Nurse 4:45)

ily reveals flutter waves and allows easy determination of the degree of AV block (Fig. 24-13). In atrial fibrillation, erratic fibrillatory waves that may be obscured on the surface ECG are readily detected by an atrial electrogram (Fig. 24-14). An atrial electrogram also is valuable in differentiating ventricular tachycardia and supraventricular tachycardia with aberrancy. Because it more clearly displays the relationship of atrial and ventricular activity, an atrial electrogram may unmask AV dissociation. AV dissociation does not confirm a ventricular origin of the arrhythmia because retrograde conduction from the ventricles to the atria may produce a P wave related to each QRS complex. As a general rule, however, AV dissociation during a wide QRS tachycardia is strong presumptive evidence of an arrhythmia's ventricular origin (Zipes, 1997).

REFERENCES

Antman EM, Braunwald E, 1997: Acute myocardial infarction. In Braunwald E (ed): Heart Disease: A Textbook of Cardiovascular Medicine, ed. 5. Philadelphia, WB Saunders

Conover MB, 1996a: Normal electrical activation of the heart. In Understanding Electrocardiography, ed. 7. St. Louis, Mosby–Year Book

Conover MB, 1996b: The 12 electrocardiogram leads. In Understanding Electrocardiography, ed. 7. St. Louis, Mosby–Year Book

Conover MB, 1996c: Bundle branch block and hemiblock. In Understanding Electrocardiography, ed. 7. St. Louis, Mosby–Year Book

Finkelmeier BA, Salinger MH, 1984: The atrial electrogram: Its diagnostic use following cardiac surgery. Critical Care Nurse 4:42

Fisch C, 1997: Electrocardiography. In Braunwald E (ed): Heart Disease: A Textbook of Cardiovascular Medicine, ed. 5. Philadelphia, WB Saunders

Gilmore SB, Woods SL, 1995: Electrocardiography and vectorcardiography. In Woods SL, Froelicher ESS, Halpenny

CJ, Motzer SU (eds): Cardiac Nursing, ed. 3. Philadelphia, JB Lippincott

Goldberger E, 1990: Electrocardiography. In Essentials of Clinical Cardiology. Philadelphia, JB Lippincott

Hendel RC, 1997. Interpreting noninvasive cardiac tests. In Alpert JS (ed): Cardiology for the Primary Care Physician, ed. 2. Philadelphia, Current Medicine

Hill NE, Goodman JS, 1987: Importance of accurate placement of precordial leads in the 12-lead electrocardiogram. Heart Lung 16:561

Hillis LD, Lange RA, Winniford MD, Page RL, 1995: Bundle branch and fascicular blocks. In Manual of Clinical Problems in Cardiology, ed. 5. Boston, Little, Brown

Hudak CM, Gallo BM, Morton PG, 1998: Patient assessment: Cardiovascular system. In Critical Care Nursing: A Holistic Approach. ed. 7. Philadelphia, Lippincott Williams & Wilkins

Huff J, 1997: Waveforms, intervals, segments, and complexes. In ECG Workout: Exercises in Arrhythmia Interpretation, ed. 3. Philadelphia, Lippincott-Raven

Moore SL, Wilkoff BL, 1991: Rhythm disturbances after cardiac surgery. Semin Thorac Cardiovasc Surg 3:24

Morton PG, 1991: Electrocardiographic assessment of right heart dysfunction. J Cardiovasc Nurs 6:34

Sgarbossa EB, Wagner G, 1998: Electrocardiography. In Topol EJ (ed): Comprehensive Cardiovascular Medicine. Philadelphia, Lippincott Williams & Wilkins

White J, 1998: Disorders of cardiac conduction and rhythm. In Porth CM (ed): Pathophysiology: Concepts of Altered Health States, ed. 5. Philadelphia, Lippincott Williams & Wilkins

Zipes DP, 1997: Specific arrhythmias: Diagnosis and treatment. In Braunwald E (ed): Heart Disease: A Textbook of Cardiovascular Medicine, ed. 5. Philadelphia, WB Saunders

25

Cardiac Arrhythmias

The ability to diagnose *cardiac arrhythmias* is an essential skill for nurses in cardiothoracic surgical settings. Clinically significant arrhythmias occur quite commonly during the early postoperative period after cardiac operations. Predisposing factors include hypothermia, metabolic abnormalities, alterations in gas exchange, withdrawal from beta-adrenergic blocking agents, inadequate protection of atrial tissue during aortic cross-clamping, underlying cardiac disease, and edema of myocardial tissue and pericardial inflammation related to surgical manipulation of the heart. Patients who undergo pulmonary or esophageal surgery also are prone to postoperative arrhythmias, particularly in association with extensive pulmonary or esophageal resection, atelectasis and hypoxemia, or perioperative myocardial infarction.

Arrhythmia identification is performed using a consistent set of criteria applied in systematic fashion. The discussion in this chapter is by no means a complete review of all cardiac arrhythmias and the nuances of diagnosis. Rather, it is confined to summary information regarding diagnosis and management of the most commonly encountered arrhythmias. Each of the selected arrhythmias is defined according to its site of origin, rate, rhythm, waveform appearance, and length of P-R and QRS duration. For the purpose of comparison, the criteria defining normal sinus rhythm are included.

NORMAL SINUS RHYTHM (FIG. 25-1)

Origin: sinus node

Rate: 60 to 100 beats per minute

Rhythm: regular

Waveform Appearance: PQRST

P-R Interval: 0.12 to 0.20 second

QRS Duration: 0.04 to 0.10 second

Normal sinus rhythm is regular with a rate that is determined by several factors, including activity of the autonomic nervous system and body temperature (Wellens, 1998). A sinus arrhythmia is present if each cardiac impulse arises normally in the sinus node but the rhythmicity is irregular, with the P-P interval varying by more than 0.16 second (Hillis et al., 1995a). The rate variation in sinus arrhythmia usually is related to respiration; the sinus rate increases during inspiration and decreases during expiration. Sinus arrhythmia is of no clinical significance and does not require treatment (Huff, 1997a).

▶ Common Arrhythmias

Premature Complexes

PREMATURE ATRIAL CONTRACTIONS (FIG. 25-2)

Origin: atrial tissue

Rhythm: irregular

Waveform Appearance: P′ (ectopic P) QRST

P-R Interval: normal or prolonged

QRS Duration: 0.04 to 0.10 second unless aberrant conduction occurs

A *premature atrial contraction* (PAC) is the discharge of an ectopic atrial focus that depolarizes the atria and interrupts the dominant rhythm. PACs occur early, usually are caused by enhanced automaticity, and may originate from one or more foci (Huff, 1997b). In addition to prematurity, the P′ wave may be altered in morphology; that is, it may be taller, shorter, notched, widened, or superimposed on the preceding T wave (Wilkinson, 1991). PACs may be interpolated (ie, produce no alteration in regularity of the cardiac rhythm), or they may be associated with a noncompensatory or full compensatory pause.

Premature atrial contractions usually are conducted to the ventricles normally, producing a QRS complex identical to that after sinus node discharge. Occasionally, PACs are conducted aberrantly. Aberrancy, defined as a transient abnormality in intraventricular conduction of a complex of supraventricular origin, is discussed in

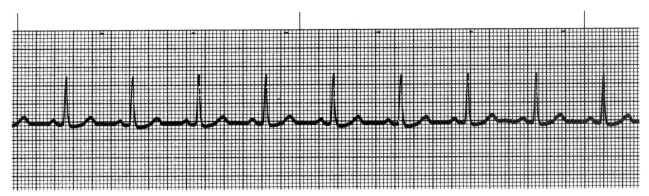

FIGURE 25-1. Normal sinus rhythm with heart rate of 84 beats per minute. (Huff J, 1997: Sinus arrhythmias. In ECG Workout: Exercises in Arrhythmia Interpretation, ed. 3, p. 50. Philadelphia, Lippincott-Raven)

further detail later in the chapter. If a PAC is very premature, ventricular tissue may still be refractory. If so, the PAC is nonconducted and no QRS complex follows the P′ wave. PACs are common after cardiac and pulmonary resection procedures. Although they are usually a precursor of supraventricular tachyarrhythmias, they otherwise have little clinical significance.

PREMATURE JUNCTIONAL CONTRACTIONS

Origin: atrioventricular (AV) nodal tissue

Rhythm: irregular

Waveform Appearance: P′ QRST, QRST, or QRST P′

P-R Interval: if P′ precedes QRS, less than 0.12 second

QRS Duration: 0.04 to 0.10 second unless aberrant conduction occurs

Premature junctional contractions (PJCs), often a precursor to junctional tachycardia, originate in the AV node. Depolarization of the atria may occur in a retrograde fashion, producing a morphologically abnormal P wave that may appear before, simultaneously with, or after the QRS complex (Hillis et al., 1995b). Alternatively, depolarization of the atria by the sinus node may occur simultaneously with or after AV nodal depolarization. In this case, a morphologically normal P wave appears before, during, or after the QRS complex. PJCs that are conducted normally through the bundles produce an appropriately narrow QRS complex. If aberrant conduction occurs, the QRS is widened. PJCs do not require treatment.

PREMATURE VENTRICULAR CONTRACTIONS (FIG. 25-3)

Origin: ventricular tissue

Rhythm: irregular

P-R Interval: none

QRS Duration: more than 0.12 second

Premature ventricular contractions (PVCs) originate from an ectopic focus or foci in the ventricles. They are characterized by abnormal width and distorted morphology of the QRS complex compared with the narrow QRS complex produced by impulses originating in the atria or AV node (Drew, 1987). PVCs may be uniform in morphology or multiformed. Often the T wave after

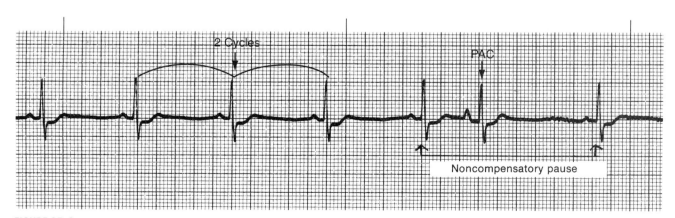

FIGURE 25-2. Normal sinus rhythm with premature atrial contraction. Note different morphology of ectopic P wave preceding premature beat and noncompensatory pause (less than two R-R intervals). (Huff J, 1997: Atrial arrhythmias. In ECG Workout: Exercises in Arrhythmia Interpretation, ed. 3, p. 94. Philadelphia, Lippincott-Raven)

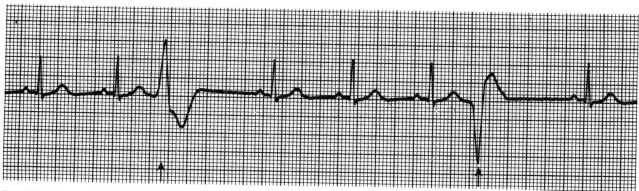

FIGURE 25-3. Normal sinus rhythm with multifocal premature ventricular contractions (PVCs). These PVCs differ in size, shape, and direction because they arise from different ectopic sites. (Huff J, 1997: Ventricular arrhythmias and bundle branch block. In ECG Workout: Exercises in Arrhythmia Interpretation, ed. 3, p. 185. Philadelphia, Lippincott-Raven)

a PVC is opposite the primary deflection of the QRS waveform. PVCs usually are followed by a full compensatory pause; that is, the R-R interval surrounding the PVC is exactly twice as long as the R-R interval between two complexes of sinus origin. Three or more consecutive PVCs are considered ventricular tachycardia (VT).

In postoperative patients, PVCs may occur transiently because of a precipitant, such as hypoxemia, hypokalemia, or hypomagnesemia. New-onset ventricular ectopy must be evaluated promptly and treated appropriately. Correction of the underlying precipitant often eradicates ventricular ectopy. Hypoxemia is treated with oxygen, pulmonary hygiene measures, or assisted ventilation. The serum potassium level is maintained above 4.0 mEq/L and the magnesium level above 1.5 mEq/L (Mackall et al., 1996). Intravenous lidocaine or temporary pacing typically is used to suppress PVCs.

Many patients with organic heart disease have underlying ventricular arrhythmias. It is important to ascertain if the frequency and morphology of PVCs in the postoperative period differ from those in the preoperative period and to reinstitute preoperative antiarrhythmic therapy. In some patients, particularly those with major ventricular wall motion abnormalities, ventricular ectopy is a sign of a chronic arrhythmic disorder and electrophysiologic evaluation is necessary to direct future therapy.

Tachyarrhythmias

Supraventricular Tachyarrhythmias

SINUS TACHYCARDIA

Origin: sinus node

Rate: 100 to 160 beats per minute

Rhythm: regular

Complex: PQRST

P-R Interval: 0.12 to 0.20 second

QRS Duration: 0.04 to 0.10 second

Sinus tachycardia is sinus rhythm with an accelerated rate. It usually is gradual in onset and termination. P waves precede each QRS complex and have a normal configuration, duration, and axis. The P-R interval often is shortened, but may be normal or even lengthened (Hillis et al., 1995a). Both the upper and lower rate limits of sinus tachycardia vary with age. In adults, a sinus rhythm at a rate greater than 100 beats per minute is considered tachycardic; sinus tachycardia rarely occurs at a rate greater than 160 beats per minute.

Sinus tachycardia usually develops secondary to a hypermetabolic state. Common causes in postoperative patients include fever, pain, anxiety, anemia, hypoxemia, and hypovolemia. The heart works less efficiently during sinus tachycardia because diastolic filling time is reduced. However, the arrhythmia rarely produces symptoms. Correction of the precipitating factor usually results in a return to normal sinus rhythm. Antiarrhythmic medications usually are not necessary. Alternatively, a beta-blocking medication (eg, propranolol or metoprolol) may be instituted to treat the arrhythmia in the absence of any detectable physiologic abnormality (Elefteriades et al., 1996).

Supraventricular tachycardia (SVT) includes several arrhythmias, all of which originate above the bifurcation of the bundle of His. Paroxysmal SVT (PSVT), atrial flutter, and atrial fibrillation are all forms of SVT. In patients who have undergone cardiac and thoracic operations, they are all points on a spectrum of postoperative supraventricular irritability (Elefteriades et al., 1996). The primary distinguishing features among the various forms of SVT are the mechanism of arrhythmogenesis and rate of atrial depolarization.

PAROXYSMAL SUPRAVENTRICULAR TACHYCARDIA

Origin: atrial tissue or AV nodal tissue

Rate:

  Atrial—160 to 250 beats per minute (atrial origin or retrograde conduction from AV nodal origin)

  Ventricular—same, or may be slower if atrial origin with block

Rhythm: regular

Complex: P'QRST, QRST, or QRSTP' (P' may be
superimposed on preceding T wave or inverted)

P-R Interval: may be shortened, prolonged, or absent

QRS Duration: 0.04 to 0.10 second

Paroxysmal SVT is the nonspecific term used to describe arrhythmias thought to arise because of reentry and includes tachycardias formerly called *paroxysmal atrial tachycardia* and *paroxysmal junctional tachycardia* (Erickson, 1991). Episodes of PSVT typically have a sudden onset and termination (Hillis et al., 1995c). AV conduction usually occurs at a 1:1 ratio, although AV block sometimes is present. Although QRS duration often is normal, it may be prolonged in the presence of aberrant conduction. PSVT is less common than atrial flutter or atrial fibrillation in postoperative patients. PSVT with block may occur as a manifestation of digoxin toxicity.

ATRIAL FLUTTER (FIG. 25-4)

Origin: atrial tissue

Rate:
  Atrial—250 to 350 beats per minute (type I);
    320 to 430 beats per minute (type II)
  Ventricular—rate dependent on degree of block

Rhythm: regularly irregular

Complex: P'P'QRST, P'P'P'QRST, or
  P'P'P'P'QRST

P-R Interval: cannot be determined

QRS Duration: 0.04 to 0.10 second

Atrial flutter is a form of SVT characterized by a rapid, regular atrial rate that may range from 250 to 430 beats per minute (Conover, 1996). In type I, or typical, atrial flutter, flutter waves occur at a rate of 250 to 350 beats per minute and often create a characteristic "sawtooth" pattern with negatively oriented P waves in the inferior leads (II, III, and aV_F) (Hillis et al., 1995d). The ventricular rate during atrial flutter depends on the conduction characteristics of the AV conduction system and usually varies from 2:1 conduction to higher degrees of

AV block (Wellens, 1998). Often, type I atrial flutter occurs with an atrial rate of 300 beats per minute, 2:1 AV block, and a ventricular rate of 150 beats per minute. Despite the high atrial depolarization rates, mechanically significant contraction of the atria often is preserved (McGuire, 1982).

Type II, or atypical, atrial flutter has elements of both atrial flutter and atrial fibrillation. The atrial rate ranges from 320 to 430 beats per minute (Conover, 1996). The flutter waves are less uniform than in type I atrial flutter, varying in morphology and spacing. QRS complexes usually are normal in duration and configuration, occurring at a rate of 75 to 150 per minute (Hillis et al., 1995d). The term *flutter-fibrillation* is sometimes used to describe type II atrial flutter.

ATRIAL FIBRILLATION (FIG. 25-5)

Origin: atrial tissue

Rate:
  Atrial—350 to 600 beats per minute
  Ventricular—variable

Rhythm: irregularly irregular

Complex:
  Atrial—chaotic fibrillatory waves
  Ventricular—QRST

P-R Interval: cannot be determined

QRS Duration: 0.04 to 0.10 second

Atrial fibrillation is the most common sustained arrhythmia affecting humans (Prystowsky & Katz, 1998). It is present in 0.4% of the general population and is particularly prevalent in specific subgroups; it occurs in 10% of people older than 60 years of age, 30% of those with idiopathic cardiomyopathy, and in approximately 60% of those undergoing mitral valve repair or replacement (Sundt & Cox, 1998). It also is the most common arrhythmia occurring in patients who undergo any form of cardiac operation. Atrial fibrillation develops when the atrial chambers can no longer sustain a regular, coordinated rhythm and multiple foci in one or both atria

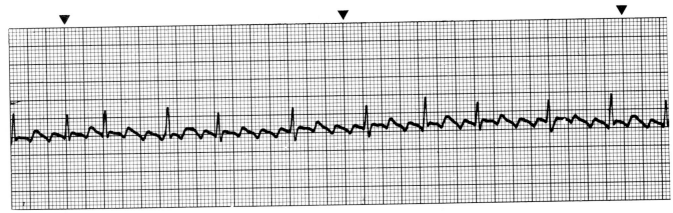

FIGURE 25-4. Atrial flutter with variable degree of block. Note "sawtooth" appearance of flutter waves. (Huff J, 1997: Atrial arrhythmias. In ECG Workout: Exercises in Arrhythmia Interpretation, ed. 3, 118. Philadelphia, Lippincott-Raven)

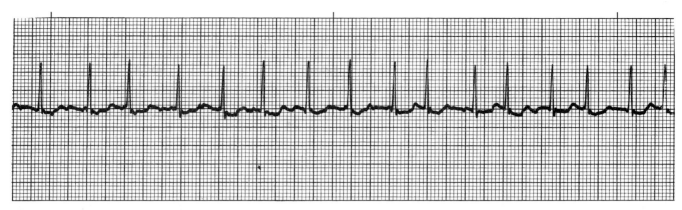

FIGURE 25-5. Atrial fibrillation with ventricular response rate of approximately 130 beats per minute. Note irregular rhythm and fibrillatory baseline without discernible P waves. (Huff J, 1997: Atrial arrhythmias. In ECG Workout: Exercises in Arrhythmia Interpretation, ed. 3, p. 115. Philadelphia, Lippincott-Raven)

begin to discharge hundreds of times per minute (Kastor, 1991). Its electrocardiographic hallmarks are a fibrillatory baseline in association with an irregularly irregular ventricular rate. Although QRS complexes are usually of normal duration, intermittent aberrant conduction is common because of the rapid and erratic rate of AV nodal depolarization. As a result, occasional widened QRS complexes are typical. It sometimes is difficult to determine if these widened complexes represent aberrancy or PVCs.

The forms of SVT described previously are common both in postoperative cardiac surgical patients and in patients who have undergone esophagectomy or major pulmonary resection, particularly pneumonectomy. Atrial fibrillation occurs most often, usually 2 to 4 days after operation. Although a number of theories have been postulated to explain the frequency of postoperative SVT, the mechanism of arrhythmogenesis remains unclear. In addition, no pharmacologic regimen has proven effective in entirely preventing its occurrence. Atrial electrograms, obtained using the atrial epicardial pacing wire, are useful for magnifying atrial activity and for helping to distinguish among the various forms of SVT and between SVT and VT (Finkelmeier & Salinger, 1984).

Although SVT usually is not a life-threatening problem, patients with compromised ventricular function or untreated myocardial ischemia may experience clinically significant hypotension. The rapid ventricular rates typically associated with all forms of SVT compromise cardiac output. The rapid rate increases myocardial oxygen consumption while at the same time shortening diastolic filling time for the coronary arteries (Elefteriades et al., 1996).

Inappropriate timing of mitral and tricuspid valve closure further impairs ventricular filling. In atrial fibrillation, mechanically effective atrial contractions are absent. Therefore, the proportion of ventricular filling that results from a properly timed atrial systole (ie, the "atrial kick") is lost and cardiac output may be reduced by 20% to 30% in some patients. Atrial fibrillation also is asso-

ciated with an increased risk for thromboembolism. Stasis of blood along endocardial surfaces of the quivering or quiescent atria predisposes to thrombus formation. Atrial thrombosis can be demonstrated in 15% of patients who have atrial fibrillation for longer than 3 days (Marino, 1998). Small fragments of thrombus can embolize from the left atrium into the systemic circulation and from the right atrium into the pulmonary vessels; cerebral, renal, splenic, peripheral, or pulmonary embolism may result (Goldberger, 1990a).

The goals of treating postoperative SVT are twofold: slowing the ventricular rate and conversion to normal sinus rhythm. Treatment may consist of (1) pharmacologic agents, (2) rapid atrial pacing, or (3) cardioversion. Often a combination of therapies is used. Digoxin is used commonly for both prophylaxis and treatment of SVT. Digoxin prolongs the effective refractory period and decreases conduction velocity in the AV node, thereby slowing the ventricular rate in atrial flutter or atrial fibrillation and prolonging the P-R interval in normal sinus rhythm. It is the only available drug that slows ventricular rate without adversely affecting myocardial contractility (Elefteriades et al., 1996).

Beta-blocking medications, particularly cardioselective agents that preferentially block beta$_1$ receptors (eg, metoprolol), or propranolol also are used commonly to prevent or treat postoperative SVT. Verapamil or diltiazem is used occasionally but may not be well tolerated in patients with compromised left ventricular function. For patients with persistent SVT, ibutilide or amiodarone may be considered.

Rapid atrial pacing sometimes is effective in converting PSVT or type I atrial flutter, particularly when used in combination with pharmacologic therapy. It is not useful in converting atrial fibrillation to normal sinus rhythm because atrial capture cannot be achieved when the atria are fibrillating. Electrical cardioversion is performed immediately for SVT that produces significant hypotension. Techniques for rapid atrial pacing and cardioversion are described in Chapter 26, Temporary Pacing and Defibrillation.

Ventricular Tachyarrhythmias

VENTRICULAR TACHYCARDIA (FIG. 25-6)

Origin: ventricular tissue

Rate: 100 to 250 beats per minute

Rhythm: regular or slightly irregular

Waveform Appearance: QRST; P waves independent of or hidden in QRS complex

P-R Interval: none

QRS Duration: more than 0.12 second

Ventricular tachycardia is an arrhythmia originating below the bifurcation of the bundle of His. It usually is exhibited electrocardiographically by wide, tall, bizarre QRS complexes that persist longer than 0.12 second (White, 1998). The heart rate is seldom faster than 200 beats per minute and does not exceed 250 beats per minute (Goldberger, 1990b). Atrial activity may occur independent of the ventricular rhythm (AV dissociation), or retrograde ventriculoatrial conduction may be present. If atrial and ventricular activity is dissociated, fusion or capture beats may occur. Fusion beats represent ventricular depolarization partially from a supraventricular focus and partially from an ectopic ventricular focus. They have a slightly shorter P-R interval than the sinus beats and a slightly different configuration than the tachycardic beats (Drew & Ide, 1994). Capture beats are ventricular depolarizations resulting from an impulse originating in the atrium. VT may be monomorphic or polymorphic and may be nonsustained or sustained. Sustained VT has a rate greater than 100 beats per minute and lasts more than 30 seconds or requires an intervention to terminate.

Ventricular tachycardia usually is not well tolerated and may produce severe hypotension or deteriorate into ventricular fibrillation (VF). It is a major cause of sudden cardiac death and accounts for approximately 50% of all cardiac-related deaths (Tchou, 1998). Therefore, VT must be treated promptly, usually with intravenous bo-

lus doses of lidocaine followed by a continuous infusion. Intravenous procainamide, bretylium, or amiodarone also may be used if lidocaine fails to suppress VT. Rapid defibrillation is performed if hemodynamic instability is present. Electrophysiologic studies may be necessary to evaluate the likelihood of arrhythmia recurrence and the need for chronic antiarrhythmic therapy.

Torsades de pointes is a form of VT characterized by QRS complexes of changing amplitude that appear to twist around the isoelectric line and that occur at rates of 200 to 250 beats per minute (Zipes, 1997). Torsades is the classic form of proarrhythmia observed during therapy with drugs that prolong ventricular repolarization, such as class III antiarrhythmic agents (eg, amiodarone or sotalol). A long cycle length preceding initiation of the arrhythmia typically characterizes drug-induced torsades de pointes (Fig. 25-7). Intravenous administration of high-dose magnesium sulfate has been demonstrated to be effective in terminating and preventing new episodes of torsades (Hohnloser, 1997). The responsible antiarrhythmic drug is discontinued and predisposing factors, such as electrolyte imbalance, are corrected.

VENTRICULAR FIBRILLATION (FIG. 25-8)

Origin: ventricular tissue

Rate: not measurable; QRS complexes not present

Rhythm: irregular

Waveform Appearance: chaotic fibrillatory waves

P-R Interval: none

QRS Duration: inconsistent

Ventricular fibrillation is a cardiac rhythm characterized by irregular, disorganized, oscillating ventricular complexes. The ventricles quiver but do not contract and there is no cardiac output (White, 1998). Death is usually instantaneous because peripheral perfusion ceases immediately and irreversible neurologic injury begins within minutes (Hillis et al., 1995e). For the patient to survive, cardiopulmonary resuscitation and defibrillation must be

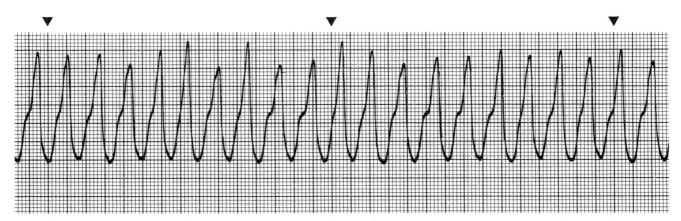

FIGURE 25-6. Ventricular tachycardia at a heart rate of 188 beats per minute; P waves are not identified. (Huff J, 1997: Ventricular arrhythmias and bundle branch block. In ECG Workout: Exercises in Arrhythmia Interpretation, ed. 3, p. 211. Philadelphia, Lippincott-Raven)

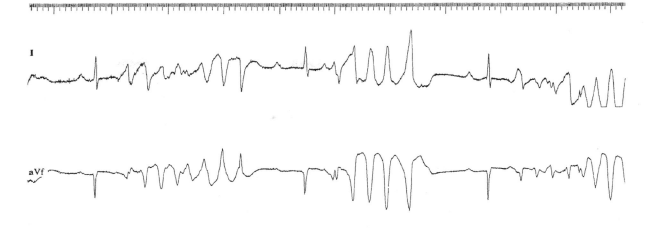

FIGURE 25-7. Typical characteristics of torsades de pointes. The initiation of the first ventricular beat of the tachycardia tends to occur after a pause; the QRS of this first beat initiates on the T wave, making it difficult to appreciate where the T wave terminates. (Tchou PJ, 1998: Ventricular tachycardia. In Topol EJ [ed]: Comprehensive Cardiovascular Medicine, p. 1935. Philadelphia, Lippincott Williams & Wilkins)

initiated immediately on detection of VF and continued until organized ventricular activity is restored.

Bradyarrhythmias

Transient bradyarrhythmias sometimes occur, particularly in the early postoperative period after cardiac surgery. Responsible factors are thought to include perioperative beta blockade, the use of intraoperative antiarrhythmic agents, and metabolic damage from cardioplegic solution (Landolfo & Smith, 1995).

SINUS BRADYCARDIA
Origin: sinus node
Rate: less than 60 beats per minute
Rhythm: regular

Complex: PQRST
P-R Interval: 0.12 to 0.20 second
QRS Duration: 0.04 to 0.10 second

Sinus bradycardia is a rhythm that originates in the sinus node but with a discharge rate less than 60 beats per minute. It can occur (1) as a normal variant, particularly in athletes or during sleep; (2) in response to vagal stimulation, such as with carotid sinus massage or vomiting; (3) as a result of medications, such as digoxin, beta-adrenergic blocking agents, or calcium channel antagonists; and (4) secondary to disease processes, such as inferior myocardial infarction or sick sinus syndrome (Jacobson, 1995).

In most patients, sinus bradycardia is well tolerated. Often, discontinuance of a precipitating medication, such as digoxin, is the only required treatment. In the immediate postoperative period when there is an

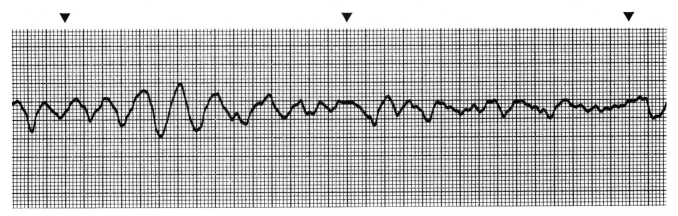

FIGURE 25-8. Ventricular fibrillation. (Huff J, 1997: Ventricular arrhythmias and bundle branch block. In ECG Workout: Exercises in Arrhythmia Interpretation, ed. 3, p. 206. Philadelphia, Lippincott-Raven)

increase in circulating catecholamines, a sinus rate less than 80 beats per minute is considered a relative bradycardia (Mackall et al., 1996). Relative bradycardia also can occur in critically ill patients in response to vasovagal reactions that may or may not be accompanied by an overt manifestation, such as nausea or vomiting (Drew & Ide, 1996a). Patients with underlying ventricular dysfunction in particular may benefit from temporarily increasing the heart rate to augment cardiac output. Either atrial, AV synchronous, or ventricular temporary pacing may be used to increase heart rate during sinus bradycardia. Atrial (if AV nodal function is normal) or AV synchronous pacing is preferable because the atrial contribution to ventricular filling is preserved. In patients without epicardial pacing wires, atropine or isoproterenol may be administered. Atropine is given as an intravenous bolus, and isoproterenol is given by continuous intravenous infusion. Both drugs, if effective, increase heart rate within several minutes. Transthoracic or transvenous pacing also may be used.

Sinus bradycardia usually is present in the early postoperative period after heart transplantation because the donor heart is no longer innervated by the autonomic nervous system. Because of the loss of vagal influence in the denervated donor heart, atropine is ineffective in treating postoperative bradycardia after heart transplantation (Hudak et al., 1998). Isoproterenol (which works directly on beta-adrenergic receptors in the myocardium) or temporary pacing is used alternatively. Sinus node dysfunction also can occur after operations to correct congenital heart defects, specifically the Mustard procedure and repair of atrial septal defect (Mackall et al., 1996).

When sinus node function is depressed, secondary pacemakers, such as the AV node, bundle of His and its branches, or the Purkinje fibers, can form stimuli to initiate the cardiac rhythm (Goldberger, 1990b). Depending on the site of impulse formation, an idiojunctional or idioventricular rhythm results.

IDIOJUNCTIONAL RHYTHM (FIG. 25-9)

Origin: AV nodal tissue
Rate: 40 to 60 beats per minute
Rhythm: regular
Waveform Appearance: P'QRST, QRST, or QRST P'
P-R Interval: if present, less than 0.12 second
QRS Duration: 0.04 to 0.10 second

Idiojunctional rhythm originates in the AV node and depolarizes the atria and ventricles almost simultaneously. It usually is transient and, in postoperative cardiac surgical patients, usually is treated with temporary atrial or AV synchronous pacing to increase heart rate.

IDIOVENTRICULAR RHYTHM

Origin: ventricular tissue
Rate: 25 to 40 beats per minute
Rhythm: regular or irregular
Waveform Appearance: QRST
P-R Interval: none
QRS Duration: greater than 0.12 second

An *idioventricular* or *ventricular escape rhythm* occurs rarely as a result of complete heart block or suppression of higher pacemakers. The combination of the excessively slow rate and the loss of AV synchrony usually produces symptomatic hypotension. Temporary AV synchronous or ventricular pacing is performed until an acceptable heart rhythm resumes or a permanent pacemaker is placed.

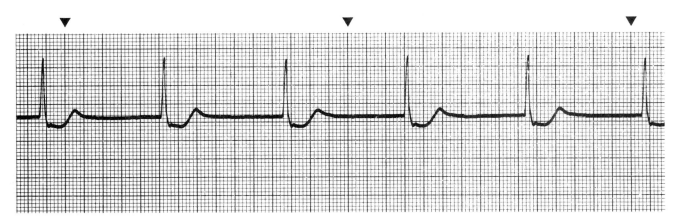

FIGURE 25-9. Junctional rhythm with heart rate of 47 beats per minute; note absence of P waves. (Huff J, 1997: AV junctional arrhythmias and AV blocks. In ECG Workout: Exercises in Arrhythmia Interpretation, ed. 3, p. 149. Philadelphia, Lippincott-Raven)

Heart Block

Heart block describes arrhythmias in which there is some degree of impairment in transmission of electrical impulses through the AV node. Acquired AV block most commonly is caused by idiopathic fibrosis, acute myocardial infarction, or drug effects (Wolbrette & Naccarelli, 1998). With advanced age, there is an increasing incidence of AV block progressing to complete heart block, most commonly appearing in the seventh decade of life (Ide & Drew, 1998). In cardiac surgical patients, heart block also can result from edema or trauma during intraoperative surgical manipulation of the heart.

FIRST-DEGREE HEART BLOCK

Origin: sinus node

Rate: 60 to 100 beats per minute

Rhythm: regular

Waveform Appearance: PQRST

P-R Interval: greater than 0.20 second

QRS Duration: 0.04 to 0.10 second

In *first-degree heart block,* all impulses are conducted through the AV node, bundle of His, and bundle branches, but at a slower-than-normal rate. The arrhythmia does not produce any abnormality in rate or rhythm. First-degree heart block may result from increased vagal tone, several pharmacologic agents (eg, digoxin or beta-blocking medications), a number of disease entities (eg, acute myocardial infarction or ischemic heart disease), or may be present in otherwise normal subjects and in well-trained athletes (Hillis et al., 1995f).

SECOND-DEGREE HEART BLOCK—MOBITZ TYPE I (FIG. 25-10)

Origin: sinus node

Rate:

Atrial—60 to 100 beats per minute

Ventricular—slightly less than atrial rate, because some atrial complexes are not conducted

Rhythm:

Atrial—P-P interval regular

Ventricular—irregular repetitive cycles of "group beating"

Waveform Appearance: PQRST, intermittent nonconducted P waves

P-R Interval: progressively lengthens until P wave is not followed by QRS, then cycle begins again

QRS Duration: 0.04 to 0.10 second

Second-degree heart block describes the condition in which some atrial impulses are conducted to the ventricles and some are not. If the P-R interval progressively lengthens from cycle to cycle until an atrial impulse is not conducted, the arrhythmia is termed *Mobitz type I,* or *Wenckebach, second-degree heart block.* After each nonconducted P wave, a new cycle begins with a normal or slightly prolonged P-R interval (McGuire, 1982). Examining multiple electrocardiographic leads is helpful in identifying four characteristic features of the Wenckebach phenomenon: (1) QRS complexes appear in groups, (2) R-R intervals tend to decrease following the pause, (3) the pause is less than two of the short cycles, and (4) there is a gradual lengthening of the P-R interval (Drew & Ide, 1996b).

SECOND-DEGREE HEART BLOCK—MOBITZ TYPE II

Origin: sinus node

Rate:

Atrial—60 to 100 beats per minute

Ventricular—slightly less than atrial rate, because some atrial complexes are not conducted

Rhythm:

Atrial—P-P interval regular

Ventricular—regular unless AV conduction ratio varies

Waveform Appearance: PQRST, intermittent nonconducted P waves

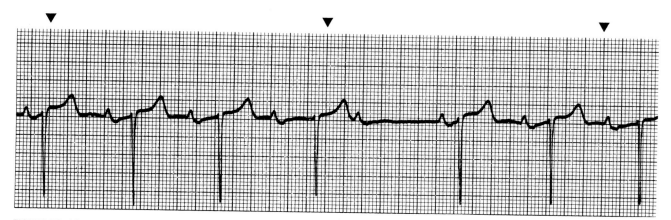

FIGURE 25-10. Mobitz I second-degree heart block. Note that P-R interval progressively lengthens (0.2 to 0.48 second) followed by nonconducted P wave and repetition of P-R interval lengthening. (Huff J, 1997: AV junctional arrhythmias and AV blocks. In ECG Workout: Exercises in Arrhythmia Interpretation, ed. 3, p. 152. Philadelphia, Lippincott-Raven)

P-R Interval: normal or prolonged, but not all P waves are conducted

QRS Duration: usually more than 0.10 second

In *Mobitz type II second-degree heart block,* some atrial impulses are conducted to the ventricles and some are not, but the P-R interval remains constant. The QRS complex almost always is widened because the block is infranodal in location, in the bundle and one or both branches or in the Purkinje fibers (Hillis et al., 1995f; Goldberger, 1990b). Mobitz type II heart block is more likely than Mobitz type I to progress to complete heart block and usually requires permanent cardiac pacing.

THIRD-DEGREE HEART BLOCK (COMPLETE HEART BLOCK) (FIG. 25-11)

Rate:

    Atrial—60 to 100 beats per minute

    Ventricular—25 to 60 beats per minute, depending on whether escape rhythm originates in AV nodal or ventricular tissue

Rhythm:

    Atrial—P-P interval regular

    Ventricular—R-R interval regular

    Atrial and ventricular activity unrelated

Waveform Appearance: QRST, P waves independent of QRS complexes

P-R Interval: none

QRS Duration: normal or wide

In *third-degree,* or *complete heart block,* no atrial impulses are conducted successfully to the ventricles. Instead, atrial and ventricular activity occurs independent of one another; that is, AV dissociation is present. Third-degree heart block is recognized by an atrial rate that is faster than the ventricular rate and the absence of a predictable relationship between the two (Gray & Mandel, 1990).

Transient heart block occasionally occurs in postoperative cardiac surgical patients, particularly those who have undergone valvular procedures. It is most likely the result of trauma and subsequent edema of the AV node (Mackall et al., 1996). In all forms of heart block, the electrocardiogram (ECG) is monitored. Possible pharmacologic precipitants, such as digoxin, are discontinued. Second- or third-degree heart block associated with significant bradycardia is treated with temporary AV synchronous or ventricular pacing. Postoperative heart block usually resolves within 1 to 2 weeks. If not, implantation of a permanent, transvenous pacemaker may be necessary.

► Differentiation of Wide QRS Tachycardias

Aberrancy is the abnormal intraventricular conduction of supraventricular impulses. Sometimes all supraventricular impulses are conducted aberrantly because of a fixed intraventricular conduction disturbance, such as right or left bundle branch block. In other cases, conduction of supraventricular impulses may be normal during sinus rhythm but become aberrant when the heart rate increases or an impulse occurs prematurely. The degree of aberrancy depends on the refractory state of the bundles when the impulse is conducted. If a premature complex is only slightly early, the complex is slightly abnormal; if it occurs earlier after the preceding complex, it may be extremely widened and bizarre. A premature complex that is very early finds all the fascicles refractory, and the impulse is not conducted.

Supraventricular tachycardia with aberrant conduction produces a widened QRS complex and altered T wave that often causes it to be mistaken for VT. Differentiation between VT and SVT with aberrancy is quite important, and yet it is often difficult for experienced physicians and nurses (Cooper & Marriott, 1989). Sometimes, the presence or absence of associated symptoms

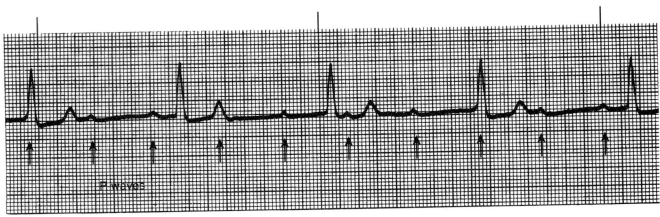

FIGURE 25-11. Complete heart block. Note presence of AV dissociation with regular ventricular rate of 38 beats per minute and regular atrial rate of 88 beats per minute. Arrows demonstrate P waves. (Huff J, 1997: AV junctional arrhythmias and AV blocks. In ECG Workout: Exercises in Arrhythmia Interpretation, ed. 3, p. 145. Philadelphia, Lippincott-Raven)

distinguishes the arrhythmias. VT usually produces hemodynamic deterioration and SVT does not. However, VT without symptoms or SVT with symptoms can occur.

The therapeutic implications of misdiagnosis are significant. VT that remains untreated can lead to hemodynamic compromise or cardiac arrest due to VF. An important clinical guideline is that as many as 95% of wide QRS complex tachycardias in patients with underlying cardiac disease represent VT (Marino, 1998). Thus, in postoperative patients, and in patients with a history of myocardial infarction or congestive heart failure, it should be assumed that wide QRS complex tachycardias are ventricular in origin. It also is important that verapamil, sometimes used to treat SVT, not be given to a patient with VT; it is ineffective in terminating VT and, more important, its negative inotropic effect is likely to cause hemodynamic instability with deterioration of the arrhythmia into VF or asystole (Drew & Ide, 1998).

The first response to the occurrence of a wide QRS tachycardia is assessment of the patient's hemodynamic status and, if necessary, initiation of resuscitative measures. In general, it is safer to err in the direction of treating aberrancy as if it were VT rather than failing to treat ventricular arrhythmias appropriately. If the patient is stable and there is a question about whether a rhythm represents VT or SVT with aberrancy, a 12-lead ECG and a long rhythm tracing are obtained. The patient is monitored closely for hemodynamic sequelae of the arrhythmia, which are treated as necessary.

A number of electrocardiographic criteria have been identified that can assist in diagnosing wide QRS tachycardias. Morphology of the QRS complex in the precordial leads is one distinguishing feature. Although an aberrantly conducted impulse can produce any form of widened QRS, a right bundle branch block (RBBB) morphology of the ectopic complexes (rSR′ in lead V_1 and qRS in V_6) is most typical (Fig. 25-12). The right bundle is the longest, thinnest fascicle of the bundle branch system and has the longest refractory period. If a supraven-

tricular impulse is conducted through the AV node before the right bundle is totally repolarized from the previous depolarization, the impulse cannot travel through the right bundle normally and the ventricular portion of the complex is widened with a RBBB configuration.

A second electrocardiographic feature suggesting SVT with aberrancy is ectopic beats that occur after a short R-R interval preceded by a long R-R interval. Refractory time of the bundles varies directly with the interval between ventricular depolarizations; the longer the R-R interval, the longer is the refractory period that follows it. The R wave after the short interval is likely to be conducted aberrantly, displaying a RBBB morphology. Aberrancy caused by R-R interval variation is termed *Ashman's phenomenon*. It often occurs in association with atrial fibrillation because of the irregularity of the rhythm, with long R-R intervals followed frequently by short R-R intervals. Ashman's phenomenon also may occur during sinus arrhythmias with pronounced R-R interval variation or with PACs that have a short coupling interval.

Aberrancy also may be suggested by recognition of a P wave superimposed on the T wave preceding the QRS complex (Petrie, 1988). SVT with aberrancy is likely if the rate and rhythm of the P wave and QRS complex are linked, suggesting that ventricular activation depends on the atrial impulse. In postoperative cardiac surgical patients, an atrial electrogram may unmask the presence of P waves preceding and linked to each QRS complex. Other electrocardiographic manifestations suggesting SVT with aberrancy are listed in Table 25-1.

Table 25-2 lists those features that favor a diagnosis of VT. Although QRS width can be greater than 0.14 second with aberrancy and less than 0.14 second with VT, in general, the wider the QRS complex, the more likely it is that the tachycardia is ventricular in origin (Wellens, 1998) (Fig. 25-13). Other characteristic electrocardiographic manifestations of isolated ventricular complexes include a left bundle branch morphology, full compensatory pauses, a fixed coupling interval, and

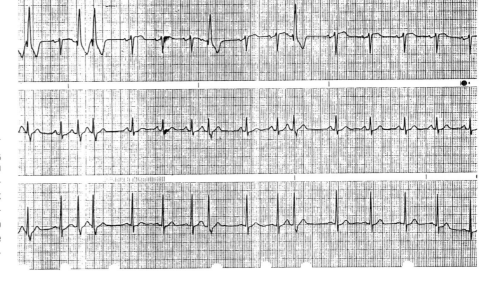

FIGURE 25-12. Simultaneous rhythm tracings of leads V_1 (*top*), II (*middle*), and V_5 (*bottom*) demonstrate sinus rhythm with aberrantly conducted premature atrial contractions. Note right bundle branch block configuration (rSR′ in V_1, qRs in V_5) of aberrant beats. Supraventricular origin is also revealed by ectopic P wave preceding wide QRS complexes. (Courtesy of Linda Hellstedt, RN, MS)

multiform complexes. If the ECG demonstrates a left bundle branch block tachycardia (negative complex in V_1), the following criteria provide further support of a ventricular origin of the tachycardia: (1) notch on the S wave downstroke in V_1 or V_2, (2) QRS onset to S nadir interval greater than 0.06 second in leads V_1 or V_2, and (3) no Q wave in lead V_6 (Drew & Ide, 1998). If the wide QRS complexes are predominantly positive in lead V_1, a QR configuration or a taller left peak notched pattern both provide strong evidence for a diagnosis of VT (Drew & Ide, 1994).

Ventricular tachycardia is most easily confirmed by identification of AV dissociation. AV dissociation has long been considered a hallmark of VT, but it does not always occur and, uncommonly, it occurs during SVT (Zipes, 1997). An atrial electrogram may reveal an independent atrial rhythm that is obscured on the surface ECG. The dissociated atrial rate usually is slower than the ventricular rate, unless an atrial tachycardia also is present (Wellens, 1998). The presence of fusion or capture beats also indicates AV dissociation and a ventricular origin of the tachycardia, but the presence of these complexes is rare (Jacobson, 1995).

REFERENCES

Conover MB, 1996: Atrial flutter. In Understanding Electrocardiography, ed. 7. St. Louis, Mosby–Year Book

Cooper J, Marriott HJ, 1989: Why are so many critical care nurses unable to recognize ventricular tachycardia in the 12-lead electrocardiogram? Heart Lung 18:243

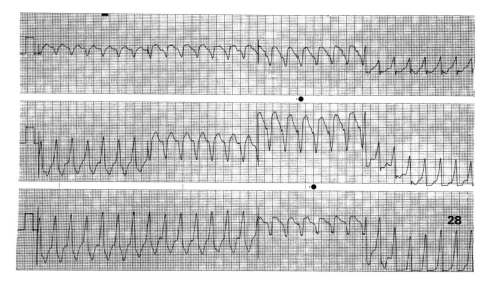

FIGURE 25-13. Twelve-lead ECG demonstrating ventricular tachycardia. Findings suggestive of the diagnosis include a QRS complex duration greater than 0.14 second and a left bundle branch block configuration. (Courtesy of Richard Davison, MD)

Drew BJ, 1987: Differentiation of wide QRS complex tachycardias. Prog Cardiovasc Nurs 2:130

Drew BJ, Ide B, 1994: Aberration versus ectopy. Prog Cardiovasc Nurs 9(3):46

Drew BJ, Ide B, 1996a: "Relative" sinus bradycardia. Prog Cardiovasc Nurs 11(3):47

Drew BJ, Ide B, 1996b: An arrhythmia known by its tracks. Prog Cardiovasc Nurs 11(2):46

Drew BJ, Ide B, 1998: Differential diagnosis of wide QRS complex tachycardia. Prog Cardiovasc Nurs 13(3):46

Elefteriades JA, Geha AS, Cohen LS, 1996: Arrhythmias. In House Officer Guide to ICU Care: Fundamentals of Management of the Heart and Lungs, ed. 2. Philadelphia, Lippincott-Raven

Erickson BA, 1991: Dysrhythmias. In Kinney MR, Packa DR, Andreoli KG, Zipes DP (eds): Comprehensive Cardiac Care, ed. 7. St. Louis, Mosby–Year Book

Finkelmeier BA, Salinger MH, 1984: The atrial electrogram: Its diagnostic use following cardiac surgery. Critical Care Nurse 4:42

Goldberger E, 1990a: Disorders of cardiac rhythm. In Essentials of Clinical Cardiology. Philadelphia, JB Lippincott

Goldberger E, 1990b: The cardiac arrhythmias. In Treatment of Cardiac Emergencies, ed. 5. St. Louis, CV Mosby

Gray RJ, Mandel WJ, 1990: Management of common postoperative arrhythmias. In Gray RJ, Matloff JM (eds): Medical Management of the Cardiac Surgical Patient. Baltimore, Williams & Wilkins

Hillis LD, Lange RA, Winniford MD, Page RL, 1995a: Sinus tachycardia, sinus bradycardia, and sinus arrhythmia. In Manual of Clinical Problems in Cardiology, ed. 5. Boston, Little, Brown

Hillis LD, Lange RA, Winniford MD, Page RL, 1995b: Premature beats. In Manual of Clinical Problems in Cardiology, ed. 5. Boston, Little, Brown

Hillis LD, Lange RA, Winniford MD, Page RL, 1995c: Paroxysmal supraventricular tachycardia. In Manual of Clinical Problems in Cardiology, ed. 5. Boston, Little, Brown

Hillis LD, Lange RA, Winniford MD, Page RL, 1995d: Atrial flutter. In Manual of Clinical Problems in Cardiology, ed. 5. Boston, Little, Brown

Hillis LD, Lange RA, Winniford MD, Page RL, 1995e: Ventricular tachycardia and ventricular fibrillation. In Manual of Clinical Problems in Cardiology, ed. 5. Boston, Little, Brown

Hillis LD, Lange RA, Winniford MD, Page RL, 1995f: Atrioventricular block. In Manual of Clinical Problems in Cardiology, ed. 5. Boston, Little, Brown

Hohnloser SH, 1997: Proarrhythmia with class III antiarrhythmic drugs: Types, risks, and management. Am J Cardiol 80(8A):82G

Hudak CM, Gallo BM, Morton PG, 1998: Organ and hemopoietic stem cell transplantation. In Critical Care Nursing, ed. 7. Philadelphia, Lippincott Williams & Wilkins

Huff J, 1997a: Sinus arrhythmias. In ECG Workout: Exercises in Arrhythmia Interpretation, ed. 3. Philadelphia, Lippincott-Raven

Huff J, 1997b: Atrial arrhythmias. In ECG Workout: Exercises in Arrhythmia Interpretation, ed. 3. Philadelphia, Lippincott-Raven

Ide B, Drew BJ, 1998: Cardiac arrhythmias with aging. Prog Cardiovasc Nurs 13:31

Jacobson C, 1995: Arrhythmias and conduction disturbances. In Woods SL, Froelicher ESS, Halpenny CJ, Motzer SU (eds): Cardiac Nursing, ed. 3. Philadelphia, JB Lippincott

Kastor JA, 1991: Supraventricular tachyarrhythmias. In Horowitz LN (ed): Current Management of Arrhythmias. Philadelphia, BC Decker

Landolfo K, Smith PK, 1995: Postoperative care in cardiac surgery. In Sabiston DC Jr, Spencer FC (eds): Surgery of the Chest, ed. 6. Philadelphia, WB Saunders

Mackall JA, Buchter CM, Thames MD, 1996: Pharmacological approach to the management of the cardiac surgical patient. In Baue AE, Geha AS, Hammond GL, et al. (eds): Glenn's Thoracic and Cardiovascular Surgery, ed. 6. Stamford, CT, Appleton & Lange

Marino PL, 1998: Tachyarrhythmias. In The ICU Book, ed. 2. Baltimore, Williams & Wilkins

McGuire LB, 1982: Cardiac rhythms. In Beckwith JR (ed): Basic Electrocardiography and Vectorcardiography. New York, Raven Press

Petrie JR, 1988: Distinguishing supraventricular aberrancies from ventricular ectopy. Focus on Critical Care 15:15

Prystowsky EN, Katz A, 1998: Atrial fibrillation. In Topol EJ (ed): Comprehensive Cardiovascular Medicine. Philadelphia, Lippincott Williams & Wilkins

Sundt TM, Cox JL, 1998: Maze III procedure for atrial fibrillation. In Kaiser LR, Kron IL, Spray TL (eds): Mastery of Cardiothoracic Surgery. Philadelphia, Lippincott Williams & Wilkins

Tchou PJ, 1998: Ventricular tachycardia. In Topol EJ (ed): Comprehensive Cardiovascular Medicine. Philadelphia, Lippincott Williams & Wilkins

Wellens HJ, 1998: The electrocardiographic diagnosis of atrial arrhythmias. In Topol EJ (ed): Comprehensive Cardiovascular Medicine. Philadelphia, Lippincott Williams & Wilkins

White J, 1998: Disorders of cardiac conduction and rhythm. In Porth CM (ed): Pathophysiology: Concepts of Altered Health States, ed. 5. Philadelphia, Lippincott Williams & Wilkins

Wilkinson DV, 1991: Supraventricular premature complexes. In Horowitz LN (ed): Current Management of Arrhythmias. Philadelphia, BC Decker

Wolbrette DL, Naccarelli GV, 1998: Sinus nodal disturbances and AV conduction disturbances. In Topol EJ (ed): Comprehensive Cardiovascular Medicine. Philadelphia, Lippincott Williams & Wilkins

Zipes DP, 1997: Specific arrhythmias: Diagnosis and treatment. In Braunwald E (ed): Heart Disease: A Textbook of Cardiovascular Medicine, ed. 5. Philadelphia, WB Saunders

26

Temporary Pacing and Defibrillation

▶ Temporary Pacing

Temporary pacing is an important modality for treating postoperative cardiac arrhythmias. Bradycardia and, in selected instances, tachycardia, often can be managed effectively with pacing therapy. Goals that can be achieved include one or more of the following: (1) augmentation of cardiac output by increasing heart rate, (2) provision of a safe minimum heart rate, (3) provision of atrioventricular (AV) synchrony, and (4) suppression of arrhythmias. Temporary pacing can be initiated and discontinued rapidly and avoids the adverse effects of antiarrhythmic medications. It may be used alone or in combination with pharmacologic therapy.

Components of the System

The components of temporary pacing systems include pacing leads, a connecting cable, and a pulse generator. The pacing leads and connecting cable provide a pathway between the external pulse generator and the myocardium. Through this pathway, stimulating current travels to the heart and sensed depolarization signals travel to the pulse generator. In patients who undergo cardiac surgical procedures, pacing leads consist of insulated, flexible wires attached to the epicardial surfaces of the right atrium and ventricle (Fig. 26-1). Atrial wires are placed by affixing the noninsulated tip of the wire to the thin-walled atrial surface with suture; for ventricular wires, the noninsulated tip is passed into the anterior ventricular myocardial wall at a spot free of fat (Elefteriades et al., 1996a). Atrial pacing wires, in addition to their therapeutic purpose, may be used diagnostically to obtain atrial electrograms for arrhythmia identification.

Atrial electrograms are discussed in Chapter 24, Twelve-Lead Electrocardiography and Atrial Electrograms.

Each pacing wire has an electrode (ie, electrically conductive material) located at its epicardial end. The electrode is positioned securely in the atrial or ventricular myocardium, yet can be removed easily when traction is applied to the external end of the pacing wire. Two electrodes are required to complete the electrical circuit, a pacing electrode and an indifferent electrode. The system is termed *bipolar* if both electrodes are attached to the chamber being paced, and *unipolar* if only the pacing electrode is attached to the chamber being paced. Bipolar systems are less susceptible to electromagnetic interference, defined as any signal, biologic or nonbiologic, that falls within a frequency spectrum that may be detected by the sensing circuitry of the pacemaker, and that may result in rate alteration or sensing abnormalities (Medtronic 5348 Technical Manual, 1997; Hayes, 1998). Placement of bipolar wires approximately 2 cm apart in the chamber to be paced and into a superficial layer of myocardium ensures proper sensing and capture if the leads remain intact (Mehta & Pae, 1997).

By convention, pacing wires attached to the atrial epicardium are brought out through the chest wall to the right of the sternotomy incision (ie, the patient's right side) and ventricular wires are brought out to the left of the incision (Fig. 26-2). A ground wire for use as an indifferent electrode usually is placed in the subcutaneous tissue. Ground wires are usually of a different color than pacing wires or are identified by a small clip attached to the wire. If emergent pacing becomes necessary in the absence of a second epicardial or a ground wire, a 21-gauge needle inserted tangentially through the subcutaneous tissue may be used alternatively as the indifferent electrode (Moreno-Cabral et al., 1988).

The pulse generator provides the power source. It is

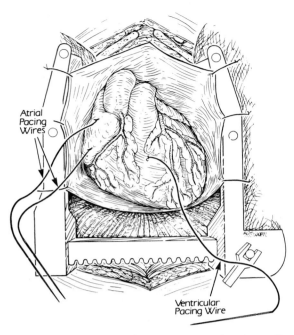

FIGURE 26-1. Placement of atrial and ventricular pacing wires on the epicardial surface of heart. (Finkelmeier BA, O'Mara SR, 1984: Temporary pacing in the cardiac surgical patient. Critical Care Nurse 4:109)

programmed to discharge electric current of sufficient strength to depolarize myocardial tissue. Pacing is achieved by connecting the epicardial wire from the cardiac chamber to be paced to the negative pole of the connecting cable. A second wire from the same chamber or a ground wire is attached to the positive terminal. The connecting cable in turn is attached to the pulse generator, with negative and positive terminals correctly matched

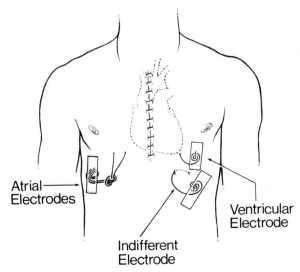

FIGURE 26-2. Position of atrial and ventricular pacing wires and indifferent electrode on chest wall after sternotomy incision has been closed. (Finkelmeier BA, O'Mara SR, 1984: Temporary pacing in the cardiac surgical patient. Critical Care Nurse 4:109)

with those of the pulse generator. Two types of external pulse generators are used for temporary pacing in cardiac surgical patients: single-chamber and dual-chamber pulse generators. Available models of temporary single-chamber (eg, Medtronic 5348) and dual-chamber (eg, Medtronic 5388) pulse generators can be used both for antibradycardia pacing and for rapid atrial pacing (RAP).

Pacing Modes

A coding system devised by the North American Society of Pacing and Electrophysiology (NASPE) and British Pacing and Electrophysiology Group (BPEG) provides standard nomenclature for describing pulse generator functions (Bernstein et al., 1987). The *NBG (NASPE/BPEG) generic) pacemaker code* comprises five categories that define pacing mode or type of pulse generator function. The letter in the first position signifies the chamber in which pacing can occur. "A" signifies atrial pacing only; "V," ventricular pacing only; and "D," pacing in both atrial and ventricular chambers. Similarly, the letter "A," "V," or "D" in the second position denotes chambers in which sensing of intrinsic cardiac activity occurs. The letter "O" signifies that sensing is not possible in either chamber. The letter in the third position designates pulse generator response to sensed cardiac activity. "I" signifies that sensed activity inhibits the pulse generator from firing; "T," that intrinsic activity produces a triggered pacing impulse; and "D," that both inhibited and triggered responses can occur. Dual response to sensed activity occurs only with dual-chamber pulse generators; a sensed event in the atrium inhibits the atrial output but triggers a ventricular output after a delay that simulates the P-R interval (Hayes, 1998). The fourth and fifth categories refer to rate modulation and antitachycardia functions and are not relevant to temporary pacing. Table 26-1 displays features of pacing modes commonly used for temporary pacing.

TABLE 26-1

Common Modes of Temporary Cardiac Pacing

Setting	NBG Pacing Mode			
	AAI	VVI	DDI	DDD
Pacing	A	V	A & V	A & V
Sensing	A	V	A & V	A & V
Atrial output	On	Off	On	On
Ventricular output	Off	On	On	On
Atrial sensitivity	On	Off	On	On
Ventricular sensitivity	Off	On	On	On
Atrial tracking	Off	Off	Off	On

A, atrial; V, ventricular.
Adapted from Medtronic 5388 Technical Manual, 1997: Minneapolis, Medtronic.

Single-Chamber Pacing

Indications

Single-chamber pacing is used to provide a consistent minimum heart rate while avoiding undesirable effects of chronotropic medications. Either atrial or ventricular pacing may be performed, using a pulse generator designed for single-chamber pacing (Fig. 26-3). If AV nodal function is normal, atrial pacing is preferable to ventricular pacing because AV synchrony and the atrial contribution to ventricular filling are preserved. An appropriately timed atrial contraction increases stroke volume by 5% to 15% in the normal heart, and is of even greater clinical significance in the presence of left ventricular hypertrophy or heart failure (Spotnitz, 1997). AV synchrony improves cardiac output through several mechanisms: (1) atrial systole increases ventricular filling; (2) the atria empty more completely, resulting in increased venous return; (3) appropriately timed closing of the mitral and tricuspid valves prevents regurgitation across open valves during ventricular systole; and (4) retrograde activation of the atria is avoided.

Temporary *atrial (AAI) pacing* is performed in patients with sinus bradycardia and normal AV nodal function. It also may be used to increase heart rate in patients with impaired left ventricular function and relative bradycardia. For patients with low cardiac output after cardiac surgery, manipulation of heart rate provides an important means of augmenting hemodynamic performance. A heart rate in the range of 90 to 100 beats per minute usually provides the best cardiac output during the early postoperative period (Geha & Whittlesey, 1996). In addition, atrial pacing occasionally is used to increase heart rate to suppress premature atrial or ventricular complexes. Pacing the atrium is ineffective in the presence of atrial flutter, atrial fibrillation, or AV nodal dysfunction; atrial capture cannot be achieved during atrial flutter or atrial fibrillation and, in the presence of a dysfunctional AV node, paced atrial impulses are not transmitted to the ventricles.

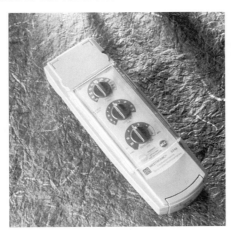

FIGURE 26-3. Medtronic 5348 single-chamber pulse generator used for temporary atrial or ventricular pacing. (Courtesy of Medtronic, Minneapolis, MN)

Single-chamber *ventricular (VVI) pacing* formerly was the most common mode of temporary pacing in cardiac surgical patients. The availability of temporary pulse generators that provide reliable dual-chamber pacing in a demand mode has greatly expanded the use of dual-chamber pacing. Single-chamber ventricular pacing currently is used primarily to ensure an adequate heart rate in the presence of intermittent AV nodal dysfunction or sinus bradycardia. Other indications for ventricular pacing include suppression of ventricular ectopy and prophylaxis against profound bradycardia during the early hours after cardiac surgery or when administering medications that slow heart rate or AV conduction. Ventricular pacing also is used when chronic atrial fibrillation, intermittent supraventricular tachycardia (SVT), or the absence of atrial epicardial wires precludes atrial or AV synchronous pacing.

Technique of Pacing

Atrial pacing is performed by attaching an atrial epicardial wire to the negative terminal of the connecting cable and another atrial wire, or a ground wire, to the positive terminal. Atrial pacing is most reliable when a bipolar system is used. Ventricular pacing can be achieved similarly with either a bipolar (two ventricular wires) or unipolar (one ventricular wire and one ground wire) system. Three settings are programmed when using a single-chamber pulse generator: rate, output, and sensitivity. The *pacing rate* is selected based on the individual patient's needs. Typically, the initial setting is 70 to 80 beats per minute for bradycardic patients; a rate of 45 to 50 beats per minute is selected for patients who are not bradycardic but who are at risk for becoming so (Elefteriades et al., 1996a).

The *output setting* controls the amplitude of the pacing pulse, measured in milliamperes (mA), delivered to the heart with each pacemaker discharge. The correct setting for pulse generator output is established by determining the patient's *stimulation threshold*, defined as the minimum intensity of current needed to produce consistent depolarization of myocardial cells. To ascertain stimulation threshold, the output dial is set between 5 and 10 mA and the pacing rate is temporarily adjusted to exceed the patient's intrinsic heart rate by approximately 10 beats per minute. When this has been accomplished, the monitor should display a 100% paced cardiac rhythm with each pacing artifact immediately followed by an appropriate depolarization (ie, 1:1 capture). While the monitor is being observed, pulse generator output is decreased gradually until a loss of capture occurs, evidenced by the appearance of a pacing artifact that is not followed by a cardiac depolarization. The output setting is increased slowly until 1:1 capture is regained; the setting at which this occurs is the patient's stimulation threshold. The rate dial is readjusted to its desired position.

Stimulation threshold varies depending on the site of electrode placement and the state of the myocardium. Because threshold can be expected to increase over time as a result of fibrosis at the electrode–myocardium interface, output is set to a value that is at least twice as high as the patient's stimulation threshold and is measured daily. However, if the patient's intrinsic heart rate is rapid or the underlying rhythm is unstable, it may be preferable to defer daily measurements after establishing a safe milliamperage setting. Epicardial wires in general are very reliable, and an arbitrary setting of 10 to 15 mA is likely to produce consistent capture for 1 to 2 weeks. If high milliamperage settings are required, pacing discharges may cause an unpleasant twinge of pain or diaphragmatic pacing, evidenced by epigastric twitching or hiccups at a rate equal to the pacing rate (Finkelmeier & O'Mara, 1984).

The *sensitivity setting* allows adjustment of the pulse generator's sensing circuitry. Depending of the selected setting, voltage of a specified level (measured in millivolts [mV]) is detected and evokes a pulse generator response. Single-chamber pulse generators are capable only of inhibition in response to a sensed cardiac event—that is, a sensed depolarization in the atrium or ventricle inhibits delivery of a pacing discharge to that chamber. Pacing modes that provide an inhibition response to sensed depolarizations are referred to as *demand* or *synchronous modes*. The *sensing threshold* is the smallest signal that is detectable by the pulse generator. The less sensitive the pulse generator, the higher the voltage of cardiac depolarization necessary for sensing by the pulse generator. To determine the sensing threshold, the pacing rate is decreased to approximately 10 beats less than the patient's intrinsic heart rate (if the intrinsic cardiac rhythm is adequate) and the pulse generator output setting is dialed fully clockwise (0.1 mA) to avoid the risk of competitive pacing. The sensitivity dial is adjusted to a fully clockwise position (0.5 mV); flashing of the sense indicator light indicates sensing of the intrinsic heart rate. Pulse generator sensitivity then is decreased gradually (by increasing the millivoltage level required for sensing) until the sense indicator light stops flashing and the pace indicator light flashes continuously, indicating generation of pacing discharges because the device's ability to sense intrinsic cardiac depolarizations has been disabled.

Pulse generator sensitivity is then increased by adjusting the dial clockwise (ie, decreasing the millivoltage of intrinsic depolarizations that inhibit pulse generator firing) until the sense indicator begins flashing. The setting at which this occurs (ie, the patient's sensing threshold) should be at least 2 mV for P wave sensing (AAI mode) and at least 4 mV for R wave sensing (VVI mode) (Medtronic 5348 Technical Manual, 1997). Because lead maturation and drug therapy can affect the sensing threshold, the sensitivity setting is adjusted to at least twice as sensitive as the threshold value (ie, one half the millivoltage) to provide a margin of safety (Medtronic 5348 Technical Manual, 1997). The rate and output dials are then readjusted to appropriate settings. Adjustment of sensitivity threshold usually is omitted if the patient's heart rate is less than 60 beats per minute.

Single-chamber pacing of either the atrium or ventricle almost always is performed using a synchronous mode (AAI or VVI) to avoid pacemaker discharge during atrial or ventricular repolarization (R on T phenomenon), respectively. The pulse generator is inhibited unless the patient's intrinsic heart rate falls below the pacing rate. Thus, pacing occurs only when the pulse generator senses absence of intrinsic cardiac activity. If the patient has an inadequate underlying ventricular rhythm (heart rate <50 beats per minute), an asynchronous setting may be desirable to avoid profound bradycardia that might occur in the event of failure of the sensing function. Turning the sensitivity dial fully counterclockwise to the asynchronous position disables the sensing circuitry, allowing the pulse generator to pace asynchronously (Medtronic 5348 Technical Manual, 1997). Except for patients with an inadequate underlying cardiac rhythm, asynchronous pacing is not used.

Dual-Chamber Pacing

Indications

Dual-chamber pacing (ie, sequential pacing of the atrium and ventricle) provides significant hemodynamic benefits in certain clinical situations. AV synchronous pacing most commonly is performed in patients in whom it is important to preserve the atrial contribution to cardiac output but in whom single-chamber atrial pacing is precluded because of AV nodal dysfunction. Compared with ventricular pacing, AV synchronous pacing has been shown to improve cardiac output in patients with normal ventricular function, as well as in those with valvular heart disease, impaired ventricular function, recent cardiac surgery, and myocardial infarction (Finkelmeier & Salinger, 1986). AV synchronous pacing is not suitable for patients with atrial flutter or atrial fibrillation because successful capture of the atria by the pulse generator is not possible.

Dual-chamber pulse generators have two sets of terminals so that pacing electrodes for both the atrium and ventricle can be attached (Fig. 26-4). Bipolar pacing is recommended for dual-chamber pacing to avoid electromagnetic interference; epicardial leads should be positioned so that the atrial and ventricular electrodes are at least 1.5 inches apart and at right angles to one another (Medtronic 5388 Technical Manual, 1997). Adjustable parameters on a dual-chamber pulse generator include heart rate, output and sensitivity for both the atrium and ventricle, and the AV interval. The atrial and ventricular output settings control the amount of current delivered to the atrium and ventricle, respectively. The desired pacing rate is selected and stimulation thresholds are determined for both the atrial and ventricular electrodes in the manner described previously. Sensing thresholds are similarly determined for the atrial and ventricular circuits and the sensitivity setting is adjusted to approximately one half the measured threshold to avoid delivery of competitive discharges. Although a more sensitive setting may be selected, it may result in inappropriate sensing of far-field signals, such as atrial sensing of R or T

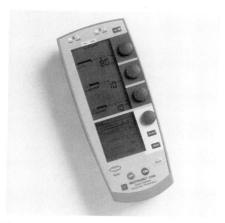

FIGURE 26-4. Medtronic 5388 dual-chamber pulse generator. (Courtesy of Medtronic, Minneapolis, MN)

waves or ventricular sensing of P waves (Medtronic 5388 Technical Manual, 1997).

The *AV interval setting* allows adjustment of the time interval between delivery of atrial and ventricular pacing discharges. The programmed AV interval simulates the P-R interval of an intrinsic cardiac depolarization. The optimal AV interval is thought to range from 150 to 175 milliseconds (msec), depending on the selected heart rate (Landolfo & Smith, 1995). Often, the AV interval setting is arbitrarily set at approximately 150 msec (0.15 second). This setting falls within the limits of the normal P-R interval (120 to 200 msec or 0.12 to 0.20 second). Programming a prolonged AV interval may result in pacing the ventricle during the vulnerable portion of ventricular repolarization, thus precipitating arrhythmias (Medtronic 5388 Technical Manual, 1997).

Pacing Modes

Dual-chamber pacing most commonly is performed using a DDI or DDD mode.

With *DDI pacing,* pacing and sensing occur in both the atrium and ventricle. Intrinsic atrial activity inhibits discharge of an atrial pacing impulse and intrinsic ventricular activity inhibits discharge of a ventricular impulse. When the intrinsic atrial rate is less than the pacing rate, the atrium is stimulated. An intrinsic or paced atrial depolarization is followed by either an intrinsic ventricular depolarization with inhibition of the ventricular pacing discharge, or a ventricular pacing discharge following the programmed AV interval. Because the only response to atrial sensing is inhibition, ventricular pacing occurs only at the programmed rate. DDI pacing may be selected when AV synchronous pacing is the primary pacing objective.

DDD pacing provides the sensing and pacing capabilities of DDI pacing plus a ventricular pacing rate that varies with changes in the rate of intrinsic atrial depolarization. This so-called *P-synchronous pacing* is achieved through atrial tracking; that is, the delivery of a triggered ventricular pacing impulse after each sensed

atrial depolarization. Changing from a DDI to a DDD mode enables the atrial tracking function. When atrial tracking is activated, each sensed intrinsic atrial event not only inhibits the scheduled atrial pacing discharge, but triggers an AV interval followed by a ventricular pacing discharge. Atrial tracking may provide an important contribution to cardiac output in selected patients.

A DDD mode is used in patients with normal sinus node function, AV nodal dysfunction, and the need for AV synchrony and rate variation according to physiologic needs. It is the most physiologic of the pacing modes, providing a composite of sensing and pacing in both the atrium and ventricle as required by the patient's underlying rhythm (Kleinschmidt & Stafford, 1991). Four different cardiac rhythms can occur as a result of normal DDD function: (1) normal sinus rhythm, (2) atrial pacing, (3) AV sequential pacing, and (4) P-synchronous pacing (Hayes, 1998). DDD pacing frequently is chosen as the mode of dual-chamber pacing in postoperative patients because both AV synchrony and physiologic increases in heart rate contribute to enhancing cardiac output.

Because DDD pacing allows sensing in the atrium to trigger a ventricular response, it is contraindicated in the presence of rapid atrial arrhythmias, such as atrial fibrillation or atrial flutter (Medtronic 5388 Technical Manual, 1997).

DDD pacing requires programming of two additional settings: the upper rate limit and the postventricular atrial refractory period (PVARP). Establishing an *upper rate limit* prevents tracking of SVT by activating a Wenckebach-type response when the sensed atrial rate exceeds the programmed upper rate limit. The upper rate limit affects only the paced ventricular rate; spontaneous SVT that is conducted normally through the AV node can result in ventricular pacing inhibition and a ventricular intrinsic rate that exceeds the upper rate limit of the pacemaker (Busch & Haskin, 1995).

The *postventricular atrial refractory period* is an interval following a ventricular event during which the pulse generator is unable to respond to sensed atrial activity with a triggered ventricular response. It prevents pacemaker-mediated tachycardia, a rapid ventricular paced rhythm that may occur when retrograde ventriculoatrial conduction is sensed and in turn triggers subsequent ventricular pacing discharges. Unless manually adjusted, the upper rate limit, AV interval, and PVARP usually are determined automatically by the selected pacing rate.

Rapid Atrial Pacing

Rapid atrial pacing is used specifically for treatment of paroxysmal atrial tachycardia or atrial flutter. The objectives of RAP are twofold: (1) conversion of the arrhythmia to normal sinus rhythm by overdrive atrial pacing, or (2) conversion to atrial fibrillation by stimulating the atrium during the vulnerable phase of atrial repolarization. Atrial fibrillation is more desirable than atrial flutter because the more rapid atrial depolarization rate increases the degree of AV block, thus slowing the ventricular rate. Also, digoxin is more effective in controlling the ventricular response rate in atrial fibrillation. In addition, atrial fibrillation induced by RAP usually is transient, lasting only briefly before converting to normal sinus rhythm (Waldo et al., 1984).

Rapid atrial pacing is performed with a single-chamber or dual-chamber pulse generator with RAP functionality. Enabling the RAP function allows delivery of pacing discharges at rates of up to 800 beats per minute. Because the generator has the capacity for such rapid pacing rates, it is essential that it be used only with atrial pacing wires. A ventricular wire is never used, even as the indifferent electrode. Ventricular pacing at such rapid rates would produce ventricular fibrillation and cardiac arrest. RAP is performed only by physicians or nurses who are thoroughly familiar with the procedure.

Two atrial wires or an atrial wire and ground wire are used for RAP. A bedside monitor always is used to allow observation of the electrocardiogram (ECG) during the procedure and a defibrillator should be readily available. The rapid atrial pulse function operates only in an asynchronous mode. The amplitude of pacing impulses delivered during RAP is adjusted using the pulse generator's output dial. An output setting of 15 to 20 mA usually is necessary to achieve atrial capture. The high threshold for atrial capture presumably is due to the relative refractoriness associated with a fast atrial rate (Zoble, 1989).

With the pulse generator appropriately attached to atrial pacing wires, pacing is initiated at a rate of 80 to 100 beats per minute to ensure that ventricular pacing does not occur. After adjusting the RAP rate setting to the desired level, a burst of RAP is delivered and terminated. Atrial capture may be evidenced by a change in P wave morphology, or may not be discernible on the ECG. Pacing usually is performed for 15 to 20 seconds and then abruptly terminated (Fig. 26-5). The sequence may be repeated several times if not initially successful in producing sinus rhythm or atrial fibrillation. Despite conversion with RAP, supraventricular arrhythmias can be expected to persist or recur as long as the responsible stimulus continues (Gray & Mandel, 1990). Therefore, RAP is accompanied by concomitant pharmacologic therapy and is most effective in patients in whom therapeutic serum digoxin levels are present.

Precautions and Common Problems

Although epicardial pacing wires almost never cause morbidity, certain precautions are important to ensure the patient's safety while the wires are in place. Most important, epicardial wires provide a direct, low-resistance current pathway to the myocardium. Therefore, the wires must be electrically isolated to prevent potential ventricular fibrillation caused by stimulation of the myocardium during the vulnerable portion of repolarization. The non-insulated external portion of the pacing wire is covered with a needle cap, finger cot, or nonconductive tape and secured to the chest when not in use. The entire pacing system must be protected from moisture. All line-powered equipment used on or in the vicinity of the patient must be properly grounded to avoid ventricular fibrillation resulting from alternating current leakage (Medtronic 5348 Technical Manual, 1997).

When temporary pacing is initiated and during any adjustments, bedside monitoring is used so that the cardiac rhythm can be observed while settings on the pulse generator are manipulated. All connections between the epicardial leads, cable, and pulse generator should be made before turning on the power. Any patient who requires temporary pacing also requires continuous cardiac monitoring, with either a bedside or a telemetry system. Lower alarm rates are set just below the programmed pacing rate so that pacing failure is detected promptly. Patients who require temporary pacing for an unstable heart rhythm or profound bradycardia should remain in a closely monitored setting until the problem resolves or a permanent pacemaker is implanted (Finkelmeier & O'Mara, 1984). An extra pulse generator should be readily available for immediate attachment in the event of pacing failure. During stimulation threshold measurements, sensing threshold measurements, and other adjustments, stimuli may be delivered inadvertently into a vulnerable period of the cardiac cycle; defibrillation equipment should be readily available (Medtronic 5348 Technical Manual, 1997). When discontinuing temporary pacing, gradual reduction of the pacing rate using the demand mode is recommended; abrupt termination of pacing stimuli may result in a period of asystole before an intrinsic rhythm ensues (Medtronic 5348 Technical Manual, 1997).

With any type of pacemaker malfunction, the first step is to assess the effect of the malfunction on the patient's hemodynamic status. If the patient is pacemaker

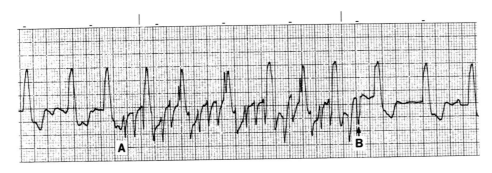

FIGURE 26-5. Electrocardiogram demonstrating successful conversion of atrial flutter with rapid atrial pacing: *A,* initiation of pacing at a rate of 450 beats per minute; *B,* termination of pacing is followed by restoration of normal sinus rhythm. (Finkelmeier BA, O'Mara SR, 1984: Temporary pacing in the cardiac surgical patient. Critical Care Nurse 4:110)

dependent, malfunction of the pacing system can lead to cardiac arrest. Cardiopulmonary resuscitation may be necessary if the problem is not corrected immediately or the pulse generator replaced with a properly functioning unit. More often, problems with temporary pacing systems do not pose an immediate threat to the patient's hemodynamic status. Still, it is important that any dysfunction be corrected promptly to ensure patient safety and obtain maximum benefit from the pacing system.

Two categories of pacemaker malfunction can occur: failure to pace and failure to sense. *Pacing failure* may be categorized as failure to discharge (ie, the absence of a pacing artifact at the programmed interval) or failure to capture, when a pacing artifact fails to initiate depolarization of the atrium or ventricle (Fig. 26-6). Pacing failure can result from a variety of factors, such as loosening of one of the system connections, the patient's stimulation threshold exceeding the current milliamperage setting, pulse generator battery depletion, or disconnection of the pacing wire from the epicardium of the heart. Occasionally, metabolic and acid–base abnormalities impede capture (Mehta & Pae, 1997).

When pacing failure occurs, all connections from the skin exit site of the pacing wire to the pulse generator itself are examined. The milliamperage setting is increased, and the pacing threshold is remeasured. If these steps fail to correct the problem, the battery and then the cable and pulse generator are replaced. It is unusual for a previously working system to fail to produce cardiac depolarizations when the milliamperage is adjusted to its maximal setting (20 mA). Inability to correct pacing failure with the aforementioned steps probably signifies that the pacing wire is no longer attached to the epicardium, even if it remains secured at the skin surface. If a second epicardial wire attached to the same cardiac chamber is in place, it may be used to replace the failed one.

If no other wire is available and the patient requires pacing, a temporary transvenous single-chamber or dual-chamber pacing catheter may be placed through the subclavian, internal jugular, or femoral vein. If emergent pacing is required, temporary pacing also can be achieved using a transcutaneous pulse generator and external chest wall electrodes. Transcutaneous pacing can be instituted quickly but is unlikely to be effective for cardiac asystole unless instituted early during resuscitation (Atlee, 1999). In dire emergencies, transthoracic pacing may be performed using a percutaneous pacing wire inserted directly into the right ventricle through a needle puncture in the anterior chest wall (Hudak et al., 1998; Spotnitz, 1997).

In patients with severe cardiogenic shock or cardiac arrest, electromechanical dissociation may occur; that is, pacing impulses and electrical depolarizations are present but they fail to produce mechanical contraction of the ventricles (Falk, 1997). This inability of the myocardium to generate a cardiac output in response to electrical stimulation is not pacing failure but rather electromechanical dissociation. It is invariably a terminal event.

Two types of *sensing failure* can occur. Undersensing occurs when the pulse generator delivers a pacing impulse before the pacing escape interval. It signifies failure to detect an intrinsic cardiac event (Fig. 26-7). Undersensing is one of the more common types of temporary pacemaker malfunction. Loss of the sensing function is often an early sign of battery depletion (Hickey & Baas, 1991). If it occurs when the sensitivity dial is adjusted to its most sensitive setting (fully clockwise), the battery, and if necessary the entire pacing system, is changed. If battery replacement does not solve the problem, the wire currently used as the indifferent lead can be replaced with another ground wire or, if possible, a pacing wire attached to the same chamber that is being paced. Changing the system from unipolar to bipolar, or vice versa, may correct the problem by providing a different, and larger, electrogram signal for sensing.

Oversensing, on the other hand, occurs when the pulse generator does not deliver a pacing impulse within the escape interval. In this case, pacing has been inappropriately inhibited by sensing of far field signals (eg, R or T wave sensing by the atrial lead or P wave sensing by the ventricular lead). The sensitivity dial can be adjusted

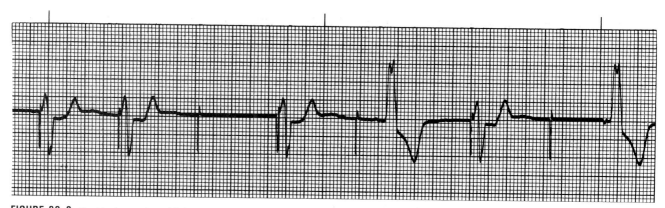

FIGURE 26-6. Ventricular pacing with intermittent failure to capture. From left to right, rhythm tracing displays two paced beats, a pacing artifact that does not produce ventricular depolarization (failure to capture), a paced beat, a pacing artifact without capture, an intrinsic beat, a paced beat, a pacing artifact without capture, and an intrinsic beat. (Huff J, 1997: Pacemakers. In ECG Workout: Exercises in Arrhythmia Interpretation, ed. 3, p. 236. Philadelphia, Lippincott-Raven)

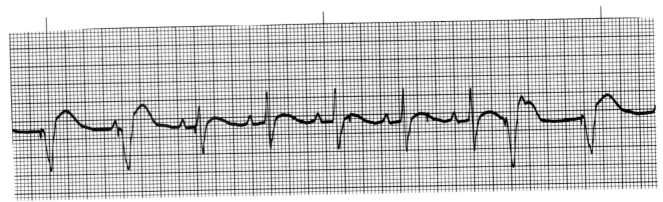

FIGURE 26-7. Undersensing is demonstrated by pacing discharges that represent failure to sense the fifth, sixth, and seventh complexes. From left to right, rhythm tracing displays two paced ventricular beats, a fusion beat (note pacing artifact at beginning of QRS complex and different QRS morphology), a sinus beat, two sinus beats with pacing artifacts in the T waves, a sinus beat, a paced beat that occurs too early, and a paced beat. (Huff J, 1997: Pacemakers. In ECG Workout: Exercises in Arrhythmia Interpretation. ed. 3, p. 240. Philadelphia, Lippincott-Raven)

to decrease pulse generator sensitivity so that oversensing does not inappropriately inhibit delivery of a pacing impulse. If this maneuver fails to correct the problem, all connections are inspected. The battery and, if necessary, the pulse generator and connecting cable, are changed.

A phenomenon known as *pacemaker syndrome* sometimes occurs with VVI pacing in patients who have alternating periods of sinus rhythm and ventricular pacing. It results from intermittent loss of AV synchrony with resultant valvular incompetence and retrograde activation of the atria (Hillis et al., 1995a). Pacemaker syndrome is characterized by a sudden decrease in blood pressure and cardiac output each time the atrial contribution to ventricular filling is lost (Finkelmeier & Salinger, 1986).

Potential problems when using a DDD pacing mode include the possibility of cross-talk between atrial and ventricular circuits and the potential for pacemaker-mediated tachycardia (Ferguson & Cox, 1991). *Crosstalk* is inappropriate sensing in one chamber of a pacing discharge or its afterpotential that was intended for the other chamber (Kleinschmidt & Stafford, 1991). Dualchamber pulse generators incorporate blanking periods to prevent cross-talk. The postatrial ventricular blanking period prevents the ventricular circuit from sensing an atrial pulse, and the postventricular atrial blanking period prevents the atrial circuit from sensing a ventricular pulse. However, the simultaneous use of a high-milliamperage (output) setting and maximum sensitivity (lowest millivoltage setting) should be avoided to prevent inappropriate sensing of far-field signals (eg, sensing of R or T waves on the atrial channel or P waves on the ventricular channel) (Medtronic 5388 Technical Manual, 1997).

Pacemaker-mediated tachycardia can occur when DDD pacing is performed in patients with intact ventriculoatrial, or retrograde, conduction pathways. It typically is initiated by a paced or spontaneous ectopic ventricular depolarization that is conducted in retrograde fashion, producing atrial depolarization. The sensed atrial depolarization triggers a paced ventricular depolarization that is again conducted to the atria, establishing an endless-loop tachycardia. The automatic, rate-dependent PVARP usually prevents pacemaker-mediated tachycardia. However, if retrograde P waves are being sensed outside the rate-dependent, automatic PVARP, the PVARP setting should be increased manually until the retrograde P waves fall inside the PVARP to avoid pacemaker-mediated tachycardia (Medtronic 5388 Technical Manual, 1997). Pacemaker-mediated tachycardia is terminated by disabling atrial sensing.

Epicardial pacing wires typically are removed the day before patient discharge from the hospital. In patients receiving anticoagulant therapy, the wires are removed before achieving therapeutic anticoagulation levels. The wires are removed with the patient in a supine position by severing the securing skin suture and applying gentle traction to the wires. Excessive pulling on epicardial wires may be painful, may cause serious damage, and should be avoided (Mehta & Pae, 1997). If an epicardial wire cannot be removed by the application of gentle traction, the entry site is swabbed with povidone-iodine or alcohol and, while applying gentle traction to the wire, it is cut off at the skin, allowing the remaining segment to retract beneath the skin surface.

It is essential that the patient be monitored for several hours after epicardial wire removal because of the rare but potentially lethal complication of cardiac tamponade caused by atrial or ventricular laceration during wire removal. Vital signs should be measured at 5, 15, and 30 minutes after removal of the epicardial wires. The patient is monitored for the presence of signs or symptoms of cardiac tamponade, including tachycardia, hypotension, tachypnea, chest pain, or a sense of foreboding. If any of these manifestations occur, the surgeon is notified immediately and examines the patient so that emergency thoracotomy can be performed if necessary to relieve the tamponade.

▶ Defibrillation

Defibrillation is the purposeful delivery of an electrical discharge to the heart to depolarize simultaneously the myocardial cells. If defibrillation is successful, the sinus node resumes its role as the dominant pacemaker and normal sinus rhythm ensues. Defibrillation is performed when emergent conversion of an arrhythmia is essential because of profound hypotension or cardiac arrest. Usually, the offending arrhythmia is ventricular tachycardia (VT) or ventricular fibrillation (VF). Occasionally, SVT with a rapid ventricular response produces hemodynamic compromise. Defibrillation is ineffective in converting asystole. However, a rhythm that appears to be asystole may in fact be a fine VF that may respond to defibrillation.

All nurses caring for cardiac surgical patients should be trained in use of a defibrillator so that response to a life-threatening arrhythmia is not delayed. Defibrillation is the single most effective resuscitative measure for improving survival in patients with cardiac arrest (Marino, 1998). Successful conversion of VT or VF is more effective than cardiopulmonary resuscitation. The probability of successful defibrillation is as high as 90% when it is performed immediately at the time of cardiac arrest (Hendrickson et al., 1997).

Electrode gel is applied to the paddles to obtain good electrical contact between the paddles and the patient and to avoid burning the skin (Elefteriades et al., 1996b). Paddles are placed on the chest, one just to the right of the sternum and the other on the left midaxillary line at approximately the fifth interspace (Fig. 26-8). This positioning places most of the heart between the two paddles. All personnel must avoid contact with the patient or bed during defibrillation to avoid accidental shock. Usually 200 joules (J) of current is used for defibrillation, followed by 300 to 360 J if the first attempt is unsuccessful (Myerburg & Castellanos, 1997). When de-

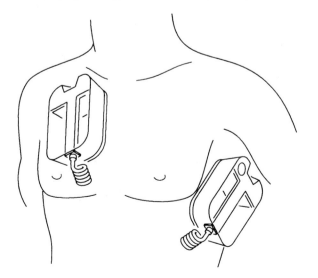

FIGURE 26-8. Standard anterolateral paddle electrode placement for transthoracic defibrillation. (Courtesy of Physio-Control Co., Redmond, WA)

fibrillation is performed using internal paddles applied directly to the surface of the heart (eg, during a cardiac operation or when the chest is opened in the intensive care unit), much lower energy levels are used.

Cardiopulmonary resuscitation is performed throughout the cardiac arrest, except during defibrillation, until a stable cardiac rhythm is achieved. Repeated electric shocks are delivered, as necessary, in conjunction with other modalities of advanced life support, until a stable cardiac rhythm is restored or a physician pronounces the patient dead. Although defibrillation has not affected temporary pacemaker function in laboratory testing, it is recommended that defibrillator paddles be placed 6 inches away from a temporary pulse generator or lead system (Medtronic Model 5388 Technical Manual, 1997).

Defibrillation synchronized to occur during ventricular depolarization, represented by the R wave of the ECG, is termed *cardioversion* or R wave synchronous defibrillation. Synchronized defibrillation reduces the likelihood of inducing VF by stimulating ventricular myocardial cells during the vulnerable portion of repolarization. Cardioversion is used only for arrhythmias with distinct R waves, such as VT, atrial flutter, or atrial fibrillation. It is effective only for reentrant atrial or ventricular arrhythmias, not for those due to abnormal automaticity (Hillis et al., 1995b). Although traditional teaching has been that synchronous cardioversion should always be used for an arrhythmia in which detectable R waves are present, emergent defibrillation may be performed in an unsynchronized mode regardless of the type of arrhythmia. The most important goal in a hemodynamically unstable patient is prompt defibrillation, and using a synchronous setting may delay response time.

Cardioversion most commonly is performed for the elective conversion of SVT, most often atrial flutter or atrial fibrillation, or VT in a patient who is hemodynamically stable. If possible, oral intake is withheld for 6 to 8 hours before the procedure. If the patient is receiving digoxin, it is withheld, if possible, before cardioversion to avoid precipitation of ventricular fibrillation in the presence of digoxin toxicity (Elefteriades et al., 1996b). Intravenous access is established, and the patient is placed in a monitored unit. Although the procedure usually is well tolerated, emergency drugs and intubation equipment should be readily accessible. Intravenous diazepam usually is administered to provide amnesia and reduce anxiety.

The cardioverter-defibrillator is placed in a synchronous setting. Electrocardiographic leads are attached to the cardioverter oscilloscope and a lead displaying a tall R wave is selected. Energy requirements vary with the type of arrhythmia. Organized rhythms (eg, VT or atrial flutter) tend to require less energy than disorganized rhythms (eg, atrial fibrillation) (Main, 1995). As little as 5 J may be used in the case of atrial flutter; 100 J or more may be necessary for atrial fibrillation (Goldberger, 1990). The charge is delivered on the first R wave after depression of the button. If the first electric shock does not convert the arrhythmia, the procedure may be repeated at a higher current setting.

Cardioversion occasionally is performed in postoperative cardiac surgical patients for SVT refractory to pharmacologic control. More commonly, cardioversion is deferred if the ventricular rate response is well controlled in hopes that spontaneous rhythm conversion occurs within several weeks. If it does not, cardioversion may be performed during a follow-up visit. In patients with long-standing atrial fibrillation due to an enlarged left atrium, cardioversion usually is not successful.

REFERENCES

Atlee JL, 1999: Cardiac pacing and electroversion. In Kaplan JA (ed): Cardiac Anesthesia, ed. 4. Philadelphia, WB Saunders

Bernstein AD, Camm AJ, Fletcher RD, et al., 1987: The NASPE/BPEG generic pacemaker code for antibradyarrhythmia and adaptive-rate pacing and antitachyarrhythmia devices. Pacing Clin Electrophysiol 10:794

Busch MM, Haskin JB, 1995: Pacemakers and implantable defibrillators. In Woods SL, Froelicher ESS, Halpenny CJ, Motzer SU (eds): Cardiac Nursing, ed. 3. Philadelphia, JB Lippincott

Elefteriades JA, Geha AS, Cohen LS, 1996a: Temporary pacemakers. In House Officer Guide to ICU Care: Fundamentals of Management of the Heart and Lungs, ed. 2. Philadelphia, Lippincott-Raven

Elefteriades JA, Geha AS, Cohen LS, 1996b: The defibrillator. In House Officer Guide to ICU Care: Fundamentals of Management of the Heart and Lungs, ed. 2. Philadelphia, Lippincott-Raven

Falk JL, 1997: Cardiopulmonary resuscitation. In Parrillo JE (ed): Current Therapy in Critical Care Medicine, ed. 3. St. Louis, CV Mosby

Ferguson TB, Cox JL, 1991: Temporary external DDD pacing after cardiac operations. Ann Thorac Surg 51:723

Finkelmeier BA, O'Mara SR, 1984: Temporary pacing in the cardiac surgical patient. Critical Care Nurse 4(1):108

Finkelmeier BA, Salinger MH, 1986: Dual-chamber cardiac pacing: An overview. Critical Care Nurse 6(5):12

Geha AS, Whittlesey D, 1996: Postoperative low cardiac output. In Baue AE, Geha AS, Hammond GL, et al. (eds): Glenn's Thoracic and Cardiovascular Surgery, ed. 6. Stamford, CT, Appleton & Lange

Goldberger E, 1990: Cardiac pacing and cardioversion. In Essentials of Clinical Cardiology. Philadelphia, JB Lippincott

Gray RJ, Mandel WJ, 1990: Management of common postoperative arrhythmias. In Gray RJ, Matloff JM (eds): Medical Management of the Cardiac Surgical Patient. Baltimore, Williams & Wilkins

Hayes DL, 1998: Pacemakers. In Topol EJ (ed): Comprehensive Cardiovascular Medicine. Philadelphia, Lippincott Williams & Wilkins

Hendrickson SC, Glower DD, Lowe JE, 1997: Cardiopulmonary resuscitation. In Edmunds LH Jr (ed): Cardiac Surgery in the Adult. New York, McGraw-Hill

Hickey CS, Baas LS, 1991: Temporary cardiac pacing. AACN Clin Issues Crit Care Nurs 2:107

Hillis LD, Lange RA, Winniford MD, Page RL, 1995a: Temporary and permanent pacing. In Manual of Clinical Problems in Cardiology, ed. 5. Boston, Little, Brown

Hillis LD, Lange RA, Winniford MD, Page RL, 1995b: Cardioversion. In Manual of Clinical Problems in Cardiology, ed. 4. Boston, Little, Brown

Hudak CM, Gallo BM, Morton PG, 1998: Patient management: Cardiovascular system. In Critical Care Nursing: A Holistic Approach, ed. 7. Philadelphia, Lippincott Williams & Wilkins

Kleinschmidt KM, Stafford MJ, 1991: Dual-chamber cardiac pacemakers. J Cardiovasc Nurs 5:9

Landolfo K, Smith PK, 1995: Postoperative care in cardiac surgery. In Sabiston DC Jr, Spencer FC (eds): Surgery of the Chest, ed. 6. Philadelphia, WB Saunders

Main CC, 1995: Sudden cardiac death and cardiac arrest. In Woods SL, Froelicher ESS, Halpenny CJ, Motzer SU (eds): Cardiac Nursing, ed. 3. Philadelphia, JB Lippincott

Marino PL, 1998: Cardiac arrest. In The ICU Book, ed. 2. Baltimore, Williams & Wilkins

Mehta SM, Pae WE Jr, 1997: Complications of cardiac surgery. In Edmunds LH Jr (ed): Cardiac Surgery in the Adult. New York, McGraw-Hill

Medtronic Model 5348 Technical Manual, 1997. Minneapolis, Medtronic

Medtronic Model 5388 Technical Manual, 1997. Minneapolis, Medtronic

Moreno-Cabral CE, Mitchell RS, Miller DC, 1988: Postoperative problems. In Manual of Postoperative Management in Adult Cardiac Surgery. Baltimore, Williams & Wilkins

Myerburg RJ, Castellanos A, 1997: Cardiac arrest and sudden cardiac death. In Braunwald E (ed): Heart Disease: A Textbook of Cardiovascular Medicine, ed. 5. Philadelphia, WB Saunders

Spotnitz HM, 1997: Practical considerations in pacemaker-defibrillator surgery. In Edmunds LH Jr (ed): Cardiac Surgery in the Adult. New York, McGraw-Hill

Waldo AL, Henthorn RW, Plumb VJ, 1984: Temporary epicardial wire electrodes in the diagnosis and treatment of arrhythmias after open heart surgery. Am J Surg 148:275

Zoble RG, 1989: Cardiac pacing. In Henning RJ, Grenvick A (eds): Critical Care Cardiology. New York, Churchill Livingstone

Cardiovascular Medications

A wide variety of medications are used in the treatment of patients with cardiovascular disease. The discussion in this chapter is limited to summary information about those medications most commonly administered to patients in cardiac surgical settings. For more detailed information concerning pharmacologic actions, precise dosing regimens, and adverse or toxic effects, the reader is referred to a textbook of clinical pharmacology.

► Inotropic Medications

Inotropic medications are those agents that affect contractility of the heart. Because positive inotropic agents increase the strength of myocardial contraction at a given point on the Starling curve, increased cardiac output occurs at the same filling pressure, or preload level. Inotropic drugs most often are used for treatment of acute ventricular dysfunction in patients with low cardiac output syndrome or cardiogenic shock. They commonly are administered in cardiac surgical patients because of the transient ventricular impairment, termed *myocardial stunning*, that may occur after operations that necessitate cardiopulmonary bypass and cardioplegic arrest of the heart. Etiology of the reversible biventricular dysfunction commonly observed in the early postoperative period is multifactorial, including preexisting cardiac disease, in-

complete operative correction of cardiac disease, myocardial edema, reperfusion injury, release of cytokines (immunoregulatory substances secreted by the cells of the immune system), and generation of nitric oxide (Bailey et al., 1997).

A number of medications are categorized as positive inotropic agents (Table 27-1). They differ in intensity of action as well as in the other cardiac and systemic effects they produce. With knowledge of the types of actions associated with each agent, choice of the most appropriate drug may be individualized to the specific patient and clinical situation. Sometimes more than one inotrope is infused to take advantage of particular actions of each agent. Often, inotropic drugs are used in combination with a pharmacologic vasodilating agent or intra-aortic balloon counterpulsation to provide concomitant afterload reduction. Most inotropic agents are given by continuous intravenous infusion. Central venous catheters and rate-regulating pumps always are used to ensure consistent delivery of a precise dosage. Constant hemodynamic monitoring and close nursing observation are necessary during administration of these potent agents. Positive inotropic agents can be categorized as (1) drugs that stimulate sympathetic, or adrenergic, receptors; (2) phosphodiesterase inhibitors; and (3) other inotropic agents. Most inotropes act by stimulating sympathetic receptors of the autonomic nervous system.

TABLE 27-1

TABLE 27-1

Commonly Used Inotropic and Vasodilating Medications

Drug	Concentration*	Infusion Rate
Inotropes		
Amrinone	250 mg	5–10 µg/kg/min
Dobutamine	250 mg	2–10 µg/kg/min
Dopamine	200 mg	1–2 µg/kg/min (dopaminergic)
		2–7 µg/kg/min (beta)
		>7 µg/kg/min (alpha/beta)
Epinephrine	2 mg	0.01–0.1 µg/kg/min
Isoproterenol	2 mg	0.01–0.1 µg/kg/min
Milrinone	50 mg	0.375–0.75 µg/kg/min
Norepinephrine	2 mg	0.05–0.2 µg/kg/min
Vasodilators		
Nitroglycerin	50 mg	0.1–5 µg/kg/min
Nitroprusside	75 mg	0.1–10 µg/kg/min

*Amount of drug in 250-mL solution.

TABLE 27-2

Adrenergic Receptor Sites Affecting Cardiovascular Function

Receptor	Site	Stimulation Response
Alpha$_1$	Vascular smooth muscle	Vasoconstriction
	Myocardium	Positive inotropic action
Alpha$_2$	Presynaptic nerve terminals	Inhibition of norepinephrine release
Beta$_1$	Myocardium	Positive inotropic action
		Positive chronotropic action
Beta$_2$	Vascular smooth muscle	Vasodilatation
	Bronchial smooth muscle	Bronchodilation
Dopaminergic	Vascular smooth muscle	Vasodilatation

Adrenergic Receptor Agonists

The heart is innervated by both subdivisions (parasympathetic and sympathetic) of the autonomic nervous system, but sympathetic, or adrenergic, stimulation plays a more significant role in regulating cardiovascular function. Parasympathetic innervation of the heart occurs through the vagus nerve, and the principal effect of vagal stimulation is slowing of the heart rate; the parasympathetic nervous system has little or no control over smooth muscle tone in blood vessels (Porth, 1998). Cardiac sympathetic fibers, widely distributed in the sinus and atrioventricular (AV) nodes and myocardium, allow increases in heart rate and cardiac contractility with increased sympathetic activity, and sympathetic fibers innervating blood vessels regulate vascular smooth muscle tone through alterations in sympathetic activity (Porth, 1998).

Adrenergic receptor sites, located at the cell surface in myocardial and vascular smooth muscle cells, convert signals from exogenous or endogenous neurotransmitters and circulating hormones into altered cellular function (Mackall et al., 1996). Adrenergic receptors include alpha-adrenergic receptors (subclassified as alpha$_1$ and alpha$_2$), beta-adrenergic receptors (beta$_1$ and beta$_2$), and dopaminergic receptors. Most body tissues have both alpha and beta receptors; dopaminergic receptors are located in blood vessels of the kidneys and other viscera. The effects of adrenergic drugs depend largely on each drug's activation of particular receptors and the number of affected receptors in a particular body tissue (Abrams, 1998a) (Table 27-2).

Alpha$_1$ receptors are located primarily on the surface of vascular smooth muscle cells. Agents that are alpha-adrenergic agonists, or stimulators, predominantly cause peripheral vasoconstriction. Evidence suggests that alpha-adrenergic receptors also are located in the myocardium and mediate a positive inotropic effect as well (Bailey et al., 1997). Beta-adrenergic agonists increase heart rate and myocardial contractility (beta$_1$) and cause peripheral vasodilatation (beta$_2$). Activation of dopaminergic receptors, which respond only to dopamine, causes vasodilatation (Abrams, 1998b).

Dopamine, epinephrine, and norepinephrine are endogenous, or naturally occurring, catecholamines that may be administered as pharmacologic inotropes to affect adrenergic receptors. Dobutamine and isoproterenol are examples of synthetic sympathomimetic drugs (ie, agents that act on adrenergic receptors in the same manner as catecholamines).

In cardiac surgical patients, dopamine is often the initial drug chosen for inotropic support. It usually is administered in a dosage range between 1 and 10 µg/kg/min and has dopaminergic, beta$_1$-adrenergic, and alpha-adrenergic effects, depending on the dosage. In low dosages, such as less than 2 µg/kg/min, dopaminergic effects predominate, causing renal vasodilatation, increased renal blood flow, and improved renal function. More commonly, dopamine is given in larger doses for its beta$_1$-adrenergic actions, which increase myocardial contractility. Activation of postsynaptic myocardial beta$_1$ receptors with resultant positive inotropic and chronotropic effects is most evident clinically at doses greater than 5 µg/kg/min (Haas & Young, 1998).

When doses of 7 to 10 µg/kg/min are administered, alpha-adrenergic (vasoconstrictive) effects of dopamine dominate, producing increased systemic vascular resistance and blood pressure (DiSesa, 1991). Because dopamine does not stimulate postsynaptic beta$_2$ receptors, the predominant effect of higher dosing is one of vasoconstriction (Haas & Young, 1998). Accordingly, a vasodilating agent usually is administered concomitantly when higher doses of dopamine are used. The major limiting factor in the use of dopamine is the frequently associated tachycardia. If the patient's heart rate is consistently greater than 110 beats per minute, substitution of another inotropic agent may be desirable. Dopamine also may cause ventricular tachyarrhythmias. Extravasation of the drug causes local tissue necrosis that can lead to digit loss.

Dobutamine, a synthetic catecholamine, also is used commonly to increase contractility. It differs from dopamine in that its physiologic actions do not vary with dosage. Dobutamine acts primarily on beta$_1$-adrenergic receptors in the myocardium and to a limited degree on beta$_2$ receptors and alpha receptors (Phelan & Klein, 1991). Unlike dopamine, dobutamine exerts no influence on dopaminergic receptors (Mackall et al., 1996). Dobutamine usually does not produce tachycardia to the same degree as dopamine but, like dopamine, it can cause ventricular arrhythmias.

Isoproterenol, another synthetic catecholamine, is a pure beta-adrenergic agonist medication. It increases heart rate (positive chronotropic action), increases contractility, decreases systemic and pulmonary vascular resistance, and causes bronchodilatation. Because isoproterenol produces pulmonary as well as systemic vasodilatation, it is a particularly useful agent in patients with chronic pulmonary hypertension or acute right ventricular failure (Elefteriades et al., 1996a). The drug may be infused safely in a peripheral catheter; a separate agent to reduce afterload is not necessary.

Isoproterenol is a good inotropic choice in bradycardic patients who can benefit from its chronotropic effect. It typically is used to provide transient chronotropic support in heart transplant recipients during the immediate postoperative period. Conversely, the use of isoproterenol is limited in some situations by the tachycardia and ventricular arrhythmias that may occur. The drug also is thought to increase myocardial oxygen consumption. Therefore, it usually is not used in the presence of acute myocardial ischemia.

Epinephrine is a naturally occurring catecholamine with both alpha- and beta-agonist actions. Beta-receptor activation predominates with low doses (0.005 to 0.02 µg/kg/min), causing decreases in systemic and pulmonary vascular resistance with increases in stroke volume and cardiac output; at higher doses, alpha activation predominates with intense vasoconstriction (Mackall et al., 1996). Epinephrine is likely to be chosen when it is desirable to increase heart rate, blood pressure, and cardiac output rapidly (Greco, 1990). Because of its alpha-adrenergic effects, a vasodilating medication usually is administered concomitantly. Epinephrine also may be given as an intravenous bolus, or occasionally through an endotracheal tube, to restore spontaneous cardiac activity in patients who experience cardiac arrest. Use of epinephrine is limited by tachycardia caused by its chronotropic effect and by its proarrhythmic potential.

Norepinephrine is the neurotransmitter released from sympathetic nerves and is the biosynthetic precursor of epinephrine (Mackall et al., 1996). Norepinephrine has both beta-adrenergic and chronotropic actions, but it is principally an alpha-adrenergic agent (Ferguson, 1991). Consequently, it increases systolic and diastolic arterial pressure secondary to peripheral vasoconstriction. Norepinephrine is not useful purely as a positive inotropic agent (Hillis et al., 1995a). Because its vasoconstrictive effect increases afterload, norepinephrine may in fact cause cardiac output to decrease and myocardial

work to increase. Therefore, it usually is reserved for profound cardiogenic shock, when other inotropic agents fail to correct severe hypotension. Norepinephrine also is used as the agent of choice to increase the profoundly low systemic vascular resistance associated with septic shock.

Phosphodiesterase-Inhibiting Agents

Amrinone and milrinone belong to a newer class of drugs, *phosphodiesterase inhibitors*. Their actions are not related to direct adrenergic receptor stimulation. Instead, they increase contractility by selectively inhibiting phosphodiesterase III, a myocardial enzyme responsible for the breakdown of cyclic adenosine monophosphate (cAMP), thereby enhancing intracellular levels of cAMP (Bailey et al., 1997; Hudak et al., 1998a). Increasing cAMP enhances the movement of calcium into cells, thus improving contractility. Amrinone and milrinone also produce peripheral vasodilatation. Therefore, cardiac output is improved both by increased contractility and decreased afterload (Bond & Underhill, 1990).

Amrinone is administered in a bolus dose of 0.75 mg/kg slowly over 2 to 3 minutes, followed by a maintenance infusion of 5 to 10 µg/kg/min (Abrams, 1998c). Studies suggest that amrinone has a synergistic effect when infused in combination with adrenergic inotropic agents (DiSesa, 1991). The major disadvantage of amrinone is a high incidence of reversible thrombocytopenia. The decrease in platelet count is dose dependent and usually occurs within 48 to 72 hours of initiating therapy (Mackall et al., 1996).

Milrinone is approximately tenfold more potent than amrinone, has a shorter half-life, is associated with a lesser risk of thrombocytopenia, and is less expensive (Smith et al., 1997, Bailey et al., 1997). For these reasons, it often is used in preference to amrinone. Milrinone is administered as a loading dose of 50 µg/kg intravenously over 10 minutes, followed by continuous infusion at 0.375 to 0.75 µg/kg/min (Abrams, 1998c).

Other Inotropic Agents

Digoxin is not useful as an inotropic agent in the acute setting, but is used for chronic inotropic support of the heart. Once a mainstay of therapy for congestive heart failure, the use of digoxin has waned in the face of newer pharmacologic agents, especially angiotensin-converting enzyme inhibitors, that, unlike digoxin, have been shown to increase life expectancy in patients with chronic heart failure (Kalkanis et al., 1998). Still, patients with impaired ventricular function often are receiving chronic digitalis therapy.

Calcium chloride sometimes is administered to provide acute inotropic support of the heart. Calcium plays an important role in excitation–contraction coupling in the myocardium by interacting with active proteins in muscle to initiate contraction (DiSesa, 1991). The inotropic effect of calcium administration depends strongly on the patient's plasma calcium concentration; if ionized plasma calcium is low, exogenous calcium administration may increase contractility but it does little to increase the inotropic state if the plasma calcium level is normal (Bailey et al., 1997).

An intravenous bolus dose of calcium (0.05 to 1.0 g) often is given in patients who become profoundly hypotensive because it stimulates myocardial contractility and increases blood pressure regardless of the cause of hypotension (Elefteriades et al., 1996b). The enhancement of contractility and resulting improvement in cardiac output is transient but may sustain the patient to allow time for initiation of other supportive therapies.

▸ Vasodilating Medications

Intravenous *vasodilating agents* frequently are used in cardiac surgical patients to reduce afterload, or the impedance to ejection of blood from the ventricle. Vasodilator therapy is based on the sensitivity of ventricular performance to changes in afterload; with fixed preload, the velocity of cardiac contraction diminishes as afterload increases (Barron & Parrillo, 1991). In the early hours after cardiac operations, left ventricular afterload, measured clinically as systemic vascular resistance, typically is elevated secondary to hypothermia and peripheral vasoconstriction. Patients with ventricular dysfunction are more affected by changes in afterload, such that small increases in systemic vascular resistance can lead to appreciable decreases in cardiac output (Mackall et al., 1996). Pharmacologic afterload reduction may be necessary to maintain adequate cardiac output and prevent worsening ventricular dysfunction due to increased left ventricular work and myocardial oxygen consumption.

Vasodilating agents also are used commonly in the early postoperative period to correct hypertension that develops as a consequence of patient emergence from anesthesia, endotracheal suctioning, resistance to mechanical ventilation, or pain (Whitman, 1991). Because of impaired coagulation after the use of cardiopulmonary bypass, postoperative hypertension must be corrected promptly to avoid excessive mediastinal bleeding.

Because both coronary artery disease and valvular heart disease more often damage the left ventricle, left ventricular dysfunction is commonly present. Consequently, it usually is left ventricular afterload that must be pharmacologically decreased. However, in disorders associated with pulmonary hypertension, such as severe mitral stenosis or postoperative right ventricular failure, an agent that lowers pulmonary vascular resistance may be necessary.

The most commonly used intravenous vasodilating agents are nitroglycerin and sodium nitroprusside (see Table 27-2). Nitroglycerin causes direct relaxation of vascular smooth muscle. It primarily produces venous dilatation at low dosages, but produces arterial dilatation at higher doses (Hillis et al., 1995b). The increased

volume of the venous capacitance vessels redistributes intravascular blood, effectively reducing preload. Although a less effective afterload-reducing agent than nitroprusside, nitroglycerin provides the added benefit of dilating coronary arteries. It thus increases blood flow through arteries affected by spasm and collateral arteries in areas of myocardium not completely revascularized by coronary artery bypass grafting (Elefteriades et al., 1996a). The coronary artery dilatation associated with nitroglycerin also makes it an effective agent for controlling acute myocardial ischemia. Sustained high doses of intravenous nitroglycerin have been associated with a loss of hemodynamic efficacy after 24 to 72 hours of administration (Barron & Parrillo, 1991).

Nitroprusside relaxes vascular smooth muscle, producing almost immediate arterial and venous dilatation. The balanced action lowers both pulmonary and systemic vascular resistances while increasing venous capacitance (Greco, 1990). The resulting reduction in systemic vascular resistance allows the left ventricle to eject blood more easily, thereby increasing cardiac output. Nitroprusside acts rapidly, has a short half-life, causes minimal change in heart rate, and can be titrated readily to achieve the desired hemodynamic effect (Hillis et al., 1995b). The drug is quite potent and can produce precipitous, severe hypotension. Also, because cyanogen, cyanide, and thiocyanate are potential toxic breakdown products, cyanate toxicity can occur when high doses (>7 μg/kg/min) are infused for a prolonged period (Landolfo & Smith, 1995). Thiocyanate levels are measured intermittently in susceptible patients or if metabolic acidosis or signs of central nervous system dysfunction develop. Because nitroprusside is degraded by exposure to light, the infusion bag is covered with an opaque wrapping to prevent product degradation during infusion.

▸ Antiarrhythmic Medications

Because of the propensity for cardiac arrhythmias in patients who undergo cardiac operations, any of a number of *antiarrhythmic agents* may be used. Several considerations are particularly relevant when administering antiarrhythmic agents to cardiac surgical patients. First, many agents have proarrhythmic actions; that is, they actually can induce arrhythmias. Second, most antiarrhythmic drugs have negative inotropic effects. Although they may be well tolerated in patients with good ventricular function, they may worsen ventricular function significantly in patients with heart disease, especially when given intravenously (Lewis, 1991). Third, drugs with short effective half-lives after intravenous administration, such as adenosine, esmolol, or lidocaine, are preferable for acute arrhythmia management because adverse effects, particularly hemodynamic alterations, are short-lived (Bailey et al., 1997). Finally, many antiarrhythmic agents alter the thresholds for defibrillation. For example, amiodarone, lidocaine, and propranolol increase the defibrillation threshold, whereas sotalol decreases the threshold (Barold

& Zipes, 1997). Antiarrhythmic agents commonly are classified in four categories according to whether they exert blocking actions predominantly on sodium, potassium, or calcium channels, and whether they block beta-adrenergic receptors (Zipes, 1997) (Table 27-3).

Class I Agents

Class I antiarrhythmic medications are membrane-stabilizing agents. They block the movement of sodium into cardiac conducting cells, thereby stabilizing the cell membrane and decreasing the formation and conduction of electrical impulses (Abrams, 1998d). Class I drugs affect impulse conduction, excitability, and automaticity to varying degrees and thus are subclassified to reflect their predominant effect (White, 1998). Class IA agents prolong action potential duration; class IB drugs shorten

TABLE 27-3

Classification of Antiarrhythmic Medications

CLASS I: MEMBRANE-ACTIVE DRUGS
IA
  Disopyramide
  Procainamide
  Quinidine
IB
  Lidocaine
  Mexiletine
  Tocainide
IC
  Flecainide
  Propafenone

CLASS II: BETA-ADRENERGIC BLOCKING DRUGS
Atenolol
Esmolol
Propranolol
Metoprolol
Nadolol
Timolol

CLASS III: REPOLARIZATION PROLONGING DRUGS
Amiodarone
Bretylium tosylate
Sotalol

CLASS IV: CALCIUM CHANNEL BLOCKING DRUGS
Diltiazem
Nifedipine
Verapamil

OTHER ANTIARRHYTHMIC DRUGS
Adenosine
Atropine
Digoxin

action duration potential; and class IC drugs primarily slow conduction (Zipes, 1997).

Class IA drugs include quinidine, procainamide, and disopyramide. Quinidine is used occasionally in cardiac surgical patients for suppression of supraventricular or ventricular arrhythmias. It has two modes of action: (1) its vagolytic effect enhances conduction through the AV node, and (2) its direct myocardial effect prolongs AV conduction, His-Purkinje conduction times, and the duration of repolarization (Q-T interval) (Hudak et al., 1998a). When using quinidine to treat supraventricular tachycardia (SVT), digoxin or a beta-blocking agent is given first to prevent undesirable acceleration of the ventricular rate due to vagolytic enhancement of AV conduction. However, quinidine administration increases the serum digitalis level, and the digoxin dose may need to be reduced in patients who have already been receiving maintenance digoxin to avoid digoxin toxicity (Mandel, 1990).

Quinidine is contraindicated in the presence of AV or intraventricular conduction disorders because it slows conduction (Bond, 1990). It rarely is given intravenously because its alpha-adrenergic blocking effects may cause vasodilatation with resultant hypotension (Buckingham & Parrillo, 1991). Because quinidine can prolong the Q-T interval, a small number of patients develop torsades de pointes, a distinctive, polymorphic ventricular tachyarrhythmia (Zipes, 1997). Approximately 30% of patients cannot tolerate quinidine therapy because of troublesome side effects, including diarrhea, nausea and vomiting, headache, and arrhythmias (Hudak et al., 1998a).

Procainamide, an agent similar to quinidine, occasionally is administered by intravenous infusion for ventricular arrhythmias refractory to lidocaine therapy. It works by decreasing rates of conduction through the conducting system and ventricular tissue (Slovis & Brody, 1991). When administered intravenously, a loading dose of 15 mg/kg (maximum 1 g) is administered at a rate of 25 to 50 mg/min, followed by a continuous infusion of 1 to 4 mg/min (Hillis et al., 1995c). Because procainamide elimination involves both liver metabolism and renal elimination, dosage is adjusted downward in patients with significant hepatic or renal disease (Bailey et al., 1997). Like quinidine, procainamide prolongs the Q-T interval and may cause serious arrhythmias, such as torsades de pointes, especially in the setting of hypokalemia or hypomagnesemia. It also can precipitate hypotension. Procainamide is not widely used for chronic oral therapy of arrhythmias because anti-nuclear antibodies develop in most patients, and in a minority a lupus-like syndrome characterized by arthralgia and rash develops (Roden, 1998).

Disopyramide, another class IA medication, is an oral agent that sometimes is used for chronic treatment of ventricular arrhythmias. Disopyramide has electrophysiologic effects similar to those of quinidine and procainamide, but negative inotropic effects limit its usefulness (Bailey et al., 1997).

Lidocaine is a class IB drug and probably is the most

commonly used antiarrhythmic agent. It is generally accepted as the drug of choice for initial treatment of significant ventricular arrhythmias. Lidocaine decreases myocardial irritability, or automaticity, in the ventricles, with little effect on atrial tissue (Abrams, 1998d). It must be given parenterally because significant first-pass hepatic metabolism occurs with oral administration, resulting in unpredictable, low plasma levels and excessive metabolites that can cause toxicity (Zipes, 1997).

Lidocaine is administered first as an intravenous bolus or loading dose (1 mg/kg) and then by continuous intravenous infusion at a rate of 1 to 4 mg/min. It acts almost immediately, and because of its short half-life, a continuous infusion is necessary to sustain drug effect. Lidocaine toxicity can cause a variety of neurologic manifestations, including slurred speech, mental confusion, lethargy, obtundation, and, occasionally, grand mal seizures (Hillis et al., 1995d). AV block with a slow junctional or ventricular rhythm is a contraindication to lidocaine use (Hudak et al., 1998a).

Mexiletine and tocainide are other class IB agents used less commonly for treatment of ventricular tachycardia. They have mechanisms of action similar to that of lidocaine. However, because they do not undergo the significant first-pass hepatic degradation that occurs with lidocaine, they can be administered orally.

Class IC agents markedly decrease conduction velocity. Flecainide and propafenone are class IC agents used infrequently for treatment of life-threatening ventricular tachyarrhythmias refractory to other agents. Flecainide has moderate negative inotropic effects and its use is limited by demonstrated proarrhythmic properties. It is used primarily in patients with supraventricular arrhythmias but no structural heart disease (Roden, 1998). Propafenone appears to have less of a proarrhythmic effect than flecainide, but it can cause conduction abnormalities, worsening of heart failure, and minor noncardiac disturbances, including dizziness, taste disturbances, and blurred vision (Zipes, 1997). The usual adult dose of propafenone is 150 to 300 mg orally every 8 hours (Bailey et al., 1997).

Class II Agents

Class II antiarrhythmic agents are beta-adrenergic blocking medications, such as propranolol, esmolol, and metoprolol. Beta-blocking medications occupy beta-adrenergic receptor sites and prevent the receptors from responding to sympathetic nerve impulses, circulating catecholamines, and beta-adrenergic drugs (Abrams, 1998e). Antiarrhythmic actions of beta-blocking drugs include decreasing (1) heart rate; (2) automaticity in the AV node; and (3) conduction velocity in the atria, AV node, His-Purkinje system, and ventricles (Loveys, 1990).

Beta-blocking agents sometimes are used for treatment of SVT. Propranolol is selected most commonly. In patients with atrial fibrillation or atrial flutter, it increases the degree of AV block and reduces heart rate (Hudak et al., 1998a). Oral propranolol is given in doses

of 10 to 80 mg every 6 hours. Intravenous propranolol may be administered to achieve more rapid ventricular rate control. However, the drug must be injected slowly (0.5 to 1.0 mg every 5 minutes, to a maximum of 3 mg) with electrocardiographic and arterial pressure monitoring because it may precipitate profound hypotension. Propranolol also may be given prophylactically in low doses (10 mg orally every 6 hours) to decrease the incidence of postoperative SVT (Landolfo & Smith, 1995). Propranolol is contraindicated in patients with underlying pulmonary disease because its inhibition of beta$_2$ receptors may cause bronchospasm.

Esmolol is an ultrashort-acting beta-blocking agent that also may be used to treat SVT. It is administered by intravenous infusion and is an attractive choice in the early postoperative period or in critically ill patients. It is more cardioselective and therefore less likely to produce bronchospasm in patients with mild chronic obstructive pulmonary disease or asthma, and its ultrashort duration of action allows easy control of the magnitude and duration of beta blockade (Marino, 1998a). A loading dose of up to 500 µg/kg is followed by a continuous infusion rate in the range of 50 to 250 µg/kg/min (Butterworth et al., 1996). Hypotension is the most common cardiovascular adverse effect of esmolol; it is most likely to occur within the first 30 minutes after initiating administration of the drug (Morton, 1994).

Metoprolol, another cardioselective beta-blocking agent, also can be given intravenously (5 mg every 5 minutes to a maximum of 15 mg [3 doses]) for treatment of postoperative supraventricular arrhythmias (Antman, 1997). Although not as rapid acting as esmolol, its effects are more sustained and the patient can be converted to an oral form of the drug.

Class III Agents

Class III antiarrhythmic agents (bretylium tosylate, amiodarone, and sotalol) prolong the action potential duration. Bretylium is sometimes given intravenously in postoperative patients for ventricular tachycardia or ventricular fibrillation refractory to suppression with lidocaine therapy. It is not effective in the treatment of atrial arrhythmias (Bailey et al., 1997). A loading dose is administered intravenously (5 to 10 mg/kg) over 10 to 12 minutes, followed by a continuous infusion of 1 to 2 mg/min (Hudak et al., 1998a). Because bretylium is excreted almost entirely by the kidneys, drug half-life is prolonged with renal insufficiency and dosage must be reduced (Abrams, 1998d). The most significant adverse effect is hypotension, which is usually orthostatic. Hypertension, sinus tachycardia, or other arrhythmias also may occur after initial administration of bretylium (Buckingham & Parrillo, 1991).

Amiodarone, an oral class III agent, generally is considered the most effective antiarrhythmic medication for prevention of recurrent ventricular tachycardia or ventricular fibrillation. It is also effective, in doses lower than those used for ventricular arrhythmias, for treatment of atrial arrhythmias and for conversion of atrial fibrillation to normal sinus rhythm (Bailey et al., 1997). Amiodarone has many pharmacologic properties, and the mechanism by which it exerts its arrhythmia-suppressing effects is unknown (Haas & Young, 1998). A unique feature of amiodarone is its extraordinarily long duration of action, with a half-life of 14 to 52 days (Hudak et al., 1998a). Because of the drug's long serum half-life, oral therapy is initiated with a loading dose (800 to 1600 mg/d) for 1 to 3 weeks. Dosage is then gradually reduced to a maintenance dose of 400 mg/d or less.

Amiodarone is a very potent medication with a number of quite serious and potentially lethal side effects. In 5% to 15% of patients receiving at least 400 mg/d for an extended period, amiodarone-induced pulmonary fibrosis develops, usually manifested by dyspnea, cough, weight loss, fever, pleuritic chest pain, and new radiographic pulmonary infiltrates (Hillis et al., 1995e; Dusman et al., 1990). This complication, which can be fatal, is more likely in patients with a longer duration of therapy, in those receiving higher maintenance doses, and in those with underlying pulmonary disease (Haas & Young, 1998). Other potential adverse effects of amiodarone include corneal microdeposits, impaired vision, hyperthyroidism, hypothyroidism, photosensitivity, skin pigmentation, neurologic toxicity, and increased hepatic enzyme levels (Hudak et al., 1998a). Because of its significant side effect profile, it usually is reserved for those patients at high risk for sudden cardiac death or with hemodynamically compromising ventricular tachyarrhythmias in whom other agents are ineffective.

Several considerations are relevant when amiodarone is given to cardiac surgical patients to treat life-threatening ventricular arrhythmias in the perioperative period. First, amiodarone has been associated with intraoperative atropine-resistant bradycardia and with vasodilatation and decreased contractility that is not responsive to pharmacologic therapy (Moore & Wilkoff, 1991). Second, life-threatening respiratory failure can develop during the early postoperative period. At particular risk are patients who have had preoperative pulmonary toxicity (Nalos et al., 1987). Because of its potential for hemodynamic instability and pulmonary toxicity, amiodarone is used most often as an alternative therapy for arrhythmias refractory to other antiarrhythmic agents (Balser, 1997). Finally, amiodarone interacts with several cardiovascular medications, such as digoxin and warfarin sodium, and downward adjustment of dosages may be required (Haas & Young, 1998). Extreme caution is necessary when initiating anticoagulant therapy with warfarin in patients who are receiving amiodarone.

Sotalol is a class III antiarrhythmic agent with beta-adrenergic blocking properties. Sotalol, like the other class III agents, may be used to suppress life-threatening ventricular tachyarrhythmias refractory to other therapy. Its cardiovascular adverse effects include hypotension, bradycardia, congestive heart failure, and proarrhythmia; fatigue, light-headedness, dyspnea, headache, nausea, vomiting, and diarrhea are other adverse effects (Hillis et al., 1995f). In patients with significant ventric-

ular impairment, the beta-blocking effects of sotalol may lead to heart failure (Bailey et al., 1997). Therapy is initiated slowly and patient response is monitored closely.

Class IV Agents

Class IV antiarrhythmic medications are calcium channel antagonists, such as verapamil, diltiazem, and nifedipine. They work by blocking movement of calcium into both conductive and contractile myocardial cells, thereby reducing automaticity of the sinus and AV nodes, slowing conduction, and prolonging the AV node refractory period (Abrams, 1998d). Calcium channel blocking agents occasionally are used to treat SVT in postoperative cardiac surgical patients. However, because these agents depress myocardial contractility to varying degrees, many of them produce heart failure in patients with impaired ventricular function. Also, intravenous verapamil can cause profound hypotension or ventricular fibrillation if given to a patient with ventricular tachycardia who is misdiagnosed as having SVT (Drew, 1991).

Diltiazem may be preferable in postoperative cardiac surgical patients because it has less of a negative inotropic effect than verapamil. The intravenous dose of diltiazem is a loading dose of 0.25 mg/kg over 2 minutes with a second dose of 0.35 mg/kg if the response is inadequate after 15 minutes, followed by a continuous infusion of 5 to 15 mg/h for up to 24 hours (Bailey et al., 1997; Abrams, 1998d).

Other Antiarrhythmic Agents

Digoxin is one of the more commonly used antiarrhythmic agents in cardiac surgical patients. Because of the prevalence of SVT (eg, atrial fibrillation and atrial flutter) after cardiac operations, prophylactic digitalization sometimes is performed in the early postoperative period. Digoxin also usually is administered as the agent of choice for treatment of SVT. It effectively lowers ventricular rate response in atrial flutter or atrial fibrillation by increasing AV block and enhances conversion to normal sinus rhythm. Digoxin also may be effective at terminating paroxysmal SVT because it enhances vagal tone, which slows impulse conduction and prolongs the effective refractory period, thereby interrupting reentrant circuits that pass through the AV node (Kalkanis et al., 1998).

The specific dosing regimen for digoxin depends on the ventricular rate, the urgency of conversion, patient age, body size, and renal function (Gray & Mandel, 1990). Typically, intravenous bolus doses (0.125- to 0.25-mg doses to a total of 1.0 to 1.5 mg over 24 hours) of digoxin are given to achieve a therapeutic serum level. Subsequent doses of 0.125 to 0.25 mg may be given intravenously until ventricular rate is less than 100 beats per minute or a total of 2 mg has been administered. Digoxin has a low therapeutic index; that is, therapeutic and toxic levels are separated only by a small margin. Cardiac arrhythmias are a common manifestation of digoxin toxicity. Although any change in heart rhythm in a patient receiving digoxin should suggest toxicity, a characteristic feature of its occurrence is the concurrent presence of enhanced automaticity and depressed conduction (heart block) (Ide & Drew, 1998). Digoxin toxicity also may cause gastrointestinal symptoms (eg, nausea or diarrhea) and visual abnormalities.

Adenosine is an ultrashort-acting, intravenous agent for treatment of paroxysmal SVT originating in the AV node. Its primary actions are depression of sinus node automaticity, slowing of AV nodal conduction, shortening of the action potential in atrial tissue, and dilatation of coronary vessels (Severson & Meyer, 1992). Adenosine has an extremely short half-life (1 to 2 seconds), making it well suited for treatment of reentry arrhythmias in which transient interruption can eliminate the arrhythmia (Bailey et al., 1997). Because adenosine rapidly slows AV nodal conduction, it also is useful in differentiating wide-complex tachycardias of uncertain origin. The usual dose is 6 mg, administered by rapid intravenous injection. Transient adverse effects lasting less than 1 minute are common and include dyspnea, flushing, headaches, and chest pressure (Morton, 1994).

Atropine is an anticholinergic, or cholinergic-blocking, medication that blocks the action of acetylcholine on the parasympathetic receptors of the autonomic nervous system. It is used to increase the sinus rate and enhance AV conduction in patients with symptomatic bradyarrhythmias. Atropine is given as an intravenous bolus dose (0.5 to 1 mg) and may be repeated every 5 minutes to a total of 2 mg (Hudak et al., 1998a; Lapsley, 1991). The drug usually has little or no effect on blood pressure; large doses cause facial flushing due to vasodilatation of blood vessels in the neck (Abrams, 1998f). Because of the loss of vagal influence in the denervated (ie, no autonomic nervous system innervation) donor heart, atropine is ineffective in treating postoperative bradycardia after heart transplantation (Hudak et al., 1998b).

Magnesium sulfate is an intracellular cation that influences cardiac automaticity, excitability, conduction, and contractility (LeClair & Carlson, 1990). Some data suggest that magnesium may help suppress torsades de pointes and atrial arrhythmias characteristic of digoxin toxicity (Roden, 1998). Magnesium deficiency is common in the postoperative period and the administration of magnesium has been shown to decrease the incidence of postoperative arrhythmias (Bailey et al., 1997). Magnesium is administered as an intravenous infusion of 1 to 2 g over 1 to 2 hours.

▶ Antianginal Medications

Three types of *antianginal medications* are used commonly to decrease the frequency of angina pectoris and improve exercise tolerance in patients with coronary artery disease: nitrates, beta-blocking agents, and cal-

cium channel antagonists. Often a combination of the three types of agents is used.

Nitrates exert a multitude of effects on the cardiovascular system that promote relief of ischemia, including (1) reduction of left ventricular preload and afterload through venous and arterial vasodilatation; (2) dilatation of epicardial coronary vessels and, in selected circumstances, enhancement of intracoronary collateral flow; (3) relief of epicardial vasoconstriction and spasm, producing a favorable redistribution of transmural coronary flow from epicardial to endocardial layers; and (4) a direct increase in left ventricular compliance (Armstrong, 1998). Nitroglycerin is effective primarily because of its dilating effects on coronary arteries. Although it does not increase coronary artery flow that is obstructed by fixed anatomic lesions, it decreases superimposed arterial spasm and dilates collateral arteries that supply jeopardized muscle (Elefteriades et al., 1996c). In addition, by reducing preload, nitroglycerin reduces myocardial wall tension and oxygen consumption.

Nitroglycerin is available in several forms. In patients with chronic stable angina, it may be administered sublingually or as an oral spray to dissipate or forestall periodic anginal episodes (Armstrong, 1998; Kutcher, 1991). To provide more extended relief from angina, a timed-release nitroglycerin patch may be applied topically or an oral, long-acting nitrate (eg, isosorbide dinitrate) may be given. Consideration must be given to using the smallest effective dose of nitrate required with long-acting nitrate therapy to minimize tolerance development (Armstrong, 1998).

In patients with unstable angina, nitroglycerin is administered by continuous intravenous infusion. Arterial pressure monitoring is performed, and dosage is titrated by mean arterial pressure and the occurrence of angina. Typically, intravenous nitroglycerin is initiated at a dose of 5 to 10 µg/min and the rate is increased until angina is eliminated or mean systolic arterial pressure is reduced by 10%; the maximally effective dose varies widely between 10 to 500 µg/min (Hillis et al., 1995g; Pratt & Roberts, 1991). Adverse effects of nitroglycerin therapy include hypotension and tachyphylaxis (Schaer, 1991). Because nitrates also can cause reflex tachycardia with a resultant increase in myocardial oxygen demand, a beta-blocking agent typically is administered concomitantly (Simandl & Cohn, 1997). The use of intravenous nitroglycerin therapy for afterload reduction has been described already.

Beta-adrenergic blocking medications decrease myocardial ischemia, and thus anginal pain, by decreasing the major determinants of myocardial oxygen demand–heart rate, left ventricular contractility, and left ventricular wall tension (Hillis et al., 1995h). Limiting or preventing sympathetically induced increases in heart rate, contractility, and systolic blood pressure minimizes increases in myocardial oxygen demand (Bailey et al., 1997).

Beta-blocking agents used for angina control include metoprolol, propranolol, atenolol, nadolol, and timolol. The agents differ in duration of action (some allow greater time intervals between doses) and cardioselectivity (ie, the degree to which beta receptors outside the heart are affected) (Elefteriades et al., 1996c). Intravenous beta-blocking agents, such as atenolol, metoprolol, or timolol, are administered for all patients with acute MI and no contraindication to their use; they are particularly useful in patients in a hyperdynamic state with tachycardia and hypertension (Marino, 1998b). Beta-adrenergic blocking medications have a mixed effect in patients with left ventricular systolic dysfunction and resultant heart failure. In patients with acute ventricular dysfunction, their negative inotropic effect may cause a further deterioration in cardiac function; conversely, long-term administration of beta-blocking agents in patients with fully compensated heart failure appears to improve cardiac performance, lessen symptoms, and improve exercise tolerance (Hillis et al., 1995h).

The third category of antianginal medication is calcium channel blocking, or antagonist, medications. These agents decrease angina by dilating coronary arteries and preventing spasm; to differing degrees, the individual calcium channel blocking agents also decrease myocardial oxygen consumption by reducing blood pressure, afterload, and contractility (Kutcher, 1991). Diltiazem, nifedipine, and verapamil are examples of calcium channel antagonists used for anginal control.

Despite the anti-ischemic effect of calcium channel blocking agents, their efficacy in the treatment of acute myocardial infarction (MI) has not been demonstrated and they may in fact increase mortality when prescribed routinely to patients with acute MI (Antman & Braunwald, 1997). Nifedipine specifically is contraindicated because of reports of associated acute MI or stroke (Schroeder, 1997). Because verapamil is a potent negative inotrope, its use is not recommended in patients with poor left ventricular function (Simandl & Cohn, 1997).

▶ Anticoagulant, Thrombolytic, and Antiplatelet Medications

Anticoagulation is accomplished with intravenous administration of heparin or, for chronic therapy, with oral administration of warfarin sodium (Coumadin). Heparin combines with antithrombin III to inactivate several clotting factors (IX, X, XI, XII) and thrombin, thus preventing thrombus formation (Abrams, 1998g). Heparin does not dissolve existing thrombus but does prevent its extension. Because heparin is inactivated by hydrochloric acid in the stomach, it must be administered intravenously or subcutaneously (Christopherson & Froelicher, 1990).

Systemic anticoagulation with heparin is necessary in all patients who undergo operations necessitating cardiopulmonary bypass. Anticoagulation throughout the period of extracorporeal circulation prevents massive thrombosis that would occur otherwise as blood is circulated outside the body and exposed to the nonbiologic surfaces of the cardiopulmonary bypass circuit. An intravenous bolus of heparin (eg, 300 U/kg) is injected directly into the right atrium just before cannulation for

cardiopulmonary bypass. Activated clotting time (ACT) is measured intermittently to ensure an adequate degree of anticoagulation, and additional bolus doses of heparin are administered as indicated. Although the optimal ACT range for cardiopulmonary bypass is not precisely defined, the ACT typically is maintained at a level between 400 and 600 seconds (normal baseline is 80 to 120 seconds) (Nolan & Zacour, 1998). Protamine sulfate, a heparin antagonist, is given after termination of cardiopulmonary bypass to reverse the anticoagulated state.

Anticoagulation also may be necessary in selected patients during the preoperative or postoperative period. The most common indication for anticoagulation during the preoperative period is retardation of thrombus formation in patients with acute MI or unstable angina. Another common indication for preoperative anticoagulation is a known or suspected source of systemic thromboembolism, such as a mechanical valvular prosthesis, deep venous thrombosis, left ventricular thrombus, or atrial fibrillation. Heparin is used instead of warfarin in the immediate preoperative period because of its shorter half-life.

Heparin therapy usually is initiated with a bolus dose of 5000 U, followed by a continuous infusion of 800-1200 U/h. The anticoagulant effect of heparin is monitored by a baseline, and then serial, measurements of partial thromboplastin time. Dosage is adjusted to achieve an activated partial thromboplastin time 1.5 to 2.5 times greater than control levels (Marino, 1998c). Intravenous heparin therapy in preoperative cardiac surgical patients is continued until the morning of surgery or, in the case of unstable angina, until the patient is transported to the operating room.

The most common adverse effect of heparin is bleeding, which usually can be treated with dose reduction or discontinuance of heparin therapy. Life-threatening hemorrhage may necessitate neutralization with protamine sulfate (Becker, 1996). Another potential complication of heparin therapy is heparin-induced thrombocytopenia, an antibody-mediated (immunoglobulin G) reduction in platelets with associated thrombosis. Because of the serious consequences of heparin-induced thrombocytopenia, serial platelet counts should be measured routinely in all patients receiving heparin therapy.

Ten to 20% of patients experience a mild thrombocytopenia after 1 to 4 days of heparin therapy, and nearly 3% of patients after 5 to 10 days acquire a more sinister form, characterized by a platelet count of less than 150,000/mm^3 and the presence of heparin-dependent antiplatelet antibodies (Brieger et al., 1998). The syndrome is manifest clinically by thrombotic events, typically producing arterial occlusion that can result in lower limb ischemia, a cerebral vascular accident, or MI. In patients with heparin-induced thrombocytopenia, heparin therapy is discontinued immediately and heparin is removed from all intravenous infusions and flush solutions.

Low–molecular-weight heparin (LMWH) (eg, enoxaprin) more recently has become available as an alternative therapy for patients requiring anticoagulation with heparin. LMWH has more anticoagulant activity and produces an anticoagulant effect at lower doses than conventional, heterogenous heparin preparations (Marino, 1998c). Its longer plasma half-life makes it possible to administer subcutaneous doses (eg, enoxaprin, 30 mg) only twice a day. The patient can self-administer the subcutaneous injections at home. Doses are weight adjusted and require no monitoring of clotting status (Nunnelee, 1997).

LMWH may be associated with a lower incidence of bleeding than standard heparin because it binds with less affinity to platelets and endothelial cells and interferes less with von Willebrand factor (Kayser, 1998). The incidence of heparin-induced thrombocytopenia is less with LMWH, but because of the strong likelihood of cross-sensitivity, patients in whom thrombocytopenia developed with standard heparin should not receive LMWH (Kayser, 1998). LMWH is considerably more costly than conventional heparin.

In postoperative cardiac surgical patients, anticoagulation usually is necessary only in those who have a prosthetic heart valve or a preexisting condition, such as chronic atrial fibrillation, that necessitates an anticoagulated state. Because the use of cardiopulmonary bypass impairs coagulation during the early postoperative period, anticoagulant therapy, usually with warfarin sodium only, is not initiated until the second postoperative day to avoid exacerbation of bleeding in the immediate postoperative period.

Warfarin sodium is an oral agent used for chronic anticoagulation. It acts by competing with vitamin K and thus inhibiting hepatic synthesis of vitamin K–dependent clotting factors (factors II, VII, IX, and X) (Christopherson & Froelicher, 1990). Warfarin does not affect circulating clotting factors or platelet function. In most patients, anticoagulation is begun with an initial dose of 5 mg. Subsequent doses are titrated according to the international normalized ratio (INR) value calculated from the prothrombin time measured each morning.

The optimal therapeutic range for the INR depends on the specific indication for anticoagulation and the perceived risk of thromboembolism. In patients with mechanical cardiac valvular prostheses, the target INR ratio also depends on the particular prosthesis. An INR between 2.0 and 2.9 appears to be sufficient for patients with St. Jude prostheses, whereas an INR between 3.0 and 3.9 is preferable for those with Medtronic-Hall or Bjork-Shiley valves; patients with ball-and-cage prostheses, multiple mechanical prostheses, or a prosthesis in the mitral position may require an INR between 4.0 and 4.9 (Garcia, 1998).

Particular care must be exercised when warfarin is administered to patients who are elderly, malnourished, have chronic liver dysfunction, or are receiving amiodarone. In these patients, prothrombin times may rise rapidly with only small doses of warfarin. The anticoagulant effect of warfarin can be reduced or reversed entirely by dose reduction or discontinuance of the drug or by replacing defective coagulation factors with fresh-frozen plasma (Becker, 1996). The administration of vitamin K also may be considered, unless there is a risk of inducing a life-threatening thrombotic complication, such as might occur in a patient with a cardiac valve prosthesis.

Contraindications to warfarin therapy include gastrointestinal ulcerations, blood dyscrasias, severe kidney or liver disease, severe hypertension, and recent surgery of the eye, spinal cord, or brain (Abrams, 1998g). Because warfarin crosses the placental barrier, it has the potential in pregnant women to cause both bleeding in the fetus and embryopathy, resulting in fetal hemorrhage, wastage, or malformation (Ginsberg & Hirsh, 1998; Badduke et al., 1991).

Thrombolytic medications are agents that destroy thrombus by stimulating conversion of plasminogen to plasmin, which in turn degrades fibrin, fibrinogen, and other procoagulant proteins (Stanley, 1991). Thrombolytic agents are used to lyse thrombus in patients with acute MI or massive pulmonary embolism. When given to patients within 4 hours of acute MI, thrombolytic agents often can restore blood flow through an acutely occluded coronary artery, thereby preventing myocardial necrosis. Similarly, thrombolytic agents rapidly dissolve pulmonary artery thrombus. They are much more effective than heparin in correcting acute hemodynamic abnormalities caused by massive pulmonary embolism (Rubin & Sherry, 1991). Commonly used thrombolytic agents include recombinant tissue plasminogen activator, streptokinase, and anisoylated plasminogen-streptokinase activator complex.

Bleeding, the major complication of thrombolytic therapy, occurs in approximately 5% of patients; the most significant form is cerebral hemorrhage, which occurs in 0.5% to 0.7% of patients treated with thrombolytic agents (Becker, 1996). Streptokinase also may cause hypotension and allergic reactions. Thrombolytic therapy is discussed in more detail in Chapter 1, Coronary Artery Disease.

The most commonly used *antiplatelet medication* is aspirin. Aspirin exerts pharmacologic action by inhibiting synthesis of thromboxane A_2, a prostaglandin that causes platelet aggregation; the prevention of thromboxane A_2 formation thereby prevents platelet aggregation and thrombus formation (Abrams, 1998g). Aspirin is commonly administered in patients with coronary artery disease. It is a mainstay of therapy for unstable angina because of its demonstrated effectiveness in reducing the incidence of MI and mortality (Hillis et al., 1995i). It also is given indefinitely to patients who have undergone coronary artery bypass grafting to promote long-term vein graft patency. The antithrombotic effect of aspirin can be achieved with doses ranging from 160 to 325 mg/d, or even less (Becker, 1996). Aspirin therapy is contraindicated in the presence of gastrointestinal bleeding or peptic ulcer disease.

Two less commonly used platelet-inhibiting agents are ticlopidine and abciximab (ReoPro). Ticlopidine interferes with the ability of platelets to aggregate by inhibiting IIb/IIIa receptors involved in binding of fibrinogen; abciximab is a monoclonal antibody that directly binds to the IIb/IIIa receptor of platelets (Bailey et al.,

1997). Because of its adverse effects (eg, neutropenia, diarrhea) and greater cost, ticlopidine is used primarily as a second-line drug in patients who cannot tolerate aspirin (Abrams, 1998g). Abciximab is used to lessen the incidence of restenosis in those who have undergone percutaneous transluminal angioplasty or intracoronary stent placement.

▶ Other Selected Medications

Diuretic Agents

Of the many available *diuretic agents,* loop diuretics are used most commonly in cardiac surgical patients. These are agents that work primarily by actions in the ascending loop of Henle in the renal medulla. Loop diuretics, which include furosemide, bumetanide, and ethacrynic acid, inhibit absorption of sodium, chloride, and potassium (Cunningham, 1990). All three agents can be given intravenously, begin to act within several minutes, and have a short duration of action. The agents differ primarily in potency and produce similar effects at equivalent doses (40 mg furosemide = 1 mg bumetanide = 50 mg ethacrynic acid) (Abrams, 1998h).

Furosemide is used most commonly and may be given routinely to postoperative cardiac surgical patients to promote diuresis of fluid retained secondary to use of cardiopulmonary bypass. It also is used to reduce preload acutely in patients with pulmonary edema. Bumetanide or ethacrynic acid may be given alternatively if furosemide does not produce the desired response. Because potassium excretion is enhanced, adequate potassium repletion is essential to avoid potentially lethal hypokalemia-induced arrhythmias. Also, all of the loop diuretics can damage the eighth cranial nerve. Ototoxicity with resultant hearing loss is most likely with high doses or rapid intravenous administration (Makoff, 1990).

Antihypertensive Agents

A variety of agents are used for chronic management of hypertension, and a complete discussion of *antihypertensive agents* is beyond the scope of this chapter. Many patients who undergo cardiac operations have been on long-term therapy for associated hypertension. These agents usually are continued until the time of surgery, but may not be necessary during the postoperative hospitalization because of hemodynamic changes associated with surgery. However, patients who required antihypertensive therapy before a cardiac operation usually require resumption of therapy, if not in the early postoperative period, then in the first several months after surgery. Many of the previously discussed vasodilators, beta-blocking agents, and calcium channel antagonists have antihypertensive actions and may be used for postoperative blood pressure control.

Angiotensin-converting enzyme inhibiting medications are used occasionally in cardiac surgical patients, but are used most commonly as a major component of therapy in patients with heart failure for afterload reduction. These agents reduce afterload by blocking the action of angiotensin-converting enzyme, which is necessary for conversion of angiotensin I to the potent vasoconstrictor, angiotensin II (Mackall et al., 1996). They also lessen sodium retention by inhibiting the release of aldosterone and lower preload by producing venous dilatation (Laurent-Bopp, 1995). Captopril (Capoten) and enalapril (Vasotec) are examples of angiotensin-converting enzyme inhibitors.

For rapid blood pressure control in the postoperative period, an intravenous agent, such as nitroprusside, nitroglycerin, or esmolol usually is administered. Two antihypertensive agents not previously discussed also may be used. Labetalol is a unique agent with both alpha- and beta-adrenergic blocking actions. It decreases systemic arterial pressure by reducing peripheral vascular resistance with little effect on cardiac output and heart rate (Hillis et al., 1995j). Hydralazine is a vasodilating agent that primarily affects arterial smooth muscle with little or no effect on venous capacitance vessels. Both drugs can be administered intravenously to produce rapid reduction of blood pressure.

REFERENCES

Abrams AC, 1998a: Adrenergic drugs. In Clinical Drug Therapy, ed. 4. Philadelphia, Lippincott Williams & Wilkins

Abrams AC, 1998b: Physiology of the autonomic nervous system. In Clinical Drug Therapy, ed. 4. Philadelphia, Lippincott Williams & Wilkins

Abrams AC, 1998c: Cardiotonic-inotropic agents used in congestive heart failure. In Clinical Drug Therapy, ed. 4. Philadelphia, Lippincott Williams & Wilkins

Abrams AC, 1998d: Antiarrhythmic drugs. In Clinical Drug Therapy, ed. 4. Philadelphia, Lippincott Williams & Wilkins

Abrams AC, 1998e: Antiadrenergic drugs. In Clinical Drug Therapy, ed. 4. Philadelphia, Lippincott Williams & Wilkins

Abrams AC, 1998f: Anticholinergic drugs. In Clinical Drug Therapy, ed. 4. Philadelphia, Lippincott Williams & Wilkins

Abrams AC, 1998g: Anticoagulant, antiplatelet, and thrombolytic agents. In Clinical Drug Therapy, ed.4. Philadelphia, Lippincott Williams & Wilkins

Abrams AC, 1998h: Diuretics. In Clinical Drug Therapy, ed. 4. Philadelphia, Lippincott Williams & Wilkins

Antman EM, 1997: Medical management of the patient undergoing cardiac surgery. In Braunwald E (ed): Heart Disease: A Textbook of Cardiovascular Medicine, ed. 5. Philadelphia, WB Saunders

Antman EM, Braunwald E, 1997: Acute myocardial infarction. In Braunwald E (ed): Heart Disease: A Textbook of Cardiovascular Medicine, ed. 5. Philadelphia, WB Saunders

Armstrong PW, 1998: Stable ischemic syndromes. In Topol EJ (ed): Comprehensive Cardiovascular Medicine. Philadelphia, Lippincott Williams & Wilkins

Badduke BR, Jamieson WR, Miyagishima RT, et al., 1991: Pregnancy and childbearing in a population with biologic valvular prostheses. J Thorac Cardiovasc Surg 102:179

Bailey JM, Levy JH, Hug CC, 1997: Cardiac surgical pharmacology. In Edmunds LH Jr (ed): Cardiac Surgery in the Adult. New York, McGraw-Hill

Balser JR, 1997: The rational use of intravenous amiodarone in the perioperative period. Anesthesiology 86:974

Barold SS, Zipes DP, 1997: Cardiac pacemakers and antiarrhythmic devices. In Braunwald E (ed): Heart Disease: A Textbook of Cardiovascular Medicine, ed. 5. Philadelphia, WB Saunders

Barron JT, Parrillo JE, 1991: Congestive heart failure: Vasodilator therapy. In Parrillo JE (ed): Current Therapy in Critical Care Medicine, ed. 2. Philadelphia, BC Decker

Becker RC, 1996: Hematologic and coagulation considerations in patients with cardiac disease. In Kvetan V, Dantzker DR (eds): The Critically Ill Cardiac Patient: Multisystem Dysfunction and Management. Philadelphia, Lippincott-Raven

Bond EF, 1990: Antiarrhythmic drugs. In Underhill SL, Woods SL, Froelicher ES, Halpenny CJ (eds): Cardiovascular Medications for Cardiac Nursing. Philadelphia, JB Lippincott

Bond EF, Underhill SL, 1990: Inotropic agents. In Underhill SL, Woods SL, Froelicher ES, Halpenny CJ (eds): Cardiovascular Medications for Cardiac Nursing. Philadelphia, JB Lippincott

Brieger DB, Mak KH, Kottke-Marchant K, et al., 1998: Heparin-induced thrombocytopenia. J Am Coll Cardiol 31:1449

Buckingham TA, Parrillo JE, 1991: Ventricular arrhythmia. In Parrillo JE (ed): Current Therapy in Critical Care Medicine, ed. 2. Philadelphia, BC Decker

Butterworth JF, Prielipp RC, MacGregor DA, Zaloga GP, 1996: Pharmacologic cardiovascular support. In Kvetan V, Dantzker DR (eds): The Critically Ill Cardiac Patient: Multisystem Dysfunction and Management. Philadelphia, Lippincott-Raven

Christopherson DJ, Froelicher ES, 1990: Anticoagulant, antithrombotic, and platelet-modifying drugs. In Underhill SL, Woods SL, Froelicher ES, Halpenny CJ (eds): Cardiovascular Medications for Cardiac Nursing. Philadelphia, JB Lippincott

Cunningham SG, 1990: Diuretics. In Underhill SL, Woods SL, Froelicher ES, Halpenny CJ (eds): Cardiovascular Medications for Cardiac Nursing. Philadelphia, JB Lippincott

DiSesa VJ, 1991: Pharmacologic support for postoperative low cardiac output. Semin Thorac Cardiovasc Surg 3:13

Drew BJ, 1991: Bedside diagnosis of wide QRS tachycardia. Critical Care Nursing Quarterly 14:19

Dusman RE, Stanton MS, Miles WM, et al., 1990: Clinical features of amiodarone-induced pulmonary toxicity. Circulation 82:51

Elefteriades JA, Geha AS, Cohen LS, 1996a: Continuous infusion agents. In House Officer Guide to ICU Care: Fundamentals of Management of the Heart and Lungs, ed. 2. Philadelphia, Lippincott-Raven

Elefteriades JA, Geha AS, Cohen LS, 1996b: Cardiac arrest and near arrest. In House Officer Guide to ICU Care: Fundamentals of Management of the Heart and Lungs, ed. 2. Philadelphia, Lippincott-Raven

Elefteriades JA, Geha AS, Cohen LS, 1996c: Additional topics. In House Officer Guide to ICU Care: Fundamentals of Management of the Heart and Lungs, ed. 2. Philadelphia, Lippincott-Raven

Ferguson DW, 1991: Cardiogenic shock. In Hurst JW (ed): Current Therapy in Cardiovascular Disease, ed. 3. Philadelphia, BC Decker

Garcia MJ, 1998: Prosthetic valve disease. In Topol EJ (ed): Comprehensive Cardiovascular Medicine. Philadelphia, Lippincott Williams & Wilkins

Ginsberg JS, Hirsh J, 1998: Use of antithrombotics during pregnancy. Chest 114:524S

Gray RJ, Mandel WJ, 1990: Management of common postop-erative arrhythmias. In Gray RJ, Matloff JM (eds): Medical Management of the Cardiac Surgical Patient. Baltimore, Williams & Wilkins

Greco SA, 1990: Vasoactive drugs. In Underhill SL, Woods SL, Froelicher ES, Halpenny CJ (eds): Cardiovascular Medications for Cardiac Nursing. Philadelphia, JB Lippincott

Haas GJ, Young JB, 1998: Acute heart failure management. In Topol EJ (ed): Comprehensive Cardiovascular Medicine. Philadelphia, Lippincott Williams & Wilkins

Hillis LD, Lange RA, Winniford MD, Page RL, 1995a: Inotropic agents. In Manual of Clinical Problems in Cardiology, ed. 5. Boston, Little, Brown

Hillis LD, Lange RA, Winniford MD, Page RL, 1995b: Vasodilators. In Manual of Clinical Problems in Cardiology, ed. 5. Boston, Little, Brown

Hillis LD, Lange RA, Winniford MD, Page RL, 1995c: Procainamide. In Manual of Clinical Problems in Cardiology, ed. 5. Boston, Little, Brown

Hillis LD, Lange RA, Winniford MD, Page RL, 1995d: Lidocaine. In Manual of Clinical Problems in Cardiology, ed. 5. Boston, Little, Brown

Hillis LD, Lange RA, Winniford MD, Page RL, 1995e: Amiodarone. In Manual of Clinical Problems in Cardiology, ed. 5. Boston, Little, Brown

Hillis LD, Lange RA, Winniford MD, Page RL, 1995f: Sotalol. In Manual of Clinical Problems in Cardiology, ed. 5. Boston, Little, Brown

Hillis LD, Lange RA, Winniford MD, Page RL, 1995g: Nitrates. In Manual of Clinical Problems in Cardiology, ed. 5. Boston, Little, Brown

Hillis LD, Lange RA, Winniford MD, Page RL, 1995h: Beta-adrenergic blocking agents. In Manual of Clinical Problems in Cardiology, ed. 5. Boston, Little, Brown

Hillis LD, Lange RA, Winniford MD, Page RL, 1995i: Anticoagulants and antiplatelet agents. In Manual of Clinical Problems in Cardiology, ed. 5. Boston, Little, Brown

Hillis LD, Lange RA, Winniford MD, Page RL, 1995j: Antihypertensive agents. In Manual of Clinical Problems in Cardiology, ed. 5. Boston, Little, Brown

Hudak CM, Gallo BM, Morton PG, 1998a: Patient management: Cardiovascular system. In Critical Care Nursing, ed. 7. Philadelphia, Lippincott Williams & Wilkins

Hudak CM, Gallo BM, Morton PG, 1998b: Organ and hemopoietic stem cell transplantation. In Critical Care Nursing, ed. 7. Philadelphia, Lippincott Williams & Wilkins

Ide B, Drew BJ, 1998: The many rhythms of digitalis toxicity. Prog Cardiovasc Nurs 13:41

Kalkanis SN, Sloane D, Strichartz GR, Lilly LS, 1998: Cardiovascular drugs. In Lilly LS (ed): Pathophysiology of Heart Disease, ed. 2. Baltimore, Williams & Wilkins

Kayser SR, 1998: Low-molecular-weight heparins in the management of cardiovascular conditions. Prog Cardiovasc Nurs 13:34

Kutcher MA, 1991: Angina pectoris: stable. In Hurst JW (ed): Current Therapy in Cardiovascular Disease, ed. 3. Philadelphia, BC Decker

Landolfo K, Smith PK, 1995: Postoperative care in cardiac surgery. In Sabiston DC Jr, Spencer FC (eds): Surgery of the Chest, ed. 6. Philadelphia, WB Saunders

Lapsley DP, 1991: Drug therapy for sudden cardiac death. In Owens PM (ed): Sudden Cardiac Death. Gaithersburg, MD, Aspen

Laurent-Bopp D, 1995: Heart failure. In Woods SL, Froelicher ES, Halpenny CJ, Motzer SU (eds): Cardiac Nursing, ed. 3. Philadelphia, JB Lippincott

LeClair HH, Carlson KK, 1990: Agents used to restore electrolyte balance. In Underhill SL, Woods SL, Froelicher ES, Halpenny CJ (eds): Cardiovascular Medications for Cardiac Nursing. Philadelphia, JB Lippincott

Lewis RP, 1991: Supraventricular arrhythmia. In Parrillo JE (ed): Current Therapy in Critical Care Medicine, ed. 2. Philadelphia, BC Decker

Loveys BJ, 1990: Beta-blocking agents. In Underhill SL, Woods SL, Froelicher ES, Halpenny CJ (eds): Cardiovascular Medications for Cardiac Nursing. Philadelphia, JB Lippincott

Mackall JA, Buchter CM, Thames MD, 1996: Pharmacological approach to the management of the cardiac surgical patient. In Baue AE, Geha AS, Hammond GL, et al. (eds): Glenn's Thoracic and Cardiovascular Surgery, ed. 6. Stamford, CT, Appleton & Lange

Makoff DL, 1990: Hypertension. In Berk JL, Sampliner JE (eds): Handbook of Critical Care, ed. 3. Boston, Little, Brown

Mandel WJ, 1990: Cardiac arrhythmias. In Berk JL, Sampliner JE (eds): Handbook of Critical Care, ed. 3. Boston, Little, Brown

Marino PL, 1998a: Tachyarrhythmias. In The ICU Book, ed. 2. Baltimore, Williams & Wilkins

Marino PL, 1998b: Early management of acute myocardial infarction. In The ICU Book, ed. 2. Baltimore, Williams & Wilkins

Marino PL, 1998c: Venous thromboembolism. In The ICU Book, ed. 2. Baltimore, Williams & Wilkins

Moore SL, Wilkoff BL, 1991: Rhythm disturbances after cardiac surgery. Semin Thorac Cardiovasc Surg 3:24

Morton PG, 1994: Update on new antiarrhythmic agents. Critical Care Nursing Clinics of North America 6:69

Nalos PC, Kass RM, Gang ES, et al., 1987: Life-threatening pulmonary complications in patients with previous amiodarone pulmonary toxicity undergoing cardiothoracic operations. J Thorac Cardiovasc Surg 93:904

Nolan SP, Zacour R, 1998: Cardiopulmonary bypass. In Kaiser LR, Kron IL, Spray TL (eds): Mastery of Cardiothoracic Surgery. Philadelphia, Lippincott Williams & Wilkins

Nunnelee JD, 1997: Low-molecular-weight heparin. J Vasc Nurs 15:94

Phelan J, Klein LW, 1991: The postoperative cardiac surgical patient. In Parrillo JE (ed): Current Therapy in Critical Care Medicine, ed. 2. Philadelphia, BC Decker

Porth CM, 1998: Control of the circulation. In Porth CM (ed): Pathophysiology: Concepts of Altered Health States, ed. 5. Philadelphia, Lippincott Williams & Wilkins

Pratt CM, Roberts R, 1991: Angina pectoris: Unstable. In Hurst JW (ed): Current Therapy in Cardiovascular Disease, ed. 3. Philadelphia, BC Decker

Roden DM, 1998: Antiarrhythmic drugs. In Topol EJ (ed): Comprehensive Cardiovascular Medicine. Philadelphia, Lippincott Williams & Wilkins

Rubin RN, Sherry S, 1991: Pulmonary embolism. In Parrillo JE (ed): Current Therapy in Critical Care Medicine, ed. 2. Philadelphia, BC Decker

Schaer GL, 1991: Unstable angina. In Parrillo JE (ed): Current Therapy in Critical Care Medicine, ed. 2. Philadelphia, BC Decker

Schroeder JS, 1997: Unstable angina and non–Q-wave myocardial infarction. In Alpert JS (ed): Cardiology for the Primary Care Physician, ed. 2. Philadelphia, Current Medicine

Severson AL, Meyer LT, 1992: Treatment of paroxysmal supraventricular tachycardia with adenosine: Implications for nursing. Heart Lung 21:350

Simandl S, Cohn PF, 1997: Chronic ischemic heart disease. In Alpert JS (ed): Cardiology for the Primary Care Physician, ed. 2. Philadelphia, Current Medicine

Slovis CM, Brody SL, 1991: Cardiac arrest and resuscitation from sudden death. In Hurst JW (ed): Current Therapy in Cardiovascular Disease, ed. 3. Philadelphia, BC Decker

Smith TW, Kelly RA, Stevenson LW, Braunwald E, 1997: Management of heart failure. In Braunwald E (ed): Heart Disease: A Textbook of Cardiovascular Medicine, ed. 5. Philadelphia, WB Saunders

Stanley R, 1991: Cardiovascular drugs. In Kinney MR, Packa DR, Andreoli KG, Zipes DP (eds): Comprehensive Cardiac Care, ed. 7. St. Louis, Mosby–Year Book

White J, 1998: Disorders of cardiac conduction and rhythm. In Porth CM (ed): Pathophysiology: Concepts of Altered Health States, ed. 5. Philadelphia, Lippincott Williams & Wilkins

Whitman GR, 1991: Hypertension and hypothermia in the acute postoperative period. Critical Care Nursing Clinics of North America 3:661

Zipes DP, 1997: Management of cardiac arrhythmias: Pharmacological, electrical, and surgical techniques. In Braunwald E (ed): Heart Disease: A Textbook of Cardiovascular Medicine, ed. 5. Philadelphia, WB Saunders

28

Complications of Cardiac Operations

Postoperative complications can occur after any cardiac operation. They not only cause morbidity, but prolong hospitalization and have a direct effect on survival probability. Patients who experience one or more complications have an up to 10 times greater probability of death compared with those without complications (Loop, 1998). Complications after cardiac operations also increase costs significantly. As much as 40% of yearly costs associated with coronary artery revascularization may be consumed by 10% to 15% of patients with serious postoperative complications (Ferraris, 1997). Although it is not possible to predict with certainty which patients will have complications in the perioperative period, certain groups of patients can be profiled for whom risk is higher than usual. Unfortunately, an increasing number of cardiac surgical patients fall into these high-risk categories.

Coronary artery bypass grafting is the most common type of cardiac operation performed in the United States. Patient selection for surgical revascularization has changed substantially owing to more effective nonsurgical therapies. Improvements in antianginal medications, percutaneous transluminal angioplasty catheters, and intracoronary stents have increased the number of patients who can be treated initially with these modalities. Therefore, patients likely to receive surgical intervention are those with more diffuse coronary artery disease and greater left ventricular dysfunction. Also, because coronary artery disease is progressive and none of the therapies is curative, patients often require surgical revascularization after previous pharmacologic therapy, angioplasty, or bypass grafting, when they are older and have more extensive disease, more ventricular impairment, and associated medical diseases.

The average age of patients undergoing cardiac operations also has risen because increased longevity in the United States has resulted in a large population of elderly people, many of whom have significant coronary artery disease. By 70 years of age, clinically diagnosable coronary atherosclerosis occurs in approximately 15% of men and 9% of women; the incidence increases to 20% in both sexes by 80 years (Loop, 1998). Elderly persons also may have aortic valve stenosis secondary to degenerative valve calcification and fibrosis, necessitating aortic valve replacement during the seventh, eighth, or ninth decade of life. Consequently, surgical intervention in septuagenarians and octogenarians is commonplace.

Another complex group of patients referred increasingly for cardiac operations are individuals who previously have undergone solid organ transplantation. Although solid organ transplant recipients usually can undergo subsequent cardiac surgical procedures safely, they are at increased risk for significant perioperative morbidity (Mitruka et al., 1997).

► Risk Factors

Most of the risk stratification analyses that have been performed examine risk factors associated with operative mortality, particularly in patients undergoing coronary artery revascularization (Ferraris, 1997). Identified risk factors for operative mortality in patients undergoing coronary artery bypass grafting include advanced age, emergency surgery, elevated serum creatinine, left main coronary artery disease, female sex, anemia, and moderate to severe left ventricular dysfunction (Loop, 1998).

Age is an important predisposing factor for operative risk. Most series report higher operative mortality rates in elderly patients, especially when surgery is performed urgently or emergently (Edwards et al., 1991). Higher complication rates also have been demonstrated consistently, probably related to generalized deterioration in the function of major organ systems and the presence of associated chronic medical problems. Significant preoperative risk factors for postoperative complications in elderly patients include prior stroke, diabetes mellitus, and a New York Heart Association class IV functional status (Deiwick et al., 1997). Neurologic complications are particularly prevalent in elderly patients (Edwards et al., 1991).

The nature and degree of underlying cardiac disease, especially the status of ventricular function, is another major determinant of operative risk. Compared with coronary artery bypass grafting, operative risk is increased in patients who require valve replacement, coronary revascularization combined with valve replacement, or ventricular aneurysmectomy (Higgins & Starr, 1991). A strong relationship also exists between emergency surgery and postoperative morbidity. Contributing factors in patients receiving emergency operations include the severity of illness; the likely presence of uncontrolled heart failure, cardiogenic shock, or ongoing myocardial infarction (MI); and the limited amount of preoperative preparation, evaluation, and monitoring (Tuman et al., 1992).

Prior heart surgery is another powerful predictor of perioperative complications (Hammermeister et al., 1990). Some patients who undergo coronary artery revascularization or valve repair or replacement require a subsequent cardiac operation, and a small percentage of patients require more than one reoperation. A previous cardiac operation adds to operative risk primarily because of the advanced nature of disease associated with the need for reoperation and the increased potential for technical problems (Tuman et al., 1992). Entry into the chest is more hazardous because the right ventricle or previously constructed bypass grafts often are adherent to the posterior table of the sternum and may be injured. In addition, the presence of adhesions (internal scarring) from a previous surgical procedure and the loss of distinct tissue planes make intraoperative dissection longer and more exacting. Perioperative bleeding and the need for blood transfusion are greater. Patients undergoing repeat operations also are more likely to require postoperative mechanical cardiac assistance (Jones et al., 1991).

Associated arterial occlusive disease is yet another factor that predisposes to postoperative morbidity. Patients undergoing coronary artery revascularization in particular are likely to have significant cerebral or peripheral occlusive lesions because atherosclerosis is a systemic vascular disease. Carotid or cerebral artery atherosclerosis increases risk for a cerebral vascular accident. Perioperative stroke also can result from embolization of atherosclerotic debris in the ascending aorta. An abdominal aortic aneurysm may rupture in the perioperative period. Occlusive arterial disease in the abdominal aorta or femoral arteries may preclude insertion through the femoral artery of an intra-aortic balloon catheter (for counterpulsation) and increases the likelihood of balloon-related complications (Finkelmeier & Finkelmeier, 1991).

Complications also are more likely in patients with associated major medical diseases, such as chronic obstructive pulmonary disease, diabetes mellitus, or renal failure. Some medications increase perioperative risk as well. Aspirin is associated with an increased incidence of postoperative bleeding, increased use of blood products, and longer intensive care unit hospitalization (Loop, 1998). Preoperative use of corticosteroids suppresses the inflammatory process and may impair wound healing.

The most common causes of operative morbidity are discussed in this chapter. Occurrences of some types of complications, such as bleeding and heart failure, are fairly predictable. Other complications, such as air embolism, iatrogenic aortic dissection, or cardiopulmonary bypass system malfunction, may occur unexpectedly. Most complications occur either during the operation or within the first 24 postoperative hours. However, by convention, operative morbidity is defined to include any complication that occurs either within 30 days of operation or before patient discharge from the hospital.

► Cardiovascular Complications

Hemorrhage

Bleeding is a common complication of cardiac operations because of intraoperative systemic anticoagulation and the use of cardiopulmonary bypass. Systemic anticoagulation with heparin is necessary to prevent massive thrombosis that would otherwise occur as blood is circulated through an extracorporeal circuit. Although protamine sulfate is given to reverse the effects of heparin when cardiopulmonary bypass is terminated, normal coagulation is not restored immediately. There is some evidence to suggest that the fibrinolytic cascade is activated to some extent during cardiopulmonary bypass and that fibrinolysis plays a role in postoperative bleeding after cardiopulmonary bypass (McGiffin & Kirklin, 1995). In addition, blood is hemodiluted by priming of the cardiopulmonary circuit with crystalloid solution. As a result, levels of coagulation factors (fibrinogen, prothrombin, and factors V and VIII) are reduced by approximately 50% (Halfman-Franey & Berg, 1991).

The surgeon achieves adequate hemostasis before closing the chest incision and transporting the patient out of the operating room. Areas that are inspected for bleeding include anastomotic suture lines; cannulation sites; conduit side branches; internal thoracic artery (also called internal mammary artery) pedicle; and thymic and epicardial tissue; and sternal wire and chest tube sites (Mahfood et al., 1991). However, bleeding may increase substantially as the patient's body temperature warms. Postoperative bleeding also is exacerbated by hypertension, a common problem in the early postoperative hours, that may occur as a paroxysmal event or be caused by pain, endotracheal suctioning, patient arousal from anesthesia, or the patient's resistance to mechanical ventilation (Whitman, 1991). Even brief periods of hypertension (eg, with systolic blood pressures of 180 to 200 mm Hg) can cause significant increases in chest tube drainage (Elefteriades et al., 1996a).

Excessive mediastinal bleeding, or hemorrhage, is characterized by sustained chest tube output greater than 100 mL/h, or greater than 300 mL in any 1 hour. It usually occurs within the first 24 postoperative hours. Certain categories of patients are more likely to experience excessive bleeding, including those who (1) have undergone one or more previous cardiac operations; (2) have liver dysfunction secondary to valvular heart disease and passive congestion; (3) have an underlying bleeding disorder; (4) have received preoperative antiplatelet therapy; (5) require lengthy operations necessitating a prolonged period of cardiopulmonary bypass; or (6) have friable tissue or an underlying pathologic process likely to be associated with hemorrhage, such as a traumatic cardiac wound, aortic dissection, or ruptured aortic aneurysm.

Postoperative bleeding is categorized as (1) mechanical (ie, surgically correctable), or (2) nonsurgical (ie, generalized bleeding related to a coagulopathy). A mechanical cause is characterized by brisk hemorrhage (>200 mL/h), normal or near-normal coagulation study results, and the appearance of blood clots in the mediastinal drainage tubes (Landolfo & Smith, 1995). More commonly, excessive bleeding is due predominantly to postoperative coagulopathy. Platelet dysfunction is partially responsible for the hemostatic derangement after cardiopulmonary bypass and is a major cause of postoperative coagulopathy (Khuri et al., 1999; Halfman-Franey & Berg, 1991). Nonsurgical bleeding also may be caused by inadequate heparin neutralization, fibrinolysis, complement activation, or decreased levels of factors V, VIII, and XIII, fibrinogen, and plasminogen (Hendren & Higgins, 1991). Coagulopathy is more common in patients who have received antiplatelet agents, thrombolytic therapy, or heparin in the preoperative period (Landolfo & Smith, 1995).

Autotransfusion of shed mediastinal blood may be performed during the first 6 to 12 hours, or longer if active bleeding continues. If necessary, autotransfusion is supplemented with allogeneic blood component therapy. Packed red blood cells, platelets, or fresh frozen plasma may be administered to replenish hemoglobin, platelets, or clotting factors, respectively. Drugs that improve platelet function (eg, desmopressin) or prevent fibrinolysis (eg, aminocaproic acid) also may be administered in selected patients to treat postoperative coagulopathy (Halfman-Franey & Berg, 1991). Uncommonly, heparin activity recurs after initial adequate reversal with protamine sulfate. This so-called *heparin rebound phenomenon* occurs because protamine sulfate, given as an antidote to heparin, is eliminated from the blood before heparin (Ellison et al., 1991). Heparin rebound is treated with protamine sulfate administration.

If bleeding is excessive or sustained, reexploration may be necessary to detect and correct a mechanical bleeding source. Although often no surgically correctable cause of bleeding is identified at the time of reexploration, surgical irrigation and the removal of clots may reduce the fibrinolytic process in the mediastinum, allowing the bleeding ends of capillaries and small vessels to thrombose (Pelletier et al., 1998). Indications for reexploration include chest tube output between 300 and 500 mL/h for the first hour, 200 and 300 mL/h for the second hour, or greater than 100 mL/h for 6 to 8 hours (Baumgartner et al., 1997). Each clinical situation should be viewed individually, however, and management of postoperative bleeding always should include correction of abnormal coagulation parameters. Reexploration for bleeding is an independent risk factor for mortality, renal failure, respiratory distress syndrome, sepsis, and atrial arrhythmias (Loop, 1998).

Occasionally, precipitous hemorrhage occurs as the result of disruption of a suture or loosening of a surgical clip. In such cases, the patient is transferred immediately to the operating room for reexploration. If hemorrhage is massive, the surgeon may need to open a portion of the sternotomy incision in the intensive care unit to obtain digital control of the bleeding source and stabilize the patient before transport to the operating room. Hemorrhage that is treated inadequately leads to hypovolemic shock, exsanguination, or cardiac tamponade.

Severe postoperative coagulopathies, such as disseminated intravascular coagulation, are rare. Disseminated intravascular coagulation is not a specific disease entity, but rather a complex event characterized by abnormal bleeding, small vessel obstruction, tissue necrosis, and end-organ damage (Becker, 1996). It occurs most often in patients with low cardiac output, intense peripheral vasoconstriction, and poor tissue perfusion.

Cardiac Tamponade

Cardiac tamponade describes a condition in which the heart is compressed by blood that has accumulated in the pericardium or anterior mediastinum. It usually represents a combination of excessive bleeding and inadequate pericardial or mediastinal drainage. To reduce the risk of cardiac tamponade, many surgeons leave the pericardium widely open and place one of the mediastinal chest tubes in the most dependent part of the pericardial sac near the left ventricle (Lee & Geha, 1996). Also, if excessive bleeding is anticipated, one of the pleural spaces may be opened intentionally to provide adequate egress for blood.

The hemodynamic changes associated with cardiac tamponade result from biventricular restriction of end-diastolic volume (Landolfo & Smith, 1995). As blood accumulates in the pericardial space or mediastinum, the abnormally positive pressure in the finite space is transmitted to the ventricular cavity, eliminating the intercavitary pressure gradients responsible for normal ventricular filling during diastole (Elefteriades et al., 1996b). The heart is unable to fill adequately and cardiac output decreases. Arterial pressure is preserved initially by alpha-adrenergic–mediated peripheral vasoconstriction but then decreases as a premortal event (Klein & Scalia, 1998).

Clinical manifestations of cardiac tamponade include hypotension; decreased cardiac output; elevation and equalization of filling pressures (central venous, pulmonary artery diastolic, and left atrial pressures); roentgenographic evidence of mediastinal widening; diminished or excessive chest tube drainage; and pulsus paradoxus. The diagnosis also should be suspected any time there is a sudden deterioration in the condition of a postoperative cardiac surgical patient, particularly in the early postoperative hours and in association with sudden diminution in the amount of chest tube drainage.

Temporizing measures to support cardiac function in the presence of tamponade include administration of fluids and inotropic medications. However, relief of the tamponade is essential to correct hemodynamic compromise. Chest tubes are stripped to evacuate clotted material and restore patency. If the rate of bleeding is so excessive that tamponade occurs despite patent chest tubes, the surgeon reopens the incision emergently to relieve tamponade and control hemorrhage with digital compression. Depending on the degree of hemodynamic instability, the lower end of the sternotomy incision may be opened in the intensive care unit as a life-saving measure.

If time allows, the patient instead is transported rapidly to the operating room. Regardless of where the incision is reopened, eventual transfer to the operating room is necessary for thorough exploration of the mediastinum and reclosure of the incision under sterile conditions.

Although tamponade most often occurs during the first 24 hours after operation, it occasionally occurs late, usually in patients with excessive postoperative bleeding, in patients being anticoagulated, or in those with postpericardiotomy syndrome (Landolfo & Smith, 1995). Late cardiac tamponade also can occur from bleeding associated with removal of an epicardial pacing wire or a left atrial catheter. For this reason, patients are monitored carefully for several hours after removal of pacing wires, and a chest tube usually remains in place until the left atrial catheter has been removed.

Myocardial Infarction

Myocardial infarction can occur after any cardiac operation but is most common after coronary artery bypass grafting. It occurs in 2% to 5% of patients who undergo coronary revascularization (Loop, 1998). Perioperative MI after coronary artery bypass grafting can be caused by one of several mechanisms. Probably most common is inadequate myocardial oxygenation during cardiopulmonary bypass, particularly in areas of muscle supplied by diseased coronary arteries. Arterial spasm may occur in an internal thoracic artery graft or in native coronary arteries regardless of whether they have received bypass grafts.

Acute graft closure of saphenous veins is unusual but can occur as a result of technical difficulties with graft construction, poor conduit quality, or inadequate runoff secondary to distal disease. Although less common, perioperative MI sometimes occurs after other types of cardiac operations. Even in the absence of coronary artery disease, profound hypotension, inadequate myocardial protection during cardiopulmonary bypass, or air or

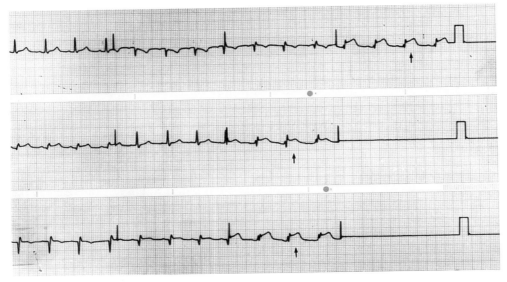

FIGURE 28-1. Twelve-lead electrocardiogram obtained in intubated and sedated patient after uneventful coronary artery bypass grafting (leads V$_5$ and V$_6$ not recorded because of presence of bandage). Marked ST segment elevation in leads V$_2$ through V$_4$ (*arrows*) represents acute anterior wall injury; subsequent emergent operative exploration revealed severe spasm of the internal thoracic artery (grafted to the left anterior descending coronary artery).

thrombotic emboli to the coronary circulation can cause an intraoperative MI.

An electrocardiogram obtained in the immediate postoperative period is particularly important because it is likely to show the first manifestations of myocardial injury in sedated, intubated patients (Fig. 28-1). In the alert postoperative patient, an MI may be manifest as chest discomfort that is similar to preoperative anginal pain. An electrocardiogram is obtained during the pain, and sublingual nitroglycerin may be ordered by the physician to assess its efficacy in abating pain.

Arterial spasm usually is treated with intravenous nitroglycerin and calcium channel antagonists. In severe cases, emergency cardiac catheterization may be performed for instillation of nitroglycerin or papaverine directly into the affected coronary artery (Landolfo & Smith, 1995). If a technical problem with one of the grafts is identified in the first 24 hours, emergent reexploration may be performed, particularly if the patient's condition is unstable. Pharmacologic and mechanical support of the heart occasionally may be necessary if cardiac function is impaired significantly.

Although it can be a major complication, most perioperative MIs are mild and are detected only by elevated isoenzymes or electrocardiographic changes. In asymptomatic or minimally symptomatic patients, treatment and the postoperative course usually are similar to that of patients without MI, except that the return to a normal activity level is more gradual. Beta-blocking and afterload reduction medications may be initiated, as well as other drug therapy that increases longevity after MI (Landolfo & Smith, 1995). If graft closure is suspected during the postoperative period, coronary angiography may be performed to assess graft patency. Although it is demoralizing for the patient and surgeon to document early graft closure, determining graft viability may be important to guide future therapy.

Ventricular Dysfunction

Left, right, or *biventricular dysfunction* can complicate cardiac operations. Some degree of transient, global, biventricular dysfunction that peaks at 2 hours after operation and resolves within 24 to 48 hours is common even in patients with normal preoperative cardiac function (Mackall et al., 1996). In patients with coronary artery disease, ventricular dysfunction is most likely in those who undergo operation within 1 week of an acute MI and in those with compromised ventricular function from previous MIs. Significant ventricular dysfunction also can complicate valvular heart surgery and usually represents an exacerbation of preexisting ventricular impairment caused by the underlying valvular heart disease.

Other causes of postoperative ventricular dysfunction include inadequate myocardial protection, intraoperative MI, long periods of cardiopulmonary bypass or ischemia (the period when the aorta is cross-clamped), and technical difficulties during the conduct of the operation (Richen-

bacher & Pierce, 1997). Because both coronary and valvular heart disease most often damage the left ventricle, perioperative left ventricular dysfunction occurs most frequently. Left ventricular dysfunction may be recognized in the operating room as failure to wean from cardiopulmonary bypass or may develop in the early postoperative hours in the intensive care unit (Mackall et al., 1996).

Ventricular dysfunction is categorized as low cardiac output syndrome or cardiogenic shock, depending on its severity. It results from alterations in those variables that affect cardiac output (ie, heart rate, preload, afterload, and contractility). Ventricular dysfunction may occur secondary to an inadequate cardiac rhythm (bradycardia or tachycardia), inadequate intravascular volume, interference with ventricular filling or emptying, increased afterload, or myocardial dysfunction (Mackall et al., 1996). Often, a combination of these factors is present.

Parameters indicative of ventricular failure include a cardiac index less than 2.0 L/min/m^2, systemic vascular resistance greater than 2100 dynes·sec·cm^{-5}, pulmonary artery diastolic pressure greater than 20 mm Hg, and urine output less than 20 mL/h. Other clinical manifestations include cold, clammy extremities; hypotension; tachycardia; diminished peripheral pulses and capillary refill; and persistent obtundation (Moreno-Cabral et al., 1988). However, residual effects of anesthesia, the patient's thermal instability, and the osmotic diuresis that follows cardiopulmonary bypass may obscure classic manifestations in the early postoperative hours (DiSesa, 1991).

Treatment is directed at manipulating heart rate, preload, afterload, and contractility to restore an adequate cardiac output. Temporary pacing may be used to increase heart rate or provide atrioventricular synchrony in the presence of sinus bradycardia or heart block, respectively. Volume replacement with crystalloid or colloid solutions, or blood products often is necessary to provide an adequate preload, particularly in the presence of postoperative bleeding, diuresis, or vasodilatation. Patients are maintained in a sedated state to minimize sympathetic overstimulation and its deleterious effects on heart rate and systemic vascular resistance (Moran & Singh, 1989).

Afterload reduction and improved myocardial contractility are achieved with a combination of vasodilating and inotropic medications (DiSesa, 1991). Intra-aortic balloon counterpulsation (IABC) may be necessary if pharmacologic afterload reduction alone is ineffective. In selected patients with cardiogenic shock refractory to pharmacologic therapy or IABC, a circulatory assist device may be necessary.

Right ventricular dysfunction is less common but may occur in patients with chronic pulmonary hypertension or secondary to left ventricular failure. Pharmacologic pulmonary vascular vasodilatation can be achieved with nitroglycerin or isoproterenol infusion or nitric oxide inhalation. Rarely, a right ventricular assist device may be necessary. Cardiac transplantation may be considered in selected patients with irreversible postoperative left ventricular, right ventricular, or biventricular dysfunction.

Cardiac Arrhythmias

Arrhythmic complications may be categorized as ventricular tachycardia (VT) or ventricular fibrillation (VF), ventricular ectopy without VT or VF, supraventricular tachycardia (SVT), and conduction disturbances. The incidence of arrhythmias in the postoperative period has been reported as 2% to 13% for ventricular arrhythmias and 11% to 54% for supraventricular arrhythmias (Mackall et al., 1996).

Ventricular tachycardia and VF are the most serious arrhythmic complications. New-onset VT may occur after surgery in as much as 3% of patients who undergo coronary artery bypass grafting; at highest risk are those patients with prior MI and severe left ventricular dysfunction (Steinberg et al., 1999). Other causes of postoperative ventricular arrhythmias include (1) perioperative myocardial ischemia, (2) hypertrophic cardiomyopathy, (3) an underlying arrhythmic disorder, (4) severe aortic valve disease, and (5) proarrhythmic effects of antiarrhythmic medications. Torsades de pointes is the classic form of drug-induced proarrhythmia observed in patients receiving antiarrhythmic agents that prolong ventricular repolarization, such as the class III antiarrhythmic drugs (eg, sotalol, amiodarone). Rarely, VT or VF occurs in the absence of a detectable precipitant.

Ventricular tachycardia that causes hemodynamic instability and VF are treated with prompt defibrillation and cardiopulmonary resuscitation as necessary. Intravenous lidocaine therapy or direct-current cardioversion is used to treat VT that is not associated with hemodynamic instability. When antiarrhythmic drug-induced proarrhythmia occurs, the responsible agent is discontinued immediately and predisposing factors, such as electrolyte disorders or bradycardia, are corrected (Hohnloser, 1997). The occurrence of sustained or recurring VT or VF in the postoperative period warrants electrophysiologic evaluation to determine inducibility, likelihood of arrhythmia recurrence, and the most effective form of chronic antiarrhythmic therapy.

Transient, nonsustained VT and ventricular ectopy are fairly common in the postoperative period and may result from any of the following factors: hypokalemia, hypomagnesemia, myocardial ischemia, hypoxemia, acidosis, digoxin toxicity, edema from surgical manipulation, or mechanical irritation from an intracardiac catheter. Usually such ectopy resolves with elimination of the precipitating cause. An intravenous lidocaine infusion may be necessary temporarily.

Supraventricular tachycardias include paroxysmal atrial tachycardia, atrial flutter, atrial fibrillation, and junctional tachycardia. Most common is atrial fibrillation, which occurs in approximately one third of patients who undergo cardiac operations (Almassi et al., 1997). Although the arrhythmogenic mechanism is unknown, etiologic factors may include inadequate protection of atrial myocardium against intraoperative ischemia, the high potassium concentration in cardioplegic solutions, and surgical manipulation of the heart. Advanced age also appears to predispose patients to development of postoperative SVT (Leitch et al., 1990; Hashimoto et al., 1991).

In most patients, SVT is tolerated without hemodynamic compromise. It usually is treated with digoxin, propranolol, or ibutilide. Digoxin or propranolol may be given prophylactically in the postoperative period to control the incidence and severity of supraventricular arrhythmias. Amiodarone also provides effective prophylaxis when administered before surgery in high-risk populations (Daoud et al., 1997). Type I atrial flutter (atrial rate ranging from 230 to 340 beats/min) usually can be converted successfully with rapid atrial pacing. In patients with compromised cardiac function, SVT may produce significant hypotension necessitating urgent cardioversion.

Atrioventricular block is most likely after valve replacement procedures and may represent edema, ischemic damage, or mechanical injury of conduction pathways secondary to surgical manipulation. Because significant second- or third-degree heart block usually is transient, it is treated with temporary pacing and usually resolves within 7 to 10 days. If the intrinsic cardiac rhythm is inadequate to support hemodynamic function, the patient remains during this time in a closely monitored intensive or intermediate care unit with easily available additional pacing and emergency equipment and medications.

Occasionally, postoperative atrioventricular block or symptomatic bradycardia persists, necessitating implantation of a transvenous permanent pacemaker. The incidence of permanent pacing ranges from 0.4% to 1.1% after coronary artery bypass grafting and from 3% to 6% after valvular operations (Gordon et al., 1998). Permanent pacemaker implantation is required in 9.7% of patients undergoing reoperative cardiac surgery; factors strongly related to the need for permanent pacing after reoperation include valve replacement, preoperative endocarditis, the number of reoperations, advanced age, and the degree of hypothermia during cardiopulmonary bypass (Lewis et al., 1998).

Patients who have undergone coronary artery bypass grafting may have new bundle branch blocks; however, complete resolution occurs in most within 2 months (Moore & Wilkoff, 1991). Cardiac arrhythmias and their management are discussed further in Chapter 22, Postoperative Patient Management, and Chapter 25, Cardiac Arrhythmias.

Cardiac Arrest

Infrequently, cardiac surgical patients experience *cardiac arrest* in the postoperative period. Precipitous cardiac arrest in a previously stable patient usually is due to an arrhythmia and is most likely to occur during the first 48 hours after surgery, when electrolyte disturbances, hypoxemia, or myocardial ischemia may be present. Rarely, cardiac arrest occurs late in the postoperative period, presumably caused by an undetected cardiac rhythm disorder. Other, less common causes of cardiac arrest in cardiac surgical patients include undetected cardiac tamponade or pulmonary embolism.

Cardiac arrest is treated with immediate institution of cardiopulmonary resuscitation and advanced life support measures. Rapid defibrillation, with subsequent shocks as necessary, is essential for VF or VT with hemodynamic instability. If timely defibrillation is not performed, the outcome of cardiac arrest, with or without cardiopulmonary resuscitation, is dismal. Successful resuscitation is possible in as much as 90% of patients if defibrillation is performed immediately at the time of cardiac arrest (Hendrickson et al., 1997). During each minute that a patient remains in VF, survival probability decreases by 7% to 10% (Ornato & Peberdy, 1998).

The likelihood of successful resuscitation also is related to the duration of cardiopulmonary resuscitation, with a duration of less than 30 minutes correlating with increased survival (Spotnitz & Spotnitz, 1996). In a cardiac surgical patient who does not respond to initial life-saving therapeutic measures, the surgeon often reopens the sternal incision to detect and relieve possible tamponade.

Postpericardiotomy Syndrome

Postpericardiotomy syndrome is an inflammatory process that can complicate operations in which the pericardial sac is opened. It occurs in approximately 18% of adults who undergo cardiac operations (Mehta & Pae, 1997). Postpericardiotomy syndrome typically appears in the first or second week after a cardiac operation, may last 3 to 5 weeks, and is usually self-limited (Edmunds, 1996). It has a variable clinical presentation but usually produces a mild illness. The diagnosis is based on clinical findings, including malaise, fever, a pericardial friction rub, chest pain, and pericardial or pleural effusion. The associated fever is low grade and persists over several days without evidence of local infection.

Treatment with aspirin, indomethacin, or other nonsteroidal anti-inflammatory medication usually results in resolution of symptoms. Antacids are administered concomitantly to reduce gastric irritation, especially in patients who also are receiving warfarin. A single dose of intravenous dexamethasone may be given. Oral corticosteroids may be necessary in more severe cases. Infrequently, postpericardiotomy syndrome leads to development of significant pericardial or pleural effusions.

Pericardial Effusion

Pericardial effusion may represent hemorrhage, as described earlier, or an increased volume of pericardial fluid secondary to postpericardiotomy syndrome. Clinical manifestations of pericardial effusion include dyspnea, fatigue, pulsus paradoxus, and unexplained hypotension. The severity of symptoms associated with pericardial effusion is determined by the volume of the effusion, the rapidity with which the fluid accumulates, and the physical characteristics of the pericardium

(Lorell, 1997). Large effusions can impede diastolic ventricular filling enough to produce cardiac tamponade.

If tamponade develops or if the effusion does not diminish with medical treatment of postpericardiotomy syndrome, it may be necessary to evacuate the pericardial fluid by means of a pericardiocentesis or surgical creation of a pericardial window. These procedures must be performed with particular care in patients who have had recent coronary artery revascularization to avoid damaging grafts that lie on the anterior surface of the heart. Also, in anticoagulated patients, the procedure may need to be delayed until the prothrombin time is lowered, either by withholding warfarin or with the administration of fresh frozen plasma.

Pulmonary Embolism

Major *pulmonary embolism* is an unusual complication after cardiac operations. However, small pulmonary emboli without associated symptoms may occur more commonly than is detected clinically. The individual or combined presence of surface thrombogenicity, hypercoagulability, and locally static blood flow in the cardiovascular system (Virchow's triad) determines the propensity for thrombus formation (Schoen, 1997). Preventive measures against pulmonary embolism include early ambulation and, in high-risk patients, prophylactic anticoagulation.

At greatest risk are patients with a prior history of deep venous thrombosis or pulmonary embolism, patients with coagulation abnormalities, or obese patients with prolonged immobility. Pulmonary emboli originate primarily in the systemic venous circulation, and most arise from the iliac and femoral veins (Fontana & Sabiston, 1995). However, clinical evidence of deep venous thrombosis often is absent. In most patients who sustain fatal pulmonary embolism no clinical features of deep venous thrombosis precede sudden cardiovascular collapse (Moossa et al., 1997).

Clinical manifestations of pulmonary embolism vary. The hemodynamic disturbance is caused not only by embolic vessel occlusion but by the release of vasoactive amines into the pulmonary circulation, with consequent pulmonary artery constriction (Elefteriades et al., 1996c). Findings may include dyspnea, tachypnea, chest pain, new-onset atrial fibrillation, signs and symptoms of deep venous thrombosis, hypotension, and tachycardia. The typical ventilatory response is hyperventilation leading to hypocarbia ($PaCO_2$ < 30 mm Hg), and hypoxemia due to ventilation–perfusion imbalance, anatomic shunting, and impaired oxygen diffusion (Jamieson, 1996). Because symptoms vary and noninvasive studies are not definitive, diagnosis may be difficult. Ventilation–perfusion scanning usually is not specific in postoperative cardiac surgical patients because postoperative atelectasis causes ventilation–perfusion shunting and cardiopulmonary bypass increases levels of interstitial fluid in the lungs. Definitive diagnosis necessitates pulmonary angiography.

On definitive or presumptive diagnosis of a pulmonary

embolus, anticoagulation is instituted, initially with heparin and then with warfarin. Supplemental oxygen or intubation and mechanical ventilation may be necessary, depending on the degree of respiratory compromise. Rarely, massive pulmonary embolism occurs, causing severe hypoxemia and right ventricular failure. Such patients are treated with mechanical ventilation, high fraction of inspired oxygen (FiO_2) and positive end-expiratory pressure levels, and inotropic support of the heart. Thrombolytic therapy, using tissue plasminogen activator, streptokinase, or urokinase, may provide dramatic clinical improvement. However, because of the risk of bleeding complications with thrombolytic therapy, its use typically is limited to critically ill patients.

In the hemodynamically compromised patient who is unresponsive to medical therapy, emergent pulmonary embolectomy may be performed. A patient who has recurrent pulmonary emboli despite therapeutic anticoagulation may require placement of a vena caval filter. Approximately 20% to 40% of patients die within 48 hours of a major pulmonary thromboembolic event (Jamieson, 1996).

▶ Noncardiac Complications

Neurologic Complications

Central neurologic deficits comprise a spectrum of clinical events ranging from isolated transient ischemic attack to fatal cerebral injury. Cerebral vascular accident is the major cause of neurologic disability after cardiac surgery (Mills & Prough, 1991). Strokes occur in 3.4% of patients who undergo cardiac operations; the incidence is higher in patients who undergo coronary artery bypass grafting combined with other procedures (11.3%) and in those older than 70 years of age (5.25%) (Almassi et al., 1999).

The etiology of perioperative strokes is poorly understood. Criteria identified at the Johns Hopkins Hospital as predictive of stroke risk in cardiac surgery patients include age older than 70 years, hypertension, diabetes, history of previous stroke, and asymptomatic carotid bruit (Goldsborough et al., 1997). The most important preoperative risk factor appears to be a history of symptoms suggestive of underlying cerebral vascular disease. In patients with neurologic symptoms or carotid bruits, preoperative ultrasound scanning of carotid arteries usually is performed. Consequently, strokes related to undetected carotid artery disease are fairly uncommon.

More often, perioperative stroke is thought to result from embolization of atherosclerotic material in the ascending aorta (Rao & Weisel, 1997). Atheroma in the ascending aorta and aortic arch can embolize as a result of manipulation, clamping, or cannulation of the aorta (Wareing et al., 1992). The incidence of significant aortic atherosclerosis increases with age from less than 10% in people younger than 60 years of age to more than 32% in those older than 80 years of age (Kohl et al., 1999). Other potential sources of embolic stroke are (1)

thrombus from the left atrium (due to stasis of blood in patients with atrial fibrillation) or ventricle (after MI); (2) air from the arterial perfusion cannula of the cardiopulmonary bypass circuit or a chamber of the heart that has been opened or vented; or (3) calcium from the aortic valve area. Stroke also can occur because of prolonged hypotension associated with left ventricular failure or because of arterial dissection that occludes cerebral blood flow.

Approximately 70% of strokes occur during surgery; the remaining 30% occur in the early postoperative period (Mills & Prough, 1991). Neurologic complications most often become apparent as the patient is allowed to awaken from general anesthesia. Less commonly, a patient who is neurologically intact in the immediate postoperative hours acquires a new deficit in the ensuing postoperative days. Stroke is diagnosed by physical examination and computed tomography of the brain. Therapy is primarily supportive; if a severe neurologic deficit is present, extensive rehabilitation may be necessary.

Seizures occasionally occur in postoperative cardiac surgical patients. Although emboli are the probable cause of most postoperative seizures, other factors, such as fluid overload, electrolyte imbalance, and hypoxemia may also precipitate seizures (Anderson et al., 1991). *Neuropsychologic dysfunction* may occur more commonly than previously recognized in patients who undergo cardiac and aortic operations. Cognitive defects as assessed by neuropsychologic testing have been demonstrated in as much as 60% of patients in the first week after coronary artery bypass grafting; the incidence of these defects decreases substantially after 2 months, but subtle changes in intellectual performance may persist (Taylor, 1998). Predictors of postoperative memory and fine motor deficits include advanced patient age and intraoperative deep hypothermia with cardioplegic arrest of 25 minutes or more (Reich et al., 1999). Typical cognitive disturbances include mild difficulties with memory, problem solving, and ability to learn.

Peripheral neurologic damage also can result from cardiac operations. Occasionally, *phrenic nerve paralysis* occurs. The phrenic nerves, which course over the pericardium, can be injured as a result of regional hypothermia used for myocardial protection or surgical trauma during harvesting of the internal thoracic artery. Paralysis and elevation of the ipsilateral diaphragm results. The consequences are variable, depending primarily on the underlying condition of the patient, particularly with regard to pulmonary function (Tripp & Bolton, 1998). Unilateral phrenic nerve paralysis usually does not produce significant problems, except in patients with marginal pulmonary function who may require prolonged ventilatory support. Bilateral injury to the phrenic nerves is manifested by difficulty in weaning from mechanical ventilation. Prolonged ventilatory support may be required. *Recurrent laryngeal nerve injury* occurs rarely, usually on the left side (Nyhan & Traystman, 1996).

Compression of the lower trunk of the brachial plexus during retraction of the sternum may produce a *brachial plexus injury* (McLaughlin, 1991). To reduce the risk of this complication, sternal retractors often are placed in a more caudad (toward the lower end of the body) position, thereby avoiding overstretching of the cephalad (toward the head) nerves. Brachial plexus injury most commonly is manifested as paresthesia involving the fourth and fifth fingers on the affected side, but it may cause weakness or pain in more severe cases. Although symptoms may persist for several months, they almost always resolve. *Horner's syndrome* may result from first rib fracture (Loop, 1998). *Meralgia paresthetica,* or *lateral cutaneous femoral nerve syndrome,* is an unusual neurologic complication characterized by paresthesia and numbness on the anterolateral aspect of the thigh (Parsonnet et al., 1991). Although the precise cause is unknown, it is presumed to occur secondary to intraoperative immobility and positioning of the legs. There is no specific treatment, and symptoms usually resolve within several months.

Respiratory Complications

Atelectasis and pleural effusion are the most common minor respiratory abnormalities. *Atelectasis* is the most common complication of operations performed under general anesthesia, with radiologic evidence present in as much as 70% of patients after thoracic operations (Moossa et al., 1997). In fact, some degree of atelectasis, particularly of the left lower lobe, is an expected postoperative finding that usually is easily treated with aggressive pulmonary hygiene measures. Significant atelectasis is most likely in patients with a long smoking history, underlying chronic obstructive pulmonary disease, or pronounced preoperative debilitation.

Pleural effusions occur particularly on the left side and in those patients in whom one or both internal thoracic arteries have been harvested for coronary artery bypass grafting. Although pleural effusions usually resolve with time, large or persistent effusions are treated with thoracentesis or chest tube drainage. A persistent effusion that is not drained may eventually cause lung entrapment, necessitating surgical decortication. *Bacterial pneumonia* occasionally occurs, usually because of colonization of the upper respiratory tract in patients who require prolonged intubation. Organism-specific antimicrobial therapy and aggressive pulmonary hygiene measures are instituted.

Acute respiratory failure is uncommon. It exists when either oxygenation, carbon dioxide removal, or both, is inadequate, that is, when the PaO_2 is less than 60 mm Hg (hypoxia) or $PaCO_2$ is greater than 50 mm Hg (hypercapnia) (Elefteriades et al., 1996c). At greatest risk are patients with severe underlying pulmonary impairment. Other patients at risk include those with marginal cardiac function and those who are in a generally debilitated state. Precipitating etiologic factors include atelectasis caused by hypoventilation and retention of secretions, pneumonia (more likely in critically ill patients who are intubated for prolonged periods or who

have other infections), and pulmonary edema (usually related to poor ventricular function). Additional contributing factors include excessive crystalloid fluid infusion, poor nutritional status, multiple blood transfusions, prolonged length of operation, and phrenic nerve dysfunction (Loop, 1998).

The most severe form of respiratory failure is *adult respiratory distress syndrome (ARDS)*. In postoperative patients, it almost always is precipitated by sepsis or shock that causes direct injury to pulmonary parenchyma, changes in capillary membrane permeability, and release of bronchoconstrictive mediators. The pathophysiologic process remains unknown, although multiple theories exist on how the alveolar capillary membrane injury occurs (Multz & Dantzker, 1997).

Adult respiratory distress syndrome is characterized by refractory hypoxemia, noncompliant lungs, and diffuse and sometimes homogeneous infiltrates throughout both lungs (Mehta & Pae, 1997). Therapy is directed at supporting respiratory function and includes mechanical ventilation, maintaining adequate oxygenation with high FiO_2 and positive end-expiratory pressure levels, and diuresis. Mortality rates associated with ARDS range from 50% to 76%; death is most likely in patients with advanced age, multisystem organ failure, or sepsis (Suchyta et al., 1992).

Gastrointestinal Complications

Gastrointestinal complications develop in less than 2% of cardiac surgical patients (Mehta & Pae, 1997). They are relatively uncommon because the abdomen is not entered and patients usually are immobilized for less than 24 to 36 hours. Although infrequent, abdominal complications can be quite serious. Mortality rates of 20% to 60% are reported and often are attributed to delayed diagnosis of abdominal sepsis with resultant multisystem organ failure (Critchlow & Fink, 1996; Krasna et al., 1988). Types of complications that may occur include gastrointestinal bleeding, ileus, pancreatitis, cholecystitis, and intestinal ischemia or infarction.

Gastrointestinal bleeding is the most common intraabdominal complication (Ohri et al., 1991). It may be detected by gradually decreasing hemoglobin levels or when the patient experiences hematemesis or bloody or black stools. Esophagoscopy or colonoscopy is performed to identify the bleeding source. Acute gastritis is the most common etiology of gastrointestinal bleeding. Bleeding also may arise from preexisting gastroduodenal ulcers. The administration of anticoagulants increases the risk of clinically significant hemorrhage from peptic disease, and nonsteroidal anti-inflammatory drugs increase the incidence of mucosal ulcerations of the stomach and duodenum (Critchlow & Fink, 1996).

Gastrointestinal bleeding caused by peptic disease is treated with histamine type 2 (H_2) receptor antagonist therapy and dietary restriction. Surgical intervention may be required for persistent bleeding or visceral perforation. Less common causes of gastrointestinal bleeding include esophagitis, ischemic bowel disease, diverticulitis, and arteriovenous malformations (Mehta & Pae, 1997).

Postoperative ileus can develop secondary to excessive analgesia and immobility. It is characterized by abdominal distention; absence of bowel sounds, flatus, or bowel movements; and radiographic evidence of dilated loops of bowel. Nasogastric suction is necessary until bowel motility is restored. An ileus must be differentiated from *small bowel obstruction*, which occurs rarely. The reason for its development during the postoperative period is unclear, but the obstruction usually is related to adhesions from a previous abdominal operation.

Acute pancreatitis is an inflammatory disorder of the pancreas in which pancreatic proteolytic enzymes (ie, trypsin, chymotrypsin, and elastase) are abnormally activated and destroy tissue in and around the pancreas (Briones, 1991). Pancreatitis is most likely in patients with low cardiac output, a previous history of pancreatitis, and in those who have received large doses of calcium chloride during the surgical procedure (Loop, 1998). Pancreatitis produces upper abdominal pain, nausea and vomiting, low-grade fevers, and elevated serum amylase levels. Diagnosis may be delayed by the subtle nature of clinical findings and nonspecific laboratory findings (Krasna et al., 1988).

Most cases of pancreatitis in postoperative cardiac surgical patients are self-limited and respond to fluid therapy and nasogastric suction (Shapiro & Gordon, 1990). *Necrotizing pancreatitis,* which occurs in less than 1% of postoperative cardiac patients, requires immediate operation with mobilization and débridement of the pancreas, wide drainage, gastrostomy, and feeding jejunostomy (Mehta & Pae, 1997). *Acute cholecystitis* occasionally occurs, manifested by fever, elevated bilirubin level and white blood cell count, and right upper quadrant pain. Cholecystectomy or tube cholecystostomy may be necessary.

Intestinal ischemia is caused by compromised blood flow to the mesenteric arteries. It is most often due to a prolonged low-flow state, particularly in association with infusion of alpha-adrenergic agents. Patients at greatest risk are those whose postoperative course is complicated by hemorrhage, low cardiac output, or other major organ system failure. Intestinal ischemia due to embolism is most likely in patients with intracardiac thrombi and arrhythmias.

Acute intestinal ischemia produces severe abdominal pain, which frequently is out of proportion to physical findings (Critchlow & Fink, 1996). Because patients typically are intubated, however, the pain may remain unrecognized. An important sign heralding development of intestinal ischemia in moribund patients is moderate to severe acidosis. Other signs include elevated white blood cell count, abdominal distention, gastrointestinal bleeding, abdominal tenderness, and evidence of sepsis. If bowel ischemia or infarction is suspected, an angiogram of the abdominal aorta may be performed or the patient may be taken directly to the operating room for an exploratory laparotomy. If only a small portion of bowel is necrotic, the involved segment is resected and the pa-

tient may survive. However, if a large portion or the entire bowel is infarcted, the condition is fatal and surgical intervention is abandoned.

Renal Failure

The incidence of *acute renal failure* after cardiac and aortic operations ranges from 2% to 15%, but the mortality rate for those in whom the complication develops is as high as 40% (Davila-Roman et al., 1999). Acute renal failure necessitating some form of dialysis occurs in 1.5% of patients after cardiac surgery; variables independently associated with its development include an elevated preoperative serum creatinine, a longer duration of cardiopulmonary bypass, a carotid bruit, and diabetes (Conlon et al., 1999).

In the postoperative setting, renal dysfunction usually is due to acute tubular necrosis precipitated by prolonged hypotension or hypovolemia. The reduced renal blood flow becomes inadequate for normal glomerular filtration. A number of factors associated with cardiopulmonary bypass can adversely affect renal blood flow, including periods of low perfusion, hypotension, vasoconstrictors (eg, norepinephrine), and microemboli (Anderson et al., 1991).

Other risk factors for development of renal failure include multiple transfusions, low cardiac output, preoperative contrast agents, nephrotoxic drugs, advanced age, prolonged cardiopulmonary bypass or aortic cross-clamp time, and preexisting renal dysfunction. An atherosclerotic ascending aorta also is an important predictor of postoperative renal dysfunction, possibly because it predisposes to atheroembolism to the kidneys or because it is a marker of widespread atherosclerosis (Davila-Roman et al., 1999).

Renal dysfunction can range from mild to severe and can be oliguric or nonoliguric (Landolfo & Smith, 1995). Impending renal failure is manifested by oliguria that is unresponsive to fluid and diuretic therapy and by rising blood urea nitrogen and serum creatinine levels. Therapy directed at converting oliguric to nonoliguric renal failure includes provision of adequate preload, maintenance of adequate systemic blood pressure, administration of diuretic agents, and low-dose dopamine infusion (Landolfo & Smith, 1995). Dialysis may become necessary to remove toxic substances, correct metabolic acidosis, and maintain normokalemia and fluid balance (Landolfo & Smith, 1995). Hemodialysis is usually the preferred method in hemodynamically stable patients. In unstable patients, continuous venovenous hemofiltration may be used alternatively to remove excess fluid.

Sepsis

Sepsis is the presence of microorganisms or their toxins in the bloodstream; *septic shock* describes the systemic response to sepsis, manifested by hypotension, hyperthermia or hypothermia, impaired organ perfusion, metabolic abnormalities, and, if the process is unchecked, progression to multiple organ failure (Luce, 1987). Characteristic hemodynamic indicators of septic shock include high cardiac output, low systemic vascular resistance, and tachycardia. Patients who require prolonged mechanical ventilation and invasive instrumentation for hemodynamic monitoring and support are at greatest risk for systemic infections. Other risk factors include premorbid infection, poor nutritional status, and a debilitated state. The most frequent causative organisms are gram-negative bacteria, notably *Escherichia coli, Klebsiella, Aerobacter, Pseudomonas, Proteus,* and *Bacteroides;* common gram-positive organisms are *Staphylococcus, Streptococcus,* and pneumococci (Curran & Anderson, 1995).

In postoperative patients who have high or persistent fevers or who deteriorate clinically for unexplained reasons, serious infection should be suspected. Cultures of blood, sputum, urine, and any draining wounds are obtained. Sometimes a septic syndrome occurs without an obvious source of infection. If an overt source cannot be identified, evaluation of the nasal sinuses and abdomen may reveal sinusitis caused by nasotracheal intubation or a covert intra-abdominal infection (eg, abscess or acalculous cholecystitis) (Zapol, 1989). Therapy for sepsis includes organism-specific antimicrobial therapy and supportive therapy to sustain adequate tissue perfusion and organ function.

Wound Complications

Sternal wound complications include sternal dehiscence and superficial or deep wound infection. Factors that have been implicated as placing patients at greater risk for sternal wound complications include operative reexploration through the same incision; closed chest massage; prolonged cardiopulmonary bypass; infection elsewhere in the body; diminished tissue perfusion secondary to low cardiac output syndrome; deliberate nonclosure of the sternal incision secondary to hemodynamic instability; and the presence of a tracheostomy, which allows colonization of bacteria close to the sternal incision. Factors that adversely affect wound healing, such as obesity, diabetes, nutritional depletion, or corticosteroids, also increase the risk of infection.

Diabetes has been established as an independent risk factor for postoperative sternal wound infection, with infection rates two to five times greater than in the nondiabetic population (Furnary et al., 1999). Harvesting of both internal thoracic arteries for grafting increases the risk, particularly in diabetic patients, who have a 14.3% incidence of deep sternal wound infection after bilateral internal thoracic artery grafting (Borger et al., 1998). Data indicate that perioperative continuous intravenous insulin infusion in diabetic patients significantly reduces perioperative blood glucose levels with a resultant significant reduction in the incidence of postoperative deep sternal wound infection (Furnary et al., 1999).

Mobilization of one or both internal thoracic arteries for bypass grafting contributes to sternal wound prob-

lems because the internal thoracic arteries provide the major source of blood supply to the sternum. Mobilization of an internal thoracic artery significantly devascularizes the sternal half from which it is harvested (Ulicny & Hiratzka, 1991). Because of the prevalence of osteoporosis in elderly women, internal thoracic artery harvesting may contribute to greater risk in this population.

Sternal dehiscence is the postoperative separation of the sutured sternal halves. At the completion of operations that necessitate median sternotomy, the surgically divided sternum is reapproximated securely using heavy suture material or wire. Normally, the sternal halves heal and the sternum regains its full strength over a course of 8 to 12 weeks. If the edges of the sternal halves fail to heal properly or if the suture or wire becomes disrupted before this can occur, sternal dehiscence results. Although usually associated with deep infection of the sternal wound, it also may occur in the absence of wound infection. At particular risk are patients with chronic obstructive pulmonary disease and excessive postoperative coughing who exert greater force on the healing sternum.

A sterile, or noninfected, sternal dehiscence is termed a *mechanical dehiscence*. A division of the sternum that is off-center (paramedian) contributes to the likelihood of dehiscence by leaving small segments of bone that can fracture or separate from the tension of the closure. Other factors contributing to mechanical dehiscence are a technically inadequate closure, erosion of wire or suture through the bone, sutures that are not tight, the type of suture material used, patient noncompliance with limitations on activities involving the upper extremities, and a failure of the bone to heal.

Mechanical dehiscence is likely to occur earlier in the postoperative course than dehiscence associated with infection. Sterile dehiscence occurs most often within several days after operation, whereas infective dehiscence is more likely to become evident 1 to 2 weeks after operation. Mechanical dehiscence is corrected by reoperation to resecure the sternal halves. Heavy bands may be applied to help maintain sternal approximation. A major concern associated with sternal dehiscence is damage to bypass grafts lying on the anterior surface of the heart from movement of the unstable sternum during respiration or at the time of operative restabilization.

Occasionally, mechanical dehiscence occurs late, usually as a result of vigorous upper extremity activity initiated before the bone is fully healed. If only a small portion of the sternum is separated and the patient has a fairly sedentary lifestyle, the surgeon may elect to follow the patient over several months to determine if sternal healing will occur. In most cases, operative reclosure is required.

Sternal wound infection may result from intraoperative contamination of the operative field, hematogenous spread of pathogens from elsewhere in the body, or postoperative wound contamination. *Staphylococcus aureus* and *Staphylococcus epidermidis* are the most common pathogenic organisms causing clean wound infections; enteric gram-negative rods are less frequent causes

(Doebbeling et al., 1990). Superficial infection involving only the subcutaneous tissue is manifested by small amounts of purulent drainage and localized areas of erythema surrounding the incision. It is treated with local drainage, wound care, and organism-specific antimicrobial therapy.

Signs of deep sternal infection are copious purulent drainage from or extensive cellulitis surrounding the sternal incision, localized tenderness, fever, sternal instability, and malaise. Deep infection of a sternal wound produces significant morbidity and prolongation of hospitalization. It frequently causes sternal dehiscence, osteomyelitis of the sternum, and mediastinitis. These infections often are associated with generalized sepsis and a mortality rate of 10% to 30% (Loop, 1998).

Treatment of deep sternal wound infection associated with dehiscence includes operative exploration for the purpose of sternal débridement and antibiotic irrigation of the mediastinal cavity. Early exploration improves the patient's outcome by reducing the damage caused by a prolonged and contained infection. An indwelling catheter may be placed in the mediastinum through which an antibiotic solution, dilute povidone-iodine, or saline is continuously infused over several days. Chest tubes are placed to evacuate the solution. If possible, primary closure is performed by reapproximating the sternal halves. The skin is often left open for secondary healing.

In the case of severe osteomyelitis, radical operative débridement of all necrotic, avascular tissue may be necessary (Ulicny & Hiratzka, 1991). The bone and cartilage are poorly vascularized structures and, once infected, are very difficult to sterilize. Much or all of the sternum and a significant amount of costal cartilage may need to be removed. The procedure is performed with ready availability of cardiopulmonary bypass because of the danger of injury to bypass grafts or entry into a cardiac chamber. Unless chronic obstructive pulmonary disease is present, most patients do not experience impairment of respiratory effort with only fibrous union or even with complete absence of the sternum. However, protection against trauma to the anterior chest is no longer present.

If a significant amount of sternum is excised, reconstruction with muscle flaps may be necessary to close the wound primarily (Fig. 28-2). Use of muscle flaps has been a major advance, markedly reducing morbidity and mortality. Applying muscle flaps brings a rich network of blood supply to the poorly vascularized bone (Jeevanandam et al., 1990). The improved blood supply is thought to increase oxygen tension and intravascular delivery of antibiotics to jeopardized tissue. Either the pectoralis major or rectus abdominis muscle may be used. An omental flap is used rarely. The omentum, which also has a rich blood supply, is harvested from the upper abdomen and placed over the mediastinal structures. In addition to enhancing regional blood supply, the presence of a muscle or omental flap eradicates empty spaces in the mediastinum that could otherwise provide pockets for accumulation of purulent material.

Mediastinitis associated with sternal wound infection necessitates intensive nursing care with meticulous at-

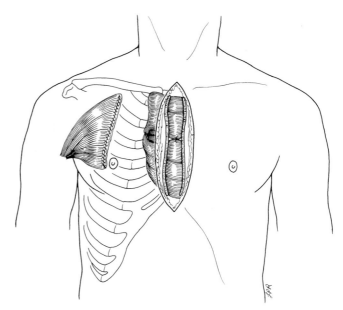

FIGURE 28-2. Pectoralis muscle flap is mobilized to reach midline and cover sternal wound. (Craver JM, Rand RP, Bostwick J III, Hatcher CR Jr, 1991: Management of postoperative mediastinitis. In Waldhausen JA, Orringer MB [eds]: Complications in Cardiothoracic Surgery, p. 128. St. Louis, Mosby–Year Book)

tention to wound management and antibiotic administration. During periods of inadequate drainage of infection and after each operative débridement, bacteremia with resultant septic shock is likely. In the presence of extensive mediastinal infection, the surgeon may elect to leave the wound open to provide adequate drainage. While the wound is left open, a large protein loss can be anticipated. Multiple operative interventions may be required for débridement and eventual wound closure. Although patients are critically ill for a prolonged period, the prognosis is in general good if cardiac function is satisfactory and the infection is adequately drained.

A potential complication of mediastinitis is infection of aortic or cardiac suture lines, especially if prosthetic material, such as felt pledgets, has been implanted during the primary cardiac operation. If prosthetic material does become infected, surgical removal of the material may be necessary to eradicate the infection. A false aneurysm of the ascending aorta also may develop secondary to indolent infection. Such an infected aneurysm, termed a *mycotic aneurysm*, may occur months or years after the infection, particularly if prosthetic material has been placed on the aorta or cardiac structures. Mycotic aneurysm is a particularly difficult problem to manage. Aortic rupture may occur if the aneurysm is treated conservatively. On the other hand, surgical resection of the aneurysm is technically difficult because of dense adhesions caused by infection in the mediastinum.

Superficial infection of the leg incision is a minor problem that usually occurs in patients who are obese, are diabetic, or have compromised peripheral arterial circulation. Leg wound infections are treated with local drainage, débridement, and frequent dressing changes. Infection of the surrounding soft tissue, termed *cellulitis,* is treated with intravenous antibiotics. Wound infections that are not promptly treated may lead to extensive cellulitis and the need for reopening the entire length of incisions on the affected leg. In severe cases, skin grafting may be necessary for reclosure.

Skin breakdown and incisional drainage do not always signify infection. They may instead represent necrosis of poorly vascularized subcutaneous fat. In addition, some patients have a local inflammatory reaction to the suture material used to close subcutaneous tissue. In such cases, small openings may appear along the incision line, from which small amounts of fluid can be expressed. Occasionally, this tissue reaction continues until the incision is surgically reopened and the offending suture material removed.

An occasional late wound complication is incisional discomfort due to sternal wires or bands in the subcutaneous tissue. The patient may be able to palpate these, and they may be painful when anything is pressed against overlying skin. In cachectic patients with minimal subcutaneous tissue, the skin may erode and infection can ensue. In such cases, it may be necessary for the surgeon to reopen the incision with the patient under general anesthesia, remove the anterior portions of the wires or bands, and bury the remaining ends before reclosing the incision. Usually, this operative correction of the problem is deferred until 6 months after the original cardiac procedure to allow full healing of the sternum before removing supportive material.

Other Complications

Urinary tract infection can occur secondary to the urethral catheter inserted at the time of operation. It is particularly likely in patients with a prolonged preoperative length of hospitalization. Most patients are asymptomatic, and their urine may clear spontaneously after catheter removal (Keys & Serkey, 1991). The infection often is detected by the routine urine culture obtained at the time of catheter removal. It also should be suspected if dysuria or an unexplained postoperative fever develops. Organism-specific antibiotic therapy is instituted.

Urinary retention occurs occasionally in men with preexisting prostatic hypertrophy. If a patient fails to void within 8 to 10 hours of catheter removal, the catheter is reinserted. If 500 mL or more residual urine is present in the bladder, the catheter is usually left in place. A second trial of catheter removal may be tried 24 to 48 hours later when the patient is more ambulatory. If a second recatheterization is necessary, a urologic consultation may be obtained. Sometimes a dilating procedure or transurethral prostatic resection may be necessary before successful catheter removal. If repeated catheterization or urologic instrumentation is necessary in patients with prosthetic valves, appropriate prophylactic antibiotics against infective endocarditis should be given.

Postoperative psychological disturbances may occur, ranging from mild depression or disorientation to agitation, hallucinations, combative behavior, or frank psychosis. Patients most likely to experience postoperative psychological sequelae include (1) those with underlying psychological disturbances, (2) those with extreme preoperative anxiety, (3) those who have a prolonged course in the intensive care unit with sleep deprivation, (4) elderly patients, and (5) those with a history of alcohol abuse. Psychological complications usually are of a very transient nature and are treated with symptomatic management. Supportive therapy to suppress agitation and protect the patient from injury is used until the psychological disturbance resolves. If the patient has been on psychotropic medications before surgery, the medications usually are resumed as soon as the patient is taking oral nourishment.

Because prophylactic antibiotics are given routinely, a postoperative *Clostridium difficile bowel infection* occasionally develops because of suppression of normal bowel flora. Protracted diarrhea with resultant dehydration can occur. Accordingly, a stool culture is obtained in postoperative patients in whom diarrhea develops. If the culture is positive for *C. difficile,* metronidazole (Flagyl) usually is administered to eradicate the infection. Oral vancomycin may be used alternatively.

An unusual problem after cardiac operations is development of *local tissue necrosis,* presumably due to the combination of pressure points, prolonged immobility on the operating table, and hypothermia. The most common site for development of tissue necrosis is the back of the head. Although the ulcerated tissue usually heals without complication, the affected area is often quite painful and alopecia is common. If this problem is noted in any postoperative patients, attempts to prevent its recurrence in other patients by different intraoperative positioning of the head or placement of pillows should be promptly investigated.

Iatrogenic aortic dissection is a rare complication of cardiac operations. Injury to the aortic intima or media can occur at the site of cannulation, partial occlusion clamp or aortic cross-clamp, or aorta–saphenous vein graft anastomoses. Risk factors for development of aortic dissection are cystic medial necrosis, hypertension, and atherosclerosis. Surgical repair of the aorta may be required.

Complications resulting from intraoperative cardiopulmonary bypass are unusual but can occur. Massive air embolism occurs in 0.1% to 0.2% of perfused patients and approximately half of these patients have permanent neurologic damage or die as a result of the complications (Edmunds, 1996). Numerous safety features are incorporated into the cardiopulmonary bypass system to prevent infusion of air into the arterial circulation, and various maneuvers to prevent air embolism (venting, positioning, aspiration, lung ventilation) are performed routinely by the surgeon and anesthesiologist before discontinuing cardiopulmonary bypass. However, air embolism can occur and cause catastrophic cerebral or coronary artery occlusion. A neurologic deficit known or suspected to be due to air embolism may be reversible if detected and treated in the first few postoperative hours.

The adverse physiologic effects imposed by cardiopulmonary bypass occasionally produce a clinical response known in its most severe form as *postperfusion syndrome*. It is characterized by pulmonary and renal dysfunction, bleeding diathesis, increased interstitial fluid, leukocytosis, fever, vasoconstriction, hemolysis, and increased susceptibility to infection (McGiffin & Kirklin, 1995). Patients subjected to prolonged duration of cardiopulmonary bypass are most likely to experience postperfusion syndrome.

Postoperative complications also can occur as a result of implanted prosthetic devices such as cardiac valves, pacemakers, and implantable cardioverter-defibrillators. Prosthetic valves can become infected (prosthetic endocarditis), become acutely regurgitant around the sewing ring (paravalvular leak), cause thromboembolism, or may be associated with anticoagulant-related hemorrhage. Pacemaker or cardioverter-defibrillator implantation can be complicated by infection, lead dislodgment, or device failure. Three predominant types of complications are associated with IABC—ischemia, infection, and hematologic derangements; identified risk factors for these complications include female sex, age, obesity, comorbidities, smoking, and duration of counterpulsation (Cook et al., 1999). Arterial complications of IABC include limb ischemia, thromboembolism, bleeding, pseudoaneurysm, aortic dissection, or arteriovenous fistula (Finkelmeier & Finkelmeier, 1991). Circulatory assist devices may cause hemorrhage, thromboembolism, or sepsis. These prosthetic devices and their associated complications are discussed in greater detail elsewhere in the text.

REFERENCES

Almassi GH, Schowalter T, Nicolosi AC, et al., 1997: Atrial fibrillation after cardiac surgery: A major morbid event? Ann Surg 226:501

Almassi GH, Sommers T, Moritz TE, et al., 1999: Stroke in cardiac surgical patients: Determinants and outcomes. Ann Thorac Surg 68:391

Anderson DR, Stephenson LW, Edmunds LH, 1991: Management of complications of cardiopulmonary bypass: Complications of organ systems. In Waldhausen JA, Orringer MB (eds): Complications in Cardiothoracic Surgery. St. Louis, Mosby–Year Book

Baumgartner FJ, Robertson J, Omari B, 1997: ICU management. In Cardiothoracic Surgery. Austin, TX, Chapman & Hall

Becker RC, 1996: Hematologic and coagulation considerations in patients with cardiac disease. In Kvetan V, Dantzker DR (eds): The Critically Ill Cardiac Patient: Multisystem Dysfunction and Management. Philadelphia, Lippincott-Raven

Borger MA, Rao V, Weisel RD, et al., 1998: Deep sternal wound infection: Risk factors and outcomes. Ann Thorac Surg 65:1050

Briones TL, 1991: The gastrointestinal system. In Alspach JG (ed): Core Curriculum for Critical Care Nursing, ed. 4. Philadelphia, WB Saunders

Critchlow JF, Fink MP, 1996: Abdominal crises in the cardiac patient. In Kvetan V, Dantzker DR (eds): The Critically Ill Cardiac Patient: Multisystem Dysfunction and Management. Philadelphia, Lippincott-Raven

Conlon PJ, Stafford-Smith M, White WD, et al., 1999: Acute renal failure following cardiac surgery. Nephrol Dial Transplant 14:1158

Cook L, Pillar B, McCord G, Josephson R, 1999: Intra-aortic balloon pump complications: A five-year retrospective study of 283 patients. Heart Lung 28:195

Curran RD, Anderson RW, 1995: Shock and circulatory collapse. In Sabiston DC Jr, Spencer FC (eds): Surgery of the Chest, ed. 6. Philadelphia, WB Saunders

Daoud EG, Strickberger SA, Man KC, et al., 1997: Preoperative amiodarone as prophylaxis against atrial fibrillation after heart surgery. N Engl J Med 337:1785

Davila-Roman VG, Kouchoukos NT, Schechtman KB, Barzilai B, 1999: Atherosclerosis of the ascending aorta is a predictor of renal dysfunction after cardiac operations. J Thorac Cardiovasc Surg 117:111

Deiwick M, Tandler R, Mollhoff T, et al., 1997: Heart surgery in patients aged eighty years and above: Determinants of morbidity and mortality. Thorac Cardiovasc Surg 45:119

DiSesa VJ, 1991: Pharmacologic support for low cardiac output. Semin Thorac Cardiovasc Surg 3:13

Doebbeling BN, Pfaller MA, Kuhns KR, et al., 1990: Cardiovascular surgery prophylaxis. J Thorac Cardiovasc Surg 99:981

Edmunds LH Jr, 1996: Cardiopulmonary bypass for open heart surgery. In Baue AE, Geha AS, Hammond GL, et al. (eds): Glenn's Thoracic and Cardiovascular Surgery, ed. 6. Stamford, CT, Appleton & Lange

Edwards FH, Taylor AJ, Thompson L, et al., 1991: Current status of coronary artery operation in septuagenarians. Ann Thorac Surg 52:265

Elefteriades JA, Geha AS, Cohen LS, 1996a: Postoperative bleeding. In House Officer Guide to ICU Care: Fundamentals of Management of the Heart and Lungs, ed. 2. Philadelphia, Lippincott-Raven

Elefteriades JA, Geha AS, Cohen LS, 1996b: Chest trauma. In House Officer Guide to ICU Care: Fundamentals of Management of the Heart and Lungs, ed. 2. Philadelphia, Lippincott-Raven

Elefteriades JA, Geha AS, Cohen LS, 1996c: Management of acute pulmonary disease. In House Officer Guide to ICU Care: Fundamentals of Management of the Heart and Lungs, ed. 2. Philadelphia, Lippincott-Raven

Ellison N, Campbell FW, Jobes DR, 1991: Postoperative hemostasis. Semin Thorac Cardiovasc Surg 3:33

Ferraris VA, 1997: Risk stratification and comorbidity. In Edmunds LH Jr (ed): Cardiac Surgery in the Adult. New York, McGraw-Hill

Finkelmeier BA, Finkelmeier WR, 1991: Iatrogenic arterial injuries resulting from invasive procedures. J Vasc Nurs 9:12

Fontana GP, Sabiston DC Jr, 1995: Pulmonary embolism: Acute pulmonary embolism. In Sabiston DC Jr, Spencer FC (eds): Surgery of the Chest, ed. 6. Philadelphia, WB Saunders

Furnary AP, Zerr KJ, Grunkemeier GL, Starr A, 1999: Continuous intravenous insulin infusion reduces the incidence of deep sternal wound infection in diabetic patients after cardiac surgical procedures. Ann Thorac Surg 67:352

Goldsborough MA, Boronicz LM, McKhann GM, Baumgartner WA, 1997: Variation in stroke occurrence by cardiac procedures. Perfusion 12:47

Gordon RS, Ivanov J, Cohen G, Ralph-Edwards AL, 1998: Permanent cardiac pacing after a cardiac operation: Predicting the use of permanent pacemakers. Ann Thorac Surg 66:1698

Halfman-Franey M, Berg DE, 1991: Recognition and management of bleeding following cardiac surgery. Critical Care Nursing Clinics of North America 3:675

Hammermeister KE, Burchfiel C, Johnson R, Grover FL, 1990: Identification of patients at greatest risk for developing major complications at cardiac surgery. Circulation 82(Suppl IV):IV-380

Hashimoto K, Ilstrup DM, Schaff HV, 1991: Influence of clinical and hemodynamic variables on risk of supraventricular tachycardia after coronary artery bypass. J Thorac Cardiovasc Surg 101:56

Hendren WG, Higgins TL, 1991: Immediate postoperative care of the cardiac surgical patient. Semin Thorac Cardiovasc Surg 3:3

Hendrickson SC, Glower DD, Lowe JE, 1997: Cardiopulmonary resuscitation. In Edmunds LH Jr (ed): Cardiac Surgery in the Adult. New York, McGraw-Hill

Higgins TL, Starr NJ, 1991: Risk stratification and outcome assessment of the adult cardiac surgical patient. Semin Thorac Cardiovasc Surg 3:88

Hohnloser SH, 1997: Proarrhythmia with class III antiarrhythmic drugs: Types, risks, and management. Am J Cardiol 80:82G

Jamieson SW, 1996: Pulmonary embolism. In Baue AE, Geha AS, Hammond GL, et al. (eds): Glenn's Thoracic and Cardiovascular Surgery, ed. 6. Stamford, CT, Appleton & Lange

Jeevanandam V, Smith CR, Rose EA, et al., 1990: Single-stage management of sternal wound infections. J Thorac Cardiovasc Surg 99:256

Jones EL, Weintraub WS, Craver JM, et al., 1991: Coronary bypass surgery: Is the operation different today? J Thorac Cardiovasc Surg 101:108

Keys TF, Serkey JM, 1991: Management and control of infectious complications. Semin Thorac Cardiovasc Surg 3:71

Khuri SF, Healey N, MacGregor H, et al., 1999: Comparison of the effects of transfusions of cryopreserved and liquid-preserved platelets on hemostasis and blood loss after cardiopulmonary bypass. J Thorac Cardiovasc Surg 117:172

Klein AL, Scalia GM, 1998: Diseases of the pericardium, restrictive cardiomyopathy and diastolic dysfunction. In Topol EJ (ed): Comprehensive Cardiovascular Medicine. Philadelphia, Lippincott Williams & Wilkins

Kohl PH, Torchiana DF, Buckley MJ, 1999: Atheroembolization in cardiac surgery: The need for preoperative diagnosis. J Cardiovasc Surg 40:77

Krasna MJ, Flancbaum L, Trooskin SZ, et al., 1988: Gastrointestinal complications after cardiac surgery. Surgery 104:773

Landolfo K, Smith PK, 1995: Postoperative care in cardiac surgery. In Sabiston DC Jr, Spencer FC (eds): Surgery of the Chest, ed. 6. Philadelphia, WB Saunders

Lee JH, Geha AS, 1996: Postoperative low cardiac output. In Baue AE, Geha AS, Hammond GL, et al. (eds): Glenn's Thoracic and Cardiovascular Surgery, ed. 6. Stamford, CT, Appleton & Lange

Leitch JW, Thomson D, Baird DK, Harris PJ, 1990: The importance of age as a predictor of atrial fibrillation and flutter after coronary artery bypass grafting. J Thorac Cardiovasc Surg 100:338

Lewis JW Jr, Webb CR, Pickard SD, et al., 1998: The increased need for a permanent pacemaker after reoperative cardiac surgery. J Thorac Cardiovasc Surg 116:74

Loop FD, 1998: Coronary artery bypass surgery. In Topol EJ (ed): Comprehensive Cardiovascular Medicine. Philadelphia, Lippincott Williams & Wilkins

Lorell BH, 1997: Pericardial diseases. In Braunwald E (ed): Heart Disease: A Textbook of Cardiovascular Medicine, ed. 5. Philadelphia, WB Saunders

Luce JM, 1987: Pathogenesis and management of septic shock. Chest 91:883

Mackall JA, Buchter CM, Thames MD, 1996: Pharmacological approach to the management of the cardiac surgical patient. In Baue AE, Geha AS, Hammond GL, et al. (eds): Glenn's Thoracic and Cardiovascular Surgery, ed. 6. Stamford, CT, Appleton & Lange

Mahfood SS, Higgins TL, Loop FD, 1991: Management of complications related to coronary artery bypass surgery. In Waldhausen JA, Orringer MB (eds): Complications in Cardiothoracic Surgery. St. Louis, Mosby–Year Book

McGiffin DC, Kirklin JK, 1995: Cardiopulmonary bypass for cardiac surgery. In Sabiston DC Jr, Spencer FC (eds): Surgery of the Chest, ed. 6. Philadelphia, WB Saunders

McLaughlin JS, 1991: Positional and incisional complications of thoracic surgery. In Waldhausen JA, Orringer MB (eds): Complications in Cardiothoracic Surgery. St. Louis, Mosby–Year Book

Mehta SM, Pae WE Jr, 1997: Complications of cardiac surgery. In Edmunds LH Jr (ed): Cardiac Surgery in the Adult. New York, McGraw-Hill

Mills SA, Prough DS, 1991: Neuropsychiatric complications following cardiac surgery. Semin Thorac Cardiovasc Surg 3:39

Mitruka SN, Griffith BP, Kormos RL, et al., 1997: Cardiac operations in solid-organ transplant recipients. Ann Thorac Surg 64:1270

Moore SL, Wilkoff BL, 1991: Rhythm disturbances after cardiac surgery. Semin Thorac Cardiovasc Surg 3:24

Moossa AR, Hart ME, Easter DW, 1997: Surgical complications. In Sabiston DC Jr (ed): Textbook of Surgery: The Biological Basis of Modern Surgical Practice, ed. 15. Philadelphia, WB Saunders

Moran JM, Singh AK, 1989: Cardiogenic shock. In Grillo HC, Austen WG, Wilkins EW Jr, et al. (eds): Current Therapy in Cardiothoracic Surgery. Toronto, Canada, BC Decker

Moreno-Cabral CE, Mitchell RS, Miller DC, 1988: Postoperative problems. In Manual of Postoperative Management in Adult Cardiac Surgery. Baltimore, Williams & Wilkins

Multz AS, Dantzker DR, 1997: Adult respiratory distress syndrome. In Parrillo JE (ed): Current Therapy in Critical Care Medicine, ed. 3. St. Louis, Mosby

Nyhan D, Traystman RJ, 1996: Neurologic disorders and heart disease. In Kvetan V, Dantzker DR (eds): The Critically Ill Cardiac Patient: Multisystem Dysfunction and Management. Philadelphia, Lippincott-Raven

Ohri SK, Desai JB, Gaer JA, et al., 1991: Intraabdominal complications after cardiopulmonary bypass. Ann Thorac Surg 52:826

Ornato JP, Peberdy MA, 1998: Cardiopulmonary resuscitation. In Topol EJ (ed): Comprehensive Cardiovascular Medicine. Philadelphia, Lippincott Williams & Wilkins

Parsonnet V, Karasakalides A, Gielchinsky I, et al., 1991: Meralgia paresthetica after coronary bypass surgery. J Thorac Cardiovasc Surg 101:219

Pelletier MP, Solymoss S, Lee A, Chie RC, 1998: Negative re-exploration for cardiac postoperative bleeding: Can it be therapeutic? Ann Thorac Surg 65:999

Rao V, Weisel RD, 1997: Intraoperative protection of organs: Hypothermia, cardioplegia, and cerebroplegia. In Edmunds LH Jr (ed): Cardiac Surgery in the Adult. New York, McGraw-Hill

Reich DL, Uysal S, Sliwinski M, et al., 1999: Neuropsychologic outcome after deep hypothermic circulatory arrest in adults. J Thorac Cardiovasc Surg 117:156

Richenbacher WE, Pierce WS, 1997: Assisted circulation of the heart. In Braunwald E (ed): Heart Disease: A Textbook of Cardiovascular Medicine, ed. 5. Philadelphia, WB Saunders

Schoen FJ, 1997: Pathologic considerations in the surgery of adult heart disease. In Edmunds LH Jr (ed): Cardiac Surgery in the Adult. New York, McGraw-Hill

Shapiro SJ, Gordon LA, 1990: General surgical complications following cardiac surgery. In Gray RJ, Matloff JM (eds): Medical Management of the Cardiac Surgical Patient. Baltimore, Williams & Wilkins

Spotnitz WD, Spotnitz HM, 1996: Cardiopulmonary resuscitation. In Baue AE, Geha AS, Hammond GL, et al. (eds): Glenn's Thoracic and Cardiovascular Surgery, ed. 6. Stamford, CT, Appleton & Lange

Steinberg JS, Gaur A, Sciacca R, et al., 1999: New-onset sustained ventricular tachycardia after cardiac surgery. Circulation 99:903

Suchyta MR, Clemmer TP, Elliott CG, et al., 1992: The adult respiratory distress syndrome. Chest 101:1074

Taylor KM, 1998: Brain damage during cardiopulmonary bypass. Ann Thorac Surg 65:S20

Tripp HF, Bolton JW, 1998: Phrenic nerve injury following cardiac surgery: A review. J Cardiac Surg 13:218

Tuman KJ, McCarthy RJ, March RJ, 1992: Morbidity and duration of ICU stay after cardiac surgery. Chest 102:36

Ulicny KS Jr, Hiratzka LF, 1991: The risk factors of median sternotomy infection: A current review. J Cardiac Surg 6:338

Wareing TH, Davila-Roman VG, Barzilai B, et al., 1992: Management of the severely atherosclerotic ascending aorta during cardiac operations. J Thorac Cardiovasc Surg 103:453

Whitman GR, 1991: Hypertension and hypothermia in the acute postoperative period. Critical Care Nursing Clinics of North America 3:661

Zapol WM, 1989: Adult respiratory distress syndrome. In Grillo HC, Austen WG, Wilkins EW Jr, et al. (eds): Current Therapy in Cardiothoracic Surgery. Toronto, Canada, BC Decker

29

Management of Critically Ill Patients

One of the most challenging aspects of cardiothoracic surgical nursing is the care of patients who are critically ill. Sometimes, patients who appear to be recovering in a routine fashion have sudden and catastrophic problems. Other patients come to operation critically ill and on life-support systems. Particularly in elderly patients and in those with underlying cardiac, pulmonary, or renal impairment, serious complications can develop and evolve into multisystem organ failure. Cardiothoracic surgical nurses play a major role in determining the ultimate outcome of these critically ill patients. The most common forms of major organ system dysfunction in cardiac surgical patients are cardiogenic shock and respiratory failure.

▶ Support of the Failing Heart

Management of Heart Failure

Acute ventricular dysfunction is a major cause of critical illness in cardiac surgical patients. Severe ventricular dysfunction, termed *cardiogenic shock*, is characterized by a cardiac index less than 1.8 L/min/m², mean pulmonary capillary wedge pressure greater than 18 mm Hg, tachycardia, and a systemic vascular resistance greater than 2400 dynes·sec·cm⁻⁵ (Ashton et al., 1997). The condition usually is fatal unless temporary augmentation of cardiac function can be provided through pharmacologic or mechanical means. Cardiogenic shock may represent left ventricular, right ventricular, or biventricular dysfunction. Because coronary artery disease and valvular heart disease most commonly damage the left ventricle, left ventricular dysfunction is most common. In the early postoperative period after cardiac operations, reversible biventricular dysfunction may be superimposed on underlying dysfunction due to incomplete operative correction of cardiac disease, myocardial edema, and reperfusion injury (Bailey et al., 1997).

Standard monitoring of the patient in cardiogenic shock includes cardiac rate and rhythm, arterial pressure, central venous pressure, pulmonary artery pressure, cardiac output, and systemic vascular resistance. Measurement of these hemodynamic parameters is discussed in detail in Chapter 23, Hemodynamic Monitoring. In addition to the various intracardiac and vascular pressures and calculated indices, assessment of adequate tissue perfusion necessitates close attention to level of consciousness (cerebral blood flow), urine output (renal blood flow), and peripheral pulses and color and temperature of extremities (peripheral blood flow).

The goals of supportive therapy are to increase cardiac output and myocardial oxygen supply while reducing myocardial work and oxygen demands. Interventions are focused on manipulation of hemodynamic parameters (ie, heart rate and rhythm, preload, afterload, and contractility) that determine cardiac output. Iatrogenic alteration of these hemodynamic parameters produces rapid and sometimes profound changes in the patient's cardiovascular physiologic state. Consequently, cardiothoracic surgical nurses require a thorough understanding of principles of cardiovascular physiology, the meaning and relationship of the various hemodynamic parameters, and the actions of commonly used pharmacologic agents.

Heart rate may be artificially manipulated by temporary pacing. A rate in the range of 90 to 100 beats per minute is considered optimal in most patients. Sinus bradycardia is treated with temporary atrial pacing. Atrioventricular (AV) synchronous pacing is used in the presence of AV nodal dysfunction to preserve the contribution to cardiac output provided by atrial systole. The "atrial kick" (ie, an appropriately timed atrial contraction) increases ventricular filling, allows more complete emptying of the atria, and prevents regurgitation across AV valves during ventricular systole. An appropriately timed atrial contraction increases stroke volume by 5% to 15% in the normal heart and is of even greater clinical significance in the presence of left ventricular impairment (Spotnitz, 1997). Ventricular pacing is used if atrial fibrillation or other supraventricular tachycardia precludes atrial or AV synchronous pacing.

Antiarrhythmic medications are administered if clinically significant supraventricular tachycardia or ventricular arrhythmias occur. Tachyarrhythmias at rates greater than 120 beats per minute compromise diastolic ventricular filling time and decrease contractility by altering myocardial oxygen supply and demand (Lee & Geha, 1996). Digoxin is used most commonly for ventricular rate control during supraventricular tachycardia. Negative inotropic effects usually preclude the use of beta-blocking agents or calcium channel antagonists in patients with acute ventricular dysfunction. Ventricular arrhythmias are common in patients with cardiogenic shock. Hypoxemia, hypokalemia, and hypomagnesemia are typical precipitants; when these are corrected, the ventricular ectopy usually resolves. If ventricular arrhythmias are related to myocardial ischemia or an underlying cardiac rhythm disorder, an intravenous infusion of lidocaine or other antiarrhythmic agent may be required.

Preload, or filling pressure, is the end-diastolic volume in the ventricle and is measured indirectly by pulmonary artery diastolic pressure, pulmonary capillary wedge pressure, or, less commonly, left atrial pressure. The relationship between cardiac muscle fiber length at the end of diastole and cardiac output is expressed in Starling's law (Hudak et al., 1998a). That is, as preload increases, cardiac output also increases until a point is reached at which a further increase in filling pressure produces a decrease in cardiac output and congestive heart failure. Preload is maintained at an optimal level for an individual patient using monitored filling pressures to guide volume replacement.

In the presence of reduced ventricular compliance and diastolic dysfunction, a higher left ventricular end-diastolic pressure (eg, 18 to 20 mm Hg) is required to achieve an adequate preload (Vander Salm & Stahl, 1997; Elefteriades et al., 1996a). Overdistention of the heart, however, must be avoided. Increases in left ventricular pressure and diameter cause proportional increases in wall tension (Laplace's law), a major determinant of myocardial oxygen consumption; in addition to increasing oxygen demand, the elevated left ventricular end-diastolic pressure also reduces oxygen supply by impeding coronary blood flow (Elefteriades et al., 1996a).

Left ventricular afterload, assessed by measurement of systemic vascular resistance, is lowered to decrease impedance to left ventricular ejection and, as a result, reduce cardiac work and oxygen consumption. Sodium nitroprusside and nitroglycerin are the mainstays of pharmacologic vasodilatation. Intra-aortic balloon counterpulsation (IABC) often is necessary as well to provide mechanical left ventricular afterload reduction. Pulmonary vascular resistance is the clinical indicator of right ventricular afterload. Nitroglycerin, isoproterenol, or prostaglandin E$_1$ infusion or nitric oxide inhalation may be used to lower pulmonary vascular resistance in patients with severe right ventricular dysfunction.

Myocardial contractility may be increased using one or more of the various intravenous inotropic agents. Dopamine, dobutamine, isoproterenol, and milrinone are commonly used inotropic agents. Dopamine is often the agent of choice. In addition to its inotropic effect, dopamine at low doses (0.5 to 2.0 μg/kg/min) stimulates renal dopaminergic receptors, thus improving renal perfusion and function (Haas & Young, 1998). Usually, vasodilating and inotropic agents are infused concomitantly to achieve the desired degree of afterload reduction and enhancement of myocardial contractility (DiSesa, 1991). The most effective combination and dosing of the various pharmacologic agents are determined empirically and modified by serial measurements of hemodynamic parameters.

Continuous intravenous infusions of inotropic and vasodilating agents must be performed with great attention to detail. Commonly, multiple drugs are administered simultaneously and doses are changed frequently. It is imperative that the nurse at the bedside know the precise dose of each agent being infused, which catheter is being used for infusion, and which drugs can be safely infused through a single catheter or through a peripheral catheter. Central venous catheters almost always are used to ensure consistent delivery of the medication and to avoid caustic effects of some agents on peripheral veins. Rate-regulating pumps are essential to maintain dosage at a constant rate. Changing intravenous solutions or tubing is performed in a manner that avoids a bolus or disruption of medication infusion with resultant precipitous hypertension or profound hypotension. Flushing a catheter through which medications are being infused is contraindicated.

Patients in cardiogenic shock usually are mechanically ventilated to reduce the work of respiration and, therefore, lower oxygen demand. Because acidosis severely depresses myocardial contractility, respiratory or metabolic acidosis, if present, should be corrected to avoid blunting the patient's response to inotropic agents (Elefteriades et al., 1996b). Sedation, with morphine, midazolam, or propofol, may be administered to minimize sympathetic overstimulation due to pain or anxiety and its deleterious effects on heart rate and systemic vascular resistance. Although serial patient repositioning is a routine component of caring for critically ill, bedridden patients, it may be precluded when severe hemodynamic instability is present because of the potential for inducing profound hypotension.

Implications of Circulatory Assist Devices

Mechanical support of the failing heart is a primary modality for treating cardiogenic shock refractory to pharmacologic therapy. Most commonly used is *intraaortic balloon counterpulsation*. The balloon-tipped catheter, usually inserted through the femoral artery in a retrograde fashion, is positioned so that the tip lies in the descending thoracic aorta, just distal to the left subclavian artery. Rhythmic inflation and deflation of the balloon in synchrony with cardiac contractions increases arterial pressure during diastole and decreases pressure during systole. IABC thus decreases myocardial oxygen consumption by reducing left ventricular afterload and improves myocardial oxygenation by augmenting coronary artery blood flow during diastole.

Interventions during IABC include monitoring and adjusting timing of balloon inflation and deflation to maximize hemodynamic benefits. Arrhythmias are treated promptly to prevent their interference with the timing of counterpulsation. Hemodynamic and clinical indicators of tissue perfusion are monitored to assess effectiveness of counterpulsation and patient readiness for weaning. Serial blood sampling (including complete blood cell count, blood urea nitrogen, creatinine, and platelet count) is performed to detect deleterious effects of IABC. An elevated white blood cell count suggests infection, increases in blood urea nitrogen and creatinine levels may represent renal dysfunction secondary to catheter-related impairment of renal artery perfusion, and a decreased platelet count (thrombocytopenia) may result from catheter-induced trauma to platelets. Antibiotics and heparin usually are administered as prophylaxis against infection and thromboembolism, respectively. The use of heparin is omitted in the early postoperative period because of the disturbances in blood coagulation mechanisms and freshness of suture lines and incisions (Elefteriades et al.,

1996b). The balloon catheter insertion site is monitored for evidence of hematoma or infection.

Three predominant types of complications are associated with IABC—ischemia, infection, and hematologic derangements; identified risk factors for these complications include female sex, age, obesity, comorbidities, smoking, and duration of counterpulsation (Cook et al., 1999). Most common is limb ischemia, which can result from thrombosis around the catheter or embolization of thrombus. Patients with underlying arterial occlusive disease and compromised blood flow to the lower extremities are at particular risk. Prevention of permanent limb dysfunction or loss depends on prompt detection and treatment of ischemia. The extremity distal to the balloon catheter is evaluated hourly, including palpation or Doppler ultrasound of peripheral pulses and assessment of capillary refill, color, temperature, and motor and sensory function.

The hallmarks of ischemia are the "six Ps": pulselessness, paresthesia, paralysis, pallor, pain, and poikilothermia (ie, decreased temperature due to environmental rather than internal temperature control). Observation of the extremity is essential because patients typically are intubated and sedated. Patients who are able to follow commands are asked to wiggle their toes and flex and extend the affected foot; the ability to do so is compared with the other foot. Often the earliest signs of ischemia are discoloration or mottling of the foot and absence of pulses. The appearance of pain, dullness to sensation, and minimal circulation indicate severe ischemia and require restoration of circulation to the extremity without delay (McCarthy & Golding, 1997).

If a patient has acute limb ischemia, compartment syndrome may develop because of associated edema. The fascia surrounding the calf muscles is fixed in size. As the muscle becomes swollen, it is compressed and becomes ischemic. Metabolic acidosis, hyperkalemia, and elevated blood urea nitrogen and creatinine levels all can result from the toxic waste products of ischemic tissue. In the presence of compartment syndrome, surgical fasciotomies (opening of the fascial compartments) may be necessary in addition to operative revascularization of the femoral artery to prevent muscle necrosis (Fig. 29-1). Other complications associated with IABC include aortic dissection, hemorrhage, false aneurysm, and arteriovenous fistula (Finkelmeier & Finkelmeier, 1991).

Ventricular assist devices (VADs) are used much less commonly but are available in some centers for use in patients with cardiogenic shock. A VAD is a sophisticated device designed to support completely one or both ventricles for days, weeks, or even months. Criteria for application of a VAD include a systolic blood pressure less than 90 mm Hg and a cardiac index less than 1.8 L/min/m² despite a left ventricular end-diastolic pressure of 25 mm Hg on maximal inotropic and IABC support (Elefteriades et al., 1996c). Several types of devices are available. The particular device to be used is determined by institutional availability, the expected duration of mechanical assistance, the potential for myocardial recovery, and the likelihood of subsequent cardiac transplantation. A Bio-Pump

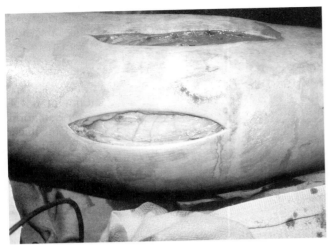

FIGURE 29-1. Fasciotomy incisions performed for relief of compartment syndrome. (Mravic PJ, Massey DM, 1992: Compartment syndrome. J Vasc Nurs 10:10)

centrifugal pump (Medtronic, Eden Prairie, MN) or BVS 5000 (Abiomed, Danvers, MA) device may be selected for short-term use when myocardial recovery is anticipated. The TCI HeartMate (Thermo Cardiosystems, Woburn, MA), Novacor (Baxter Healthcare Corporation, Novacor Division, Oakland, CA), and Thoratec (Thoratec, Berkeley, CA) VADs are devices designed for long-term use, providing a bridge to cardiac transplantation.

Operation of a VAD is performed by a perfusionist or nurse with specialized training. The most common complications occurring early after VAD implantation are bleeding, right heart failure, air embolism with stroke, and progressive multiorgan system failure; thromboembolism, infection, and catastrophic device failure are complications more likely to occur later (Haas & Young, 1998). IABC and VADs are discussed in more detail in Chapter 30, Circulatory Assist Devices.

Cardiopulmonary Arrest

Cardiopulmonary arrest is the cessation of spontaneous respiration and effective cardiac contractions. It can result from a respiratory arrest, a cardiac arrhythmia, or a hemodynamic catastrophe. Cardiopulmonary arrest continues to be associated with a high mortality rate and a significant incidence of postresuscitation neurologic impairment. The likelihood of successful cardiopulmonary resuscitation is directly related to the duration of resuscitation, with a duration of less than 30 minutes correlating with increased survival (Spotnitz & Spotnitz, 1996).

Cardiopulmonary resuscitation is initiated immediately on detection of cardiac arrest. A self-inflating bag with a fraction of inspired oxygen (FiO_2) of 100% is used to ventilate the patient manually by means of a face mask. Chest compressions are performed at a rate of 80 to 100 per minute with the duration of compressions comprising 50% of the compression–release cycle (Marino,

1998a). Electrocardiographic monitoring is established. Immediate defibrillation, using 200 joules (J) of current, is recommended for ventricular fibrillation or ventricular tachycardia with hemodynamic instability (Mistovich et al., 1997). If unsuccessful, defibrillation is repeated a second time with 200 to 300 J; subsequent shocks with up to 360 J are delivered if the arrhythmia persists.

Rapid defibrillation is essential because restoration of an adequate cardiac rhythm is more effective therapy than cardiopulmonary resuscitation. The outcome of cardiac arrest, with or without cardiopulmonary resuscitation, is dismal if timely defibrillation is not performed. The likelihood of successful resuscitation is as high as 90% if defibrillation is performed immediately at the time of cardiac arrest (Hendrickson et al., 1997). The probability of survival decreases by 7% to 10% each minute that a patient remains in ventricular fibrillation (Ornato & Peberdy, 1998). Although defibrillation is not effective therapy for asystole, sometimes what appears on the oscilloscope as asystole is actually a fine ventricular fibrillation that may be successfully converted with defibrillation.

Endotracheal intubation is performed to provide a secure airway, and manual ventilation through the endotracheal tube is continued. Intravenous bolus doses of antiarrhythmic medications, such as lidocaine, procainamide, or bretylium, are administered to stabilize the cardiac rhythm. A continuous infusion of an appropriate antiarrhythmic medication is begun. Lidocaine is the initial drug of choice to treat ventricular tachycardia and to maintain a stable rhythm after defibrillation for ventricular fibrillation (Spotnitz & Spotnitz, 1996). Occasionally, the heart rhythm is so unstable that multiple episodes of ventricular tachycardia or ventricular fibrillation occur. In this situation, defibrillator patches may be secured to the chest wall so that defibrillation can be repeated as necessary without delay.

Most cardiac surgical patients have temporary pacing wires placed at the time of operation. If bradycardia is present, a pulse generator is connected and single- or dual-chamber pacing is performed as indicated to maintain a stable cardiac rhythm. In the absence of pacing wires, a bolus dose of atropine may be given or an isoproterenol infusion initiated. Occasionally, electromechanical dissociation occurs—that is, a cardiac rhythm is present but the electrical depolarization produces no mechanical contraction of the ventricles (Falk, 1997). Electromechanical dissociation almost always signifies impending death.

Central venous access is established to ensure effective delivery of pharmacologic agents during the low-flow state of artificial circulation (Landolfo & Smith, 1995). A central venous catheter usually is used for continuous infusion of cardiotonic medications and a peripheral catheter for bolus doses of drugs or fluids. Blood samples are obtained for immediate arterial blood gas and serum electrolyte analysis. If venous access cannot be established quickly, epinephrine, lidocaine, or atropine can be administered through the endotracheal tube followed by several rapid insufflations to disperse the drug; the dose is 2 to 2.5 times the recommended intravenous dose diluted in 10 mL saline or water (Hendrickson et al., 1997). The intracardiac route for the administration of epinephrine is considered as a last resort if venous and endotracheal routes are unavailable.

Although cardiopulmonary resuscitation may be life saving, external cardiac compression can cause serious complications, particularly in patients who have recently undergone sternotomy. Most common in postoperative patients is sternal dehiscence and infection, which can lead to osteomyelitis and mediastinitis. Other complications of external cardiac massage include rib fractures, hemopericardium, hemothorax, pneumothorax, laceration of abdominal viscera (especially the liver), and myocardial contusion (Hendrickson et al., 1997).

▶ Management of Respiratory Failure

Acute Respiratory Distress

Acute respiratory distress is the inability to sustain respiration that is sufficient to maintain adequate blood oxygen saturation. Tachypnea, diaphoresis, dyspnea, and tachycardia are common early manifestations. The patient often attempts to remain in a sitting position, resisting efforts to lower the head of the bed. Initially anxious and agitated, the patient gradually becomes more somnolent as the problem worsens. If not corrected, respiratory and cardiac arrest soon follow.

Immediately on noticing a deterioration in the patient's respiratory status, oxygen saturation is measured using a pulse oximeter, and arterial blood gases and a portable chest roentgenogram are obtained. The lung fields are auscultated carefully. If rales are heard, intravenous diuretic therapy may be indicated to remove excess fluid. Endotracheal suctioning may be necessary if diminished breath sounds or rhonchi, representing atelectasis or the presence of secretions, respectively, are present. Suctioning must be performed with great caution in nonintubated patients with evidence of respiratory distress. Supplemental oxygenation is provided and the electrocardiogram is monitored during the procedure. Endotracheal intubation and mechanical ventilation are usually necessary to treat acute respiratory distress.

Continuous positive airway pressure (CPAP), delivered through a tightly fitting face mask, is used occasionally to provide temporary support in nonintubated patients with acute respiratory failure. However, if ventilation is compromised enough to warrant a CPAP mask, intubation almost invariably becomes necessary. In addition, the masks are uncomfortable for alert patients and often are tolerated poorly. Air leakage is common and gastric overdistention can result in vomiting and aspiration (MacIntyre, 1997).

Intubation and Mechanical Ventilation

Endotracheal intubation is performed through the mouth or nose. Orotracheal intubation is technically easier and is performed when immediate intubation is

necessary. Because tubes with a larger diameter can be used for oral intubation, less airway resistance is created and more effective suctioning can be performed; nasotracheal tubes, on the other hand, are more comfortable for the patient, permit better oral hygiene, and can be more effectively stabilized (Pierson, 1988). Complications of orotracheal intubation include dental trauma, tube occlusion in awake patients, and damage to the posterior larynx; nasotracheal tubes can cause epistaxis, paranasal sinusitis, and necrosis of the nasal mucosa (Marino, 1998b) (Fig. 29-2).

Endotracheal tubes are designed with a balloon that can be inflated around the tube to allow positive-pressure ventilation through the tube. Almost all endotracheal tubes have low-pressure cuffs that are inflated to the point of a minimal leak during peak inspiration. Routine cuff deflation usually is not necessary when a minimal leak technique is used. Characteristics of a good-quality endotracheal tube cuff include (1) low sealing pressure, (2) cuff pressure distributed over a large contact area, (3) large volumes of air accepted with minor increases in balloon tension, (4) maintenance of a good seal during inspiration and expiration, and (5) no distortion to the tracheal wall (Neagley, 1991).

Secure fixation of the endotracheal tube prevents dislodgment or damage to the tracheal wall and requires periodic replacement of soiled or moist tape. When intubation is prolonged, the tube is stabilized using a technique that prevents local pressure necrosis of skin on the nose or mouth. Oral hygiene measures are performed

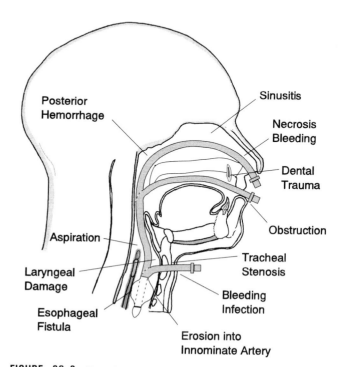

FIGURE 29-2. Potential complications of endotracheal intubation. (Adapted from Marino PL, 1998: The ventilator-dependent patient. In The ICU Book, ed. 2, p. 450. Baltimore, Williams & Wilkins)

as needed. During the period that the patient is intubated, suctioning with appropriate oxygenation is performed at least every 2 hours. The injection of small amounts (2 to 3 mL) of saline into the endotracheal tube, followed by ventilation and suctioning, may facilitate loosening and mobilization of tenacious secretions. In patients with copious secretions or continued significant atelectasis, bronchoscopy may be performed through the endotracheal tube to achieve more effective lavage and aspiration of secretions.

Critically ill patients almost always require mechanical ventilation for support of respiratory function. Even in the presence of normal respiratory function, mechanical ventilation may be helpful in unstable patients to conserve energy that would otherwise be expended on the work of breathing. Management of ventilators nearly always is handled by respiratory therapists. However, nurses require a basic understanding of the principles and types of mechanical ventilation.

There are two components to providing adequate respiration for patients on mechanical ventilators: oxygenation (the maintenance of a satisfactory arterial oxygen pressure [PaO_2]) and ventilation (the maintenance of a satisfactory arterial carbon dioxide pressure [$PaCO_2$]) (Elefteriades et al., 1996d). Maintaining oxygenation at a level sufficient to preserve aerobic metabolism is the more common problem in critically ill patients. Arterial PaO_2 can decrease to approximately 60 mm Hg before oxygen-carrying capacity begins to decrease significantly. Accordingly, a PaO_2 of 60 mm Hg is probably adequate for patients without compromised blood flow to key organs; a PaO_2 of 75 mm Hg is adequate for all patients (Elefteriades et al., 1996d). Ventilation, or the removal of carbon dioxide, depends directly on the minute volume (ie, the respiratory rate times the tidal volume of each breath). For patients on mechanical ventilators, the $PaCO_2$ usually is maintained at approximately 40 mm Hg. Effective CO_2 removal rarely is a problem when using mechanical ventilation in patients with respiratory failure. Common arterial blood gas abnormalities and corrective ventilator adjustments are listed in Table 29-1.

Most ventilators are volume controlled—that is, a preset volume of oxygenated air is delivered by positive pressure through an endotracheal or tracheostomy tube into the tracheobronchial tree. The level of ventilator support is determined by the clinical circumstances and ranges from partial ventilatory support, in which the patient is obliged to contribute to the work of breathing, to total ventilator support, in which the patient is rendered unable to contribute to the work of breathing (Shapiro & Lichtenthal, 1999). Intermittent mandatory ventilation (IMV) most often is selected as the mode of ventilation. With IMV, the ventilator delivers a preset number of breaths each minute at a given tidal volume. Between these mandatory breaths, the patient can breathe spontaneously, generating a tidal volume that varies according to ventilatory effort.

Positive end-expiratory pressure (PEEP) almost always is used in conjunction with mechanical ventilation.

TABLE 29-1	
Interventions for Common Arterial Blood Gas Abnormalities	
Abnormality	**Ventilator Adjustment**
High $PaCO_2$	Increase tidal volume
	Increase respiratory rate
Low $PaCO_2$	Decrease tidal volume
	Decrease respiratory rate
High PaO_2	Decrease FiO_2
	Decrease PEEP (if > 5 cm)
Low PaO_2	Increase FiO_2
	Increase PEEP

PEEP, positive end-expiratory pressure; $PaCO_2$, partial pressure of arterial carbon dioxide; PaO_2, partial pressure of arterial oxygen; FiO_2, fraction of inspired oxygen.

PEEP is positive pressure applied at the end of expiration; it compensates for the loss of physiologic PEEP provided by the glottis in the nonintubated patient. A pressure of 5 cm H_2O is the standard amount used to keep small airways open. However, because PEEP decreases intrapulmonary shunting, larger amounts may be used in selected situations to improve oxygenation and decrease the FiO_2 level. An additional physiologic effect of PEEP is that it increases intrathoracic pressure, which in turn decreases venous return to the heart. Therefore, the addition of PEEP may require increasing preload to prevent a decrease in cardiac output with resultant hypotension.

Pressure support ventilation may be used with the IMV mode to overcome the resistance of breathing spontaneously through an endotracheal tube and ventilator tubing. At the onset of each spontaneous breath, the negative pressure generated by the patient opens a valve that delivers the inspired gas at a preselected pressure, usually 5 to 10 cm H_2O (Marino, 1998c). Pressure support decreases the work of spontaneous breathing in mechanically ventilated patients who have an intact respiratory drive (Hudak et al., 1998b). Because of the significant complications associated with prolonged endotracheal intubation, tracheostomy usually is performed if the duration of intubation exceeds 10 to 14 days. A tracheostomy frees the patient's nose and mouth of an endotracheal tube. If level of consciousness and the swallowing mechanism are not impaired, oral feedings may be resumed.

Prolonged mechanical ventilation exposes the patient to the risks of nosocomial infections, airway injuries, debilitation, stress ulceration, and adverse cardiac events (Mehta & Pae, 1997). Radiographic evidence of pneumothorax occurs in 5% to 15% of ventilator-dependent patients (Marino, 1998b). Unilateral or bilateral pneumothoraces are particularly likely when high levels of PEEP are used (Fig. 29-3). Once alveolar rupture occurs, positive pressure during mechanical inhalation forces air through the rent into the pleural space. Tension pneumothorax is likely, with precipitous hypotension, tachycardia, and hypoxemia. Prompt chest tube thoracostomy is performed to relieve the tension component. Usually, the chest tube is left in place to suction drainage until positive-pressure ventilation is discontinued.

Adult Respiratory Distress Syndrome

Adult respiratory distress syndrome (ARDS) is a clinical syndrome that follows acute injury to the alveolar capillary membrane. It is the most severe form of respiratory failure. ARDS is characterized by refractory hypoxemia, noncompliant lungs, and diffuse and sometimes homogeneous infiltrates throughout both lungs (Mehta & Pae, 1997). The pathophysiologic process leading to ARDS remains unknown, although there are multiple theories of how the alveolar capillary membrane injury occurs (Multz & Dantzker, 1997) (Table 29-2). In postoperative patients, ARDS usually develops secondary to sepsis. The inflammatory reaction associated with cardiopulmonary bypass is a contributing factor in that extracorporeal perfusion initiates a massive inflammatory response and the production and release of a host of vasoactive substances capable of increasing pulmonary capillary permeability (Mehta & Pae, 1997).

A major goal in the treatment of ARDS is restoration of adequate oxygenation. Frequently, high levels of FiO_2 are necessary to maintain a PaO_2 greater than 60 mm Hg. However, prolonged administration of an oxygen concentration greater than 50% may cause clinically significant pulmonary oxygen toxicity. Ten to 20 cm of PEEP commonly is applied when ventilating patients with ARDS. PEEP improves lung compliance and recruits alveolar units

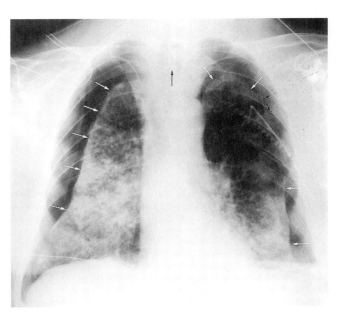

FIGURE 29-3. Anteroposterior roentgenogram demonstrating bilateral pneumothroaces secondary to mechanical ventilation with high levels of positive end-expiratory pressure. Note clearly visible edges of the partially collapsed lungs (*white arrows*) and the absence of lung markings external to lung edges. A tracheostomy tube also is apparent (*black arrow*). (Courtesy of Robert M. Vanecko, MD)

TABLE 29-2
Major Risk Factors for Adult Respiratory Distress Syndrome
Sepsis
Aspiration
Trauma
Pneumonia
Multiple transfusions

Adapted from Multz AS, Dantzker DR, 1997: Adult respiratory distress syndrome. In Parillo JE (ed): Current Therapy in Critical Care Medicine, ed. 3. St. Louis, Mosby.

that may have collapsed at low lung volumes (Multz & Dantzker, 1997). The enhanced oxygenation provided by PEEP allows the use of lower, and less toxic, FiO_2 levels. An arterial PaO_2 of 50 to 59 mm Hg may be tolerated when severe lung injury is present to avoid using a potentially deleterious level of FiO_2 or PEEP (Shapiro & Lichtenthal, 1999). Bilateral prophylactic chest tubes may be inserted when high levels of PEEP are used.

Diuretic therapy is used adjunctively to improve oxygenation, particularly if bilateral rales indicative of fluid overload are present. Even in the absence of clinical evidence of pulmonary edema, diuresis may help by lowering the hydrostatic capillary pressure. A lower pulmonary capillary wedge pressure (one that continues to provide adequate cardiac output and renal perfusion) reduces fluid movement into the interstitial tissue through capillary membranes that are made more permeable by respiratory failure (Todd, 1994). Bronchodilators are used to relieve bronchospasm, secretions are removed by frequent suctioning, and broad-spectrum antibiotics are administered to prevent infection (Mehta & Pae, 1997). In anemic patients, oxygenation may be improved by blood replacement therapy. Although transfusion with allogeneic blood often can be avoided in stable patients, blood is transfused more liberally in critically ill patients. The extra oxygen-carrying capacity provided by a normal hemoglobin level plays an important role in patients with marginal organ system function.

Hemodynamically stable patients who can tolerate repositioning are turned every 2 hours. Because pulmonary blood flow preferentially travels to dependent areas and ventilation is better in upright areas, prolonged periods in one position increase ventilation–perfusion mismatching. Especially in obese patients, oxygenation also is improved by placing the bed in a reversed Trendelenburg position (with the head elevated) so that the diaphragm is not subjected to pressure from the pendulous abdomen.

Weaning From Prolonged Ventilatory Support

Weaning is attempted when the ventilated patient demonstrates the capacity for self-ventilation, as evidenced by adequate respiratory parameters. Vital capacity and negative inspiratory force are the two measurements that best represent the patient's readiness for weaning and extubation. In addition, the patient should be alert enough to protect the airway and demonstrate a gag reflex by coughing during suctioning. Failure to wean may be due to inadequate gas exchange at the alveolar level or inadequate ventilation. The most common causes of inadequate gas exchange are pulmonary edema and ARDS; causes of inadequate ventilation are numerous, including cachexia, respiratory muscle weakness, and chronic lung disease (Vander Salm & Stahl, 1997). Common impediments to weaning are listed in Table 29-3.

In patients who have required prolonged ventilation, the weaning process often takes days or weeks. Before weaning is initiated, the patient should be receiving adequate calories to meet metabolic demands, and complicating factors, such as infection or hemodynamic instability, must be under control. If the patient is otherwise stable, weaning often can be performed in an intermediate care or "step-down" unit. Nursing observation must be adequate, however, to monitor the patient's tolerance of progressive reductions in ventilatory support. Oximetry monitoring usually is performed during the weaning process to detect impending respiratory distress.

Most commonly, weaning consists of gradual reduction of the IMV rate over a period of days or weeks. The addition of pressure support (ie, 5 to 10 cm H_2O positive pressure delivered during inspiration of spontaneous breaths) may facilitate weaning by reducing or eliminating the imposed work of breathing through a narrow endotracheal tube (MacIntyre, 1997). Pressure support during weaning is thought to increase endurance of respiratory muscles by decreasing the physical work and

oxygen demands during spontaneous breathing (Hudak et al., 1998b).

For patients who are difficult to wean, other techniques may prove more successful. Although various regimens may be used, a consistent schedule is designed to allow periods of rest interspersed with periods in which the patient must increasingly perform the work of breathing. Nursing care and visiting periods are coordinated with the weaning schedule so that the patient has adequate sleeping and resting periods. In patients who have had significant respiratory failure, weaning requires a great deal of patience and cannot be rushed to exceed the patient's endurance. Gradual retraining of the respiratory muscles is necessary before a sustained, coordinated pattern of respiratory effort is restored.

If the patient has required mechanical ventilation for more than 2 weeks, a tracheostomy tube usually will have been placed. When the patient has demonstrated the ability to sustain adequate respiration, supplemental oxygenation or humidification through a tracheostomy collar or T-shaped adaptor may be attempted. Removal of the tracheostomy tube usually is preceded by serial downsizing and changing from a cuffed to noncuffed tube. Nursing observation is essential after tracheostomy tube removal. The presence of granulation tissue due to prolonged intubation may lead to respiratory insufficiency within minutes or hours of removing the tube. Absence of a leak around the tube when the cuff is deflated suggests possible upper airway obstruction. Once the tube has been removed, the tracheostomy stoma closes over 24 to 48 hours. Insertion of another tube through the stoma usually is not possible after this time.

► Other Considerations in Critically Ill Patients

Nutritional Support

Critical illness significantly alters the body's metabolism. One major effect is increased metabolism with mobilization of fat and protein to provide energy and substrate for immune responses and healing (Zimmerman & Junker, 1997). Carbohydrate stores are available for only 8 to 12 hours, after which the body uses amino acids from protein and, to some degree, fatty acids for energy (Hudak et al., 1998c). Providing adequate nutrition is essential to patient recovery. Malnutrition increases susceptibility to pulmonary complications and has a number of adverse cardiac effects, including decreases in heart rate, arterial pressure, stroke volume, and cardiac index; in addition, both diaphragmatic and myocardial atrophy parallel losses in lean body mass (Zimmerman & Junker, 1997). Ventilator dependency, prolonged hospitalization, and operative mortality can result if nutrition is not maintained at an adequate level.

Supplemental nutrition is instituted in any patient who cannot be fed orally because of prolonged intubation, a diminished level of consciousness, or other factors. Nutritional maintenance rather than repletion is the de-

---

TABLE 29-3

Impediments to Weaning From Mechanical Ventilation

Pulmonary
  Atelectasis
  Retention of secretions
  Pneumonia
  ARDS
  Chronic lung disease
Cardiovascular
  Low cardiac output
  Pulmonary edema
Musculoskeletal
  Diaphragm and chest wall muscle weakness
  Sternal separation
Neurologic
  Central nervous system dysfunction
  Phrenic nerve paralysis
Other
  Sepsis
  Malnutrition
  Cachexia
  Anemia
  Pain

sired goal in critically ill patients because of the potential complications of overfeeding (Berry & Braunschweig, 1998). Overfeeding can increase carbon dioxide production and also can be associated with metabolic complications, such as hyperglycemia (Trujillo et al., 1999). Supplemental nutrition can be provided either directly into the gastrointestinal tract or intravenously. Enteral feedings through the gastrointestinal tract in general are preferred to avoid potential infectious complications associated with a central intravenous catheter used for parenteral nutrition. Enteral feedings also are preferable because progressive atrophy and disruption of intestinal mucosa becomes evident after just a few days of complete bowel rest and is not prevented by intravenous nutrition (Marino, 1998d). Enteral feedings are thought to maintain gut integrity, thus reducing bacterial translocation (movement of enteric pathogens across the bowel mucosa and into the systemic circulation) and infection (Berry & Braunschweig, 1998).

A percutaneous endoscopic gastrostomy (PEG) may be performed for placement of a feeding tube in the stomach. More commonly, a small feeding tube is placed in the duodenum or jejunum. Placing the tube distal to the pylorus is thought to lessen the risk of gastroesophageal reflux and possible aspiration associated with feedings delivered directly into the stomach through a gastrostomy tube. A nasogastric route usually is chosen if feedings will be necessary for only a short time. A soft, small-caliber tube is used with a weighted tip that aids passage into the duodenum. Proper tube position is confirmed by a chest roentgenogram before feedings are instituted. Alternatively, a jejunostomy tube is inserted by the nasogastric route over a guidewire and using fluoroscopy, or is placed through a small incision in the abdominal wall.

A variety of enteral feedings are available. Commercially prepared nutritional solutions deliver 1 to 2 calories/mL and contain carbohydrate, fat, protein, vitamins, and minerals; the dietary formula is selected based on the patient's ability to digest and absorb major nutrients, the total nutrient requirements, and fluid and electrolyte restrictions (Hudak et al., 1998c). The feeding regimen is introduced gradually, with serial increases in volume and concentration of solution, to avoid diarrhea. Diarrhea develops in approximately 30% of patients receiving enteral tube feedings (Marino, 1998d). Development of diarrhea necessitates temporary cessation of feedings until the problem abates. Because of the small lumen of distal feeding tubes, they become easily clogged and cannot be used for solid medications.

Central parenteral alimentation, also called total parenteral nutrition (TPN), is used when enteral feedings are not tolerated or advisable. A catheter is placed in the subclavian or jugular vein for continuous infusion. TPN solutions contain 15% to 35% glucose; 3.5% to 5% amino acids; and electrolyte, vitamin, and trace mineral additives (Hudak et al., 1998c). Because the solutions are hypertonic, they must be infused into a central vein where rapid blood flow dilutes the solution to lessen the risk of inflammation and venous thrombosis. An intravenous lipid emulsion solution (long-chain triglycerides rich in linoleic acid) is administered as well to prevent essential fatty acid deficiency (Marino, 1998e).

Because of the risk of infection, the catheter is used solely for the TPN infusion and care is taken to maintain sterility of the solution and the catheter insertion site. Meticulous technique to avoid bacteremia is imperative, particularly in patients with prosthetic cardiac valves (Elefteriades et al., 1996e). The catheter is changed every 5 to 7 days or if the patient becomes febrile or has signs of infection at the insertion site. Peripheral parenteral nutrition may be used to supplement nutrition in patients with marginal caloric intake. Solutions used for peripheral intravenous administration, which contain 5% to 10% dextrose, 3.5% amino acids, and isotonic lipids, have a lesser risk of infection and are less expensive (Hudak et al., 1998c).

Prevention of Infection

Infection is a major problem in critically ill patients. The multitude of invasive catheters and tubes in combination with the patient's debilitated state provides a fertile setting for nosocomial pathogens. The most serious nosocomial infections in critically ill patients are bacteremia, pneumonia, and surgical wound infection (Cooper & Larson, 1992). Intravenous catheters are one of the most common sources of infection (Fig. 29-4). Risk factors for catheter-related infection include the underlying disease process, duration of catheter use (ie, >3 days), location of insertion, the number of lumens in the catheter, and insertion technique (Murray & Torres, 1999). To reduce the incidence of catheter-induced infection, established protocols should be in place that guide nursing practices for inspection, dressing changes, and routine replacement of catheters. Typically, peripheral cannulae are changed every 2 to 3 days and arterial catheters every 4 days. Central venous and pulmonary artery catheters are changed every 5 to 7 days.

Urethral drainage catheters are a second common source of nosocomial infection in critically ill patients. Bacteriuria occurs in 80% of patients who have indwelling urethral catheters for 10 days or more (Landolfo & Smith, 1995). Pathogenic bacteria can enter the bladder at the time of catheterization, by retrograde migration along the outer surface of the catheter, or in urine that refluxes into the bladder from the drainage tubing (Yanelli & Gurevich, 1988).

A third major source of infection is prolonged endotracheal intubation. An endotracheal tube bypasses the defense mechanisms of the nasopharynx and allows organisms to enter the sterile tracheobronchial tree. Bacterial colonization occurs after several days of endotracheal intubation, and bacterial pneumonia develops in 5% to 40% of patients (Zapol, 1989). Aspiration also can occur as a result of an altered level of consciousness, abnormal swallowing, or a depressed gag or cough reflex (Recker, 1992). Surgical incisions are another possible site for infection. Most serious is deep infection of the sternal wound with sternal dehiscence and mediastinitis. Deep sternal wound

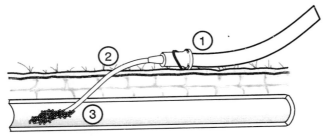

FIGURE 29-4. Routes of infection with indwelling intravenous catheters include (1) microbe entry into the catheter lumen through stopcocks or catheter hubs; (2) migration of microbes from the skin along the subcutaneous tract created by an indwelling catheter; and (3) entrapment of microorganisms circulating in the blood into the fibrin meshwork surrounding the intravascular segment of the catheter. (Marino PL, 1998: The indwelling vascular catheter. In The ICU Book. ed. 2, p. 83. Baltimore, Williams & Wilkins)

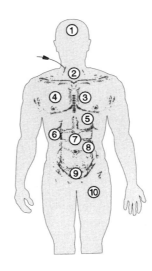

① Sinusitis
② Catheter sepsis
    Drug fever
③ Wound infection
④ Pneumonia
    Pulmonary embolism
⑤ Acute myocardial infarction
    Endocarditis
    Pericarditis
⑥ Acalculous cholecystitis
⑦ Perforated ulcer
    Pancreatitis
⑧ Translocation
    Enterocolitis
    Bowel infarction
⑨ Urosepsis
⑩ Deep vein thrombosis

FIGURE 29-5. Potential sources of nosocomial infection. (Marino PL, 1998: The febrile patient. In The ICU Book. ed. 2, p. 488. Baltimore, Williams & Wilkins)

infection can arise from direct contamination of the wound, from the bloodstream, or from extension of an adjacent infection; staphylococcal organisms are the most common pathogenic agents (Mehta & Pae, 1997).

Sepsis (ie, the presence of microorganisms or their toxins in the bloodstream) is the most serious consequence of infection. The incidence of sepsis in critically ill patients is increasing in the United States and, presumably, in other countries (Murray & Torres, 1999). It is the most common cause of death in intensive care unit patients and the 13th most common cause of death in the United States (Curran & Anderson, 1995). The most common pathogens for sepsis are gram-negative enteric organisms (eg, *Klebsiella*, *Pseudomonas aeruginosa*, and *Escherichia coli*), staphylococci, and enterococci (Marino, 1998f).

When clinical evidence of sepsis develops, attempts are made to determine the source of the infection (Fig. 29-5). Blood, urine, sputum, and drainage from any wounds are cultured to identify the source and responsible organism. Because indwelling central venous catheters are a common source of sepsis, insertion sites are changed and the withdrawn catheter tip is cultured. Sometimes, the source of the infection is not easily identified. Physical findings may be masked in the critically ill patient, who typically is heavily sedated or has an impaired level of consciousness. Common covert sources of infection in such patients include sinusitis caused by nasotracheal intubation or an undetected intra-abdominal process such as acalculous cholecystitis or abscess (Zapol, 1989). Broad-spectrum antibiotics are begun empirically and modified according to culture results as they become available.

The initial symptoms of sepsis are nonspecific, including malaise, tachycardia, hyperthermia or hypothermia, tachypnea, and either leukocytosis (increased white blood cell count) or leukopenia (decreased white blood cell count) (Hollenberg & Parrillo, 1997). Septic shock is the body's systemic response to sepsis and is manifest by hypotension, impaired organ perfusion, lactic acidosis, and multiple organ failure. The hallmark of septic shock is hypotension associated with a high cardiac output and low systemic vascular resistance. Increased capillary permeability sequesters fluid and proteins in the interstitial space, thus decreasing the effective intravascular circulating volume (Hudak et al., 1998d).

Therapy for septic shock is directed at supporting adequate organ perfusion while the infection is eradicated. The profound vasodilatation associated with septic shock usually necessitates infusion of large volumes of fluid to maintain adequate preload and arterial pressure. In addition, a continuous intravenous infusion of a vasopressor agent, such as norepinephrine, may be necessary to increase systemic vascular resistance. Septic shock is associated with a mortality rate of 30% to 70% (Murray & Torres, 1999; Hollenberg & Parrillo, 1997).

Electrolyte and Metabolic Imbalances

Hypokalemia is one of the most common metabolic imbalances in critically ill patients and a common cause of ventricular arrhythmias. It can occur secondary to urinary diuresis, diarrhea, vomiting, decreased intake, or alkalosis. Intravenous or oral potassium supplementation is often necessary to maintain the serum potassium level in a range of 3.5 to 5.0 mEq/L.

Hyperkalemia most often occurs in association with renal failure, acidosis, or overzealous intravenous potassium supplementation. Electrocardiographic manifestations of hyperkalemia include peaked T waves, widened QRS complexes, disappearance of the P wave, heart block, and conduction abnormalities that may be life threatening (Savino & Cheung, 1997). The cardiac rhythm may be difficult to distinguish from ventricular tachycardia. Serum potassium levels between 5 and 6 mEq/L usually can be treated by withholding potassium supplementation and by diuresis. If the serum potassium level exceeds 6.0 mEq/L or if electrocardiographic or neuromuscular manifestations of hyperkalemia are present, medical treatment should be instituted immediately (Arieff, 1997). Either intravenous insulin (with glucose to prevent hypoglycemia) or sodium bicarbonate is administered to shift potassium into the cells, thus lowering the serum concentration. Calcium also may be administered. Calcium does not lower serum potassium levels but counteracts the cardiac and neuromuscular effects of hyperkalemia. Patients with renal failure may require administration of sodium polystyrene sulfonate (Kayexelate) to treat hyperkalemia. Kayexelate is a potassium-binding resin that may be given by nasogastric tube or in the form of a retention enema.

Continuous venovenous hemofiltration (CVVH) may be used when pharmacologic therapy is ineffective. CVVH is one method of continuous hemofiltration, a form of therapy that mimics the native kidney in removing fluid and solute slowly over time (Craig, 1998). The CVVH system consists of a large-bore, double-lumen venous access catheter; a filter; an extra corporeal circuit; and a blood pump. Incorporation of a blood pump in the extracorporeal circuit allows the blood to be propelled through the circuit at a flow rate that is independent of the patient's mean arterial blood pressure; this differs from continuous arteriovenous hemofiltration (CAVH), in which blood is propelled not by a pump, but rather by the hydrostatic force of arterial blood pressure (Headrick, 1998). Large volumes of fluid can be removed in a manner that is better tolerated than hemodialysis in hemodynamically unstable patients with renal failure. Removal of nitrogenous waste products, however, is less efficient.

Blood urea nitrogen and creatinine levels may become seriously elevated in the presence of renal failure. Elective hemodialysis may be necessary if the blood urea nitrogen and creatinine levels reach 100 and 10 mg/dL, respectively; indications for immediate hemodialysis include manifestations of severe uremia (neurologic disturbances or gastrointestinal bleeding), refractory hyperkalemia, severe metabolic acidosis, and fluid overload (Moreno-Cabral et al., 1988).

Hyperglycemia can occur in critically ill patients due to diabetes, metabolic derangements, parenteral alimentation, and stress. Accordingly, serial blood samples are measured to determine blood glucose levels and guide corrective therapy. Urinary ketones also are monitored. Hyperglycemia usually is treated using a sliding scale protocol for insulin administration. Hypoglycemia is uncommon unless iatrogenically produced; it is treated with bolus doses of intravenous glucose. Other common metabolic disorders include hypomagnesemia, which may cause cardiac arrhythmias, and hypophosphatemia, which can produce depression of ventricular function and dysfunction of white blood cells and platelets (Landolfo & Smith, 1995).

Disturbances in the acid–base balance also occur frequently because of the many pathophysiologic processes that can increase the body's acid or base production or elimination. Inadequate alveolar ventilation that results in carbon dioxide retention is termed *respiratory acidosis,* and excessive alveolar ventilation that decreases $PaCO_2$ is termed *respiratory alkalosis.* Metabolic acidosis is that which is caused by excess ingestion of acid or acid precursors, increased production of metabolic acids, impaired acid excretion, or a decrease in bicarbonate (Felver, 1995). Metabolic alkalosis occurs because of a loss of acid or an excessive intake of bicarbonate.

Problems Associated With Immobility

Critically ill patients are confined to bed rest and often endure prolonged periods of passive immobility. In low cardiac output states, blood flow to the skin is marginal. Frequent turning may not be possible in hemodynamically unstable patients. As a result, decubitus ulcers are likely to develop on any body part that is exposed to prolonged pressure. Ulceration occurs when pressure exceeding mean capillary perfusion pressure is applied to an area of the body over time. Shearing forces and infection are other contributing factors in decubitus ulcer development. Pressure decubitus ulcers are a source of further morbidity and are associated with significant increases in hospital costs and length of stay (Allman et al., 1999). Prolonged wound care usually is necessary once an ulcer develops, and skin grafting may eventually be required. Infection of a decubitus ulcer can lead to sepsis. Special oscillating mattresses, positional changes, and other nursing measures to relieve local skin pressure are an important component of caring for critically ill patients.

Immobility also increases the risk for deep venous thrombosis and atelectasis with resultant pneumonia. Anticoagulation with heparin and vigorous pulmonary hygiene are used to prevent deep venous thrombosis and respiratory complications, respectively. Other deleterious effects of immobility include a loss of bone mass, atrophy of skeletal muscle, urolithiasis, urinary tract infections, and psychological disturbances, such as insomnia, anxiety, and depression (Molnar, 1998).

▶ Support of the Family

Nurses who specialize in cardiothoracic surgical nursing routinely care for patients who are critically ill and, sometimes, dying. It is imperative that families of such patients receive adequate emotional support. Occasionally, a previously stable patient sustains a catastrophic event. This information is difficult to convey to family members. The news is profoundly shocking, and the family needs time to absorb the information. As soon as a patient has a major hemodynamic problem or experiences cardiac arrest, a team member begins communicating with the family. Often, when the patient's condition is unstable, the primary physician is unable to leave the patient's bedside (or operating room) and the task is delegated to an appropriate physician or nurse member of the team. Ideally, the team member already has an established relationship with the family. The designated liaison person remains in communication with the family until the immediate life-threatening situation resolves. Simple measures such as arranging for a priest to administer sacramental rites or contacting other family members mean a great deal to the family during this time.

Cardiothoracic surgical services often have a designated advanced practice nurse who functions as the liaison in communicating with families, particularly when the patient is critically ill. This person should have excellent communication skills, including the ability to translate highly technical information into lay terms and to summarize probable outcomes in a compassionate manner. Availability of a liaison does not negate the need for each nurse at the bedside to communicate openly with the family. It is natural that families seek information from those who are caring directly for the patient. Providing accurate information to family members in a caring manner is an integral component of the role of the nurse at the bedside. At the same time, questions should be referred appropriately to the managing physician to ensure that the information that families receive is consistent and accurate. Although each person attempts to convey information as honestly and completely as possible, the same information can take on different connotations depending on what portions are stressed and the manner in which the information is communicated.

Patients frequently remain critically ill for days, weeks, and sometimes even months. During this time, it is important that the family, physicians, and nursing staff all are working together in the best interest of the patient. Some family members prefer to spend as much time as possible with the patient and participate actively in providing care. Direct care activities, such as brushing teeth, bathing, or combing the hair for the patient, may decrease anxiety and provide a sense of control for family members (Hudak et al., 1998e). Others may find waiting at the hospital too stressful or may be unable to remain at the hospital because of dependents at home or other responsibilities. In these cases, it may be necessary to communicate by phone to provide regular communication about the patient's condition and significant treatments and events. Although phone communication makes it more difficult to assess family members' understanding of information and the level of coping, regular communication with the family is an important adjunct to daily care of the patient and must not be overlooked.

Families require a tremendous amount of emotional support to withstand the stress of being suspended between hope for patient recovery and grief in anticipation of patient death. It may be several days or sometimes weeks before it is evident whether a patient can survive. The managing physician should discuss prognostic implications with the family regularly and thoroughly. As long as aggressive supportive measures are used, it is appropriate that hope for recovery is expressed by all staff who provide care to the patient. When survival is no longer realistically anticipated, the managing physician discusses this openly with the family. If the patient's critical illness and suffering have been lengthy and death be-

comes increasingly likely, it is natural for loved ones to want the waiting to come to an end. However, these feelings commonly evoke a great deal of guilt and it is quite difficult for family members to assume an active decision-making role in taking steps that hasten the patient's death. Many patients have prepared advance directives to be followed in the event of loss of decision-making ability. Advance directives communicate the patient's wishes in the event of terminal illness or a permanently comatose state (ie, living will), and also designate another person to act on the patient's behalf if the patient is unable to do so (ie, durable power of attorney for health care) (Hudak et al., 1998f).

The overriding concern for the dying patient is to maximize comfort and minimize suffering. Medical and nursing care plans should reflect that a decision has been made to change the goal of therapy from prolonging life to easing death. Interventions are reevaluated in light of whether they make the process of dying more or less difficult for the patient. Patients who die in critical care units are nearly always comatose at this stage, and it is often the family members who need emotional support and comfort. The nurses at the bedside play a key role in providing support for the family during and immediately after the patient's death.

Assessment skills are vital to providing appropriate emotional support. The manner in which families grieve varies considerably depending on a host of factors, including cultural norms, circumstances of the death, age and vitality of the patient, individual personalities of family members, and the relationship between patient and family and between the family members themselves. Although some families are effusive in their grief, others keep their emotions in check. Even when death is expected, family members sometimes react with shock and disbelief. Other common reactions include crying, screaming, hitting the wall or floor, hugging one another, sitting impassively, or abruptly leaving the area.

Occasionally, family members may become hostile or abusive to nursing or medical staff, particularly if prior relations between family and staff have been strained or if the death occurs unexpectedly. Family members who have had a strained or turbulent relationship with the patient may be unable to confront negative feelings for the deceased patient and instead direct the negativity toward staff members. It may be helpful for a patient representative or social worker who has not directly participated in the patient's care to remain available to the family. Family members may be able to verbalize to these people feelings that they are unable to express directly to the staff members. Value judgments should not be made about how an individual family grieves; rather, the nurse guides the family members through the initial phase of the grieving process while allowing them to deal with the death in their own manner.

Interventions are aimed at providing comfort. Protocols should be established so that necessary administrative details can be handled with minimal bother to the family. Typical interventions include offering the services of a hospital chaplain, providing water or coffee, or sitting with the family. If the family is large or if one family member is requiring a great deal of attention, it may be necessary to have two people available to the family during this time. For many family members, it is very important to spend a few moments with the deceased patient before leaving the hospital. Every attempt should be made to accommodate the family and to make the patient appear as natural to the family as possible.

REFERENCES

Allman RM, Goode PS, Burst N, et al., 1999: Pressure ulcers, hospital complications, and disease severity: Impact on hospital costs and length of stay. Advances in Wound Care 12:22

Arieff AI, 1997: Life-threatening electrolyte and metabolic disorders. In Parrillo JE (ed): Current Therapy in Critical Care Medicine, ed. 3. St. Louis, Mosby

Ashton RC, Mehmet CO, Rose EA, 1997: Surgery for acute myocardial infarction-cardiogenic shock. In Edmunds LH Jr (ed): Cardiac Surgery in the Adult. New York, McGraw-Hill

Bailey JM, Levy JH, Hug CC, 1997: Cardiac surgical pharmacology. In Edmunds LH Jr (ed): Cardiac Surgery in the Adult. New York, McGraw-Hill

Berry JK, Braunschweig CA, 1998: Nutritional assessment of the critically ill patient. Critical Care Nursing Quarterly 21:33

Cook L, Pillar B, McCord G, Josephson R, 1999: Intra-aortic balloon pump complications: A five year retrospective study of 283 patients. Heart Lung 28:195

Cooper B, Larson E, 1992: Infection control issues for critical care units: An overview and challenge—physician and nurse perspective. Heart Lung 21:317

Craig M, 1998: Continuous venous to venous hemo filtration: Implementing and maintaining a program: Examples and alternatives. Crit Care Cl N Amer 10:219

Curran RD, Anderson RW, 1995: Shock and circulatory collapse. In Sabiston DC Jr, Spencer FC (eds): Surgery of the Chest, ed. 6. Philadelphia, WB Saunders

DiSesa VJ, 1991: Pharmacologic support for low cardiac output. Semin Thorac Cardiovasc Surg 3:13

Elefteriades JA, Geha AS, Cohen LS, 1996a: Hemodynamic management. In House Officer Guide to ICU Care: Fundamentals of Management of the Heart and Lungs, ed. 2. Lippincott-Raven

Elefteriades JA, Geha AS, Cohen LS, 1996b: The intra-aortic balloon pump. In House Officer Guide to ICU Care: Fundamentals of Management of the Heart and Lungs, ed. 2. Lippincott-Raven

Elefteriades JA, Geha AS, Cohen LS, 1996c: Cardiac assist devices. In House Officer Guide to ICU Care: Fundamentals of Management of the Heart and Lungs, ed. 2. Lippincott-Raven

Elefteriades JA, Geha AS, Cohen LS, 1996d: Respirators and respiratory management. In House Officer Guide to ICU Care: Fundamentals of Management of the Heart and Lungs, ed. 2. Lippincott-Raven

Elefteriades JA, Geha AS, Cohen LS, 1996e: Additional topics. In House Officer Guide to ICU Care: Fundamentals of Management of the Heart and Lungs, ed. 2. Lippincott-Raven

Falk JL, 1997: Cardiopulmonary resuscitation. In Parrillo JE (ed): Current Therapy in Critical Care Medicine, ed. 3. St. Louis, Mosby

Felver L, 1995: Acid–base balance and imbalances. In Woods SL, Froelicher ES, Halpenny CJ, Motzer SU (eds): Cardiac Nursing, ed. 3. Philadelphia, JB Lippincott

Finkelmeier BA, Finkelmeier WR, 1991: Iatrogenic arterial injuries resulting from invasive arterial procedures. J Vasc Nurs 9:12

Haas GJ, Young JB, 1998: Acute heart failure management. In Topol EJ (ed): Comprehensive Cardiovascular Medicine. Philadelphia, Lippincott Williams & Wilkins

Headrick CL, 1998: Adult/pediatric CVVH: The pump, the patient, the circuit. Crit Care Cl N Amer 10:197

Hendrickson SC, Glower DD, Lowe JE, 1997: Cardiopulmonary resuscitation. In Edmunds LH Jr (ed): Cardiac Surgery in the Adult. New York, McGraw-Hill

Hollenberg SM, Parrillo JE, 1997: Septic shock. In Parrillo JE (ed): Current Therapy in Critical Care Medicine, ed. 3. St. Louis, Mosby

Hudak CM, Gallo BM, Morton PG, 1998a: Heart failure. In Critical Care Nursing: A Holistic Approach, ed. 7. Philadelphia, Lippincott Williams & Wilkins

Hudak CM, Gallo BM, Morton PG, 1998b: Patient management: Respiratory system. In Critical Care Nursing: A Holistic Approach, ed. 7. Philadelphia, Lippincott Williams & Wilkins

Hudak CM, Gallo BM, Morton PG, 1998c: Patient management: Gastrointestinal system. In Critical Care Nursing: A Holistic Approach, ed. 7. Philadelphia, Lippincott Williams & Wilkins

Hudak CM, Gallo BM, Morton PG, 1998d: Hypoperfusion states. In Critical Care Nursing: A Holistic Approach, ed. 7. Philadelphia, Lippincott Williams & Wilkins

Hudak CM, Gallo BM, Morton PG, 1998e: The family's experience with critical illness. In Critical Care Nursing: A Holistic Approach, ed. 7. Philadelphia, Lippincott Williams & Wilkins

Hudak CM, Gallo BM, Morton PG, 1998f: Legal issues in critical care. In Critical Care Nursing: A Holistic Approach, ed. 7. Philadelphia, Lippincott Williams & Wilkins

Landolfo K, Smith PK, 1995: Postoperative care in cardiac surgery. In Sabiston DC Jr, Spencer FC (eds): Surgery of the Chest, ed. 6. Philadelphia, WB Saunders

Lee JH, Geha AS, 1996: Postoperative care of the cardiovascular surgical patient. In Baue AE, Geha AS, Hammond GL, et al. (eds): Glenn's Thoracic and Cardiovascular Surgery, ed 6. Stamford, CT, Appleton & Lange

MacIntyre NR, 1997: Mechanical ventilation strategies. In Parrillo JE (ed): Current Therapy in Critical Care Medicine, ed. 3. St. Louis, Mosby

Marino PL, 1998a: Cardiac arrest. In The ICU Book, ed. 2. Baltimore, Williams & Wilkins

Marino PL, 1998b: The ventilator-dependent patient. In The ICU Book, ed. 2. Baltimore, Williams & Wilkins

Marino PL, 1998c: Patterns of assisted ventilation. In The ICU Book, ed. 2. Baltimore, Williams & Wilkins

Marino PL, 1998d: Enteral nutrition. In The ICU Book, ed. 2. Baltimore, Williams & Wilkins

Marino PL, 1998e: Parenteral nutrition. In The ICU Book, ed. 2. Baltimore, Williams & Wilkins

Marino PL, 1998f: Infection, inflammation, and multiorgan injury. In The ICU Book, ed. 2. Baltimore, Williams & Wilkins

McCarthy PM, Golding LA, 1997: Temporary mechanical circulatory support. In Edmunds LH Jr (ed): Cardiac Surgery in the Adult. New York, McGraw-Hill

Mehta SM, Pae WE, 1997: Complications of cardiac surgery. In Edmunds LH Jr (ed): Cardiac Surgery in the Adult. New York, McGraw-Hill

Mistovich JJ, Benner RW, Margolis GS, 1997: Electrical therapy. In Advanced Cardiac Life Support. Upper Saddle River, NJ, Prentice-Hall

Molnar HM, 1998: Intra-aortic balloon pump: Nursing implications for patients with an iliac artery approach. Am J Crit Care 7:300

Moreno-Cabral CE, Mitchell RS, Miller DC, 1988: Postoperative problems. In Manual of Postoperative Management in Adult Cardiac Surgery. Baltimore, Williams & Wilkins

Multz AS, Dantzker DR, 1997: Adult respiratory distress syndrome. In Parrillo JE (ed): Current Therapy in Critical Care Medicine, ed. 3. St. Louis, Mosby

Murray MJ, Torres NE, 1999: Critical care medicine for the cardiac patient. In Kaplan JA (ed): Cardiac Anesthesia, ed. 4. Philadelphia, WB Saunders

Neagley SR, 1991: The pulmonary system. In Alspach JG (ed): Core Curriculum for Critical Care Nursing, ed. 4. Philadelphia, WB Saunders

Ornato JP, Peberdy MA, 1998: Cardiopulmonary resuscitation. In Topol EJ (ed): Comprehensive Cardiovascular Medicine. Philadelphia, Lippincott Williams & Wilkins

Pierson DJ, 1988: Endotracheal intubation. In Luce JM, Pierson DJ (eds): Critical Care Medicine. Philadelphia, WB Saunders

Recker D, 1992: Caring for the long-term critical care patient. Critical Care Nurse 12:40

Savino JS, Cheung AT, 1997: Cardiac anesthesia. In Edmunds LH Jr (ed): Cardiac Surgery in the Adult. New York, McGraw-Hill

Shapiro BA, Lichtenthal PR, 1999: Postoperative respiratory management. In Kaplan JA (ed): Cardiac Anesthesia, ed. 4. Philadelphia, WB Saunders

Spotnitz HM, 1997: Practical considerations in pacemaker-defibrillator surgery. In Edmunds LH Jr (ed): Cardiac Surgery in the Adult. New York, McGraw-Hill

Spotnitz WD, Spotnitz HM, 1996: Cardiopulmonary resuscitation. In Baue AE, Geha AS, Hammond GL, et al. (eds): Glenn's Thoracic and Cardiovascular Surgery, ed. 6. Stamford, CT, Appleton & Lange

Todd TR, 1994: Ventilatory support of postoperative surgical patients. In Shields TW (ed): General Thoracic Surgery, ed. 4. Baltimore, Williams & Wilkins

Trujillo EB, Robinson MK, Jacobs DO, 1999: Nutritional assessment in the critically ill. Critical Care Nurse 19:67

Vander Salm TJ, Stahl RF, 1997: Early postoperative care. In Edmunds LH Jr (ed): Cardiac Surgery in the Adult. New York, McGraw-Hill

Yannelli B, Gurevich I, 1988: Infection control in critical care. Heart Lung 17:596

Zapol WM, 1989: Adult respiratory distress syndrome. In Grillo HC, Austen WG, Wilkins EW Jr, et al. (eds): Current Therapy in Cardiothoracic Surgery, Toronto, Canada, BC Decker

Zimmerman JE, Junker CD, 1997: Nutrition in the critically ill. In Parrillo JE (ed): Current Therapy in Critical Care Medicine, ed. 3. St. Louis, Mosby

30

Circulatory Assist Devices

irculatory assist devices that temporarily augment or substitute for the native heart contribute significantly to the management of patients with severe ventricular dysfunction. Use of mechanical circulatory assistance is considered when hemodynamic data indicate progressive ventricular failure despite adequate preload, optimal cardiac rate and rhythm, and maximal pharmacologic interventions to reduce afterload and improve contractility. As the technical capabilities of circulatory assist devices have improved, indications for clinical use have expanded correspondingly. A wide spectrum of devices are now available that can provide partial or complete circulatory support on a short-term or extended basis for patients with severe ventricular failure (Table 30-1).

Available circulatory assist devices may be categorized as (1) intra-aortic balloon pumps, (2) short-term circulatory support devices, and (3) ventricular assist devices (VADs) designed for extended use. Intra-aortic balloon counterpulsation (IABC), available for nearly three decades, is used widely in a variety of clinical circumstances to decrease myocardial work and increase myocardial oxygenation. Short-term circulatory support devices are used much less frequently, primarily in patients with postcardiotomy (ie, after cardiac surgery) shock. VADs designed for extended therapy also are used in a relatively small number of patients and are available in only a limited number of medical centers. Nevertheless, they have become a standard form of therapy for patients with severe ventricular failure when myocardial recovery is anticipated or cardiac transplantation is planned.

On an investigational basis, VADs are being used as temporary support in patients with cardiogenic shock associated with acute myocardial infarction, myocarditis, or

heart failure. Some VADs also are being used experimentally as an alternative to cardiac transplantation in patients with irreversible ventricular dysfunction and ineligibility for transplantation. Total artificial hearts designed for permanent replacement of the native ventricles remain under clinical investigation as well. The terms *bridge to transplantation, bridge to recovery,* and *destination therapy* often are used to convey the intended purpose of a circulatory assist device.

Decisions about patient selection for mechanical assistance, timing for initiation of therapy, and the most appropriate type of device demand a great deal of judgment on the part of the managing cardiothoracic surgeon or cardiologist. Factors that must be considered include the nature of the underlying cardiac pathologic process, prognosis for recovery of native heart function with medical or surgical therapy, patient age, associated medical problems, eligibility for cardiac transplantation, and potential complications of device therapy. Because of the limited supply of donor hearts relative to demand, devices used as bridges to transplantation must be suitable for maintenance of the circulation for a year or more.

▶ Intra-aortic Balloon Counterpulsation

Intra-aortic balloon counterpulsation was introduced into clinical use in 1967 by Kantrowitz and associates (Kantrowitz et al., 1968). Since that time, its use as a therapeutic modality has become widespread owing to development of sophisticated hemodynamic monitoring, introduction of percutaneous catheter insertion techniques, and biomedical engineering advances that improved balloon catheters and control consoles (Pae et al.,

TABLE 30-1

Types of Circulatory Assist Devices

Type	Function	Typical Duration
Intra-aortic balloon counterpulsation (IABC)	Support left ventricular function by reducing afterload and increasing coronary blood flow	Days
Nonpulsatile extracorporeal centrifugal pump	Substitute for left, right, or both ventricles during periods of severe ventricular dysfunction	Days
Extracorporeal membrane oxygenation system (ECMO)	Circulate and oxygenate blood as substitute for heart and lungs	Days
Temporary pulsatile ventricular assist device*	Substitute for one or both ventricles during periods of severe ventricular dysfunction	Weeks or months
Permanent pulsatile ventricular assist device†	Permanent left ventricular substitute when irreversible dysfunction present	Months to years
Total artificial heart†	Permanent orthotopic replacement for both ventricles when irreversible dysfunction present	Months to years

*Some devices provide left ventricular support only.
†Investigational use in patients with irreversible ventricular dysfunction who are not candidates for cardiac transplantation.

1996). IABC generally is considered the most appropriate initial mode of circulatory support because of its physiologic effectiveness and relative ease and safety of applicability.

Principles of Counterpulsation

Counterpulsation is the phasic displacement of intra-aortic blood to increase arterial pressure during diastole and decrease pressure during systole. It is achieved using a balloon-tipped catheter positioned in the descending thoracic aorta just distal to the left subclavian artery (Fig. 30-1). A console attached to the catheter emits a driving gas into the intra-aortic balloon lumen to produce rhythmic balloon inflations and deflations timed to occur in synchrony with the patient's cardiac contractions (Fig. 30-2). Using either the electrocardiogram or arterial pressure waveform for timing, balloon inflation occurs during diastole and deflation occurs during the isovolumetric phase of cardiac systole.

Counterpulsation provides two distinct hemodynamic benefits: (1) augmented diastolic arterial pressure, and (2) decreased end-diastolic pressure (Fig. 30-3). Balloon inflation during diastole mechanically displaces a volume of blood equal to that of the balloon proximally and distally in the aorta, producing elevation of the diastolic arterial pressure. Coronary blood flow is also increased because most coronary artery filling occurs during diastole.

Deflation of the balloon decreases aortic end-diastolic pressure (ie, left ventricular afterload) by creating a "space" in the aorta. Consequently, there is less resistance to forward flow during the subsequent left ventricular contraction. This results in a reduction in systolic wall tension, an increase in stroke volume, and an overall increase in cardiac output. The reduced preload also lowers the resistance to coronary artery filling, which allows for better subendocardial perfusion. Thus, IABC de-

creases myocardial oxygen consumption by reducing the afterload against which the left ventricle must eject and improves oxygen supply to the myocardium by augmenting coronary flow during diastole, thereby enhancing subendocardial perfusion.

Indications

Intra-aortic balloon counterpulsation is a valuable adjunct in the care of both preoperative and postoperative cardiac surgical patients (Table 30-2). It is used primarily when pharmacologic therapy alone is unsuccessful in treatment of perioperative ventricular dysfunction or unstable angina. A trend toward increased perioperative IABC use as well as toward increased preoperative prophylactic placement has been observed and is attributed both to liberalized indications for IABC use and a higher percentage of surgical patients with left ventricular dysfunction (Mehlhorn et al., 1999). In a study of nearly 7000 patients undergoing coronary artery bypass grafting in Massachusetts, IABC was used during the perioperative period in 13.4% of patients, although risk-adjusted rates of use varied widely across hospitals from 7.8% to 20.8% (Ghali et al., 1999).

The most frequent indication for IABC is postoperative left ventricular dysfunction, manifested in the operating room as an inability to wean from cardiopulmonary bypass (CPB) or in the postoperative unit as low cardiac output or the more severe form of ventricular dysfunction, cardiogenic shock. Two to 12% of patients who undergo myocardial revascularization or valvular heart operations require IABC for postoperative ventricular dysfunction (Naunheim et al., 1992). Most often, IABC is initiated in the operating room when left ventricular dysfunction becomes apparent as the surgeon prepares to separate the patient from CPB after the heart operation is completed. Intra-aortic balloon catheter insertion is considered if

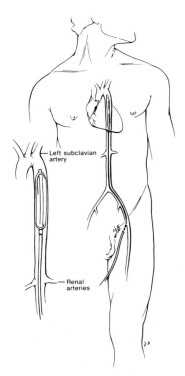

Left subclavian
artery

Renal
arteries

FIGURE 30-1. Intra-aortic balloon catheter has been inserted percutaneously through femoral artery and positioned in descending thoracic aorta; catheter tip lies just distal to left subclavian artery. (Hudak CM, Gallo BM, Morton PG, 1998: Patient management: Cardiovascular system. In Critical Care Nursing, ed. 7, p. 285. Philadelphia, Lippincott Williams & Wilkins)

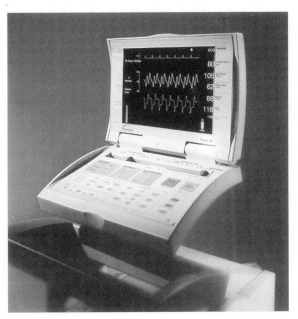

FIGURE 30-2. Display screen and keypad of the Datascope System 98 intra-aortic balloon pump; the console is beneath the keypad. (Courtesy of Datascope Corporation, Fairfield, NJ)

Systole   Diastole

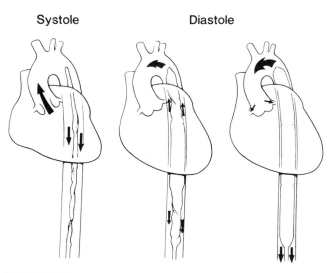

FIGURE 30-3. Hemodynamic benefits of counterpulsation. Balloon deflation decreases afterload and left ventricular work; balloon inflation augments diastolic blood flow. (Jorge E, Pierce WS, 1987: Mechanical support or replacement of the heart. In McGoon DC [ed]: Cardiac Surgery, ed. 2, p. 363. Philadelphia, FA Davis)

moderate doses of inotropic drugs are insufficient to improve cardiac performance, especially in patients with preoperative left ventricular impairment and in those with evolving myocardial infarction, destabilizing arrhythmias, or uncorrected mitral valve insufficiency (Vander Salm & Stahl, 1997).

Less commonly, left ventricular dysfunction necessitating balloon catheter placement develops in the early postoperative hours. Postcardiotomy shock is characterized by a systolic pressure less than 90 mm Hg, cardiac index less than 2.0 L/min/m², left or right atrial pressure greater than 20 mm Hg, urine output less than 30 mL/h, and persistent lactic acidosis. IABC is used to provide temporary support while the left ventricle recovers, typically over the course of 2 to 3 days. If postoperative ventricular dysfunction is irreversible and the patient is a suitable candidate for cardiac transplantation, IABC may provide sufficient support until a donor heart becomes available. More commonly, the degree of ventricular dysfunction in such patients and the lengthy waiting period for donor organs necessitates subsequent implantation of a VAD designed for extended therapy.

The most common preoperative indication for IABC is acute coronary syndrome. Because IABC augments coronary artery perfusion, it is quite effective in treating unstable angina not controlled by pharmacologic management. The decreased cardiac workload and increased flow through diseased coronary arteries almost always eliminates even refractory angina (Elefteriades et al., 1996). Particularly in patients in whom operative risk can be lessened by delaying surgery (eg, those with postinfarction angina), IABC provides a valuable treatment alternative.

In preoperative patients with precarious coronary artery anatomy (eg, severe left main coronary artery stenosis), IABC may be initiated prophylactically to pro-

Clinical Indications for Intra-aortic Balloon Counterpulsation

PREOPERATIVE SUPPORT

Acute coronary syndrome
Postinfarction cardiogenic shock
End-stage heart failure, awaiting transplantation
Postinfarction ventricular septal defect or mitral regurgitation

POSTOPERATIVE SUPPORT

Low cardiac output state
Reversible cardiogenic shock

vide protection of coronary blood flow during induction of anesthesia and the pre-CPB period (Elefteriades et al., 1996a). IABC also may be used to treat acute myocardial ischemia in nonsurgical patients. Many patients with acute coronary syndromes are treated with percutaneous coronary intervention rather than surgical intervention. As might be expected, IABC is being used increasingly in patients with acute myocardial ischemia or infarction who undergo percutaneous coronary intervention (Mehlhorn et al., 1999).

Another use of IABC in nonsurgical patients is cardiogenic shock resulting from acute myocardial infarction. Cardiogenic shock develops in approximately 15% of patients with myocardial infarction (Hudak et al., 1998). Counterpulsation can provide life-sustaining support in patients with coronary artery lesions amenable to revascularization; most patients demonstrate temporary hemodynamic and clinical improvement (Bates et al., 1998). Unfortunately, IABC is less useful if coronary artery anatomy is unsuitable for revascularization. Despite initial hemodynamic improvement with IABC, most patients with inoperable coronary artery disease remain device dependent and die in the hospital (Pae et al., 1996). If revascularization is not possible but cardiac transplantation is a treatment option, IABC may be replaced with a long-term form of circulatory assist device as a bridge to transplantation.

Other patients who benefit from IABC therapy include those with acute ventricular septal defect or mitral regurgitation that occurs secondary to acute myocardial infarction. In patients with ventricular septal defect, the afterload reduction achieved with counterpulsation decreases left ventricular peak systolic pressure, thereby decreasing the left-to-right shunt. In patients with mitral regurgitation, IABC increases coronary artery perfusion and decreases ischemic ventricular dysfunction, regurgitant flow across the mitral valve into the left atrium, and pulmonary capillary wedge pressure (Richenbacher & Pierce, 1997).

Intra-aortic balloon counterpulsation sometimes is used in combination with CPB. Counterpulsation continued during CPB may provide a pulsatile component to blood flow, although beneficial effects remain unproven. If IABC is continued during CPB, an intrinsic rate mode is used during the period of cardioplegic arrest because timing from the electrocardiogram or arterial pressure waveform is not possible. More commonly, counterpulsation is suspended during CPB. A standby mode is safe during CPB because the patient is systemically anticoagulated. Occasionally, IABC is used in combination with a nonpulsatile VAD (eg, a centrifugal pump) to provide a pulsatile component to blood flow.

There are very few contraindications to IABC therapy. Balloon counterpulsation is contraindicated in patients with aortic regurgitation because balloon inflation raises intra-aortic diastolic pressure and may increase regurgitation of blood through an incompetent aortic valve. IABC also is contraindicated in the presence of aortic dissection because counterpulsation may cause propagation of the dissection. Occasionally, intra-aortic balloon catheter insertion is precluded by severe peripheral arterial occlusive disease.

Techniques

Most balloon catheters are inserted into the common femoral artery using a percutaneous technique. The femoral artery with the stronger pulse is selected for insertion of the catheter. Doppler arterial pressure measurements may be performed to assess arterial circulation to the lower extremities, especially in preoperative patients with a high likelihood for perioperative ventricular dysfunction and balloon catheter insertion. In such cases, an arterial catheter may be inserted into the femoral artery with better perfusion before the operation to be used for pressure monitoring and to allow easy percutaneous balloon catheter insertion during the operation.

A cutdown technique may be necessary for balloon catheter insertion when it is not possible to palpate femoral pulses owing to peripheral arterial occlusive disease, cardiogenic shock, or CPB, and when attempted percutaneous insertion has failed (Richenbacher & Pierce, 1991). Although a cutdown technique formerly necessitated insertion of a graft sewn in end-to-side fashion to the artery, direct insertion of the catheter into the artery without a graft now is possible because of the smaller diameter of current catheters and sheath delivery systems.

With standard femoral artery placement, the balloon catheter is positioned with the cephalad end just distal to the origin of the left subclavian artery. The balloon catheter is placed in this position so that the balloon is as close as possible to the aortic valve without impeding blood flow through the arch vessels. Proper positioning allows peripheral flow around the balloon, and reduces the possibility of emboli to the cerebral circulation. The balloon, when inflated, should nearly occlude the aortic lumen (Franco, 1999). However, the balloon should not obstruct the left subclavian artery. Proper balloon catheter position is confirmed by chest roentgenogram and observation of the left radical artery pressure waveform.

In approximately 5% of patients, femoral artery placement of a balloon catheter is precluded or contraindicated (Mueller et al., 1998; Hazelrigg et al., 1992). Femoral artery insertion may not be possible in the presence of (1) extensive arterial occlusive disease or a previous peripheral arterial reconstructive procedure, (2) abdominal aortic aneurysm, (3) arterial injury during attempted insertion, or (4) ischemia in the ipsilateral (same side) leg.

When balloon catheter insertion is required for failure to wean from CPB and femoral cannulation is not possible or desirable, a transthoracic approach may be used; that is, the balloon catheter may be inserted directly through the aortic arch downward into the descending thoracic aorta. Transthoracic balloon catheter placement can be associated with significant morbidity and is used infrequently. Possible complications related to transthoracic catheter placement include graft and mediastinal infection; balloon rupture and malposition; postoperative bleeding secondary to cannulation; and cerebral, coronary, mesenteric, renal, spinal cord, or extremity embolization (Mueller et al., 1998).

Occasionally, IABC is used for extended periods in hospitalized patients waiting for cardiac transplantation. In these instances, the iliac artery may be used for balloon catheter placement to allow the patient to sit in a chair and ambulate, thus preventing deconditioning and avoiding the consequences of immobility (Molnar, 1998). Infrequently, the axillary artery or, rarely, the abdominal aorta is used as an alternative site for balloon catheter insertion (McCarthy & Golding, 1997).

Device Function

Most IABC systems use helium as the driving gas to produce balloon inflation. Optimal timing of inflation and deflation is critical to maximize coronary artery perfusion and lessen myocardial work. Timing is adjusted by comparing arterial pressure waveform morphologies while augmenting every other cardiac cycle (ie, a console setting of 1:2, or one counterpulsation to two cardiac contractions).

Properly timed inflation should begin just after aortic valve closure, represented on the arterial pressure waveform by the dicrotic notch. Because of the delay between actual cardiac events and transmission of the resulting pressure changes to the arterial pressure transducer, inflation timed to appear on the oscilloscope at the onset of the dicrotic notch actually occurs correctly after valve closure. Appropriately timed inflation thus produces a V-shaped configuration at the dicrotic notch (Fig. 30-4). Early balloon inflation causes premature closing of the aortic valve, lengthening of diastole, and impedance of left ventricular ejection. Stroke volume may be decreased, and left ventricular end-diastolic volume and pressure increased as a result. Late inflation unnecessarily shortens diastolic augmentation (Laurent-Bopp & Shinn, 1995) (Fig. 30-5).

Deflation should occur as late as possible to maintain the duration of the augmented diastolic blood pressure, but before the aortic valve opens and the ventricle ejects (McCarthy & Golding, 1997). Appropriate timing of de-

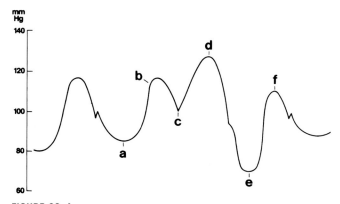

FIGURE 30-4. Arterial pressure tracing with 1:2 intra-aortic balloon counterpulsation demonstrates appropriately timed balloon inflation and deflation: *a*, unassisted aortic end diastolic pressure; *b*, unassisted systole; *c*, onset of balloon inflation; *d*, diastolic augmentation; *e*, assisted end-diastolic pressure; *f*, assisted systole. Note that both the end-diastolic and systolic pressures of the assisted cardiac cycle are lower than those of the unassisted cycle. (Courtesy of Datascope Corporation, Montvale, NJ)

flation is evidenced by lowering of end-diastolic pressure of the augmented cardiac cycle compared with the patient's unassisted cardiac cycle; systolic pressure after the assisted cardiac cycle should be lower or at least not higher than unassisted systolic pressure (Quaal, 1993) (see Fig. 30-4). Early deflation allows retrograde flow from the coronary and brachial arteries to fill the space created by balloon deflation, compromising forward flow into these vessels. In addition, the beneficial effects of afterload reduction are diminished. Late deflation impedes the subsequent left ventricular ejection and increases intraventricular wall stress (see Fig. 30-5). Failure to achieve counterpulsation may indicate retention of the balloon within the sheath, incomplete unwrapping

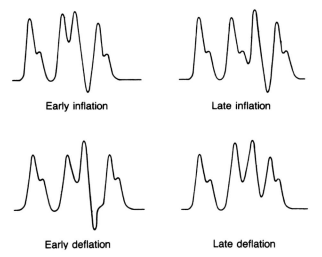

FIGURE 30-5. Waveforms representing early and late inflation and early and late deflation of intra-aortic balloon. (Hudak CM, Gallo BM, Morton PG, 1998: Patient management: Cardiovascular system. In Critical Care Nursing, ed. 7, p. 287. Philadelphia, Lippincott Williams & Wilkins)

of the balloon, an empty helium tank, or mechanical failure of the console (Lee, 1990).

In nonsurgical or preoperative patients, a continuous intravenous heparin or dextran infusion usually is administered to prevent clotting or platelet aggregation along the balloon catheter. Anticoagulant therapy is not administered immediately after cardiac surgery because blood coagulation mechanisms have been disturbed by intraoperative anticoagulation and extracorporeal circulation and because of the potential for exacerbation of bleeding from suture lines. If counterpulsation is required beyond the first or second postoperative day, a heparin infusion may be initiated in the absence of active bleeding, after chest tube drainage subsides and clotting parameters return to normal.

Weaning from IABC is accomplished by reducing the frequency of counterpulsations from every cardiac contraction to every other, and then to every third. When the patient is able to sustain an adequate cardiac output with a 1:3 ratio of counterpulsation or with the device momentarily in a standby mode, the balloon catheter is removed. Regardless of the patient's need for balloon augmentation, the balloon is never left motionless in the aorta; at least a 1:3 ratio of counterpulsation is continued until the catheter is removed from the aorta to reduce thrombosis along the catheter and possible embolization. Balloon catheters inserted percutaneously usually can be removed in the intensive care unit except in cases of a high percutaneous insertion site, morbid obesity, or limb ischemia (Pae et al., 1996). If the balloon catheter was inserted by direct cutdown technique or through a transthoracic approach, an operative procedure is necessary for catheter removal.

Associated Complications

Although IABC rarely is a direct cause of death, the mortality rate in patients receiving IABC therapy is high because of the types of underlying cardiac disease associated with the need for mechanical support. The overall hospital mortality rate for patients receiving IABC ranges from 26% to 50% and is higher in older patients, women, and patients with more severe ventricular dysfunction (McCarthy & Golding, 1997). Survival rates in cardiac surgical patients also are affected by timing of balloon catheter placement. Survival is improved with preoperative initiation of IABC in high-risk patients with unstable angina, left main coronary artery stenosis, and left ventricular dysfunction, suggesting that more liberal and earlier use of IABC in high-risk patients is advisable (Arafa et al., 1998; Gutfinger et al., 1999).

Intra-aortic balloon counterpulsation can be associated with significant morbidity. The reported incidence of complications varies from 6% to 49% (Richenbacher & Pierce, 1997). Risk factors for development of a major complication include female sex, peripheral arterial occlusive disease, diabetes mellitus, cigarette smoking, advanced age, obesity, and cardiogenic shock (McCarthy & Golding, 1997). The most common cause of morbidity is arterial injury secondary to insertion or the presence of an indwelling balloon catheter in the aorta. Vascular complications of IABC occur in 9% to 29% of patients and include thrombosis, embolization, aortic dissection, hemorrhage, false aneurysm, arteriovenous fistula, and embolization (Arafa et al., 1999; Finkelmeier & Finkelmeier, 1991).

Limb-threatening ischemia is the most common complication of intra-aortic balloon catheters. Because of the systemic nature of atherosclerosis, many patients with coronary artery disease have peripheral arterial (aortoiliac or femoropopliteal) occlusive lesions. Some degree of limb ischemia has been reported in as many as 47% of patients with balloon catheters in place (McCarthy & Golding, 1997). Significant limb ischemia occurs in approximately 5% to 18% of patients (Mehlhorn et al., 1999; Naunheim et al., 1992). Primary mechanisms for its development include arterial injury during catheter insertion, thromboembolism, and arterial spasm. Obstruction by the catheter also is a contributing factor because of the balloon catheter's large diameter and the relative lack of collateral arterial supply to the leg.

If ischemia is detected, the balloon catheter is removed unless the patient is dependent on counterpulsation. Although transient ischemia may resolve with balloon catheter removal, patients with significant limb ischemia may require surgical intervention for thrombus removal or bypass of the occluded arterial segment. In patients in whom continued counterpulsation is necessary, the balloon catheter is replaced with another catheter inserted in the opposite femoral artery. Alternatively, the balloon catheter is left in place and a femorofemoral or axillary-femoral bypass graft is performed to increase blood supply to the ischemic leg.

Hemorrhage can occur because of femoral artery injury or perforation of the aorta, particularly if balloon advancement is traumatic. An increasing number of patients who require IABC for acute coronary syndrome have been treated with thrombolytic therapy or heparin. Insertion of a balloon catheter in these circumstances increases the likelihood of bleeding complications but may be unavoidable if other means of controlling myocardial ischemia are unsuccessful.

Insertion and advancement of the balloon catheter can cause aortic dissection, particularly if repeated attempts at insertion are necessary or if the patient has associated peripheral arterial occlusive disease. Although aortic dissection occurs in less than 5% of patients, most patients in whom this complication develops do not survive (Richenbacher & Pierce, 1997). Difficulty in advancing the catheter or failure to achieve counterpulsation may be indicative of aortic dissection if the balloon is lying in the false lumen. Appropriate augmentation, however, does not rule out the existence of dissection. Development of iatrogenic dissection necessitates prompt balloon catheter removal. False aneurysm (pseudoaneurysm) and arteriovenous fistula are other types of arterial injury that occasionally develop at the insertion site after the balloon catheter has been removed.

In addition to vascular complications, wound infection or sepsis may complicate IABC therapy. Local wound infection occurs in 2% to 3% of patients and septicemia in up to 1% (McCarthy & Golding, 1997). Balloon rupture occurs rarely and usually is evidenced by the appearance of blood in the catheter shaft. It is thought to be related to rough handling during insertion or prolonged contact between the balloon and a calcified atherosclerotic plaque (Richenbacher & Pierce, 1991). A ruptured balloon should be deflated forcibly and removed immediately. A ruptured balloon catheter left motionless in the aorta can lead to thrombus formation along the catheter with subsequent embolization; in addition, blood entering the ruptured balloon lumen becomes clotted, making catheter removal difficult or impossible without damage to the femoral artery or an operative procedure. If continued counterpulsation is required, another balloon catheter is introduced over a guidewire that has been inserted through the original balloon catheter before its removal.

▶ Ventricular Assist Devices

Although IABC is the most commonly used form of mechanical circulatory assistance, it augments cardiac function only, improving the myocardial oxygen supply-and-demand ratio and supporting systemic perfusion to a modest degree (Richenbacher & Pierce, 1997). Unlike IABC, *ventricular assist devices* are true pumps that temporarily support or substitute for the left ventricle (LVAD), right ventricle (RVAD), or both ventricles (bi-VAD). VADs are an evolving, highly technical, and expensive form of therapy available only in selected centers. They are used in a variety of settings, including intensive care units for patients with acute ventricular dysfunction (ie, cardiogenic shock), as well as cardiothoracic nursing units and even patients' homes for extended support in patients with chronic ventricular dysfunction due to end-stage heart failure.

Ventricular assist devices serve two primary pur-

poses: (1) partial or complete support of the systemic circulation, pulmonary circulation, or both; and (2) effective ventricular decompression (Anstadt & Lowe, 1995; Richenbacher & Pierce, 1997). With an LVAD, blood is diverted from the left atrium or left ventricle to the device and returned to the ascending aorta; with an RVAD, blood is diverted from the right atrium to the device and returned to the pulmonary artery. VADs differ from conventional CPB in that they do not provide oxygenation of the blood. Instead, blood circulates through the pulmonary vasculature normally and is oxygenated by the patient, not by the device. Extracorporeal membrane oxygenation (ECMO) is a form of circulatory assist device that does provide oxygenation of blood in addition to circulatory support. ECMO is used rarely in adults and is described later in the chapter.

Ventricular assist devices also differ from conventional CPB in the duration of time they can be safely used. Whereas standard intraoperative CPB is designed to be used only for the duration of a typical cardiac operation (less than 6 to 8 hours), VADs can provide circulatory support and ventricular decompression for a few days or many months, depending on the specific device. In fact, successful VAD use for more than a year is not uncommon. Previously high rates of morbidity and mortality associated with long-term VAD use have declined through design improvements, more judicious patient selection, and greater clinical experience (Piccione, 1997). Researchers at several institutions also are investigating permanent devices for use in patients with profound left ventricular or biventricular failure and no anticipated hope of myocardial recovery or transplantation.

Types of Devices

The VADs described in this chapter are categorized according to whether they are designed for short-term or long-term support. Other features that help to characterize VADs and distinguish them from one another in-

---

TABLE 30-3

Comparison of Ventricular Assist Devices

	Bio-Medicus Pump	ABIOMED BVS	HeartMate Implantable Pneumatic	HeartMate Vented Electric	Novacor Left Ventricular Assist System	Thoratec Ventricular Assist Device
Pump type	Centrifugal	Pneumatic	Pneumatic	Electric	Electric	Pneumatic
Blood flow	Nonpulsatile	Pulsatile	Pulsatile	Pulsatile	Pulsatile	Pulsatile
Ventricle	Either or both	Either or both	Left only	Left only	Left only	Either or both
Duration	Short-term	Short-term	Long-term	Long-term	Long-term	Long-term
Pump location	External	External	Implanted	Implanted	Implanted	External
Drive system	Console	Console	Console	Wearable	Wearable	Console
Anticoagulation	Heparin or warfarin sodium	Heparin or warfarin sodium	Aspirin or dipyridamole	Aspirin or dipyridamole	Heparin or warfarin sodium	Heparin or warfarin sodium

clude (1) the type of blood flow (ie, nonpulsatile or pulsatile); (2) the type of pump (ie, centrifugal, pneumatic, electrical, or axial-flow); (3) whether the pump is external (extracorporeal) or implantable (intracorporeal); (4) whether the device supports one or both ventricles; and (5) whether the drive system is contained in a console or is portable (Table 30-3). Selection of the most appropriate type of VAD is tailored to the underlying nature of cardiac disease, expected duration of ventricular dysfunction, and long-term prognosis.

Short-Term Circulatory Assistance

Short-term circulatory assistance for postcardiotomy shock commonly is provided with a *centrifugal pump system*. The centrifugal circuits used for intraoperative CPB (eg, Bio-Medicus, Medtronic Bio-Medicus, Eden Prairie, MN) can be modified easily to provide extended, nonpulsatile circulatory support (Fig. 30-6). Centrifugal circulatory assistance used for postoperative support differs from conventional, intraoperative CPB in that the patient's pulmonary arterial circulation is not bypassed. That is, although standard CPB systems include an oxygenator, the system is modified when used as a postoperative circulatory assist device to provide circulatory support only with oxygenation of blood by the patient. Centrifugal pumps require transcutaneous cannulation, some degree of anticoagulation, and a means to reduce heat loss from the extracorporeal circuit (McCarthy & Golding, 1997). Left, right, or biventricular circulatory support may be provided.

The primary advantages of using a centrifugal pump for short-term circulatory assistance are its easy applicability, widespread availability, and familiarity to surgeons and perfusionists in institutions where cardiac surgery is performed routinely. However, the system necessitates continuous monitoring, activates and destroys some blood elements, and is associated with significant morbidity when use is prolonged. Also, patients essentially are limited to bed rest with no potential for physi-

cal conditioning. Sustained immobility increases the risk for formation of thrombus, respiratory complications, or other problems that may preclude eventual cardiac transplantation (Molnar, 1998; McCarthy et al., 1991). Therefore, use usually is limited to a week or less to limit untoward complications. Bleeding, thromboembolism, and hemolysis are the primary complications of centrifugal pump devices (Goldstein et al., 1998; Haas & Young, 1998; Killen et al., 1991).

The *ABIOMED system* (ABIOMED, Inc., Danvers, MA) is a pulsatile circulatory assist device designed for short-term (eg, 5 days or less) mechanical support in the postoperative period. It also has been used to provide temporary circulatory assistance for patients with acute myocarditis (Chen et al., 1999). The ABIOMED is a dual-chamber pneumatic, or air-driven, device that has an extracorporeal pumping chamber (prosthetic atrium and ventricle in combination) connected by transcutaneous cannulae to the inflow and outflow sites (Fields & Mentzer, 1992) (Fig. 30-7). The vertically oriented pump houses an upper gravity-filled atrial chamber and a lower air-driven ventricular chamber separated by a polyurethane trileaflet valve to maintain unidirectional flow (Franco, 1999). The ABIOMED can provide complete temporary left, right, or biventricular support. It is easy to use, can provide mechanical circulatory support for up to several weeks, and does not require the continuous presence of a perfusionist (Chen et al., 1999). Systemic anticoagulation with heparin is necessary during ABIOMED use.

Rarely, *extracorporeal membrane oxygenation* is used in adults to provide short-term (2 to 3 days) circulatory support for patients with postcardiotomy cardiogenic shock. ECMO, like standard CPB, provides total circulatory support and oxygenation of blood, typically using a centrifugal pump and a membrane oxygenator. However, also like CPB, ECMO activates blood elements causing coagulation and inflammatory problems (Franco, 1999). Survival with ECMO has been poor in adults with postcardiotomy shock and its use is associated with significant complications, including hemolysis, renal failure, and bleeding (Tjan et al., 1999). Consequently, the use of ECMO in adults remains controversial.

Long-Term Circulatory Assistance

In patients who are candidates for transplantation, it is preferable to use a device that is more suited to the prolonged waiting period typically associated with organ transplantation. Systems that have Food and Drug Administration (FDA) approval for clinical use in providing physiologic long-term circulatory support of the heart as a bridge to transplantation include (1) the HeartMate Left Ventricular Assist System (LVAS) (Thermo Cardiosystems, Inc., Woburn, MA); (2) the Novacor LVAS (Baxter Healthcare Corporation, Novacor Division, Oakland, CA); and (3) the Thoratec Ventricular Assist Device (Thoratec Laboratories Corporation, Berkeley, CA). The HeartMate and Novacor LVASs are both im-

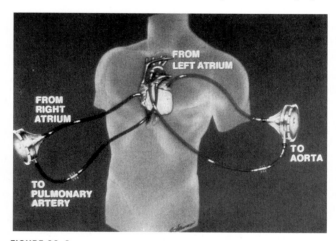

FIGURE 30-6. A centrifugal pump may be used for short-term left ventricular, right ventricular, or biventricular support of the heart. (Courtesy of Medtronic Bio-medicus, Inc., Eden Prairie, MN, 2000)

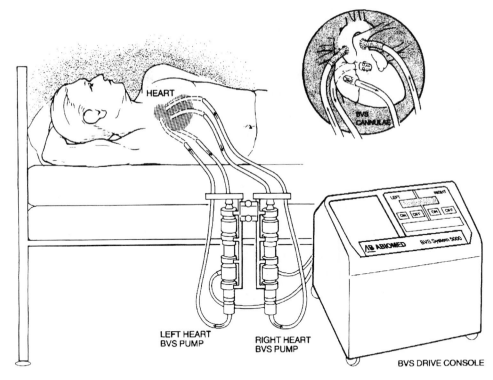

FIGURE 30-7. ABIOMED BVS 5000 biventricular support system. (Courtesy of Abiomed Cardiovascular, Inc., Danvers, MA)

plantable devices, whereas the Thoratec VAD is an external device.

Devices designed for long-term support are more complex and costly. Although most VADs require the patient to be connected to a cumbersome extracorporeal drive system, miniaturization of control and power supply components has resulted in a new generation of wearable LVADs that make it possible for selected patients to undergo rehabilitation, discharge to home, and return to work (Goldstein et al., 1998). Because of their portability, suitability for long-term use, and the shortage of donor organs, VADs with wearable drive systems are being investigated as permanent alternatives to transplantation.

The *HeartMate Left Ventricular Assist System* is designed for assistance of the left ventricle only and has a fully implantable pulsatile blood pump. Two types of HeartMate LVASs are available: an implantable pneumatic (IP) device that is operated by pneumatic energy and a more recently approved vented electric (VE) device operated by electrical energy. During normal operation, the HeartMate LVAS unloads the left ventricle and supports cardiac output at physiologic levels (Hunt & Frazier, 1998). Extensive experience has been obtained with the HeartMate LVAS, which to date has been implanted in nearly 1000 patients worldwide at more than 120 clinical centers in 18 different countries (Poirier, 1999).

Implantation of a HeartMate LVAS requires a median sternotomy and the use of CPB. The inflow conduit is inserted in the apex of the left ventricle and the outflow conduit is secured to the side of the ascending aorta. Both inflow and outflow conduits contain porcine valves that ensure unidirectional flow of blood from the left ventricle to the pump and from the pump to the ascending aorta. The implantable pump is placed below the left diaphragm, either within the peritoneal cavity or in a surgically created pocket in the left upper quadrant of the abdominal wall under the left rectus muscle and on top of the posterior rectus fascia (Poirier, 1999). A drive line brought out through the abdominal wall connects the implanted pump to the external system controller console (IP) or to an external system controller and battery pack (VE) (Fig. 30-8).

Compared with the HeartMate IP, the HeartMate VE has improved portability and longer battery life, allowing patients with the device to be discharged home while waiting for transplantation (Chillcott et al., 1998). Electrical power is obtained from two batteries that the patient carries in a shoulder holster; these batteries provide sufficient energy to power the system from 5 to 10 hours, depending on the activity level (Poirier, 1999). A back-up hand pump is used in emergency situations to maintain adequate blood flow in the event of an interruption in operation of the system (Poirier, 1999). An advantage of the HeartMate IP and VE devices is that only minimal anticoagulation with aspirin or another platelet inhibitor is required, owing to the unique blood-contacting surfaces that line the blood pump and are textured to encourage the deposition of circulating cells (Hunt & Frazier, 1998)(Figure 30–9). The Novacor LVAS and Thoratec VAD have smooth blood-contacting surfaces that necessitate anticoagulant therapy.

The *Novacor Left Ventricular Assist System* is an electrical VAD. Like the Heartmate LVAS, the Nova-

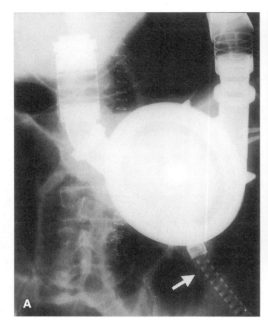

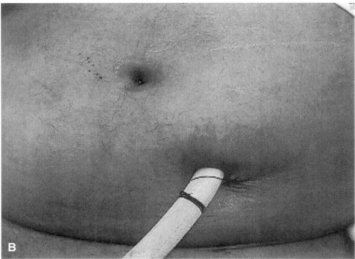

FIGURE 30-8. (A) Abdominal radiograph shows implanted HeartMate IP LVAS and drive line (*arrow*). **(B)** Drive line exiting abdominal wall. (Courtesy of Robert Mentzer, MD)

cor LVAS is an implantable device designed exclusively for support of the left ventricle (Fig. 30-10). Implantation of a Novacor LVAS also necessitates a sternotomy and the use of CPB. Inflow and outflow cannulae are inserted in the apex of the left ventricle and aorta, respectively. The pump usually is implanted in a pocket in the left upper quadrant of the abdomen (Murali, 1999). A percutaneous drive line connects the implanted Novacor LVAS pump to the external control unit or drive console.

In 1993, the Novacor LVAS was converted from a console-operated system into a wearable system (Hunt & Frazier, 1998). A compact controller and rechargeable power system worn on the patient's belt allow unrestricted mobility and potential discharge from the hospital. Systemic anticoagulation is necessary while the Novacor LVAS is in place, initially with heparin and then with warfarin sodium and aspirin. As of 1997, Novacor LVAS implantation had been performed in nearly 800 patients, 58% of whom subsequently underwent transplantation (Murali, 1999).

The *Thoratec VAD* is a pneumatic device with an external, pulsatile pumping chamber. Its main components are the extracorporeal blood pump(s), cannulae, and a large console. Thoratec VADs can be used to provide complete temporary left, right, or biventricular support. The Thoratec VAD is implanted through a median sternotomy incision, but CPB is not always required (Hunt & Frazier, 1998). For left ventricular support, the inflow cannula is placed in either the left atrium or the left ventricle. Left atrial cannulation avoids significant injury to an already damaged left ventricle and is technically easier. Ventricular cannulation, on the other hand, provides more effective left

ventricular decompression. It is ideally suited for patients in whom the VAD is used as a bridge to transplantation because recovery of the native ventricle is not anticipated (negating the issue of damage from cannulation) and ventricular cannulation avoids damage to the native atrium, which will be anastomosed to the transplanted heart.

The cannulae exit the chest below the costal margin and are connected to the pneumatic pump, which is placed on the anterior surface of the abdomen and attached by tubing to an external control console. If biventricular support is necessary, two pneumatic pumps, with appropriate cannulation, are used (Fig. 30-11). While the Thoratec VAS is in place, systemic anticoagulation with heparin or warfarin is required.

A Thoratec system is advantageous when biventricular support is required or anticipated because both an RVAD and LVAD can be placed. Because the devices are extracorporeal, Thoratec VADs also are preferable for patients with small body surface areas. Patients may be ambulatory, but their mobility is limited by the size of the drive console and the positioning of the pumps externally on the abdomen (Hunt & Frazier, 1998). A wearable system has become available for clinical investigation at selected institutions (El-Banayosy et al., 1999).

Principles of Function and Clinical Indications

Proper patient selection for VAD therapy is crucial to survival outcomes, and several factors are taken into consideration before initiating VAD use. All of the devices can cause serious, potentially fatal complications,

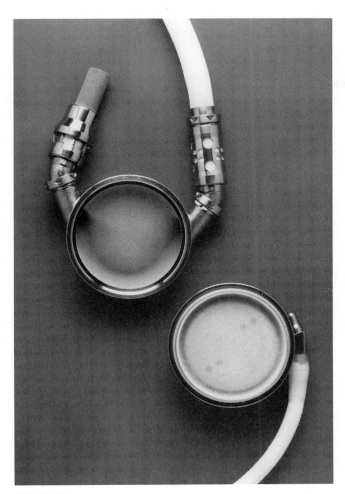

FIGURE 30-9. Interior of HeartMate Left Ventricular Assist System blood pump demonstrating textured blood-contacting surfaces. (Courtesy of Thermo Cardiosystems, Inc, Woburn, MA).

While an LVAD is operational, the heart can continue to contract. Pharmacologic agents that affect myocardial contractility, preload, and afterload may be used to maximize intrinsic cardiac function as well as device function. In patients with a pulmonary artery catheter in place, cardiac output can be measured by thermodilution technique and theoretically reflects the combined output of the LVAD and the ventricle itself. Acceptable cardiac output when an LVAD is in place depends on adequate filling (determined by right ventricular function and adequate intravascular volume) and proper emptying (affected by afterload).

Although there is no way to synchronize LVAD function with right-sided cardiac activity, filling of a left-sided VAD usually is not a problem unless the patient has elevated pulmonary vascular resistance and right ventricular failure. If so, an RVAD or right-sided centrifugal pump may be used to provide biventricular support. An LVAD is unlikely to sustain a patient successfully if inadequate filling of the device is the result of significant hemorrhage.

Indications for VAD implantation continue to be refined as more experience is gained in their use. The primary indications for use of a VAD are (1) to allow time for recovery of cardiac function in patients with what is considered to be reversible postcardiotomy shock, (2) to provide a bridge of cardiovascular support until cardiac transplantation, and (3) investigationally, as a bridge to recovery or as a permanent form of ventricular support (ie, destination therapy) (Table 30-4).

Short-term circulatory support most commonly is used in patients in whom cardiogenic shock develops after cardiac surgery (Table 30-5). Approximately 1% of patients who undergo cardiac operations experience

and some of the devices are quite costly. More conservative, less hazardous pharmacologic therapy and IABC should be considered first. Also, a VAD does not correct the underlying cardiac disease. Careful consideration must be given to a patient's eligibility for future cardiac transplantation or the likelihood of myocardial recovery. In addition, timeliness of VAD insertion is one of the most important factors for a successful outcome. If patients qualify as candidates for VAD placement, every hour that passes without adequate myocardial and systemic perfusion potentiates the risk for secondary organ dysfunction and eventual multiorgan failure (Schmid et al., 1998).

Most acquired forms of cardiac disease affect left ventricular function predominantly. Consequently, it is the left ventricle that more often requires mechanical support. Hemodynamic stability can be attained with isolated mechanical support of the left ventricle in more than 90% of patients, even in those with substantial right ventricular dysfunction, if there is effective replacement of left-sided heart function and treatment of pulmonary hypertension (Goldstein et al., 1998).

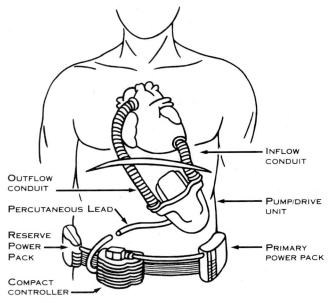

FIGURE 30-10. Novacor Left Ventricular Assist System. (Courtesy of Baxter Healthcare Corporation, Novacor Division, Oakland, CA)

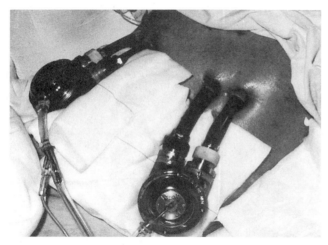

FIGURE 30-11. Right and left Thoratec ventricular assist devices in patient awaiting cardiac transplantation. (Courtesy of Robert Mentzer, MD)

postcardiotomy cardiogenic shock that is unresponsive to IABC and inotropic pharmacologic therapy (Richenbacher & Pierce, 1997). Heart failure in this group of patients often is due to temporary dysfunction (ie, "stunned myocardium") and may improve with time and temporary circulatory support.

Patients placed on a VAD because of inability to wean from CPB after a cardiac operation should be those in whom repair of the underlying cardiac disorder has been accomplished successfully. With appropriate candidate selection, VADs provide a valuable treatment modality to increase survival in this moribund group of patients. Approximately 45% of patients who probably otherwise would die can be weaned successfully from ventricular support, and 55% of weaned patients are discharged from the hospital; the overall survival rate is 25% (Pae et al., 1992). Patients most likely to recover are those with isolated left ventricular failure or predominant right with only mild left ventricular failure. Age is also an important factor in predicting successful outcomes. Early experience with the use of postcardiotomy devices for cardiac recovery showed that patients younger than 60 years of age had a survival rate of 21% to 31%, patients older than 60 years of age had a survival rate of 12%, and only 6% of patients older than 70 years of age survived (Arabia & Copeland, 1999).

Ventricular assist devices also provide a safe and ef-

TABLE 30-4

Clinical Indications for Ventricular Assist Device Placement

Postcardiotomy shock
Bridge to transplantation
Bridge to recovery*
Destination therapy*

*Under clinical investigation.

TABLE 30-5

Hemodynamic Indications for Ventricular Assist Device Placement*

Cardiac index <2.0 L/min/m^2
Systolic arterial pressure <90 mm Hg
Systemic vascular resistance >2100 dynes·sec·cm^{-5}
Left or right atrial pressure >20 mm Hg
Urine output <30 mL/h

*Despite optimal pharmacologic therapy and intra-aortic balloon counterpulsation.

fective way of supporting hemodynamic function in patients with end-stage heart failure who have already been or who are likely to be accepted as candidates for heart transplantation. In most patients with chronic dilated or ischemic cardiomyopathy, isolated left ventricular support with an LVAD allows adequate stabilization of the patient; less commonly, biventricular support is required (Tjan et al., 1999). As waiting time for transplantation has increased, availability of devices designed for long-term support has become more important.

In some centers, as many as 30% to 50% of patients who undergo cardiac transplantation are bridged to transplantation with a VAD (Haas & Young, 1998). Sometimes, LVAD placement is required urgently in patients awaiting transplantation for treatment of acute cardiogenic shock. However, there is a trend toward earlier LVAD implantation for patients with chronic heart failure awaiting transplantation, before irreversible end-organ dysfunction occurs (Piccione, 1997). In transplant candidates with slowly progressive cardiac deterioration, elective VAD placement may be considered to improve hemodynamic stability, reverse end-organ hypoperfusion, improve nutritional status, and allow physical rehabilitation before transplantation (Argenziano & Oz, 1998) (Fig. 30-12).

With LVAD support, patients can recover from secondary organ dysfunction, such as liver or renal failure; perform substantial amounts of physical activity; and largely overcome the sequelae of chronic heart failure (Loebe et al., 1999). Selected patients with wearable VADs can even be discharged to home, where they can resume a reasonable quality of life with an acceptable incidence of adverse events (Rose et al., 1999). An extensive education program for patients, families, and community emergency personnel is necessary for patients who are discharged from the hospital with a wearable VAD. All must demonstrate an understanding of proper maintenance of the system and required procedures in the event of system failure.

Of patients who receive an LVAD as a bridge to transplantation, 68% survive to undergo transplantation, and of those who receive transplants, 70% survive to be discharged (Kormos & Griffith, 1998). Patients who require only left ventricular assistance have much better rates of transplantation and discharge; patients with implantable LVASs have a better survival

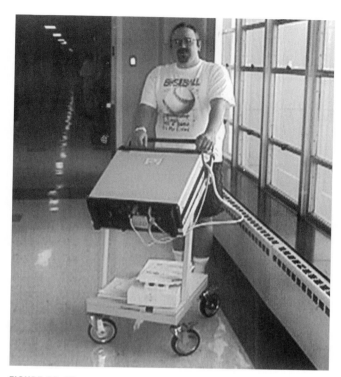

FIGURE 30-12. Patient with HeartMate IP LVAS. VAD implantation allows patients with end-stage heart failure to undergo physical reconditioning prior to the transplant procedure. (Courtesy of Robert Mentzer, MD)

rate, presumably because they can be supported safely for a longer duration, allowing complete physical rehabilitation before transplantation (Hunt & Frazier, 1998).

An investigational indication for VAD use is as a "bridge to recovery" in carefully selected patients with severe cardiogenic shock secondary to idiopathic dilated cardiomyopathy, acute inflammatory myocarditis, or myocardial infarction. Extended periods of left ventricular support have been associated with significant myocardial recovery in some patients. VADs also are being used investigationally as destination therapy in patients who are not candidates for cardiac transplantation. There are an estimated 3 million patients with congestive heart failure in the United States (Kaplon et al., 1999). Because only approximately 2500 donor hearts become available in the United States each year, it is essential that other effective forms of treatment for patients with end-stage heart failure be developed. Because of the shortage of donor organs, the lack of effective pharmacologic therapy, and the encouraging clinical outcomes with the current generation of VAD's, wearable LVADs are being evaluated as an alternative to transplantation.

The Ramdomized Evaluation of Mechanical Assistance for the Treatment of Congestive Heart Failure (REMATCH) trial is in progress to compare a wearable LVAD with optimal medical treatment for patients with end-stage heart failure who are ineligible for cardiac transplantation. The trial will provide data about the long-term effects of LVADs on survival, quality of life, and costs, as well as information about device reliability and the long-term safety profile of LVADs (Rose et al., 1999).

Associated Complications

Ventricular assist devices can be associated with significant morbidity regardless of which device is used. Bleeding, thromboembolism, and infection are the most prevalent complications associated with mechanical circulatory support (El-Banayosy et al., 1999). Complications more likely to occur early include bleeding, right heart failure, air embolism with stroke, and progressive multiorgan system failure; thromboembolism, infection, and catastrophic device failure more often occur later (Haas & Young, 1998). VADs do not yet offer an alternative to transplantation; long-term durability of the pump chamber and valves is undetermined and the infection rate exceeds 30% in most centers (Tjan et al., 1999).

Excessive bleeding can be a major problem, particularly in patients who require a VAD in the early postoperative period when hemostasis is impaired. Patients with end-stage heart failure requiring mechanical ventricular support are at greater risk for bleeding because of underlying hepatic dysfunction and associated coagulopathy. Bleeding rates may be as high as 60% because of coagulopathy due to hepatic dysfunction, the extensive surgical procedure required for implantation, and the combined effects of CPB and blood pump rheology on platelet activation (Hunt & Frazier, 1998). Significant bleeding is more likely in patients requiring biventricular assistance. Bleeding is of less concern when VADs are used for long-term support in patients waiting for transplantation. However, significant bleeding can occur at the time of device explantation. Dense adhesions between the device and intrathoracic organs may cause diffuse hemorrhage when the device is removed (Arabia & Copeland, 1999).

Thromboembolism is a potential problem because of the large artificial surface in contact with blood (Reedy et al., 1990). VADs, like most biomechanical devices, activate the clotting cascade because of the device–blood interface (Kaplon et al., 1999). Thromboembolism may occur in as many as 10% to 35% of patients with mechanical circulatory devices; the incidence is less in patients with HeartMate devices because of the textured surface of the blood–device interface (Haas & Young, 1998).

Patients with VADs are prone to nosocomial and device-related infections. Infection rates range from 30% to 40%; the longer the device remains implanted, the higher is the incidence of infection (Arabia & Copeland, 1999; Hunt & Frazier, 1998). Pneumonia and mediastinitis occur frequently. Infections related to the drive line also are common and usually are manageable with local wound care and antibiotics (Goldstein et al., 1998). Although infections usually do not preclude patients from undergoing device removal and transplantation, they can profoundly debilitate patients with underlying heart failure and limit physical rehabilitation before transplantation; fungal and drug-resistant infections are particularly problematic (Haas & Young, 1998).

► Total Artificial Heart

Total artificial hearts under clinical investigation include the Cardiowest artificial heart and Penn State pneumatic artificial heart. These devices are pulsatile, biventricular cardiac replacement systems that necessitate excision of both native ventricles for orthotopic placement. Neither the Cardiowest nor the Penn State total artificial heart is FDA approved yet. The devices are expensive and potential complications include bleeding, thromboembolism, mechanical failure, and infection (Goldstein et al., 1998).

REFERENCES

Anstadt MP, Lowe JE, 1995: Assisted circulation. In Sabiston DC Jr, Spencer FC (eds): Surgery of the Chest, ed. 6. Philadelphia, WB Saunders

Arabia FA, Copeland JG, 1999: Bridge to transplantation with left ventricular assist devices and total artificial heart. In Franco KL, Verrier ED (eds): Advanced Therapy in Cardiac Surgery. Hamilton, Canada, BC Decker

Arafa OE, Pedersen TH, Svennevig JL, et al., 1998: Intraaortic balloon pump in open heart operations: 10-year follow-up with risk analysis. Ann Thorac Surg 65:741

Arafa OE, Pedersen TH, Svennevig JL, et al., 1999: Vascular complications of the intraaortic balloon pump in patients undergoing open heart operations: 15-year experience. Ann Thorac Surg 67:645

Argenziano M, Oz MC, 1998: Left ventricular assist devices. In Rose EA, Stevenson LW (eds): Management of End-Stage Heart Disease. Philadelphia, Lippincott Williams & Wilkins

Bates ER, Stomel JR, Hochman JS, Ohman EM, 1998: The use of intra-aortic balloon counterpulsation as an adjunct to reperfusion therapy in cardiogenic shock. Int J Cardiol 65(Suppl 1):S37

Chen JM, Spanier TB, Gonzalez JJ, et al., 1999: Improved survival in patients with acute myocarditis using external pulsatile mechanical ventricular assistance. J Heart Lung Transplant 18:351

Chillcott SR, Atkins PJ, Adamson RM, 1998: Left ventricular assist as a viable alternative for cardiac transplantation. Critical Care Nursing Quarterly 20:64

El-Banayosy A, Korfer R, Arusoglu L, et al., 1999: Bridging to cardiac transplantation with the Thoratec Ventricular Assist Device. Thorac Cardiovasc Surg 47(Suppl 2):307

Elefteriades JA, Geha AS, Cohen LS, 1996: The intra-aortic balloon pump. In House Officer Guide to ICU Care: Fundamentals of Management of the Heart and Lungs, ed. 2. Philadelphia, Lippincott-Raven

Fields BL, Mentzer RM Jr, 1992: Extended circulatory support for cardiac failure. Cardiac Surgery: State of the Art Reviews 6:439

Finkelmeier BA, Finkelmeier WR, 1991: Iatrogenic arterial injuries resulting from invasive procedures. J Vasc Nurs 9:12

Franco KL, 1999: Temporary mechanical support. In Franco

KL, Verrier ED (eds): Advanced Therapy in Cardiac Surgery. Hamilton, Canada, BC Decker

Ghali WA, Ash AS, Hall RE, Moskowitz MA, 1999: Variation in hospital rates of intra-aortic balloon pump use in coronary artery bypass operations. Ann Thorac Surg 67:441

Goldstein DJ, Oz MC, Rose EA, 1998: Implantable left ventricular assist devices. N Engl J Med 339:1522

Gutfinger DE, Ott RA, Miller M, et al., 1999: Aggressive preoperative use of intra-aortic balloon pump in elderly patients undergoing coronary artery bypass grafting. Ann Thorac Surg 67:610

Haas GJ, Young JB, 1998: Acute heart failure management. In Topol EJ (ed): Comprehensive Cardiovascular Care. Philadelphia, Lippincott Williams & Wilkins

Hazelrigg SR, Auer JE, Seifert PE, 1992: Experience in 100 transthoracic balloon pumps. Ann Thorac Surg 54:528

Hudak CM, Gallo BM, Morton PG, 1998: Patient management: Cardiovascular system. In Critical Care Nursing: A Holistic Approach, ed. 7. Philadelphia, Lippincott Williams & Wilkins

Hunt SA, Frazier OH, 1998: Mechanical circulatory support and cardiac transplantation. Circulation 97:2079

Kantrowitz A, Tjonneland S, Freed PS, et al., 1968: Initial clinical experience with intra-aortic balloon pumping in cardiogenic shock. JAMA 203:113

Kaplon RJ, Gillinov AM, Smedira NG, et al., 1999: Vitamin K reduces bleeding in left ventricular assist device recipients. J Heart Lung Transplant 18:346

Killen DA, Piehler JM, Borkon AM, Reed WA, 1991: Bio-Medicus ventricular assist device for salvage of cardiac surgical patients. Ann Thorac Surg 52:230

Kormos RL, Griffith BP, 1998: Ventricular assist. In Kaiser LR, Kron IL, Spray TL (eds): Mastery of Cardiothoracic Surgery. Philadelphia, Lippincott Williams & Wilkins

Laurent-Bopp D, Shinn JA, 1995: Shock. In Woods SL, Froelicher ES, Halpenny CJ, Motzer SU (eds): Cardiac Nursing, ed. 3. Philadelphia, JB Lippincott

Lee ME, 1990: Mechanical support of the circulation. In Gray RJ, Matloff JM (eds): Medical Management of the Cardiac Surgical Patient. Baltimore, Williams & Wilkins

Loebe M, Muller J, Hetzer R, 1999: Ventricular assistance for recovery of cardiac failure. Curr Opin Cardiol 14:234

McCarthy PM, Golding LAR, 1997: Temporary mechanical circulatory support. In Edmunds LH Jr (ed): Cardiac Surgery in the Adult. New York, McGraw-Hill

McCarthy PM, Portner PM, Tobler HG, et al., 1991: Clinical experience with the Novacor ventricular assist system. J Thorac Cardiovasc Surg 102:578

Mehlhorn U, Kroner A, de Vivie ER, 1999: 30 years clinical intra-aortic balloon pumping: Facts and figures. Thorac Cardiovasc Surg 47:298

Molnar HM, 1998: Intra-aortic balloon pump: Nursing implications for patients with an iliac artery approach. Am J Crit Care 7:300

Mueller DK, Stout M, Blakeman BM, 1998: Morbidity and mortality of intra-aortic balloon pumps placed through the aortic arch. Chest 114:85

Murali S, 1999: Mechanical circulatory support with the Novacor LVAS: Worldwide clinical results. Thorac Cardiovasc Surg 47:321

Naunheim KS, Swartz MT, Pennington DG, et al., 1992: Intraaortic balloon pumping in patients requiring cardiac operations. J Thorac Cardiovasc Surg 104:1654

Pae WE Jr, Miller CA, Matthews Y, Pierce WS, 1992: Ventricular assist devices for postcardiotomy cardiogenic shock. J Thorac Cardiovasc Surg 104:541

Pae WE Jr, Pierce WS, Sapirstein JS, 1996: Intra-aortic balloon counterpulsation, ventricular assist pumping, and the artificial heart. In Baue AE, Geha AS, Hammond GL, et al. (eds): Glenn's Thoracic and Cardiovascular Surgery, ed. 6. Stamford, CT, Appleton & Lange

Piccione W, 1997: Mechanical circulatory assistance: Changing indications and options. J Heart Lung Transplant 16:S25

Poirier VL, 1999: Worldwide experience with the TCI Heartmate system: Issues and future perspective. Thorac Cardiovasc Surgeon 47:316

Quaal SJ, 1993: Conventional timing using the arterial waveform. In Comprehensive Intra-aortic Balloon Counterpulsation, ed. 2. St. Louis, CV Mosby

Reedy JE, Ruzevich SA, Noedel NR, et al., 1990: Nursing care of the ambulatory patient with a mechanical assist device. Journal of Heart Transplantation 9:97

Richenbacher WE, Pierce WS, 1991: Management of complications of intra-aortic balloon counterpulsation. In Waldhausen JA, Orringer MB (eds): Complications in Cardiothoracic Surgery. St. Louis, Mosby–Year Book

Richenbacher WE, Pierce WS, 1997: Assisted circulation of the heart. In Braunwald E (ed): Heart Disease: A Textbook of Cardiovascular Medicine, ed. 5. Philadelphia, WB Saunders

Rose EA, Moskowitz AJ, Packer M, et al., 1999: The REMATCH trial: Rationale, design and end points. Ann Thorac Surg 67:723

Schmid C, Deng M, Hammel D, et al., 1998: Emergency versus elective/urgent left ventricular assist device implantation. J Heart Lung Transplant 17:1024

Tjan TDT, Schmid C, Deng MC, et al., 1999: Evolving short-term and long-term mechanical assist for cardiac-failure: A decade of experience in Munster. Thorac Cardiovasc Surg 47:293

Vander Salm TJ, Stahl RF, 1997: Early postoperative care. In Edmunds LH Jr (ed): Cardiac Surgery in the Adult. New York, McGraw-Hill

Cardiothoracic Transplantation and Trauma

Heart, Lung, and Heart-Lung Transplantation

Current accomplishments in transplantation of the heart and lungs derive from research dating to the beginning of the 20th century. As early as 1905, Alexis Carrel performed experimental heart transplantation in a dog (Carrel & Guthrie, 1905). Investigations regarding technical and immunologic aspects of thoracic transplantation have continued since that time. Ongoing laboratory research and the collective clinical experience of many physicians and scientists during the past several decades have led to significant improvements in achieving long-term survival and quality of life after thoracic organ transplantation (Table 31-1). Although many researchers have contributed to the field, Norman Shumway and Richard Lower are recognized particularly for their sustained research and clinical contributions leading to current success in cardiac transplantation. James Hardy and Joel Cooper have been pioneers in the development of lung transplantation.

Data from the Registry of the International Society for Heart and Lung Transplantation (ISHLT) demonstrate the growth that has occurred in the field of thoracic transplantation. The Sixteenth Official Report of the ISHLT, published in 1999, reports data on 48,541 heart transplants from 304 programs, 5347 single-lung, and 3751 double- or bilateral lung transplants from 153 programs, and 2510 heart-lung transplants from 124 programs (Hosenpud et al., 1999). Essential to the success achieved by these thoracic organ transplantation programs throughout the world are dedicated and expert transplant teams, comprising specially trained surgeons, cardiologists, pulmonologists, nurses, and other professionals providing expertise in the social, psychological, nutritional, rehabilitation, and financial implications of transplantation. As with other types of solid-organ transplantation, a major limitation to further growth in thoracic transplantation is the scarcity of donors relative to the number of potential recipients.

▶ Heart Transplantation

Cardiac transplantation has become a standard therapeutic option for the treatment of end-stage heart failure and currently is the only form of treatment that achieves long-term survival. The first successful heart transplantation was reported by Christiaan Barnard in 1967 (Barnard, 1967). Despite technical accomplishment of the procedure, organ rejection prevented long-term survival of patients. It was not until the early 1980s that results improved dramatically because of the availability of the immunosuppressive agent, cyclosporine. From that

TABLE 31-1
Factors Leading to Improved Long-Term Outcomes After Thoracic Organ Transplantation

- More knowledgeable donor and recipient selection
- Early referral and management of candidates by transplantation specialists
- Improved preservation of donor lungs
- Use of ventricular assist devices that provide an effective "bridge to transplantation" and allow preconditioning of cardiac transplantation candidates
- Pretransplantation rehabilitation of lung transplantation candidates
- Improved immunosuppressive therapy to control rejection

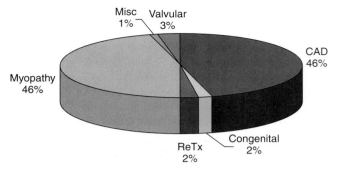

FIGURE 31-1. Indications for cardiac transplantation in adults. Coronary artery disease (CAD) and cardiomyopathy together account for 92% of transplant in adults. Misc, miscellaneous; ReTx, retransplantation.

point forward, the number of transplantation programs, as well as the number of transplantations performed each year, increased steadily until reaching a plateau imposed by the finite number of donor hearts available. The 1999 ISHLT Registry Report demonstrates a declining number of transplantations performed annually from a peak of approximately 4000 several years ago to just under 3000 transplantations in the most recent year for which data are available (Hosenpud et al., 1999).

Recipient Selection

Ischemic heart disease and cardiomyopathy are the two primary indications for cardiac transplantation in adults and together represent most cases (Fig. 31-1). Less commonly, cardiac transplantation is performed in adults with severe ventricular failure secondary to congenital heart disease or valvular heart disease.

Ischemic heart disease has become a major indication for cardiac transplantation owing to the widespread prevalence and progressive nature of coronary artery disease. Most patients considered for transplantation have ischemic cardiomyopathy, a form of chronic heart failure caused by severe left ventricular or biventricular dysfunction. Ischemic cardiomyopathy is characterized by an ejection fraction less than 40%, multifocal wall motion abnormalities due to coronary atherosclerosis, significant disability, and a 5-year survival rate of only approximately 40% (Rodkey et al., 1998). Infrequently, patients with ischemic heart disease require cardiac transplantation not for severe heart failure but rather for intractable angina or refractory ventricular arrhythmias.

Dilated cardiomyopathy (DCM) is the other major indication for cardiac transplantation in adults. It is the most common form of nonischemic cardiomyopathy in the United States, accounting for 87% of all cases (American Heart Association, 1998). DCM is characterized primarily by dilatation and impaired systolic function of the left ventricle. Patients with DCM severe enough to warrant transplantation, however, usually have right ventricular failure as well.

Although the cause or causes of DCM remain unclear, a number of clinical conditions are known to be associated with its development, including alcohol and cocaine abuse, metabolic abnormalities, and the cardiotoxicity of anticancer drugs (Wynne & Braunwald, 1997). Frequently, no specific etiologic factor is identified and the condition is termed *idiopathic DCM*.

Regardless of etiology, patients considered for cardiac transplantation usually have severe, chronic ventricular dysfunction known as end-stage heart failure. Approximately 60,000 patients eventually have end-stage heart failure that is unresponsive to maximal medical therapy and, for many of these people, cardiac transplantation is the only hope for long-term survival (Goldstein & Rose, 1998). The use of angiotensin-converting enzyme inhibitor and beta-adrenergic blocking medications has been shown to improve functional status and prolong survival in patients with end-stage heart failure. However, even with advances in pharmacologic therapy, patients with severe ventricular dysfunction have a 1- to 2-year mortality rate approaching 50% (Renlund, 1998).

Selecting patients who will benefit most from cardiac transplantation is crucial because of the significant implications of receiving a transplanted heart and because of the tremendous disparity between the large number of potential recipients and the limited number of available donor organs. Cardiac transplantation is considered for patients with severe heart failure; a New York Heart Association III or IV functional class; severe symptoms despite optimal pharmacologic therapy; and no other therapeutic options, such as coronary artery revascularization or valve replacement. Typically, potential candidates have a projected life expectancy of 1 to 2 years, a left ventricular ejection fraction less than 20%, and severely impaired exercise tolerance ($VO_2 <$ 15 mL/kg/min during formal exercise testing). Psychological stability and ability to comply with the management protocol after transplantation are other important considerations in candidate selection. Table 31-2 lists typical inclusion and exclusion criteria for heart transplant recipients.

TABLE 31-2

Recipient Criteria for Heart Transplantation

ACCEPTANCE CRITERIA

New York Heart Association functional class III or IV on maximized
  therapy
Life expectancy 1 to 2 years
Age < 65 to 70 years
Stable family support system
Ability to adhere to complex medical regimen

EXCLUSION CRITERIA

Refractory elevation of pulmonary vascular resistance
Active malignancy
Recent pulmonary infarction
Active infection
Active peptic ulcer disease
Irreversible end-organ failure
Active substance abuse
Psychological instability

Heart transplantation is contraindicated in the presence of factors that make success unlikely. Most of these factors are relative contraindications only and are viewed as one factor among many considered in making an overall judgment about the risk/benefit ratio of transplantation for an individual patient. For example, most transplant programs limit candidates to patients younger than 65 years of age because of significantly poorer survival outcomes in elderly patients. Organ dysfunction is another relative contraindication. Some degree of organ dysfunction (eg, kidney, liver, or brain) secondary to cardiac disease frequently is present in potential recipients, but usually is considered reversible with successful transplantation and therefore does not necessarily preclude candidacy. However, significant end-organ dysfunction, such as irreversible renal failure or hepatic failure, is a contraindication to performing cardiac transplantation unless renal or liver transplantation, respectively, is planned.

Insulin-dependent diabetes usually is considered a contraindication only in those patients with end-organ damage, such as nephropathy, retinopathy, or neuropathy (Fleischer & Baumgartner, 1997). However, immunosuppression can exacerbate diabetes and diabetic patients have a propensity for accelerated atherosclerosis that can cause progressive coronary artery disease in the transplanted heart. Other relative contraindications include severe obesity, osteoporosis, and a prior malignancy with an uncertain prognosis for recurrence (Hunt & Frazier, 1998).

A few absolute contraindications to heart transplantation remain. An absolute contraindication to orthotopic cardiac transplantation is severe, irreversible pulmonary hypertension. Because a transplanted heart has a normal, thin-walled right ventricle, acute right ventricular failure is likely to occur if the heart is implanted in a recipient with elevated pulmonary vascular resistance. Consequently, patients with fixed pulmonary vascular resistance greater than 6 Wood units usually are excluded from consideration for heart transplantation. If elevated pulmonary vascular resistance is reversible, as demonstrated by lowering of pulmonary vascular resistance to an acceptable range in response to nitroprusside or inhaled nitric oxide, cardiac transplantation may be considered. Patients with fixed pulmonary hypertension may be suitable candidates for combined heart-lung transplantation.

The necessity for lifelong immunosuppression precludes cardiac transplantation in other patients. Infection with the human immunodeficiency virus (HIV) probably is the only infection that currently is considered a permanent contraindication to transplantation (Hunt & Frazier, 1998). However, any active systemic infection precludes candidacy until the infection is eliminated because postoperative immunosuppression could lead to overwhelming sepsis. Recent pulmonary infarction (ie, within 6 to 8 weeks) is a contraindication because it could evolve into a necrotizing pneumonia or lung abscess with the initiation of immunosuppression. Active peptic ulcer disease is a contraindication because immunosuppressive therapy is likely to exacerbate gastrointestinal irritation and produce gastrointestinal bleeding.

Patients with diffuse, advanced peripheral or cerebral arterial occlusive disease usually are not suitable candidates for cardiac transplantation. Candidacy also is precluded in people with active substance abuse and in those with significant psychological disorders. Addiction to cigarettes, drugs, or alcohol is indicative of an inability to comply with the complex medical regimen that is essential after transplantation.

In critically ill patients who require continuous intravenous inotropic support or mechanical circulatory assistance, transplantation is likely to be life saving and the decision to proceed is relatively straightforward unless contraindications to transplantation are present. In patients with severe heart failure who do not require hospitalization, determination of suitability and precise timing for transplantation are more difficult. Severe heart failure is a complex clinical syndrome and identifying all patients at high risk for death during continued medical therapy is not yet possible (Young, 1999; Renlund, 1998).

One of the strongest predictors of outcome in patients with severe heart failure is patient response to medical therapy. Mortality is highest in patients with symptoms and hemodynamic abnormalities of severe heart failure that persist despite optimal medical therapy (Gronda et al., 1999). Cardiopulmonary stress testing also has become an important diagnostic modality for selection of potential transplantation candidates. It has gained widespread acceptance because VO_2 levels less than 15 mL/kg/min are associated with poor outcomes in patients with heart failure receiving maximized pharmacologic therapy (Beniaminovitz & Mancini, 1999; Young, 1999).

Patients in whom transplantation is considered undergo an extensive evaluation. Usually, coronary angiography and right heart catheterization will already have been performed in potential candidates, and those with DCM are likely to have undergone endomyocardial biopsy. If pulmonary hypertension is present, right heart catheterization may need to be repeated to determine if elevated pulmonary vascular resistance is reversible. Additional components of the transplantation evaluation usually include chest radiography, echocardiography, exercise testing with VO_2 measurement, hematologic and biochemical laboratory evaluation, a panel of infectious disease serologies, and a psychological profile. Selected patients may require abdominal ultrasound, carotid and lower extremity Doppler flow studies, esophagogastroduodenoscopy, or screening studies for malignancy (Fleischer & Baumgartner, 1997).

The decision to list a patient for cardiac transplantation is based on evaluation of all objective data, as well as the transplant physicians' subjective assessment of the patient's disease progression and anticipated prognosis. Once candidacy is determined, the transplant center registers the patient as a potential recipient with the United Network for Organ Sharing (UNOS), the organization responsible for maintaining a national computerized registry of candidates and for coordinating organ sharing among regional organ procurement organizations. Donor hearts are allocated based on ABO blood type compatibility, body size match between donor and recipient, length of time on the waiting list, and the status of medical urgency for the transplant (Table 31-3).

TABLE 31-3

United Network for Organ Sharing (UNOS) Status Grouping for Allocation of Donor Hearts

Status	Severity of Illness
1A	Candidate admitted to listing transplant center hospital with at least one of the following devices or therapies: • VAD implanted for ≤ 30 days, TAH, IABC, or ECMO* • Mechanical circulatory support for > 30 days and device-related complication* • Mechanical ventilation* • Continuous infusion of intravenous inotrope and continuous hemodynamic monitoring of left ventricular filling pressure† • Life expectancy < 7 days†
1B	Candidate with at least one of the following devices or therapies: • VAD implanted for > 30 days • Continuous infusion of intravenous inotropes
2	Candidate does not meet criteria for status 1A or 1B listing
7	Candidate is temporarily ineligible to receive transplant

VAD, ventricular assist device; TAH, total artificial heart; IABC, intra-aortic balloon counterpulsation; ECMO, extracorporeal membrane oxygenator.
*Must be recertified every 14 days.
†Valid for 7 days.
From UNOS, 1999: Amended UNOS Policy 3.7 (Allocation of Thoracic Organs), Effective August 16, 1999, Richard, VA.

Recipient Management

The commitment to undergo cardiac transplantation is a major undertaking that involves not only the recipient but the entire family support system. Implications for the pretransplantation waiting period and posttransplantation lifestyle are profound. Development of a close, supportive relationship between the transplant team and the candidate is essential. Extensive teaching and counseling are integral components of preparing the patient for transplantation and are initiated as soon as candidacy is considered.

The mean waiting period for a recipient is over 8 months, with more than one half of patients waiting longer than a year for a donor organ (Fleisher & Baumgartner, 1998). During the waiting period, therapeutic interventions are performed as indicated to maintain the patient's hemodynamic function, physical conditioning, and psychological status at an optimal level. Pharmacologic therapy (eg, afterload reducing, inotropic, and diuretic agents) is used to support hemodynamic function. Antiarrhythmic medications or implantation of an implantable cardioverter-defibrillator may become necessary in patients who are determined to be at high risk for sudden death from malignant ventricular arrhythmias. Sudden death is the most common cause of death in patients awaiting heart transplantation, especially during the first 3 months after referral for transplantation (Fleischer & Baumgartner, 1997). Anticoagulant therapy also is recommended to reduce the risk of pulmonary or systemic embolization arising from thrombus associated with atrial fibrillation, poorly contractile ventricles, or peripheral venous stasis.

Worsening heart failure may cause hemodynamic deterioration that manifests as significant azotemia, refractory sodium and water overload, persistent hypotension, altered mental status, or even gastrointestinal distress (Renlund, 1998). In many patients, intermittent or continued hospitalization is necessary to treat refractory heart failure with intravenous diuretic and inotropic agents and to provide mechanical circulatory support with intra-aortic balloon counterpulsation or a ventricular assist device. Intra-aortic balloon counterpulsation often is used initially for mechanical support, but it is designed for short-term use only and usually does not provide adequate support for patients with severe ventricular dysfunction. More often, mechanical support with a ventricular assist device becomes necessary as a "bridge to transplantation" when pharmacologic therapy alone is inadequate to sustain a patient until a donor heart becomes available.

Ventricular assist devices are used increasingly in patients awaiting transplantation because they can provide adequate hemodynamic support for periods much longer than the median waiting time, improve quality of life during the waiting period, and increase survival (Chillcott et al., 1998). Available long-term ventricular assist devices include the HeartMate Left Ventricular Assist System (LVAS; Thermo Cardiosystems, Inc., Woburn, MA) and the Novacor LVAS (Baxter Healthcare Corporation, Novacor Division, Oakland, CA) for left ventricular support, and the Thoratec Ventricular Assist Device (Thoratec Laboratories Corporation, Berkeley, CA) for either single or biventricular support. These devices restore hemodynamic stability, allow patient mobility and functional improvement (sometimes in the home), and seldom produce complications that prohibit successful transplantation. More than 75% of transplant candidates survive to transplantation after mechanical circulatory support, and survival after transplantation appears to be similar to or only slightly worse than that in patients without prior device use (Renlund, 1998). Ventricular assist devices are described in further detail in Chapter 30, Circulatory Assist Devices.

Because of the long waiting period for transplantation, recipients undergo periodic reassessment to determine if cardiac function has improved sufficiently to delay transplantation or if modifications in therapeutic interventions are necessary. A right heart catheterization is repeated every 3 to 6 months to ensure continued acceptable pulmonary vascular resistance (Renlund, 1998). Maximal oxygen consumption and left ventricular ejection fraction also are measured periodically. Panel-reactive antibodies (PRA) are measured intermittently during the waiting period and after any transfusion of blood; if blood transfusion is required, leukocyte-removing filters are used to minimize anti-human leukocyte antigen (HLA) antibody formation. Elevated PRA levels are associated with hyperacute rejection and graft failure.

Donor Selection and Management

The most significant limiting feature in cardiac transplantation is the inadequate number of donors compared with the number of patients waiting for transplantation. In the United States alone, an estimated 40,000 patients per year could benefit from heart transplantation, whereas less than 2500 patients receive donor hearts. The number of patients who are added to the waiting list each month is consistently higher than the number of patients who are transplanted. Consequently, waiting times for transplantation are long and there is a 25% mortality rate among patients waiting for transplantation (Kaplon et al., 1999). Because of the scarcity of acceptable donors, the mortality rate in most programs is higher among patients waiting for transplantation than in those undergoing the procedure.

Allocation of available donor hearts is complex and sometimes controversial. Although UNOS is the national network for organ procurement and allocation, individual transplant centers interact with regional organ procurement organizations that allocate donated organs based on criteria established by UNOS. Because of the limited ischemic times allowed for heart allografts (usually <4 hours), allocation is prioritized geographically, with preference to local recipients, or when no local recipients exist, to those within areas in succeeding 500-mile radii from the hospital where the donor is located.

Donors most often are young adults who die of closed-head trauma, penetrating head trauma, or intracerebral hemorrhage. Acceptance criteria for donors in general include age less than 65 years and no evidence of malignancy, septicemia, or antibodies to HIV, hepatitis B, or hepatitis C (Goldstein & Rose, 1998). A donor must have a compatible ABO blood type (Rh factor not important) and be of similar size and weight to the recipient. In general, donor weight should be at least 70% of recipient weight. An upper limit in donor size is less important unless the size discrepancy between donor and recipient is exceedingly large (Renlund, 1998). Blood, urine, and sputum cultures are obtained from the donor to ensure the absence of active infection. If the recipient has tested positive for anti-HLA antibodies (PRA ≥ 10% to 15%), a negative T-cell cross-match is mandatory before transplantation to avoid possible hyperacute rejection (Fleischer & Baumgartner, 1997).

Once initial eligibility for organ donation is ascertained, every effort is made to ensure that the potential donor has no underlying cardiac disease or injury that would preclude adequate cardiac function in the recipient after transplantation. Although some compromise based on clinical judgment often must be made, organs ideally are obtained from donors with no history of prior cardiac disease or prolonged cardiopulmonary resuscitation and no chest trauma (Baldwin, 1996). Indicators used to determine acceptable cardiac function include a normal electrocardiogram and adequate hemodynamic parameters without excessive doses of inotropic medications. An echocardiogram also is obtained to detect clinically unsuspected wall motion abnormalities, decreased ventricular function, or congenital defects. Because of the prevalence of coronary artery disease, coronary angiography is often performed in older donors (male donors >45 years and female donors >50 years).

Appropriate donor management before organ procurement is essential and must be directed at protecting all usable organs. Ideally, the lungs, kidneys, liver, and pancreas are procured in addition to the heart. Arterial and central venous pressure monitoring, as well as a urethral drainage catheter, are important to titrate therapy to preserve function of potential donor organs. Mechanical ventilation is maintained to support respiratory function and to ensure adequate blood oxygen saturation levels. Physiologic stability often is tenuous and of limited duration in a brain-dead donor. Volume replacement and vasopressor agents usually are required to manage the diabetes insipidus associated with severe neurologic injury. However, prolonged administration of large doses of vasopressors may be detrimental to myocardial function. The need for such agents also may reflect underlying ventricular dysfunction in the donor heart.

Organ procurement often is performed at a distant hospital and, almost always, the heart is only one of several organs procured. The various organs are used for multiple recipients and usually are procured by separate teams of transplant surgeons for use in different facilities. Another team is used for preparation of the transplant recipient to expedite the process and reduce allograft ischemic time.

Coordination of timing among the various procurement teams and between each of the procurement and recipient teams is essential. If organ procurement is well coordinated among the multiple transplant teams and the donor coordinator, a maximal number of recipients can benefit from each donor with excellent results.

Usually, the heart is procured through a median sternotomy incision. The donor heart is inspected carefully to assess contractile function and to detect the presence of a wall motion abnormality. After systemic anticoagulation with heparin, the superior vena cava is ligated and transected and the inferior vena cava is transected. The ascending aorta is cross-clamped and cardioplegic solution is administered into the coronary circulation. Cold saline solution is poured into the pericardial well surrounding the heart to facilitate rapid cooling. The donor heart is then excised by transecting the right and left pulmonary veins, aorta, and right and left pulmonary arteries (Fig. 31-2).

When cardiac function ceases in the donor after cardioplegic arrest, so does the supply of oxygenated blood to myocardial tissue. The heart remains without oxygen until circulation to coronary arteries is restored after implantation of the organ in the recipient. An ischemic time, defined as the time of aortic cross-clamping in the donor until release of the aortic cross-clamp in the recipient, of 4 hours in general is considered acceptable, although some risk is incurred with each hour of donor heart ischemia (Renlund, 1998). Therefore, the transplant procedure must be accomplished expediently. Cardioplegic arrest and immersion of the heart in cold saline (0°C to 7°C) provide topical hypothermia to protect the heart from damage during the ischemic time.

Transplantation Procedures

Over 95% of cardiac transplantations are orthotopic transplantations. In an orthotopic transplantation, the recipient's heart is removed and the donor heart is implanted in its place in normal anatomic position in the thorax. The operation performed through a median sternotomy incision. Cardiopulmonary bypass and hypothermia are used to maintain circulation, protect the brain, and oxygenate the recipient while the native heart is excised. Cardiopulmonary bypass usually is initiated after the donor allograft has been brought into the operating room unless the recipient is unstable.

In the standard technique for allograft implantation, the recipient heart is removed by transecting the aorta, pulmonary artery, and the right and left atria, leaving the posterior and lateral walls of the atria and the atrial septum intact. The allograft is implanted by anastomosing the donor left atrium, right atrium, pulmonary artery, and aorta to the recipient's arterial cuffs, pulmonary artery, and aorta (Fig. 31-3). When these anastomoses are completed, the surgeon performs

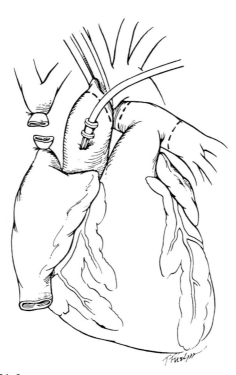

FIGURE 31-2. Donor cardiectomy. The superior vena cava and inferior vena cava have been transected. The pulmonary veins (on posterior surface of the heart) are not shown in this illustration. Dotted lines indicate standard incisions for transecting aorta and pulmonary arteries. (Fleischer KJ, Baumgartner WA, 1998: Transplantation: Heart. In Kaiser LR, Kron IL, Spray TL [eds]: Mastery of Cardiothoracic Surgery, p. 502. Philadelphia, Lippincott Williams & Wilkins)

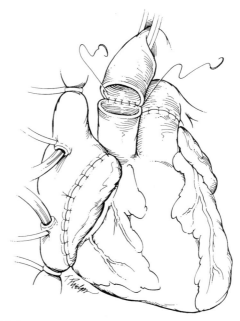

FIGURE 31-3. Orthotopic implantation of the cardiac allograft. The atrial and pulmonary artery anastomoses have been completed. The aortic anastomosis is being constructed. (Fleischer KJ, Baumgartner WA, 1998: Transplantation: Heart. In Kaiser LR, Kron IL, Spray TL [eds]: Mastery of Cardiothoracic Surgery, p. 506. Philadelphia, Lippincott Williams & Wilkins)

maneuvers to ensure that no air remains in the transplanted heart before removing the aortic cross-clamp. Suture lines are inspected to ensure hemostasis, the aortic cross-clamp is removed, and the heart is reperfused. Upon achieving a regular rhythm and good contractility, the patient is weaned from cardiopulmonary bypass and the cannulae are removed.

An alternative implantation technique for orthotopic cardiac transplantation substitutes superior and inferior vena caval anastomoses for the right atrial anastomosis described previously. When this technique is used, the recipient right atrium is excised leaving small cuffs around the superior and inferior venae cavae. Implantation of the donor heart is then performed with end-to-end anastomoses between recipient and donor superior and inferior venae cavae, as well as left atrial, pulmonary artery, and aortic anastomoses. Bicaval anastomoses better preserve donor atrial anatomy and may be associated with improved preservation of the atrial contribution to cardiac output, and, at least theoretically, a decreased incidence of left atrial thrombus formation. Whether this technique results in better overall heart function remains to be determined.

Rarely, heterotopic transplantation is performed. A heterotopic transplantation is one in which the recipient heart is left in place and the donor heart is inserted into the thorax adjacent to the native heart. The donor and recipient hearts are joined with anastomoses between the donor left atrium and recipient left atrium, donor right atrium and recipient right atrium, donor and recipient aortas, and donor and recipient pulmonary arteries. A

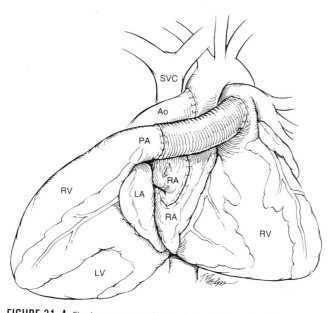

FIGURE 31-4. Final appearance of heterotopically transplanted heart. An interposition graft often is necessary for the pulmonary artery anastomosis to permit the allograft to reside in the right hemithorax. SVC, superior vena cava; Ao, aorta; PA, pulmonary artery; RV, right ventricle; LA, left atrium; RA, right atrium; LV, left ventricle. (Fleischer KJ, Baumgartner WA, 1998: Transplantation: Heart. In Kaiser LR, Kron IL, Spray TL [eds]: Mastery of Cardiothoracic Surgery, p. 509. Philadelphia, Lippincott Williams & Wilkins)

synthetic graft often is implanted between the native and donor pulmonary arteries (Fig. 31-4). Heterotopic transplantation may be indicated in selected situations when the donor heart is small in relation to the recipient or in the presence of severe pulmonary hypertension.

Postoperative Considerations

Early postoperative care of cardiac transplant recipients is similar to that for patients undergoing other types of cardiac surgery. Inotropic and vasodilating drugs are required frequently in the early postoperative hours to support cardiac function. Because the transplanted heart has no innervation from the autonomic nervous system, it does not receive direct sympathetic and parasympathetic stimulation. Thus, the transplanted heart is unresponsive to carotid sinus massage, Valsalva maneuver, or atropine; instead, it relies on circulating catecholamines for a positive chronotropic response to stresses, such as hypovolemia, hypoxia, or anemia (Fleischer & Baumgartner, 1997). Intravenous catecholamines, such as isoproterenol or dobutamine, often are necessary in the early period after transplantation to increase heart rate and support cardiac function.

Because of the serious consequences of infection in immunosuppressed patients, efforts are made to reduce those factors that increase the risk of infection. Most centers no longer practice rigorous protective isolation with positive-pressure air filtration systems, but instead rely primarily on proper handwashing regimens and the use of masks (Fleischer & Baumgartner, 1998). Recipients are segregated from potentially infectious patients. Intravenous and other invasive catheters typically are removed within 1 to 2 days in patients who are hemodynamically stable. Antibiotics are used sparingly to avoid overgrowth of more resistant bacteria. Patients often can be transferred out of the intensive care unit after 2 or 3 days and are ready for discharge from the hospital after 7 to 10 days.

One of the most important considerations in postoperative care is the immunosuppression regimen. Organ rejection remains a significant problem despite immunosuppression because of immunologic differences between donor and recipient hearts; immunosuppressive therapy is required for the remainder of the patient's life. A careful balance must be maintained between inadequate suppression of the patient's immunologic defense mechanisms with possible allograft rejection and death, and too much immunosuppression leading to potential overwhelming opportunistic infection or malignancy. Current immunosuppressive regimens do not completely prevent rejection but rather only prolong the life of the allograft (Young, 1999).

The basic strategy of immunosuppression after transplantation is early induction with intense immunosuppression followed by gradual reduction to long-term maintenance levels (Fleischer & Baumgartner, 1997). Because each of the immunosuppressive agents is associated with significant adverse effects, multiple agents are administered so that adequate immunosuppression can be achieved using low doses of individual agents. Although specific drug regimens vary significantly, most transplant centers use a prophylactic triple-drug regimen to suppress the body's immunologic defenses: either cyclosporine or tacrolimus, either azathioprine or mycophenolate mofetil, and corticosteroids. In some centers, an anti–T-cell agent (ie, antithymocyte globulin, antilymphocyte globulin, or monoclonal anti–T-cell antibodies) is also administered during the perioperative period.

Cyclosporine and the more recently introduced drug, tacrolimus, work early in the rejection cascade by restricting T-cell proliferation through limitation of calcium-dependent gene transcription factors (Griffith & Magee, 1996). Tacrolimus (formerly called FK506) is similar to cyclosporine not only in its mechanisms of actions but in its pharmacokinetic characteristics and adverse effects; potential advantages of tacrolimus may include the need for less corticosteroid therapy and shorter hospitalizations (Abrams, 1998). Many medications can affect serum levels of cyclosporine and tacrolimus, which must be measured frequently to avoid levels that are too low (with resultant rejection) or too high (with resultant toxicity).

Azathioprine works nonspecifically to inhibit lymphocyte proliferation and corticosteroids act at various levels by inhibiting the release of interleukin-1 and interleukin-6 from macrophages (Griffith & Magee, 1996). Mycophenolate mofetil is an inhibitor of the de novo pathway for purine biosynthesis. Its use in heart transplant recipients has increased, based on data demonstrating reduction in mortality and rejection in the first year after cardiac transplantation when mycophenolate is substituted for aziathioprine (Kobashigawa et al, 1998).

Immunosuppressive therapy can be associated with significant complications. Heart transplant recipients, like all immunosuppressed patients, are at increased risk for development of malignancies. Skin malignancies and lymphoma are most common. Primary complications associated with cyclosporine therapy are nephrotoxicity with resultant renal dysfunction and hypertension necessitating chronic antihypertensive therapy. In approximately 3% to 10% of cardiac transplant recipients, end-stage renal failure develops and requires dialysis or renal transplantation, and 50% to 90% of patients have moderate to severe systemic hypertension (Fleischer & Baumgartner, 1998). Corticosteroids can lead to infection, hyperlipidemia, hypertension, osteoporosis, and diabetes. Chronic steroid therapy also increases the risk of peptic ulcer disease and erosive gastritis because it increases the secretion of hydrochloric acid and pepsinogen (Hudak et al., 1998).

Mortality and Morbidity

Operative mortality rates for patients undergoing cardiac transplantation have remained stable in the late 1990s despite expansion of indications to include higher-risk patients (eg, those on ventricular assist devices or with associated medical illnesses). Early operative mortality rates (< 30 days) range from 5% to 10%. Most deaths during the first month after transplantation are due to acute rejection, nonspecific graft failure, or multisystem organ failure (Hunt & Frazier, 1998).

The current 1-year survival rate after cardiac transplantation is 79%, and there is a constant mortality rate of 4% per year from years 1 through 15; the patient half-life, or time until 50% of patients are still surviving, is 8.8 years (Hosenpud et al., 1999). Survival prognosis is lower in older patients, and the cohort of patients who are older than 65 years has a significantly reduced survival probability (Hunt & Frazier, 1998). Most patients return to a New York Heart Association class I functional status with no limitations in activities.

The three major types of morbidity associated with heart transplantation are rejection, infection, and coronary artery vasculopathy. Acute rejection and infection are the primary causes of death during the first year after transplantation. *Hyperacute rejection* is a rejection episode that occurs almost immediately after reperfusion of the transplanted heart because of preformed, donor-specific antibodies in the recipient. Its occurrence has been reduced greatly by preoperative screening for alloreactive antibodies and prospective, donor-specific cross-matching in sensitized recipients (Joseph et al., 1999). Although hyperacute rejection occurs rarely, it usually is so severe that retransplantation is necessary to achieve patient survival.

The more common form of rejection (ie, *acute rejection*) has become less prevalent with the addition of cyclosporine to the immunosuppressive regimen. Still, approximately 55% of patients have an episode of rejection during the first year, and 80% of these episodes occur during the first 3 months after transplantation (Goldstein & Rose, 1998). Rejection occurring early after transplantation tends to be more fulminant and life threatening than late-occurring rejection (Renlund, 1998). Serial transvenous endomyocardial biopsies are performed to monitor for evidence of rejection and to assess adequacy of the immunosuppressive regimen. These biopsy specimens, obtained from the right ventricular endomyocardium during right-sided heart catheterization, provide a very accurate method of diagnosing cellular rejection.

Rejection often is asymptomatic, but subtle signs and symptoms may be present, including decreased cardiac output, atrial flutter or fibrillation, elevated white blood count, and low-grade fever (Hudak et al., 1998). An increased dosage of oral or intravenous steroids usually is effective in treating asymptomatic or mild rejection. Anti–T-cell therapy is administered for rejection episodes that recur, are refractory to corticosteroid therapy, or are associated with hemodynamic compromise. Although most rejection episodes can be managed with corticosteroid therapy alone, rejection remains a major cause of mortality for transplant recipients.

Infection is the other major cause of death in transplant recipients during the first postoperative year and remains a potential risk thereafter. The risk of infection is highest during the first year because the frequency of rejection, and thus degree of immunosuppression, is highest during the early period after transplantation. Most infections result from opportunistic bacterial, viral, or fungal organisms in the individual or environment. Opportunistic pathogens, such as herpes simplex and herpes zoster virus, cytomegalovirus (CMV), *Candida albicans,* and *Aspergillus fumigatus,* usually are harmless but pose serious threats to patients with compromised immune systems (Hudak et al., 1998). Bacterial and viral infections account for more than 80% of infections after cardiac transplantation; fungi and protozoa, although causing less than 15% of infections after transplantation, can be associated with the worst prognosis (Renlund, 1998).

Because of the prevalence of infectious complications, cardiac transplant recipients receive antibiotic prophylaxis against bacterial infection (eg, vancomycin and aztreonam in the perioperative period), viral infection (annual influenza A and B vaccines and perioperative CMV prophylaxis), protozoal infection (daily trimethoprimsulfamethoxazole during the first year), and fungal infection (daily nystatin for 3 months) (Goldstein & Rose, 1998). Mortality caused by infectious complications accounts for 15% of early and 40% of late deaths in cardiac transplant recipients (Fleischer & Baumgartner, 1998).

After the first year, *coronary allograft vasculopathy* becomes the leading cause of death in transplant recipients. All solid-organ grafts are prone to chronic rejection, and coronary allograft vasculopathy is analogous to bronchiolitis obliterans in lung grafts and chronic rejection in renal allografts (Hunt & Frazier, 1998). The development of allograft vasculopathy in the transplanted heart is the major factor limiting long-term survival. It affects recipients of all ages, including children (Miller & Miller, 1999).

Coronary angiographic studies demonstrate the presence of allograft vasculopathy in as many as 40% to 50% of cardiac transplant recipients within 5 years of transplantation (Allen-Auerbach et al., 1999). Although several postoperative risk factors have been implicated, including CMV infection, hypercholesterolemia, immunosuppressive therapy, and histocompatibility mismatch, the pathogenesis of coronary artery disease in the transplanted heart remains incompletely defined (Labarrere, 1999). A number of features unique to allograft coronary vasculopathy distinguish it from conventional, atherosclerotic coronary artery disease. These include concentric rather than eccentric involvement of the arterial wall, diffuse involvement along the entire length of the vessel rather than focal or segmental disease, development within months to years rather than decades, and occurrence in young recipients or in hearts from young donors (Miller & Miller, 1999).

Detection of early disease development while patients are asymptomatic is thought to be important in preventing irreversible damage to the transplanted heart. The diagnosis of coronary artery vasculopathy still is based primarily on coronary angiography. However, surveillance coronary angiography is not very sensitive because allograft arteriopathy is a more diffuse and concentric process, and the disease usually is well advanced by the time vasculopathy manifests as ischemia on functional studies (Young, 1999; Kapadia et al., 1999). Intravascular ultrasound of coronary arteries is used as an adjunct to post-transplantation conventional coronary angiography to monitor the develop-

ment of transplant vasculopathy. Although its use is restricted to major epicardial vessels, it is the most sensitive invasive tool for diagnosis.

Treatment of coronary artery disease in a transplanted heart is complicated by two factors. First, the vasculopathy affecting transplanted hearts tends to be more diffuse and less amenable to conventional revascularization (ie, percutaneous coronary intervention or coronary artery bypass grafting). Second, allograft vasculopathy usually is a clinically silent disease process. Because the transplanted heart is denervated, most patients do not experience angina. The problem may become evident only after myocardial infarction and substantial irreversible damage have occurred, producing congestive heart failure, arrhythmias, or sudden death. The outlook for patients with advanced allograft vasculopathy is poor and retransplantation remains the most definitive treatment (Goldstein & Rose, 1998).

Cardiac retransplantation is performed infrequently. The primary indications are (1) early primary failure of the allograft resulting from preservation, technical, or immunologic problems; (2) intractable or recurrent acute rejection; and (3) coronary allograft vasculopathy (McCurry et al., 1999). In patients with primary graft failure or intractable rejection, the survival rate for repeat transplantation is significantly worse than that associated with primary transplantation. In carefully selected patients with coronary allograft vasculopathy, the survival outcome after retransplantation is comparable with that of primary transplantation. Significant risk factors for death after cardiac retransplantation include an initial diagnosis of ischemic cardiomyopathy and a shorter interval between transplantations (John et al., 1999).

The question of whether donor hearts should be used preferentially for first-time transplantation or for retransplantation raises difficult ethical issues. The decision for retransplantation continues to be made selectively on an individual patient basis. In view of the severely limited donor organ supply in relation to demand, the issues associated with cardiac retransplantation are likely to become increasingly complex as the number of long-term survivors of cardiac transplantation continues to increase.

▶ Lung Transplantation

Lung transplantation has become an increasingly important therapeutic option for treatment of end-stage pulmonary disease. It offers the potential for prolonged survival and improved quality of life in patients with otherwise terminal disease. Improved donor and recipient selection and lung preservation techniques, superior immunosuppression protocols, and newer antibiotic regimens have improved results dramatically (Sundaresan & Patterson, 1996; Patterson & Cooper, 1995). Nevertheless, lung transplantation continues to be associated with significant morbidity and mortality and is reserved for patients who have a limited life expectancy with other forms of therapy.

Development of Lung Transplantation

The first human lung transplantation was performed by James Hardy in 1963 (Hardy et al., 1963). As with cardiac transplantation, long-term patient survival was not achieved despite technical accomplishment of the operation. The current era of successful lung transplantation began in 1983 when Joel Cooper and associates performed successful single-lung transplantation for a patient with pulmonary fibrosis; the patient survived 6 years before succumbing to complications of renal failure (Toronto Lung Transplant Group, 1986; Sundaresan & Patterson, 1996).

Initial clinical success with single-lung transplantation was achieved in patients with restrictive lung disease, most commonly pulmonary fibrosis. Cooper and associates demonstrated that replacing one of the diseased lungs dramatically improves pulmonary function in patients with restrictive lung disease because the poor compliance and increased vascular resistance in the remaining native lung cause the transplanted lung to be preferentially ventilated and perfused.

Single-lung transplantation initially was not considered applicable for the more common obstructive form of pulmonary disease. In the early experience with lung transplantation, single-lung transplantation for obstructive disease often resulted in preferential ventilation of the native lung, with resultant mediastinal shift toward and crowding of the transplanted lung, and ventilation-perfusion mismatching. Consequently, double-lung transplantation was developed to provide a treatment alternative for patients with obstructive lung disease.

Cooper and associates performed the first double-lung transplantation for obstructive lung disease in 1986 (Cooper et al., 1989). However, early double-lung transplantation procedures were associated with considerable morbidity. Airway problems related to the tracheal anastomosis (eg, dehiscence and stenosis) were common late sequelae. To avoid these complications, the operative technique was modified to include bilateral bronchial anastomoses instead of a single tracheal anastomosis. In 1990, a bilateral sequential technique was developed and reported with excellent results (Bavaria et al., 1997).

With increased clinical experience, single-lung transplantation proved successful in patients with obstructive as well as restrictive pulmonary disease (Marinelli et al., 1992). Oversizing the donor to the recipient and careful graft preservation to minimize reperfusion injury prevented hyperinflation of the native lung, crowding of the transplant lung, and the ventilation-perfusion imbalance noted in the early single-lung transplants for obstructive disease (Sundaresan & Patterson, 1996).

Indications for Transplantation

Lung transplantation is indicated for several forms of end-stage pulmonary diseases, broadly categorized in Table 31-4. Although indications for single-lung and bi-

---

TABLE 31-4

Pulmonary Diseases Treated With Lung Transplantation

OBSTRUCTIVE PULMONARY DISEASE (EMPHYSEMA)
Chronic obstructive pulmonary disease
Alpha$_1$-antitrypsin deficiency emphysema

RESTRICTIVE PULMONARY DISEASE
Idiopathic pulmonary fibrosis

SEPTIC PULMONARY DISEASE
Cystic fibrosis

PULMONARY VASCULAR DISEASE
Primary pulmonary hypertension
Eisenmenger's syndrome

Adapted from Sundaresan RS, Patterson GA, 1996: Lung transplantation. In Baue AE, Geha AS, Hammond GL, et al. (eds): Glenn's Thoracic and Cardiovascular Surgery, ed. 6. Stamford, CT, Appleton & Lange.

---

lateral lung transplantation overlap considerably, each of the procedures is best suited to particular types of pulmonary and pulmonary vascular diseases. Emphysema is the most common indication for single-lung transplantation, accounting for 45% of procedures, and cystic fibrosis is the most common indication for bilateral lung transplantation, comprising 33% of procedures (Fig. 31-5) (Hosenpud et al., 1999). Other indications for single- or bilateral lung transplantation include idiopathic pulmonary fibrosis, alpha$_1$-antitrypsin deficiency, and primary pulmonary hypertension.

Chronic obstructive pulmonary disease and alpha$_1$-antitrypsin deficiency are forms of emphysema, or obstructive pulmonary disease. *Emphysema* is the fifth leading cause of death in North America and the most common indication for lung transplantation worldwide (Waddell & Keshavjee, 1998). It is characterized by a chronic elevation in airway resistance, with a decrease in expiratory flow rates (forced expiratory volume in 1 second [FEV_1], forced vital capacity [FVC], and FEV_1 : FVC ratio) and air trapping (increased total lung capacity) (Sundaresan & Patterson, 1996). *Alpha$_1$-antitrypsin deficiency* is a congenital subtype of emphysema characterized by development of severe bullous emphysema in the fourth or fifth decade of life.

Clinical manifestations of end-stage emphysema include dyspnea, orthopnea, hypoxemia, and hypercarbia. Although emphysema is quite debilitating, associated mortality may be less than with other forms of end-stage pulmonary disease, especially in young patients (Hosenpud et al., 1998). Patients with obstructive pulmonary disease and an FEV_1 of 25% to 30% of the predicted normal value have a 60% to 70% survival rate at 3 years (Trulock, 1997). The decision making surrounding transplantation for emphysema also is affected by availability of lung volume reduction surgery as an alternative therapy. Lung volume reduction is an effective procedure for

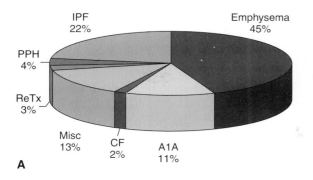

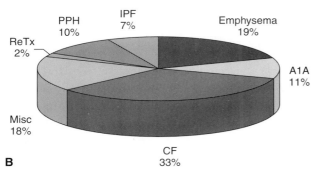

FIGURE 31-5. Indications for (**A**) single-lung transplantation and (**B**) bilateral/double lung transplantation in adults. IPF, idiopathic pulmonary fibrosis; PPH, primary pulmonary hypertension; ReTx, retransplantation; Misc, miscellaneous; CF, cystic fibrosis; A1A, alpha₁-antitrypsin deficiency.

the relief of dyspnea in selected patients with advanced emphysema and may obviate or delay lung transplantation (Sundaresan et al., 1996). Thus, lung transplantation for advanced emphysema is recommended in patients who are ideal transplantation candidates with no other therapeutic options.

Idiopathic pulmonary fibrosis is the most common type of interstitial pulmonary disease in patients considered for lung transplantation. The disease is characterized by excessive interstitial deposition of collagen, resulting in a significant loss of pulmonary compliance; diminished lung volumes and expiratory flow rates; and a reduction in diffusing capacity (Sundaresan & Patterson, 1996). Median survival usually is less than 5 years from the time of diagnosis. Clinical manifestations of pulmonary fibrosis include dyspnea requiring supplemental oxygen, digital clubbing, and eventual pulmonary hypertension.

Lung transplantation is considered for patients who fail to respond to medical treatment, with worsening exercise-induced desaturation, resting hypoxia, and a sustained downward trend in vital capacity (Trulock, 1997). Patients with pulmonary fibrosis who have deteriorated to the point of requiring consideration for lung transplantation usually have a rapid downhill course and do not survive a lengthy wait for a suitable donor organ (Patterson & Cooper, 1995). This group of pa-

tients has the highest mortality rate among those waiting for lung transplantation.

Cystic fibrosis is the most common cause of end-stage obstructive lung disease in the first three decades of life. It is an inherited disease characterized by excessive thick, viscid secretions and poor ciliary clearance with resultant mucous plugging and chronic pulmonary sepsis (Sundaresan & Patterson, 1996). A pattern of recurrent pulmonary infections may begin early in life and eventually results in airway destruction and impaired gas exchange; eventual colonization with *Pseudomonas* species, hemoptysis, and recurrent pneumothorax secondary to bronchiectasis are relatively common pulmonary sequelae (Mendeloff, 1998).

Patients with cystic fibrosis tend to be small, malnourished, and hypoxemic; display digital clubbing; have copious pulmonary secretions; and often have undergone thoracic operations for complications of the disease, such as pneumothorax or hemoptysis (Sundaresan & Patterson, 1996). More than 90% of patients with cystic fibrosis die of chronic suppurative, obstructive lung disease, with the median survival in the United States being 29 years of age (Mendeloff, 1998).

Lung transplantation is a final therapeutic option to restore patients with advanced cystic fibrosis to a nearly normal state of health. At present, it is the only definitive treatment for patients with advanced disease (Zuckerman & Kotloff, 1998). Longitudinal studies suggest that patients with an FEV_1 less than 30% of the normal predicted value have a 2-year mortality rate exceeding 50%; hypoxemia (PO_2 <55 mm Hg) and hypercapnia (PCO_2 >50 mm Hg) also portend a high mortality rate within 2 years (Rubin, 1999; Trulock, 1997). Because of the bleak natural history of the disease, patients with cystic fibrosis derive the clearest survival benefit from lung transplantation (Hosenpud et al., 1998).

Primary pulmonary hypertension is the most common form of pulmonary vascular disease leading to lung transplantation. It is an idiopathic process affecting small pulmonary arteries, causing luminal obliteration and a sustained elevation in pulmonary vascular resistance and right ventricular afterload; the disease most often affects young people, and particularly women (Sundaresan & Patterson, 1996). The natural history of primary pulmonary hypertension is somewhat variable, but in general carries a poor prognosis; the 1-year survival rate from the time of diagnosis is 68%, and median survival is 2.8 years (Sundaresan, 1998a).

Whereas lung transplantation formerly was the only therapeutic option to achieve long-term survival in patients with primary pulmonary hypertension, therapeutic advances, including warfarin anticoagulation, calcium channel blocking therapy, and chronic prostacyclin, have improved survival and functional status with medical management (Rich & McLaughlin, 1998). Transplantation is recommended in those patients in whom right ventricular failure develops despite optimal medical therapy.

Single- versus Bilateral Lung Transplantation

The decision to recommend single- or bilateral lung transplantation is based partially on the anticipated effect of leaving native lung behind. A single-lung transplant is acceptable for many patients with chronic obstructive pulmonary disease and for most patients with pulmonary fibrosis but is undesirable for patients with end-stage infectious lung disease (Egan & Detterbeck, 1998).

Single-lung transplantation is the most commonly performed type of lung transplantation. It is well suited for patients with idiopathic pulmonary fibrosis. The diminished compliance and elevated pulmonary vascular resistance in the native lung allow preferential ventilation and perfusion of the allograft. Single-lung transplantation is technically easier than bilateral lung transplantation, allows two recipients to benefit from a single donor, and has been used successfully in patients with all types of lung disease except cystic fibrosis and bronchiectasis (Arcasoy & Kotloff, 1999).

Either single- or bilateral lung transplantation may be performed for obstructive lung disease, including emphysema and alpha$_1$-antitrypsin deficiency (Meyers & Patterson, 1998). Whether single- or bilateral lung transplantation is preferable remains somewhat controversial. Single-lung transplantation is a technically simpler operation and therefore is well suited to minimize potential perioperative morbidity in older patients at higher risk for complications; it also is preferable for patients with a smaller body habitus (Sundaresan et al., 1996). The scarcity of donor organs also favors the use of single-lung transplantation to allow the second donor lung to be used for a second recipient.

Bilateral lung transplantation may be preferable for younger candidates (eg, <55 years) because it is associated with improved postoperative pulmonary function and exercise tolerance, and in those with a larger body habitus (Bavaria et al., 1997; Sundaresan et al., 1996). Both single- and bilateral lung transplantation appear to offer satisfactory transplantation options in patients with emphysema. The choice should be individualized to the patient, based on patient age, body habitus, and relevant clinical factors.

Bilateral lung transplantation is necessary for patients with cystic fibrosis and other forms of bronchiectasis that necessitate removal of both infected lungs (Arcasoy & Kotloff, 1999). Single-lung transplantation is not appropriate in septic pulmonary diseases because the native, diseased lung would provide a continued source for infection of the lung allograft, particularly because of the immunosuppressive therapy necessary after transplantation.

Either single- or bilateral lung transplantation may be performed for patients with irreversible pulmonary hypertension. Both have been demonstrated to provide suitable transplantation alternatives. Bilateral lung transplantation is associated with a slightly higher perioperative risk, but long-term outcomes for single- and bilateral lung transplantation appear equivalent and the use of a single lung permits greater utility of cadaveric organs (McCurry & Keenan, 1998).

Recipient Selection and Management

Patients considered for lung transplantation must demonstrate progressive lung disease, as evidenced by decreased exercise tolerance or deteriorating pulmonary function studies. The transplant surgeon and pulmonologist base the decision to recommend transplantation on a number of factors, including natural history and prognosis of the underlying disease, patient response to medical therapy, trend in clinical status over time, objective measurements of pulmonary function, and the degree of disability.

Lung transplantation is most appropriate when pulmonary or pulmonary vascular disease has advanced to the point that transplantation offers a better prognosis than medical therapy. However, it must be considered early enough so that the patient can survive the long waiting period for a donor organ and undergo the operation with an acceptable mortality risk. As waiting time for donor organs has increased, patients with end-stage lung disease are being listed earlier. Still, the number of patients in the United States who die while on the waiting list for a donor lung continues to increase (Egan & Detterbeck, 1998). Because of the average waiting time of up to 2 years, transplantation should be considered early enough so that survival with relatively stable pulmonary function during this period can be anticipated. Typical criteria for lung transplantation candidacy are given in Table 31-5.

Contraindications to candidacy for lung transplantation include dysfunction of major organs other than the lung (particularly renal failure), infection with HIV, active malignancy within the past 2 years, hepatitis B antigen positivity, and hepatitis C with biopsy-proven histologic evidence of liver disease (Maurer et al., 1998). Ventilator dependence is a relative contraindication to lung transplantation because of the demonstrated higher

---

TABLE 31-5

Recipient Criteria for Lung Transplantation

ACCEPTANCE CRITERIA

End-stage pulmonary disease unresponsive to other forms of therapy
Adequate cardiac function without significant coronary artery disease
Estimated life expectancy between 1 and 2 years
Ambulatory with potential for rehabilitation
Adequate nutritional status
Stable psychological status and family support system
Ability to adhere to complex medical regimen

EXCLUSION CRITERIA

Active infection
Malignancy
Acute illness
Renal, hepatic, or cardiac failure
Substance abuse (cigarettes, alcohol, drugs)
Psychological instability

mortality rate after transplantation. Many, if not most, transplant centers exclude those patients referred for lung transplantation evaluation who are receiving mechanical ventilation (O'Brien & Criner, 1999). However, patients accepted for transplantation sometimes require mechanical ventilation during the waiting period because of respiratory failure, and successful transplantation has been performed in several such patients (Low et al., 1992).

Because older patients have a significantly worse survival prognosis after transplantation, it is recommended that single-lung transplantation be restricted to candidates younger than 65 years of age, bilateral lung transplantation to those younger than 60 years, and heart-lung transplantation to those younger than 55 years (Maurer et al., 1998). Many patients with end-stage pulmonary disease are treated with corticosteroid therapy and are unable to tolerate weaning without clinical deterioration. Although formerly considered a contraindication to lung transplantation, low-dose corticosteroid therapy no longer precludes consideration for transplantation. Available data suggest that low-dose prednisone does not increase the risk of airway complications and actually may enhance early bronchial circulation in the allograft (Sundaresan & Patterson, 1996). Prior thoracic surgery, pleurodesis, or pleurectomy do not necessarily preclude transplantation, although they increase technical difficulty of extracting the native lung and the operative risk of the transplantation procedure (Trulock, 1997).

As with cardiac transplantation candidates, potential candidates for lung transplantation undergo a series of diagnostic studies. These include pulmonary function testing, chest radiograph, electrocardiogram, hematologic and biochemical laboratory studies, exercise testing, and nutritional and psychosocial evaluations. Depending on the assessed risk for coronary artery or other cardiovascular disease, cardiovascular studies may include stress echocardiography, radionuclide ventriculography, or coronary angiography. High-resolution computed tomography of the thorax is performed in patients with parenchymal disease, pleural disease, or previous thoracic surgical procedures (Maurer et al., 1998). Patients with emphysema, pulmonary fibrosis, or septic lung disease participate in a rigorous cardiopulmonary rehabilitation program during the waiting period to increase strength and exercise tolerance; patients with pulmonary hypertension are not enrolled in rehabilitation because they have an increased risk of sudden death during exercise (Sundaresan & Patterson, 1996).

Donor Selection and Management

As with other forms of solid-organ transplantation, lung transplantation is limited primarily by the lack of suitable donor lungs. Despite the continued growth of the candidate pool, the availability of suitable donor lungs has remained relatively fixed at a level increasingly insufficient to meet demand (Arcasoy & Kotloff, 1999). Currently, there are between 5000 and 6000 cadaveric

organ donors annually in the United States. Lung recovery is possible only in approximately 20% of these donors because of susceptibility of the lungs to trauma, aspiration, and infection (Waddell & Keshavjee, 1998). Because of this, the annual lung transplantation rate has reached a plateau, median recipient waiting time has doubled to approximately 18 months, and an increasing number of candidates die while waiting for transplantation (Arcasoy & Kotloff, 1999; Maurer et al., 1998).

Donor lungs are allocated according to ABO blood type compatibility and the candidate's length of time on the UNOS waiting list. Patients waiting for single- and bilateral lung transplantation are grouped together for allocation purposes. If a patient eligible to receive a donor organ needs only a single lung, the other donor lung is allocated to another patient waiting for a single lung. Unlike heart transplantation, no priority is given for severity of illness or clinical status. However, patients with a diagnosis of pulmonary fibrosis are assigned 90 days of waiting time when listed for transplantation because of their known high mortality rate while waiting for transplantation.

Evaluation of a potential donor includes examination of the chest radiograph, assessment of gas exchange and compliance, bronchoscopy, and visual inspection of both lungs at the time of procurement with palpation for masses or evidence of pneumonia or major contusion (Egan & Detterbeck, 1998). Current criteria for acceptable donor lungs include a normal chest radiograph; a less than 20-pack/year history of cigarette smoking, absence of purulent secretions or evidence of gross aspiration at bronchoscopy, and a PO_2 greater than 300 mm Hg while receiving 100% FIO_2 with 5-cm positive end-expiratory pressure (Waddell & Keshavjee, 1998).

After removal of the heart from the donor, the two lungs are extracted and transported en bloc (as a unit); if the lungs are to be used for recipients at different centers, they are separated after extraction. Preservation of the lung allograft typically is achieved by bolus administration of prostaglandin E_1 before inflow occlusion and cross-clamp application, pulmonary artery flush with a preservation solution (eg, cold Euro-Collins solution) extraction of the lungs semi-inflated with 100% oxygen, transportation of the grafts under hypothermic conditions, and protection during implantation with ice slush topical cooling (Sundaresan & Patterson, 1996).

Transplantation Procedures

As with cardiac transplantation, the recipient is taken to the operating room and prepared for implantation of the lung allograft concomitantly with procurement of the donor organ. An epidural catheter usually is inserted before anesthesia induction for postoperative pain management, except in patients who require cardiopulmonary bypass with systemic anticoagulation. The use of cardiopulmonary bypass has decreased dramatically since the early days of lung transplantation (Meyers & Patterson, 1998). Cardiopulmonary bypass almost never is required for single-lung transplantation for emphysema, but is used frequently during transplantation for pulmonary vascular disease. It occasionally is necessary when single-lung transplantation is performed for idiopathic pulmonary fibrosis, particularly if secondary pulmonary hypertension is present (Sundaresan & Patterson, 1996).

Single-lung transplantation is performed through a posterolateral thoracotomy incision using single-lung ventilation. The native lung is excised and the donor lung implanted with bronchial, pulmonary artery, and left atrial (containing the pulmonary vein orifices) anastomoses. Bilateral lung transplantation is performed through a transverse thoracosternotomy, and the lungs are implanted separately and sequentially (Fig. 31-6). The thoracosternotomy incision provides ready access to both hilar regions and allows improved exposure for disrupting adhesions (Mendeloff, 1998). The most damaged lung is excised first, with single-lung ventilation to the contralateral lung while the first donor lung is implanted. When airway and vascular anastomoses have been completed, the newly implanted lung is ventilated while the other native lung is removed and the second donor lung implanted.

A technique has been developed more recently for *transplantation of pulmonary lobes from living donors.* The procedure, which has been performed almost exclusively in patients with cystic fibrosis, involves implanting lower lobes from two blood group–compatible living donors (Arcasoy & Kotloff, 1999). This approach has been advocated when the patient's prognosis is poor and there is little probability of obtaining cadaveric donor organs; however, it is not recommended for patients in extremis (Trulock, 1997).

Mortality and Morbidity

The operative mortality rate for lung transplantation is less than 10% in most experienced centers (Patterson, 1998). One-year and five-year actuarial survival after lung transplantation is 71% and 43%, respectively, with a median survival of 3.7 years (Arcasoy & Kotloff, 1999). Independent predictors of adverse outcome after lung transplantation include preoperative ventilator support, retransplantation, diagnosis other than emphysema, and older recipient age (Hosenpud et al., 1999).

As with heart transplant recipients, triple-drug immunosuppressive therapy typically is administered. Standard regimens consist of cyclosporine or tacrolimus, azathioprine or mycophenolate, and prednisone (Arcasoy & Kotloff, 1999). *Acute rejection* occurs during the early postoperative period in nearly all lung transplant recipients. It has a typical presentation of dyspnea, low-grade fever, perihilar infiltrate, hypoxia, and increased white blood count (Patterson & Cooper, 1995). Acute rejection usually can be managed effectively with an increased dosage of steroids. Anti–T-cell therapy may be required for more persistent rejection episodes. Refractory or recurrent acute rejection also may prompt conversion from cyclosporine to tacrolimus (Mentzer et al, 1998; Garrity et al., 1999).

The rate of death is highest in the year after transplantation, with infection and primary graft failure representing the leading causes of early death (Arcasoy & Kotloff, 1999). *Infectious complications,* particularly pneumonia, are prevalent. Bacterial pathogens are the greatest threat in the perioperative period, but fungal infection with *Candida* or *Aspergillus* species or viral in-

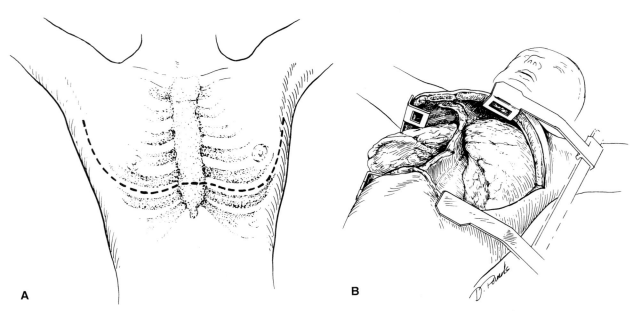

FIGURE 31-6. (A) Skin incision for bilateral lung transplantation using a "clamshell" or bilateral thoracosternotomy incision. **(B)** The incision offers excellent exposure of both pleural spaces as well as exposure of the pericardial sac and its contents. (Egan TM, Detterbeck FC, 1998: Technique of lung transplantation. In Kaiser LR, Kron IL, Spray TL [eds]: Mastery of Cardiothoracic Surgery, p. 174. Philadelphia, Lippincott Williams & Wilkins)

fection with herpes or CMV also can occur (Trulock, 1997). The rate of infection is several times higher than among recipients of other organs and most likely is related to exposure of the allograft to the external environment (Arcasoy & Kotloff, 1999). *Graft dysfunction*, characterized by pulmonary infiltrates, poor oxygenation, and a histologic pattern of diffuse alveolar damage or organizing pneumonia, can range in clinical severity from a very mild lung injury to adult respiratory distress syndrome (Trulock, 1997).

The most significant long-term complication after lung transplantation is chronic allograft dysfunction, thought to be synonymous with chronic rejection. This so-called *bronchiolitis obliterans syndrome* is characterized clinically by a progressive deterioration in pulmonary function with or without pathologic evidence of obliterative bronchiolitis (Kroshus et al., 1997). The pathogenesis of the allograft dysfunction is unclear, but, as previously mentioned, it is analogous to chronic rejection observed with other solid-organ transplants. It remains the major cause of death and disability in long-term survivors and the most challenging limitation of lung transplantation.

Development of bronchiolitis obliterans appears to be inevitable in all lung transplant recipients who survive long enough. It affects more than 50% of patients late after transplantation and accounts for 57% of deaths after the first year (Hosenpud et al., 1998). Bronchiolitis obliterans frequently does not respond to medical treatment and the resulting fibrosis, once established, is irreversible and usually fatal (Smith et al., 1998). Although specific symptoms are lacking, patients typically experience worsening respiratory debilitation, with the characteristic physiologic hallmark being airflow limitation as evidenced by progressive decline in several spirometric parameters (Sundaresan, 1998b).

With the increasing number of lung transplant recipients and improved survival, the issue of retransplantation is emerging and may be considered in selected patients. The best intermediate-term functional results have been achieved in patients receiving retransplantation in transplant centers with more experience, in nonventilated patients, and in patients who undergo retransplantation more than 2 years after the primary transplantation (Novick & Stitt, 1998).

▶ Heart-Lung Transplantation

Heart-lung transplantation is performed most often for congenital heart disease, pulmonary hypertension, or cystic fibrosis (Hosenpud et al., 1999) (Fig. 31-7). The number of heart-lung transplantations appears to be decreasing as applicability of single- and bilateral lung transplantation has broadened to include more forms of pulmonary and pulmonary vascular disease. Heart-lung transplantation, first performed in 1981 by Bruce Reitz and associates, initially was considered the most appropriate form of transplantation for pulmonary or cardiac diseases associated with irreversible pulmonary hyperten-

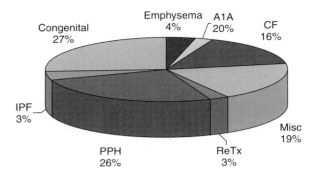

FIGURE 31-7. Indications for heart-lung transplantation in adults. IPF, idiopathic pulmonary fibrosis; PPH, primary pulmonary hypertension; ReTx, retransplantation; Misc, miscellaneous; CF, cystic fibrosis; A1A, alpha$_1$-antitrypsin deficiency.

sion (Reitz et al., 1982). Since then, single- and bilateral lung transplantation have been shown to be associated with hemodynamic improvement and right ventricular functional recovery in most patients with pulmonary hypertension.

Potential recipients for heart-lung transplantation are those with progressively disabling cardiopulmonary or pulmonary disease who possess the capacity for full rehabilitation after transplantation (Yuh et al., 1997). Indications overlap considerably for bilateral lung and heart-lung transplantation and the choice of procedure varies regionally. Although heart-lung transplantation still accounts for approximately one third of total heart-lung and bilateral lung transplants in the Eastern Hemisphere (predominantly Europe), it represents only 10% of Western Hemisphere (predominantly North America) procedures (Hosenpud et al., 1999). Given the paucity of donor organs, the role of heart-lung transplantation for pulmonary hypertension in the United States has become limited to patients with associated coronary artery disease; significant left ventricular dysfunction; or complex, uncorrectable congenital heart defects (Trulock, 1997).

Candidates waiting for heart-lung transplantation are registered on the UNOS waiting list for each organ. If the patient first becomes eligible to receive a heart, the lungs are allocated from the same donor; if the patient first becomes eligible to receive lungs, the heart from the same donor is allocated only if no suitable status IA isolated heart candidate is eligible to receive the heart (UNOS, 1999). The donor heart and lungs are extracted together as a block. Through a median sternotomy incision and using cardiopulmonary bypass, the recipient's native heart and lungs are excised. The donor heart-lung block is then implanted with anastomoses between recipient and donor trachea (airway), right atrium or venae cavae (inflow), and aorta (outflow). Early morbidity and mortality after heart-lung transplantation is caused most commonly by infection and graft failure; mortality after the first year usually is due to bronchiolitis obliterans, infection, or malignancy (Yuh et al., 1997).

As with lung transplantation, bronchiolitis obliterans remains the most serious limitation to long-term survival after heart-lung transplantation. Chronic rejection in the lungs (ie, bronchiolitis obliterans) and in the heart (ie, allograft vasculopathy) can occur separately, and often lung rejection occurs before and without cardiac rejection. Cardiac allograft vasculopathy also can occur, but the incidence of both acute cardiac rejection and cardiac allograft vasculopathy is much lower in heart-lung recipients than in heart recipients; less than 5% of late deaths are related to cardiac allograft vasculopathy (Kriett & Jamieson, 1996).

Rarely, *"domino-donor" transplantation* may be performed in which the healthy heart of the heart-lung recipient is procured for implantation in a second recipient awaiting cardiac transplantation. The domino-donor procedure avoids the loss of a relatively healthy heart. Proponents assert that hearts conditioned to the elevated pulmonary vascular resistance associated with end-stage lung disease are theoretically ideal for cardiac recipients with moderate pulmonary hypertension (Fleischer & Baumgartner, 1998).

REFERENCES

Abrams AC, 1998: Immunosuppressants. In Clinical Drug Therapy, ed. 5. Philadelphia, Lippincott Williams & Wilkins

Allen-Auerbach M, Schoder H, Johnson J, et al., 1999: Relationship between coronary function by positron emission tomography and temporal changes in morphology by intravascular ultrasound (IVUS) in transplant recipients. J Heart Lung Transplant 18:211

American Heart Association, 1998: 1999 Heart and Stroke Statistical Update. Dallas, American Heart Association

Arcasoy SM, Kotloff RM, 1999: Medical progress: Lung transplantation. N Engl J Med 340:1081

Baldwin JC, 1996: Preservation of intrathoracic organs for transplantation. In Baue AE, Geha AS, Hammond GL, et al. (eds): Glenn's Thoracic and Cardiovascular Surgery, ed. 6. Stamford, CT, Appleton & Lange

Barnard CN, 1967: A human cardiac transplant: An interim report of a successful operation performed at Groote Schuur Hospital, Cape Town. S Afr Med J 41:1271

Bavaria JE, Kotloff R, Palevsky H, et al., 1997: Bilateral versus single lung transplantation for chronic obstructive pulmonary disease. J Thorac Cardiovasc Surg 113:520

Beniaminovitz A, Mancini DM, 1999: The role of exercise-based prognosticating algorithms in the selection of patients for heart transplantation. Curr Opin Cardiol 14:114

Carrel A, Guthrie CC, 1905: The transplantation of veins and organs. Am Med 10:1101

Chillcott SR, Atkins PJ, Adamson RM, 1998: Left ventricular assist as a viable alternative for cardiac transplantation. Critical Care Nursing Quarterly 20:64

Cooper JD, Patterson GA, Grossman R, et al., 1989: Double-lung transplant for advanced chronic obstructive lung disease. American Review of Respiratory Disease 139:303

Egan TM, Detterbeck FC, 1998: Technique of lung transplantation. In Kaiser LR, Kron IL, Spray TL (eds): Mastery of Cardiothoracic Surgery. Philadelphia, Lippincott Williams & Wilkins

Emery RW, Joyce LD, 1991: Directions in cardiac assistance. J Card Surg 6:400

Fleischer KJ, Baumgartner WA, 1997: Heart transplantation. In Edmunds LH Jr (ed): Cardiac Surgery in the Adult. New York, McGraw-Hill

Fleischer KJ, Baumgartner WA, 1998: Transplantation: Heart. In Kaiser LR, Kron IL, Spray TL (eds): Mastery of Cardiothoracic Surgery. Philadelphia, Lippincott Williams & Wilkins

Garrity ER, Hertz MI, Trulock EP, et al., 1999: Editorial: Suggested guidelines for the use of tacrolimus in lung-transplant recipients. J Heart Lung Transplant 18:175

Goldstein DJ, Rose EA, 1998: Cardiac allotransplantation. In Rose EA, Stevenson LW (eds): Management of End-Stage Heart Disease. Philadelphia, Lippincott Williams & Wilkins

Griffith BP, Magee MJ, 1996: Cardiac transplantation. In Baue AE, Geha AS, Hammond GL, et al. (eds): Glenn's Thoracic and Cardiovascular Surgery, ed. 6. Stamford, CT, Appleton & Lange

Gronda EG, Barbieri P, Frigerio M, et al., 1999: Prognostic indices in heart transplant candidates after the first hospitalization triggered by the need for intravenous pharmacologic circulatory support. J Heart Lung Transplant 18:654

Hardy JD, Webb WR, Dalton TL Jr, Walker GR Jr, 1963: Lung homotransplantation in man: Report of the initial case. JAMA 186:1063

Hosenpud JD, Bennett LE, Keck BM, et al., 1998: Effect of diagnosis on survival benefit of lung transplantation for end-stage lung disease. Lancet 351:24

Hosenpud JD, Bennett LE, Keck BM, et al., 1999: The Registry of the International Society for Heart and Lung Transplantation: Sixteenth official report—1999. J Heart Lung Transplant 18:611

Hudak CM, Gallo BM, Morton PG, 1998: Organ and hemopoietic stem cell transplantation. In Critical Care Nursing: A Holistic Approach, ed. 7. Philadelphia, Lippincott Williams & Wilkins

Hunt SA, Frazier OH, 1998: Mechanical circulatory support and cardiac transplantation. Circulation 97:2079

John R, Chen JM, Weinberg A, et al., 1999: Long-term survival after cardiac retransplantation: A twenty-year single-center experience. J Thorac Cardiovasc Surg 117:543

Joseph J, Trehan S, Taylor DO, 1999: Advances in immunosuppression. In Franco KL, Verrier ED (eds): Advanced Therapy in Cardiac Surgery. Hamilton, Canada, BC Decker

Kapadia SR, Nissen SE, Tuzcu EM, 1999: Impact of intravascular ultrasound in understanding transplant coronary artery disease. Curr Opin Cardiol 14:140

Kaplon RJ, Gillinov AM, Smedira NG, et al., 1999: Vitamin K reduces bleeding in left ventricular assist device recipients. J Heart Lung Transplant 18:346

Kobashigawa J, Miller L, Renlund D, et al, 1998: A randomized active-controlled trial of mycophenolate mofetil in heart transplant recipients. Mycophenolate Mofetil Investigators. Transplantation 66:507

Kriett JM, Jamieson SW, 1996: Heart and lung transplantation. In Baue AE, Geha AS, Hammond GL, et al. (eds): Glenn's Thoracic and Cardiovascular Surgery, ed. 6. Stamford, CT, Appleton & Lange

Kroshus TJ, Kshettry VR, Savik K, et al., 1997: Risk factors for the development of bronchiolitis obliterans syndrome after lung transplantation. J Thorac Cardiovasc Surg 114:195

Labarrere CA, 1999: Relationship of fibrin deposition in microvasculature to outcomes in cardiac transplantation. Curr Opin Cardiol 14:133

Low DE, Trulock EP, Kaiser LR, et al., 1992: Lung transplantation of ventilator dependent patients. Chest 101:8

Marinelli WA, Hertz MI, Shumway SJ, et al., 1992: Single lung transplantation for severe emphysema. J Heart Lung Transplant 11:577

Maurer JR, Frost AE, Estenne M, et al., 1998: International guidelines for selection of lung transplant candidates. J Heart Lung Transplant 17:703

McCurry KR, Keenan RJ, 1998: Controlling perioperative morbidity and mortality after lung transplantation for pulmonary hypertension. Semin Thorac Cardiovasc Surg 10:139

McCurry KR, Kormos RL, Griffith BP, 1999: Cardiac retransplantation. In Franco KL, Verrier ED (eds): Advanced Therapy in Cardiac Surgery. Hamilton, Canada, BC Decker

Mendeloff EN, 1998: Lung transplantation for cystic fibrosis. Semin Thorac Cardiovasc Surg 10:202

Mentzer RM Jr, Jaharia MS, Lasley RD, et al, 1998: Tacrolimus as a rescue immunosuppressant after heart and lung transplantation. Transplantation 65:109

Meyers BF, Patterson GA, 1998: Technical aspects of adult lung transplantation. Semin Thorac Cardiovasc Surg 10:213

Miller LW, Miller EM, 1999: Allograft coronary artery disease. In Franco KL, Verrier ED (eds): Advanced Therapy in Cardiac Surgery. Hamilton, Canada, BC Decker

Novick RJ, Stitt L, 1998: Pulmonary retransplantation. Semin Thorac Cardiovasc Surg 10:227

O'Brien GO, Criner GJ, 1999: Mechanical ventilation as a bridge to lung transplantation. J Heart Lung Transplant 18:255

Patterson GA, 1998: Adult lung transplantation. Semin Thorac Cardiovasc Surg 10:190

Patterson GA, Cooper JD, 1995: Lung transplantation. In Pearson FG, Deslauriers J, Ginsberg RJ, et al. (eds): Thoracic Surgery. New York, Churchill Livingstone

Reitz BA, Wallwork JL, Hunt SA, et al., 1982: Heart-lung transplantation. Successful therapy for patients with pulmonary vascular disease. N Engl J Med 306:557

Renlund DG, 1998: Cardiac transplantation. In Topol EJ (ed): Comprehensive Cardiovascular Medicine. Philadelphia, Lippincott Williams & Wilkins

Rich S, McLaughlin VV, 1998: Lung transplantation for pulmonary hypertension: Patient selection and maintenance therapy while awaiting transplantation. Semin Thorac Cardiovasc Surg 10:135

Rodkey SM, Ratliff NB, Young JB, 1998: Cardiomyopathy and myocardial failure. In Topol EJ (ed): Comprehensive Cardiovascular Disease. Philadelphia, Lippincott Williams & Wilkins

Rubin BK, 1999: Emerging therapies for cystic fibrosis lung disease. Chest 115:1120

Smith MA, Sundaresan S, Mohanakumar T, et al., 1998: Effect of development of antibodies to HLA and cytomegalovirus mismatch on lung transplantation survival and development of bronchiolitis obliterans syndrome. J Thorac Cardiovasc Surg 116:812

Sundaresan RS, Patterson GA, 1996: Lung transplantation. In Baue AE, Geha AS, Hammond GL, et al. (eds): Glenn's Thoracic and Cardiovascular Surgery, ed. 6. Stamford, CT, Appleton & Lange

Sundaresan RS, Shiraisi Y, Trulock EP, et al., 1996: Single or bilateral lung transplantation for emphysema? J Thorac Cardiovasc Surg 112:1485

Sundaresan S, 1998a: The impact of bronchiolitis obliterans on late morbidity and mortality after single and bilateral lung transplantation for pulmonary hypertension. Transplantation Review 12:222

Sundaresan S, 1998b: Bronchiolitis obliterans. Semin Thorac Cardiovasc Surg 10:221

Toronto Lung Transplant Group, 1986: Unilateral lung transplantation for pulmonary fibrosis. N Engl J Med 314:1140

Trulock EP, 1997: Lung transplantation. Am J Respir Crit Care Med 155:789

United Network for Organ Sharing (UNOS), 1999: Amended UNOS Policy 3.7 (Allocation of Thoracic Organs) Richmond, VA

Waddell TK, Keshavjee S, 1998: Lung transplantation for chronic obstructive pulmonary disease. Semin Thorac Cardiovasc Surg 10:191

Wynne J, Braunwald E, 1997: The cardiomyopathies and myocarditides. In Braunwald E (ed): Heart Disease: A Textbook of Cardiovascular Medicine, ed. 5. Philadelphia, WB Saunders

Young JB, 1999: Progress and controversy in cardiac transplantation: Commentary on patient selection, management, and determinants of outcome. Curr Opin Cardiol 14:111

Yuh DD, Robbins RC, Reitz BA, 1997: Transplantation of the heart and lungs. In Edmunds LH Jr (ed): Cardiac Surgery in the Adult. New York, McGraw-Hill

Zuckerman JB, Kotloff RM, 1998: Lung transplantation for cystic fibrosis. Clin Chest Med 19:535

Cardiac and Thoracic Trauma

The incidence of *chest trauma* continues to increase, largely owing to the prevalence of accidents associated with high speed and rapid deceleration and with violent acts of aggression. Trauma is the leading cause of death in people younger than 40 years of age and the third leading cause of death from all diseases; chest injuries are responsible for 25% of these deaths (Calhoon & Trinkle, 1997). Young adult men are affected disproportionately by chest trauma. They are more likely to have automobile and motorcycle accidents, to incur injuries while performing heavy labor, and to be victims of physical violence (Cohn & Braunwald, 1997). In addition to the increased number of trauma victims, improvements in emergency transport systems allow more patients to reach hospitals where appropriate diagnosis and treatment can occur.

Chest trauma is categorized as either blunt or penetrating. Blunt chest trauma consists of those injuries to thoracic structures that are caused by application of external force to the thorax without penetration of the chest wall. Blunt trauma most often is associated with motor vehicle accidents but also can result from falling or crushing accidents or assaults with blunt objects. In high-speed accidents, injury results from the application of shearing force to contiguous fixed and nonfixed intrathoracic structures as the person rapidly decelerates. In low-speed accidents, the injury is likely to be caused by localized crushing. Penetrating chest trauma consists of injuries to thoracic structures caused by an object that penetrates the chest wall. The incidence of penetrating thoracic injuries, and gunshot wounds in particular, has increased during the past two decades.

▶ Types of Injuries

Bony Injuries

Rib fractures are the most common chest injury, particularly in older people with more brittle bones. Fractures frequently occur in the fifth through ninth ribs, often at the posterior angle (Rodriguez, 1990a; McElvein & Novick, 1991). Clinical manifestations of rib fracture are pain localized to the area of injury, point tenderness, and splinting. The diagnosis is confirmed by posteroanterior and lateral chest roentgenograms. However, because linear rib fractures are easily missed on standard chest roentgenograms, a rib fracture should be assumed in the presence of characteristic clinical findings even if the fracture is not evident radiographically (Wisner, 1995). Treatment is palliative; pain medications are prescribed, and, if necessary, intercostal nerve blocks may be used to provide local anesthesia. It is important that pain control is adequate to prevent hypoventilation with resultant atelectasis and retention of secretions. Healing of rib fractures takes 3 to 6 weeks.

If more than one rib is fractured, respiratory function may be compromised. Elderly patients with multiple rib fractures are likely to acquire significant atelectasis and pneumonia that, if untreated, may lead to severe respiratory distress (Wisner, 1995). Such patients may require admission to the hospital for observation, supplemental oxygenation, pulmonary hygiene, or ventilatory support. Contrary to popular belief, application of a chest binder or taping of the chest wall is not indicated because these splinting devices impede deep breathing and predispose to atelectasis (Baker, 1990).

Fracture of the first or second rib may have clinical significance. A great deal of force is required to fracture these ribs because they are well protected by the clavicle, scapula, humerus, and soft tissue (Rodriguez, 1990a). For this reason, the possibility of associated internal injuries should be considered when the first or second rib is fractured. Serious injury to intrathoracic structures also is more likely when multiple ribs are fractured. Upper rib fractures may be associated with aortic injury; spleen and liver injuries are frequently associated with fracture of multiple lower ribs.

Flail chest is the term used to describe an injury in which multiple consecutive ribs or costal cartilages are fractured in several places (Fig. 32-1). The dislocated segment moves paradoxically to the remainder of the bony structure of the chest wall during respiration. With inspiration, the flail segment hinders the creation of ipsilateral negative inspiratory force and, with expiration, it lags behind and impedes the development of positive airway pressure (Mayberry & Trunkey, 1997). Although the injured ribs usually heal without treatment, the lung on the injured side may be significantly hypoventilated if the size of the flail segment is large. Mechanical ventilation with positive end-expiratory pressure (PEEP) may be necessary for stabilization of the bony thorax if the injury is associated with respiratory insufficiency. In such cases, it is usu-

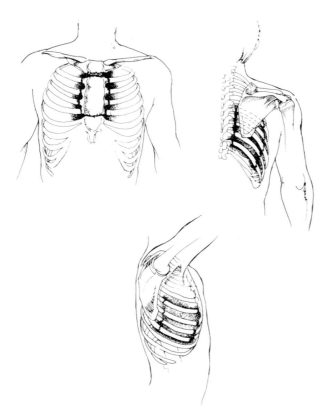

FIGURE 32-1. Typical sites of flail chest injury. (Campbell DB, 1992: Trauma to the chest wall, lung, and major airways. Semin Thorac Cardiovasc Surg 4:235)

ally underlying pulmonary contusion, rather than abnormal chest movements, that causes the respiratory failure.

Fracture of the sternum usually is caused by impact of a victim's chest against a steering wheel (Rodriguez, 1990a). Most sternal fractures occur in the upper or middle body of the sternum (Mayberry & Trunkey, 1997). The fracture may be identified by palpation, local swelling and discoloration, pain, and its appearance on a lateral roentgenogram (McElvein & Novick, 1991). Unless the fracture produces severe displacement of the sternal edges, open reduction and fixation usually are not required. Sternal fracture is most significant because of its frequent association with myocardial contusion. Accordingly, patients usually are admitted for observation and cardiac monitoring. Less commonly, sternal fracture is accompanied by tracheobronchial or great vessel injury.

Fractures of the scapula and clavicle are relatively uncommon. Although treatment for both is palliative, they often are associated with injury to underlying structures. In contrast to other fractures of the bony thorax, a fractured clavicle may be treated with an external support brace. A figure-of-eight soft harness usually is applied for 6 to 8 weeks to produce sustained hyperextension of the shoulders.

Aortic Transection

Aortic transection describes traumatic laceration of the aorta. The most common injury of the great vessels, it usually is caused by severe blunt chest trauma associated with rapid deceleration or severe chest compression. It is a leading cause of immediate death in motor vehicle accidents and falls (Turney & Rodriguez, 1990). Most aortic lacerations occur secondary to high-speed (>20 miles/h) motor vehicle accidents; the incidence is higher in car occupants if they are driving, not wearing a seat belt, and are ejected (Warren et al., 1996). Other causes of aortic transection include kicks, falls from heights, and crush injuries (Miller & Calhoon, 1998).

Traumatic aortic injury almost always occurs at one of two sites: (1) the thoracic isthmus, just distal to the left subclavian artery at the location of the ligamentum arteriosum; or (2) just distal to the aortic valve (Fig. 32-2). Injury is more likely at these locations because the segment of aorta between the aortic valve and thoracic isthmus is not tethered. The heart and descending aorta, on the other hand, are relatively fixed in position by contiguous structures. Transection just distal to the left subclavian artery is produced most often by rapid horizontal deceleration, such as occurs with high-speed motor vehicle accidents. Rapid vertical deceleration, as occurs with a fall from a building or airplane, is likely to cause disruption of the ascending aorta.

Approximately 80% of people with aortic transection, and almost all with transection of the ascending aorta, die at the scene of the accident. However, if aortic adventitia or periaortic fibrous tissue remains intact, blood is contained in the aorta and the victim may survive for a period. The prognosis for these early survivors depends on timely

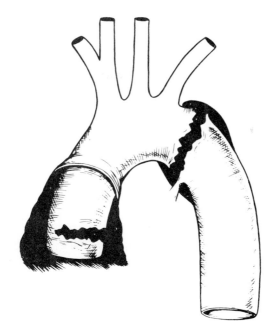

FIGURE 32-2. Schematic representation of aorta demonstrating the two common sites of aortic transection. (Turney SZ, Rodriguez A, 1990: Injuries to the great thoracic vessels. In Turney SZ, Rodriguez A, Cowley RA [eds]: Management of Cardiothoracic Trauma, p. 232. Baltimore, Williams & Wilkins)

diagnosis of the injury. Precipitous adventitial rupture with death from exsanguination is most likely in the first few hours after injury (Turney & Rodriguez, 1990). Without definitive treatment, half of those who survive the initial injury die within 24 hours and almost 75% die within 1 week (Sweeney et al., 1997). Therefore, it is essential to consider the diagnosis of aortic transection in any victim of a deceleration-type injury, particularly if other injuries indicative of major chest trauma are present.

A fracture of the sternum, clavicle, first rib, or multiple ribs suggests that there has been a blow to the chest forceful enough to tear the aorta. Roentgenographic signs of bleeding into the pericardial or pleural spaces provide additional evidence of aortic transection. Mediastinal widening is the most common radiographic finding. Obliteration of the aortic knob, pleural effusion representing hemothorax, and tracheal deviation also may be present. Interpretation of roentgenographic mediastinal widening is difficult because the chest roentgenogram almost always is obtained with portable equipment using an anteroposterior projection. In anteroposterior chest films, there is some magnification of the mediastinal shadow because of technique. Also, the absence of a widened mediastinum does not rule out the diagnosis. Other signs and symptoms of aortic transection that may be present include shock and a difference in blood pressure measurements between upper and lower extremities.

Aortography remains the gold standard for diagnosis of aortic transection. If the type of accident, clinical manifestations, or radiographic findings suggests aortic injury, an aortogram is obtained to confirm the diagnosis. If aor-

tography is not immediately available and the patient is stable hemodynamically, contrast-enhanced computed tomographic (CT) scanning of the chest may be used to aid in diagnosis by revealing the presence of a periaortic hematoma. However, CT scanning may not demonstrate an intimal tear that has not yet caused a periaortic hematoma and thus is inadequate to rule out the diagnosis (Elefteriades et al., 1996a; McLean et al., 1991).

Transesophageal echocardiography also may be used for diagnosis, especially in patients with other critical injuries. Often, the diagnosis of aortic transection is delayed because of associated injuries, some of which may require emergent operative treatment. Failure to establish the diagnosis usually results in precipitous death of the patient. Because it can be performed rapidly at the bedside, intraoperative transesophageal echocardiography may be particularly useful to establish or rule out aortic injury in patients requiring emergent treatment for other life-threatening injuries (Miller & Calhoon, 1998).

Once the diagnosis is established, surgical repair of the aorta is performed immediately, unless severe associated injuries take precedence. If hemothorax is present, repair of the aortic transection is of highest priority. If no hemothorax is present and there is evidence of active bleeding elsewhere (eg, in the abdomen), other surgical interventions may take priority, particularly because systemic anticoagulation will be necessary if cardiopulmonary bypass is used during the aortic repair.

Surgical repair of the aorta is performed through a left thoracotomy incision for aortic transection in the classic location at the thoracic isthmus. The aorta is clamped above and below the area of transection, and the injured segment is resected and replaced with a prosthetic graft (Fig. 32-3). Cardiopulmonary bypass usually is not required for repair of a transection of the descending thoracic aorta. Also, cardiopulmonary bypass necessitates systemic anticoagulation, which is contraindicated in the presence of active bleeding or associated injuries. Prognosis for patient survival is good if repair is undertaken before adventitial rupture. Complications of the operative repair include bleeding, renal failure, and paraplegia due to ischemic injury to the spinal cord while blood flow through the descending aorta is interrupted. Several techniques are described in the surgical literature for intraoperative protection of spinal cord blood flow and monitoring of spinal cord ischemia. Despite these measures, the development of paraplegia as an operative complication remains unpredictable. The incidence is variable, ranging from 5% to 25% in reported series (Miller & Calhoon, 1998; Cowley et al., 1990; Mattox, 1989).

Rarely, in patients with undiagnosed aortic transection, the adventitia remains intact and a chronic traumatic aneurysm develops at the site of the transection. The aneurysm may exist for many years before it is detected when a chest roentgenogram is performed for another reason or the patient experiences symptoms of aneurysm enlargement. Because of the propensity for sudden rupture, operative repair of chronic traumatic aneurysm is recommended even in the absence of symptoms (Finkelmeier et al., 1982).

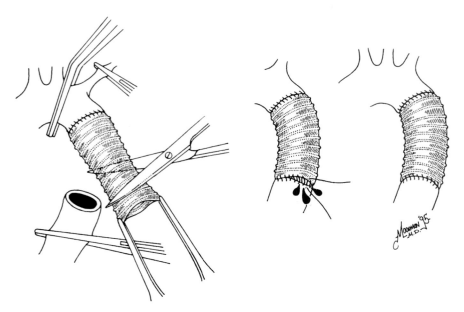

FIGURE 32-3. Operative repair of aortic transection at the classic location just distal to the left subclavian artery. (Miller OL, Calhoon JH, 1998: Acute traumatic aortic transection. In Kaiser LR, Kron IL, Spray TL [eds]: Mastery of Cardiothoracic Surgery. p. 485. Philadelphia, Lippincott Williams & Wilkins)

Cardiac Injuries

Penetrating Wounds

Cardiac injuries are usually the result of penetrating wounds that occur during acts of aggression. The incidence of penetrating cardiac wounds has increased dramatically over the past several decades, as has the relative frequency of injuries caused by gunshot wounds compared with stab wounds (Crawford, 1997). Gunshot wounds are more often lethal because they produce a larger defect in the pericardium and more destruction of myocardial tissue. As a result, exsanguination is more likely than with stab wounds. Conversely, as many as 80% of patients with stab wounds present with manifestations of cardiac tamponade because the small pericardial laceration typically produced by a long, narrow instrument seals from clot or mediastinal fatty tissue (Brown & Grover, 1997) (Fig. 32-4). Penetrating cardiac wounds also can result from inward displacement of ribs or sternal fragments associated with chest injury or, uncommonly, from intravascular or intracardiac catheters that have fractured and become impaled in the wall of a great vessel or cardiac chamber (Cohn & Braunwald, 1997).

Any portion of the heart can be damaged by traumatic injury. The right ventricle is the most frequently injured cardiac chamber, although one third of injuries involve multiple cardiac structures (Brown & Grover, 1997). Typically, patients with penetrating cardiac injuries have clinical manifestations of either hemorrhagic shock or cardiac tamponade (Crawford, 1997). As with aortic transection, patients with injuries to the heart frequently die before reaching the hospital. However, the clinical presentation is quite variable, ranging from acute cardiovascular collapse with cardiopulmonary arrest to complete hemodynamic stability (Asensio et al., 1996).

If the patient arrives at the hospital with cardiac arrest or in extremis (ie, with severe hypotension refractory to volume resuscitation), it may be necessary for the surgeon to open the patient's chest in the emergency department. A left anterolateral thoracotomy incision is made and a rib retractor is used to separate the ribs. Because massive hemorrhage is likely, digital or clamp compression of the bleeding site and rapid infusion of large volumes of blood or other fluid is mandatory. Most victims of penetrating cardiac injury are young, otherwise healthy people and aggressive treatment, including emergency department thoracotomy, results in the survival of a significant number of patients whose condition does not permit the delay associated with transport to an operating room (Crawford, 1997). In the event of severe internal damage to the heart, however, the likelihood of survival is remote. If bleeding cannot be controlled quickly, exsanguination, tamponade, or cardiac failure results in the patient's death.

If the patient survives long enough to be transported to the operating room, surgical exploration is performed with repair of the traumatic defect. A median sternotomy incision usually is used because it provides excellent exposure of the heart and great vessels. Repair of injured cardiac valves, coronary arteries, or septa requires trained personnel and equipment for providing extracorporeal circulation (cardiopulmonary bypass) during the operation. However, most people with cardiac injuries who survive to be transported to a hospital do not have internal cardiac damage but rather a laceration confined to the atrial or ventricular wall. This type of cardiac injury often can be repaired without cardiopulmonary bypass by clamping the injured tissue and suturing the laceration. Delay in operation, rather than lack of cardiopulmonary bypass capability in the institution, is the major cause of death in these patients (Lockhart, 1986).

Sometimes, the diagnosis of cardiac injury is elusive; the classic clinical manifestations may not be present, particularly if blood from the heart drains through a peri-

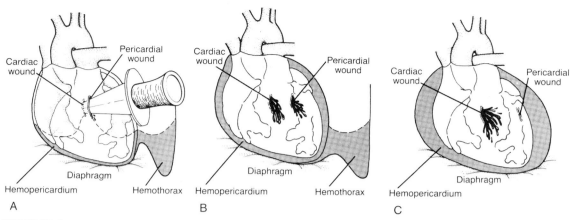

FIGURE 32-4. Penetrating injury to the heart (**A**), with open (**B**) and sealed (**C**) pericardial wound. (Symbas PN, 1989: Penetrating wounds of the heart. In Cardiothoracic Trauma, p. 31. Philadelphia, WB Saunders)

cardial laceration into the pleural space (Wall et al., 1998). Cardiac injury should be considered in any person with a history of a penetrating wound to the chest, upper abdomen, or neck. A heart wound is particularly likely if the entrance wound of a penetrating object is between the two midclavicular lines (Rodriguez, 1990b) (Fig. 32-5). Blood in the left pleural space provides further evidence of cardiac or vascular injury. Gunshot wounds anywhere in the vicinity of the chest always should be suspected of injuring the heart because of the unpredictable trajectory of bullets in the body (Elefteriades et al., 1996b).

In all patients who have sustained major chest trauma, the heart is carefully auscultated for the presence of murmurs. An echocardiogram may be performed if in-

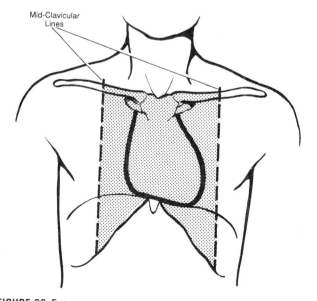

FIGURE 32-5. Injury to the heart should be considered in any patient with a penetrating wound between the anterior midclavicular lines (*shaded area*). (Rodriguez A, 1990: Initial patient evaluation and indications for thoracotomy. In Turney SZ, Rodriguez A, Cowley RA [eds]: Management of Cardiothoracic Trauma, p. 9. Baltimore, Williams & Wilkins)

ternal cardiac injury is suspected. Availability of transesophageal echocardiography has enhanced rapid and accurate diagnosis of cardiac injuries in hemodynamically stable patients. The demonstration of the presence or absence of fluid in the pericardial cavity usually correlates with the presence or absence of a cardiac wound (Symbas & Justicz, 1996). Transesophageal echocardiography can be performed in the emergency department in approximately 15 minutes, provides information that can be interpreted immediately, has minimal risks, and does not necessitate administration of contrast medium (Shapiro et al., 1991). Using this bedside technique, intracardiac septal defects, valvular damage, or the presence of foreign bodies can be diagnosed (Follette, 1991).

Patients who undergo repair of a lacerated cardiac chamber wall should be assessed carefully for injury to internal structures of the heart. If possible, intraoperative transesophageal echocardiography is performed once the external injury has been repaired and the patient is stable hemodynamically (Crawford, 1997). Occasionally, a penetrating object perforates the atrial or ventricular septum or damages one of the cardiac valves without producing hemodynamic compromise. The internal injury may not be detected when the external laceration is repaired. If an internal cardiac defect is identified but the patient demonstrates no adverse hemodynamic effects, the surgeon may elect to defer intracardiac repair for several weeks until tissues surrounding the lacerated area have matured and become more firm. This makes the repair technically easier and safer for the patient.

Retention of a projectile object in the heart may result from a direct injury to the heart or from an injury to a systemic vein with migration of the missile into the heart (Symbas & Justicz, 1996). Foreign bodies that penetrate the heart and are free-floating in one of the cardiac chambers should be removed. Retained objects may embolize, predispose to endocarditis, or erode into cardiac chambers or vessels (Crawford, 1997). If the object is embedded in myocardium, however, the surgeon may elect not to remove the object unless its presence causes arrhythmias, infection, or pericardial effusion.

Myocardial Contusion

Myocardial contusion is histopathologic injury of the heart muscle secondary to blunt trauma. Contusion injury may vary considerably in extent and character, ranging from small areas of petechiae or ecchymosis to full-thickness contusion of the myocardial wall (Symbas & Justicz, 1996). Myocardial contusion is particularly likely in accidents in which there is a blow to the anterior chest, such as when a person is propelled against the steering wheel of a car (Fig. 32-6). Because the right ventricle is the most anterior chamber of the heart, it is injured most often. Myocardial contusion usually produces no significant symptoms and often goes unrecognized (Cohn & Braunwald, 1997). It is detected by the same electrocardiographic, echocardiographic, and enzymatic changes representative of acute myocardial infarction. A pericardial rub may be present.

If myocardial contusion is suspected, the patient is observed in the hospital with continuous electrocardiographic monitoring. Although no specific electrocardiographic abnormality is pathognomonic for myocardial contusion, nearly any type of electrocardiographic change can occur as a result of the injury (Unkle et al., 1989). Treatment is similar to that for myocardial infarction, including electrocardiographic monitoring, rest, supplemental oxygen, and mild fluid restriction. In severe cases, contusion can produce significant clinical sequelae, including conduction disturbances, arrhythmias, pericardial effusion, myocardial rupture, or cardiogenic shock. Late complications of myocardial contusion include constrictive pericarditis and ventricular aneurysm.

Tracheal and Bronchial Injuries

Laceration or transection of the trachea or a major bronchus is uncommon but can be lethal. The injury most often is due to blunt trauma. The mainstem bronchus at the level of the carina is the most frequent site of injury (Pezzella et al., 1998). Severity of tracheal or bronchial injury can vary from a partial tear to complete disruption. Severe tracheobronchial injuries frequently are associated with injury to surrounding structures (eg, the esophagus, thoracic great vessels, larynx, cervical spine, or recurrent laryngeal nerves) (Mathisen & Grillo, 1991).

Patients with complete *tracheal transection* present with profound respiratory distress, stridor, hemoptysis, hoarseness, and cyanosis. The injury causes a massive air leak that is likely to produce a tension pneumothorax. A continuous air leak remains after chest tube placement, and significant subcutaneous emphysema usually is present. Hypoventilation, with resultant impaired carbon dioxide removal, occurs because an effective tidal volume of air cannot be moved in and out of the tracheobronchial tree. Hypoxemia usually is present as well secondary to associated pulmonary contusion or the marked reduction in minute volume. The chest roentgenogram reveals pneumothorax, hemothorax, and mediastinal emphysema.

The first priority in the treatment of tracheal or bronchial injury is establishment of a patent airway using an endotracheal tube or, if necessary, by performance of a tracheostomy. Immediate intubation of the severed distal segment may be life saving (Pezzella et al., 1998). Chest tube thoracostomy is used to evacuate air and blood from the pleural space. Depending on location and severity of the tear, it may be impossible to reexpand the lung until integrity of the airway is restored.

In most cases, a tracheal or bronchial laceration requires surgical treatment. Bronchoscopy is performed to define the location and extent of the injury. Injuries to the upper trachea commonly are repaired through a cervical incision. Injuries to the lower trachea, carina, and right bronchus are repaired through a right posterolateral thoracotomy incision; a left thoracotomy approach is used for left bronchial tears (Weissberg & Utkin, 1991). The

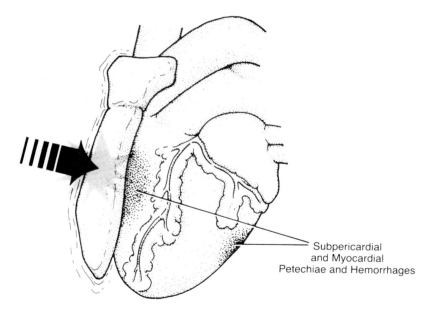

Subpericardial
and Myocardial
Petechiae and Hemorrhages

FIGURE 32-6. Blunt trauma to the anterior chest resulting in myocardial contusion. (Symbas PN, 1989: Contusion of the heart. In Cardiothoracic Trauma, p. 57. Philadelphia, WB Saunders)

lacerated tissue is repaired, and, if heavy contamination is present, the area is drained. With severe injuries, survival is most likely in young adults who better tolerate the profound hypoxemia associated with the injury and who have a more resilient tracheobronchial tree.

Pulmonary Injuries

There are two types of pulmonary injuries: laceration and contusion. *Pulmonary laceration,* or tearing of the parenchyma (lung tissue), is associated with leakage of air and blood into the pleural space. Pulmonary lacerations often can be treated by placement of a chest tube to drain the pleural space until the laceration heals. However, if significant bleeding or a large air leak persists, surgical exploration is performed to repair the laceration and to explore for other intrathoracic injuries. Most parenchymal injuries can be repaired by oversewing of the injured tissue or nonanatomic segmental resection with a stapling device (Wall et al., 1998). Massive tissue destruction, involvement of the hilum, or uncontrolled hemorrhage occasionally necessitates pneumonectomy. Sometimes a penetrating object, such as a bullet, remains in the parenchyma. Surgical removal of the object may be necessary if it is large or sharp and centrally located, or if it causes infection or hemoptysis.

Uncommonly, parenchymal lung injury leads to *systemic air embolism.* This phenomenon can occur when air from a disrupted bronchus enters an adjacent injured pulmonary vein, travels through the left side of the heart, and is ejected into the systemic circulation, where it can cause myocardial infarction or stroke. Systemic air embolism most often occurs in patients who have sustained a central penetrating lung injury, but also has been recognized in patients with pulmonary contusion from blunt trauma (Boyd & Glassman, 1997). The condition is thought to occur more commonly than is clinically recognized and usually is fatal.

Systemic embolism is most likely when positive-pressure ventilation is instituted, making it easier for air exiting a bronchus to find routes of egress into pulmonary veins, and when the patient is hypovolemic, because lower pressure in the pulmonary veins facilitates air entry into rather than bleeding from the veins (Elefteriades et al., 1996b). It also may occur during chest tube thoracostomy or thoracotomy when air from outside the chest can enter a disrupted pulmonary vein. Precipitous hemodynamic instability, cardiac arrest, or neurologic symptoms after institution of positive-pressure ventilation or opening of the chest suggest the diagnosis. Treatment includes placing the patient in the Trendelenburg position and urgent thoracotomy. The pulmonary hilum is occluded and air is vented from the left side of the heart, aorta, and coronary arteries; injured bronchial and venous structures are repaired, if possible, or pulmonary resection is performed (Boyd & Glassman, 1997).

Pulmonary contusion is injury of the lung parenchyma itself. It occurs when hemorrhage and extravasation of plasma and protein into alveolar and interstitial spaces produce atelectasis and consolidation (Hudak et al., 1998). Contusion occurs most often in association with a blast injury, such as an explosion, or with rapid deceleration. A localized infiltrate usually is apparent on the initial chest roentgenogram, tends to progress over the next several days, and resolves within 1 week. One or both lungs may be affected.

Treatment of pulmonary contusion includes fluid restriction, diuresis, antibiotics, pulmonary hygiene, and, if necessary, mechanical ventilation. The goal of restricting hydration is not always achieved because lung injury often is accompanied by other major body injuries that necessitate vigorous fluid resuscitation. Excessive overhydration can lead to pulmonary edema in the contused segments (Elefteriades et al., 1996b). Diminished ventilation of the contused portions of lung tissue produces significant arteriovenous shunting with resultant hypoxemia. Severe pulmonary contusion may be followed by adult respiratory distress syndrome. Mechanical ventilation with adjunctive PEEP is considered the most effective method for improving functional residual capacity, keeping alveoli open, and improving oxygenation.

Pneumothorax and Hemothorax

Pneumothorax

Pneumothorax and hemothorax are common sequelae of intrathoracic injuries. *Pneumothorax* (ie, the presence of air in the pleural space) occurs when air enters one of the pleural cavities, either from the lung or from outside the body. Pneumothorax associated with blunt chest trauma most often is due to laceration of the pulmonary parenchyma by the sharp ends of fractured rib segments. With penetrating trauma, it is usually the penetrating object that injures the lung. Rarely, pneumothorax is caused by a bronchial or tracheal tear.

The abnormal communication between the airways and pleural space allows inspired air to leak through the opening and become trapped between visceral and parietal pleurae. The degree of pneumothorax is determined by the rate of air leakage. The size of a pneumothorax is described according to the estimated percentage of lung collapse (eg, a 100% pneumothorax denotes complete collapse of the lung). Chest tube thoracostomy almost always is necessary unless the pneumothorax is small (<15% to 20%) and does not increase in size over time. If mechanical ventilation is necessary because of associated injuries, the increased airway pressure and use of PEEP may aggravate or perpetuate air leakage (Wiles, 1990).

A large or untreated air leak can produce a tension pneumothorax (ie, complete collapse of the ipsilateral lung and shifting of the mediastinum to the opposite side). Tension pneumothorax can be fatal if untreated. The increased intrathoracic pressure compresses the superior and inferior venae cavae, compromising venous return to the heart and thereby decreasing cardiac output. Hypotension and distended neck veins caused by tension pneumothorax may lead to a misdiagnosis of cardiac tamponade; careful auscultation of the lungs to detect a lack of breath sounds over the affected hemithorax provides the diagnosis (Wall et al., 1998). Treatment of tension pneumothorax is immediate thoracentesis or chest tube thoracostomy.

Less commonly, parenchymal air leakage does not produce pneumothorax; instead, air travels along the pleural surfaces to enter the mediastinum or subcutaneous tissue. The abnormal presence of air in these locations is termed *mediastinal emphysema* or *subcutaneous emphysema*, respectively.

Fractured rib segments or penetrating objects also can create a perforation in the chest wall. *Sucking chest wound* describes a chest wall injury that allows air to move freely in and out of the pleural space during respiration. Uncommon except in military trauma, sucking chest wounds can be life threatening. The injury significantly disturbs the normal physiology of ventilation. Pleural and atmospheric pressures equilibrate, removing the gradient responsible for moving air in and out of the tracheobronchial tree. If the pressure changes produce "to-and-fro" movement of the mediastinum, venous return to the heart also may be compromised. The presence of a sucking chest wound can be detected by the audible sound of air moving in and out of the pleural space with each respiration (Elefteriades et al., 1996b). Treatment includes chest tube thoracostomy to evacuate the pneumothorax and an occlusive dressing over the open wound to prevent continued entry of air into the pleural cavity.

Hemothorax

Hemothorax is the presence of blood in the pleural space. Some degree of hemothorax occurs in virtually all cases of chest trauma. Significant hemothorax can result from injury to the heart, one of the major vascular structures in the thorax, or pulmonary parenchymal or intercostal blood vessels. Massive hemorrhage into one or both pleural spaces is the most common cause of shock in patients with chest trauma. It usually is caused by laceration of the heart or great vessels. Because nearly the entire blood volume can be emptied into one hemithorax, death from exsanguination occurs unless the bleeding source is tamponaded (Elefteriades et al., 1996b).

Hemothorax appears on a chest roentgenogram as an opacity at the base of the lung, if the film is taken with the patient in an erect position. When the film is taken with the patient in a supine position, as is often the case with victims of chest trauma, hemothorax produces a hazy shadow superimposed over the entire lung field. The radiographic diagnosis of hemothorax necessitates careful observation of the roentgenogram. One liter of fluid may be just detectable to the astute observer, and even 2 liters may produce only a subtle increase in density of the affected hemithorax (Elefteriades et al., 1996b).

Except in cases of initial massive or continuing bleeding, hemothorax often can be treated effectively with chest tube drainage. Only 10% of patients require thoracotomy (Rodriguez, 1990a). However, if blood loss from the chest tube does not diminish within several hours of tube place-

ment, exploratory thoracotomy usually is performed to identify and ligate the bleeding vessel or vessels. Because hypovolemia rather than impaired pulmonary function is the key physiologic abnormality associated with massive hemothorax, volume replacement with blood and crystalloid is essential (Elefteriades et al., 1996b).

It is important also that accumulated blood in the pleural space be thoroughly evacuated. An adequately sized chest tube (eg, 36 French) with sufficient drainage holes should be inserted promptly (Mattox & Wall, 1997). Retained hemothorax occurs in 5% to 30% of patients with chest trauma (Richardson et al., 1996). If a moderate amount of blood remains in the pleural space, it becomes fibrous, entrapping the lung and inhibiting full lung expansion. In addition, blood provides an excellent medium for the growth of bacteria and may lead to empyema (ie, infection of the pleural space). Blood that is not drained within 1 week after occurrence of a hemothorax usually is too gelatinous to be evacuated by tube thoracostomy. Video-assisted thoracoscopy or thoracotomy may be necessary for removal of the clotted blood. Decortication, or removal of the fibrinous, visceral pleura, often is required as well to allow full reexpansion of the lung.

Esophageal Perforation

Esophageal perforation is a tear or disruption in the wall of the esophagus. It may be caused by penetrating wounds of the chest, ingestion of a caustic substance or foreign body, instrumentation, or severe vomiting. Rarely, it results from blunt chest trauma. Classic manifestations of esophageal perforation are severe chest pain and the presence of mediastinal or subcutaneous air on the roentgenogram. Other signs and symptoms include subcutaneous emphysema, dysphagia, fever, shock, neck swelling, pleural effusion, hemoptysis, and hematemesis.

Diagnosis is based on these findings and a corroborative clinical history. A contrast swallow study or esophagoscopy is performed to confirm the diagnosis. Treatment of esophageal perforation is surgical exploration to drain the area of infection and repair the perforation. Although small cervical perforations without significant contamination may respond to nonoperative management, most cervical tears require débridement, closure, and drainage, and almost all intrathoracic perforations require surgical exploration, repair or excision, and drainage (Pezzella et al., 1998). Saliva and gastric contents are diverted by nasogastric suction catheters placed above and below the anastomosis or by surgical division of the esophagus. Appropriate antibiotic therapy is essential to control mediastinal infection.

If diagnosis of esophageal perforation is delayed, mediastinitis soon develops from leakage of esophageal contents into the mediastinum. Sepsis ensues and death is likely unless surgical treatment is undertaken promptly. Primary repair of the esophagus rarely is possible when surgical intervention is performed more than 24 hours after injury. In these cases, the esophagus is divided and an esophagostomy is performed; the proximal esophageal segment is brought through the skin of the neck as a fistula so that saliva can drain externally into an esophagostomy pouch. The distal esophageal lumen is sutured closed and a drainage catheter placed. Enteral or intravenous alimentation is necessary until the infection has cleared and the esophagus can be reconstructed.

Injury to the Diaphragm

Laceration of the diaphragm can result either from blunt or penetrating chest or abdominal trauma. It commonly is caused by rib fractures or by rapid deceleration associated with increased intra-abdominal pressure. Although acute diaphragmatic rupture may be an isolated injury, it more commonly is associated with other injuries, such as rib, extremity, or pelvic fractures; splenic rupture; liver laceration; or gastrointestinal tract contusion or perforation (Mansour, 1997). Injury to the diaphragm almost always occurs on the left side, probably because the liver protects the right diaphragm and because of the preponderance of right-handed assailants who are most likely to cause left-sided wounds in their victims. The primary symptom associated with diaphragmatic injury is abdominal, chest, or shoulder pain. If the rent is large enough to allow herniation of an abdominal viscus, the stomach, colon, or small bowel may migrate through the rent into the thorax, producing symptoms of gastrointestinal distress. Auscultation of the chest may reveal diminished breath sounds on the side of the tear or the presence of bowel sounds in the chest.

On a supine chest roentgenogram, abdominal viscera may be apparent in the thorax. If the patient has a nasogastric tube in place, its tip may appear in the thorax as well. Diaphragmatic injury also should be suspected when there is unexplained difficulty in maintaining adequate ventilation. Sometimes positive-pressure mechanical ventilation prevents herniation of abdominal viscera through the diaphragmatic injury. Respiratory decompensation may occur when mechanical ventilation is terminated and normal negative-pressure ventilation precipitates herniation (Wiles, 1990). If the diagnosis is made soon after the injury, repair of a diaphragmatic laceration can be performed through a laparotomy incision. An abdominal approach allows the surgeon to thoroughly explore the abdomen for associated injuries, which frequently are present (Rodriguez, 1990c).

Small diaphragmatic perforations may remain undetected because they produce no associated signs and symptoms at the time of injury. However, the pressure of abdominal contents against the weakened diaphragmatic site of injury can produce gradual enlargement of the opening with eventual herniation of abdominal contents into the thorax. As the volume of herniated contents increases, the patient may experience chest or abdominal pain, shortness of breath, or acute bowel obstruction. In such cases, or if the diagnosis is missed for other reasons, a traumatic diaphragmatic hernia may be detected months or years after the injury.

Before late operative repair, a gastrointestinal contrast study often is performed to determine which portion of the gastrointestinal tract has herniated through the diaphragmatic opening. If colon is present in the thorax, a preoperative cleansing bowel preparation may be performed to reduce the risk of intrathoracic contamination should bowel perforation occur during the operative procedure. A thoracotomy is used for repair of a delayed traumatic diaphragmatic hernia because adhesions usually are present between intrathoracic segments of abdominal viscera and lung (Ganzel & Gray, 1991). A thoracotomy incision allows structures to be mobilized safely and returned through the diaphragmatic rent to the abdominal cavity. The diaphragm is then repaired.

▶ Acute Management of the Chest Trauma Victim

Most chest injuries require only conservative therapy, such as chest tube insertion for evacuation of pneumothorax or hemothorax. Exploratory thoracotomy and operative repair of internal structures are necessary only in a small percentage of cases. However, when life-threatening internal injuries are present, survival depends on rapid diagnosis and immediate interventions to maintain airway patency, adequate ventilation, and hemodynamic stability. Although there is a trimodal (ie, early, hospital, and delayed) pattern of death, the greatest number of trauma deaths occur during the early period after injury (Pezzella et al., 1998). Protocols developed by the Advanced Trauma Life Support (ATLS) Committee on Trauma of the American College of Surgeons provide systematic management guidelines for the acute management of trauma victims (American College of Surgeons Committee on Trauma, 1993).

Because the organs responsible for circulation and respiration are contained in the thorax, it is essential to evaluate cardiac and pulmonary function rapidly and diagnose injury to the heart, great vessels, or lungs. Chest trauma can produce a number of life-threatening physiologic abnormalities (Fig. 32-7). Massive hemothorax or cardiac tamponade may result from injury to the heart or a major blood vessel. Airway obstruction can be caused by a foreign object or by laceration or transection of the trachea or a major bronchus. Tension pneumothorax can occur secondary to tracheobronchial or pulmonary parenchymal disruption. Severe impairment of ventilation can occur if a penetrating object creates a sucking chest wound.

General resuscitation principles are implemented in providing immediate care to the victim of chest trauma. These include (1) establishing and maintaining a reliable airway, (2) providing adequate ventilation, and (3) supporting circulation. With severe injuries, it frequently is necessary to begin cardiopulmonary resuscitation in the field. If spinal cord injury is a possibility, the head and neck are immobilized to prevent further damage. In unconscious or severely injured patients, intubation is performed to ensure a patent airway. In the presence of an

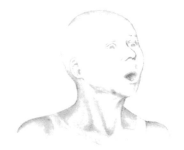

UPPER AIRWAY (LARYNGEAL) OBSTRUCTION

Marked restlessness
Anxious facies
Ashen-gray color or cyanosis
Stridor (crowing respiration)
Indrawing at suprasternal notch, around clavicles,
  in intercostal spaces, and at epigastrium

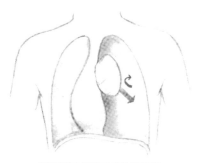

TENSION PNEUMOTHORAX

Progressive cyanosis
Respiratory embarrassment
Tracheal displacement away from affected side
Hyperresonant percussion note
Distant or absent breath sounds
Shock

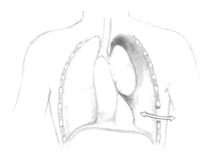

OPEN PNEUMOTHORAX

Cyanosis
Respiratory embarrassment
Sucking wound of the chest
Shock

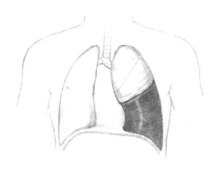

MASSIVE HEMOTHORAX

Cyanosis
Respiratory embarrassment
Dullness of percussion
Absent or distant breath sounds
Unrelenting shock if hemothorax increases

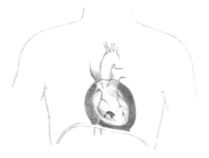

CARDIAC TAMPONADE

Neck veins distended
Falling or absent blood pressure
Patient in variable degrees of shock or in extremis
Venous pressure elevated (pathognomonic)
Muffled or distant heart tones

FIGURE 32-7. The major life-threatening injuries associated with thoracic trauma and associated manifestations. (Hood RM, 1989: Pre-hospital management, initial evaluation, and resuscitation. In Hood RM, Boyd AD, Culliford AT [eds]: Thoracic Trauma, p. 14. Philadelphia, WB Saunders)

injury to the larynx or trachea, emergent cricothyroidotomy (surgical intubation of the trachea through the cricothyroid membrane) may be necessary to ensure a reliable airway (Wisner, 1995). A self-inflating bag or mechanical volume respirator is used to provide ventilation to patients who are unable to sustain self-ventilation adequately. The chest and neck are palpated to detect subcutaneous emphysema, and chest wall motion is observed to identify the presence of a flail segment. The lung fields are auscultated to detect tension pneumothorax and the need for emergency tube thoracostomy.

Chest tubes are inserted in either or both sides of the thorax if absent breath sounds suggest the presence of significant air or fluid in the pleural spaces.

Chest compressions are begun immediately if cardiac arrest has occurred. At the same time, maneuvers are initiated to correct the cause of the cardiovascular collapse. Cardiac arrest associated with chest trauma usually is due to hemorrhagic shock or cardiac tamponade. Chest compressions alone are of little value until intravascular volume is restored or cardiac tamponade is relieved. *Hemorrhagic shock* is manifest by hypotension, low cardiac output, low central venous pressure, and decreased urine output (Rodriguez, 1990b). Rapid volume replacement, autotransfusion, and control of bleeding are the mainstays of correcting hemorrhagic shock. A crystalloid solution, such as lactated Ringer's solution, is infused through one or more large-bore intravenous catheters until compatible blood for transfusion is available. Chest tube drainage systems with autotransfusion capabilities are used to salvage and transfuse blood drained from the chest. External hemorrhage should be controlled by digital pressure (Warren et al., 1996). Emergent thoracotomy may be necessary to control massive intrathoracic bleeding.

Cardiac tamponade occurs when accumulated blood in the pericardial sac or mediastinal space causes equalization of fluid pressures within the cardiac chambers. Because blood flow into and through the heart depends on the interchamber pressure gradients that normally exist, adequate filling of the heart cannot occur when these gradients disappear (Elefteriades et al., 1996b). Recognition of acute cardiac tamponade is essential. The diagnosis is suggested by hypotension that (1) is out of proportion to blood loss, (2) is associated with distended neck veins, and (3) persists despite volume replacement and vasopressive medications. Other signs include distant heart sounds and pulsus paradoxus. Abdominal ultrasonography, with the transducer positioned in the subxiphoid area, can be used to diagnose hemopericardium rapidly in the emergency department (Mattox & Wall, 1997).

Cardiac tamponade is treated by a procedure to drain the pericardium or mediastinum and relieve cardiac compression. Volume administration is performed to increase the gradient between the venae cavae and right atrium, and thus cardiac filling, while preparing to evacuate the pericardial fluid (Elefteriades et al., 1996b). Depending on clinical circumstances, blood may be evacuated through pericardiocentesis, a subxiphoid incision, sternotomy, or thoracotomy. Injured intrathoracic structures are then repaired operatively as indicated.

Life-threatening injuries to internal viscera sometimes are present without evidence of any external wounds (blunt trauma) or with only a small entry wound (penetrating trauma). Both the chest and back should be examined carefully for a penetrating wound. Identification of entry and exit sites suggests the path through the chest of a penetrating object and which internal structures are likely to be injured. Chest trauma frequently is accompanied by other injuries, such as head injury, extremity or pelvic fractures, and injury to abdominal viscera. Therefore, initial medical management includes identification and prioritization of severity of the various injuries in consultation with appropriate surgical specialists.

In moribund trauma victims, a thoracotomy sometimes is performed in the emergency department as a therapeutic measure to control hemorrhage or relieve tamponade. Urgent thoracotomy in the emergency department is most successful when applied to victims of isolated, penetrating trauma to the heart (especially stab wounds) who have not irreversibly lost signs of cerebral viability (Mattox & Wall, 1997). Although thoracotomy in the emergency depart-

ment can be life saving in some patients, in others it offers no realistic probability of salvaging the patient and exposes physicians and nurses at the bedside to infectious risks (eg, hepatitis and human immunodeficiency virus). Victims found without signs of life and without vital signs in the field have no meaningful hope of survival (Brown & Grover, 1997). Because of the dismal survival results, thoracotomy in the emergency department usually is not appropriate in the following groups of patients: (1) those without signs of life at the time of initial prehospital field assessment, and (2) those with cardiac arrest after blunt chest trauma (Lorenz et al., 1992).

REFERENCES

American College of Surgeons Committee on Trauma, 1993: Advanced Trauma Life Support. American College of Surgeons, Chicago

Asensio JA, Stewart BM, Murray J, et al., 1996: Penetrating cardiac injuries. Surg Clin North Am 76:685

Baker JL, 1990: Management of thoracic trauma by the emergency physician. In Turney SZ, Rodriguez A, Cowley RA (eds): Management of Cardiothoracic Trauma. Baltimore, Williams & Wilkins

Boyd AD, Glassman LR, 1997: Trauma to the lung. Chest Surg Clin N Am 7:263

Brown J, Grover FL, 1997: Trauma to the heart. Chest Surg Clin N Am 7:325

Calhoon JH, Trinkle JK, 1997: Pathophysiology of chest trauma. Chest Surg Clin N Am 7:199

Cohn PF, Braunwald E, 1997: Traumatic heart disease. In Braunwald E (ed): Heart Disease: A Textbook of Cardiovascular Medicine, ed. 5. Philadelphia, WB Saunders

Cowley RA, Turney SZ, Hankins JR, et al., 1990: Rupture of the thoracic aorta caused by blunt trauma. J Thorac Cardiovasc Surg 100:652

Crawford FA Jr, 1997: Penetrating cardiac injuries. In Sabiston DC Jr (ed): Textbook of Surgery: The Biological Basis of Modern Surgical Practice, ed. 15. Philadelphia, WB Saunders

Elefteriades JA, Geha AS, Cohen LS, 1996a: Thoracic imaging in acute disease. In House Officer Guide to ICU Care: Fundamentals of Management of the Heart and Lungs, ed. 2. Philadelphia, Lippincott-Raven

Elefteriades JA, Geha AS, Cohen LS, 1996b: Chest trauma. In House Officer Guide to ICU Care: Fundamentals of Management of the Heart and Lungs, ed. 2. Philadelphia, Lippincott-Raven

Finkelmeier BA, Mentzer RM Jr, Kaiser DL, et al., 1982: Chronic traumatic aneurysm. J Thorac Cardiovasc Surg 84:257

Follette DM, 1991: Penetrating cardiac injuries: A look to the future. Ann Thorac Surg 51:701

Ganzel BL, Gray LA, 1991: Diaphragmatic injuries. In Webb WR, Besson A (eds): Thoracic Surgery: Surgical Management of Chest Injuries, vol. 7. St. Louis, Mosby–Year Book

Hudak CM, Gallo BM, Morton PG, 1998: Trauma. In Critical Care Nursing: A Holistic Approach, ed. 7. Philadelphia, Lippincott Williams & Wilkins

Lockhart CG, 1986: Thoracic trauma. Critical Care Quarterly 9:32

Lorenz HP, Steinmetz B, Lieberman J, et al., 1992: Emergency thoracotomy: Survival correlates with physiologic status. J Trauma 32:780

Mansour KA, 1997: Trauma to the diaphragm. Chest Surg Clin N Am 7:373

Mathisen DJ, Grillo HC, 1991: Airway trauma: Laryngotracheal trauma. In Webb WR, Besson A (eds): Thoracic Surgery: Surgical Management of Chest Injuries, vol. 7. St. Louis, Mosby–Year Book

Mattox KL, 1989: Fact and fiction about management of aortic transection. Ann Thorac Surg 48:1

Mattox KL, Wall MJ Jr, 1997: Newer diagnostic measures and emergency management. Chest Surg Clin N Am 7:213

Mayberry JC, Trunkey DD, 1997: The fractured rib in chest wall trauma. Chest Surg Clin N Am 7:373

McElvein RB, Novick WM, 1991: Chest wall fractures. In Webb WR, Besson A (eds): Thoracic Surgery: Surgical Management of Chest Injuries, vol. 7. St. Louis, Mosby–Year Book

McLean TR, Olinger GN, Thorsen MK, 1991: Computed tomography in the evaluation of the aorta in patients sustaining blunt chest trauma. J Trauma 31:254

Miller OL, Calhoon JH, 1998: Acute traumatic aortic transection. In Kaiser LR, Kron IL, Spray TL (eds): Mastery of Cardiothoracic Surgery. Philadelphia, Lippincott Williams & Wilkins

Pezzella AT, Silva WE, Lancey RA, 1998: Cardiothoracic trauma. Curr Probl Surg 35:647

Richardson JD, Miller FB, Carrillo EH, Spain DA, 1996: Complex thoracic injuries. Surg Clin North Am 76:725

Rodriguez A, 1990a: Injuries of the chest wall, the lungs, and the pleura. In Turney SZ, Rodriguez A, Cowley RA (eds): Management of Cardiothoracic Trauma. Baltimore, Williams & Wilkins

Rodriguez A, 1990b: Initial patient evaluation and indications for thoracotomy. In Turney SZ, Rodriguez A, Cowley RA (eds): Management of Cardiothoracic Trauma. Baltimore, Williams & Wilkins

Rodriguez A, 1990c: Injuries to the diaphragm. In Turney SZ, Rodriguez A, Cowley RA (eds): Management of Cardiothoracic Trauma. Baltimore, Williams & Wilkins

Shapiro MJ, Yanofsky SD, Trapp J, et al., 1991: Cardiovascular evaluation in blunt thoracic trauma using transesophageal echocardiography (TEE). J Trauma 31:835

Sweeney MS, Young J, Frazier OH, et al., 1997: Traumatic aortic transections: Eight-year experience with the "clamp-sew" technique. Ann Thorac Surg 64:384

Symbas PN, Justicz AG, 1996: Cardiac trauma. In Kvetan V, Dantzker DR (eds): The Critically Ill Cardiac Patient: Multisystem Dysfunction and Management. Philadelphia, Lippincott-Raven

Turney SZ, Rodriguez A, 1990: Injuries to the great thoracic vessels. In Turney SZ, Rodriguez A, Cowley RA (eds): Management of Cardiothoracic Trauma. Baltimore, Williams & Wilkins

Unkle DW, Smejkal R, O'Malley KF, 1989: Myocardial contusion without creatine kinase-MB elevation. Heart Lung 18:539

Wall MJ, Hirshberg A, Mattox KL, 1998: Pitfalls in the care of the injured patient. Curr Probl Surg 35:1019

Warren RL, Hilgenberg AD, McCabe DJ, 1996: Blunt and penetrating trauma to the great vessels. In Baue AE, Geha AS, Hammond GL, et al. (eds): Glenn's Thoracic and Cardiovascular Surgery, ed 6. Stamford, CT, Appleton & Lange

Weissberg D, Utkin V, 1991: Airway trauma: Tracheobronchial trauma. In Webb WR, Besson A (eds): Thoracic Surgery: Surgical Management of Chest Injuries, vol. 7. St. Louis, Mosby–Year Book

Wiles CE III, 1990: Critical care of chest trauma. In Turney SZ, Rodriguez A, Cowley RA (eds): Management of Cardiothoracic Trauma. Baltimore, Williams & Wilkins

Wisner D, 1995: Trauma to the chest. In Sabiston DC Jr, Spencer FC (eds): Surgery of the Chest, ed. 6. Philadelphia, WB Saunders

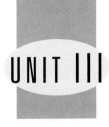

UNIT III

Thoracic Surgery

SURGICAL DISEASES
OF THE CHEST

Pulmonary, Tracheal, and Pleural Diseases

► Lung Cancer

Carcinoma of the lung was relatively uncommon until the early 20th century. Since that time, however, the incidence has increased dramatically. Lung cancer is now one of the most common malignant diseases and a major health problem throughout the world. An estimated 171,500 new cases of lung cancer are diagnosed in the United States annually, and lung cancer is now the leading cause of death from cancer in both men and women (Landis et al., 1998). The incidence of lung cancer is even higher elsewhere in the world; Hungary and the former Czechoslovakia have the two highest lung cancer death rates (Benfield & Russell, 1996).

Lung cancer develops most often in late middle age or in elderly people. Although it continues to occur more frequently in men, the incidence in women has been climbing steadily. The ratio of men to women was formerly 8:1; it is now less than 2:1 (Shields et al., 1994). The incidence rates of lung cancer vary considerably by race and ethnicity; in the United States, the highest incidence rates for lung cancer in men are among African Americans, and among women, in Alaskan natives and African Americans (Parker et al., 1998).

Etiologic Factors

A number of factors are associated with an increased incidence of lung cancer. Cigarette smoking is believed to be the most significant etiologic factor. It is thought to be responsible for approximately 80% of lung cancer cases (Baldini & Strauss, 1997). Although smoking among adults has declined substantially in the United States since the late 1960s, the downward trend appears to have leveled off. Currently, more than 48 million adult and 4.1 million adolescent Americans are smokers (American Heart Association, 1998). The prevalence of smoking among women is expected to surpass that in men by the year 2000; among women, smoking rates are highest among young girls and those with less education (Baldini & Strauss, 1998).

The risk for development of lung cancer is directly related to the number of cigarettes smoked per day, the duration of smoking, the depth of inhalation, and the amount of tar and nicotine in the cigarettes smoked; heavy smokers have 25 times as many lung cancers as nonsmokers (Benfield & Russell, 1996). Cigarette smoking also markedly increases risk imposed by other environmental carcinogens. Although cessation of smoking is associated with a progressively declining risk, previous smokers continue at higher risk for the remainder of their lives (Mulshine & Tockman, 1992).

A causal association also has been demonstrated between exposure to environmental tobacco smoke and the risk of lung cancer. In epidemiologic studies of women who have never smoked, a significant excess risk of lung cancer has been demonstrated among those with exposure to environmental tobacco smoke from spouses; this risk increases with the number of cigarettes smoked by the spouse and the duration of the marriage (Hackshaw, 1998). Heavy environmental pollution (eg, air pollution, toxic waste hazards) also increases the risk for development of lung cancer (Woodward & Boffetta, 1997). Lung cancer is more common in urban areas and in people with chronically diseased and scarred lungs. Specifically identified industrial carcinogens that predispose to lung cancer include asbestos, radioactive material, arsenic, and nickel (Shields et al., 1994).

Genetic factors also contribute to development of lung cancer. Epidemiologic studies consistently demonstrate an excess of lung cancer in some families that cannot be accounted for by chance or common environmental exposure (Sellers et al., 1991). Genetic risk appears to augment environmental carcinogens, supporting an ecogenetic etiology; that is, a genetic predisposition is present but requires the environmental factor (eg, smoking) to induce the disease (Miller, 1995). People in whom lung cancer develops are at increased risk for development of a second primary lung tumor, particularly if cigarette smoking is continued. The risk for development of a second lung cancer in patients who have survived resection of a non-small cell lung tumor is approximately 1% to 2% per patient per year; the risk in survivors of small cell lung cancer is approximately 6% per patient per year (Johnson, 1998).

Histologic Cell Types

Bronchogenic carcinoma, which arises from the epithelial lining of the bronchi, is by far the most common form of lung cancer and accounts for approximately 90% of cases. Far less common are bronchoalveolar carcinoma, originating in the lung parenchyma itself, and mesothelioma, which arises in the pleura. Bronchogenic carcinoma is categorized broadly as non-small cell or small cell carcinoma. Non-small cell lung tumors, which comprise 75% to 80% of lung cancer, are divided into three major histologic cell types: (1) adenocarcinoma, (2) squamous or epidermoid carcinoma, and (3) large cell carcinoma. Some lung tumors have a mixed histologic type (eg, both squamous and adenocarcinomatous features). Pathologic determination of cell type has significant therapeutic importance. Nearly all surgical candidates have one of the three major types of non-small cell tumors, whereas patients with small cell tumors are rarely surgical candidates because of advanced disease at presentation. Chemotherapy is the primary therapeutic modality for small cell lung cancer (Shields, 1996).

Adenocarcinoma comprises approximately 50% of lung tumors (D'Amico & Sabiston, 1995). Its increasing incidence has caused it to surpass squamous cell carcinoma as the most common form of lung cancer. Adenocarcinoma occurs more commonly in women. It is the histologic subtype most likely to occur in nonsmokers in whom lung cancer develops (Sridhar & Raub, 1992). Adenocarcinoma usually originates in the lung periphery, arising from the epithelium of distal bronchi to form a small nodule. The tumors characteristically grow at an intermediate rate, more slowly than small cell tumors but faster than squamous cell lesions (Shields et al., 1994).

Adenocarcinoma tends to metastasize to mediastinal, periaortic, axillary, supraclavicular, or neck lymph nodes; pleural involvement also is common, as are extrathoracic metastases, typically to the adrenal glands, liver, bone, or brain (Benfield & Russell, 1996). Some adenocarcinomas occur in conjunction with areas of scarring or chronic interstitial fibrosis. These so-called *scar carcinomas* most frequently arise in the peripheral portions of the upper lobes, particularly in the apical segment (Auerbach & Garfinkel, 1991).

Bronchoalveolar cancer may represent a highly differentiated form of adenocarcinoma, although many pathologists regard it as a separate and distinct histologic form (Shields et al., 1994). It is an unusual form of lung cancer that spreads along alveolar walls. The incidence of bronchoalveolar carcinoma has increased worldwide (Benfield & Russell, 1996). The increase in adenocarcinoma and bronchoalveolar carcinoma actually may represent a decrease in cell types strongly linked to smoking (ie, squamous cell and small cell), owing to the increased use of filters and decreased nicotine content in cigarettes and a decreased quantity of smoking (Auerbach & Garfinkel, 1991; Sridhar & Raub, 1992). Bronchoalveolar carcinoma also is referred to as alveolar cell carcinoma, bronchioloalveolar carcinoma, and bronchiolar carcinoma.

Squamous cell carcinoma comprises 30% to 35% of lung cancer. It almost always occurs in people with a long smoking history. Squamous cell tumors usually are located centrally in major bronchi, usually the lobar or first segmental bronchus of the upper lobes or the superior segment of the lower lobes (Zaman, 1995). Squamous tumors are relatively slow growing. They often remain within the thorax, spreading by direct extension and invasion of hilar, mediastinal, and supraclavicular lymph nodes. Metastases occur late and even then are limited for some time to peribronchial or hilar lymph nodes (Zaman, 1995). The tumor frequently is detected late in the disease when bronchial obstruction leads to atelectasis or pneumonia.

Large cell carcinoma, comprising 7% to 10% of lung cancer, includes undifferentiated tumors and giant cell and clear cell variants. Approximately half of large cell undifferentiated tumors arise in subsegmental or larger bronchi, and half are peripheral and subpleural in location (Benfield & Russell, 1996). Large cell carcinomas typically are large, rapidly growing, bulky tumors with areas of necrosis.

Small cell carcinoma accounts for 20% to 25% of lung cancer. Most people in whom small cell tumors develop have a smoking history, especially women. Women who smoke appear to have a higher risk for development of small cell lung cancer than men who smoke (Baldini & Strauss, 1997). Small cell lung cancer is highly malignant and is characterized by a rapid tumor doubling time, early and widespread dissemination, and relatively short patient survival. Most tumors are located centrally. More than two thirds of patients have clinically evident distant metastases at the time of diagnosis (Govindan & Ihde, 1997). Because of the rapid systemic spread, surgical resectability is uncommon.

Rarely, patients have multiple primary lung carcinomas. *Synchronous tumors* are separate primary lung tumors occurring simultaneously in different locations. They may have different histologic cell types or the same cell type. *Metachronous tumors* are primary lung tumors that develop as separate occurrences separated by an interval of time. Given the prevalence of bronchogenic cancer and the fact that inhaled carcinogens affect large areas of respiratory epithelium, it is presumed that metachronous tumors would occur more commonly if survival from primary lung cancer were not so limited (Fleisher et al., 1991). The predominant histologic cell type in patients with synchronous or metachronous lung tumors is squamous cell (Rosengart et al., 1991).

Tumor Location and Routes of Extension

Lung neoplasms occur more commonly in the right lung, and usually in the upper lobes (Shields et al., 1994). The location of the tumor usually is categorized as central, peripheral, or apical. Lesions are termed central if they involve the mainstem, lobar, or segmental bronchi and peripheral if they originate in distal bronchi, bronchioles, or lung parenchyma. Central lesions are associated with a poorer prognosis because the tumor often spreads to hilar and mediastinal lymph nodes before detection. Peripheral lesions occasionally are detected on a routine chest roentgenogram while the patient is still without symptoms. A tumor in the extreme apex of either lung is referred to as a superior sulcus tumor. Because of their location, superior sulcus tumors invade the pleura and adjacent structures, producing classic signs and symptoms (McLauglin, 1996). Superior sulcus tumors also are called Pancoast tumors, named for the physician who described the clinical and radiologic characteristics of the tumor.

Lung tumors can disseminate by three routes. The first is by direct extension. Tumors can grow directly into pulmonary parenchyma, across fissures, along a bronchus, and into adjacent structures in the thorax, such as the pleura, chest wall, or mediastinal organs. Second, lung tumors spread through the lymphatic system. Even small tumors may be associated with hilar or mediastinal lymph node metastasis. Undifferentiated small cell lesions are most likely to spread in this manner, followed by undifferentiated large cell, adenocarcinoma, and squamous cell tumors (Shields et al., 1994). The third route of metastasis is hematologic spread. Tumor cells invade branches of the pulmonary veins in the lung and are disseminated to distant structures through the vascular system. The most common sites of lung cancer metastasis are demonstrated in Figure 33-1.

Clinical Manifestations

Occasionally, a lung neoplasm is detected before development of symptoms when a chest roentgenogram taken for another purpose displays an abnormal shadow. However, 90% to 95% of patients with lung cancer are symptomatic at the time of diagnosis (Shields, 1996). The clinical signs and symptoms depend on size and location of the tumor, extent of spread to adjacent or distant structures, and occurrence of associated hormonal syndromes. Bronchopulmonary symptoms, such as cough, hemoptysis, and respiratory infection, are common secondary to the presence of the tumor causing bronchial irritation, obstruction, or ulceration (Shields, 1996). Cough occurs in most patients. Patients often have persistent upper respiratory tract infections or pneumonia due to bronchial obstruction. Other pulmonary manifestations include dyspnea, wheezing, and lung abscess (Maddaus & Ginsberg, 1995). Nonspecific symptoms associated with lung cancer include weight loss, anorexia, and malaise.

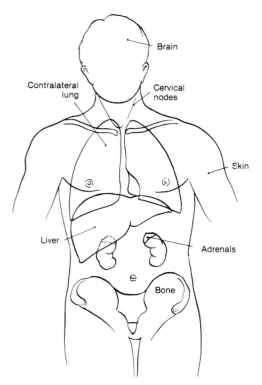

FIGURE 33-1. Common sites of metastasis in patients with carcinoma of the lung. (Beahrs OH, Myers MH [eds], 1992: American Joint Committee on Cancer: Manual for Staging of Cancer, ed. 4, p. 122. Philadelphia, JB Lippincott)

If the tumor has spread beyond the lung itself to involve pleura, chest wall, mediastinal structures, or nerves, the patient may experience corresponding symptoms. Compression of the recurrent laryngeal nerve may cause hoarseness; brachial nerve compression may produce persistent arm or shoulder pain; esophageal compression may result in dysphagia; pleural invasion may cause pleural effusion; and extensive mediastinal spread can produce superior vena cava syndrome, manifested by swelling of the face and upper extremities and venous distention in the neck and anterior chest wall.

Pancoast's syndrome describes the characteristic clinical manifestations associated with superior sulcus tumors (ie, severe pain and Horner's syndrome). Localized pain typically begins in the shoulder. The pain becomes unremitting with time and spreads to the medial area of the scapula, then along the ulnar distribution of the arm to involve the elbow (T1 distribution) and the medial forearm and hand (C8 distribution) (McLaughlin, 1996). Horner's syndrome (ie, ptosis, pupillary constriction, vasodilatation, and anhidrosis [absence of sweat secretion]) occurs on the affected side of the face and upper extremity. Extrathoracic manifestations of lung cancer, such as elevated liver enzyme levels, Cushing's syndrome, excessive antidiuretic hormone production, hypercalcemia, hypoglycemia, and carcinoid syndrome, can occur because of distant metastases or the secretion of endocrine-like substances by the tumor (termed *paraneoplastic syndrome*).

Diagnosis

Diagnostic modalities for evaluation of lung cancer are used to achieve two objectives: (1) identification of the histologic cell type of the tumor, and (2) determination of the extent of tumor metastasis to adjacent structures, the lymphatic system, or distant structures. The most common and probably most important diagnostic study for lung cancer is the chest roentgenogram. Although it does not establish cell type, it does give essential information regarding the location and nature of a lung tumor. Both posteroanterior and lateral films are obtained to provide a three-dimensional view of the chest. Comparison with past chest radiographs provides important information about initial onset of the lesion and its rate of growth. If the tumor has invaded the chest wall, the chest roentgenogram may demonstrate rib destruction.

Computed tomographic (CT) scanning, a technique for imaging cross-sectional anatomy, is performed routinely in patients with suspected lung cancer to detect and evaluate mediastinal lymphadenopathy (ie, abnormal enlargement of mediastinal lymph nodes) that may represent malignant invasion. CT scanning also may demonstrate invasion of the vertebral bodies; reveal the presence of small, undetected pleural effusions; or suggest encirclement of vital structures by the tumor (Shields, 1997). When a chest CT scan is obtained for evaluation of a patient with lung cancer, the upper abdomen is included in the scan so that occult liver or adrenal metastasis may be detected. Positron emission tomography (PET) scanning with [18F]fluorodeoxyglucose (FDG) has proven helpful in characterizing radiographic lung lesions, staging known lung cancer, and identifying recurrent disease after treatment (Lowe & Naunheim, 1998). PET-FDG imaging is very sensitive for detection of cancer in patients who have indeterminate lesions on CT scanning and is thought to be more accurate than CT in evaluating hilar and mediastinal lymph node status (Al-Sugair & Coleman, 1998).

Direct evaluation of the tracheobronchial tree using a fiberoptic bronchoscope is performed in all patients suspected of having lung cancer. Bronchoscopy allows a thorough examination of segmental and subsegmental bronchi. Bronchoscopic visualization of the affected area may reveal the tumor itself exposed in bronchial mucosa or changes in the bronchial wall or lumen size caused by tumor infiltration or external compression (Shields, 1996). In addition, tissue for histologic evaluation or cells for cytologic examination may be obtained by (1) biopsy of a small piece of bronchial tissue, (2) brushing the surface of the lesion, or (3) aspirating fluid washed over the suspect area. A transbronchial fine-needle aspiration of mediastinal lymph nodes may be performed when rigidity is present and when enlarged lymph nodes have been identified by CT examination (Shields, 1997).

Cytologic evaluation of sputum (sputum cytology) may be performed in patients with large tumors involving a main bronchus. Tumors most likely to produce a positive sputum cytology are those that are centrally located, large, or a squamous cell type (Shields, 1996). A transthoracic needle biopsy is performed occasionally to obtain tissue from lesions located in the lung periphery. Although transthoracic needle biopsy often is successful in establishing a diagnosis, there is a significant incidence of false-negative results. Because thoracotomy usually is necessary to prove absence of malignancy, transthoracic needle biopsy is most useful to obtain a diagnosis in patients who are not candidates for surgical resection. If none of these diagnostic measures yields a definitive diagnosis of lung cancer, or if surgical exploration is likely in any case, an exploratory thoracotomy may be performed before definitive confirmation of malignancy. Thoracoscopy is used to obtain tissue if less invasive diagnostic efforts have been unsuccessful. A frozen section pathologic evaluation can be performed during the procedure. If malignant disease is detected, the operation can be converted to a thoracotomy for pulmonary resection.

A number of diagnostic studies may be useful in detecting tumor metastasis to lymph nodes or distant structures. Mediastinoscopy or, less commonly, mediastinotomy, often is performed for biopsy of mediastinal lymph nodes. Mediastinoscopy is the most sensitive and specific modality for pathologic staging of the mediastinum (Krasna et al., 1999). Metastasis to mediastinal lymph nodes is present in nearly one half of patients with non-small cell lung cancer (Nakanishi et al., 1997). If lymph nodes in the supraclavicular fossa (scalene nodes) are palpable, an incisional biopsy of the enlarged node may be performed to obtain tissue for histologic examination. Brain, liver, or bone scans may be performed in patients in whom distant metastasis is suspected. Diagnostic studies used in the evaluation of thoracic surgical diseases are described in further detail in Chapter 36, Diagnostic Evaluation of Thoracic Diseases.

Staging of Lung Cancer

To classify extent of disease, direct therapy, and provide more accurate prognostic information, standard nomenclature for pathologic classification was developed by the American Joint Committee on Cancer Staging and End Results Reporting (Beahrs & Myers, 1978). The classification system has since been expanded and revised into the currently used *International Staging System,* which consists of a three-letter code: the first letter, "T," categorizes tumor size; the second, "N," the presence and extent of nodal involvement; and the third, "M," the presence of distant metastases (Mountain, 1986, 1997) (Table 33-1).

Depending on TNM designation, the stage of the patient's disease is categorized (Table 33-2). Stage 0 (also called *occult*) lung cancer is present when cytologic examination of sputum reveals malignant cells but there is no identifiable lesion on the chest roentgenogram. Occult neoplasm is rare and nearly always represents in situ or early invasive squamous cell carcinoma (Pairolero et al., 1989). The other stages signify progressively larger and more invasive tumors. Stage I disease is confined to the lung parenchyma and visceral pleura; stage II tumors have metastasized to or directly invaded intrapleural but not mediastinal lymph nodes; stage IIIA is defined by ipsilateral (ie, same side) mediastinal node metastases or

---

TABLE 33-1

International Staging System for Lung Cancer: TNM Definitions

PRIMARY TUMOR (T)

TX	Primary tumor cannot be assessed, or tumor proven by the presence of malignant cells in sputum or bronchial washings but not visualized by imaging or bronchoscopy
T0	No evidence of primary tumor
Tis	Carcinoma *in situ*
T1	Tumor ≤3 cm in greatest dimension, surrounded by lung or visceral pleura, without bronchoscopic evidence of invasion more proximal than the lobar bronchus (ie, not in the main bronchus)
T2	Tumor with any of the following features of size or extent: >3 cm in greatest dimension Involves main bronchus, ≥2 cm distal to the carina Invades the visceral pleura Associated with atelectasis or obstructive pneumonitis that extends to the hilar region but does not involve the entire lung
T3	Tumor of any size that directly invades any of the following: chest wall (including superior sulcus tumors), diaphragm, mediastinal pleura, parietal pericardium; or tumor in the main bronchus <2 cm distal to the carina but without involvement of the carina; or associated atelectasis or obstructive pneumonitis of the entire lung
T4	Tumor any size that invades any of the following: mediastinum, heart, great vessels, trachea, esophagus, vertebral body, carina; or tumor with a malignant pleural or pericardial effusion, or with satellite tumor nodule(s) within the ipsilateral primary tumor lobe of the lung

NODAL INVOLVEMENT (N)

NX	Regional lymph nodes cannot be assessed
N0	No regional lymph node metastasis
N1	Metastasis to ipsilateral peribronchial or ipsilateral hilar lymph nodes, and intrapulmonary nodes involved by direct extension of the primary tumor
N2	Metastasis to ipsilateral mediastinal or subcarinal lymph nodes
N3	Metastasis to contralateral mediastinal, contralateral hilar, ipsilateral or contralateral scalene, or supraclavicular lymph node(s)

DISTANT METASTASIS (M)

MX	Presence of distant metastasis cannot be assessed
M0	No distant metastasis
M1	Distant metastasis present

From Mountain CF, 1997: Revisions in the international system for staging lung cancer. Chest 111:1710.

---

direct invasion of potentially resectable structures; stage IIIB connotes involvement of scalene or contralateral lymph nodes, malignant pleural effusion, or invasion of unresectable structures; and stage IV is characterized by distant metastasis (Ponn & Federico, 1998).

Stage I lung cancer is considered early disease with a favorable prognosis after surgical resection; stage II tu-

TABLE 33-2

International Staging System for Lung Cancer: Stage Grouping

Stage	TNM Subset
0	Carcinoma *in situ*
IA	T1 N0 M0
IB	T2 N0 M0
IIA	T1 N1 M0
IIB	T2 N1 M0
	T3 N0 M0
IIIA	T3 N1 M0
	T1 N2 M0
	T2 N2 M0
	T3 N2 M0
IIIB	T4 N0 M0
	T4 N1 M0
	T4 N2 M0
	T1 N3 M0
	T2 N3 M0
	T3 N3 M0
	T4 N3 M0
IV	Any T any N M1

From Mountain CF, 1997: Revisions in the international system for staging lung cancer. Chest 111:1710.

mors are intermediate; and stage III and IV tumors are considered advanced with a poor prognosis (Martini et al., 1992). However, within each stage there may be marked differences in postoperative 5-year survival rates; for example, in stage I, T2 N0 M0 tumors have a 5-year survival rate that is 10% or more below that of T1 N0 M0 tumors (Maddaus & Ginsberg, 1995). The most recent refinement of the International Staging System recognizes this difference by subcategorizing T1 N0 M0 tumors as stage IA disease and T2 N0 M0 tumors as stage IB disease. Staging categories may be determined at the completion of the diagnostic evaluation (clinical), at the time of thoracotomy (surgical), or by examination of the resected specimen (pathologic) (Shields, 1997).

Although the TNM staging system provides useful prognostic information about non-small cell lung tumors, it is not as useful for small cell lung cancer. Instead, small cell tumors usually are categorized broadly as limited or extensive disease. Limited small cell cancer is defined as disease confined to one hemithorax with or without contralateral hilar or ipsilateral supraclavicular lymph node involvement; extensive small cell lung cancer signifies that the disease has spread beyond these limits (Shields, 1997).

Treatment

Despite intensive research and treatment efforts during the past several decades, survival prognosis for patients diagnosed with lung cancer continues to be poor. Only 10% to 13% of patients survive 5 years after diagnosis (Burt et al., 1996). For non-small cell lung cancer, the treatment of choice is surgical resection of the tumor and surrounding lymphatic tissue. The selection of the specific operative procedure depends on location and size of the tumor, whether spread to regional lymph nodes has occurred, involvement of extrapulmonary structures, and the patient's age and general medical condition, particularly pulmonary and cardiovascular function.

Surgical treatment of lung cancer is performed predominantly in patients with stage I or stage II non-small cell lung tumors (Fig. 33-2). A curative procedure in these patients necessitates a pulmonary resection that completely eradicates the tumor yet leaves the patient with adequate lung function. Pulmonary resection procedures always are accompanied by sampling of the ipsilateral superior mediastinal and subcarinal lymphatic stations or by a systematic mediastinal lymph node dissection (Shields, 1997). Lobectomy (removal on an entire lobe) in general is considered the minimum definitive pulmonary resection because it is an anatomic resection that removes the regional lymph nodes located along the

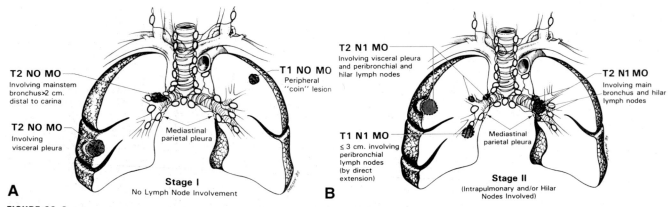

FIGURE 33-2. (**A**) Stage I lung cancer includes T1 N0 M0 (stage IA) and T2 N0 M0 (stage IB) tumors. (**B**) Stage II includes T1 N1 M0 (stage IIA) and T2 N1 M0 (stage IIB) tumors; not shown in this illustration, but also included in stage IIB, are T3 N0 M0 tumors. (Mountain CF, 1986: A new international staging system for lung cancer. Chest 4:230S)

lobar bronchus and ensures an adequate tumor-free parenchymal margin (Kaiser, 1998).

In patients whose pulmonary function precludes lobectomy, it may be possible to accomplish complete resection with removal of only the tumor itself and minimal surrounding lung tissue, if the lesion is small and located in the periphery. This procedure, termed a *wedge resection,* sacrifices the least amount of normal lung tissue. If an entire segment of a lobe is removed, the procedure is termed a *segmentectomy.* More commonly, lung tumors are positioned in such a way that a curative resection necessitates performance of a lobectomy. In some instances, right-sided lung tumors necessitate removal of two of the three lobes (ie, a bilobectomy) for curative resection.

Removal of an entire lung, or pneumonectomy, may be necessary if the tumor is centrally located or involves more than one lobe. A pneumonectomy sacrifices considerably more lung tissue but usually is tolerated well in patients with adequate pulmonary function. Patients with moderate impairment of pulmonary function, however, may be unable to withstand loss of an entire lung. A sleeve resection (ie, removal of a lobe with its attaching bronchus and reimplantation of the remaining lobe) is performed in selected situations, primarily when a tumor is located at a major lobar orifice and impaired pulmonary function precludes pneumonectomy (Martini & Ginsberg, 1995; Van Schil et al., 1991).

Curative pulmonary resection is possible in a limited number of stage IIIA lung tumors (eg, peripheral tumors that have invaded the parietal pleura, pericardium, diaphragm, or chest wall or are located in the main bronchus within 2 cm of the carina). If a tumor has invaded structures adjacent to the lung, an extended resection, including the chest wall or diaphragm, may be performed concomitantly with the pulmonary resection. In patients with parietal pleura or chest wall invasion and no evidence of mediastinal lymph node involvement (ie, N2 disease), the operative approach includes resection of overlying parietal pleura and en bloc chest wall resection in addition to the appropriate pulmonary resection (Burt et al., 1996; Albertucci et al., 1992). Prognosis appears to be influenced less by spread to the chest wall than by the presence of tumor in lymph tissue (Allen et al., 1991). Depending on the size and location of the defect created by the removal of rib segments, reconstruction of the chest wall with placement of prosthetic material may be necessary.

Pulmonary resection also may include removal of a portion of the pericardium or diaphragm if either has been invaded by tumor. If the tumor encroaches on the carina of the mainstem trachea, curative resection usually is considered technically infeasible. A sleeve pneumonectomy (ie, carinal resection and reconstruction in combination with pneumonectomy) may be considered for carefully selected patients with bulky central tumors involving the carina or tracheobronchial angle (Burt et al., 1996; Mathisen & Grillo, 1991).

In stage IIIA tumors with N2 (ipsilateral mediastinal or subcarinal lymph node) involvement, surgical resection is possible only rarely. In general, surgical resection is performed in this subset of patients only when mediastinal lymph node involvement, or N2 disease, is not detected before surgery but rather is detected by pathologic diagnosis at the time of thoracotomy. Although many physicians consider N2 disease incurable, some surgeons advocate complete resection with extensive mediastinal lymph node dissection when N2 disease is detected at thoracotomy, in the belief that these patients have a better prognosis than those with mediastinal lymph node metastasis that is clinically apparent (Nakanishi et al., 1997).

Long-term results of surgical treatment for non-small cell lung tumors depend primarily on the stage of the tumor as determined by pathologic staging. The 5-year survival rate after surgical resection of stage I (T1 N0 M0 or T2 N0 M0) non-small cell lung cancer is approximately 75%; stage II (T1 N1 M0 or T2 N1 M0) disease is associated with a 39% to 49% 5-year survival rate after surgical resection (Burt et al., 1996). Few patients with stage IIIA non-small cell lung cancer are treated surgically. Pulmonary resection procedures are discussed in more detail in Chapter 38, Surgical Treatment of Pulmonary Diseases.

Although surgical treatment is the most effective therapy for non-small cell lung cancer, only 30% to 40% of newly diagnosed patients are candidates for curative resection (Carney, 1998). In most patients, the extent of disease at the time of diagnosis precludes surgical treatment. Evidence of extrapulmonary tumor spread, such as paralysis of the recurrent laryngeal nerve, superior vena cava syndrome, phrenic nerve paralysis, pleural effusion containing malignant cells, extrathoracic metastases, or involvement of the main pulmonary artery, contraindicates pulmonary resection. Pulmonary resection also may be precluded by a prohibitive operative risk in patients with marginal cardiopulmonary reserve. Small cell lung cancer seldom is treated with surgical resection, except as one component of multimodal therapy in patients with early stage disease.

Radiation therapy may be used as an adjunct to surgical resection or as the primary treatment modality when pulmonary resection is not a viable option. For most types of lung cancer, radiation therapy alone is unlikely to be curative. Radiation therapy often is administered after surgical resection if histologic examination of lymph nodes sampled at the time of operation reveals malignant cells. Preoperative radiation seldom is performed because it delays operation and increases operative morbidity. In patients with Pancoast tumors, however, preoperative radiation may be successful in converting a nonresectable tumor into one that can be removed surgically.

Brachytherapy may be considered for tumors that prove to be surgically nonresectable at thoracotomy because of invasion of adjacent structures or inability of the patient to tolerate the necessary pulmonary resection. Brachytherapy is the direct application of radioactive sources either into a tumor (interstitial) or into a naturally occurring cavity (intracavitary), such as the bronchus (Armstrong, 1995). It delivers a higher tumor dose compared with external-beam radiation, while sparing normal tissue outside the tumor (Hilaris & Mastoras, 1998). Brachytherapy is used uncommonly and it is unclear whether it provides any benefit over external-beam radiation in controlling local spread or increasing survival. The most effective application appears to be endobronchial brachytherapy to provide palliative treatment of obstructive symptoms and hemoptysis in patients with inoperable tumors (Gaspar, 1998).

Chemotherapy is the primary form of therapy used in patients with small cell lung cancer. Combination chemotherapy, with either platinum plus etoposide or cyclophosphamide, Adriamycin, and vincristine, appears to offer the best chance for improved survival (Clark & Ihde, 1998). Thoracic irradiation may be used as adjunctive therapy depending on the stage of the tumor. Prophylactic brain irradiation sometimes is performed as well to lessen the disabling effects of brain metastasis. Surgical resection sometimes is performed along with the other two modalities for patients with resectable small cell tumors and limited-stage disease. Although the role of surgical resection in patients with small cell lung cancer is controversial, it may reduce the frequency of local recurrences and surgical staging may be of clinical significance (Lassen & Hansen, 1999). Despite intensive research with various multimodal treatment regimens for small cell lung cancer, survival prognosis remains poor. Median survival time for patients with limited-stage disease ranges from 14 to 16 months, and a small proportion may be cured; median survival usually is less than 1 year for those with extensive-stage disease (Shepherd, 1997). Survival beyond 5 years occurs in only 3% to 8% of all patients with small cell lung cancer (Elias, 1997).

For non-small cell lung tumors, chemotherapy usually is reserved for patients with stage II or III disease. Response rates are higher when combination chemotherapy is used as compared with single-agent therapy. Combinations of paclitaxel, gemcitabine, and vinorelbine with cisplatin have been shown to improve survival in patients with advanced-stage disease compared with cisplatin alone or in combination with etoposide (Bunn & Kelly, 1998). Both chemotherapy and radiation are limited by their lack of differentiation between malignant and normal cells; adverse effects can have a significant impact on the patient's quality of life and must be taken into consideration when evaluating the benefits and risks of these treatment modalities (Scott, 1998).

Basic research in the molecular pathogenesis and immunology of lung cancer has suggested that gene therapy may affect treatment of lung cancer in the future. Preliminary results of phase I lung cancer gene therapy clinical trials have demonstrated safety of gene therapy and offer promise of an important future role for gene therapy in the treatment of lung malignancies (Swisher & Roth, 1998).

▶ Other Intrathoracic Malignancies

Metastatic Lung Neoplasms

The lung is a common site of metastasis for many malignancies originating elsewhere. *Pulmonary metastases* typically develop in the periphery of the lung and, because bronchial involvement is uncommon, many patients remain relatively asymptomatic for long periods (Holmes, 1995). Surgical resection of pulmonary metas-

tases sometimes is undertaken in patients in whom it can be expected to affect survival favorably. Factors taken into consideration when selecting patients for surgical therapy include (1) the histologic cell type and behavior of the primary tumor, (2) the presence of other metastatic lesions, and (3) the disease-free interval between treatment of the primary tumor and development of the pulmonary metastasis. However, the presence of more than one lesion or a short disease-free interval does not necessarily preclude surgical resection if the primary tumor has been treated adequately and pulmonary metastases can be resected completely while preserving adequate pulmonary function (Martini & McCormack, 1998).

Tracheal Tumors

Primary tumors of the trachea are rare. In adults, more than 90% of primary tumors of the trachea and carina are malignant and most are squamous cell carcinoma or adenoid cystic carcinoma (Pearson et al., 1995). Tracheal tumors can extend up and down the trachea and metastasize into regional lymph nodes, mediastinal structures, and lung parenchyma. The diagnosis often is not made until the tumor is advanced and the patient experiences airway obstruction. Common manifestations of tracheal tumors are hemoptysis (41%), cough (37%), and signs of progressive airway obstruction, including dyspnea on exertion (54%), wheezing and stridor (35%), and, uncommonly, dysphagia or hoarseness (7%) (Mathisen & Grillo, 1996). Curative resection usually is precluded by an advanced stage of the tumor at the time of diagnosis, but tumor resection and tracheal reconstruction may be performed if the tumor is not extensive and has not metastasized. Radiation therapy also may be used.

Mesothelioma

Mesothelioma is an unusual neoplasm that originates in the pleura. Any portion of the parietal, visceral, or mediastinal pleura may be the site of origin of the tumor, which grows selectively along the pleural surfaces. Extension into the lung parenchyma is unusual. Benign mesothelioma and localized malignant mesothelioma are rare. Most common is a diffuse, malignant variety that is associated with a history of exposure to asbestos.

The latency period between asbestos exposure and development of malignant mesothelioma is 20 to 40 years, and the younger the age at first exposure, the higher the cumulative lifetime risk (Cohen et al., 1995). Because of the long latency period and the fact that measures to limit asbestos were not instituted until the 1970s, the incidence of malignant mesothelioma is expected to continue to rise into the first or second decade of the 21st century (Rusch, 1995). At least 20% of mesotheliomas in the United States are not associated with asbestos exposure, suggesting that additional carcinogens might play a role in patients without asbestos exposure (Pass et al., 1998).

Diffuse malignant mesothelioma occurs most often in men between the ages of 50 and 70 years (Sugarbaker &

Garcia, 1998). Common clinical manifestations include an insidious onset of shortness of breath or nonpleuritic chest pain referred to the upper abdomen or shoulder and a large pleural effusion occupying 50% or more of the hemithorax (Light, 1997). Although abnormalities on the chest roentgenogram or CT scan may be suggestive, definitive diagnosis of mesothelioma is based on biopsy and histologic examination of pleural tissue, usually obtained by thoracoscopy or thoracotomy. All forms of treatment for mesothelioma, and particularly the role of surgical resection, are controversial because none has proven efficacy in prolonging survival.

One of two surgical procedures may be performed: pleurectomy (removal of the parietal pleura) or extrapleural pneumonectomy (resection of the parietal pleura and ipsilateral lung). Of the two procedures, pleurectomy carries a lower operative risk but does not provide complete removal of all gross disease, as does extrapleural pneumonectomy. Radiation and chemotherapy sometimes are used adjunctively to surgical resection. Because none of the available treatment modalities definitively improves survival, many physicians advocate supportive care only in lieu of more aggressive therapy, with chemical sclerosis to relieve the effusion component of the disease (LoCicero, 1996). Trimodal therapy, consisting of extrapleural pneumonectomy followed by combination chemotherapy and radiation therapy, may prolong survival in patients with resectable mesothelioma tumors of an epithelial cell type (Sugarbaker & Garcia, 1998). Regardless of the type of therapy, malignant mesothelioma is usually a fatal disease. Most patients die within 1 to 2 years of diagnosis.

▶ Benign Lung Neoplasms

Benign lung neoplasms are uncommon, comprising only 5% of all lung tumors (Zaman, 1995). The most frequently occurring benign tumor is hamartoma, which also is referred to as chondroma. It occurs more often in men, and in 90% of cases arises in the lung periphery (Shields & Robinson, 1994). Most hamartomas do not produce symptoms, and although they may increase in size, growth usually is slow (Hansen et al., 1992). The tumor often is detected as an incidental finding on a chest roentgenogram. Hamartomas do not require treatment except in the rare instance of symptoms due to bronchial compression, such as atelectasis or infection. However, surgical removal may be necessary to differentiate definitively hamartoma from a malignant tumor. Other less common benign lung neoplasms include fibroma, pulmonary hemangioma, leiomyoma, and papilloma.

▶ Infectious Problems

Pulmonary Infection

Widespread availability of broad-spectrum antibiotics has greatly decreased the incidence of serious *pulmonary infections*. Most susceptible to pulmonary infection are peo-ple who are immunocompromised by disease or immunosuppressive therapy, and hospitalized patients who are critically ill and require mechanical ventilation. The population of immunocompromised patients has grown substantially, principally because of (1) an increased number of transplant recipients who must take immunosuppressive medications to prevent organ rejection, (2) aggressive chemotherapy protocols used to treat lymphoproliferative and neoplastic disorders, and (3) the significant incidence of acquired immunodeficiency syndrome (AIDS) (Van Trigt, 1995). These people are subject to a variety of bacterial, fungal, and parasitic infections.

People who abuse intravenous drugs also are at greater risk for pulmonary infections. Several factors directly related to intravenous substance abuse contribute to development of pulmonary infections, including (1) vomiting and aspiration due to the respiratory depression associated with drug overdose; (2) septic pulmonary emboli secondary to tricuspid valve endocarditis or injection site thrombophlebitis; and (3) the frequency of associated alcoholism, malnourishment, substandard housing, and AIDS (Hoover et al., 1988). Pulmonary infections only occasionally are treated with surgical therapy.

The most common type of pulmonary infection encountered in cardiothoracic surgical patients is hospital-acquired (nosocomial) *pneumonia*. Organisms most frequently causing pneumonia in hospitalized patients include *Pseudomonas aeruginosa, Staphylococcus aureus, Enterobacter* species, *Klebsiella pneumoniae,* and *Escherichia coli* (Mark & Rizk, 1996). Affected patients usually are critically ill and require mechanical ventilatory support. Frequently, pneumonia occurs concomitantly with another pulmonary pathophysiologic process. For example, pneumonia is present in 50% to 75% of patients with adult respiratory distress syndrome (Lynch, 1997). Diagnosis usually is based on radiologic evidence of a pulmonary infiltrate and identification of pathogenic organisms in an aspirated sputum culture. Pneumonia is treated with organism-specific antibiotic therapy. A pneumonitis that does not resolve is suggestive of bronchial obstruction secondary to tumor. Uncommonly, pneumonia leads to development of a lung abscess.

Pulmonary tuberculosis, once thought nearly eradicated, is reemerging as a significant infectious health problem, particularly in poverty areas and in immunocompromised patients. It is a major cause of morbidity and mortality worldwide, resulting in the greatest number of deaths due to any one single infectious agent (Hirsch et al., 1999). More than eight million active cases of tuberculosis occur globally each year, accounting for nearly three million deaths per year (Lynch & Toews, 1997). Currently, approximately two billion people worldwide are infected with tuberculosis, and in many countries, it is the most common preventable cause of death (Pomerantz & Brown, 1998). The disease is most common in South America, Africa, and Asia (Moran, 1995). Although tuberculosis remains relatively uncommon in the United States, the number of reported cases has been increasing during the 1990s. Reasons for the increase in tuberculosis include the appearance of AIDS with its immunocompromised hosts, immigration patterns, some complacency in the medical community, and an increase in poverty areas with associated overcrowding and poor sanitation (Pomerantz, 1996).

Pulmonary tuberculosis is caused by the organism *Mycobacterium tuberculosis*. The bacilli responsible for pulmonary tuberculosis are most often airborne and the disease is highly contagious, especially in closed populations of susceptible people (Shields, 1994). The most common pattern of mycobacterial infection is reinfection or postprimary tuberculosis (formerly called *adult tuberculosis*). It begins as a segmental pneumonia in the apical or posterior segment of an upper lobe or the superior segment of a lower lobe; the pneumonic infiltrate progresses to caseous necrosis, cavity formation, drainage into an adjacent bronchus, and expectoration of debris and viable mycobacteria from the cavity (Moran, 1995).

Characteristic symptoms of tuberculosis include fever, chills, night sweats, a persistent cold, weight loss, fatigue, cough, and hemoptysis. The diagnosis is confirmed by isolating *M. tuberculosis* from sputum or lung tissue. Medical treatment consists of various antituberculous chemotherapeutic agents, administered in combination to produce an effective bactericidal combination with minimal side effects. An example of an appropriate pharmacologic regimen is isoniazid and rifampin for 9 months with ethambutol or streptomycin for the first 2 to 8 weeks (Shields, 1994). The development of drug-resistant tuberculous organisms has increased and is of particular concern in hospitals and other institutional settings. Multidrug-resistant tuberculosis, defined as disease that is resistant to both isoniazid and rifampin, requires treatment with a minimum of four drugs; the regimens are highly toxic, difficult to tolerate, and, particularly in patients infected with human immunodeficiency virus, can be associated with a high mortality rate (Lynch & Toews, 1997). Surgical therapy occasionally is required for drug-resistant infections or to treat complications of tuberculosis, such as massive hemoptysis or empyema.

Pulmonary mycotic, or *fungal*, *infections* result from the inhalation of fungus. The most common pulmonary fungal infections in the United States are histoplasmosis, coccidioidomycosis, blastomycosis, cryptococcosis, aspergillosis, sporotrichosis, mucormycosis, candidiasis, and paracoccidioidomycosis; although millions of people probably have sustained primary subclinical fungal infections, most have no clinical infection or only a slight clinical infection that clears rapidly with no long-lasting effects (Grover & Hopeman, 1995).

Serious fungal pulmonary infection occurs most often in the population of immunocompromised persons who become infected with opportunistic fungal agents. Diagnosis often can be established using transbronchial biopsy or CT-guided transthoracic needle biopsy techniques. Most often, pulmonary fungal infections are treated effectively with medical therapy and surgical treatment is not required. Most fungal diseases respond to treatment with appropriate antimycotic drugs, especially amphotericin B (Van Trigt, 1995). Pulmonary resection is required rarely for pulmonary fungal infection that is unresponsive to medical treatment or for removal of lung tissue destroyed by infection. Several types of fungal infections can produce a pulmonary nodule similar in appearance to a malignant lesion.

Lung Abscess

The formation of a local area of infection and tissue destruction in the pulmonary parenchyma is termed a *lung abscess* (Fig. 33-3). Lung abscess can develop as a result of (1) aspiration of esophageal contents or other foreign matter into the tracheobronchial tree, (2) pneumonia, (3) infection elsewhere in the body, (4) pulmonary embolism, or (5) bronchial obstruction by tumor or a foreign body.

Aspiration is the most common cause of lung abscess, especially in the presence of alcohol abuse, neurologic disorders, general anesthesia, or prolonged intubation. Oral or gastric feeding of patients with diminished levels of consciousness or of those who are in a supine position also predisposes to aspiration and lung abscess. Because aspiration usually occurs when the patient is supine, lung abscesses typically develop in lung segments with dependent bronchial orifices in that posture, specifically the posterior segments of the right upper lobe and the superior segments of the left or right lower lobes (Hodder et al., 1995). The responsible pathogens, derived from the mixed flora of the mouth, are most commonly *Staphylo-*

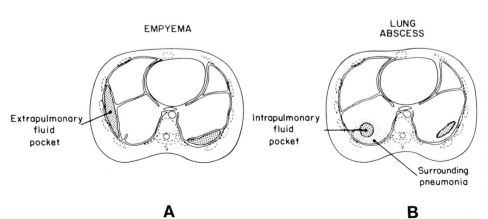

EMPYEMA

Extrapulmonary fluid pocket

LUNG ABSCESS

Intrapulmonary fluid pocket

Surrounding pneumonia

A

B

FIGURE 33-3. Schematic of chest computed tomographic scan demonstrating difference between (**A**) empyema, an extrapulmonary process, and (**B**) lung abscess, an intrapulmonary process. (Cohen RG, DeMeester TR, Lafontaine E, 1995: The pleura. In Sabiston DC Jr, Spencer FC [eds]: Surgery of the Chest, ed. 6, p. 550. Philadelphia, WB Saunders)

coccus, fusiform bacilli, alpha-nonhemolytic *Streptococcus, Peptococcus,* or *Bacteroides fragilis* (Hood, 1994a).

Unchecked necrosis of infected tissue in a lung abscess eventually produces erosion into a bronchus or the pleural space. Communication with a bronchus allows the lung abscess to be partially drained by expectoration of suppurative material. Erosion into the pleural space (ie, a bronchopleural fistula) produces an empyema. Lung abscesses usually are treated with pulmonary hygiene interventions and organism-specific antimicrobial therapy. Most lung abscesses respond promptly to treatment and resolve completely in 3 to 5 months (Hodder et al., 1995). Surgical procedures to drain infected material or remove necrotic lung tissue are required rarely.

Empyema Thoracis

Empyema thoracis is infection of the pleural space (see Fig. 33-3). Approximately 50% of empyemas result from pyogenic (ie, pus-producing) pneumonia; other common causes are infection after an operation on the esophagus, lungs, or mediastinum, and extension of a subphrenic abscess. Empyema occurs in 5% of patients who undergo pneumonectomy and in 10% of those who undergo completion pneumonectomy (Gharagozloo et al., 1998). *S. aureus,* gram-negative bacteria, and anaerobic organisms are the most common pathogens causing empyemas (LoCicero, 1996; Cohen et al., 1995). In most patients, the pleural space is infected with more than one organism.

The pathologic evolution of an empyema comprises three stages: (1) an exudative phase, in which pleural fluid is thin and lung reexpansion is easily achieved; (2) the fibrinopurulent phase, characterized by large quantities of frank pus, deposition of fibrin on the visceral and parietal pleura, and fixation of the lung so that it becomes less expandable; and (3) the organizing phase, in which a very thick exudate and inelastic "peel" cover the visceral and parietal pleural surfaces (Webb & Harrison, 1996). Common clinical manifestations of empyema include fever, chest pain, dyspnea, and cough. An empyema that remains untreated eventually may result in dissection of pus through the soft tissues of the chest wall and the skin (termed an *empyema necessitatis*) or, alternatively, a bronchopleural fistula with spontaneous drainage of pus into the tracheobronchial tree (Deslauriers, 1995).

Treatment of empyema comprises two major objectives, adequate drainage of infected material and lung reexpansion. Specific treatment modalities vary, however, depending on a number of factors, including the source of the empyema, the condition of underlying lung and its ability to reexpand, and the presence or absence of a bronchopleural fistula. Chest tube thoracostomy or rib resection and open drainage may be performed to drain the pleural space (Fig. 33-4). Thoracoscopy sometimes is performed for direct visualization and débridement of the empyema cavity, followed by cyclic irrigation and drainage (Ridley & Braimbridge, 1991). Decortication (ie, an operation to remove an infected or constrictive fibrinous peel) may be necessary to achieve lung reexpansion.

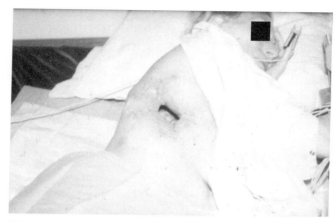

FIGURE 33-4. Bronchial dehiscence and empyema developed in this patient 2 weeks after a right completion pneumonectomy for a metachronous primary lung tumor. To allow open drainage of the infected hemithorax, a Clagett window (ie, a window thoracostomy) has been created. Through an H-shaped incision, 2-inch segments of the fourth, fifth, sixth, and seventh ribs have been removed; skin flaps were then fully mobilized, turned inward, and sutured to the parietal pleura on the undersurface of the chest wall. (Courtesy of Sudhir Sundaresan, MD)

Although antibiotics are important in treating pneumonia that might lead to empyema, their value in treating established empyema is unproven.

Failure of the lung to reexpand leaves a residual space that invariably becomes reinfected. Occasionally, it may be necessary to obliterate a residual space surgically. A thoracoplasty is the surgical collapsing of the chest wall to obliterate the space surrounding the nonexpanded lung. Alternatively, a pectoralis muscle flap may be performed, in which extrathoracic muscle is transposed to fill the residual space. In patients with postpneumonectomy empyema, treatment is complicated by the absence of residual lung to fill the hemithorax and the frequent presence of a bronchopleural fistula.

Bronchiectasis

Bronchiectasis is a disease characterized by localized or diffuse dilatation and destruction of bronchi. Pathogenesis of the condition is infection, followed by obstruction, followed by destruction of the involved bronchi (Sealy, 1989). Although formerly a prevalent pulmonary problem, it now is reported commonly only in certain geographic locations and ethnic groups, specifically in New Zealand, Nigeria, Australia, and India, and among Polynesians and Alaskan natives (Hodder et al., 1995).

The diagnosis is suggested by a clinical history of multiple respiratory infections with cough, abundant sputum production, or hemoptysis. Bronchoscopy and bronchography are performed to confirm the diagnosis and identify bronchiectatic segments. The mainstay of medical treatment is vigorous pulmonary hygiene, including postural drainage. Surgical resection of the involved portions of lung may be indicated in patients with localized bronchiectasis that can be resected completely and recurrent pneumonia, continuing copious sputum, or hemoptysis despite medical therapy.

▶ Abnormalities of the Pleural Space

Pneumothorax

Pneumothorax is the abnormal accumulation of air in the pleural space. It can occur (1) as a spontaneous event; (2) secondary to blunt or penetrating chest trauma; (3) as a result of an invasive intrathoracic procedure (eg, central venous catheter placement, transthoracic needle biopsy, or thoracentesis); (4) because of parenchymal disruption associated with pulmonary resection procedures; or (5) secondary to the use of high levels of positive end-expiratory pressure (PEEP) in mechanically ventilated patients.

Pneumothorax most often results from the rupture of an air-filled pseudocyst, or bleb, in the lung. A bleb is a small group of alveoli with abnormally thin walls, usually located in the lung periphery. Large pseudocysts, or bullae, commonly develop in individuals with emphysematous lung disease. A disruption in the visceral covering of the pseudocyst allows air from the tracheobronchial tree to leak into the pleural space. As air accumulates in the pleural space, the ipsilateral lung is increasingly compressed. If air continues to fill the pleural space, it eventually compresses mediastinal structures, shifting them toward the opposite hemithorax. This condition is termed *tension pneumothorax*. Unrelieved tension pneumothorax causes severe hemodynamic compromise because of inability of the compressed venae cavae to deliver blood into the heart. Cardiac filling decreases, causing decreased cardiac output and profound hypotension.

Primary spontaneous pneumothorax is presumed to occur because of idiopathic rupture of a peripheral lung bleb. The condition most often occurs in healthy young men with an asthenic (slight) body build. Smoking substantially increases the risk for development of a spontaneous pneumothorax, particularly in men (Bense, 1992). The disease is slightly more common on the right side, and simultaneous bilateral pneumothoraces occur in 10% of patients (Cohen et al., 1995). Rarely, recurrent cyclic pneumothoraces occur in women in association with the onset of menstruation. The physiologic mechanism of this so-called *catamenial pneumothorax* remains obscure (Fonseca, 1998).

Pneumothorax is manifested by pleuritic chest pain. A small spontaneous pneumothorax may be treated with activity restriction and observation. Indications for chest tube thoracostomy and closed drainage include a moderate-sized pneumothorax (>25%) on the first radiograph, tension pneumothorax, disease in the contralateral lung, significant persisting symptoms, or progression of the pneumothorax as demonstrated on successive radiographs (LoCicero, 1996). If a tension component is present, immediate evacuation of air from the pleural space is necessary and may be accomplished by thoracentesis with

a large-bore catheter (followed by chest tube thoracostomy) or emergent chest tube insertion. Usually, the alveolar rent gradually seals and the air leak abates within 1 to 2 days.

A patient who has experienced a spontaneous pneumothorax is at increased risk for development of another one subsequently. Approximately 20% of patients experience recurrent pneumothorax, usually on the ipsilateral side. Once a second pneumothorax has occurred, the risk for a third is even greater. The most common treatment for recurrent pneumothoraces is mechanical pleurodesis; that is, mechanical abrasion of the pleural surfaces to produce inflammation with resultant adhesion formation. Pleurodesis usually can be accomplished using video-assisted thoracoscopy. If pseudocysts are detected at the time of operation, they may be surgically resected. Occasionally, pleurodesis is performed after the first episode of spontaneous pneumothorax if the air leak persists despite conservative measures or if the patient's lifestyle is such that a subsequent pneumothorax could be life threatening (eg, working in a hyperbaric chamber, scuba diving, or piloting small aircraft requiring use of a pressurized mask).

Secondary spontaneous pneumothorax, or that which develops secondary to another condition, occurs most commonly in older people with emphysema or other forms of chronic obstructive pulmonary disease. The predominant symptom in this group of patients is severe shortness of breath that, because of impaired pulmonary function, can progress to frank respiratory failure (LoCicero, 1996). Chest tube drainage is initiated promptly and may be necessary for several weeks until the air leak resolves. Patients with secondary spontaneous pneumothorax have a recurrence rate similar to that for primary spontaneous pneumothorax (Cohen et al., 1995).

Patients receiving mechanical ventilation with high levels of PEEP (15 to 20 cm) also are at risk for acquired pneumothoraces, which may develop bilaterally. Such patients usually are critically ill and are likely to die of the hemodynamic sequelae of tension pneumothorax if the air is not evacuated promptly. A vigorous air leak may persist and chest tube drainage with negative suction usually is required until mechanical ventilation is discontinued. Pneumothorax also can occur secondary to infections in the lung (bacterial, viral, mycotic, or parasitic), pleural space (empyema), or abdomen (eg, subphrenic abscess) (Beauchamp, 1995).

Patients with AIDS are at risk for secondary pneumothoraces, frequently in association with *Pneumocystis carinii* pneumonia. Treatment of pneumothorax in the presence of an immunocompromised state requires special considerations. Healing of visceral pleura and resolution of the air leak is very slow. Chest tube drainage frequently is required for weeks, or even months. Under most other circumstances, pneumothorax is treated with closed water-seal drainage until the air leak completely resolves. However, because of the persistence of air leaks in immunocompromised patients, a Heimlich (one-way flutter) valve (Becton Dickinson, Franklin Lakes, NJ) may be used in place of a conventional water-seal drainage system so that the patient can be treated on an outpatient basis. Heimlich valves, chest tubes, and pleural drainage systems are described in further detail in Chapter 42, Pleural Thoracostomy Drainage.

Surgical pleurodesis is undesirable for prevention of recurrent pneumothorax in patients with AIDS because of the significant morbidity associated with an operation. Chemical pleurodesis, also called pleural sclerosis, may be performed instead. The installation of a sclerosing solution through a chest tube produces an inflammatory response that causes the visceral and parietal pleural surfaces to become adherent. Such adherence, termed *pleural symphysis,* serves to obliterate the potential pleural space so that the lung is unable to collapse.

Pleural Effusion

Pleural effusion is the abnormal accumulation of fluid between the parietal pleura, which lines the inside of the chest wall, and the visceral pleura, which covers the lungs. Under normal conditions, fluid flows from systemic capillaries in the parietal pleura into the pleural space. The fluid is absorbed rapidly by pulmonary capillaries in the visceral pleura and pulmonary lymphatics. Only several milliliters of fluid is present normally in the pleural cavity. If a disturbance in the normal equilibrium of fluid entering and leaving the pleural space occurs, the pleural space fills with fluid and the ipsilateral lung is compressed. Disturbances causing pleural effusion include increased capillary permeability (eg, from inflammation or tumor implants), increased hydrostatic pressure (eg, due to congestive heart failure), decreased oncotic pressure (eg, caused by hypoalbuminemia), increased negative intrapleural pressure (eg, due to atelectasis), and decreased lymphatic drainage (eg, due to lymphatic obstruction caused by tumor) (Rusch, 1995).

Thoracentesis commonly is performed for diagnostic purposes. The fluid obtained is categorized as either transudative or exudative, according to the protein and lactate dehydrogenase (LDH) content of the fluid. Transudative pleural effusions are caused by an imbalance in formation and reabsorption of pleural fluid. Congestive heart failure and pulmonary embolism are examples of conditions that cause transudative pleural effusions. Transudative pleural effusion is managed primarily by treating the underlying disease process.

Exudative pleural effusions are caused by pathologic processes that either increase permeability of the pleural surface to protein or decrease lymphatic flow. Because lymphatic drainage is important in clearing protein that enters the pleural space from the parietal and visceral pleural surfaces, exudative effusions are characterized by a higher ratio of pleural fluid protein to serum protein. An effusion is considered an exudate if the pleural fluid protein to serum protein ratio is greater than 0.5 and the pleural fluid LDH to serum LDH ratio is greater than 0.6 (Rusch, 1995). Other descriptive information that may help determine the etiology of a pleural effusion includes the color, odor, and character of the fluid as well as analysis of the fluid for white blood cell count and differential, glucose, and pH values. Gram and acid-fast bacillus stains and pleural fluid cultures are performed if infection is suspected; if malignancy is likely, pleural fluid cytology or a pleural biopsy is performed.

Pleural effusion can result from a number of nonmalignant disease processes but occurs more often secondary to malignancy (Table 33-3). Local inflammation and increased capillary permeability associated with tumor implants increase fluid transudation, and lymphatic obstruction impairs its reabsorption (LoCicero, 1996). Approximately 75% of malignant pleural effusions are associated with lung cancer (30%), breast cancer (25%), or lymphoma (20%) (Light, 1997). Lung cancer is the most common cause of malignant effusion, due to contiguous spread of lung tumors and their propensity to invade the pulmonary vasculature and embolize to the visceral pleura (Sahn, 1998).

Palliative treatment of malignant pleural effusion is undertaken to relieve the associated respiratory distress, which often is the only or most troublesome symptom in a patient who is otherwise able to remain fairly active. Most often, thoracentesis or chest tube thoracostomy is performed to evacuate fluid and provide symptomatic relief. Video-assisted thoracoscopy may be performed if loculated areas of fluid are present. Through the thoracoscope, adhesions that prevent free drainage of fluid can be disrupted. Prompt evacuation of the effusion is important to achieve lung reexpansion. Because malignant effusions are exudative, the visceral pleura becomes coated with a proteinaceous material. If the effusion remains for an extended period, the lung becomes trapped and incapable of reexpansion.

Because of the underlying malignancy, fluid can be expected to reaccumulate. Intermittent thoracentesis or

---

TABLE 33-3

Causes of Pleural Effusion

Malignancy
Congestive heart failure
Pulmonary embolism
Cirrhosis of the liver with ascites
Nephrotic syndrome
Infections
    Tuberculosis
    Histoplasmosis
Immunologic diseases
    Rheumatoid disease
    Systemic lupus erythematosus
Postpericardiotomy syndrome
Chylothorax
Hemothorax

tube thoracostomy is uncomfortable for the patient and can cause pneumothorax, hypoproteinemia, or empyema (Flye, 1989). *Chemical pleural sclerosis* often is performed to prevent reaccumulation of fluid. As in treatment of pneumothorax, the objective of pleural sclerosis is inflammation of the pleural surfaces with resultant pleural symphysis so that fluid accumulation cannot recur. Although pleural sclerosis does not affect progression of malignant disease, it provides palliation from the dyspnea produced by recurring effusions.

Chemical sclerosis typically is performed through the chest tube by injection of a caustic agent after the effusion has been drained and the lung has reexpanded. Full lung expansion is important so that visceral and parietal pleural layers can become adherent to one another. Formerly, tetracycline was the standard agent used for chemical sclerosis. Because it is no longer commercially available, other agents, such as talc, doxycycline (an antibiotic in the tetracycline class), or bleomycin (a chemotherapeutic agent), may be selected. After fluid instillation, the chest tube is clamped for several hours. During this period, the patient is repositioned from side to back to side to allow distribution of the sclerosing solution over the entire pleural surface.

Chemical pleurodesis effectively controls pleural effusions in 70% to 90% of properly selected patients (Light, 1997). Surgical procedures for prevention of effusion recurrence, such as mechanical abrasion (pleurodesis) or removal of the parietal pleura (pleurectomy), usually are not performed for malignant pleural effusions because of the significant morbidity associated with a thoracic operation in a patient with a limited life expectancy.

An alternative therapy for intractable, symptomatic pleural effusion is the implantation of a pleuroperitoneal shunt. The Denver pleuroperitoneal shunt (Denver Biomaterials, Inc., Golden, CO) consists of a pumping chamber that contains a one-way valve and connects fenestrated catheters placed in the pleural space and peritoneum (Fig. 33-5). The shunt drains fluid from the pleural space into the peritoneal cavity, where it is reabsorbed. Because pleural pressure is lower than peritoneal pressure, drainage of fluid through the shunt requires frequent manual compression of the pumping chamber, which is placed in subcutaneous tissue over the anterolateral costal margin of the chest wall (Ponn et al., 1991). Placement of the shunt usually can be performed using local anesthesia and sedation.

Chylothorax

Chylothorax is the presence of chyle, or fluid from the thoracic duct, in the pleural space. The thoracic duct is the largest lymphatic channel, conveying most of the lymph in the body into the circulatory system (Rodgers, 1998) (Fig. 33-6). Its primary function is the transport of digestive fat from the liver and intestinal tract into the venous system (Miller, 1994). If the thoracic duct, which courses through the thorax close to the esophagus, be-

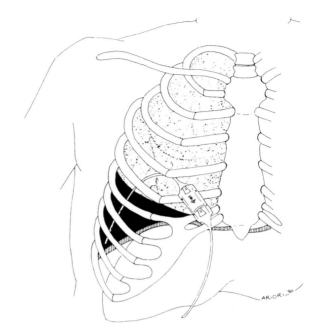

FIGURE 33-5. Schematic illustrating pleuroperitoneal shunt. (Ponn RB, Blancaflor J, D'Agostino RS, et al., 1991: Pleuroperitoneal shunting for intractable pleural effusions. Ann Thorac Surg 51:606. Reprinted with permission of the Society of Thoracic Surgeons)

comes disrupted or obstructed, chyle can enter the pleural space. Chylothorax occasionally occurs as a complication of a thoracic operation, caused by laceration of the thoracic duct or its major divisions. Although it can occur after any operation in the thorax, it is most common after esophagectomy or a cardiac operation that necessitates considerable mediastinal dissection (Rodgers, 1998). Chylothorax also can result from obstructed lymphatic flow secondary to lymphoma or other malignancy.

Chylothorax is distinguished from other types of pleural effusions by the characteristic milky appearance of the fluid. Treatment consists of chest tube thoracostomy drainage and dietary management to limit chyle formation. Restricting dietary intake to low-fat enteral formulas supplemented with medium-chain triglycerides may be recommended, but the most effective treatment is total parenteral nutrition and nothing by mouth (Malthaner & McKneally, 1995). In postoperative thoracic surgical patients, reexploration of the thorax with ligation of the thoracic duct may occasionally be necessary if significant chylous drainage persists.

▶ Other Disorders

Massive Hemoptysis

Hemoptysis, or expectoration of blood, can occur as a manifestation of a number of pathologic cardiovascular and pulmonary conditions. Most often, it occurs in small quantities. Occasionally, massive hemoptysis, defined as

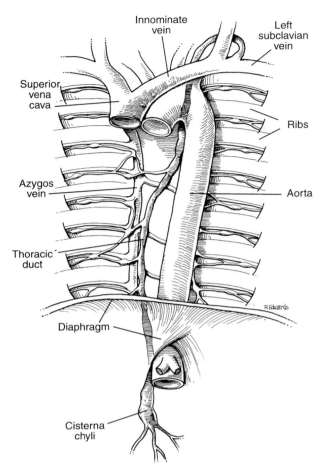

Innominate vein

Left subclavian vein

Superior vena cava

Ribs

Azygos vein

Aorta

Thoracic duct

R Edwards

Diaphragm

Cisterna chyli

FIGURE 33-6. The most common anatomic pattern of the thoracic duct. (Rodgers BM, 1998: The thoracic duct and the management of chylothorax. In Kaiser LR, Kron IL, Spray TL [eds]: Mastery of Cardiothoracic Surgery, p. 213. Philadelphia, Lippincott Williams & Wilkins)

expectoration of more than 600 mL of blood over a 24-hour period, occurs. Massive hemoptysis is a life-threatening condition. If untreated, the patient is likely to die of suffocation secondary to hemorrhage into the tracheobronchial tree. The patient usually succumbs to impaired oxygenation before enough bleeding occurs to cause hemodynamic instability.

Bronchoscopy is performed, preferably during the period of active bleeding, to localize the site of bleeding. When bronchoscopy is performed during active bleeding, rigid bronchoscopy with general anesthesia is recommended. Rigid bronchoscopy is advantageous because the bronchoscope's larger conduit size allows snug cannulation of the nonbleeding lung for ventilation, suction of blood and clots, good visibility, and the passage of suction cannulae and balloon catheters (Guimaraes, 1995). Often, an endobronchial blocker, which consists of a balloon-tipped catheter, is used to occlude the lumen of the affected bronchus, thus preventing blood from spilling into other parts of the tracheobronchial tree. Emergent pulmonary angiography may be performed with selective embolization of the responsible artery.

Thoracotomy with resection of involved pulmonary parenchyma also may be necessary because of the significant incidence (80%) of recurrent massive hemoptysis (Garzon, 1989).

Foreign Body Aspiration

Aspiration of foreign bodies is relatively uncommon in adults, except in people with diminished ability of the glottis to protect the airway. Specifically, aspiration is most likely after heavy ingestion of alcohol or other consciousness-altering drug and in people with decreased levels of consciousness. Aspirated items are usually organic material, such as gum, hard candy, nuts, or boluses of food. Inorganic material that may be aspirated includes such items as needles, teeth, dentures, beer can tabs, or other objects that may be placed in the mouth.

Aspiration of a foreign object into the larynx causes coughing, gagging, choking, and cyanosis, and aspiration into the subglottis or trachea produces a harsh stridor and paroxysmal coughing; if an object passes into a bronchus, it may produce only minimal symptoms, such as an expiratory wheeze and coughing bouts with exercise (Smitheringale, 1995). A small object in a distal airway can produce pneumonia, either from contamination or airway obstruction and atelectasis. Sometimes aspiration is a presumptive diagnosis based on clinical history and the type of pneumonia that is present. Because the most direct pathway into the tracheobronchial tree is through the right mainstem bronchus, aspiration pneumonia occurs typically in the right upper lobe. If there is suspicion of a lodged foreign object in the tracheobronchial tree, rigid bronchoscopy is performed. Perforation of the airway can occur before or during removal of a foreign object that has sharp edges.

Congenital Anomalies

Pulmonary sequestration is a mass of nonfunctioning pulmonary tissue, either in the substance of the lung (intralobar) or in an extralobar location, that lacks a normal communication with the tracheobronchial tree (La Quaglia, 1995). It is a congenital lung anomaly detected rarely in adults. The condition may cause chronic pulmonary infections. Treatment is surgical resection of the sequestration.

A *pulmonary arteriovenous malformation* is a congenital anomalous communication between a pulmonary artery and vein, resulting in right-to-left shunting of blood. Clinical manifestations of pulmonary arteriovenous malformations include hemoptysis, congestive heart failure, and abnormally low arterial oxygen saturation. Systemic embolization of thrombus originating in the abnormal vessel can occur with resultant stroke or brain abscess (La Quaglia, 1995). A pulmonary arteriovenous malformation usually is apparent on the chest roentgenogram as a solitary pulmonary nodule, typically with two large vascular markings (Miller, 1996). The abnormal vessel usually can be treated effectively with selective embolization during angiography. Surgical resection may be necessary for large malformations and for localized lesions that have recurred or that have not responded to embolic therapy (La Quaglia, 1995).

Broncholithiasis

Broncholithiasis is an unusual disorder in which hilar lymph nodes become enlarged and calcified. The cause of calcification most often is a prior granulomatous infection, particularly histoplasmosis or tuberculosis (Grover & Hopeman, 1995; Faber, 1989). Cough and hemoptysis are common manifestations, caused by bronchial compression or erosion by a calcified lymph node. The patient may expectorate fragments of the eroding broncholith (calcified lymph node) (Hood, 1994b). In selected patients, bronchoscopy may be performed for removal or laser eradication of a broncholith. However, because the broncholith frequently is embedded in bronchial tissue with intense inflammation and fibrosis, removal through bronchoscopy can result in significant bleeding or bronchial perforation. Thoracotomy may be required for removal of the broncholith and the surrounding bronchial and lung tissue.

REFERENCES

Albertucci M, DeMeester TR, Rothberg M, et al., 1992: Surgery and the management of peripheral lung tumors adherent to the parietal pleura. J Thorac Cardiovasc Surg 103:8

Allen MS, Mathisen DJ, Grillo HC, et al., 1991: Bronchogenic carcinoma with chest wall invasion. Ann Thorac Surg 51:948

Al-Sugair A, Coleman RE, 1998: Applications of PET in lung cancer. Semin Nucl Med 28:303

American Heart Association, 1998: 1999 Heart and Stroke Statistical Update. Dallas, American Heart Association

Armstrong JG, 1995: Non-small cell lung cancer/brachytherapy. In Pearson FG, Deslauriers J, Ginsberg RJ, et al. (eds): Thoracic Surgery. New York, Churchill Livingstone

Auerbach O, Garfinkel L, 1991: The changing pattern of lung carcinoma. Cancer 68:1973

Baldini EH, Strauss GM, 1997: Women and lung cancer: Waiting to exhale. Chest 112(4 Suppl):229S

Beahrs OH, Myers MH (eds), 1978: The Manual for Staging Cancer, ed. 2. American Joint Committee on Cancer. Philadelphia, JB Lippincott

Beauchamp G, 1995: Spontaneous pneumothorax and pneumomediastinum. In Pearson FG, Deslauriers J, Ginsberg RJ, et al. (eds): Thoracic Surgery. New York, Churchill Livingstone

Benfield JR, Russell LA, 1996: Lung carcinomas. In Baue AE, Geha AS, Hammond GL, et al. (eds): Glenn's Thoracic and Cardiovascular Surgery, ed. 6. Stamford, CT, Appleton & Lange

Bense L, 1992: Spontaneous pneumothorax. Chest 101:891

Bunn PA, Kelly K, 1998: New chemotherapeutic agents prolong survival and improve quality of life in non-small cell lung cancer: A review of the literature and future directions. Clin Cancer Res 4:1087

Burt M, Martini N, Ginsberg RJ, 1996: Surgical treatment of lung carcinoma. In Baue AE, Geha AS, Hammond GL, et al. (eds): Glenn's Thoracic and Cardiovascular Surgery, ed. 6. Stamford, CT, Appleton & Lange

Carney DN, 1998: New agents in the management of advanced non-small cell lung cancer. Semin Oncol 25:83

Clark R, Ihde DC, 1998: Small-cell lung cancer: Treatment progress and prospects. Oncology 12:647

Cohen RG, DeMeester TR, Lafontaine E, 1995: The pleura. In Sabiston DC, Spencer FC (eds): Surgery of the Chest, ed. 6. Philadelphia, WB Saunders

D'Amico TA, Sabiston DC Jr, 1995: Carcinoma of the lung. In Sabiston DC Jr, Spencer FC (eds): Surgery of the Chest, ed. 6. Philadelphia, WB Saunders

Deslauriers J, 1995: Empyema and bronchopleural fistula. In Pearson FG, Deslauriers J, Ginsberg RJ, et al. (eds): Thoracic Surgery. New York, Churchill Livingstone

Elias AD, 1997: Small cell lung cancer: State-of-the-art therapy in 1996. Chest 112(4 Suppl):251S

Faber LP, 1989: Broncholithiasis. In Grillo HC, Austen WG, Wilkins EW, et al. (eds): Current Therapy in Cardiothoracic Surgery. Toronto, Canada, BC Decker

Fleisher AG, McElvaney G, Robinson CL, 1991: Multiple primary bronchogenic carcinomas: Treatment and follow-up. Ann Thorac Surg 51:48

Flye MW, 1989: Malignant pleural effusion. In Grillo HC, Austen WG, Wilkins EW, et al. (eds): Current Therapy in Cardiothoracic Surgery. Toronto, Canada, BC Decker

Fonseca P, 1998: Catamenial pneumothorax: A multifactorial etiology. J Thorac Cardiovasc Surg 116:872

Garzon AA, 1989: Massive hemoptysis: Surgical and tamponade therapy. In Grillo HC, Austen WG, Wilkins EW, et al. (eds): Current Therapy in Cardiothoracic Surgery. Toronto, Canada, BC Decker

Gasper LE, 1998: Brachytherapy in lung cancer. J Surg Oncol 67:60

Gharagozloo F, Trachiotis G, Wolfe A, et al., 1998: Pleural space irrigation and modified Clagett procedure for the treatment of early postpneumonectomy empyema. J Thorac Cardiovasc Surg 116:943

Govindan R, Ihde DC, 1997: Practical issues in the management of the patient with small cell lung cancer. Chest Surg Clin North Am 7:167

Grover FL, Hopeman AR, 1995: Mycotic infection. In Pearson FG, Deslauriers J, Ginsberg RJ, et al. (eds): Thoracic Surgery. New York, Churchill Livingstone

Guimaraes CA, 1995: Massive hemoptysis. In Pearson FG, Deslauriers J, Ginsberg RJ, et al. (eds): Thoracic Surgery. New York, Churchill Livingstone

Hackshaw AK, 1998: Lung cancer and passive smoking. Stat Methods Med Res 7:119

Hansen CP, Holtveg H, Francis D, et al., 1992: Pulmonary hamartoma. J Thorac Cardiovasc Surg 104:674

Hilaris BS, Mastoras DA, 1998: Contemporary brachtherapy approaches in non-small cell lung cancer. J Surg Oncol 69:258

Hirsch CS, Johnson JL, Ellner JJ, 1999: Pulmonary tuberculosis. Curr Opin Pulm Med 5:143

Hodder RV, Cameron R, Todd TR, 1995: Infections/bacterial infections. In Pearson FG, Deslauriers J, Ginsberg RJ, et al. (eds): Thoracic Surgery. New York, Churchill Livingstone

Holmes EC, 1995: Pulmonary metastases. In Pearson FG, Deslauriers J, Ginsberg RJ, et al. (eds): Thoracic Surgery. New York, Churchill Livingstone

Hood RM, 1994a: Bacterial infections of the lung. In Shields TW (ed): General Thoracic Surgery, ed. 4. Baltimore, Williams & Wilkins

Hood RM, 1994b: Bronchial compressive diseases. In Shields TW (ed): General Thoracic Surgery, ed. 4. Baltimore, Williams & Wilkins

Hoover EL, Hsu H, Webb H, et al., 1988: The surgical management of empyema thoracis in substance abuse patients: A 5-year experience. Ann Thorac Surg 46:563

Johnson BE, 1998: Second lung cancers in patients after treatment for an initial lung cancer. J Natl Cancer Inst 90:1335

Kaiser LR, 1998: Right-sided pulmonary resections. In Kaiser LR, Kron IL, Spray TL (eds): Mastery of Cardiothoracic Surgery. Philadelphia, Lippincott Williams & Wilkins

Krasna MJ, Reed CE, Nugent WC, et al., 1999: Lung cancer staging and treatment in multidisciplinary trials: Cancer and leukemia group B cooperative group approach. Ann Thorac Surg 68:201

Landis SH, Murray T, Bolden S, Wingo PA, 1998: Cancer statistics: 1998. CA Cancer J Clin 48:6

La Quaglia MP, 1995: Congenital anomalies. In Pearson FG, Deslauriers J, Ginsberg RJ, et al. (eds): Thoracic Surgery. New York, Churchill Livingstone

Lassen U, Hansen HH, 1999: Surgery in limited stage small cell lung cancer. Cancer Treat Rev 25:67

Light RW, 1997: Pleural diseases, pleural effusions. In Khan MG, Lynch JP (eds): Pulmonary Disease Diagnosis and Therapy: A Practical Approach. Baltimore, Williams & Wilkins

LoCicero J, 1996: Benign and malignant disorders of the pleura. In Baue AE, Geha AS, Hammond GL, et al. (eds): Glenn's Thoracic and Cardiovascular Surgery, ed. 6. Stamford, CT, Appleton & Lange

Lowe VJ, Naunheim KS, 1998: Positron emission tomography in lung cancer. Ann Thorac Surg 65:1821

Lynch JP, 1997: Bacterial pneumonia. In Khan MG, Lynch JP (eds): Pulmonary Disease Diagnosis and Therapy: A Practical Approach. Baltimore, Williams & Wilkins

Lynch JP, Toews GB, 1997: Fungal, mycobacterial, and viral pulmonary infections. In Khan MG, Lynch JP (eds): Pulmonary Disease Diagnosis and Therapy: A Practical Approach. Baltimore, Williams & Wilkins

Maddaus M, Ginsberg RJ, 1995: Cancer/diagnosis and staging. In Pearson FG, Deslauriers J, Ginsberg RJ, et al. (eds): Thoracic Surgery. New York, Churchill Livingstone

Malthaner RA, McKneally MF, 1995: Anatomy of the thoracic duct and chylothorax. In Pearson FG, Deslauriers J, Ginsberg RJ, et al. (eds): Thoracic Surgery. New York, Churchill Livingstone

Mark JB, Rizk NW, 1996: Pneumonia, bronchiectasis, and lung abscess. In Baue AE, Geha AS, Hammond GL, et al. (eds): Glenn's Thoracic and Cardiovascular Surgery, ed. 6. Stamford, CT, Appleton & Lange

Martini N, Burt ME, Bains MS, et al., 1992: Survival after resection of stage II non-small cell lung cancer. Ann Thorac Surg 54:460

Martini N, Ginsberg RJ, 1995: Cancer/surgical management. In Pearson FG, Deslauriers J, Ginsberg RJ, et al. (eds): Thoracic Surgery. New York, Churchill Livingstone

Martini N, McCormack PM, 1998: Evolution of the surgical management of pulmonary metastases. Chest Surg Clin North Am 8:13

Mathisen DJ, Grillo HC, 1991: Carinal resection for bronchogenic carcinoma. J Thorac Cardiovasc Surg 102:16

Mathisen DJ, Grillo HC, 1996: The trachea: Tracheostomy, tumors, strictures, tracheomalacia, and tracheal resection and reconstruction. In Baue AE, Geha AS, Hammond GL, et al. (eds): Glenn's Thoracic and Cadiovascular Surgery, ed. 6. Stamford, CT, Appleton & Lange

McLauglin JS, 1996: Superior sulcus tumors. In Baue AE, Geha AS, Hammond GL, et al. (eds): Glenn's Thoracic and Cardiovascular Surgery, ed. 6. Stamford, CT, Appleton & Lange

Miller AB, 1995: Cancer/epidemiology. In Pearson FG, Deslauriers J, Ginsberg RJ, et al. (eds): Thoracic Surgery. New York, Churchill Livingstone

Miller JI, 1994: Chylothorax. In Shields TW (ed): General Thoracic Surgery, ed. 4. Baltimore, Williams & Wilkins

Miller JI, 1996: Benign tumors of the lower respiratory tract. In Baue AE, Geha AS, Hammond GL, et al. (eds): Glenn's Thoracic and Cardiovascular Surgery, ed. 6. Stamford, CT, Appleton & Lange

Moran JF, 1995: Surgical treatment of pulmonary tuberculosis. In Sabiston DC Jr, Spencer FC (eds): Surgery of the Chest, ed. 6. Philadelphia, WB Saunders

Mountain CF, 1986: A new international staging system for lung cancer. Chest 89:2255

Mountain CF, 1997: Revisions in the international system for staging lung cancer. Chest 111:1710

Mulshine ML, Tockman MS, 1992: Considerations in population-based screening for the early detection of lung cancer. In Bernal SD, Hesketh PJ (eds): Lung Cancer Differentiation: Implications for Diagnosis and Treatment. New York, Marcel Dekker

Nakanishi R, Osaki T, Nakanishi K, et al., 1997: Treatment strategy for patients with surgically discovered N2 stage IIIA non-small cell lung cancer. Ann Thorac Surg 64:332

Parker SL, Davis KJ, Wingo PA, et al., 1998: Cancer statistics by race and ethnicity. Ca Cancer J Clin 48:31

Pairolero PC, Trastek VF, Payne WS, 1989: Occult neoplasia. In Grillo HC, Austen WG, Wilkins EW, et al. (eds): Current Therapy in Cardiothoracic Surgery. Toronto, Canada, BC Decker

Pass HI, Donington JS, Wu P, et al., 1998: Human mesotheliomas contain the simian virus-40 regulatory region and large tumor antigen DNA sequences. J Thorac Cardiovasc Surg 116:854

Pearson FG, Cardoso P, Keshavjee S, 1995: Upper airway tumors. In Pearson FG, Deslauriers J, Ginsberg RJ, et al. (eds): Thoracic Surgery. New York, Churchill Livingstone

Pomerantz M, 1996: Surgical treatment of tuberculosis and other pulmonary mycobacterial infections. In Baue AE, Geha AS, Hammond GL, et al. (eds): Glenn's Thoracic and Cardiovascular Surgery, ed. 6. Stamford, CT, Appleton & Lange

Pomerantz M, Brown JM, 1998: Surgery of pulmonary mycobacterial disease. In Kaiser LR, Kron IL, Spray TL (eds): Mastery of Cardiothoracic Surgery. Philadelphia, Lippincott Williams & Wilkins

Ponn RB, Blancaflor J, D'Agostino RS, et al., 1991: Pleuroperitoneal shunting for intractable pleural effusions. Ann Thorac Surg 51:605

Ponn RB, Federico JA, 1998: Mediastinoscopy and staging. In Kaiser LR, Kron IL, Spray TL (eds): Mastery of Cardiothoracic Surgery. Philadelphia, Lippincott Williams & Wilkins

Ridley PD, Braimbridge MV, 1991: Thoracoscopic debridement and pleural irrigation in the management of empyema thoracis. Ann Thorac Surg 51:461

Rodgers BM, 1998: The thoracic duct and the management of chylothorax. In Kaiser LR, Kron IL, Spray TL (eds): Mastery of Cardiothoracic Surgery. Philadelphia, Lippincott Williams & Wilkins

Rosengart TK, Martini N, Ghosn P, Burt M, 1991: Multiple primary lung carcinomas: Prognosis and treatment. Ann Thorac Surg 52:773

Rusch VW, 1995: Pleural effusion: Benign and malignant. In Pearson FG, Deslauriers J, Ginsberg RJ, et al. (eds): Thoracic Surgery. New York, Churchill Livingstone

Sahn SA, 1998: Malignancy metastatic to the pleura. Clin Chest Med 19:351

Scott CB, 1998: Issues in quality of life assessment during cancer therapy. Semin Radiat Oncol 8(4 Suppl 1):5

Sealy WC, 1989: Bronchiectasis. In Grillo HC, Austen WG, Wilkins EW, et al., (eds): Current Therapy in Cardiothoracic Surgery. Toronto, Canada, BC Decker

Sellers TA, Potter JD, Bailey-Wilson JE, et al., 1991: Lung cancer detection and prevention: Evidence for an interaction between smoking and genetic predisposition. Cancer Res 52(Suppl):2694S

Shepherd FA, 1997: The role of chemotherapy in the treatment of small cell lung cancer. Chest Surg Clin North Am 7:113

Shields TW, 1994: Pulmonary tuberculosis and other mycobacterial infections of the lung. In Shields TW (ed): General Thoracic Surgery, ed. 4. Baltimore, Williams & Wilkins

Shields TW, 1996: Diagnosis and staging of lung cancer. In Baue AE, Geha AS, Hammond GL, et al. (eds): Glenn's Thoracic and Cardiovascular Surgery, ed. 6. Stamford, CT, Appleton & Lange

Shields TW, 1997: Lung cancer and the solitary pulmonary nodule. In Khan MG, Lynch JP (eds): Pulmonary Disease Diagnosis and Therapy: A Practical Approach. Baltimore, Williams & Wilkins

Shields TW, Robinson PG, 1994: Benign tumors of the lung. In Shields TW (ed): General Thoracic Surgery, ed. 4. Baltimore, Williams & Wilkins

Shields TW, Robinson PG, Radosevich JA, 1994: Lung cancer: Etiology, carcinogenesis, molecular biology, and pathology. In Shields TW (ed): General Thoracic Surgery, ed. 4. Baltimore, Williams & Wilkins

Smitheringale A, 1995: Foreign bodies in the respiratory tract. In Pearson FG, Deslauriers J, Ginsberg RJ, et al. (eds): Thoracic Surgery. New York, Churchill Livingstone

Sridhar KS, Raub WA, 1992: Present and past smoking history and other predisposing factors in 100 lung cancer patients. Chest 101:19

Sugarbaker DJ, Garcia JP, 1998: Multimodality therapy for malignant pleural mesothelioma. Chest 112(Suppl 4):272S

Swisher SG, Roth JA, 1998: Gene therapy for human lung cancers. Surg Oncol Clin North Am 7:603

Van Schil PE, de la Riviere AB, Knaepen PJ, et al., 1991: TNM staging and long-term follow-up after sleeve resection for bronchogenic tumors. Ann Thorac Surg 52:1096

Van Trigt P, 1995: Lung infections and diffuse interstitial lung disease. In Sabiston DC Jr, Spencer FC (eds): Surgery of the Chest, ed. 6. Philadelphia, WB Saunders

Webb WR, Harrison LH, 1996: Pleural space problems and thoracoplasty. In Baue AE, Geha AS, Hammond GL, et al. (eds): Glenn's Thoracic and Cardiovascular Surgery, ed. 6. Stamford, CT, Appleton & Lange

Woodward A, Boffetta P, 1997: Environmental exposure, social class, and cancer risk. IARC Sci Publ 138:361

Zaman MB, 1995: Cancer/pathology. In Pearson FG, Deslauriers J, Ginsberg RJ, et al. (eds): Thoracic Surgery. New York, Churchill Livingstone

34

Esophageal Diseases

▶ Normal Esophageal Function

The esophagus is a hollow tube that extends from the oropharynx to the stomach, passing through the neck, through the thoracic cavity, and into the abdomen. Typically, it is described as having upper (cervical), middle (thoracic), and lower (abdominal) portions, which have different sources of arterial blood supply and lymphatic drainage. The organ has an outer longitudinal and inner circular layer of muscle and differs from the remainder of the gut in that it has no serosal layer. Like each of the other compartments of the gastrointestinal tract, the esophagus has its own distinctive pH environment, enzyme content, and propulsive ability and is coupled to its adjoining compartments by a unique valve at each end (Stein et al., 1992a).

The esophagus serves three physiologic functions: (1) transmission of food from the oropharynx to the stomach, (2) control of reflux of stomach contents into the lower esophagus, and (3) prevention of aspiration of esophageal contents into the tracheobronchial tree. Sphincters located at the upper and lower ends control movement of food and fluids into and out of the esophagus. The upper esophageal sphincter (UES), also called the cricopharyngeal sphincter, is composed primarily of the cricopharyngeus muscle. Except during swallowing, the UES remains in tonic contraction, preventing passage of air from the pharynx into the esophagus and reflux of esophageal contents into the pharynx (Patti et al., 1997). The lower esophageal sphincter (LES) is not anatomically distinct. However, esophageal muscle at the junction of the stomach clearly acts as a physiologic sphincter, maintaining closure of the distal esophagus except during swallowing, vomiting, or belching.

The esophagus is innervated by both the parasympathetic and sympathetic systems. Parasympathetic innervation, particularly that from the vagus nerves, controls opening and closing of the sphincters as well as peristalsis of the muscle layers. Sympathetic innervation, composed of mediastinal branches from the thoracic sympathetic trunk and recurrent sympathetic branches from the celiac axis, appears to have little functional importance (Orringer, 1991).

Normal esophageal function depends on complex coordination of neural and muscular activity. Contraction of the UES during swallowing begins an orderly downward wave of positive pressure that propels ingested food through the length of the esophagus and into the stomach. Esophageal peristalsis consists of three types of contractions: primary peristalsis is progressive and is triggered by voluntary swallowing, secondary peristalsis is generated by distention or irritation and is also progressive, and tertiary contractions are nonprogressive (ie, simultaneous) and may occur either after voluntary swallowing or spontaneously between swallows (Orringer, 1997a). Esophageal peristaltic pressure varies from 20 to 100 mm Hg.

▶ Benign Disorders

Disorders of the esophagus are among the most poorly understood and difficult to treat diseases of the thorax. Although most patients with benign esophageal diseases experience only minor, intermittent symptoms that are easily managed with medications or lifestyle modifications, surgical intervention sometimes is required to improve esophageal function or correct anatomic abnor-

441

malities (Watson et al., 1998). In a small subset of patients with end-stage esophageal disease, esophageal resection with replacement may be necessary.

Motility Disorders

Common among the "benign" or nonmalignant diseases of the esophagus are *motility disorders,* or pathologic conditions characterized by abnormalities of peristalsis, sphincter dysfunction, or a combination of the two. Failure of the propulsive ability of the esophagus hampers forward movement of food and predisposes to regurgitation; sphincter dysfunction exposes the esophagus to the luminal contents of the stomach, causing symptoms and eventual mucosal injury (Stein et al., 1992a). Primary motility disorders of the esophagus may involve the UES and swallowing mechanism (oropharyngeal dysphagia), the body of the esophagus (transport dysphagia), or the LES (esophagogastric dysphagia) (Duranceau, 1996). Impaired esophageal motility also may occur secondary to various collagen disorders (eg, scleroderma), alcohol abuse, and diabetes, or as a response to infection or caustic injury of the esophagus (Wilkins, 1994; Duranceau et al., 1991).

Achalasia is the best characterized primary esophageal motility disorder of the esophagus and the one most commonly treated with surgical therapy. It is a degenerative neural abnormality confined entirely to the esophagus and with an unknown etiology. The disorder is characterized by absent peristalsis in the body of the esophagus, normal or increased resting pressures in the LES, and incomplete or absent relaxation of the LES in response to swallowing (Duranceau, 1995). Achalasia has a peak incidence in the third decade of life; it occurs equally in men and women and in whites more often than in African Americans (Heitmiller, 1998).

Because the LES fails to relax appropriately in persons with achalasia, undigested food is retained in the esophagus. The predominant symptom is dysphagia, which occurs in almost all patients. Regurgitation, epigastric discomfort, and weight loss also are common. Patients with achalasia eat slowly, use large volumes of water to wash food into the stomach, and may have to resort to unusual maneuvers such as twisting the upper torso, elevating the chin, or extending the neck to force food downward (Orringer, 1997b). Halitosis is often present because of the retention of undigested food in the esophagus. Pulmonary complications of aspiration, including pneumonitis, asthma-like syndrome, and pulmonary abscesses, occur in later stages of the disease (Duranceau, 1995). Achalasia also is considered a risk factor for development of squamous cell carcinoma of the esophagus, which develops in an estimated 5% of people with achalasia at an average of 20 years after diagnosis of the motility disorder (Koshy & Nostrant, 1997).

Diagnosis of achalasia is accomplished by esophageal manometry studies, contrast radiologic examination (barium swallow), and esophagoscopy. Manometric evaluation is the gold standard, and demonstrates a zone of high intraesophageal pressure in the LES and aperistalsis in the body of the esophagus. The barium contrast study reveals dilatation of the upper esophagus, a narrowed distal esophagus, and delayed emptying (Fig. 34-1). Esophagoscopy is performed to rule out the presence of an occult malignancy as the cause of dysphagia.

There is no curative therapy for achalasia. The aperistalsis in the body of the esophagus usually is irreversible, although peristalsis is partially restored in a few patients after the sphincter pressure is reduced (Mittal & Balaban, 1997). Available therapies are directed at relieving symptoms caused by LES obstruction while protecting against gastroesophageal reflux (Heitmiller, 1998). Pharmacologic therapy is largely unsuccessful in relieving symptoms of achalasia. The primary nonsurgical therapy used to relieve obstructive symptoms is forceful dilatation of the LES performed with a pneumatic dilating instrument. A balloon-tipped dilator is advanced into the esophagus under fluoroscopic guidance and positioned so that the balloon is astride the gastroesophageal junction. Once properly positioned, the balloon is inflated, producing sharp, localized, severe pain as evidence of proper dilatation (Wilkins, 1994).

Pneumatic dilatation relieves dysphagia and regurgitation in approximately 60% to 80% of patients (Heitmiller, 1998; Koshy & Nostrant, 1997). The procedure is complicated by gastroesophageal reflux in some patients. Iatrogenic perforation of the esophagus is an occasional complication of the pneumatic dilatation. It is suspected if there is prolonged pain or excessive blood on the dilator; if suspected, a contrast esophageal swallow study is performed promptly to confirm the diagnosis (Wilkins, 1994). A second and newer nonsurgical therapy for achalasia is the direct injection, during endoscopy, of the nerve toxin, botulinum toxin, to lessen LES obstruction (Pasricha et

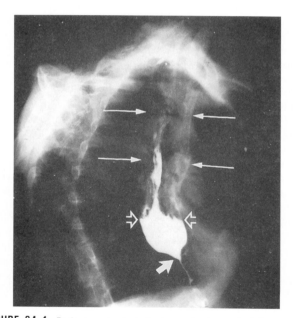

FIGURE 34-1. Barium contrast study demonstrating typical features of achalasia. Note dilated esophageal body (*long arrows*), fluid level of barium in esophagus (*short open arrows*), and characteristic "bird's beak" deformity (*short solid arrow*) produced by distal esophageal narrowing. (Courtesy of Robert M. Vanecko, MD)

al., 1995). The therapeutic response to botulinum toxin lasts 8 to 14 months, after which the treatment must be repeated (Heitmiller, 1998).

The surgical treatment for achalasia is esophagomyotomy. The operation consists of division of the muscular layer of the gastroesophageal junction to allow more complete emptying of the esophagus. Some surgeons recommend performance of a concomitant antireflux procedure to prevent iatrogenic gastroesophageal reflux through the ablated sphincter. A variety of operative techniques comprise the "antireflux procedures"; they are delineated in Chapter 39, Surgical Treatment of Esophageal Diseases. In the absence of therapy for achalasia, or if therapy is inadequate or complicated by acid reflux, the esophagus undergoes progressive dilatation and eventual marked tortuosity occurs, resulting in the condition known as end-stage achalasia (Banbury et al., 1999). The term "sigmoid esophagus" is used to describe the radiographic appearance of end-stage achalasia.

Diffuse esophageal spasm is another disorder of impaired esophageal motility. The disorder, which has an unknown etiology, is characterized by repetitive, sustained, nonperistaltic, high-pressure contractions in the body of the esophagus. The elevated esophageal wall tension results in chest pain and the disordered segmental peristalsis produces dysphagia (Heitmiller, 1998). Chest pain associated with diffuse esophageal spasm often mimics pain produced by myocardial ischemia. Because both types of pain are relieved with nitroglycerin, esophageal spasm is sometimes mistaken for angina. Regurgitation and weight loss are other common manifestations of esophageal spasm (Wilkins, 1994). Diagnosis of diffuse esophageal spasm is achieved with manometry and contrast radiologic examination. Calcium channel antagonist medications, specifically nifedipine, and nitroglycerin often are effective in relieving associated symptoms. Either pneumatic dilatation or endoscopic injection of botulinum toxin also may be performed (Heitmiller, 1998). Occasionally, an esophagomyotomy, extended from the gastroesophageal junction to the arch of the aorta (called a long myotomy), is necessary to relieve spasm. However, this procedure is considered only if all other lesser form of therapy fail.

Oropharyngeal dysphagia, or impaired function of the swallowing mechanism (UES), is usually caused by a neuromuscular disorder such as Parkinson's disease, cerebral vascular accident, muscular dystrophy, or myasthenia gravis. Clinical manifestations of oropharyngeal dysphagia include discomfort during meals and bronchopulmonary complications of aspiration (Duranceau, 1995). Medical therapy is based on treatment of the underlying disorder. Surgical therapy is not helpful for most forms of oropharyngeal dysfunction.

Esophageal Diverticulum

An *esophageal diverticulum* is an epithelial-lined, blind pouch leading from the main lumen of the esophagus (Trastek, 1994). Esophageal diverticula usually are classified according to location (cervical, thoracic, or epiphrenic), pathogenesis (pulsion or traction), or morphology (true or false) (Altorki, 1998). The three major types of esophageal diverticula are (1) pharyngoesophageal pulsion, or Zenker's diverticulum; (2) epiphrenic pulsion diverticulum; and (3) parabronchial traction diverticulum. Pulsion diverticula result from forces within the esophageal mucosa acting against an area of resistance; almost all are related to an esophageal motility disorder. Traction diverticula are caused by forces exerted from outside the esophagus, such as inflammatory disease in the mediastinal lymph nodes. Traction diverticula are rare and of little clinical significance.

Zenker's diverticulum is the most common type of esophageal diverticulum and the form most likely to necessitate surgical therapy. Zenker's diverticula originate near the cricopharyngeus muscle and usually occur in adults older than 40 years of age. The exact nature of the cricopharyngeal motor disorder that results in formation of a Zenker's diverticulum remains unclear, but it is believed to be the consequence of pharyngo-cricopharyngeal incoordination. Early in its development, the diverticulum is small and varies in size with the phase of swallowing. Once established, a diverticulum enlarges rapidly and descends dependently because of constant distention with ingested material (Trastek, 1994). In severe cases, the sac may retain several hundred milliliters of undigested food and fluid and extend to or below the level of the aortic arch (Skinner & Belsey, 1988a).

Progressive symptoms occur owing to esophageal obstruction and unimpeded emptying of the diverticulum into the upper esophagus. Dysphagia is the most frequent symptom, occurring in 80% to 90% of patients (Ferraro & Duranceau, 1994). Other characteristic symptoms include foul breath, noisy deglutition (swallowing), spontaneous regurgitation, and coughing or choking episodes. If untreated, continuous saliva and food spillage may cause aspiration pneumonia; local complications, such as inflammation, perforation, abscess formation, or tracheoesophageal fistula, also may occur (Duranceau et al., 1991).

Diagnosis of a Zenker's diverticulum is achieved with a contrast (barium) esophagogram. Because of the risk of aspiration associated with Zenker's diverticulum, surgical treatment is indicated in most patients in the absence of a compelling medical contraindication (Altorki, 1998). For small diverticula, cricopharyngeal esophagomyotomy usually is sufficient to relieve symptoms. Diverticulopexy or diverticulectomy may be performed for larger diverticula. Diverticulopexy consists of suspending the diverticulum in an inverted position so that it drains into the esophagus rather than filling with ingested material. Diverticulectomy is surgical resection of the diverticulum.

Hiatal Hernia

The esophagus normally passes from the thorax into the abdomen through an opening in the diaphragm known as the esophageal hiatus. The distal esophagus is tethered in place by the phrenoesophageal membrane, which extends from the transversus abdominis muscle and the diaphragm to connective tissue of the intrathoracic esophageal submucosa (Skinner, 1994). *Hiatal hernia* is an anatomic deformity of the esophageal hiatus that allows translocation of the gastroesophageal junction or part of the stomach into the thorax.

Most common is *type I*, or *sliding hiatal hernia*. It is thought to occur in as many as 10% of adults in North America (Skinner, 1995). A sliding hiatal hernia is characterized by stretching of the phrenoesophageal membrane, resulting in protrusion of a small portion of gastric cardia through the esophageal hiatus (Fig. 34-2). It produces no symptoms or complications itself, but often is associated with regurgitation of acidic gastric contents into the distal esophagus, a condition termed *gastroesophageal reflux* and described in detail later. Treatment of type I hiatal hernia is not necessary except for complications of the condition.

In *type II*, or *paraesophageal hernia,* a defect in the phrenoesophageal membrane allows herniation of peritoneum with protrusion of a portion or all of the stomach into the thoracic low-pressure compartment (see Fig. 34-2). In contrast to sliding hiatal hernias, paraesophageal hernias may cause symptoms even without associated gastroesophageal reflux, including early satiety, vomiting after a large meal, epigastric distress, dysphagia, and gurgling noises within the chest (Skinner, 1995). Surgical repair of paraesophageal hernias is recommended because of the risk of (1) gastric obstruction, infarction, or strangulation; (2) bleeding; or (3) acute intrathoracic dilatation (Skinner, 1994).

Gastroesophageal Reflux Disease

Gastroesophageal reflux is the regurgitation of acidic gastric contents into the distal esophagus. Some degree of reflux occurs normally and is considered physiologic;

the refluxed material quickly returns to the stomach, producing no symptoms or injury to esophageal mucosa (Skinner, 1994). Pathologic reflux is said to exist when the frequency and degree of reflux, and delayed clearing of refluxed material, are sufficient to produce symptoms or esophageal injury. The mechanism for pathologic gastroesophageal reflux remains ill defined. The etiology is thought to be multifactorial, with contributing factors including the caustic materials that are refluxed, a breakdown in the defense mechanisms of the esophagus, and a functional abnormality that results in reflux (Scott & Gelhot, 1999).

Pathologic *gastroesophageal reflux disease (GERD)* accounts for approximately 75% of esophageal disease and affects 0.4% of people in the United States (Stein et al., 1992b). Symptomatic gastroesophageal reflux commonly is associated with the presence of a hiatal hernia. Many people with hiatal hernias, however, are asymptomatic and, conversely, pathologic gastroesophageal reflux may be present in the absence of a demonstrable hiatal hernia (Cooper, 1997). Gastroesophageal reflux also may occur in association with scleroderma, a progressive systemic disease that produces fibrosis of esophageal smooth muscle, resulting in absence of peristalsis in the lower two thirds of the esophagus (Mansour & Malone, 1988). It is the most common collagen vascular disease affecting esophageal function, with esophageal involvement reported in 50% to 80% of patients (Heitmiller, 1998).

The predominant symptom of GERD is epigastric or substernal discomfort, commonly termed *heartburn*. As many as 10% of Americans have episodes of heartburn (pyrosis) every day and 44% have symptoms at least once a month (Scott & Gelhot, 1999). Two distinct patterns of reflux are observed. Some patients have an increased amount of reflux during daytime activities but

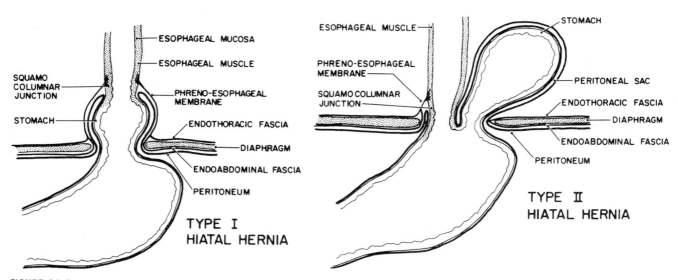

FIGURE 34-2. Diagrammatic representation of type I and type II hiatal hernia. In a type I hiatal hernia, the phreno-esophageal membrane is intact; in a type II hiatal hernia, a defect in the phrenoesophageal membrane permits herniation of the peritoneal sac. (Skinner DB, 1981: Hiatal hernia and gastroesophageal reflux. In Sabiston DC Jr [ed]: Davis-Christopher Textbook of Surgery, ed. 12, p. 823. Philadelphia, WB Saunders)

do not experience it while reclining at night; in others, the regurgitation of gastric contents occurs primarily when they are reclining (Skinner, 1994).

Although the presence of typical symptoms virtually establishes the diagnosis of GERD, 24-hour esophageal pH monitoring may be used to provide a quantitative assessment of the degree of reflux and the relationship of reflux episodes to clinical symptoms (Cooper, 1997). A monitor is placed in the esophagus above the lower esophageal sphincter and used to record esophageal pH. Concurrently, the patient records the time and situation in which symptoms occur, in the hope that symptoms can be correlated with the lowering of esophageal pH that occurs with reflux (Scott & Gelhot, 1999).

Treatment of GERD is aimed at alleviating symptoms and decreasing the damaging effects of regurgitated gastric juice on the esophagus. Dietary modifications include avoidance of particular foods and beverages that precipitate symptoms in the individual patient, typically such items as coffee, acidic beverages, or fatty foods. Remaining upright for several hours after meals and keeping the head of the bed elevated are other measures that often help reduce the degree of reflux. Obesity and cigarette smoking may worsen symptoms associated with GERD. Obesity increases intra-abdominal pressure, resulting in an increased transsphincteric gradient, and cigarette smoking can decrease LES pressure and increase the frequency of reflux episodes (Naunheim & Baue, 1996). Consequently, physicians usually recommend weight reduction in obese patients and smoking cessation.

Four categories of pharmacologic agents are used in the treatment of GERD (Table 34-1). Long-term continuation of full prescription doses of medications is important because approximately 80% of patients have symptoms or endoscopic evidence of relapse within 6 months when therapy is discontinued or tapered (Katz & Castell, 1997). If medical therapy is unsuccessful in eliminating persistent symptoms of reflux, an antireflux operation may be necessary to restore competency to the LES. Continued reflux of gastric contents into the esophagus eventually causes tissue ulceration that can lead to bleeding, perforation, or stricture formation. In as many as 20% of patients with GERD, serious complications develop, including ulcerative esophagitis, peptic stricture, or the premalignant condition, Barrett's esophagus (Katz & Castell, 1997).

Barrett's esophagus is a condition in which columnar epithelium replaces the normal squamous cell lining in the distal esophagus. It is more common in white men, with a mean age at detection of 55 years (Bremner & Bremner, 1997). The columnar metaplasia is thought to occur as a response to reflux of gastric acid into the esophagus with ulceration and destruction of squamous epithelium and consequent replacement by columnar epithelium (Wolfe & Sebastian, 1995). Patients with Barrett's esophagus commonly describe more severe symptoms and a longer duration of reflux disease, and excessive acid reflux into the distal esophagus usually can be demonstrated with 24-hour pH monitoring (DeMeester, 1997a).

Barrett's esophagus is not simple reepithelialization of injured esophageal lining but rather the metaplastic transformation into a heterogeneous collection of cell types and patterns. The mucosal abnormality is significant because of the increased incidence of esophageal adenocarcinoma after its development. The risk for development of adenocarcinoma in patients with Barrett's esophagus is 30 to 125 times that of the normal population (DeMeester, 1997b). Younger age at onset and longer duration of symptoms appear to increase the risk of malignancy (Scott & Gelhot, 1999). Patients with Barrett's esophagus also are at increased risk for progression of the mucosal abnormality up the esophagus, stricture formation, or hemorrhage from a Barrett's ulcer (Stein et al., 1992b).

Accordingly, detection of Barrett's esophagus prompts intensive medical therapy and, if necessary, a surgical antireflux procedure. Endoscopy with systematic biopsy specimens from the entire columnar-lined esophagus should be performed to detect carcinoma or high-grade dysplasia at an early stage when treatment has a better chance of preventing late cancer death (Cameron, 1998). Patients with Barrett's esophagus without dysplasia or with only low-grade dysplasia require serial endoscopic examinations with multiple surveillance biopsies to monitor the status of dysplastic changes.

The management of patients with Barrett's esophagus and high-grade dysplasia is somewhat controversial because of the difficulty in distinguishing high-grade dysplasia from adenocarcinoma in endoscopic biopsy tissue samples. An estimated 10% to 52% of patients who undergo operation after an endoscopic biopsy diagnosis of high-grade dysplasia are determined to have an invasive esophageal carcinoma on pathologic examination of the resected esophagus (Cameron, 1998).

Some physicians recommend elimination of reflux

TABLE 34-1

Pharmacologic Treatment of Gastroesophageal Reflux Disease

Category	Medications	Action
Cytoprotective agents	Sucralfate	Improve mucosal resistance
Antacids		Neutralize gastric contents
Acid suppressors	Cimetidine, ranitidine	Minimize secretions
Prokinetic agents	Cisapride	Strengthen the lower esophageal sphincter, enhance esophageal clearance, accelerate gastric emptying, and minimize gastroduodenal reflux
Proton pump inhibitors	Omeprazole, lansoprazole	Potent inhibition of gastric acid secretion

and continued frequent endoscopic surveillance for patients with Barrett's esophagus associated with high-grade dysplasia. Others consider high-grade dysplasia a marker of early adenocarcinoma in most patients and advocate esophagectomy in patients deemed medically fit to tolerate the procedure (Hagen, 1997). High-grade dysplasia is rarely associated with lymphatic spread because tumor has not penetrated the basement membrane. Delaying treatment until the occurrence of deeper esophageal wall invasion with probable lymphatic spread markedly decreases the patient's probability of survival (Rice, 1999). Increased awareness of the association between gastroesophageal reflux and esophageal adenocarcinoma and the institution of surveillance protocols for patients with Barrett's esophagus have led to a larger group of patients referred for treatment of early-stage esophageal cancer (Nigro et al., 1999).

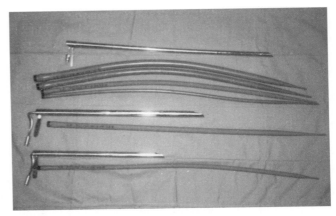

FIGURE 34-3. Various sizes of mercury-weighted bougies used for esophageal dilatation; also displayed are rigid esophagoscopes used for introduction of the bougies. (Courtesy of Sudhir Sundaresan, MD)

Esophageal Stricture

Esophageal stricture, a localized zone of luminal narrowing, due to circumferential fibrosis, usually occurs at the gastroesophageal junction as a complication of gastroesophageal reflux. An estimated 90% of esophageal strictures in North America are peptic esophageal strictures caused by gastroesophageal reflux (Duranceau, 1995). An esophageal stricture is likely to produce dysphagia, which may vary from mild to severe, depending on lumen size and length of the stricture. In contrast to motility disorders, esophageal stricture imposes a fixed mechanical obstruction. The degree of dysphagia tends to vary according to size of the food bolus and is progressive, beginning with solid foods and progressing to liquids.

The diagnostic evaluation of patients with esophageal stricture includes esophagoscopy with tissue biopsy to rule out malignancy and determine feasibility of dilating the stricture. Manometric evaluation also is performed to quantitate reflux, assess motility, and exclude other diseases. Esophageal dilatation is used in most patients with peptic esophageal strictures as an initial form of therapy because of its low cost, safety, minimal morbidity, and high degree of efficacy (Ferguson, 1994). Depending on severity of symptoms, it may be necessary for the patient to undergo occasional or even regular dilatation of the stricture.

The process of mechanically dilating narrowed esophageal segments is termed *bougienage*. Soft, moderately severe strictures are commonly dilated using mercury-weighted dilating instruments, called *bougies* (Fig. 34-3). With the patient in a sitting position to permit gravity to assist movement of the dilator through the stricture, bougienage is performed during single or multiple sessions in a stepwise fashion, with sequential use of bougies of increasing diameter (Ferguson, 1994). Alternatively, bougienage may be performed by passing a guidewire into the stomach through an endoscope; progressively larger bougies are then advanced over the guidewire and through the narrowed esophageal segment. Surgical therapy may become necessary for esophageal stricture associated with severe reflux that is unresponsive to conservative therapy or for stricture that

recurs. The stricture usually is vigorously dilated during the operation; an antireflux procedure is then performed to eliminate the source of the peptic injury allowing subsequent healing of the esophagus.

Schatzki's ring (also called *distal esophageal web*) is a sharply defined submucosal band of collagen in the distal esophagus. Although it occurs at the same location as stricture caused by reflux, it is a distinct entity. The etiology of Schatzki's ring has not been established and its incidence is impossible to determine because most patients with this abnormality are asymptomatic (Orringer, 1997c). The presence of Schatzki's ring may be associated with dysphagia, which usually can be treated effectively with intermittent bougienage. Uncommonly, Schatzki's ring also is associated with symptomatic gastroesophageal reflux, necessitating pharmacologic therapy or, rarely, a surgical antireflux procedure with intraoperative dilatation of the ring.

Other Benign Disorders

Benign neoplasms of the esophagus are rare. Approximately 60% of benign tumors and cysts of the esophagus are leiomyomas, 20% are cysts, and 5% are polyps; the remaining benign lesions occur with an incidence of less than 2% (Orringer, 1997d). Leiomyomas usually occur in young or middle-aged adults and in the middle or distal esophagus. They often cause no symptoms and are detected only incidentally at autopsy. When present, symptoms are related to size of the tumor and may include dysphagia, chest pain, or, rarely, hemorrhage (Duranceau, 1995).

► Esophageal Injuries

Caustic Injury

Caustic injury to the esophagus can occur as a result of accidental or purposeful ingestion of a poisonous agent.

Chemical agents most commonly associated with corrosive burns of the esophagus include alkaline caustics, acids or acid-like corrosives, and household bleaches (Wolfe & Sebastian, 1995). Approximately 50% of ingestion in adults and almost all ingestion in children is accidental (Handy & Reed, 1996). Damage begins almost instantaneously when the caustic substance contacts esophageal submucosa. The site and severity of injury depend primarily on the character, quantity, and concentration of the ingested substance; solid lye substances tend to lodge in the oropharynx or upper esophagus, whereas concentrated liquid caustics damage not only the esophagus but may injure the stomach and distal intestinal tract (Talbert, 1997). Esophagoscopy is performed to determine the severity of injury.

Caustic injury of the esophagus progresses through three phases: (1) inflammation, edema, and necrosis; (2) tissue sloughing, mucosal ulceration, and development of granulation tissue; and (3) cicatrization (scarring) and stricture formation (Vanecko & Shields, 1994) (Fig. 34-4). Salvage of native esophageal function is crucial because of the significant morbidity associated with esophageal replacement. In addition, caustic esophageal strictures significantly increase the risk for development of esophageal cancer. One to 4% percent of all esophageal cancers occur in an esophagus injured by caustic agents; the average interval from injury to cancer development is approximately 40 years (Wolfe & Sebastian, 1995).

Management of patients with caustic burns is directed at limiting the severity of esophageal necrosis, scarring, and stricture formation. Antibiotics and corticosteroids are recommended during the acute injury phase to reduce the severity of stricture formation (Vanecko & Shields, 1994). Bougienage is used later to dilate strictures. More severe cases may be treated with placement of an intraesophageal stent. In extreme cases, caustic agents may produce esophageal perforation, necessitating emergent esophagectomy.

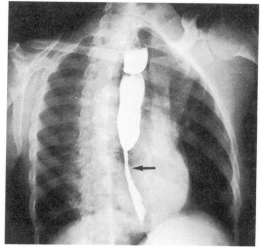

FIGURE 34-4. Barium swallow study in a patient with a history of lye ingestion. This right anterior oblique projection demonstrates a long esophageal stricture (*arrow*). (Courtesy of Robert M. Vanecko, MD)

Perforation

Perforation of the esophagus may occur as a consequence of iatrogenic injury, barogenic mechanisms, trauma, or foreign body ingestion. Iatrogenic causes account for most perforations; 43% of perforations occur secondary to instrumentation during esophagoscopy, pneumatic dilatation, bougienage, and sclerotherapy (Handy & Reed, 1996). Less commonly, iatrogenic perforation occurs as a complication of an operative procedure or, rarely, after difficult nasogastric tube insertion. Iatrogenic perforations frequently occur in the cervical portion of the esophagus because of the lack of rigid surrounding structures. Perforations are most likely to occur in a diseased esophagus (eg, in association with stricture, tumor, or achalasia).

Barogenic rupture is the cause of approximately 15% of esophageal perforations (Handy & Reed, 1996). Barogenic rupture of the esophagus is also known as spontaneous rupture or Boerhaave's syndrome. The term *spontaneous* is a misnomer because the injury always is preceded by an event that acutely raises intraluminal esophageal pressure above a critical level (Skinner & Belsey, 1988b). The most common precipitant is severe vomiting. Esophageal rupture also may result from other events that cause a sudden rapid increase in intraesophageal pressure, such as chewing on pressurized soda containers, hyperemesis gravidarum, weight lifting, convulsions, blunt abdominal trauma, defecation, and laughing fits (Bjerke, 1994a).

Traumatic perforation usually is due to a penetrating knife or gunshot wound. Injuries to the cervical esophagus occur at equal frequency with bullet or knife wounds, but gunshot wounds, especially high-velocity bullets, remain the most common cause of intrathoracic and abdominal esophageal injury (Bjerke, 1994b). The esophagus is almost never injured from blunt trauma because of its protected location within the thorax.

Perforation of the esophagus typically causes fever and severe chest, epigastric, or back pain. Depending on location of the perforation, other symptoms such as hematemesis, tachycardia, dysphagia, and dyspnea may be present. The diagnosis is suggested by these symptoms in association with a clinical history of esophageal instrumentation, severe vomiting, swallowing of a foreign body, or penetrating trauma. Because the esophageal laceration allows swallowed air to escape into the neck or mediastinum, subcutaneous emphysema or pneumomediastinum often is apparent on the chest roentgenogram. A left pleural effusion also may be evident. Diagnosis of esophageal perforation is confirmed by a contrast swallow study.

A perforation in the esophagus allows gastric juices, saliva, and bacteria to seep into the mediastinum, where they track along mediastinal planes. The leakage of ingested material and gastrointestinal secretions results in a chemical insult to surrounding tissues, leading to mediastinitis; the oral bacterial flora involving aerobic and anaerobic organisms causes a mixed necrotizing superinfection in a closed space adjacent to vital organs of the mediastinum and upper abdomen (Handy & Reed, 1996). Prompt treatment is imperative to control the inevitable mediastinitis and overwhelming sepsis. Intravenous antibiotic therapy is instituted, and operative exploration is performed to débride infected tissue and drain the area.

In patients with perforations of the cervical esophagus, drainage of the area usually is sufficient to allow healing of the esophageal tissue. Perforations in the thoracic or lower esophagus usually require suture repair of the esophagus. If treatment is delayed or infection extensive, esophageal repair may not be possible. Instead, it may be necessary to perform an esophageal diversion procedure, followed by esophageal reconstruction after the infection resolves. If the perforation is not diagnosed and treated in a timely fashion, the condition usually is fatal.

Esophageal diversion consists of dividing the esophagus, using the proximal end to create an esophagocutaneous fistula, and suturing closed the distal esophagus. Gastric drainage and enteral feeding tubes are placed to decompress the stomach and provide alimentation, respectively. Rarely, undiagnosed esophageal perforation produces a localized, contained periesophageal abscess rather than mediastinitis. In such patients, the abscess may cause manifestations of chronic infection (anemia, weight loss, inanition) that lead to its eventual diagnosis and treatment.

Foreign Body Obstruction

Foreign body obstruction occurs most frequently in young children. Occasionally, a foreign object becomes lodged in the esophagus of an adult. Common items that may be swallowed inadvertently and remain in the esophagus include coins, chicken and fish bones, boluses of meat, safety pins, and dentures (Boyd, 1995). The esophagus is vulnerable to retention of a swallowed foreign body because of weak peristalsis and multiple narrowings. An object also may become lodged because a sharp edge impinges on esophageal mucosa. Objects usually lodge in one of the three normal areas of esophageal narrowing: (1) at the esophageal entrance in the area of the cricopharyngeus muscle; (2) in the mid-portion, where the esophagus is indented by the crossing of the left mainstem bronchus and aortic arch; or (3) at the LES (Rothberg et al., 1994).

Clinical manifestations of a foreign body lodged in the esophagus include chest pain, dysphagia, and a sensation of having "something stuck." If the esophagus is totally obstructed, drooling of saliva or aspiration may occur. The presence of a foreign object usually can be demonstrated radiographically, either with a plain chest roentgenogram or a contrast swallow study. Although most ingested foreign bodies pass spontaneously, 10% to 20% require endoscopic removal and 1% require surgical treatment (Handy & Reed, 1996).

Removal of foreign bodies usually is performed using a flexible or rigid esophagoscope. Particular care is necessary to avoid iatrogenic esophageal perforation when removing objects with sharp points that have become embedded in the esophagus wall (Boyd, 1995). Surgical removal is indicated if a sharp object is not removable with esophagoscopy or a blunt object has not advanced through the gastrointestinal tract for 3 days; drug-filled condoms are removed surgically to avoid the risk of rupture (Handy & Reed, 1996). Prolonged impaction of a foreign object may lead to perforation with mediastinitis, localized abscess formation, or aspiration pneumonia.

▶ Esophageal Cancer

Esophageal cancer is relatively rare in the United States but is common in other parts of the world, such as China. The etiology of esophageal cancer appears to be multifactorial and varies with geography and cell type. The geographic variation in annual incidence is remarkable, ranging from less than 5 cases per 100,000 in the United States to over 500 cases per 100,000 in certain high-risk areas located in Iran, China, and Russia (Kirby & Rice, 1997). Esophageal cancer is more prevalent in men between 50 and 70 years of age and in African Americans. Malignant neoplasms may occur in the upper, middle, or lower esophagus. The histologic cell type is, with rare exceptions, either adenocarcinoma (most common in the distal esophagus) or squamous cell carcinoma (most common in the upper and middle esophagus). Unusual neoplasms of the esophagus include small cell carcinoma, sarcoma, and metastatic tumors, particularly melanoma.

The epidemiologic profile of esophageal cancer has been changing in North America and Western Europe (Kelsen, 1997). Although squamous cell carcinoma of the esophagus remains uncommon, an alarming increase has been reported in the incidence of adenocarcinoma of the lower esophagus and gastroesophageal junction, particularly among white men (Casson, 1998; Altorki et al., 1996). The incidence of adenocarcinoma has risen faster than that of any other malignancy and has surpassed squamous cell carcinoma to become the most common esophageal malignancy (Nigro et al., 1999).

Adenocarcinoma of the esophagus occurs in younger patients than squamous cell carcinoma and is less likely to be associated with tobacco or alcohol abuse. Barrett's esophagus, a known complication of gastroesophageal reflux disease, is the primary risk factor for development of adenocarcinoma of the distal esophagus and gastroesophageal junction. The relationship between Barrett's esophagus and esophageal cancer links one of the most deadly malignancies with the most common upper gastrointestinal disorder in Western civilization (Nigro et al., 1999). Other conditions that produce chronic esophageal irritation or strictures, such as lye burns, achalasia, and peptic reflux esophagitis, also are thought to predispose to esophageal carcinoma (Bains & Shields, 1994).

Smoking and heavy alcohol consumption are risk factors for *squamous cell carcinoma*. Smokers have a risk for development of squamous cell carcinoma that is 5 to 10 times higher than that of the general population, and the risk increases considerably when excessive alcohol consumption is combined with smoking (Kirby & Rice, 1994). The smoking-related risk is strongly dose dependent and is not confined only to cigarettes; cigar and pipe smokers exhibit a higher risk relative to nonsmokers (Altorki et al., 1996).

Cancer of the esophagus spreads by direct invasion into surrounding structures and through lymphatic and hematogenous routes to distant structures. Early and widespread lymphatic dissemination is likely because of the unique esophageal lymphatic anatomy that exposes lymphatics to carcinoma at the earliest stage of invasion, just after the carcinoma breaches the basement membrane and invades the lamina propria (Rice, 1999) (Fig. 34-5). A network of lymphatic vessels draining into regional lymph nodes extends throughout the esophageal mucosa. Neoplasms in the upper and middle third of the esophagus tend to involve the tracheobronchial tree, aorta, and left recurrent laryngeal nerve, whereas tumors in the lower third of the esophagus may invade the diaphragm, pericardium, lung, or stomach. Metastasis to the liver, lung, or bone is not unusual.

Although squamous cell carcinoma continues to be diagnosed largely at an advanced stage when regional or distant metastasis has already occurred, esophageal adenocarcinoma sometimes is diagnosed at an early stage because of increased endoscopic surveillance of patients with Barrett's esophagus, who are known to be at high risk. As a result, new information is being learned about the early behavior and spread of esophageal adenocarcinoma. Tumor depth through the esophageal wall is a strong predictor of the probability of lymph node metastases, the likelihood of distant node involvement, and the risk of recurrent disease (Nigro et al., 1999). Less than 10% of patients with tumors limited to the esophageal mucosa (intramucosal) have regional lymph node involvement but lymph node involvement increases to 50% of patients once the tumor penetrates the muscularis mucosa (submucosal) and 80% when the tumor invades the muscularis propria (intramuscular) (Nigro et al., 1999).

Esophageal carcinoma is a devastating illness, both because of its lethal nature and because of its profound impact on quality of life. Clinical manifestations are identical whether the cell type is squamous cell or adenocarcinoma. Dysphagia, the most common symptom, does not occur until late in the disease because the esophagus lacks a serosal coat and can distend to accommodate an intraluminal growth without noticeably impeding deglutination (Altorki et al., 1996). As the disease progresses, the tumor increasingly obstructs the esophageal lumen. The patient loses weight, becomes cachectic, and eventually may be unable to tolerate any oral food or liquids and may not even be able to swallow saliva. Aspiration, with resultant pneumonia, is common. Most patients are diagnosed only after the development of symptoms, late in the course of the disease. A symptomatic tumor that obstructs the esophagus usually has spread beyond the esophageal musculature to involve periesophageal tissue or adjacent organs and has metastasized to regional lymph nodes or distant sites (Rice, 1999).

The presence of an esophageal tumor is suggested by narrowing and irregularity of the esophageal lumen on a barium contrast swallow study. A tissue biopsy, obtained during esophageal endoscopy (esophagoscopy), confirms the diagnosis. If the lesion is in the upper esophagus, bronchoscopy is performed as well to detect malignant extention to the tracheobronchial tree. Therapy for esophageal cancer remains somewhat controversial because no particular treatment or combination of treatments has proven effective in improving survival rates. It is estimated that cure is possible in fewer than 10% of patients with carcinoma of the esophagus (Ginsberg & Waters, 1994). Prognosis for survival is particularly poor if the tumor is located in the upper one third of the esophagus.

Surgical intervention may be undertaken for one of several purposes: (1) to resect the tumor for curative purposes, (2) to restore the patient's ability to eat and drink, or (3) to divert esophageal contents (saliva) through an

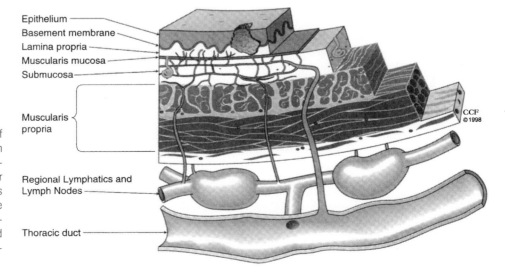

FIGURE 34-5. The lymphatic anatomy of the esophagus. Lymphatics are found in the lamina propria just below the basement membrane. An intramucosal tumor with invasion of the lamina propria is demonstrated in this illustration. (Rice TW, 1999: Commentary: Esophageal carcinoma confined to the wall—the need for immediate definitive therapy. J Thorac Cardiovasc Surg 117:26)

Epithelium
Basement membrane
Lamina propria
Muscularis mucosa
Submucosa
Muscularis propria
Regional Lymphatics and Lymph Nodes
Thoracic duct

CCF
© 1998

esophageal fistula and provide an alternative route for alimentation. Esophagogastrectomy with esophagogastrostomy (removal of the diseased esophageal segment and reattachment of stomach to proximal esophagus) is the most common type of surgical resection for esophageal carcinoma. It is performed using either a transhiatal approach (ie, through abdominal and cervical incisions) or a right thoracotomy incision (Ivor-Lewis procedure). Alternatively, the esophagus may be resected and replaced with a harvested segment of large bowel (esophagogastrectomy with colon interposition).

For early-stage esophageal tumors, complete surgical resection may be curative, with 5-year survival rates approaching 70%; for most patients with locally advanced tumors, however, the overall survival rate remains less than 20% at 5 years (Kennedy & Casson, 1999a). Surgical treatment of esophageal cancer is discussed further in Chapter 39, Surgical Treatment of Esophageal Diseases.

Chemotherapy, radiation, or both may be used as adjuncts to surgical therapy. Several studies have reported favorable survival results with adjuvant treatment before surgical resection in patients with squamous cell tumors in the upper third of the esophagus (Hoffman et al., 1998; Tsujinaka et al., 1999). However, improvement in prognosis has yet to be demonstrated in prospective, randomized, controlled trials of multimodal therapy (Lehnert, 1999). Preoperative adjuvant therapy may facilitate surgical resection by reducing tumor size and increasing the probability of technical success in removing all tumor cells, particularly with squamous cell tumors above the level of the carina (DeMeester, 1997c; Naunheim et al., 1992). Preoperative thoracoscopic lymph node staging has been recommended to help determine appropriate candidates for adjuvant chemotherapy or radiation therapy (Krasna, 1998).

Regardless of whether cure is possible, palliative therapy is important to relieve bothersome symptoms produced by esophageal obstruction. A number of palliative therapies may be useful to lessen obstruction and restore swallowing. In selected situations, tumor resection with restoration of esophageal continuity may be performed to relieve dysphagia and associated aspiration and to prevent hemorrhage from an ulcerating tumor or septic complications from a tumor associated with perforation or infection (Skinner & Belsey, 1988c). A procedure to bypass the obstructed esophagus without resection of the tumor (retrosternal gastric bypass) may be performed if the tumor is technically unresectable because of local extension to adjacent structures. Palliative surgical procedures are associated with considerable morbidity. Alternatively, esophageal dilatation may be performed or a stent may be placed in the lumen of the esophagus across the obstructed segment. Enteral alimentation through a gastrostomy or jejunostomy tube may be provided in patients who are no longer able to take oral nourishment because of obstruction from the tumor.

Radiation therapy, alone or in combination with chemotherapy, may be used for palliation. Current palliative strategies combining external-beam radiation with sensitizing chemotherapy (and including nutritional support, dilatation, or stenting) are associated with improved swallowing in 60% to 80% of patients (Kennedy & Casson, 1999b). Endoscopic palliative procedures include photodynamic laser therapy and brachytherapy. Photodynamic therapy consists of intravenous infusion of a photosensitive substance; laser therapy is then performed by means of esophagoscopy to create an opening in the occluded esophagus large enough for the passage of secretions and ingested food. Brachytherapy is a form of radiation therapy in which radioactive isotopes are implanted directly into the tumor.

Patients with incurable esophageal cancer have markedly limited life spans. Therefore, palliative interventions must be carefully planned to restore swallowing capability and improve quality of life without imposing excessive morbidity and lengthy hospitalization. Ideally, palliative therapy maximizes the number of days that a patient is able to take adequate oral nutrition while spending as little time in the hospital as possible (Low & Pagliero, 1996).

REFERENCES

Altorki NK, 1998: Excision of esophageal diverticula. In Kaiser LR, Kron IL, Spray TL (eds): Mastery of Cardiothoracic Surgery. Philadelphia, Lippincott Williams & Wilkins

Altorki NK, Skinner DB, Minsky BD, et al., 1996: Carcinoma of the esophagus. In Baue AE, Geha AS, Hammond GL, et al. (eds): Glenn's Thoracic and Cardiovascular Surgery, ed. 6. Stamford, CT, Appleton & Lange

Bains MS, Shields TW, 1994: Squamous cell carcinoma of the esophagus. In Shields TW (ed): General Thoracic Surgery, ed. 4. Baltimore, Williams & Wilkins

Banbury MK, Rice TW, Goldblum JR, 1999: Esophagectomy with gastric reconstruction for achalasia. J Thorac Cardiovasc Surg 117:1077

Bjerke HS, 1994a: Boerhaave's syndrome and barogenic injuries of the esophagus. Chest Surg Clin North Am 4:819

Bjerke HS, 1994b: Penetrating and blunt injuries of the esophagus. Chest Surg Clin North Am 4:811

Boyd AD, 1995: Endoscopy: Bronchoscopy and esophagoscopy. In Sabiston DC Jr, Spencer FC (eds): Surgery of the Chest, ed. 6. Philadelphia, WB Saunders

Bremner CG, Bremner RM, 1997: Barrett's esophagus. Surg Clin North Am 77:1115

Cameron AJ, 1998: Management of Barrett's esophagus. Mayo Clin Proc 73:457

Casson AG, 1998: Thoracic approaches to esophagectomy. In Kaiser LR, Kron IL, Spray TL (eds): Mastery of Cardiothoracic Surgery. Philadelphia, Lippincott Williams & Wilkins

Cooper JD, 1997: Current role of esophageal function studies. Semin Thorac Cardiovasc Surg 9:157

DeMeester TR, 1997a: Management of Barrett's esophagus free of dysplasia. Semin Thorac Cardiovasc Surg 9:279

DeMeester TR, 1997b: Management of adenocarcinoma arising in Barrett's esophagus. Semin Thorac Cardiovasc Surg 9:290

DeMeester TR, 1997c: Esophageal carcinoma. Semin Surg Oncol 13:217

Duranceau A, 1996: Esophageal dysmotility. In Baue AE, Geha AS, Hammond GL, et al. (eds): Glenn's Thoracic and Cardiovascular Surgery, ed. 6. Stamford, CT, Appleton & Lange

Duranceau A, 1995: Disorders of the esophagus in the adult.

In Sabiston DC Jr, Spencer FC (eds): Surgery of the Chest, ed. 6. Philadelphia, WB Saunders

Duranceau A, Lafontaine ER, Deschamps C, 1991: Complications of operations for esophageal motor disorders. In Waldhausen JA, Orringer MB (eds): Complications in Cardiothoracic Surgery. St. Louis, Mosby–Year Book

Ferguson MK, 1994: Medical and surgical management of peptic esophageal strictures. Chest Surg Clin North Am 4:673

Ferraro P, Duranceau A, 1994: Esophageal diverticula. Chest Surg Clin North Am 4:741

Ginsberg RJ, Waters PF, 1994: Surgical palliation of inoperable carcinoma of the esophagus. In Shields TW (ed): General Thoracic Surgery, ed. 4. Baltimore, Williams & Wilkins

Hagen JA, 1997: Management of Barrett's esophagus with dysplasia. Semin Thorac Cardiovasc Surg 9:285

Handy JR, Reed CE, 1996: Esophageal injury: Perforation, chemical burns, foreign bodies, and bleeding. In Baue AE, Geha AS, Hammond GL, et al. (eds): Glenn's Thoracic and Cardiovascular Surgery, ed. 6. Stamford, CT, Appleton & Lange

Heitmiller RF, 1998: Surgery of achalasia and other motility disorders. In Kaiser LR, Kron IL, Spray TL (eds): Mastery of Cardiothoracic Surgery. Philadelphia, Lippincott Williams & Wilkins

Hoffman PC, Haraf DJ, Ferguson MK, et al., 1998: Induction chemotherapy, surgery, and concomitant chemoradiotherapy for carcinoma of the esophagus: A long-term analysis. Ann Oncol 9:647

Katz PO, Castell DO, 1997: Current medical treatment and indications for surgical referral for gastroesophageal reflux disease (GERD). Semin Thorac Cardiovasc Surg 9:169

Kelsen D, 1997: Multimodality therapy for adenocarcinoma of the esophagus. Gastroenterol Clin North Am 26:635

Kennedy R, Casson AG, 1999a: Esophageal cancer: Surgery. In Casson AG, Johnston MR (eds): Key Topics in Thoracic Surgery. Oxford, UK, Bios

Kennedy R, Casson AG, 1999b: Esophageal cancer: Palliation. In Casson AG, Johnston MR (eds): Key Topics in Thoracic Surgery. Oxford, UK, Bios

Kirby TJ, Rice TW, 1994: The epidemiology of esophageal carcinoma. Chest Surg Clin North Am 4:217

Koshy SS, Nostrant TT, 1997: Pathophysiology and endoscopic/balloon treatment of esophageal motility disorders. Surg Clin North Am 77:971

Krasna MJ, 1998: Advances in staging of esophageal carcinoma. Chest 113:107S

Lehnert T, 1999: Multimodal therapy for squamous cell carcinoma of the oesophagus. Br J Surg 86:727

Low DE, Pagliero KM, 1996: Palliative treatment of carcinoma of the esophagus. In Baue AE, Geha AS, Hammond GL, et al. (eds): Glenn's Thoracic and Cardiovascular Surgery, ed. 6. Stamford, CT, Appleton & Lange

Mansour KA, Malone CE, 1988: Surgery for scleroderma of the esophagus: A 12-year experience. Ann Thorac Surg 46:513

Mittal RK, Balaban DH, 1997: The esophagogastric junction. N Engl J Med 336:924

Naunheim KS, Baue AE, 1996: Medical and surgical treatment of hiatal hernia and gastroesophageal reflux. In Baue AE, Geha AS, Hammond GL, et al. (eds): Glenn's Thoracic and Cardiovascular Surgery, ed. 6. Stamford, CT, Appleton & Lange

Naunheim KS, Petruska PJ, Roy TS, et al., 1992: Preoperative chemotherapy and radiotherapy for esophageal carcinoma. J Thorac Cardiovasc Surg 103:887

Nigro JJ, Hagen JA, DeMeester TR, et al., 1999: Prevalence and location of nodal metastases in distal esophageal adenocarcinoma confined to the wall: Implications for therapy. J Thorac Cardiovasc Surg 117:16

Orringer MB, 1991: Complications of esophageal resection and reconstruction. In Waldhausen JH, Orringer MB (eds): Complications in Cardiothoracic Surgery. St. Louis, Mosby–Year Book

Orringer MB, 1997a: The esophagus. In Sabiston DC Jr (ed): Textbook of Surgery: The Biological Basis of Modern Surgical Practice, ed. 15. Philadelphia, WB Saunders

Orringer MB, 1997b: Disorders of esophageal motility. In Sabiston DC Jr (ed): Textbook of Surgery: The Biological Basis of Modern Surgical Practice, ed. 15. Philadelphia, WB Saunders

Orringer MB, 1997c: Diverticula and miscellaneous conditions of the esophagus. In Sabiston DC Jr (ed): Textbook of Surgery: The Biological Basis of Modern Surgical Practice, ed. 15. Philadelphia, WB Saunders

Orringer MB, 1997d: Tumors of the esophagus. In Sabiston DC Jr (ed): Textbook of Surgery: The Biological Basis of Modern Surgical Practice, ed. 15. Philadelphia, WB Saunders

Pasricha PJ, Ravich WJ, Hendrix TR, et al., 1995: Intrasphincteric botulinum toxin for the treatment of achalasia. N Engl J Med 322:774

Patti MG, Gantert W, Way LW, 1997: Surgery of the esophagus: Anatomy and physiology. Surg Clin North Am 77:959

Rice TW, 1999: Commentary: Esophageal carcinoma confined to the wall—the need for immediate definitive therapy. J Thorac Cardiovasc Surg 117:26

Rothberg M, Johnson S, DeMeester TR, 1994: Anatomy of the esophagus. In Shields TW (ed): General Thoracic Surgery, ed. 4. Baltimore, Williams & Wilkins

Scott M, Gelhot AR, 1999: Gastroesophageal reflux disease: Diagnosis and management. Am Fam Physician 59:1161

Skinner DB, 1994: Gastroesophageal reflux. In Shields TW (ed): General Thoracic Surgery, ed. 4. Baltimore, Williams & Wilkins

Skinner DB, 1995: Esophageal hiatal hernia—the condition: Clinical manifestations and diagnosis. In Sabiston DC Jr, Spencer FC (eds): Surgery of the Chest, ed. 6. Philadelphia, WB Saunders

Skinner DB, Belsey RH, 1988a: The pharynx, cricopharyngeus, and Zenker's diverticulum. In Management of Esophageal Disease. Philadelphia, WB Saunders

Skinner DB, Belsey RH, 1988b: Spontaneous rupture and Boerhaave's syndrome. In Management of Esophageal Disease. Philadelphia, WB Saunders

Skinner DB, Belsey RH, 1988c: Palliation for advanced esophageal cancer. In Management of Esophageal Disease. Philadelphia, WB Saunders

Stein HJ, DeMeester TR, Hinder RA, 1992a: The concept of outpatient physiologic monitoring to diagnose functional foregut disorders. Curr Probl Surg 24:425

Stein HJ, DeMeester TR, Hinder RA, 1992b: Evaluation and surgical management of the gastroesophageal reflux disease. Curr Probl Surg 24:482

Talbert JL, 1997: Corrosive strictures of the esophagus. In Sabiston DC Jr (ed): Textbook of Surgery: The Biological Basis of Modern Surgical Practice, ed. 15. Philadelphia, WB Saunders

Trastek VF, 1994: Esophageal diverticula. In Shields TW (ed): General Thoracic Surgery, ed. 4. Baltimore, Williams & Wilkins

Tsujinaka T, Shiozaki H, Yamamoto M, et al., 1999: Role of preoperative chemoradiation in the management of upper third thoracic esophageal squamous cell carcinoma. Am J Surg 177:503

Vanecko RM, Shields TW, 1994: Esophageal trauma. In Shields TW (ed): General Thoracic Surgery, ed. 4. Baltimore, Williams & Wilkins

Watson TJ, DeMeester TR, Kauer WKH, et al., 1998: Esophageal replacement for end-stage benign esophageal disease. J Thorac Cardiovasc Surg 115:1241

Wilkins EW Jr, 1994: Motor disturbances of deglutition. In Shields TW (ed): General Thoracic Surgery, ed. 4. Baltimore, Williams & Wilkins

Wolfe WG, Sebastian MW, 1995: Benign and malignant tumors of the esophagus. In Sabiston DC Jr, Spencer FC (eds): Surgery of the Chest, ed. 6. Philadelphia, WB Saunders

Diseases of the Mediastinum and Chest Wall

The *mediastinum* is an extrapleural space that lies between the right and left thoracic cavities. Traversing through it are the aerodigestive tract; the great vessels of the arterial, venous, and lymphatic circulation; and the autonomic nervous system (DeCamp et al., 1996). Surrounding the mediastinum are the thoracic inlet (superior), the diaphragm (inferior), the parietal pleura (lateral), the sternum (anterior), and the vertebral column (posterior). The mediastinum commonly is described as comprising three anatomic regions: anterior mediastinum, visceral mediastinum, and paravertebral sulci (ie, potential spaces along each side of the vertebral bodies and adjacent ribs) (Fig. 35-1).

35

▶ Disorders of the Mediastinum

Mediastinal Masses

Although most mediastinal masses represent metastatic spread of tumors originating elsewhere, primary neoplasms and cysts of the mediastinum can occur and are the focus of this discussion. The most common *primary mediastinal masses* are cysts (21%), neurogenic tumors (20%), thymomas (19%), lymphomas (13%), and germ cell tumors (10%) (Davis & Sabiston, 1997). The incidence of these various mediastinal tumors and cysts differs with the age of the patient group under consideration (Shields, 1991a). Approximately two thirds of all mediastinal tumors are benign (Strollo et al., 1997a).

Many mediastinal lesions arise in characteristic locations in the mediastinum (Table 35-1). Most mediastinal masses occur in the anterior region. Of these, thymoma,

lymphoma, and germ cell tumors are most common. Masses occurring in the visceral mediastinum are usually lymphomas or cysts. Tumors that originate in the paravertebral sulci are usually neurogenic, arising from sympathetic ganglia (ganglioma, ganglioneuroblastoma, and neuroblastoma), intercostal nerves (neurofibroma, neurilemoma, and neurosarcoma), or paraganglia cells (paraganglioma) (Davis et al., 1995). Vascular tumors and lymphatic lesions also may occur in the paravertebral sulci (Shields, 1994).

Clinical Manifestations

Almost half of patients with mediastinal lesions are asymptomatic and have a negative physical examination (Darling, 1999a). Patients with malignant neoplasms are more often symptomatic (85%) than are those with benign lesions (46%) (Davis et al., 1995). In the adult, most normal mediastinal structures are mobile enough to conform to distortion from pressure; malignant disease, on the other hand, is often accompanied by both distortion and fixation of vital structures (Shields, 1991a). Consequently, symptoms of obstruction and compression are observed more commonly in association with malignant lesions.

The most common symptoms of large tumors are chest or back pain, cough, and dyspnea. Other less commonly reported symptoms include dysphagia, hoarseness, Horner's syndrome, superior vena cava (SVC) syndrome, palpitations, malaise, and weakness (DeCamp et al., 1996). Tumor location affects the type of presenting symptoms. Anterior masses are most likely to produce SVC syndrome, middle (visceral) mediastinal masses are most likely to cause cardiac tamponade, and posterior (paravertebral sulci) masses are most likely to produce

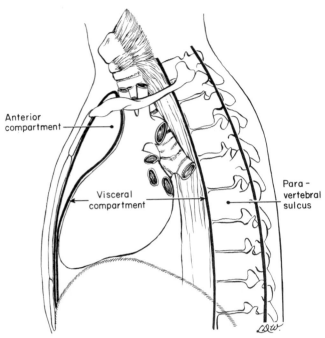

FIGURE 35-1. Mediastinal compartments as viewed from the left side. (Shields TW, 1994: Primary lesions of the mediastinum and their investigation and treatment. In Shields TW [ed]: General Thoracic Surgery, ed. 4, p. 1725. Baltimore, Williams & Wilkins)

Shields TW, 1994: Primary lesions of the mediastinum and their investigation and treatment. In Shields TW (ed): General Thoracic Surgery, ed. 4. Baltimore, Williams & Wilkins.

spinal cord compression syndromes (Davis et al., 1995). Signs and symptoms that occur also are related to the lesion's size and the presence of infection or associated disease states (Shields, 1991a).

Mediastinal tumors sometimes produce hormones or antibodies that cause systemic syndromes (eg, thyrotoxicosis due to mediastinal goiter or hypercalcemia caused by mediastinal parathyroid adenoma) (Davis et al., 1995). Serum levels of human chorionic gonadotropin may be elevated in the presence of malignant germ cell tumors, and serum alpha-fetoprotein elevation indicates a tumor that contains nonseminomatous elements (Hainsworth & Greco, 1991). Malignant lesions also are sometimes associated with constitutional symptoms, such as fatigue, weight loss, fever, and chills.

Diagnosis and Treatment

Mediastinal lesions usually are detected because of an abnormal shadow or mediastinal configuration on the chest roentgenogram. Because primary mediastinal masses often are associated with characteristic locations, identification of the anatomic subdivision within which a mass is found provides important descriptive information and often is helpful in differential diagnosis. Posteroanterior and lateral chest films are used to determine the lesion's location in the anterior, visceral, or posterior (paravertebral sulci) region of the mediastinum. The chest roentgenogram also provides important information about lesion size and relative density (solid or cys-

tic), the presence and pattern of calcification, and displacement or alteration of anatomic structures in the mediastinum and adjacent regions (Davis et al., 1995).

A computed tomographic (CT) scan almost always is obtained to define more accurately the character and size of the mass, its location, and the proximity or involvement of contiguous structures. CT scanning provides a sensitive method of distinguishing between fatty, vascular, cystic, and soft tissue masses (Shields, 1991a). Magnetic resonance imaging also may be useful in evaluation of mediastinal masses, particularly in providing definition of posterior mediastinal tumors when spinal cord compression is suspected.

For many mediastinal tumors, surgical resection is the

primary therapy, regardless of benignancy or malignancy. However, definitive diagnosis of a mediastinal tumor before surgical exploration is desirable because some tumors are treated primarily with other modalities. Tissue for histologic examination may be obtained by mediastinotomy, mediastinoscopy, video-assisted thoracoscopy, or thoracotomy. Fine-needle aspiration biopsy sometimes can provide a definitive cytologic diagnosis. Immunohistochemical and molecular pathologic techniques now permit accurate classifications of lymphomas from limited tissue specimens; a histologic diagnosis may be made from a core of tissue obtained using a larger-gauge, or cutting, needle (Darling, 1999a).

Specific Neoplasms and Cysts

Thymomas are tumors derived from thymic epithelial cells. They are the most common primary tumor of the anterior mediastinum and occur most often in adults older than 40 years of age (Strollo et al., 1997b; Shields, 1991b). Thirty to 50% of patients with thymoma have associated myasthenia gravis, and 10% to 15% of patients with myasthenia have a thymoma (Darling, 1999b; Trastek, 1998). Myasthenia gravis is discussed later in this chapter.

Most patients with thymoma are asymptomatic, although one third experience chest pain, cough, dyspnea, or other symptoms related to compression or invasion of adjacent structures (Strollo et al., 1997a). Thymomas may be either benign or malignant. In contrast to most neoplasms, benignancy or malignancy of a thymoma cannot be established by histologic examination of tumor cells. Instead, the determination of malignancy is made primarily by gross examination of the tumor at the time of surgical resection.

Staging by the surgeon is supplemented by the pathologist's histologic examination for evidence of microscopic spread not evident under gross inspection. Complete surgical resection is the treatment of choice for all patients, except those with grossly nonresectable disease or with evidence of tumor spread beyond the thorax (Shields, 1991b). All thymomas, except completely encapsulated stage I (benign) tumors, should be treated with postoperative adjuvant radiation therapy in the hope of reducing the incidence of local recurrence (Kohman, 1997). *Thymic carcinomas* and *thymic carcinoids* are rare malignancies of the thymus with a propensity for local invasion and distant metastases (Strollo et al., 1997a).

Lymphomas are malignant tumors of the lymphoid tissues. They are one of the most common mediastinal tumors and may manifest as a primary mediastinal lesion or, more frequently, as generalized disease (Strollo et al., 1997b). Lymphomas are broadly categorized as Hodgkin's lymphoma or non-Hodgkin's lymphoma. In most patients with lymphoma, the mediastinum is involved at some point during the course of the disease; infrequently, it is the sole site of disease at the time of diagnosis (Davis et al., 1995). Chemotherapy is the mainstay of treatment for lymphoma, although radiation therapy or bone marrow transplantation may be used depending on stage of the disease and the patient's

response to chemotherapy (Darling, 1999a). Surgical excision of a residual mass may be necessary infrequently.

Germ cell tumors include teratoma, seminoma, and nonseminomatous germ cell tumor. Most of these tumors occur in men between 20 and 35 years of age. *Teratoma* is a benign neoplasm composed of multiple tissue elements foreign to the area in which the tumor is found (Davis & Sabiston, 1997). Mediastinal teratomas are usually cystic and frequently contain skin, hair, smooth muscle, teeth, bone, or fat. Teratoma is treated by surgical resection of the tumor. Complete excision is usually possible, and prognosis after tumor removal is excellent (Trastek & Pairolero, 1991).

Malignant germ cell tumors are categorized histologically as seminoma or nonseminomatous germ cell tumor. *Seminoma* is histologically identical to malignant germinal tumor of testicular origin. Combination chemotherapy (cisplatin, bleomycin, etoposide, vinblastine) and large-volume radiation therapy is the primary form of therapy (Darling, 1999a). Surgical resection is performed infrequently for small residual masses. Therapy is curative in most patients, with long-term survival rates of 60% to 80% (Strollo et al., 1997a).

Nonseminomatous germ cell tumors are those that contain areas of embryonal carcinoma, teratocarcinoma, choriocarcinoma, or endodermal sinus tumor (Hainsworth & Greco, 1991). They are more aggressive than seminomas and are associated with a less favorable prognosis. Invasion of adjacent structures, including the chest wall, may occur, as well as metastases to regional lymph nodes and distant sites (Strollo et al., 1997a). Nonseminomatous tumors are treated primarily with cisplatin-based chemotherapy.

Mediastinal cysts may be bronchogenic, pericardial, or enteric. Bronchogenic cysts are most common. They are closed sacs thought to result from an abnormal budding process that occurs during early development of the foregut (St.-Georges et al., 1991). Despite the benignancy of mediastinal cysts, they frequently produce symptoms such as chest pain, dyspnea, or cough. Surgical resection is recommended to alleviate symptoms and prevent complications (Duranceau & Deslaurier, 1991).

Neurogenic tumors represent approximately 20% of all adult and 35% of all pediatric mediastinal neoplasms (Strollo et al., 1997b). They include (1) neurilemomas (schwannomas) and neurofibromas, arising from the nerve sheath; (2) ganglioneuromas, ganglioneuroblastomas, and neuroblastomas, originating from the sympathetic ganglia; (3) paraganglionic tumors, such as pheochromocytomas and chemodectomas; and (4) tumors of peripheral neuroectodermal origin (DeCamp et al., 1996). Although most neurogenic tumors arising in children are malignant, those that occur in adults are most often benign (Davis et al., 1995). Because of their characteristic shape, the term *dumbbell tumor* is commonly used to denote neurogenic tumors that extend into the spinal column. Neurogenic tumors usually are treated with surgical resection. Adjunctive treatment, usually radiation therapy, is recommended for malignant tumors.

Superior Vena Cava Syndrome

The SVC is the major vessel draining venous blood from the head, neck, upper extremities, and upper thorax into the right atrium. It is confined in a tight compartment in the anterosuperior mediastinum, immediately adjacent and anterior to the trachea and right mainstem bronchus, and is surrounded by lymph nodes draining the entire right and lower portion of the left chest (McFadden & Jamplis, 1994). *Superior vena cava syndrome* is a condition in which venous flow through the SVC is obstructed either as a result of extrinsic compression of the vessel or internal occlusion from thrombus or a foreign body.

In approximately 90% of cases, SVC syndrome occurs secondary to malignant disease (DeCamp et al., 1996). By far the most common etiology is bronchogenic lung cancer, usually originating in the right upper lobe. Mediastinal tumors, lymphoma, or metastatic disease from other organs also can cause SVC syndrome. Non-malignant conditions that can lead to SVC syndrome include granulomatous diseases, such as histoplasmosis or tuberculosis; mediastinal infection; mediastinal goiter; and the presence of an indwelling central venous catheter or pacemaker lead.

Superior vena cava obstruction causes increased pressure in veins that normally drain into the vessel and stimulates formation of extensive venous collateral circulation. SVC syndrome usually develops insidiously over weeks or months. The most prominent feature is swelling of the face, neck, and upper extremities caused by engorgement of veins that normally empty into the SVC. Venous distention usually is apparent in the neck vessels as well as in collateral veins in the upper extremities and chest wall. Plethora (ie, red, florid complexion) and cyanosis of the face may be present, particularly when the patient is recumbent (Stea & Kinsella, 1991). Symptoms include dyspnea (50%), cough (30%), and, uncommonly, chest pain, syncope, headache, or confusion (Grondin & Johnston, 1999). Severity of symptoms is affected by the rapidity with which obstruction occurs and, therefore, the degree to which collateral pathways have developed. With processes that slowly cause obstruction, manifestations develop insidiously; with rapid or sudden occlusion, the clinical presentation is often striking, with rapid development of cerebral edema and intracranial thrombosis that may lead to coma or death (Davis et al., 1995). Because venous drainage through the inferior vena cava is not impeded, the trunk and lower extremities are not affected by SVC syndrome.

A percutaneous needle biopsy is often performed to establish a cytologic diagnosis if SVC syndrome is presumed to be caused by a malignant process (Davis et al., 1995). Invasive diagnostic procedures, such as bronchoscopy or mediastinoscopy, also may be necessary and usually can be performed safely despite increased venous pressure. A definitive diagnosis usually is considered essential before initiating therapy. SVC syndrome of malignant etiology usually is treated with radiation therapy or chemotherapy. Chemotherapy has proven preferable to radiation therapy in selected patients with chemosensitive tumors.

However, in the presence of edema, it may induce vomiting, resulting in potential airway obstruction. The malignant processes that cause SVC syndrome are usually inoperable. SVC syndrome is usually not life threatening unless it develops rapidly or is associated with neurologic manifestations. In such unusual cases, emergent treatment, usually radiation therapy, is performed.

In patients with SVC syndrome secondary to benign disease, bed rest with head elevation is helpful in producing gradual improvement of symptoms. Diuretics and corticosteroids also may be administered, particularly to reduce cerebral edema that may lead to central nervous system dysfunction. If the cause of venous obstruction is thrombus, thrombolytic therapy may be effective in restoring blood flow through the SVC. Venous thrombectomy or a surgical procedure to bypass the obstructed SVC also may be considered.

Fibrosing Mediastinitis

Fibrosing mediastinitis is an unusual granulomatous reaction and immune response in the mediastinum, precipitated by a specific agent and resulting in varying degrees of sclerosis. It is thought to occur most often in association with the fungal infection, histoplasmosis. In many cases, however, fibrosis is the only histologic diagnosis that can be established (Hood, 1994). The process typically begins with a granulomatous reaction in mediastinal lymph nodes and surrounding tissue and can progress to more generalized inflammation and fibrosis. A biopsy of mediastinal tissue usually is performed for diagnostic purposes.

Extensive mediastinal fibrosis can lead to compression of structures contained in the mediastinum, including the venae cavae, trachea, main bronchi, and pulmonary vessels (Scott et al., 1996). Associated clinical manifestations include chest pain, dysphagia, dyspnea, and SVC syndrome. Treatment of fibrosing mediastinitis is primarily supportive. Surgical therapy may become necessary to treat complications of the condition.

▶ Myasthenia Gravis

Myasthenia gravis is an autoimmune disorder in which antibodies are produced against acetylcholine receptors of the muscle endplate, resulting in impaired neuromuscular transmission (Krucylak & Naunheim, 1999). Normal neuromuscular transmission occurs when a nerve impulse stimulates the release of the neuromuscular transmitter acetylcholine from the nerve side of the neuromuscular junction; acetylcholine interacts with specific acetylcholine receptors on the muscle endplate and the resultant opening of calcium channels and calcium influx stimulates muscular contraction (Heitmiller, 1999). In patients with myasthenia gravis, the reduction in functional acetylcholine receptors impairs neuromuscular transmission, causing progressive weakness and easy fatigability of voluntary muscles. The disease affects women more commonly than men, with a peak age at onset of 20 to 30 years in women, and of older than 50 years in men (Hagen & Cooper, 1997).

Clinical Manifestations

Myasthenia gravis is characterized by weakness of skeletal muscles and can involve almost any muscle group in the body. Ocular muscle involvement, resulting in ptosis and diplopia, is present in approximately one half of patients at the time of diagnosis and occurs in 90% of patients as the disease progresses (Hagen & Cooper, 1997). Extremity musculature is symmetrically affected, with preferential involvement of proximal (shoulder and upper extremity) muscle groups (Heitmiller, 1999). Other clinical manifestations that may occur include dysphagia, respiratory distress, impaired chewing, dysarthria, nasal speech, facial weakness (transverse smile or involuntary grimace), atrophic tongue, and difficulty supporting the head with neck muscles (Wechsler, 1995). The most serious symptoms are those of respiratory distress. When weakness of respiratory muscles is such that mechanical ventilatory support is required, the patient is said to be in crisis (Heitmiller, 1999).

Clinical manifestations of myasthenia gravis may develop insidiously or appear precipitously. Symptoms are more prominent with repetitive activity and diminish with rest (DeCamp et al., 1996). Pregnancy, stress, allergies, or menses may affect the degree of symptoms. Although the disorder may be confined to the ocular muscles, more than 80% of patients have generalized weakness within 1 year of onset of ocular disturbances (Wechsler, 1995).

Diagnosis and Treatment

Diagnostic confirmation of myasthenia gravis commonly is achieved by performing a Tensilon test, which consists of administering intravenous edrophonium (Tensilon), a short-acting anticholinesterase agent. Most patients with myasthenia gravis experience marked, immediate improvement after receiving the drug (DeCamp et al., 1996).

Treatment of myasthenia gravis usually includes both medical therapy and a surgical procedure, thymectomy. Pharmacologic therapy used to treat myasthenia includes long-acting anticholinesterase drugs, such as neostigmine (Prostigmin) and pyridostigmine (Mestinon), and immunosuppressive agents (steroids, azathioprine, cyclosporine, and immune globulin) (Heitmiller, 1999). Plasmapheresis may be used to provide transient clinical improvement before thymectomy. The clinical course of the disease and response to treatment are difficult to predict and episodic remissions do occur.

For reasons that are incompletely understood, significant clinical improvement usually can be achieved with surgical removal of the thymus gland from the mediastinum (Fig. 35-2). Thymectomy always is performed in

patients with myasthenia gravis if a thymoma is present. As previously stated, a thymoma is present in 10% to 15% of patients with myasthenia gravis. In the absence of thymoma, the indications and timing for thymectomy are somewhat controversial. It is performed most commonly in patients with generalized symptoms, including ptosis, dysarthria, dysphagia, and weakness of the respiratory muscles. Long-term benefits of thymectomy are difficult to identify precisely because of uncertainty about the natural history of untreated myasthenia gravis, the unpredictable rate of disease progression, and the occurrence of spontaneous remission (Hagen & Cooper, 1997). Most patients experience clinical improvement after thymectomy and complete remission is reported in 44% (Bril et al., 1998). Clinical improvement, however, may not occur for 1 to 2 years after operation.

▶ Chest Wall Disorders

Tumors of the Chest Wall

Tumors of the chest wall are unusual. Those that do occur may involve the soft tissues, the bony structures, or both, and may arise from any of a variety of cell types (Table 35-2). Approximately 50% are malignant, and of those, approximately half are primary tumors originating from tissues comprising the chest wall (ie, bone, soft tissue, nerve, or muscle) (Compeau & Johnston, 1999a).

Benign bony tumors include fibrous dysplasia, chondroma, osteochondroma, and eosinophilic granuloma. Fibrous dysplasia is most common, usually affecting posterior and lateral ribs. It usually produces a lesion

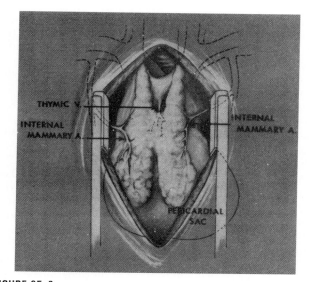

FIGURE 35-2. Anatomic location of thymus gland in anterior mediastinum overlying pericardium and great vessels. Arterial supply is predominantly from the internal thoracic (mammary) artery; venous drainage is into the innominate vein. (Trastek VF, Shields TW, 1994: Surgery of the thymus gland. In Shields TW [ed]: General Thoracic Surgery, ed. 4, p. 1771. Baltimore, Williams & Wilkins)

TABLE 35-2

Primary Chest Wall Tumors

BENIGN
Bony skeleton
  Fibrous dysplasia
  Chondroma
  Osteochondroma
  Eosinophilic granuloma
Soft tissue
  Fibroma
  Lipoma

MALIGNANT
Bony skeleton
  Chondrosarcoma
  Osteogenic sarcoma
  Myeloma
  Ewing's sarcoma
Soft tissue
  Fibrous histiocytoma
  Rhabdomyosarcoma

that expands slowly and painlessly until the periosteum is stretched or the rib is fractured (McCormack, 1996). Chondroma, a tumor of the costal cartilage, usually occurs as a small, slowly enlarging, sometimes painful lesion in the anterior chest wall. Although benign, chondromas can recur after excision and sometimes undergo malignant degeneration. Osteochondroma, a rare tumor of young adults, arises from the rib cortex and causes a painless protuberance of the rib. Eosinophilic granuloma is a painful bony lesion, frequently accompanied by constitutional symptoms of fever and malaise. Benign tumors that may originate in the chest wall soft tissue include fibroma and lipoma.

Malignant neoplasms may originate in the chest wall or may represent metastases from lung, pleura, mediastinum, muscle, or breast (Pairolero, 1994). The most common primary malignant tumor of the chest wall is chondrosarcoma. It occurs most often in the anterior chest wall and in young adults, usually men. Typically a solitary lesion, 80% arise in the upper four ribs and 20% in the sternum (Compeau & Johnston, 1999a). Osteogenic sarcoma, usually found in the long bones of young adults, uncommonly occurs in the ribs; it is more virulent and associated with earlier hematogenous spread than chondrosarcoma and carries a poor prognosis (McCormack, 1996). Myeloma, accounting for 20% of malignant chest wall neoplasms, usually occurs in older men as one manifestation of the generalized disease of multiple myeloma (McCormack, 1996). Ewing's sarcoma is seen predominantly in children, particularly boys. Fibrous histiocytoma and rhabdomyosarcoma are examples of malignant soft tissue tumors.

The first indication of a chest wall tumor is a visible or palpable mass that often is asymptomatic. Approxi-

mately two thirds of benign and almost all malignant lesions become painful as the neoplasm enlarges (Pairolero, 1995). CT scanning is particularly useful in defining the extent of the tumor and determining the presence of extension into adjacent structures. Magnetic resonance imaging also may be helpful in delineating spinal cord involvement. A definitive diagnosis is achieved with needle, incisional, or excisional biopsy. Advances in histopathology now enable pathologists to provide a more accurate tumor diagnosis, particularly from smaller tissue specimens (Compeau & Johnston, 1999a).

Surgical resection is the treatment of choice for most benign tumors because of pain, a mass effect produced by the lesion, and the potential for some benign lesions to undergo malignant degeneration. Most primary and some secondary malignant neoplasms also are treated with surgical resection. Even if cure is not anticipated, palliative resection may be performed to reduce pain caused by the lesion or to remove an infected, bleeding, or ulcerated tumor that is malodorous or disfiguring. A wide excision is performed for malignant lesions; a wide excision, defined as including a margin of at least 4 cm of normal tissue on all sides of the mass, is essential to obtain local control of the malignant process (Compeau & Johnston, 1999a).

If a significant portion of chest wall is removed, chest wall reconstruction may be necessary to maintain adequate respiratory function and to protect the thoracic viscera (Pairolero, 1994). In some cases, a muscle flap alone may provide adequate coverage of soft tissues. In others, a synthetic prosthesis may be necessary to restore the chest wall adequately. Depending on the type of tumor, radiation therapy or chemotherapy may be used adjunctively.

Pectus Deformities

Pectus deformities are structural abnormalities of the anterior chest wall. The etiology of the deformities is unknown. An increased familial incidence exists and pectus deformities are slightly more common in boys. *Pectus excavatum (funnel chest)* is the most common developmental deformity of the chest. As many as two thirds of patients with Marfan's syndrome may have associated pectus excavatum (Landolfo & Sabiston, 1995). Pectus excavatum is characterized by inward depression of the lower sternum and adjacent cartilages (Fig. 35-3). The deformity usually is apparent soon after birth, progresses during childhood, and becomes even more pronounced during adolescence (Fonkalsrud, 1996).

Pectus excavatum primarily affects posture, typically producing slouching, sunken chest, and rounded shoulders. The degree of deformity varies from slight to severe. Moderate to severe pectus excavatum causes displacement of the heart into the left chest and impingement of pulmonary expansion during inspiration (Fonkalsrud, 1996). However, the significance of the deformity in producing physiologic alterations in cardiorespiratory function is controversial.

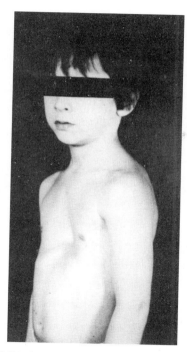

FIGURE 35-3. Child with pectus excavatum deformity. (Sandza JF Jr, Clark RE, 1982: The chest wall. In Ellis FH Jr, Goldsmith HS [eds]: Goldsmith Practice of Surgery, rev. ed. p. 22. Philadelphia, Harper & Row)

Far less common is *pectus carinatum (pigeon breast)*, a deformity consisting of outward protrusion of the sternum. Pectus carinatum produces a rigid chest with increased anteroposterior diameter locked into a position of nearly full inspiration; respiratory efforts are inefficient and gradual loss of lung compliance, progressive emphysema, and superimposed pulmonary infection may result (Fonkalsrud, 1996).

In both types of pectus deformity, the primary consequence is the psychological effect of cosmetic disfigurement. However, pectus deformities are progressive and, when severe, are believed by some to contribute to cardiac arrhythmias and exercise intolerance. The primary indication for surgical repair is cosmetic improvement (Compeau & Johnston, 1999b). Many pectus deformities are repaired surgically in early childhood (ages 2 to 5 years) and most are repaired before the adolescent growth spurt. Rarely, a pectus repair is performed during adolescence or early adulthood.

REFERENCES

Bril V, Kojic J, Isle WK, Cooper JD, 1998: Long-term clinical outcome after transcervical thymectomy for myasthenia gravis. Ann Thorac Surg 65:1520

Compeau C, Johnston MR, 1999a: Chest-wall tumors. In Casson AG, Johnston MR (eds): Key Topics in Thoracic Surgery. Oxford, Bios

Compeau C, Johnston MR, 1999b: Pectus deformities. In Casson AG, Johnston MR (eds): Key Topics in Thoracic Surgery. Oxford, Bios

Darling G, 1999a: Mediastinum and mediastinal masses. In Casson AG, Johnston MR (eds): Key Topics in Thoracic Surgery. Oxford, Bios

Darling G, 1999b: Thymoma. In Casson AG, Johnston MR (eds): Key Topics in Thoracic Surgery. Oxford, Bios

Davis RD Jr, Oldham HN Jr, Sabiston DC Jr, 1995: The mediastinum. In Sabiston DC Jr, Spencer FC (eds): Surgery of the Chest, ed. 6. Philadelphia, WB Saunders

Davis RD Jr, Sabiston DC Jr, 1997: The mediastinum. In Sabiston DC Jr (ed): Textbook of Surgery: The Biological Basis of Modern Surgical Practice, ed. 15. Philadelphia, WB Saunders

DeCamp MM, Swanson SJ, Sugarbaker DJ, 1996: The mediastinum. In Baue AE, Geha AS, Hammond GL, et al. (eds): Glenn's Thoracic and Cardiovascular Surgery, ed. 6. Stamford, CT, Appleton & Lange

Duranceau AC, Deslauriers J, 1991: Foregut cysts of the mediastinum in the adult. In Shields TW (ed): The Mediastinum. Philadelphia, Lea & Febiger

Fonkalsrud EW, 1996: Chest wall abnormalities. In Baue AE, Geha AS, Hammond GL, et al. (eds): Glenn's Thoracic and Cardiovascular Surgery, ed. 6. Stamford, CT, Appleton & Lange

Grondin S, Johnston MR, 1999: Superior vena cava syndrome. In Casson AG, Johnston MR (eds): Key Topics in Thoracic Surgery. Oxford, Bios

Hagen JA, Cooper JD, 1997: Surgical management of myasthenia gravis. In Sabiston DC Jr (ed): Textbook of Surgery: The Biological Basis of Modern Surgical Practice, ed. 15. Philadelphia, WB Saunders

Hainsworth JD, Greco FA, 1991: General features of malignant germ cell tumors and primary seminomas of the mediastinum. In Shields TW (ed): The Mediastinum. Philadelphia, Lea & Febiger

Heitmiller RF, 1999: Myasthenia gravis: Clinical features, pathogenesis, evaluation, and medical management. Semin Thorac Cardiovasc Surg 11:41

Hood RM, 1994: Bronchial compressive diseases. In Shields TW (ed): General Thoracic Surgery, ed. 4. Baltimore, Williams & Wilkins

Kohman LJ, 1997: Controversies in the management of malignant thymoma. Chest 112:296S

Krucylak PE, Naunheim KS, 1999: Preoperative preparation and anesthetic management of patients with myasthenia gravis. Semin Thorac Cardiovasc Surg 11:47

Landolfo KP, Sabiston DC Jr, 1995: Disorders of the sternum and the thoracic wall: Congenital deformities of the chest wall. In Sabiston DC Jr, Spencer FC (eds): Surgery of the Chest, ed. 6. Philadelphia, WB Saunders

McCormack P, 1996: Chest wall tumors. In Baue AE, Geha AS, Hammond GL, et al. (eds): Glenn's Thoracic and Cardiovascular Surgery, ed. 6. Stamford, CT, Appleton & Lange

McFadden PM, Jamplis RW, 1994: Superior vena cava syndrome. In Shields TW (ed): General Thoracic Surgery, ed. 4. Baltimore, Williams & Wilkins

Pairolero PC, 1994: Chest wall tumors. In Shields TW (ed): General Thoracic Surgery, ed. 4. Baltimore, Williams & Wilkins

Pairolero PC, 1995: Surgical management of neoplasms of the chest wall. In Sabiston DC Jr, Spencer FC (eds): Surgery of the Chest, ed. 6. Philadelphia, WB Saunders

Scott SM, Takaro T, Davis RD, 1996: Thoracic infections caused by actinomycetes, fungi, opportunistic organisms, and echinococcus. In Baue AE, Geha AS, Hammond GL, et al. (eds): Glenn's Thoracic and Cardiovascular Surgery, ed. 6. Stamford, CT, Appleton & Lange

Shields TW, 1991a: Primary mediastinal tumors and cysts and their diagnostic investigation. In Shields TW (ed): The Mediastinum. Philadelphia, Lea & Febiger

Shields TW, 1991b: Thymic tumors. In Shields TW (ed): The Mediastinum. Philadelphia, Lea & Febiger

Shields TW, 1994: Primary lesions of the mediastinum and their investigation and treatment. In Shields TW (ed): General Thoracic Surgery, ed. 4. Baltimore, Williams & Wilkins

St.-Georges R, Deslauriers J, Duranceau A, et al., 1991: Clinical spectrum of bronchogenic cysts of the mediastinum and lung in the adult. Ann Thorac Surg 52:6

Stea B, Kinsella TJ, 1991: Superior vena cava syndrome: Clinical features, diagnosis, and treatment. In Shields TW (ed): The Mediastinum. Philadelphia, Lea & Febiger

Strollo DC, Rosado de Christenson ML, Jett JR, 1997a: Primary mediastinal tumors: Part I. Tumors of the anterior mediastinum. Chest 112:511

Strollo DC, Rosado de Christenson ML, Jett JR, 1997b: Primary mediastinal tumors: Part II. Tumors of the middle and posterior mediastinum. Chest 112:1344

Trastek VF, 1998: Thymectomy. In Kaiser LR, Kron IL, Spray TL (eds): Mastery of Cardiothoracic Surgery. Philadelphia, Lippincott Williams & Wilkins

Trastek VF, Pairolero PC, 1991: Benign germ cell tumors of the mediastinum. In Shields TW (ed): The Mediastinum. Philadelphia, Lea & Febiger

Wechsler AS, 1995: Surgical management of myasthenia gravis. In Sabiston DC Jr, Spencer FC (eds): Surgery of the Chest, ed. 6. Philadelphia, WB Saunders

PREOPERATIVE EVALUATION
AND PREPARATION

36

Diagnostic Evaluation of Thoracic Diseases

Thoracic diseases encompass a wide variety of neoplastic, infectious, and acquired disorders. Any of a number of diagnostic modalities may be important in establishing a diagnosis and guiding therapeutic interventions. Those studies performed most commonly in patients who undergo thoracic surgical procedures are the focus of this chapter.

► Roentgenographic Studies

Chest Roentgenograms

The *chest roentgenogram* is the most commonly used diagnostic study in the evaluation of diseases of the thorax. It is the primary diagnostic imaging modality for evaluation of pulmonary tumors and of less common intrathoracic tumors occurring in the mediastinum or chest wall. Although the roentgenogram does not distinguish malignancy and benignancy or determine histologic cell type, it provides essential information about lo-

cation and characteristics of a tumor and involvement of adjacent structures. Lesion size, relative density (solid or cystic), the presence and pattern of calcification, and displacement or alteration of normal structures are demonstrated (Davis et al., 1995). Comparison with previous chest roentgenograms can help determine onset of an abnormality and its rate of growth. Chest roentgenograms also are important in determining the extent of benign, diffuse pulmonary disease. They may detect other intrathoracic abnormalities as well, such as thoracic aortic aneurysm, pleural effusion, or pneumothorax.

The standard method for obtaining a chest roentgenogram is with the patient in an upright position and during a full inspiration. Posteroanterior and lateral projections are obtained to provide a three-dimensional view of the chest. The lateral roentgenogram demonstrates certain areas of the thorax better than the posteroanterior projection. It may reveal findings not apparent on the posteroanterior roentgenogram, such as small mediastinal lesions, masses in the anterior portions of the lung adjacent to the mediastinum, and lesions in the vertebral column or behind the heart (Miller, 1994).

A posteroanterior roentgenogram obtained during expiration may be helpful in the diagnosis of small pneumothoraces. A pneumothorax appears larger on an expiratory study because lung volume is reduced during maximal forced expiration; expiration also increases radiographic density of the lung, thus enhancing the contrast between the appearance of lung tissue and air in the pleural space (Cohen et al., 1995). A lateral decubitus roentgenogram may be useful to demonstrate the presence and mobility of fluid in the pleural space (Freundlich & Bragg, 1992). It is taken with the patient lying on the right or left side.

Computed Tomography

Computed tomography (CT) is a technique for imaging cross-sectional anatomy. Although chest roentgenograms remain the primary radiologic method for identifying intrathoracic abnormalities, CT imaging provides additional valuable information in their evaluation. The diagnostic advantages of CT imaging include cross-sectional depiction of anatomy; superior contrast sensitivity; and the capability to view the entire dynamic range of lung, soft tissue, and bone densities from a single CT exposure (Gutierrez et al., 1998).

Computed tomographic imaging often is performed as a routine part of the diagnostic evaluation in patients with lung cancer. First, it may substantially supplement information obtained radiographically about a tumor by providing more precise characterization of the size, contour, extent, and tissue composition of the suspect lesion (Sagel & Slone, 1998). Second, CT imaging is important in staging lung cancer because it better evaluates mediastinal lymphadenopathy (ie, enlarged lymph nodes).

Computed tomographic imaging is more accurate than chest radiography in the detection of enlarged mediastinal and hilar lymph nodes and can differentiate enlarged lymph nodes from normal or enlarged vascular structures (Glazer et al., 1998). Although it does not definitively establish the presence of malignant cells in mediastinal lymph tissue, it better delineates enlarged or multiple lymph nodes that might represent mediastinal metastasis. CT imaging also is useful in demonstrating malignant tumor invasion of vertebral bodies or soft tissue. Chest CT imaging in patients with lung cancer usually includes imaging of the upper abdomen to detect occult adrenal or liver metastasis.

Computed tomographic scanning also is useful in detecting small pleural effusions that may not be detectable on a chest roentgenogram. In addition, it allows (1) determination of the extent and localization of loculated fluid for accurate chest tube placement, (2) assessment of pleural morphology (irregular thickening or focal masses), (3) evaluation of underlying lung disease, and (4) differentiation between parenchymal and pleural disease (using intravenous contrast material) (Collins & Stern, 1999). High-resolution CT is a special CT imaging technique that

optimizes the spatial resolution of lung anatomy. It has become established as a useful technique for the detection and characterization of diffuse lung disease that is nonspecific or not apparent on chest radiographs and conventional CT imaging (Gutierrez et al., 1998).

Chest CT imaging, along with magnetic resonance imaging (MRI), is the imaging modality of choice in patients with primary mediastinal tumors (Fig. 36-1). It accurately localizes and characterizes pathologic processes in the mediastinum and provides a sensitive method of distinguishing between fatty, vascular, cystic, and soft tissue masses (McLoud, 1989; Shields, 1991). CT or MRI also can differentiate other entities that may resemble a mediastinal mass, including esophageal lesions, diaphragmatic herniations, pancreatic pseudocysts, and mediastinitis (Davis et al., 1995). Depending on the indication, intravenous contrast medium may be administered during CT imaging to enhance the distinction between vascular structures and surrounding tissue. In patients with tracheal disease, CT imaging is valuable in assessing the local extent of malignant disease; it has limited usefulness in assessing benign tracheal stenosis, except in selected situations (Donahue & Mathisen, 1998).

Positron Emission Tomography

Positron emission tomography (PET) is a newer form of tomography that has proven useful in the diagnosis and staging of lung cancer. PET imaging is performed after administration of a tracer, most commonly [18F]fluorodeoxyglucose (FDG), which serves as a marker of glucose metabolism. FDG becomes trapped in malignant cells, thereby helping to distinguish a focal abnormality as benign or malignant. FDG PET scanning is very sensitive (approximately 95%) for detection of cancer in patients with indeterminate lesions on CT; the specificity (approximately 85%) is somewhat less because some inflammatory processes, such as active granulomatous infections, accumulate FDG avidly (Al-Sugair & Coleman, 1998).

The high sensitivity of FDG PET imaging provides a noninvasive modality for demonstrating benignancy. Also, because malignant cells have increased metabolism, the relative uptake of FDG by tumor cells can be used as a marker of tumor aggressiveness and correlates with tumor growth rate (Lowe & Naunheim, 1998). The study is performed with the patient in a fasting state to minimize competitive inhibition of FDG uptake by glucose.

Other Roentgenographic Studies

Roentgenographic studies of the trachea are useful in defining the presence and extent of a tracheal lesion; most lesions in the upper trachea can be demonstrated on lateral films of the neck with the chin raised (Donahue & Mathisen, 1998). *Bronchography* consists of imaging the chest after injecting contrast medium into the trachea and insufflating it into the dependent lung by manual pulmonary inflation (Le Roux & Rocke, 1989). The pro-

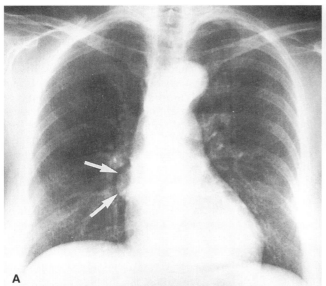

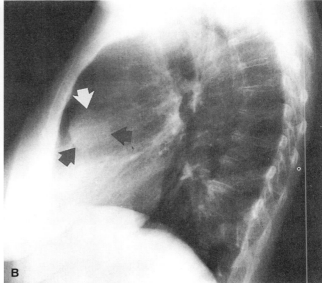

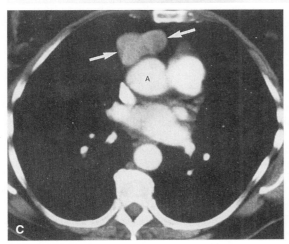

FIGURE 36-1. Radiographic and CT imaging of benign thymoma in the mediastinum. (**A**) PA chest radiograph shows a rounded mass overlying the right heart border. The visualized margins are well circumscribed (*arrows*). (**B**) Lateral chest radiograph demonstrates location of mass in anterior mediastinum (*arrows*). (**C**) CT image after administration of intravenous contrast material demonstrates peanut-shaped mass of fairly homogeneous attenuation (*arrows*); the mass is located anterior to the ascending aorta (*A*) above the right ventricular outflow tract, a typical location for thymomas. (Collins J, Stern EJ, 1999: Mediastinal masses. In Chest Radiology: The Essentials, p. 75. Philadelphia, Lippincott Williams & Wilkins)

cedure, which requires the use of general anesthesia, is performed infrequently in the United States except to define the extent and distribution of bronchiectasis before surgical resection.

Contrast radiologic studies of the esophagus using barium sulfate are performed to evaluate esophageal abnormalities, such as tumor, stricture, or diverticulum. A solid-column technique is the simplest and most reliable method for examining the esophageal wall (Balfe et al., 1994). The patient rapidly swallows radiopaque barium sulfate and fluoroscopic images are obtained. The esophageal lumen is outlined by the barium, allowing detection of esophageal abnormalities (eg, tumor or achalasia) or esophageal displacement by adjacent mediastinal structures, such as enlarged lymph nodes or an enlarged left atrium (Matthay & Sostman, 1990). Cine or videotape recordings of the barium swallow and swallowing of both a solid and a liquid bolus increase accuracy of the study (Watson & DeMeester, 1996). Videoradiology is particularly helpful to detect pharyngeal or upper esophageal abnormalities because of the rapidity with which swallowing occurs.

A double-contrast radiologic technique commonly is used to evaluate the esophageal mucosa. In this technique, the patient swallows a low-density (radiolucent) substance (usually gas-producing granules) that produces carbon dioxide in the stomach that refluxes into and distends the esophageal lumen, as well as a very–high-density agent (radiopaque barium sulfate) that coats the mucosal features (Balfe et al., 1994).

▶ Magnetic Resonance Imaging

Magnetic resonance imaging may be performed in selected patients with thoracic abnormalities. MRI uses radio waves modified by a magnetic field to produce somewhat different images than those obtained by CT scanning (Miller, 1994). The patient is placed in a strong magnetic field and subjected to short pulses of radiofrequency energy; radio signals elicited from the patient's body are compiled into images that reveal certain attributes of body tissues (Hendee, 1994). Whereas CT scanning is limited to the axial plane, MRI can supply images on the coronal and sagittal planes (Fig. 36-2). MRI is particularly useful in the evaluation of superior sulcus tumors, chest wall abnormalities, and thoracic masses abutting the spine with potential for involvement of the spinal cord (Gutierrez et al., 1998). It also may be performed to evaluate complex mediastinal masses and to diagnose suspected thoracic vascular abnormalities (eg, aortic dissection and coarctation of the aorta).

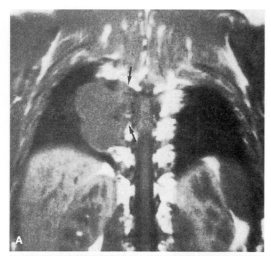

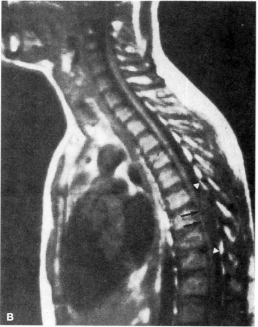

FIGURE 36-2. MRI in a patient with a malignant schwannoma. Coronal (**A**) and sagittal (**B**) planes allow evaluation of the intraspinal component (*arrows*) of this neurogenic tumor of the posterior mediastinum. (Ricci C, Rendina EA, Venuta F, et al., 1990: Diagnostic imaging and surgical treatment of dumbbell tumors of the mediastinum. Ann Thorac Surg 50:588)

► Laboratory Procedures

Cytologic examination of body fluid or exudate is performed to detect and identify malignant cells. *Sputum cytology* most often is performed in patients with large bronchogenic tumors. Centrally located tumors, larger peripheral tumors, and tumors with a squamous cell type are most likely to yield malignant cells in a sputum sample (Shields, 1996). To obtain sputum samples, the patient is asked to expectorate into a specimen cup, usually immediately on arising in the morning. Samples are obtained on 3 consecutive days to increase accuracy.

A *culture of sputum, lung tissue, or pleural fluid* may be performed if an infectious pulmonary disease is suspected. Sputum cultures are performed most frequently. A cooperative patient with a productive cough usually is able to expectorate adequate sputum for culture preparation. In others, aerosol treatments or endotracheal suctioning may be necessary to obtain an adequate sputum sample for culture. Lung tissue is obtained by needle or incisional biopsy, and pleural fluid is obtained by thoracentesis. In addition to routine culture studies, smears of exudate or fluid may be prepared using special staining techniques for detection of tuberculosis, fungi, or parasites (Sommers & Sommers, 1994). A Gram stain usually is performed in conjunction with a culture to provide a preliminary estimation of the quantity and type of bacteria present in a specimen. Gram stain findings allow initiation of appropriate antimicrobial therapy before availability of the culture results.

Skin tests may be applied for detection of several infectious pulmonary diseases. The purified protein derivative (PPD) skin test is used commonly as a screening test for tuberculosis. A positive test produces an area of indurated, erythematous swelling at the injection site after 48 to 72 hours (Pomerantz, 1996). Definitive diagnosis of pulmonary tuberculosis, however, necessitates isolation of mycobacterial organisms from sputum or lung tissue (Moran, 1995). Skin tests also may be performed to detect fungal pulmonary infections, such as coccidioidomycosis or histoplasmosis. As with tuberculosis, a positive skin test is suggestive only; definitive diagnosis must be established by culture isolation of the organism.

► Functional Assessment Studies

Pulmonary Function Testing

Pulmonary function testing often is performed before surgery to assess lung function and predict a patient's ability to withstand a planned thoracic operation, particularly pulmonary resection. No single best test exists to evaluate pulmonary function in a patient being considered for pulmonary resection and no absolute values contraindicate resection; rather, the surgeon uses a combination of studies to make a judgment about whether a patient has a prohibitive mortality or morbidity risk (Kaiser, 1998).

The most frequently performed test of pulmonary

function is forced vital capacity (FVC), measured using a spirometer. The FVC maneuver is a means of quantifying both volume and flow of respiration. FVC is the maximal volume of air expelled by forced exhalation after maximal inspiration. Flow is represented by forced expiratory volume in 1 second (FEV_1), which is the average flow exhaled in the first second (Enright & Hodgkin, 1991). Reliability of results depends on the patient's ability to cooperate fully with the various breathing maneuvers.

Forced vital capacity and FEV_1 are each compared with a "normal" value for the patient derived from studies of large groups of people with normal pulmonary function and taking into account the patient's age, sex, height, and race (Siddiqui & Knight, 1989). The measured value is then expressed as a percentage of the predicted normal value for that patient. In general, an FEV_1 of greater than 2 liters is associated with minimal perioperative risk; increased risk is associated with an FEV_1 between 1 and 2 liters, and the risk becomes prohibitive with an FEV_1 of less than 0.5 liter (Smith & Wolfe, 1995). In addition, the $FEV_1:FVC$ ratio is derived by comparing FEV_1 with FVC. The FEV_1, FVC, and the $FEV_1:FVC$ ratio are the best indicators of chronic obstructive pulmonary disease, the most common form of lung disease. Obstructive pulmonary disease is the most important pulmonary risk factor in surgical patients, and the degree of expiratory obstruction is related directly to the risk of postoperative complications (Smith & Wolfe, 1995).

Arterial blood gases usually are measured during pulmonary function testing to identify arterial hypoxemia or carbon dioxide retention that warrants further testing or predicts significant risk in preoperative patients. The baseline $PaCO_2$ is particularly useful; a $PaCO_2$ greater than 45 mm Hg is associated with increased postoperative morbidity, which may be lessened with preoperative bronchodilating therapy, breathing exercises, and antibiotics (Lumb, 1995). Patients with resting hypercarbia usually have cor pulmonale and can rarely tolerate pneumonectomy (Ginsberg, 1995). Preoperative arterial blood gas measurements also provide baseline values for comparison with postoperative measurements. Diffusion capacity is a useful measurement in the evaluation of patients in whom interstitial pulmonary disease, such as sarcoidosis or pulmonary fibrosis, is suspected. It is a measure of the capacity of the pulmonary membrane to transfer gas between alveolar air and pulmonary capillary blood (Boomsma & Glassroth, 1994).

Esophageal Manometry

Esophageal manometry is the recording of intraluminal pressures in the esophagus. It is used primarily for definition of esophageal motility disorders, particularly achalasia, scleroderma, and esophageal spasm (Watson & DeMeester, 1996). Although esophageal dysmotility also can be detected with barium radiography, manometric studies provide precise measurement of the frequency, amplitude, duration, and velocity of the peristaltic waves as well as the resting pressure of the

esophageal sphincters and their response to deglutition (Balfe et al., 1994).

Manometric testing consists of recording pressures simultaneously at various levels in the esophagus to evaluate the esophageal body and upper and lower sphincters (Duranceau, 1994) (Fig. 36-3). The study commonly is performed using an esophageal catheter assembly with a series of microtransducers embedded in the catheter itself. Baseline pressures are recorded at the lower and upper esophageal sphincters and in the esophageal body, and various swallowing and provocative maneuvers are performed to assess esophageal peristalsis and sphincter function. An *acid perfusion test* may be combined with esophageal manometry to determine if atypical chest symptoms are related to esophageal dysfunction (Cooper, 1997). This portion of the study consists of attempting to reproduce clinical symptoms of heartburn by infusing hydrochloric acid solution into the distal esophagus through a catheter attached to the manometric probe.

Esophageal pH measurement is an important component of motility studies. Because of the distinct differences in esophageal and gastric pH levels, pH measurements in the distal esophagus, in combination with various provocative maneuvers, are used to diagnose gas-

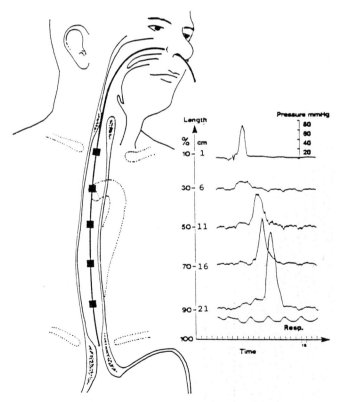

FIGURE 36-3. Diagrammatic representation demonstrating position of transducers during standard esophageal manometry and typical pressure response in the esophageal body during swallowing. Transducers are 5 cm apart, and the proximal transducer is 1 cm below the upper esophageal sphincter. (Stein HJ, DeMeester TR, Hinder RA, 1992: Evaluation and surgical management of motor disorders of the esophageal body and lower esophageal sphincter. Curr Probl Surg 24:460)

troesophageal reflux and evaluate the patient's response to medical therapy. The pH measurements provide information about competence of the lower esophageal sphincter, as well as the ability of the esophagus to clear refluxed material.

The diagnostic value of standard manometry and pH measurement is limited by the intermittent and unpredictable occurrence of motor abnormalities and symptoms in patients with esophageal motility disorders (Stein et al., 1992). As a result, ambulatory esophageal motility and pH monitoring were developed. A catheter containing two or more electronic pressure transducers is placed in the esophagus and connected to a digital data recorder. Intraluminal pressures and pH are recorded for 24 hours, during which the patient maintains a diary of activities and oral intake. Monitoring esophageal motor activity over an entire circadian cycle and under a variety of physiologic conditions multiplies the amount of data on which the diagnosis can be based, increases the probability of diagnosing an intermittent abnormality, and allows correlation of symptoms with esophageal motor function data (Watson & DeMeester, 1996).

▶ Endoscopic Examinations

Bronchoscopy

Bronchoscopy, or endoscopic inspection of the tracheobronchial tree, is useful in the diagnosis of many types of pulmonary disease. Bronchoscopy most commonly is performed in patients with lung cancer to assist with diagnosis and staging. In patients with central lung lesions that are presumed to be endobronchial, bronchoscopy allows visual inspection of abnormal bronchial mucosa and procurement of tissue for histologic evaluation. Bronchoscopic inspection may reveal a visible tumor in the bronchial mucosa or changes in the bronchial wall or lumen size due to the tumor, its infiltration in the layers of the bronchial wall, or external compression of the bronchus (Shields, 1996). Bronchoscopic examination also typically is performed in the operating room as a final assessment by the thoracic surgeon just before pulmonary resection for lung cancer.

Bronchoscopy is performed as well in all patients with tracheal stenosis, usually in the operating room just before corrective surgery (Donahue & Mathisen, 1998). It also commonly is used to establish a diagnosis in patients with nonspecific symptoms of pulmonary disease, such as persistent cough, hemoptysis, or unexplained wheezing, especially if unilateral (McElvein, 1996). In patients with massive hemoptysis, immediate bronchoscopic examination during an acute episode of bleeding is extremely useful to localize definitively the site of bleeding (Elefteriades et al., 1996).

There are two types of bronchoscopes: the fiberoptic bronchoscope, which usually is used for diagnostic bronchoscopic examinations, and the rigid bronchoscope. Advantages of flexible fiberoptic bronchoscopes include the ability to pass the bronchoscope readily with little discomfort to the patient and excellent visualization of the segmental bronchi, especially of the upper lobes (Boyd, 1995). Fiberoptic bronchoscopy usually is performed using local anesthesia and intravenous sedation. Before the procedure, oral intake is withheld for 6 to 8 hours. An anticholinergic agent and cough suppressant often are administered in addition to a sedating medication. A topical anesthetic agent is sprayed into the back of the throat and may also be injected through the neck directly into the trachea. Supplemental oxygen is administered before, during, and after the procedure and the patient is monitored with an electrocardiogram, noninvasive blood pressure monitor, and pulse oximetry (LoCicero, 1998).

The bronchoscope is passed through the nose, mouth, or an endotracheal tube into the trachea and advanced into the right and left bronchi. Flexible bronchoscopes have a circumference small enough to allow spontaneous respiration around the scope or ventilation through the endotracheal tube. Segmental bronchi may be directly visualized, and computer-assisted imaging using a microcamera incorporated into the bronchoscope allows intraluminal images to be projected on a screen in the operating room. Photographs of endobronchial abnormalities can be taken during the procedure to document the appearance of identified abnormalities (Fig. 36-4).

During bronchoscopy, tissue or cells may be obtained for histologic or cytologic analysis and for culture. Three methods are available for obtaining specimens from the endobronchial surface: (1) biopsy, (2) brushing, or (3) lavage. A biopsy is performed using a forceps passed through the bronchoscope to pluck a small piece of bronchial mucosa. Because the surface of the tumor may be necrotic, several pieces of tissue are sampled to obtain enough tissue for histologic detail (Sommers & Sommers, 1994). Bronchial brushing consists of rubbing a brush over the surface of a lesion to gather cellular material. A bronchial lavage is performed by instilling sterile saline over a suspect lesion and aspirating the fluid into a collection receptacle. Fiberoptic bronchoscopy rarely causes complications. Those that do occur usually are related to preoperative medications, cardiopulmonary dysfunction, technical difficulties, or biopsy (Kirby & Ginsberg, 1991).

A *transbronchial needle biopsy* may be performed during bronchoscopy to obtain lung or lymph tissue. A needle encased in a sheath is passed through the bronchoscope and then advanced to penetrate the trachea or bronchus to aspirate cells (Fig. 36-5). Lymph nodes in the subcarinal area or adjacent to the trachea and mainstem bronchi may be sampled using a transbronchial technique when rigidity is present and when enlarged lymph nodes have been identified by CT examination (Shields, 1997). In patients with acute forms of pulmonary disease, a transbronchial biopsy of lung tissue obviates the need for diagnostic open lung biopsy, a procedure that can be associated with considerable morbidity.

In addition to its diagnostic value, bronchoscopy frequently is used therapeutically for (1) serial deep bronchial lavage and suctioning in patients with persistent atelectasis or copious secretions, (2) removal of an

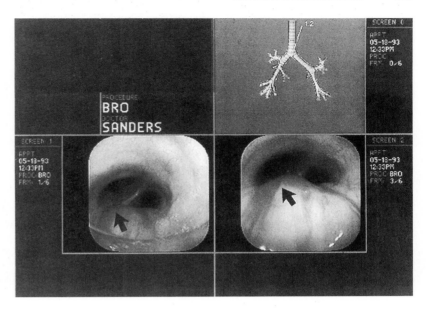

FIGURE 36-4. Images recorded during video-assisted bronchoscopy. The diagrammatic representation of the tracheobronchial tree in screen 0 (*upper right*) is used to designate the location of the endobronchial images displayed in screens 1 (*bottom left*) and 2 (*bottom right*). The endobronchial images reveal an abnormal area (*arrows*) at the bifurcation of the right and left mainstem bronchi. Histologic examination of tissue obtained from this area revealed adenocarcinoma. (Courtesy of Axel W. Joob, MD)

aspirated foreign body, (3) facilitation of endotracheal intubation, and (4) control of bleeding in the presence of massive hemoptysis. Rigid bronchoscopy is performed infrequently, primarily for therapeutic procedures. Indications for rigid bronchoscopy include massive hemoptysis, foreign body removal, dilatation of strictures, and evaluation of tracheal lesions (Warren & Faber, 1994). General anesthesia is used for rigid bronchoscopy or for flexible bronchoscopy performed concomitantly with thoracotomy.

Esophagoscopy

Esophagoscopy, or endoscopic inspection of the esophagus, is performed to examine the esophagus directly and to obtain tissue for histologic examination in patients with symptoms of esophageal disease. Esophagoscopy is technically more difficult than bronchoscopy and carries a greater risk of serious complications; the esophagus is a thin-walled tube that is easily perforated, particularly at its upper cervical constriction and just above the diaphragm (Boyd, 1995). The most common indications for esophagoscopy are the evaluation of noncardiac chest pain, persistent gastroesophageal reflux, recurrent aspiration pneumonia, dysphagia, odynophagia (painful swallowing), and an abnormal esophageal radiograph (Srivastava & Craig, 1994).

Esophagoscopy allows direct visualization of the esophageal mucosa to evaluate esophageal masses, strictures, and mucosal abnormalities, such as esophagitis and Barrett's mucosa. Tissue biopsy samples also may be extracted for histologic evaluation. In patients with gastroesophageal reflux, esophagoscopic assessment identifies the presence of a hiatal hernia and demonstrates visible inflammatory or ulcerative changes in the esophageal mucosa (Cooper, 1997). Esophagoscopy also is useful in diagnosis of esophageal perforation and for determina-

tion of severity of damage after caustic injuries of the esophagus.

Before esophagoscopy, food and fluids are withheld for 6 to 8 hours. A longer period of fasting may be required in patients with disorders that interfere with esophageal emptying, such as achalasia or gastric outlet obstruction. Premedication with a narcotic analgesic and a minor tran-

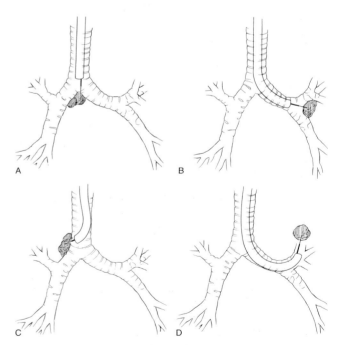

FIGURE 36-5. Transbronchial needle aspiration of subcarinal lymph nodes (**A**), a mass at the bifurcation of the left mainstem bronchus (**B**), a nodal mass at the right tracheobronchial angle (**C**), and a central mass in the left upper lobe (**D**). (Warren WH, Faber LP, 1994: Bronchoscopic evaluation of the lungs and tracheobronchial tree. In Shields TW [ed]: General Thoracic Surgery, ed. 4, p. 258. Baltimore, Williams & Wilkins)

quilizer usually is administered so that the patient is comfortably sedated, but not stuporous or combative (Rice, 1996). The patient receives supplemental oxygen and is monitored in the same manner as a patient undergoing bronchoscopy. A flexible, fiberoptic esophagoscope is used most commonly. Fiberoptic esophagoscopic evaluation usually is performed with the patient lying in a left lateral decubitus position to allow oral secretions to drain out of the mouth easily during the procedure (LoCicero, 1998). The endoscope is passed through the mouth; as it is advanced into the esophagus, the interior of the esophagus and gastroesophageal junction is visualized directly.

Rigid esophagoscopy (ie, using a rigid rather than fiberoptic esophagoscope) may be preferable in selected situations, such as to procure deep biopsy samples or assess abnormalities of the pharynx, cricopharyngeus (primary muscle of the upper esophageal sphincter), and upper esophagus (Watson & DeMeester, 1996). Rigid esophagoscopy is performed using general anesthesia. In addition to diagnostic uses, esophagoscopy sometimes is performed for therapeutic purposes, such as removal of foreign bodies lodged in the esophagus, sclerosing of esophageal varices, dilatation of strictures, and placement of intraluminal tubes (Heitmiller & Mathisen, 1989). Aspiration is the most common complication and is best prevented by an adequate length of fasting before the procedure. Less frequently, esophagoscopy causes esophageal perforation. If the patient complains of pain after the procedure, a contrast study using dilute barium is obtained to determine if perforation has occurred (LoCicero, 1998).

▶ Invasive Procedures for Tissue Sampling

Mediastinal Lymph Node Biopsy

The lymph nodes draining the lungs may be divided into two groups: (1) pulmonary lymph nodes, or those contained within the visceral pleura; and (2) mediastinal lymph nodes. In patients with lung cancer, the presence of tumor cells in mediastinal lymph nodes represents extrapulmonary spread, that is, N2 disease (Fig. 36-6). Metastasis to mediastinal lymph nodes is found in approximately 20% to 40% of patients with non-small cell lung cancer and is one of the most important factors in predicting an adverse outcome (Okada et al., 1998). Mediastinal lymph node biopsy is the most sensitive way of staging mediastinal lymph node metastasis.

Some surgeons recommend *mediastinal lymph node biopsy* selectively when there is a greater likelihood of mediastinal lymph node metastasis. The most common indication for mediastinal lymph node biopsy is lymphadenopathy or the suggestion of nodal involvement on a CT scan; other indications include factors known to increase risk for mediastinal node metastasis, such as central tumors, known adenocarcinoma, the need for pneumonectomy, and superior sulcus tumors (Ponn & Federico, 1998).

Others advocate routine mediastinal lymph node biopsy before pulmonary resection because of the prognostic significance and treatment implications of lymph node invasion and the inability to differentiate benign and malignant nodes reliably with noninvasive studies. Also, intrathoracic lymphatic anatomy does not reliably predict the pattern of lymphatic metastasis from pulmonary tumors. Lymph node involvement does not occur in a predictable, orderly sequence beginning in the intrapulmonary lymph nodes and progressing to mediastinal and then scalene lymph nodes; instead, metastasis to mediastinal lymph nodes frequently occurs without tumor invasion of ipsilateral (same side) pulmonary lymph nodes (Keller, 1998).

Mediastinal lymph node biopsy is performed before thoracotomy because pulmonary resection usually is not performed if metastasis to mediastinal lymphatic tissue already has occurred. It also may be performed to diagnose a suspected malignant tumor definitively before institution of nonsurgical therapies, such as irradiation or chemotherapy. Depending on location of the tumor and its presumed anatomic lymphatic drainage, lymph node

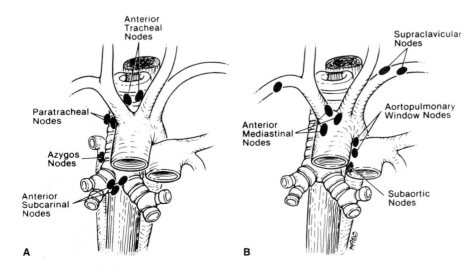

FIGURE 36-6. Mediastinal lymph nodes. (**A**) Nodes accessible through mediastinoscopy. (**B**) Nodes requiring incisional biopsy (mediastinotomy, thoracoscopy, or thoracotomy). (Mackenzie JW, Nosher JL, 1994: Invasive diagnostic procedures. In Shields TW [ed]: General Thoracic Surgery, ed. 4, p. 267. Baltimore, Williams & Wilkins)

tissue may be procured from the mediastinum by mediastinoscopy, mediastinotomy, or occasionally, video-assisted thoracoscopy (VATS), which is discussed later in the chapter.

Transcervical mediastinoscopy is performed using general anesthesia. A small transverse incision is made in the suprasternal notch. The surgeon primarily uses finger dissection to create a tunnel in the pretracheal fascia, anterior to the trachea and beneath the innominate artery, through which the mediastinoscope is advanced (Mackenzie & Riley, 1996) (Fig. 36-7). Lymph nodes along the trachea and either main bronchus are bluntly dissected from the airway surface and removed using instruments passed through the mediastinoscope. Removal of whole lymph nodes theoretically lessens the likelihood of tumor implantation during the procedure, but may not be possible because of the large size, friability, or adherence of lymph nodes (Ponn & Federico, 1998). In such cases, a piece of lymph tissue is extracted using a forceps. Although complications are uncommon, mediastinoscopy can cause hemorrhage, injury to a major airway, esophageal perforation, pneumothorax, or recurrent laryngeal nerve injury (Kirby & Ginsberg, 1991).

Mediastinotomy, also called a *Chamberlain procedure,* is the direct surgical exposure of mediastinal lymph nodes. The procedure is performed when it is necessary to sample nodes that are inaccessible through a standard transcervical mediastinoscopy. Mediastinotomy provides access for biopsy of nodes in the superior mediastinum, the anterior and superior hilum, and the upper anterior portions of the lung (Boyd & Glassman, 1998). A small incision is made over the second costal cartilage on the appropriate side (Fig. 36-8). Through this incision, the mediastinum, pulmonary vessels, and phrenic nerve also can be examined for direct tumor invasion (Ponn & Federico, 1998).

Percutaneous Transthoracic Needle Biopsy

A *percutaneous transthoracic needle biopsy* is a procedure performed occasionally to obtain lung tissue for histologic examination in patients with lesions located in the lung periphery. Except for pulmonary lesions fixed to the chest wall, transthoracic needle biopsy almost always is performed by an invasive radiologist and guided by fluoroscopy or CT scanning. Fluoroscopy is used for easily visualized lesions, especially when the lesion is located in the lower lung fields; CT scanning is used when lesions are not well localized on the chest roentgenogram or are located close to the heart, major blood vessels, or hilum of the lung (Wolverson, 1996). A needle is inserted through the chest wall and guided into the lesion. As the needle tip is moved inside the lesion, cells are aspirated for cytologic evaluation. A chest roentgenogram is obtained after the procedure to detect iatrogenic pneumothorax.

Transthoracic needle biopsy is most useful for establishing a diagnosis in those patients who, because of type of disease or general medical status, are not candidates for surgical resection but in whom a definitive diagnosis is necessary to direct nonsurgical therapy. The use of percutaneous needle biopsy in patients who are candidates for surgical resection is controversial. Because there is a significant incidence of false-negative results, the procedure does not eliminate the possibility of a pulmonary malignancy. Therefore, thoracotomy for definitive identification and removal of the lesion usually is considered necessary even when needle biopsy has yielded no diagnosis of malignancy. Because surgical resection is the treatment of choice in the event of a positive diagnosis, the procedure rarely alters the course of therapy. Contraindications to needle biopsy of the lung include pulmonary hypertension and pulmonary cysts or bullae. Pneumothorax and hemoptysis are potential complications of the procedure.

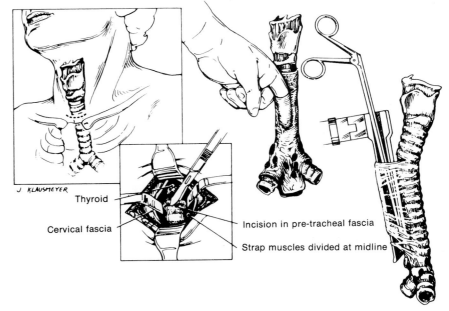

FIGURE 36-7. Mediastinoscopy. A transverse incision is made just above the sternum. Finger dissection is used to create a tunnel within the pretracheal fascia through which the mediastinoscope is advanced. Identified lymph nodes are biopsied with an instrument passed through the mediastinoscope. (Mackenzie JW, Riley DJ, 1996: Diagnostic and staging procedures: Mediastinal evaluation, scalene lymph node biopsy, mediastinoscopy, and mediastinotomy. In Baue AE, Geha AS, Hammond GL, et al [eds]: Glenn's Thoracic and Cardiovascular Surgery, ed. 6, p. 185. Stamford, CT, Appleton & Lange)

Thyroid

Cervical fascia

Incision in pre-tracheal fascia

Strap muscles divided at midline

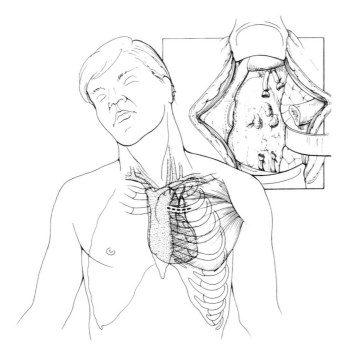

FIGURE 36-8. Anterior mediastinotomy. (*Left*) Location of incision. (*Right*) Cartilage resected, vessels ligated, and mediastinum exposed. (Boyd AD, Glassman LR, 1998: Thoracic incisions. In Kaiser LR, Kron IL, Spray TL [eds]: Mastery of Cardiothoracic Surgery, p. 34. Philadelphia, Lippincott Williams & Wilkins)

Thoracentesis

Thoracentesis is aspiration of fluid or air from the pleural space using a needle or catheter inserted through the chest wall. In the presence of unexplained pleural effusion, diagnostic thoracentesis may be performed to obtain pleural fluid for laboratory analysis. Measurement of lactate dehydrogenase, total protein, pH, glucose, white blood cell count, and amylase provide important clues about etiology of a pleural effusion.

In most cases of malignant pleural effusion, cytologic analysis of pleural fluid determines the site and histologic type of the primary tumor (Serre et al., 1990). Pleural fluid for cytology should be fresh. Because cells in fluid swell and degenerate over time, fluid withdrawn during an initial thoracentesis in a patient with suspected malignant disease is less satisfactory for cytologic study than a fluid sample removed several days later (Sommers & Sommers, 1994). Percutaneous needle biopsy of the pleura for suspected malignant disease has been replaced largely by pleural biopsy during VATS, as described in the following section.

Video-Assisted Thoracoscopy

Video-assisted thoracoscopy is a more recent addition to the armamentarium of procedures for diagnosis of intrathoracic diseases. It consists of using endoscopic in-

struments and microcameras to provide visualization of and access to intrathoracic organs without a thoracotomy incision (Lewis et al., 1992). Diagnostic procedures that may be performed through thoracoscopy include biopsies of pleura, mediastinal lymph nodes or neoplasms, lung, and pericardium. Although thoracoscopy first was performed early in the 20th century, inadequate visibility and instrumentation limited its usefulness. The introduction of video imaging techniques in the late 1980s, along with special instruments that allow more precise operative techniques, allowed rapid expansion of the applicability of VATS (Mack, 1998; Lewis et al., 1992; McKeown et al., 1992).

In patients with pleural abnormalities, thoracoscopy is thought to achieve a higher degree of accuracy than needle biopsy of the pleura because pleural metastases can vary in location according to the type of tumor (Armengod et al., 1990). Thoracoscopy allows direct visualization of all pleural surfaces and sampling of multiple sites. It also may be performed for definitive diagnosis of idiopathic pleural effusions when thoracentesis fails to establish a diagnosis (Mack et al., 1992). Thoracoscopy may be used instead of mediastinotomy for biopsy of mediastinal lymph nodes located in the aortopulmonary window. Biopsy for the diagnosis of anterior mediastinal masses also can be performed using a thoracoscopic approach (Mack, 1998).

A pericardial biopsy using VATS may be indicated for diagnosis of unexplained pericardial effusion or pericarditis. A small portion of pericardial tissue may be resected concomitantly to allow drainage of associated pericardial effusion. However, in the presence of persistent, recurring pericardial effusion, an extensive pericardiectomy performed through a thoracotomy usually is necessary to ensure chronic drainage. VATS also may be performed to obtain lung parenchymal biopsies in patients with interstitial lung diseases when less invasive methods fail to yield a diagnosis (Ferson et al., 1996).

Thoracoscopy is performed using general anesthesia and a scope similar to that used for mediastinoscopy. Patients are informed and prepared for possible thoracotomy if the desired procedure cannot be accomplished through thoracoscopy. The patient is placed in a lateral decubitus position. Usually, three small incisions are necessary for insertion of the thoracoscope and operating instruments. One incision is made in the sixth or seventh intercostal space in the midaxillary line for insertion of the thoracoscope; the second and third incisions are made in the third to sixth intercostal spaces along the anterior and posterior axillary lines to allow insertion and manipulation of instruments (Lewis et al., 1992) (Fig. 36-9). Strategic positioning of the thoracoscopic camera and endoscopic instruments is important to maximize visualization and ensure success of the procedure (Landreneau et al., 1992).

A single-lung ventilation technique is used during VATS; that is, the patient is intubated with a double-lumen endotracheal tube and only the contralateral (opposite) lung is ventilated. Single-lung ventilation allows collapse of the lung on the operative side, thereby pro-

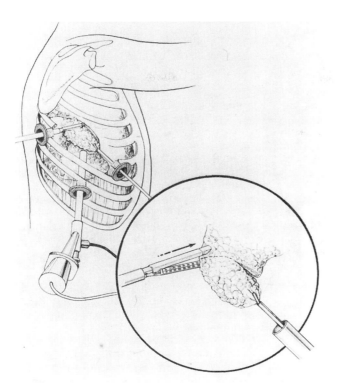

FIGURE 36-9. Video-assisted thoracoscopy for wedge resection. Thoracoscope is inserted through 6th or 7th intercostal space in midaxillary line and two additional ports are used for passage and manipulation of instruments. Inset demonstrates wedge resection of lung using stapling and grasping instruments. (Mack MJ, 1998: Video-assisted thoracic surgery. In Kaiser LR, Kron IL, Spray TL [eds]: Mastery of Cardiothoracic Surgery, p. 96. Philadelphia, Lippincott Williams & Wilkins)

Thoracoscopy is used therapeutically for procedures such as pleurodesis for treatment of spontaneous pneumothorax, thoracic sympathectomy, empyema evacuation, creation of a pericardial window, and wedge resection. It is contraindicated in two groups of patients: (1) those who are unable to tolerate single-lung anesthesia, and (2) those with complete obliteration of the pleural space due to adhesions (Lewis et al., 1992).

Incisional Biopsies

Open lung biopsy is a technique for obtaining lung tissue for examination through a small thoracotomy incision. Typically, candidates for open lung biopsy are patients in whom surgical therapy through a conventional thoracotomy is not anticipated but in whom less invasive procedures have failed to establish a diagnosis. An incisional biopsy allows procurement of larger tissue samples than can be obtained through needle aspiration techniques. The need for open lung biopsy through thoracotomy has been reduced substantially by the ability to procure adequate lung tissue samples using VATS. However, it remains a valuable diagnostic modality in patients who are unable to undergo thoracoscopy because of an inability to tolerate single-lung anesthesia or the presence of an obliterated pleural space. Open lung biopsy is most appropriate for patients with parenchymal lung disease in whom the diagnosis obtained by biopsy is likely to lead to a change in therapy and who have a reasonable survival prognosis (Kramer et al., 1998).

Open lung biopsy is performed using general anesthesia. The location of the incision depends on the area of the lung from which the biopsy will be obtained. A short anterior thoracotomy incision often is used. A transaxillary thoracotomy or vertical axillary thoracotomy may be performed alternatively, depending on the disease process as determined by radiographic examina-

viding maximal exposure and avoiding injury to intrathoracic structures. At the conclusion of the biopsy, the ipsilateral lung is reinflated. Chest tube thoracostomy drainage is required for several days after the procedure.

FIGURE 36-10. Scalene node biopsy is performed through a 2- to 3-cm incision above the clavicle (*left*); fat pad containing scalene lymph nodes is excised (*top right*) guided by anatomic landmarks (*bottom right*). (Mackenzie JW, Riley DJ, 1996: Diagnostic and staging procedures: Mediastinal evaluation, scalene lymph node biopsy, mediastinoscopy, and mediastinotomy. In Baue AE, Geha AS, Hammond GL, et al [eds]: Glenn's Thoracic and Cardiovascular Surgery, ed. 6, p. 184. Stamford, CT, Appleton & Lange)

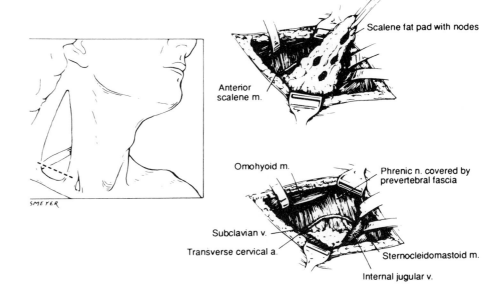

tion (Mackenzie & Nosher, 1994). Although open lung biopsy is a relatively minor surgical procedure, it necessitates general anesthesia and an incision in the thorax. It may be associated with significant morbidity because of the serious illnesses typically present in patients who require the procedure.

Scalene lymph node biopsy is performed for diagnosis of suspected sarcoidosis or lung carcinoma in patients who have palpable supraclavicular lymph nodes. Lymph nodes in the anterior scalene fat pad may contain pathologic tissue because they drain lymphatic fluid from the lungs and mediastinum. A small supraclavicular incision, using local anesthesia, allows access to the scalene fat pad, which is excised from the anterior surface of the anterior scalene muscle (Fig. 36-10).

Exploratory thoracotomy may be necessary in selected instances when less invasive procedures fail to provide definitive diagnosis of an intrathoracic abnormality or if a diagnosis does not obviate the need for thoracotomy. For example, exploratory thoracotomy is indicated in the case of a lung tumor that is thought to be malignant and surgically resectable, even if prior diagnostic studies fail to establish the certainty of malignancy. Exploratory thoracotomy for diagnosis usually is avoided if a lung lesion does not appear to be resectable.

REFERENCES

Al-Sugair A, Coleman RE, 1998: Applications of PET in lung cancer. Semin Nucl Med 28:303

Armengod AC, Saumench J, Moya J, 1990: Points to consider when choosing a biopsy method in cases of pleuritis of unknown origin, with special reference to thoracoscopy. In Deslauriers J, Lacquet LK (eds): Thoracic Surgery: Surgical Management of Pleural Diseases. St. Louis, CV Mosby

Balfe DM, Deyoe L, Ling D, Siegel MJ, 1994: The esophagus. In Putman CE, Ravin CE (eds): Textbook of Diagnostic Imaging, ed. 2. Philadelphia, WB Saunders

Boomsma JD, Glassroth J, 1994: Pulmonary gas exchange. In Shields TW (ed): General Thoracic Surgery, ed. 4. Baltimore, Williams & Wilkins

Boyd AD, 1995: Endoscopy: Bronchoscopy and esophagoscopy. In Sabiston DC Jr, Spencer FC (eds): Surgery of the Chest, ed. 6. Philadelphia, WB Saunders

Boyd AD, Glassman LR, 1998: Thoracic incisions. In Kaiser LR, Kron IL, Spray TL (eds): Mastery of Cardiothoracic Surgery. Philadelphia, Lippincott Williams & Wilkins

Cohen RG, DeMeester TR, Lafontaine E, 1995: The pleura. In Sabiston DC Jr, Spencer FC (eds): Surgery of the Chest, ed. 6. Philadelphia, WB Saunders

Collins J, Stern EJ, 1999: Chest wall, pleural, and diaphragm. In Chest Radiology: The Essentials. Philadelphia, Lippincott Williams & Wilkins

Cooper JD, 1997: Current role of esophageal function studies. Semin Thorac Cardiovasc Surg 9:157

Davis RD Jr, Oldham HN Jr, Sabiston DC Jr, 1995: The mediastinum. In Sabiston DC Jr, Spencer FC (eds): Surgery of the Chest, ed. 6. Philadelphia, WB Saunders

Donahue DM, Mathisen DJ, 1998: Tracheal resection and reconstruction. In Kaiser LR, Kron IL, Spray TL (eds): Mastery of Cardiothoracic Surgery. Philadelphia, Lippincott Williams & Wilkins

Duranceau A, 1994: Physiology and physiologic studies of the esophagus. In Shields TW (ed): General Thoracic Surgery, ed. 4. Baltimore, Williams & Wilkins

Elefteriades JA, Geha AS, Cohen LS, 1996: Management of acute pulmonary disease. In House Officer Guide to ICU Care, ed. 2. Philadelphia, Lippincott-Raven

Enright PL, Hodgkin JE, 1991: Pulmonary function tests. In Respiratory Care, ed. 3. Philadelphia, JB Lippincott

Ferson PF, Landreneau RJ, Keenan RJ, 1996: Thoracoscopy: General principles and diagnostic procedures. In Baue AE, Geha AS, Hammond GL, et al. (eds): Glenn's Thoracic and Cardiovascular Surgery, ed. 6. Stamford, CT, Appleton & Lange

Freundlich IM, Bragg DG, 1992: Introduction. In Freundlich IM, Bragg DG (eds): A Radiologic Approach to Diseases of the Chest. Baltimore, Williams & Wilkins

Ginsberg RJ, 1995: Preoperative assessment of the thoracic surgical patient: A surgeon's viewpoint. In Pearson FG, Deslauriers J, Ginsberg RJ, et al. (eds): Thoracic Surgery. New York, Churchill Livingstone

Glazer HS, Semenkovich JW, Gutierrez FR, 1998: Mediastinum. In Lee JK, Sagel SS, Stanley RJ, Heiken JP (eds): Computed Body Tomography With MRI Correlation, ed. 3. Philadelphia, Lippincott Williams & Wilkins

Gutierrez FR, Woodard PK, Fleishman MJ, et al., 1998: Thorax: Techniques and normal anatomy. In Lee JK, Sagel SS, Stanley RJ, Heiken JP (eds): Computed Body Tomography with MRI Correlation, ed. 3. Philadelphia, Lippincott Williams & Wilkins

Heitmiller RF, Mathisen DJ, 1989: Esophagoscopy. In Grillo HC, Austen WG, Wilkins EW, et al. (eds): Current Therapy in Cardiothoracic Surgery. Toronto, Canada, BC Decker

Hendee WR, 1994: The imaging process. In Putman CE, Ravin CE (eds): Textbook of Diagnostic Imaging, ed. 2. Philadelphia, WB Saunders

Kaiser LR, 1998: Right-sided pulmonary resections. In Kaiser LR, Kron IL, Spray TL (eds): Mastery of Cardiothoracic Surgery. Philadelphia, Lippincott Williams & Wilkins

Keller SM, 1998: Mediastinal lymph node dissection. In Kaiser LR, Kron IL, Spray TL (eds): Mastery of Cardiothoracic Surgery. Philadelphia, Lippincott Williams & Wilkins

Kirby TJ, Ginsberg RJ, 1991: Complications of endoscopy: Bronchoscopy, esophagoscopy, and mediastinoscopy. In Waldhausen JA, Orringer MB (eds): Complications in Cardiothoracic Surgery. St. Louis, Mosby–Year Book

Kramer MR, Berkman N, Mintz B, et al., 1998: The role of open lung biopsy in the management and outcome of patients with diffuse lung disease. Ann Thorac Surg 65:198

Landreneau RJ, Mack MJ, Hazelrigg SR, et al., 1992: Video-assisted thoracic surgery: Basic technical concepts and intercostal approach strategies. Ann Thorac Surg 54:800

Le Roux BT, Rocke DA, 1989: Bronchography. In Grillo HC, Austen WG, Wilkins EW, et al. (eds): Current Therapy in Cardiothoracic Surgery. Toronto, Canada, BC Decker

Lewis RJ, Caccavale RJ, Sisler GE, McKenzie JW, 1992: One hundred consecutive patients undergoing video-assisted thoracic operations. Ann Thorac Surg 54:421

LoCicero J, 1998: Endoscopy: Bronchoscopy and esophagoscopy. In Kaiser LR, Kron IL, Spray TL (eds): Mastery of Cardiothoracic Surgery. Philadelphia, Lippincott Williams & Wilkins

Lowe VJ, Naunheim KS, 1998: Positron emission tomography in lung cancer. Ann Thorac Surg 65:1821

Lumb PD, 1995: Perioperative pulmonary physiology. In Sabiston DC Jr, Spencer FC (eds): Surgery of the Chest, ed. 6. Philadelphia, WB Saunders

Mack MJ, 1998: Video-assisted thoracic surgery. In Kaiser LR, Kron IL, Spray TL (eds): Mastery of Cardiothoracic Surgery. Philadelphia, Lippincott Williams & Wilkins

Mack MJ, Aronoff RJ, Acuff TE, et al., 1992: Present role of thoracoscopy in the diagnosis and treatment of diseases of the chest. Ann Thorac Surg 54:403

Mackenzie JW, Nosher JL, 1994: Invasive diagnostic procedures. In Shields TW (ed): General Thoracic Surgery, ed. 4. Baltimore, Williams & Wilkins

Mackenzie JW, Riley DJ, 1996: Diagnostic and staging procedures: Mediastinal evaluation, scalene lymph node biopsy, mediastinoscopy, and mediastinotomy. In Baue AE, Geha AS, Hammond GL, et al. (eds): Glenn's Thoracic and Cardiovascular Surgery, ed. 6. Stamford, CT, Appleton & Lange

Matthay RA, Sostman HD, 1990: Chest imaging. In George RB, Light RW, Matthay MA, Matthay RA (eds): Chest Medicine, ed. 2. Baltimore, Williams & Wilkins

McElvein RB, 1996: Bronchoscopy: Transbronchial biopsy and bronchoalveolar lavage. In Baue AE, Geha AS, Hammond GL, et al. (eds): Glenn's Thoracic and Cardiovascular Surgery, ed. 6. Stamford, CT, Appleton & Lange

McKeown PP, Conant P, Hubbel DS, 1992: Thoracoscopic lung biopsy. Ann Thorac Surg 54:490

McLoud TC, 1989: Radiologic assessment. In Grillo HC, Austen WG, Wilkins EW, et al. (eds): Current Therapy in Cardiothoracic Surgery. Toronto, Canada, BC Decker

Miller WT, 1994: Roentgenographic evaluation of the lungs and chest. In Shields TW (ed): General Thoracic Surgery, ed. 4. Baltimore, Williams & Wilkins

Moran JF, 1995: Surgical treatment of pulmonary tuberculosis. In Sabiston DC Jr, Spencer FC (eds): Surgery of the Chest, ed. 6. Philadelphia, WB Saunders

Okada M, Tsubota N, Yoshimura M, Miyamoto Y, 1998: Proposal for reasonable mediastinal lymphadenectomy in bronchogenic carcinomas: Role of subcarinal nodes in selective dissection. J Thorac Cardiovasc Surg 116:949

Pomerantz M, 1996: Surgical treatment of tuberculosis and other pulmonary mycobacterial infections. In Baue AE, Geha AS, Hammond GL, et al. (eds): Glenn's Thoracic and Cardiovascular Surgery, ed. 6. Stamford, CT, Appleton & Lange

Ponn RB, Federico JA, 1998: Mediastinoscopy and staging. In Kaiser LR, Kron IL, Spray TL (eds): Mastery of Cardiothoracic Surgery. Philadelphia, Lippincott Williams & Wilkins

Rice TW, 1996: Esophagoscopy and endoscopic esophageal ultrasonography. In Baue AE, Geha AS, Hammond GL, et al. (eds): Glenn's Thoracic and Cardiovascular Surgery, ed. 6. Stamford, CT, Appleton & Lange

Sagel SS, Slone RM, 1998: Lung. In Lee JK, Sagel SS, Stanley RJ, Heiken JP (eds): Computed Body Tomography With MRI Correlation, ed. 3. Philadelphia, Lippincott Williams & Wilkins

Serre G, Daste G, Vincent C, et al., 1990: Diagnostic approach to the patient with pleural effusion: Cytologic analysis of pleural fluid. In Deslauriers J, Lacquet LK (eds): Thoracic Surgery: Surgical Management of Pleural Diseases. St. Louis, CV Mosby

Shields TW, 1991: Primary mediastinal tumors and cysts and their diagnostic investigation. In Shields TW (ed): The Mediastinum. Philadelphia, Lea & Febiger

Shields TW, 1996: Diagnosis and staging of lung cancer. In Baue AE, Geha AS, Hammond GL, et al. (eds): Glenn's Thoracic and Cardiovascular Surgery, ed. 6. Stamford, CT, Appleton & Lange

Shields TW, 1997: Lung cancer and the solitary pulmonary nodule. In Khan MG, Lynch JP (eds): Pulmonary Disease Diagnosis and Therapy: A Practical Approach. Baltimore, Williams & Wilkins

Siddiqui AK, Knight L, 1989: Pulmonary function tests. In Braun SR (ed): Concise Textbook of Pulmonary Medicine. New York, Elsevier

Smith PK, Wolfe WG, 1995: Preoperative assessment of pulmonary function: Quantitative evaluation of ventilation and blood gas exchange. In Sabiston DC Jr, Spencer FC (eds): Surgery of the Chest, ed. 6. Philadelphia, WB Saunders

Sommers HM, Sommers KE, 1994: Laboratory investigations in the diagnosis of pulmonary diseases. In Shields TW (ed): General Thoracic Surgery, ed. 4. Baltimore, Williams & Wilkins

Srivastava AK, Craig RM, 1994: Endoscopy of the esophagus. In Shields TW (ed): General Thoracic Surgery, ed. 4. Baltimore, Williams & Wilkins

Stein HJ, DeMeester TR, Hinder RA, 1992: Evaluation and surgical management of motor disorders of the esophageal body and lower esophageal sphincter. Curr Probl Surg 24:447

Warren WH, Faber LP, 1994: Bronchoscopic evaluation of the lungs and tracheobronchial tree. In Shields TW (ed): General Thoracic Surgery, ed. 4. Baltimore, Williams & Wilkins

Watson TJ, DeMeester TR, 1996: The esophagus: Anatomy and functional evaluation. In Baue AE, Geha AS, Hammond GL, et al. (eds): Glenn's Thoracic and Cardiovascular Surgery, ed. 6. Stamford, CT, Appleton & Lange

Wolverson MK, 1996: Thoracic imaging. In Baue AE, Geha AS, Hammond GL, et al. (eds): Glenn's Thoracic and Cardiovascular Surgery, ed. 6. Stamford, CT, Appleton & Lange

37

Preoperative Management and Counseling

*P*reoperative management of thoracic surgical patients includes both physical and psychological preparation for the planned operation. Although much of the preparatory management is standard, some important differences exist depending on the specific disease necessitating surgical intervention. Thoracic surgical diseases can be broadly categorized into three groups: (1) diseases of the lungs, (2) esophageal diseases, and (3) diseases of the mediastinum. Because patients usually are admitted to the hospital on the day of a planned thoracic operation, most of the evaluation and preparation for surgery must be completed on an outpatient basis.

▶ Preoperative Evaluation

The preoperative nursing evaluation complements that performed by the physician and provides baseline information that enhances interpretation of postoperative findings. It also allows the nurse to establish a relationship with the patient and family and identify potential problems that may occur during the perioperative period. Information for the preoperative evaluation is obtained from the patient record, interview with and physical examination of the patient, and diagnostic studies.

Patient Interview

Ideally, an advanced practice nurse performs the outpatient *preoperative patient assessment*. If a nurse practitioner has this responsibility, he or she may perform the preadmission history and physical examination as well. The preoperative assessment begins with an interview to gain information about the clinical history and to assess the patient's understanding of the illness, emotional readiness for the planned procedure, and family support system. Several components of the clinical history are of particular importance in preoperative patients: (1) the current illness and associated symptoms, (2) the presence of coexisting medical diseases, (3) the current medication regimen and any known allergies, and (4) the patient's functional status. The patient's occupation and personal habits, such as smoking, alcohol use, exercise, and diet, also are ascertained.

Factors that influence perioperative risk may be identified during the preoperative interview. In addition to cardiopulmonary disease, recent weight loss greater than 10%, age greater than 70 years, and the type and stage of tumor in patients with malignant disease seem to be the most significant prognostic factors for adverse events (Ginsberg, 1995). A history of cigarette smoking is pertinent in any patient undergoing a thoracic operation. Because cigarette smoking is a risk factor for both lung and esophageal cancer, a long smoking history is common. Alcohol abuse (a risk factor for squamous cell esophageal cancer) or sequelae of alcohol abuse (eg, hepatic disease or cardiomyopathy) may be present in patients with esophageal tumors. Exposure to environmental carcinogens or tuberculosis and travel to regions endemic for specific pulmonary infections are other relevant features of the clinical history.

Current Illness and Associated Symptoms

Most patients who undergo thoracic operations have malignant disease of the lungs, esophagus, or mediastinum. Associated constitutional symptoms, such as weight loss, anorexia, and malaise, frequently are present. Other significant signs and symptoms may be noted, depending on the type of underlying disease (Table 37-1). Lung cancer is the most common diagnosis in preoperative thoracic surgical patients. Ninety to 95% of patients with lung cancer are symptomatic at the time of diagnosis (Shields, 1996). Clinical manifestations may include cough, persistent upper respiratory tract infections, hemoptysis, dyspnea, or wheezing.

Patients with benign or malignant esophageal disease commonly have some degree of dysphagia. They may experience pain, choking, or vomiting with eating; may need to eat very slowly or take liquids with food; and may have difficulty in maintaining body weight (Stein et al., 1992). In those patients with esophageal cancer, nutritional depletion often has occurred and cachexia may be evident. Associated symptoms also are common in adults with primary mediastinal neoplasms or cysts (Cohen et al., 1991). Lesions in the mediastinum typically produce manifestations related to mechanical effects of compression or invasion of structures adjacent to the mass (Davis et al., 1995). Symptoms also may result from endocrine or other biochemical products secreted by the tumor.

Associated Medical Diseases

Associated medical diseases are common in patients who require thoracic surgery and can significantly affect operative outcome (Table 37-2). Most thoracic operations are performed in middle-aged and elderly patients. Pulmonary and cardiovascular disease are prevalent in this population. Systemic diseases, such as diabetes mellitus, hypertension, and renal insufficiency, also are common (Allen & Pairolero, 1996).

The presence and severity of existing pulmonary disease have a major impact on operative risk, particularly in patients who will undergo pulmonary resection. Chronic obstructive pulmonary disease is the most common form of pulmonary impairment in thoracic surgical patients. Less commonly, pulmonary function is impaired by pulmonary fibrosis or a previous pulmonary resection for lung cancer.

TABLE 37-1

Clinical Manifestations in Preoperative Thoracic Surgical Patients

Pulmonary Disease	Esophageal Disease	Mediastinal Disease
Cough	Dysphagia	Chest or back pain
Sputum production	Heartburn	Cough
Hemoptysis	Regurgitation	Dyspnea
Respiratory infection	Weight loss	Dysphagia
Dyspnea	Aspiration	Superior vena cava syndrome
Wheezing	Halitosis	Hoarseness
Chest pain	Choking	
Hoarseness		
Weight loss		

TABLE 37-2

Common Associated Medical Problems in Thoracic Surgical Patients

Chronic obstructive pulmonary disease
Coronary artery disease
Peripheral arterial occlusive disease
Hypertension
Diabetes mellitus

Coexistent cardiovascular disease, present in many older patients, also can increase operative risk significantly. Manifestations of organic heart disease that are well tolerated before surgery may become more serious during the perioperative period as a result of inadequate gas exchange, with resultant hypoxemia and hypercarbia (Wilson, 1996). Patients at increased risk for complications include those with underlying coronary artery disease and unstable angina, recent myocardial infarction, congestive heart failure, uncontrolled hypertension, or critical aortic stenosis (Hillis et al., 1995).

Other Relevant Data

During the preoperative interview, the nurse also assesses the patient's understanding of the clinical problem and planned therapy, level of anxiety, and coping ability. Appropriate preoperative counseling is based on this assessment. The patient's living arrangements and social support system are reviewed so that suitable discharge planning can be initiated. Many patients who undergo thoracic operations are elderly with limited social and financial resources. Early identification of discharge needs helps alleviate patient anxiety during the perioperative period and facilitates efficient use of hospital and community support resources.

Physical Assessment

Physical examination of the thoracic surgical patient focuses particularly on the pulmonary and cardiovascular systems. The lungs are auscultated to provide baseline data regarding respiratory rate, breath sounds, or the presence of adventitious sounds. Heart sounds are auscultated, and the cardiac rate, rhythm, and any extra sounds or murmurs are noted. Blood pressure, temperature, and weight are measured, and peripheral pulses are palpated. The carotid arteries are auscultated to detect bruits that might represent carotid artery stenosis. In patients who will undergo thymectomy, baseline respiratory parameters are measured. The findings from this preoperative examination provide important baseline values for comparison with postoperative findings.

Functional status is assessed to evaluate the patient's ability to increase activity appropriately in the postoperative period. Functional capacity is particularly important in patients who will undergo pulmonary resection. It facilitates the surgeon's determination of the patient's ability to withstand removal of a portion of lung or an entire lung. Functional status in patients with lung disease may be categorized using the Karnofsky Scale of Performance (Table 37-3). The patient also may be asked to climb one or more flights of stairs, accompanied by a surgeon or nurse who monitors oxygen saturation and pulse rate and directly evaluates the presence and severity of dyspnea on exertion. This assessment provides helpful information to supplement data obtained from standard pulmonary function testing.

Diagnostic Studies

Standard laboratory studies obtained before operations on the thorax include a complete blood cell count, urinalysis, blood clotting studies, blood chemistry survey, electrocardiogram, and chest roentgenogram. These baseline studies typically are performed within 1 week of the planned operation and are essential to detect any abnormalities that could increase operative risk or alter the plan of therapy. In patients with signs or symptoms of ischemic heart disease, exercise stress testing may be performed to detect myocardial ischemia before proceeding with a planned thoracic operation. Arrhythmias or congestive heart failure also may require diagnostic evaluation and treatment before operation.

Room air arterial blood gases typically are measured to identify arterial hypoxemia or carbon dioxide retention and to provide a baseline for comparison with postoperative measurements. Arterial hypercapnia ($PaCO_2 >$ 45 mm Hg) is considered an indicator of significantly increased risk of respiratory failure and operative death; arterial hypoxemia also is correlated with an increased risk of complications (Todd & Ralph-Edwards, 1995). In patients with pulmonary neoplasms, a stool specimen may be obtained to test for the presence of blood. Occult blood in the stool might indicate that the lung lesion is not a primary tumor but rather an adenocarcinoma of the bowel that has metastasized to the lung.

In patients who will undergo pulmonary resection, pulmonary function testing usually is performed to assess the patient's ability to withstand removal of a portion of functional lung tissue. Pulmonary function testing identifies patients at higher risk for pulmonary complications and allows implementation of prophylactic interventions in the preoperative period (Lumb, 1995). The most commonly measured parameters are forced vital capacity (FVC) and forced expiratory volume in 1 second (FEV_1), which quantitate volume and flow of respiration. FVC measures the total volume of air that can be forcefully expelled after maximal inspiration. FEV_1 measures the average flow exhaled in the first second.

Measurements of FEV_1, FVC, and the FEV_1:FVC ratio are the best indicators of obstructive lung disease, the most important pulmonary cause of surgical risk. In general, an FEV_1 of greater than 2 L is associated with minimal perioperative risk; increased risk is associated with an FEV_1 between 1 and 2 L, and operative risk becomes prohibitive with an FEV_1 of less than 0.5 L (Smith & Wolfe, 1995). Other variables suggesting significant risk of postoperative morbidity and mortality include a VO_2max less than 15 mL/kg/min and elevated pulmonary artery pressures (Kaiser, 1998).

Patients with intrathoracic lesions often have undergone bronchoscopy, chest computed tomography, or magnetic resonance imaging as part of the diagnostic evaluation. In patients with diseases of the esophagus, esophagoscopy, contrast swallow studies, or esophageal manometry may have been performed. These diagnostic modalities are described in detail in Chapter 36, Diagnostic Evaluation of Thoracic Diseases.

▶ Preoperative Regimen

General Guidelines

Most medications, with the exception of anticoagulant and antiplatelet agents, are continued throughout the preoperative period until the time of surgery. This includes maintenance antihypertensive, antiarrhythmic, antianginal, and antiseizure agents (Reves et al., 1995). Digoxin sometimes is administered prophylactically before major pulmonary or esophageal resection procedures because of the prevalence of postoperative supraventricular tachycardia. Although the etiology is unclear, postoperative supraventricular tachycardia is common, particularly in elderly patients (Shields, 1994). Achieving a therapeutic serum digoxin level before operation may not prevent occurrence of tachyarrhythmias, but it is believed by some to facilitate control of the ventricular response rate if the arrhythmia occurs.

A preoperative dose of antibiotics may be administered to reduce the likelihood of perioperative infection, although many surgeons administer several postoperative doses only. A broad-spectrum agent, such as a

---

TABLE 37-3

Karnofsky Scale of Performance

Clinical Status	Percentage
Normal, no evidence of disease	100
Minor signs or symptoms of disease	90
Normal activity with effort	80
Cares for self, cannot do normal activities	70
Cares for self with occasional assistance	60
Requires frequent assistance and medical care	50
Disabled, requires special care and assistance	40
Severely disabled, hospitalization indicated	30
Hospitalization with active supportive treatment	20
Moribund, fatal processes progressing rapidly	10

Adapted from Shields TW, 1994: Presentation, diagnosis, and staging of bronchial carcinoma and of the asymptomatic solitary pulmonary nodule. In Shields TW (ed): General Thoracic Surgery, ed. 4. Baltimore, Williams & Wilkins.

cephalosporin, typically is selected. If the patient is allergic to penicillin, an alternative agent, such as vancomycin, is used. Wound contamination is most likely to occur during the operation. Potential sources of microorganisms include a preexisting infection, the patient's skin, and operating room personnel and equipment. The most frequently encountered causative pathogens for infection of surgical wounds are *Staphylococcus aureus* and *Staphylococcus epidermidis* (Doebbling et al., 1990). Pulmonary infections after noncardiac thoracic operations usually are due to *Hemophilus influenzae*, pneumococcus, or *S. aureus* (Kaiser, 1995).

Two units of cross-matched blood usually are reserved for potential intraoperative use. Transfusion of allogeneic (ie, from genetically unlike human donors) blood is performed judiciously. Blood is a limited commodity and despite the screening of donor blood for viral agents, a small risk exists for transmitting viral infection. Specifically, human immunodeficiency virus, human T-cell lymphotropic virus, hepatitis C virus, and hepatitis B virus can be transmitted through allogeneic blood transfusion (Schreiber et al., 1996). Other risks of blood transfusion include both hemolytic and nonhemolytic reactions, graft-versus-host disease, recipient alloimmunization, and hypervolemia (Stammers, 1999).

Patients are instructed to abstain from any oral intake after midnight on the evening before the planned procedure. A preoperative shower, using an antibacterial soap, is prescribed for the evening before and morning of the operation. The patient is instructed to thoroughly cleanse the chest and axillae. Shaving of the chest is performed in the operating room.

Before transporting the patient to the operating room, a preoperative medication usually is administered to reduce anxiety, provide perioperative amnesia, suppress physiologic stress responses, and facilitate induction of anesthesia. One or more of several types of drugs may be administered, including (1) sedatives, hypnotics, and tranquilizers; (2) opioids; (3) anticholinergic agents; or (4) antihistamines and antacids (Wong & Brunner, 1994). The type and dosage are prescribed by the anesthesiologist, based on the patient's age, underlying pulmonary disease, associated medical diseases, and level of anxiety. Administration of the preoperative medication is carefully timed to reduce patient apprehension at the time of transfer yet maintain a level of consciousness sufficient for the patient to cooperate with preparatory interventions in the operating room.

Special Considerations

In patients with underlying pulmonary disease, the preoperative regimen may include interventions that are instituted several weeks before a planned operation. Particularly if pulmonary resection is planned, therapies such as smoking cessation, bronchial hygiene treatments, or administration of bronchodilating medications or antibiotics, when indicated, may significantly improve pulmonary function.

Smoking cessation is of prime importance. It permits recovery of mucociliary function and allows bronchitic effects of tobacco smoke to abate (Metzler, 1989). Even a smoke-free period of 1 to 2 weeks increases a patient's ability to clear secretions during the postoperative period. An aggressive bronchial hygiene regimen, which may include bronchodilating medications, also aids in removing retained secretions. In some patients, prolonged preoperative pulmonary rehabilitation significantly improves pulmonary function and allows surgical intervention that otherwise would be contraindicated (Ginsberg, 1995). Preoperative nutritional assessment and therapy also are important. Improving nutritional intake to restore body weight to within 10% of ideal body weight can decrease postoperative morbidity and mortality.

In diabetic patients, insulin dosage is reduced on the day of operation. Typically, one half of the usual dose is given and blood glucose levels are measured frequently during surgery. In patients who have been receiving chronic corticosteroid therapy, parenteral corticosteroids are administered immediately before the operation and are continued after surgery until oral corticosteroid therapy is resumed. If exogenous glucocorticoids are not given, patients who have been receiving steroids are at risk for development of acute adrenal insufficiency and circulatory shock because of suppressed adrenal function that is insufficient to meet the stress of a surgical procedure (Murray & Torres, 1999). Patients undergoing thymectomy for treatment of myasthenia gravis require careful titration of pharmacologic therapy during the preoperative period. Achieving relative stability of the disease before thymectomy is important to minimize postoperative complications (Mathisen, 1991). Usually, a neurologist directs the patient's preoperative medication regimen.

For selected procedures, such as esophageal resection with colon interposition, a special preoperative regimen is necessary to cleanse the bowel of fecal material and normal bacterial flora. Bowel cleansing reduces the likelihood of perioperative infection caused by bacteria normally present in the bowel. The regimen usually consists of several days of dietary restrictions and oral antibiotics.

► Preoperative Counseling

A wide continuum of learning needs and emotional responses is encountered in preoperative patients. Although typically described as "preoperative teaching," the purpose of *preoperative counseling* is twofold: (1) provision of adequate information about the perioperative course, and (2) provision of psychological support sufficient to allay anxiety and promote effective coping. The provision of concrete objective information is effective in reducing negative emotional responses during threatening procedures. When the impending procedure is described from the patient's point of view in unambiguous, concrete, and objective terms, coping is facilitated because differences between expectations and the actual experience are decreased and the patient's understanding of the experience is increased (Clark, 1997).

TABLE 37-4

Content of Preoperative Education

Preoperative Phase	Postoperative Phase
Members of the team	Units in which patient will stay
Dietary restrictions	Visiting for family
Antibacterial shower	Overview of catheters and monitoring devices
Disposition of belongings	Patient participation in recovery process
Preoperative sedation	Pulmonary hygiene measures
Time and length of operation	Pain control
Waiting area for family	Activity guidelines
	Progression of ambulation

A factor meriting special consideration is that many patients undergo thoracic operations soon after a malignant disease has been discovered or suspected. The time available for preoperative instruction after hospital admission is limited and patients are likely to have significant anxiety. Therefore, preoperative counseling is initiated during a preoperative outpatient visit by an advanced practice nurse or a nurse from the unit where the patient will recover after surgery. Preoperative teaching is designed to complement information the patient receives from the surgeon and anesthesiologist regarding the planned operation and its potential benefits and risks. Specific content varies depending on protocols for the particular operation, surgeon, and institution.

Typically, preoperative instruction includes a description of the projected events that will occur during each phase of the hospitalization, with special emphasis on the perioperative period (Table 37-4). Detailed information about discharge from the hospital and recovery at home are deferred until after the operation. Studies demonstrate that patients remember only 29% to 72% of information provided to them, and that the more information presented, the lower the recall rate (Houts et

al., 1998). Often, the teaching session is supplemented with written materials, particularly if the patient and family have differing needs for information. Audiovisual materials also are helpful adjuncts to teaching and provide a reference throughout the patient's hospitalization.

Expectations for the patient's participation in the recovery process are discussed during preoperative counseling. Patient instruction about the pulmonary hygiene regimen, progressive ambulation, and pain management is particularly important in thoracic surgical patients. Effective coughing is necessary to promote lung expansion, mobilize secretions, and prevent the side effects of retained secretions, atelectasis and pneumonia (Hudak et al., 1998). The patient is instructed in deep breathing and coughing techniques. Usually an incentive spirometry device is used in the postoperative period to facilitate effective lung expansion (Fig. 37-1). Typically, the patient is instructed to use the device every 1 to 2 hours to take and sustain a series of deep inspirations. Preoperative breathing exercises strengthen respiratory musculature, and instructions on deep breathing and effective coughing (using diaphragmatic and accessory muscles) improve postoperative cooperation (Smith & Wolfe, 1995; Ginsberg, 1995).

Patients also are informed about the planned progression of activity after surgery. Early and progressive ambulation is important to reduce the morbidity associated with immobility. If adequately prepared, the patient can participate more effectively in this regimen. It also is important to discuss postoperative pain management before thoracic operations. Because major chest wall muscles usually are divided, thoracotomy incisions are particularly painful. Several methods of analgesia are available to provide adequate postoperative pain control. Most often, an epidural catheter is placed at the time of operation and used for pain management during the first several days. Alternatively, patient-controlled intravenous dosing or conventional intermittent parenteral dosing of opioid medications may be used.

Provision of psychological support is an integral part

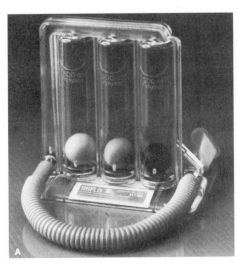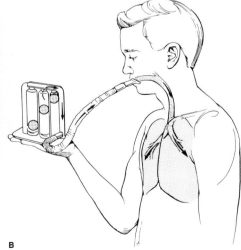

FIGURE 37-1. (A) An incentive spirometry device such as the Triflo II is used to promote lung expansion in the postoperative period. **(B)** Preoperative instruction typically includes allowing the patient to practice using the device. (Courtesy of Sherwood Services AG, The Kendall Company, Mansfield, MA)

of nursing care during the immediate preoperative period. Anxiety, along with fear, uncertainty, loss of control, and decreased self-esteem, are common in patients confronted with the need for hospitalization and surgery (Breemhaar et al., 1996). Manifestations of anxiety in preoperative patients include a variety of psychophysiologic symptoms, such as increased tension, a sense of helplessness, decreased self-assurance, and focusing on the perceived object of fear (Carty, 1991).

Effective interventions for preoperative anxiety include (1) allowing the patient to verbalize concerns, (2) providing factual information to reduce fear that is based on distorted perceptions, and (3) providing reassurance about the nurses' and physicians' commitment to the patient's well-being. Sometimes, patients are severely anxious about an impending thoracic operation. If the patient's need for support exceeds what the nurse realistically can provide, psychiatric consultation may be necessary. Principles used to guide preoperative education and psychologic support are discussed more fully in Chapter 10, Education and Psychological Support for the Patient and Family.

REFERENCES

Allen MS, Pairolero PC, 1996: Postoperative care and complications in the thoracic surgery patient. In Baue AE, Geha AS, Hammond GL, et al. (eds): Glenn's Thoracic and Cardiovascular Surgery, ed. 6. Stamford, CT, Appleton & Lange

Breemhaar B, van den Borne HW, Mullen PD, 1996: Inadequacies of surgical patient education. Patient Education and Counseling 28:31

Carty JL, 1991: Psychosocial aspects. In Alspach JG (ed): Core Curriculum for Critical Care Nursing, ed. 4. Philadelphia, WB Saunders

Clark CR, 1997: Creating information messages for reducing patient distress during health care procedures. Patient Education and Counseling 30:247

Cohen AJ, Thompson L, Edwards FH, Bellamy RF, 1991: Primary cysts and tumors of the mediastinum. Ann Thorac Surg 51:378

Davis RD, Oldham HN Jr, Sabiston DC Jr, 1995: The mediastinum. In Sabiston DC Jr, Spencer FC (eds): Surgery of the Chest, ed. 6. Philadelphia, WB Saunders

Doebbeling BN, Pfaller MA, Kuhns KR, et al., 1990: Cardiovascular surgery prophylaxis. J Thorac Cardiovasc Surg 99:981

Ginsberg RJ, 1995: Preoperative assessment of the thoracic surgical patient: A surgeon's viewpoint. In Pearson FG, Deslauriers J, Ginsberg RJ, et al. (eds): Thoracic Surgery. New York, Churchill Livingstone

Hillis LD, Lange RA, Winniford MD, Page RL, 1995: Noncardiac surgery in patients with coronary artery disease. In Manual of Clinical Problems in Cardiology, ed. 5. Boston, Little, Brown

Houts PS, Bachrach R, Witmer JT, et al., 1998: Using pictographs to enhance recall of spoken medical instructions. Patient Education and Counseling 35:83

Hudak CM, Gallo BM, Morton PG, 1998: Patient management: Respiratory system. In Critical Care Nursing: A Holistic Approach, ed. 7. Philadelphia, Lippincott Williams & Wilkins

Kaiser AB, 1995: Use of antibiotics in cardiac and thoracic surgery. In Sabiston DC Jr, Spencer FC (eds): Surgery of the Chest, ed. 6. Philadelphia, WB Saunders

Kaiser LR, 1998: Right-sided pulmonary resections. In Kaiser LR, Kron IL, Spray TL (eds): Mastery of Cardiothoracic Surgery. Philadelphia, Lippincott Williams & Wilkins

Lumb PD, 1995: Perioperative pulmonary physiology. In Sabiston DC Jr, Spencer FC (eds): Surgery of the Chest, ed. 6. Philadelphia, WB Saunders

Mathisen DJ, 1991: Thymectomy: Avoidance and management of complications. In Waldhausen JA, Orringer MB (eds): Complications in Cardiothoracic Surgery. St. Louis, Mosby–Year Book

Metzler MH, 1989: Pre- and postoperative respiratory care. In Braun SR (ed): Concise Textbook of Pulmonary Medicine. New York, Elsevier

Murray MJ, Torres NE, 1999: Critical care medicine for the cardiac patient. In Kaplan JA (ed): Cardiac Anesthesia, ed. 4. Philadelphia, WB Saunders

Reves JG, Greeley WJ, Grichnik K, et al., 1995: Anesthesia and supportive care for cardiothoracic surgery. In Sabiston DC Jr, Spencer FC (eds): Surgery of the Chest, ed. 6. Philadelphia, WB Saunders

Schreiber GB, Busch MP, Kleinman SH, et al., 1996: The risk of transfusion-transmitted viral infections. N Engl J Med 334:1685

Shields TW, 1994: General features and complications of pulmonary resections. In Shields TW (ed): General Thoracic Surgery, ed. 4. Baltimore, Williams & Wilkins

Shields TW, 1996: Diagnosis and staging of lung cancer. In Baue AE, Geha AS, Hammond GL, et al. (eds): Glenn's Thoracic and Cardiovascular Surgery, ed. 6. Stamford, CT, Appleton & Lange

Smith PK, Wolfe WG, 1995: Preoperative assessment of pulmonary function: Quantitative evaluation of ventilation and blood gas exchange. In Sabiston DC Jr, Spencer FC (eds): Surgery of the Chest, ed. 6. Philadelphia, WB Saunders

Stammers AH, 1999: Extracorporeal devices and related technologies. In Kaplan JA (ed): Cardiac Anesthesia, ed. 4. Philadelphia, WB Saunders

Stein HJ, DeMeester TR, Hinder RA, 1992: Evaluation and surgical management of motor disorders of the esophageal body and lower esophageal sphincter. Curr Probl Surg 24:447

Todd TR, Ralph-Edwards AC, 1995: Perioperative management. In Pearson FG, Deslauriers J, Ginsberg RJ, et al. (eds): Thoracic Surgery. New York, Churchill Livingstone

Wilson RS, 1996: Anesthesia for thoracic surgery. In Baue AE, Geha AS, Hammond GL, et al. (eds): Glenn's Thoracic and Cardiovascular Surgery, ed. 6. Stamford, CT, Appleton & Lange

Wong HY, Brunner EA, 1994: Preanesthetic evaluation and preparation. In Shields TW (ed): General Thoracic Surgery, ed. 4. Baltimore, Williams & Wilkins

THORACIC OPERATIONS

Surgical Treatment of Pulmonary Diseases

The pulmonary disease most commonly treated with surgery is carcinoma of the lung. Less often, pulmonary surgery is performed to remove a malignant tumor that has metastasized to the lung from outside the thorax or to treat benign forms of pulmonary disease.

► Carcinoma of the Lung

By far the most common form of lung cancer is bronchogenic carcinoma, which arises from the epithelial lining of the bronchi. *Bronchogenic lung cancer* is categorized as non-small cell lung cancer, including the histologic cell types adenocarcinoma, squamous or epidermoid carcinoma, and large cell carcinoma, or as small cell lung cancer. Uncommon forms of lung cancer include bronchoalveolar carcinoma, which originates in the lung parenchyma, and mesothelioma, which arises in the pleura.

Bronchogenic lung cancer usually occurs in the form of a solitary tumor. Lesions that involve the mainstem, lobar, or segmental bronchi are considered central, and those that originate in distal bronchi, bronchioles, or lung parenchyma are termed peripheral. Most centrally located tumors are squamous cell carcinoma; adenocarcinoma usually originates in the lung periphery. Malignant lung tumors occur more commonly in the right lung and usually in the upper lobes (Shields, 1994a). A Pancoast, or superior sulcus tumor, is a bronchogenic carcinoma that arises in the superior pulmonary sulcus (extreme apex of the lung), or thoracic inlet, and invades lymphatic tissue in the endothoracic fascia (Urschel, 1993) (Fig. 38-1).

Malignant lung tumors can spread by any of three routes. First, they may directly invade contiguous lung tissue and adjacent structures, such as the pleura, diaphragm, chest wall, or mediastinal organs. Second, lung tumors often spread to lymph nodes in the pulmonary hilum or mediastinum and are disseminated through the lymphatic system. Third, tumor cells can invade pulmonary veins in the lungs and spread to distant organs through the vascular system.

Indications for Surgical Treatment

For *non-small cell bronchogenic lung cancer*, the treatment of choice is surgical resection of the tumor and surrounding lymphatic tissue. However, the ability to remove a lung tumor surgically depends on location and size of the tumor, presence of tumor cells in regional lymph nodes, and whether tumor has invaded nearby structures, such as the great vessels or trachea. Incomplete resection of a malignant tumor does not enhance survival and has little or no palliative benefit (Shields, 1993).

To determine a tumor's suitability for resection before surgical treatment, a determination is made of the patient's clinical stage of the disease. The International Staging System provides standard nomenclature for categorizing the extent of disease in patients with lung cancer (Mountain, 1986, 1997). It consists of a three-letter code, with the first letter, "T," designating tumor size; the second, "N," the presence and extent of lymph node involvement; and the third, "M," the presence of distant metastasis.

Once TNM status is determined, the stage of disease is categorized as stage I (A or B), II (A or B), III (A or B), or IV. Staging of the disease enables the physician to

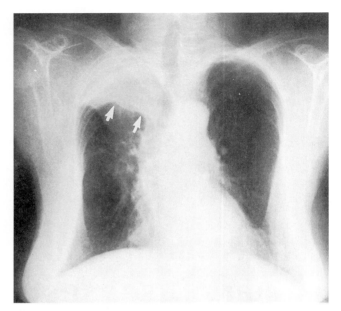

FIGURE 38-1. Chest radiograph demonstrating right Pancoast tumor (*arrows*). (Courtesy of Robert Vanecko, MD)

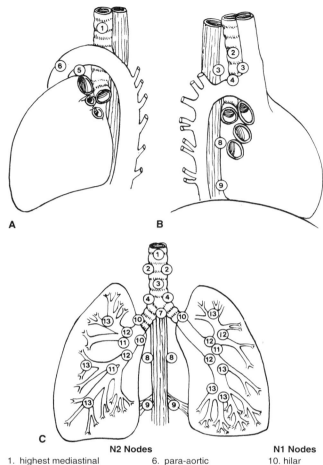

N2 Nodes		N1 Nodes
1. highest mediastinal	6. para-aortic	10. hilar
2. upper paratracheal	7. subcarinal	11. interlobar
3. pretracheal, retrotracheal	8. paraesophageal	12. lobar
4. lower paratracheal	9. pulmonary ligament	13. segmental
5. suboartic		

FIGURE 38-2. Left lateral (**A**), right lateral (**B**), and anterior (**C**) views demonstrating sites of lymph node metastasis in carcinoma of the lung. (Beahrs OH, Myers MH [eds], 1992: American Joint Committee on Cancer: Manual for Staging of Cancer, ed. 4, p. 122. Philadelphia, JB Lippincott)

select the most appropriate therapy and provide prognostic information. Stage I lung cancer is considered early disease, stage II cancer is intermediate, and stages III and IV represent advanced disease (Martini et al., 1992). TNM definitions and staging of lung cancer are described in more detail in Chapter 33, Pulmonary, Tracheal, and Pleural Diseases.

A lung tumor is assessed initially by its appearance on the chest roentgenogram. The roentgenogram demonstrates tumor size, location, and involvement of contiguous structures, such as the chest wall. The roentgenogram also may provide suggestive evidence of tumor involvement of mediastinal lymph nodes. Computed tomographic (CT) scanning, a technique for imaging cross-sectional anatomy, also is performed to detect and evaluate mediastinal lymphadenopathy (ie, lymph node enlargement) that may represent malignant invasion. Other significant findings that may be demonstrated on a CT scan include invasion of the vertebral bodies, the presence of small, undetected pleural effusions, or encirclement of vital structures by the tumor (Shields, 1997).

Mediastinoscopy or, less commonly, mediastinotomy often is performed before thoracotomy to obtain mediastinal lymph node tissue for histologic evaluation. The presence of tumor cells in mediastinal lymph nodes represents N2 as opposed to N1 disease, in which only pulmonary lymph nodes contain tumor (Fig. 38-2). Except in selected situations, pulmonary resection usually is not recommended once tumor cells have spread to mediastinal lymphatic tissue. Surgical treatment of lung cancer also is not beneficial in the presence of distant metastasis. Consequently, a patient with signs or symptoms suggestive of distant metastasis undergoes scans of all potential metastatic sites (eg, brain, upper abdomen, and bones) (Shields, 1993).

Surgical resection is the treatment of choice for patients with stage I and II lung cancer and improves outcome in a small subset of patients with stage IIIA disease (D'Amico & Sabiston, 1995) (Table 38-1). Surgical resection for stage IIIA lung cancer usually is performed in patients with peripheral tumors (T3 N1 M0) that are categorized as stage IIIA because they have invaded the parietal pleura, diaphragm, or chest wall. Tumors categorized as stage IIIA because of confirmed N2 disease (ie, tumor invasion of ipsilateral mediastinal or subcarinal lymph nodes) usually are not treated surgically.

Treatment, however, is somewhat controversial for stage IIIA, N2 lung tumors when mediastinal lymph node metastasis is not detectable by clinical staging, but rather is determined only by pathologic diagnosis at the time of thoracotomy. For this subset of patients, some surgeons recommend complete resection with extensive mediastinal lymph node dissection, based on a belief

TABLE 38-1

Primary Malignant Lung Tumors Treated with Surgical Resection

NON-SMALL CELL

Stage	TNM Classification
Stage IA	T1 N0 M0
Stage IB	T2 N0 M0
Stage IIA	T1 N1 M0
Stage IIB	T2 N1 M0
	T3 N0 M0
Stage IIIA*	T3 N1 M0
Stage IIIA†	T1 N2 M0
	T2 N2 M0
	T3 N2 M0

SMALL CELL

As one component of multimodal therapy in selected patients with isolated tumors and limited regional disease

*In selected patients if complete resection of tumor is possible.
†In selected patients when N2 disease is not clinically apparent but is detected at thoracotomy.

TABLE 38-2

Potential Contraindications to Pulmonary Resection for Lung Cancer

EVIDENCE OF EXTRAPULMONARY SPREAD
Paralysis of recurrent laryngeal nerve
Superior vena cava syndrome
Phrenic nerve paralysis
Pleural effusion with malignant cells

TECHNICAL CONSIDERATIONS
Involvement of the main pulmonary artery
Involvement of the tracheal carina

MEDICAL CONDITIONS
Marginal pulmonary function
Unstable angina or recent myocardial infarction
Congestive heart failure

DISTANT METASTASIS

Preoperative Evaluation

The objective of pulmonary resection for lung cancer is to remove all visible tumor completely with regional lymph nodes that may contain malignant cells. In planning the resection, consideration is given to whether the tumor has spread to lymph nodes or invaded extraparenchymal structures, such as the chest wall, diaphragm, or pericardium. The pulmonary resection should be as conservative as possible without compromising the complete removal of local and regional disease within the thorax (Kaiser, 1998a; Shields, 1993).

Preoperative pulmonary function testing and assessment of the patient's current functional status are performed to predict how much lung tissue can be removed safely. There is no single best test of pulmonary function and no absolute values that contraindicate resection; rather, the surgeon uses a combination of studies to make a judgment about whether a patient has a prohibitive risk for mortality or morbidity (Kaiser, 1998b). Measurements commonly used to assess a patient's ability to withstand pulmonary resection include forced expiratory volume in 1 second (FEV_1), the ratio of FEV_1 to forced vital capacity, diffusion capacity, and baseline arterial blood gases. Patient age and the presence of associated medical conditions, particularly cardiovascular disease, also influence a patient's ability to withstand a major thoracic operation. The pulmonary resection is then planned based on the amount of lung tissue that must be removed to eradicate visible tumor and the amount of lung tissue loss the patient can withstand.

Because of the association between smoking and lung cancer, many patients who require pulmonary resection have underlying obstructive pulmonary disease. In patients with severe pulmonary impairment, preoperative interventions, such as smoking cessation, intensive pulmonary hygiene, antibiotics (for existing infection),

that prognosis in these patients is more favorable than in those with clinically apparent mediastinal involvement (Nakanishi et al., 1997). Pulmonary resection is not performed in patients with stage IIIB or stage IV lung cancer.

Unfortunately, surgical resection is possible in only 30% to 40% of newly diagnosed patients with non-small cell lung tumors (Carney, 1998). Most patients have regional lymph node involvement or distant metastasis that precludes resection by the time the diagnosis is made. Pulmonary resection also may be prohibited by the patient's general medical condition, particularly in the presence of severe underlying pulmonary impairment or cardiovascular disease. Table 38-2 lists potential contraindications to pulmonary resection in patients with lung cancer.

Small cell lung tumors seldom are treated with surgical resection. Small cell lung cancer has distinct biologic and clinical characteristics that distinguish it from other types of lung cancer (Mentzer et al., 1993a). Most important from a surgical perspective is a rapid doubling time that results in early tumor dissemination. Consequently, only a limited number of patients with small cell lung cancer have a single tumor and no evident metastases. Surgical resection may be appropriate in selected patients with small cell lung cancer as an adjunct to combination chemotherapy for removal of residual disease. Appropriate candidates for adjuvant surgical resection are those patients with an isolated small cell tumor nodule and limited regional disease. Although the role of surgical resection in small cell lung cancer is controversial, it sometimes is beneficial in reducing local recurrences and in providing surgical staging of disease (Lassen & Hansen, 1999).

bronchodilator therapy, and pulmonary rehabilitation, are performed before surgical treatment to reduce perioperative risk (Reilly et al., 1993). Often these interventions can improve pulmonary function significantly.

Types of Pulmonary Resections

The various types of pulmonary resection operations are named according to the amount of lung tissue that is removed. The lungs are divided by fissures into lobes: three on the right and two on the left. The lobes are subdivided into bronchopulmonary segments: 10 in the right lung and 8 in the left lung (Shields, 1994b). Depending on tumor location, either a lobectomy or pneumonectomy usually is performed.

Lobectomy is the most commonly performed pulmonary resection for lung cancer. It is the procedure of choice when a tumor is confined to a lobe and neither N1 (lobar or hilar) nor N2 (mediastinal) lymph node metastasis is present that would preclude complete removal of all diseased tissue (Shields, 1993). Even for small, peripheral tumors, lobectomy is preferable to a limited pulmonary resection (eg, wedge resection or segmentectomy). Lobectomy remains the definitive procedure because it is an anatomic resection that removes the regional lymph nodes located along the lobar bronchus and ensures an adequate tumor-free parenchymal margin (Kaiser, 1998b). A *bilobectomy* (ie, removal of two of the three lobes of the right lung) may be performed to conserve either the right upper or lower lobe. Indications for bilobectomy include tumor extending across an interlobar fissure, absence of a fissure, an endobronchial tumor, or a tumor that has invaded the bronchus intermedius (D'Amico & Sabiston, 1997). When bilobectomy of the right middle and lower lobes is performed, they can be removed en bloc (as a whole) because of the common origin of these lobes from the bronchus intermedius (Kaiser, 1998b).

In patients with small, peripheral tumors and marginal pulmonary function, a *limited pulmonary resection* may be necessary to ensure sufficient residual lung parenchyma for adequate ventilation. A *wedge resection* is the removal of a peripheral piece of lung tissue containing the tumor. It sacrifices the least amount of normal lung parenchyma. A *segmentectomy* is the anatomic removal of the pulmonary artery, vein, bronchus, and parenchyma of a particular segment of the lung (Somers & Faber, 1996). Although any segment can be resected, segmentectomy of the upper lobes is performed most commonly (Shields, 1993).

Wedge resection and segmentectomy are considered limited pulmonary resections because it is not possible to remove all adjacent lobar lymph nodes. Although long-term survival after limited resection is similar to that for lobectomy in patients with stage I lung cancer, those who undergo limited resection are more likely to have local recurrence of disease (Mentzer et al., 1993b). As a result, limited pulmonary resection is considered by many to be an inadequate operation for treatment of bronchogenic carcinoma if the patient can tolerate lobectomy

(Warren, 1998). Thus, limited resections usually are reserved for elderly patients or those with marginal cardiopulmonary status who have a stage IA tumor (ie, tumor ≤3 cm and surrounded by lung or visceral pleura without bronchoscopic evidence of invasion) more proximal than the lobar bronchus (ie, not in the main bronchus). If pulmonary function is so marginal that the necessary surgical resection would not be tolerated, operative therapy is precluded. An alternative treatment modality (eg, irradiation) may be performed for palliation of symptoms.

A *pneumonectomy*, or removal of an entire lung, is required when lobectomy does not provide complete resection and when the loss of an entire lung can be tolerated (D'Amico & Sabiston, 1995). Most patients with good pulmonary function are able to withstand removal of one lung. However, pneumonectomy is associated with a higher mortality rate and greater morbidity than other pulmonary resections (Klemperer & Ginsberg, 1999). Also, in patients with a long smoking history, pulmonary or cardiac function may be impaired to the degree that removal of an entire lung is contraindicated. The decision regarding whether a patient will tolerate pneumonectomy is based on preoperative pulmonary function testing and functional status.

Five to 8% of patients with lung cancer have tumors that are best suited to bronchoplastic techniques, most commonly lobectomy combined with sleeve resection (Lowe et al., 1995). A *sleeve resection lobectomy* enables the surgeon to avoid performing a pneumonectomy when tumor extends into a lobar bronchus. The procedure consists of resecting the lobe en bloc with a portion of the common airway; the transected airway is then reconstructed to restore lung continuity (Mentzer et al., 1993b) (Fig. 38-3). Candidates for sleeve resection lobectomy are patients with (1) a tumor that is centrally located, (2) metastatic lymph nodes near a main bronchus, or (3) compromised pulmonary function that precludes pneumonectomy (Van Schil et al., 1991). Bronchoplastic techniques may be used for resection of tumors of the upper and lower lobes on both the right and left sides, but are most applicable for localized tumors originating in the right upper lobe orifice (Tedder & Lowe, 1992). Long-term survival in patients who undergo sleeve resection for treatment of non-small cell lung cancer is comparable with that achieved with conventional pneumonectomy (Suen et al., 1999; Lowe et al., 1995).

Sometimes tumor invasion necessitates surgical resection of structures contiguous to the lungs and bronchi. Any of the pulmonary resection procedures can be combined with en bloc removal of structures beyond the visceral pleura into which the tumor has extended (Shields, 1993). An *extrapleural pneumonectomy* is the removal of not only an entire lung but also the parietal pleura surrounding the lung, as well as portions of the diaphragm and pericardium. Approximately 5% of resectable lung tumors extend beyond the lung to involve the pleura, soft tissues, or osseous structures of the chest wall (Downey et al., 1999). In such cases, an en bloc chest wall resection may be performed along with the pulmonary resec-

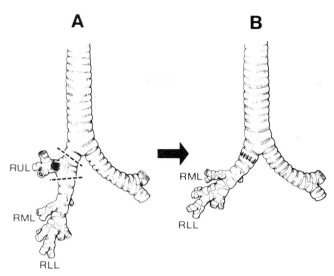

FIGURE 38-3. Schematic representation of bronchoplastic technique during sleeve lobectomy. (**A**) Tracheobronchial tree with tumor in orifice of right upper lobe (RUL) bronchus; right mainstream bronchus is divided (*dotted lines*), and RUL is removed en bloc. (**B**) Bronchial continuity is restored by reconstructing right mainstem bronchus. RML, right middle lobe; RLL, right lower lobe. (Mentzer SJ, Myers DW, Sugarbaker DJ, 1993: Sleeve lobectomy, segmentectomy, and thoracoscopy in the management of carcinoma of the lung. Chest 103:416S)

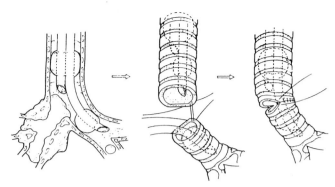

FIGURE 38-4. Schematic representation of right sleeve (carinal) pneumonectomy, including ipsilateral pneumonectomy accompanied by resection and anastomosis of the distal trachea and contralateral bronchus. (*Left*) Tumor involving tracheal carina; double-lumen endotracheal tube has been placed for ventilation of the left lung during the procedure. (*Middle*) After excision of the carina, the double-lumen tube is withdrawn into the trachea and the left lung is ventilated through a tube inserted across the operative field into the left main bronchus. (*Right*) The double-lumen endotracheal tube is repositioned in the left main bronchus and the anastomosis of the distal trachea to the left bronchus is completed. (Tsuchiya R, Goya T, Naruke T, Suemasu K, 1990: Resection of tracheal carina for lung cancer. J Thorac Cardiovasc Surg 99:782)

tion. Tumors extending to the proximal main bronchus, carina, or distal trachea may be amenable to resection by *tracheal sleeve pneumonectomy* (ie, carinal or bronchial resection and reconstruction in combination with pneumonectomy) (Klemperer & Ginsberg, 1999) (Fig. 38-4).

Completion pneumonectomy is the name given to resection of a remaining lobe or lobes after a prior lobectomy or bilobectomy of the lung. It may be indicated for second primary cancers, local recurrent tumor, pulmonary metastases, or benign inflammatory conditions (Klemperer & Ginsberg, 1999). Completion pneumonectomy is performed uncommonly. It is technically complex because adhesions from the prior pulmonary resection in the same hemithorax make mobilization of the residual lung difficult and blood loss greater (Gregoire et al., 1993). However, completion pneumonectomy can be performed with an acceptable mortality rate (5%) and may provide a second chance for cure in patients with cancer; patients who have received irradiation previously are at higher risk for perioperative morbidity (Regnard et al., 1999).

The Operative Procedure

On arrival in the operating room, an epidural catheter typically is placed for postoperative infusion of opioid analgesic agents. Single-lung ventilation is used for pulmonary resection operations, as well as for many other types of thoracic operations. The most frequently used technique for single-lung ventilation uses a specially designed double-lumen endotracheal tube that is posi-

tioned to allow isolated ventilation of each main bronchus (Fig. 38-5). During the operative procedure, ventilation is delivered only to the nonoperative lung; the lung to be resected is nonventilated, collapsed, and atelectatic during the procedure (Reves et al., 1995).

Fiberoptic bronchoscopy usually is performed before thoracotomy to identify any previously undetected endobronchial abnormalities. The bronchoscope is inserted into the tracheobronchial tree after induction of general anesthesia and used to examine thoroughly the segmental bronchi. Bronchoscopic visualization may reveal tumor exposed in bronchial mucosa or changes in the bronchial wall or lumen size caused by tumor infiltration or external compression (Shields, 1996).

Pulmonary resection is performed most commonly through a thoracotomy incision. After positioning the patient in a lateral decubitus position with the operative lung up, the skin of the operative field is shaved, cleansed with an antibiotic solution to reduce skin flora, and draped to create a sterile field. Typically, a posterolateral incision is performed (Fig. 38-6). Subcutaneous tissue along the course of the incision is divided, as well as the latissimus dorsi and serratus anterior muscles (Crawford & Kratz, 1995). The fifth or sixth interspace is incised for upper lobe or lower lobe resection, respectively. One or more ribs may be surgically divided or a small segment of rib is removed (ie, the rib is "shingled") to facilitate spreading the chest wall for adequate exposure.

In patients with limited pulmonary reserve, some pulmonary resection operations may be performed alternatively using a muscle-sparing incision (Fig. 38-7). The term *muscle-sparing* denotes that the serratus anterior

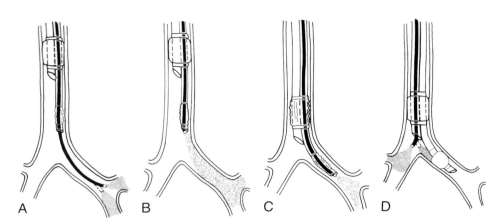

FIGURE 38-5. Fibrerscopic placement and positioning of left-sided, double-lumen endotracheal tube. (**A**) The fiberscope is passed into the left main stem bronchus to evaluate its patency and length. (**B**) The fiberscope is pulled back. (**C**) The tracheal cuff is deflated and the fiberscope and double-lumen tube are advanced together into the left main stem bronchus; the distal end of the tube is positioned about 5 mm above the orifice of the left upper lobe bronchus. (**D**) The bronchial and tracheal cuffs of the double-lumen tube are inflated using a minimal leak technique. (Ovassapian A, 1994: Conduct of anesthesia. In Shields TW [ed]: General Thoracic Surgery, ed. 4, p. 311. Baltimore, Williams & Wilkins)

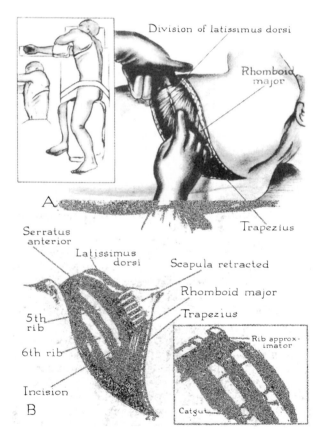

FIGURE 38-6. Posterolateral thoracotomy incision. (**A**) Skin incision extends from just below the nipple posteriorly to 1 inch below the tip of the scapula and then upward between the scapula and spine; when latissimus dorsi and serratus anterior muscles are divided, shoulder girdle glides upward and scapula retracts to expose rib cage. (**B**) Closure of the incision is begun by approximating ribs with rib approximator and securing them with heavy sutures. (Crawford FA Jr, Kratz JM, 1995: Thoracic incisions. In Sabiston DC Jr, Spencer FC [eds]: Surgery of the Chest, ed. 6, p. 214. Philadelphia, WB Saunders)

and latissimus dorsi muscles are retracted without being surgically divided when the chest wall is opened. A retractor is used to displace the serratus muscle anteriorly and the latissimus posteriorly to expose the underlying ribs (Boyd & Glassman, 1998). A muscle-sparing thoracotomy incision appears to decrease pain and reduce shoulder girdle disability in the early postoperative period (Hazelrigg et al., 1991). Splinting and hypoventilation secondary to pain may be less pronounced than after a standard thoracotomy incision in which major chest wall muscles are divided.

Initially, the pleural space is entered and, using blunt or sharp dissection, the lung is freed from the chest wall and diaphragm in areas where it is tethered by adhesions. The final determination of resectability is made after entry into the chest cavity when the lung and pleural space are inspected carefully by the surgeon. Despite preoperative clinical staging, factors that preclude curative resection occasionally are identified after opening the thorax, such as (1) undetected pleural seeding (metastasis); (2) extensive, fixed mediastinal lymph node involvement; (3) nonresectable direct extension of the tumor beyond the lung; or (4) inability to control safely the blood supply to the lung (Shields, 1993).

If a histologic diagnosis was not established before the operation, a biopsy specimen may be obtained for frozen-section examination before the pulmonary resection is performed. Guided by digital palpation of the lung, the surgeon directs a biopsy needle device through the lung parenchyma into the lesion. Four or five samples of tissue are plucked from different sites within the lesion. Tissue specimens also may be tested for tuberculosis or other bacterial or fungal infection if an infectious process is suspected.

For performance of a lobectomy, the fissure separating the involved lobe from the other lobe or lobes is divided carefully. All pulmonary artery and vein branches supplying the lobe to be resected are identified, ligated, and divided. The lobar bronchus is then isolated, stapled, and divided distal to the staple line, separating the lobe

The segment is then bluntly dissected from surrounding segments of the lobe. Vascular and small airway connections to other segments are clamped, ligated, and divided, and the segment is removed. A wedge resection is performed by excising only the portion of lung containing the tumor and closing the remaining lung edge with staples or sutures (Fig. 38-8).

After lobectomy, segmentectomy, or wedge resection, two chest tubes are inserted into the pleural space through separate incisions. Pleural chest tubes are important to allow full reexpansion of the operative lung and to evacuate blood and air from the pleural space. Negative suction is applied to facilitate lung expansion. The apposition of parietal and visceral pleural surfaces that occurs when the lung is fully expanded enhances cessation of bleeding and air leakage from the operative lung.

After pneumonectomy, usually either no chest tube is placed or a chest tube is placed and clamped. At the conclusion of the operation, pressure in the operative hemithorax is adjusted by thoracentesis to maintain the mediastinum in a midline position. Avoidance of a chest tube after pneumonectomy lessens the risk of empyema (ie, infection of the pleural space). Infection is more likely after pneumonectomy because of the residual empty space after the lung has been removed from the hemithorax. This is in contrast to lesser pulmonary resection procedures in which the remaining ipsilateral lung almost always expands to fill the hemithorax.

Patients with N2 disease (mediastinal lymph node invasion) confirmed during surgical resection usually are

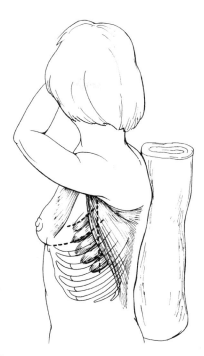

FIGURE 38-7. Muscle-sparing incisions. Location of axillary (*upper*), standard (*middle*), and vertical incisions. (Boyd AD, Glassman LR, 1998: Thoracic incisions. In Kaiser LR, Kron IL, Spray TL [eds]: Mastery of Cardiothoracic Surgery, p. 33. Philadelphia, Lippincott Williams & Wilkins)

from remaining lung. Removal of the lobe is completed by dividing any remaining tissue connections to the other lobe or lobes. The remaining bronchial stump is assessed carefully to ensure that it is airtight and hemostasis is achieved. A careful inspection of mediastinal lymph node stations is performed. Lymphatic spread may occur even with small tumors and affects both prognosis and the need for adjunctive therapy. Therefore, ipsilateral superior mediastinal and subcarinal lymphatic stations are sampled or a systematic mediastinal lymph node dissection is performed (Shields, 1997).

A pneumonectomy is performed by severing the lung from its vascular (pulmonary artery and veins) attachments and airway (bronchus). After exposing the hilar structures, the pulmonary artery and veins are identified, ligated, and divided. The mainstem bronchus is clamped, divided, and closed with sutures or a stapling device. The lung is removed from the hemithorax. The remaining bronchial segment is covered with adjacent tissue (eg, pleura, pericardial fat, or pericardium) to help prevent disruption of the closure (Shields, 1994c). Care is taken to avoid leaving a bronchial segment that is either devascularized or excessively long because both factors predispose to postpneumonectomy empyema (ie, infection of the hemithorax) (Deschamps et al., 1999). As during lobectomy, mediastinal lymph nodes are inspected and sampled. Hemostasis is achieved and the chest wall is closed.

A segmentectomy is performed by identifying, ligating, and dividing the segmental arteries, veins, and bronchus.

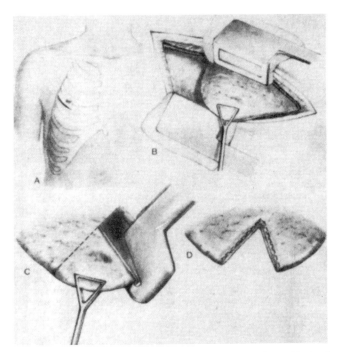

FIGURE 38-8. Wedge resection of peripheral lung parenchyma. Mechanical stapling device is used to excise wedge and close lung edges. (Hood RM, 1984: Stapling techniques involving lung parenchyma. Surg Clin North Am 3:474)

treated adjunctively with radiation therapy or chemotherapy. Radiation therapy also may be used in postoperative patients who have local recurrence after pulmonary resection.

Results

The risk of operative death is 6% to 7% after pneumonectomy and 1% to 2% after lobectomy or lesser resection (Kaiser, 1998b). Postoperative complications are infrequent. Most common are respiratory complications (eg, atelectasis, pneumonia, or respiratory failure). Other complications of pulmonary resection include cardiac arrhythmias, prolonged air leak, bronchopleural fistula, persistent air space, and empyema (Piccione & Faber, 1991). These complications are discussed in detail in Chapter 43, Complications of Thoracic Operations.

Despite curative resection, many patients die of recurrent carcinoma. Even in patients with stage I disease, who are presumed to have no lymph node or distant metastasis, local recurrence or distant disease sometimes occurs (Deschamps et al., 1990). Most deaths occur within the first 12 to 24 months after resection; patients rarely die of the original disease more than 5 years after operation (Shields, 1994d). Postoperative adjuvant therapy (irradiation or chemotherapy) has not been demonstrated to increase the number of long-term survivors; although it may control local recurrence, almost all patients who die of their disease do so with the presence of distant metastasis (D'Amico & Sabiston, 1997; Shields, 1993). In addition, patients with lung cancer have an increased risk for development of a second primary lung cancer.

Long-term results of surgical treatment vary primarily according to the TNM stage of the patient's disease at the time of operation. Cure of disease is most likely in patients with stage I lung cancer; that is, those with smaller, more peripheral tumors without nodal involvement or distant metastases (T1 N0 M0 or T2 N0 M0). Approximately 70% of patients with stage I tumors survive 5 years after surgical resection (Flehinger et al., 1992). The most favorable survival rates (80% to 85%) are in patients with stage IA tumors (T1 N0 M0) (D'Amico & Sabiston, 1997). Patients with stage IB tumors (T2 N0 M0) have a 5-year survival rate that is 10% or more below that of patients with stage IA tumors (Maddaus & Ginsberg, 1995). Stage IIA (T1 N1 M0) and stage IIB (T2 N1 M0) tumors, which are larger and more invasive, are associated with a 40% to 50% 5-year survival rate after surgical resection (Burt et al., 1996). Cure with surgical resection occurs in only a small percentage of patients with stage IIIA lung tumors. In those patients who do undergo surgical treatment, long-term survival is variable, depending on the presence and location of lymph node metastasis and the size of the tumor. The overall 5-year survival rate after surgical resection in patients with stage IIIA tumors and mediastinal lymph node involvement (N2 disease) is 27% (Suzuki et al., 1999).

▶ Other Pulmonary Diseases

Metastatic Lung Tumors

Pulmonary resection has become a widely accepted therapy for resection of *pulmonary metastasis* from a primary tumor located elsewhere in the body. Most pulmonary metastases do not cause symptoms but rather are detected incidentally on chest radiographic studies (Rusch, 1995). Surgical removal of metastatic lesions is associated with prolonged survival in patients with selected histologic types of tumors. Other factors taken into consideration when selecting candidates for resection of metastatic pulmonary disease include (1) presence of any other metastatic lesions, (2) tumor doubling time, (3) availability of adjuvant therapy (ie, irradiation or chemotherapy), and (4) the disease-free interval. However, neither the presence of more than one lesion nor a short disease-free interval necessarily precludes resection of pulmonary metastases, provided the primary tumor has been treated adequately and the pulmonary lesions can be resected completely while preserving adequate pulmonary function (Martini & McCormack, 1998).

Unilateral metastatic lesions are approached using a thoracotomy incision. If lesions are present in both lungs, a median sternotomy or clamshell thoracotomy may be used to allow entry into both pleural spaces and bilateral wedge resections of the lesions. Although metastatic lesions can be resected using video-assisted thoracoscopy, a disadvantage of this approach is that lesions not apparent on a preoperative CT scan may not be detected at the time of operation. Because long-term survival appears to be directly related to the resection of all gross disease, it is imperative that the surgeon systematically inspect and palpate the lungs to ensure that all tumor is identified and removed (Rusch, 1995). Thus, although video-assisted thoracoscopy may be useful for diagnosis and staging of pulmonary metastases, thoracotomy is recommended for therapeutic resection of metastatic lesions.

Benign Lung Disease

Benign lung tumors, such as hamartoma or fibroma, frequently are removed surgically because of an inability to determine benignity definitively without thoracotomy and removal of the tumor for histologic evaluation. Less commonly, a benign tumor is removed because it produces pneumonia or atelectasis secondary to bronchial compression.

Pulmonary resection also is performed occasionally for *benign pulmonary diseases,* such as bronchiectasis, hemoptysis, radiation necrosis, or lung abscess. Bronchiectasis is a disease characterized by localized or diffuse dilatation and destruction of bronchi. Surgical removal of bronchiectatic lung segments may become necessary in patients with complications of the condition, such as recurrent pneumonia, hemoptysis, or copious sputum production. Pulmonary resection also may be necessary to remove lung tissue destroyed by infection (eg, lung abscess, aspergillosis, tuberculosis, or empyema) or radiation necrosis. Pneumonectomy for infectious disease (eg, tuberculosis, aspergillosis, or extensive lung abscesses) is performed infrequently in North America and is associated with higher morbidity and mortality than pneumonectomy performed for malignancy (Klemperer & Ginsberg, 1999).

Rarely, pulmonary resection is performed for treatment of a congenital abnormality, such as pulmonary sequestration or a pulmonary arteriovenous malformation. *Pulmonary sequestration* is an abnormality in which a segment or lobe has no communication with the normal tracheobronchial tree and the arterial blood supply is from a systemic vessel (Reynolds, 1994). The anomaly can cause recurrent pulmonary infection or hemoptysis. Definitive treatment of pulmonary sequestration is removal of the involved segment or lobe with its anomalous blood supply. *Pulmonary arteriovenous malformation* describes an anomalous communication between a pulmonary artery and vein that can lead to hemoptysis, hemothorax, or systemic embolism. Surgical excision of the fistula and surrounding tissue is recommended.

Severe Chronic Obstructive Pulmonary Disease

Emphysema, along with other *chronic obstructive lung diseases,* affects 13.5 million people in the United States and is the fastest-growing cause of morbidity and mortality (Morse, 1998). The two primary surgical therapies for end-stage emphysema are lung volume reduction surgery and lung transplantation. *Lung volume reduction* is a relatively new surgical procedure for the treatment of debilitating emphysema. Also called *bilateral pneumectomy,* the purpose of lung volume reduction is to relieve thoracic distention and improve respiratory mechanics in severely affected patients by excising 20% to 30% of the volume of each lung (Cooper et al., 1995). The operation consists of removing lung tissue that has been identified with preoperative high-resolution CT scanning or quantitative lung perfusion scanning as most diseased (O'Brien & Criner, 1998). Using a median sternotomy incision, targeted lung tissue is excised using a stapling device fitted with strips of bovine pericardium to buttress staple lines and eliminate air leakage through the staple holes (Cooper et al., 1995).

Although the physiologic improvements after lung volume reduction are significantly less than those seen after lung transplantation, volume reduction has the potential to provide functional improvement to a larger number of patients because of wider availability (O'Brien & Criner, 1998). Also, unlike lung transplantation, it does not necessitate chronic immunosuppression and does not expose the patient to bronchiolitis obliterans, the predominant long-term complication of lung transplantation. Lung transplantation is discussed in Chapter 31, Heart, Lung, and Heart-Lung Transplantation. Surgical treatment of pneumothorax secondary to emphysema is discussed in Chapter 40, Surgery of the Pleura, Trachea, Chest Wall, and Mediastinum.

REFERENCES

Boyd AD, Glassman LR, 1998: Thoracic incisions. In Kaiser LR, Kron IL, Spray TL (eds): Mastery of Cardiothoracic Surgery. Philadelphia, Lippincott Williams & Wilkins

Burt M, Martini N, Ginsberg RJ, 1996: Surgical treatment of lung carcinoma. In Baue AE, Geha AS, Hammond GL, et al. (eds): Glenn's Thoracic and Cardiovascular Surgery, ed. 6. Stamford, CT, Appleton & Lange

Carney DN, 1998: New agents in the management of advanced non-small cell lung cancer. Semin Oncol 25:83

Cooper JD, Trulock EP, Triantafillou AN, et al., 1995: Bilateral pneumectomy (volume reduction) for chronic obstructive pulmonary disease. J Thorac Cardiovasc Surg 109:106

Crawford FA Jr, Kratz JM, 1995: Thoracic incisions. In Sabiston DC Jr, Spencer FC (eds): Surgery of the Chest, ed. 6. Philadelphia, WB Saunders

D'Amico TA, Sabiston DC Jr, 1995: Carcinoma of the lung. In Sabiston DC Jr, Spencer FC (eds): Surgery of the Chest, ed. 6. Philadelphia, WB Saunders

D'Amico TA, Sabiston DC Jr, 1997: Carcinoma of the lung. In Sabiston DC Jr, Spencer FC (eds): Textbook of Surgery: The Biological Basis of Modern Surgical Practice, ed. 15. Philadelphia, WB Saunders

Deschamps C, Pairolero PC, Allen MS, et al., 1999: Early complications: Bronchopleural fistula and empyema. Chest Surg Clin North Am 9:587

Deschamps C, Pairolero PC, Trastek VF, Payne WS, 1990: Multiple primary lung cancers. J Thorac Cardiovasc Surg 99:769

Downey RJ, Martini N, Rusch VW, et al., 1999: Extent of chest wall invasion and survival in patients with lung cancer. Ann Thorac Surg 68:188

Flehinger BJ, Kimmel M, Melamed MR, 1992: The effect of surgical treatment on survival from early lung cancer. Chest 101:1013

Gregoire J, Deslauriers J, Guojin L, Rouleau J, 1993: Indications, risks, and results of completion pneumonectomy. J Thorac Cardiovasc Surg 105:918

Hazelrigg SR, Landreneau RJ, Boley TM, et al., 1991: The effect of muscle-sparing versus standard posterolateral thoracotomy on pulmonary function, muscle strength, and postoperative pain. J Thorac Cardiovasc Surg 101:394

Kaiser LR, 1998a: Pneumonectomy. In Kaiser LR, Kron IL, Spray TL (eds): Mastery of Cardiothoracic Surgery. Philadelphia, Lippincott Williams & Wilkins

Kaiser LR, 1998b: Right-sided pulmonary resections. In Kaiser LR, Kron IL, Spray TL (eds): Mastery of Cardiothoracic Surgery. Philadelphia, Lippincott Williams & Wilkins

Klemperer J, Ginsberg RJ, 1999: Morbidity and mortality after pneumonectomy. Chest Surg Clin North Am 9:515

Lassen U, Hansen HH, 1999: Surgery in limited stage small cell lung cancer. Cancer Treat Rev 25:67

Lowe JE, Tedder M, Sabiston DC Jr, 1995: Bronchoplastic techniques in the surgical management of benign and malignant pulmonary lesions. In Sabiston DC Jr, Spencer FC (eds): Surgery of the Chest, ed. 6. Philadelphia, WB Saunders

Maddaus M, Ginsberg RJ, 1995: Cancer/diagnosis and staging. In Pearson FG, Deslauriers J, Ginsberg RJ, et al. (eds): Thoracic Surgery. New York, Churchill Livingstone

Martini N, Burt ME, Bains MS, et al., 1992: Survival after resection of stage II non-small cell lung cancer. Ann Thorac Surg 54:460

Martini N, McCormack PM, 1998: Evolution of the surgical

management of pulmonary metastases. Chest Surg Clin North Am 8:13

Mentzer SJ, Reilly JJ, Sugarbaker DJ, 1993a: Surgical resection in the management of small-cell carcinoma of the lung. Chest 103:349S

Mentzer SJ, Myers DW, Sugarbaker DJ, 1993b: Sleeve lobectomy, segmentectomy, and thoracoscopy in the management of carcinoma of the lung. Chest 103:415S

Morse CJ, 1998: Volume lung reduction surgery: A review. Critical Care Nursing Quarterly 21:1

Mountain CF, 1986: A new international staging system for lung cancer. Chest 89:2255

Mountain CF, 1997: Revisions in the international system for staging lung cancer. Chest 111:1710

Nakanishi R, Osaki T, Nakanishi K, et al., 1997: Treatment strategy for patients with surgically discovered N2 stage IIIA non-small cell lung cancer. Ann Thorac Surg 64:332

O'Brien GM, Criner GJ, 1998: Surgery for severe COPD: Lung volume reduction and transplantation. Postgrad Med 103:179

Piccione W Jr, Faber LP, 1991: Management of complications related to pulmonary resection. In Waldhausen JA, Orringer MB (eds): Complications in Cardiothoracic Surgery. St. Louis, Mosby–Year Book

Regnard JF, Icard P, Magdeleinat P, et al., 1999: Completion pneumonectomy: Experience in eighty patients. J Thorac Cardiovasc Surg 117:1095

Reilly JJ Jr, Mentzer SJ, Sugarbaker DJ, 1993: Preoperative assessment of patients undergoing pulmonary resection. Chest 103:342S

Reves, JG, Greeley WJ, Grichnik K, et al., 1995: Anesthesia and supportive care for cardiothoracic surgery. In Sabiston DC Jr, Spencer FC (eds): Surgery of the Chest, ed. 6. Philadelphia, WB Saunders

Reynolds M, 1994: Congenital lesions of the lung. In Shields TW (ed): General Thoracic Surgery, ed. 4. Baltimore, Williams & Wilkins

Rusch VW, 1995: Pulmonary metastectomy: Current indications. Chest 107:322S

Shields TW, 1993: Surgical therapy for carcinoma of the lung. Clin Chest Med 14:121

Shields TW, 1994a: Lung cancer: Etiology, carcinogenesis, molecular biology, and pathology. In Shields TW (ed): General Thoracic Surgery, ed. 4. Baltimore, Williams & Wilkins

Shields TW, 1994b: Surgical anatomy of the lungs. In Shields TW (ed): General Thoracic Surgery, ed. 4. Baltimore, Williams & Wilkins

Shields TW, 1994c: General features and complications of pulmonary resections. In Shields TW (ed): General Thoracic Surgery, ed. 4. Baltimore, Williams & Wilkins

Shields TW, 1994d: Surgical treatment of non-small cell bronchial carcinoma. In Shields TW (ed): General Thoracic Surgery, ed. 4. Baltimore, Williams & Wilkins

Shields TW, 1996: Diagnosis and staging of lung cancer. In Baue AE, Geha AS, Hammond GL, et al. (eds): Glenn's Thoracic and Cardiovascular Surgery, ed. 6. Stamford, CT, Appleton & Lange

Shields TW, 1997: Lung cancer and the solitary pulmonary nodule. In Khan MG, Lynch JP (eds): Pulmonary Disease Diagnosis and Therapy: A Practical Approach. Baltimore, Williams & Wilkins

Somers J, Faber LP, 1996: Limited pulmonary resection. In Baue AE, Geha AS, Hammond GL, et al. (eds): Glenn's Thoracic and Cardiovascular Surgery, ed. 6. Stamford, CT, Appleton & Lange

Suen HC, Meyers BF, Guthrie T, et al., 1999: Favorable results after sleeve lobectomy or bronchoplasty for bronchial malignancies. Ann Thorac Surg 67:1557

Suzuki K, Nagai K, Yoshida J, et al., 1999: The prognosis of surgically resected N2 non-small cell lung cancer: The importance of clinical N status. J Thorac Cardiovasc Surg 118:145

Tedder M, Lowe JE, 1992: Complications following bronchoplastic procedures. In Wolfe WG (ed): Complications in Thoracic Surgery. St. Louis, Mosby–Year Book

Urschel HC, 1993: New approaches to Pancoast and chest wall tumors. Chest 103:360S

Van Schil PE, de la Riviere AB, Knaepen PJ, et al., 1991: TNM staging and long-term follow-up after sleeve resection for bronchogenic tumors. Ann Thorac Surg 52:1096

Warren WH, 1998: Pulmonary resections: Limited resections and segmentectomy. In Kaiser LR, Kron IL, Spray TL (eds): Mastery of Cardiothoracic Surgery. Philadelphia, Lippincott Williams & Wilkins

Surgical Treatment of Esophageal Diseases

A variety of diseases can affect the esophagus and impair normal physiologic function. Those that may require surgical intervention are the focus of this chapter and include gastroesophageal reflux, motility disorders, esophageal diverticula, cancer of the esophagus, and esophageal perforation.

► Gastroesophageal Reflux

Gastroesophageal reflux disease (GERD) is the most common functional abnormality of the esophagus requiring surgical intervention. Heartburn, the predominant symptom of GERD, affects as many as 10% of Americans every day and 44% at least once a month (Scott & Gelhot, 1999). Although some degree of gastroesophageal reflux is considered physiologic, pathologic reflux is said to exist when symptoms or esophageal injury develop because of an increase in frequency or amount of reflux or because of delayed clearing of refluxed material. The precise mechanism for pathologic reflux is unknown. Symptomatic GERD commonly is associated with the presence of a hiatal hernia. However, hiatal hernias often are asymptomatic and, conversely, pathologic gastroesophageal reflux may be present in the absence of a demonstrable hiatal hernia (Cooper, 1997).

Continued reflux of gastric contents eventually produces esophageal tissue ulceration and can lead to bleeding, perforation, or stricture formation. The esophagitis tends to become a relapsing, chronic condition; it recurs in 50% to 80% of patients within 6 to 12 months of discontinuation of pharmacologic therapy for GERD (Scott & Gelhot, 1999). In addition, GERD can cause destruction of the normal squamous cell lining of the lower esophageal sphincter (LES), which is then replaced with columnar epithelium. This condition, termed *Barrett's esophagus,* predisposes the patient to development of adenocarcinoma of the distal esophagus. Other abnormalities of the distal esophagus also have been linked to Barrett's esophagus, including Barrett's stricture and Barrett's ulcer (Pera et al., 1992).

The diagnosis of GERD often can be based on the classic presentation of symptoms. Ambulatory pH monitoring is considered the diagnostic gold standard for patients with GERD, and endoscopy is useful for diagnosing the complications of GERD, such as Barrett's esophagus, esophagitis, and stricture (Scott & Gelhot, 1999). Pharmacologic therapy to treat GERD includes cytoprotective agents (eg, sucralfate) to improve mucosal resistance, antacids to neutralize gastric contents, acid suppressors (eg, histamine H_2-receptor antagonists) to minimize secretions, and prokinetic agents (eg, cisapride) to enhance esophageal clearance, accelerate gastric emptying, and minimize gastroduodenal reflux (Naunheim & Baue, 1996). Dietary modifications and elevating the head of the bed also may help alleviate symptoms. Surgical treatment is indicated in patients who have intractable symptoms despite medical therapy or in those who have complications of reflux, such as ulcerative esophagitis or stricture.

Antireflux operations comprise a number of surgical procedures that have been developed and modified over the years. They may be performed as primary treatment for GERD or concomitantly with surgical procedures to correct hiatal hernia or with procedures that may be complicated by gastroesophageal reflux (eg, esophagomyotomy). The modern antireflux repairs all share the anatomic goal of restoring a competent physiologic valve mechanism in the lower esophagus and the functional goal of relieving symptoms while preserving the patient's ability to eat and drink normally and belch and vomit when necessary (Cox & Sundt, 1997). None of the antireflux operations provides optimal results for all presentations of hiatal hernia and gastroesophageal reflux, and surgical results are even less predictable in patients who require reoperation for a failed prior repair (Pearson, 1997).

Commonly performed antireflux procedures include the Nissen fundoplication, the Belsey Mark IV procedure, and the Hill repair. All are designed to restore the factors that normally are important in controlling reflux; that is, an intra-abdominal segment of distal esophagus and the distal esophagus at a narrow diameter as it enters the gastric pouch (Skinner, 1994). Restoration of distal esophagus to the abdominal compartment reduces reflux of gastric contents upward into the esophagus because pressure in the abdominal compartment is positive and that in the thorax is negative. Maintaining a narrowed diameter of distal esophagus is accomplished by plication, or folding stomach tissue around a portion or all of the circumference of the distal esophagus. Factors that influence the choice of antireflux procedure include (1) whether an endoscopic approach or thoracic or abdominal incision is preferable, (2) whether the patient has had a prior antireflux procedure, (3) whether concomitant esophageal resection or esophagomyotomy is anticipated, and (4) the patient's body habitus (Skinner, 1995).

A *Nissen fundoplication* performed using a laparoscopic approach is likely to be chosen for patients with uncomplicated GERD (Rice & Gagner, 1997). Laparoscopic techniques have provided a significant advancement in the surgical treatment of GERD. Candidates best suited for a laparoscopic approach are those who are thin, who have not had prior abdominal surgery, and who do not have a large hiatal hernia (Allen, 1997). A Nissen fundoplication also can be performed through an abdominal incision for patients who are not candidates for a laparoscopic approach. After mobilizing the distal esophagus and proximal stomach, the fundus of the stomach is wrapped around the distal esophagus (Fig. 39-1).

A *Belsey Mark IV operation* is performed using a left lateral thoracotomy incision. Because a transthoracic approach provides exposure of the entire intrathoracic esophagus, it may be preferable for patients with a previous failed repair, for patients in whom inflammation and esophageal shortening are anticipated, in obese patients in whom transabdominal exposure is difficult, and when there is an associated primary motor disorder of the esophagus (Block & Cooper, 1997). In a Belsey Mark IV procedure, the gastric fundus is wrapped around approximately three fourths the circumference of the distal esophagus and the wrapped segment is placed beneath the diaphragm. The *Hill repair* consists of securing the posterior aspect of the gastroesophageal junction within the abdominal compartment (gastropexy) and partially wrapping the stomach around the distal esophagus. It is performed using a laparoscopic approach for primary surgical treatment of GERD or through an abdominal incision for reoperative repairs. The hallmark of the Hill repair is the secure fixation of the gastroesophageal junction to its normal intra-abdominal location (Hill et al., 1997).

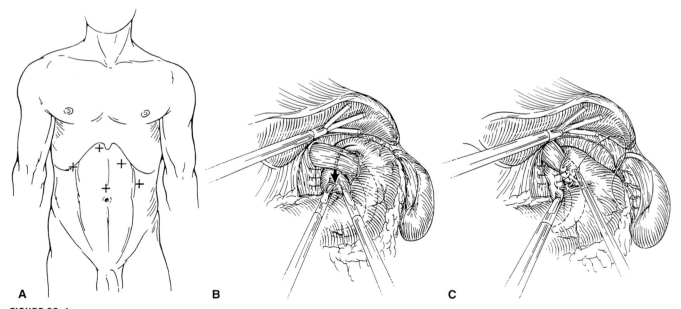

FIGURE 39-1. Laparoscopic Nissen fundoplication. (**A**) Sites for access port placement for laparoscopic fundoplication. (**B**) Using thoracoscopic instruments, the esophagus is mobilized and sutures are placed in the crus (diaphragmatic attachments) to narrow the hiatal opening to a normal caliber. The stomach is then brought posteriorly around the distal esophagus. (**C**) The fundoplication is completed by placing and tying interrupted sutures that incorporate both sides of the fundus and the esophagus. (Ferguson MK, 1996: Atlas of esophageal surgery. In Bell RH Jr, Rikkers LF, Mulholland MW [eds]: Digestive Tract Surgery: A Text and Atlas, p. 107. Philadelphia, Lippincott-Raven)

Between 85% and 90% of patients with normal esophageal motility and without esophageal stricture experience good or excellent results from an antireflux operation (Ferguson, 1998). Regardless of the specific type of antireflux procedure, prolonged postoperative follow-up for at least 5 years is essential to evaluate success in restoring the patient's ability to eat without difficulty and vomit when necessary and to ensure the sustained absence of reflux symptoms (Block & Cooper, 1997). Complications of the various antireflux procedures include (1) esophageal or gastric perforation, (2) paraesophageal herniation, (3) splenic injury, (4) disruption of the gastric wrap, (5) dysphagia, and (6) recurrent gastroesophageal reflux. "Gas-bloat" syndrome, a symptom complex characterized by bloating, abdominal pain, and an inability to belch and vomit, is a complication that appears to be unique to total fundoplication (Nissen procedure) (Ferguson, 1998).

▶ Motility Disorders

Motility disorders are pathologic abnormalities of the esophagus characterized by abnormalities of peristalsis, sphincter dysfunction, or a combination of the two. They may affect the upper esophageal sphincter, the body of the esophagus, or the LES.

Achalasia

The motility disorder most commonly treated with surgical therapy is *achalasia*, a degenerative neural abnormality that primarily involves the smooth muscle of the body of the esophagus. Achalasia is characterized by absent peristalsis in the body of the esophagus, normal or increased resting pressures in the LES, and incomplete or absent relaxation of the LES in response to swallowing (Duranceau, 1995). The neurologic defect responsible for its development remains poorly understood (Ferguson, 1991). Achalasia almost always causes dysphagia and also may be associated with regurgitation of solid foods, epigastric discomfort, and weight loss. Pulmonary complications of aspiration, including pneumonitis, asthma-like syndrome, and pulmonary abscesses, occur in later stages of the disease (Duranceau, 1995). Achalasia also is considered a risk factor for development of squamous cell carcinoma of the esophagus; it develops in an estimated 5% of people with achalasia at an average of 20 years after diagnosis of the motility disorder (Koshy & Nostrant, 1997).

Nonsurgical therapy consists of either forceful dilatation of the esophageal lumen at the level of the LES using a pneumatic dilator or the direct injection during endoscopy of the nerve toxin botulinum toxin to lessen LES obstruction. Alternatively, achalasia may be treated with a surgical procedure designed to improve the transport of a swallowed bolus through the esophagus (Stein et al., 1992a). Although some surgeons recommend surgical treatment as initial therapy for patients with symptomatic achalasia, more commonly it is reserved for those in whom nonsurgical therapies are considered ill advised or have been unsuccessful.

Esophagomyotomy is the surgical procedure performed for treatment of achalasia. The operation consists of division of the muscular layer of the gastroesophageal junction to diminish LES pressure (Fig. 39-2). Esophagomyotomy is performed most commonly through a thoracotomy incision or using a video-assisted thoracoscopic approach. A nasogastric tube is passed to decompress the stomach and single-lung ventilation (ie, sustained deflation of the ipsilateral lung) is performed to improve exposure. The esophagus is mobilized carefully, avoiding damage to the vagus nerve that passes along the esophageal wall.

A longitudinal incision is made in the distal esophagus, dividing the circular muscle layer to the level of the mucosa. Opinion varies among surgeons concerning the appropriate proximal and distal extent of the incision. In the most common operative technique, the *Heller myotomy*, the incision begins proximally a short distance above the gastroesophageal junction and extends just onto the stomach with an overall incision length of approximately 7 cm. Controversy also exists over the need to perform a concomitant antireflux procedure to prevent postoperative gastroesophageal reflux that may result from surgical alteration of LES anatomy (Ferguson, 1991). Some surgeons recommend extending the esophageal myotomy incision onto the stomach to minimize the likelihood of persistent LES obstruction, and a fundoplication is performed to minimize gastroesophageal reflux (Heitmiller, 1998). The fundoplication must be incomplete (eg, Belsey Mark IV repair). Owing to the lack of esophageal peristalsis in patients with achalasia, a complete circumferential wrap would be overly competent, resulting in postoperative dysphagia.

If therapy for achalasia is inadequate or complicated by acid reflux, the disease progresses to end-stage achalasia, characterized by progressive dilatation and eventual marked tortuosity of the esophagus (Banbury et al., 1999). Most patients with end-stage achalasia have disabling dysphagia. The only treatment for patients with such advanced disease is resection of the dilated esophagus with colon interposition or gastric reconstruction.

Diffuse Esophageal Spasm

Another motility disorder, *diffuse esophageal spasm,* also may be treated with esophagomyotomy. In this rare disorder, LES relaxation occurs appropriately, but nonperistaltic, sustained repetitive contractions occur in the body of the esophagus, producing chest pain, dysphagia, and, less commonly, regurgitation. Pharmacologic treatment is the mainstay of therapy for diffuse esophageal spasm and successfully relieves symptoms in most patients. Because tension and anxiety may play a role in pathogenesis of this disorder, treatment of these underlying factors also may decrease symptoms (Duranceau, 1996). Surgical treatment is considered only for patients with severe symptoms not relieved with medical therapy.

Esophagomyotomy for diffuse esophageal spasm is

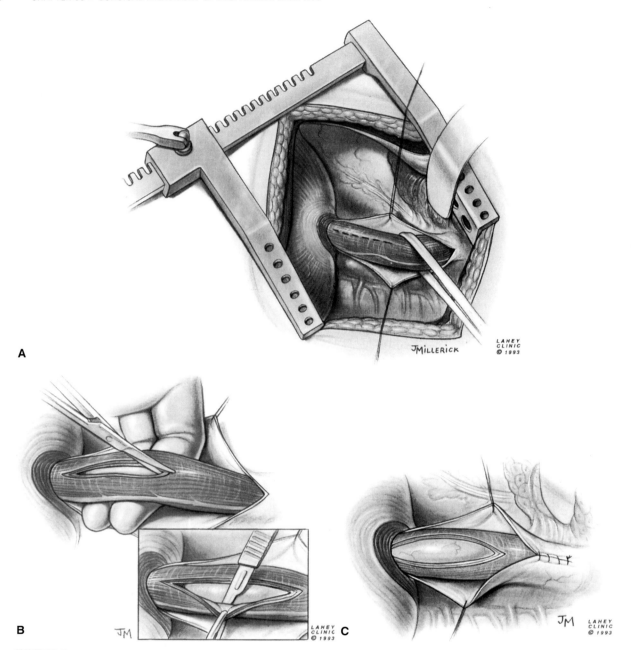

FIGURE 39-2. Esophagomyotomy. (**A**) Transthoracic exposure of distal esophagus through the seventh interspace or the bed of the eighth rib; mediastinal pleura has been opened and the esophagus is encircled. Proposed site of myotomy is indicated by dashed line. (**B**) After incising the esophageal muscle with a scalpel (not shown), the myotomy is extended cephalad and the muscle is dissected off of the esophageal submucosa. (**C**) The myotomy has been completed and the gastroesophageal junction has been returned to its normal subdiaphragmatic position. (Streitz JM Jr, 1994: Modified Heller esophagomyotomy. In Shields TW [ed]: General Thoracic Surgery, ed. 4, pp. 1439–1441. Baltimore, Williams & Wilkins)

similar to that for achalasia except that the incision is extended proximally to the apex of the intrathoracic esophagus (Wilkins, 1994). Because myotomy of the distal esophageal body markedly reduces contraction amplitude, the incision is extended distally across the gastroesophageal junction to reduce resistance to emptying of the surgically altered esophagus (Stein et al., 1992a). An antireflux procedure may be necessary to prevent postoperative gastroesophageal reflux.

► Esophageal Diverticulum

An *esophageal diverticulum* is an epithelial-lined blind pouch leading from the main lumen of the esophagus (Trastek, 1994). It is formed by localized herniation of esophageal mucosa through the outer muscular layer. Esophageal diverticula are categorized according to location and etiology as (1) pharyngoesophageal pulsion, (2) epiphrenic pulsion, or (3) parabronchial traction diverticula. Pulsion diverticula develop as a result of forces in the esophageal mucosa acting against an area of resistance, as occurs with esophageal motility disorders. Traction diverticula are caused by forces exerted from outside the esophagus, such as inflammatory disease in the mediastinal lymph nodes.

Most common is a pharyngoesophageal pulsion, or Zenker's diverticulum, which extends from the main lumen of the esophagus at or just below the cricopharyngeus muscle (primary component of the upper esophageal sphincter). The exact etiology of Zenker's diverticulum remains unclear, but it is believed to be the consequence of pharyngo-cricopharyngeal incoordination. Once the diverticulum forms, it enlarges and descends dependently owing to constant distention with ingested food (Trastek, 1994). Progressive symptoms of dysphagia, foul breath, noisy swallowing, and regurgitation are typical.

For small Zenker's diverticula, *cricopharyngeal esophagomyotomy* usually is recommended to prevent continued filling of the diverticulum with ingested material. Cricopharyngeal esophagomyotomy is performed through an incision in the neck. The pharynx and cervical esophagus are exposed by retracting the sternocleidomastoid muscle and carotid sheath laterally and the trachea and larynx medially (Stein et al., 1992b). A vertical, partial-thickness incision is made in the cricopharyngeus muscle, dividing the muscle fibers down to the mucosal layer of the esophageal wall. Typically, the incision begins at the neck of the diverticulum and extends distally onto the esophagus. As with any esophagomyotomy, complete division and lateral dissection of the muscular layer is performed so that the mucosa bulges diffusely through the divided muscle layer.

For larger diverticula, either pharyngoesophageal diverticulopexy or diverticulectomy may be performed. *Diverticulopexy* consists of suturing the diverticulum in an inverted position to prevent its distention with food and allow free drainage of its contents into the esophagus. The procedure uses the same surgical exposure as for cricopharyngeal esophagomyotomy. If a diverticulum is so large that it would be redundant if suspended or if its walls are thickened, diverticulectomy is performed instead (Stein et al., 1992b). A *diverticulectomy* consists of amputating the diverticulum from the esophagus (Fig. 39-3). Esophagomyotomy is performed concomitantly.

Less common than Zenker's diverticulum is an epiphrenic pulsion diverticulum (ie, a herniation of esophageal mucosa through muscular fibers just above the level of the diaphragm). Surgical therapy (diverticulectomy) sometimes is necessary for an epiphrenic diverticulum if it is associated with progressive symptoms or enlargement. The diverticulum is exposed through a thoracotomy incision and amputated from the esophagus. An extended esophagomyotomy also is performed. This type of diverticulum frequently is associated with a sliding hiatal hernia, which is repaired along with performance of an antireflux procedure (Trastek, 1994).

The third type of esophageal diverticulum, parabronchial traction diverticulum, may develop from in-

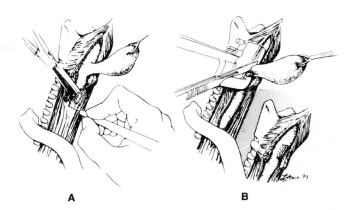

A   **B**

FIGURE 39-3. Cervical esophagomyotomy and concomitant resection of Zenker's diverticulum. (**A**) After mobilization of the diverticulum, the esophagomyotomy is performed. (**B**) The base of the diverticulum is then stapled and amputated. (Orringer MB, 1980: Extended cervical esophagomyotomy for cricopharyngeal dysfunction. J Thorac Cardiovasc Surg 80:672)

flammation and scarring of adjacent tracheobronchial lymph nodes due to granulomatous diseases. Traction diverticula are rare in the Western world and almost always are of little or no clinical significance (Altorki, 1998). Treatment, when required, consists of surgical excision of the diverticulum and adjacent inflammatory mass (Trastek, 1994).

▶ Esophageal Cancer

Esophageal cancer is a relatively unusual disease in the United States but is common in other parts of the world. Malignant neoplasms may occur in the upper, middle, or lower esophagus or in the gastroesophageal junction. Most tumors of the upper or middle esophagus are squamous cell carcinoma, and those in the distal esophagus or gastroesophageal junction are usually adenocarcinoma. Esophageal cancer is more prevalent in men between 50 and 70 years of age and in African Americans. The etiology of esophageal cancer appears to be multifactorial and varies with geography and cell type. Barrett's esophagus is the primary risk factor for adenocarcinoma of the distal esophagus and gastroesophageal junction; smoking and heavy alcohol consumption are risk factors for squamous cell carcinoma of the esophagus.

The epidemiologic profile of esophageal cancer in North America and Europe has been changing during the past decade. Although squamous cell carcinoma remains uncommon, adenocarcinoma of the lower esophagus and gastroesophageal junction has become more common, particularly among white men (Casson, 1998; Altorki et al., 1996). The incidence of adenocarcinoma has risen faster than that of any other malignancy and has surpassed squamous cell carcinoma to become the most common esophageal malignancy (Nigro et al., 1999). In the mid-20th century, only 2% to 4% of esophageal cancers were adenocarcinoma; it now accounts for more than 50% of esophageal cancer (Cameron, 1998). The reason for this epidemiologic change is unknown.

Because the esophagus distends easily, symptoms of esophageal cancer (eg, dysphagia, weight loss, chest pain) occur late in the course of the disease. Consequently, the tumor may not be detected until extensive local, regional, or distant spread has occurred (Naunheim et al., 1992). Also, the esophagus differs from other gastrointestinal viscera in that it does not have a serosal covering but consists only of muscle and a mucosal lining. The lack of an outer serosal layer and the extensive submucosal lymphatic connections of the esophagus favor early metastatic spread. Tumor depth through the esophageal wall is a strong predictor of the probability of lymph node metastases and distant lymph node involvement (Nigro et al., 1999).

Esophageal carcinoma is a devastating illness that carries a dismal prognosis regardless of treatment modality. Therapy is influenced by the knowledge that in most patients, local tumor invasion or distant metastatic disease precludes cure (Orringer, 1997). Because no single or combination therapy has significantly improved long-term survival, treatment of esophageal cancer is somewhat controversial. Operative intervention is appropriate only in carefully selected patients. It can impose significant morbidity, but if successful, may alleviate the severe dysphagia that accompanies advanced disease, which ultimately can preclude even the swallowing of saliva.

The morbidity associated with surgical therapy in patients with esophageal cancer is related to several factors. First, an operation on the esophagus is a major surgical procedure, necessitating a thoracotomy, abdominal incision, or both. Second, patients frequently are nutritionally compromised at the time of operation because of the dysphagia produced by esophageal obstruction. Wound healing, specifically that of the esophageal anastomosis, may be impaired. Third, many patients with squamous cell esophageal tumors have abused alcohol or cigarettes, both of which are independent risk factors for development of the disease. Associated cardiovascular, pulmonary, or hepatic disease may be present.

Surgical therapy for cancer of the esophagus may be undertaken for one of several purposes, including (1) resection for cure, (2) relief of esophageal obstruction, or (3) diversion of esophageal contents.

Esophageal Resection

Esophageal resection for cancer historically has been associated with disappointing results; because of the tendency for early lymphatic and hematogenous metastasis, tumor resection may not significantly increase long-term survival. However, cure is sometimes achieved when esophageal resection is performed in the early stage of the disease. Chemotherapy, irradiation, or both may be used as adjuncts to surgical therapy. Preoperative adjuvant therapy may facilitate surgical resection by reducing tumor size and increasing the probability of technical success in removing all tumor cells, particularly with squamous cell tumors above the level of the carina

(DeMeester, 1997; Naunheim et al., 1992). Others favor surgical resection without preoperative adjuvant therapy.

Resection of an esophageal tumor is undertaken if there is no lymphatic or hematologic evidence of distant spread and the patient is medically able to withstand a major operation. The size and extent of the primary lesion and potential involvement of contiguous structures also influence the ability to perform operative resection. Bronchoscopy always is performed before surgery if the tumor is at or above the level of the tracheal carina to exclude involvement of an airway by the tumor (Casson, 1998). Because of the poor prognosis associated with tumors in the upper one third of the esophagus, surgical resection seldom is performed except in patients who demonstrate a favorable response to preoperative chemotherapy.

There is no single accepted approach to esophagectomy; the choice of operation for esophageal carcinoma depends on the site of the tumor, the general condition of the patient, and the experience and preference of the surgeon (Casson, 1998). Attempts to improve the rate of cure with surgical resection have focused on (1) subtotal esophagectomy (ie, removing almost all of the esophagus); (2) en bloc resection (ie, removing all tumor in a resected block of tissue, surrounded by normal tissue on all sides); and (3) more complete lymphadenectomy (lymph node removal) (Ribet et al., 1992).

Surgical resection of esophageal tumors consists of removal of the tumor plus an adequate margin of tumor-free tissue above and below the tumor. Nearly all of the esophagus usually is removed during resection because of the tendency for tumors to spread in both directions along the length of the esophagus. For tumors in the upper or middle third of the esophagus, only esophagus is resected; for tumors of the lower third or gastric cardia, a portion of stomach is resected in addition to esophagus (DeMeester, 1997). Depending on the operative technique, adjacent lymph nodes also may be removed.

Because the remaining proximal and distal esophageal segments provide insufficient length for direct reattachment without excessive tension on the anastomosis, a replacement conduit is necessary to bridge the defect. One of three visceral structures can be used to replace the resected segment of esophagus: (1) stomach, (2) colon, or (3) jejunum. Although the stomach is used most commonly, each replacement conduit is associated with particular advantages in specific clinical situations. The determination of which organ to use is based on the location and length of esophagus that must be replaced and the blood supply and freedom from disease of the replacement viscera.

The most accessible and widely used visceral structure for esophageal replacement is the stomach (Hiebert, 1996; Huang, 1994). Advantages of using stomach as the replacement viscera include (1) its rich blood supply and submucosal collateral circulation; (2) its thick, resilient muscular wall; and (3) the ability to mobilize the stomach to reach superiorly to any level of the chest or neck for esophageal substitution (Orringer, 1996).

Sometimes it is not possible to use the stomach to replace resected esophagus because it has been damaged from caustic burn, scar, ulceration, or previous operation (Hiebert, 1996).

Alternatively, a segment of colon or jejunum may be used as a conduit to replace resected esophagus. Colon or jejunum interposition requires three anastomoses, increasing the likelihood of anastomotic complications. Most surgeons reserve colon interposition for cases in which stomach cannot be used. Jejunum interposition is performed rarely; the primary indication for using jejunum is reconstruction of the cervical esophagus.

Esophagectomy With Esophagogastrostomy

An operation to remove esophagus and replace it with stomach is called *esophagectomy* (removal of a portion of the esophagus) *with esophagogastrostomy* (reattachment of the fundus of the stomach to the remaining proximal esophageal segment)(Fig. 39-4). If a portion of stomach is removed along with the lower esophagus, the procedure is termed an *esophagogastrectomy with esophagogastrostomy*. Esophagectomy with esophagogastrostomy may be performed by one of two approaches: a transhiatal approach or a transthoracic approach.

In a transhiatal approach, the upper abdomen is explored through a midline abdominal incision to detect visible local metastatic disease. If none is apparent, the stomach is mobilized widely (ie, freed from tethering attachments) with care taken to preserve its blood supply. Through a separate incision in the left side of the neck, the cervical esophagus is exposed. Working primarily through the abdominal incision, the surgeon inserts his or her hand through the diaphragmatic hiatus (para-esophageal opening in the diaphragm) into the mediastinum (Fig. 39-5).

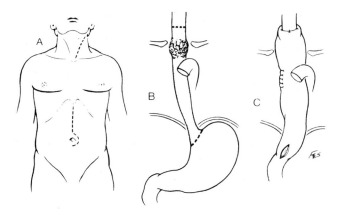

FIGURE 39-4. Esophagectomy and esophagogastrostomy using transhiatal approach. (**A**) Incisions. (**B**) Extent of esophageal resection (between dashed lines). (**C**) The stomach has been pulled upward into the mediastinum, and the gastric fundus has been anastomosed to the remaining cervical esophageal segment; a pyloromyotomy has been performed to facilitate gastric emptying. (Ellis FH Jr, 1980: Esophagogastrectomy for carcinoma: Technical considerations based on anatomic location of lesion. Surg Clin North Am 60:275)

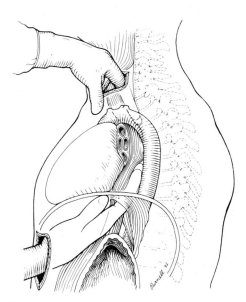

FIGURE 39-5. Technique of transhiatal esophagectomy; working through incisions in the upper abdomen and neck, the surgeon uses his or her fingers to bluntly free the esophagus from surrounding mediastinal attachments. (Shriver CD, Burt M, 1992: Transhiatal esophagectomy. Semin Thorac Cardiovasc Surg 4:309)

The surgeon uses blunt dissection (fingers or blunt instruments) to free blindly (with limited visualization) the esophagus from surrounding tissue. This technique is possible because only small blood vessels and tissue attach the esophagus to surrounding structures in the mediastinum. When the esophagus is entirely mobilized, the cervical esophagus is stapled and divided. The esophagus is pulled downward and out through the abdominal incision. The proximal stomach is stapled and divided, and the diseased esophageal segment is removed.

Next, the gastric fundus is maneuvered upward through the diaphragmatic hiatus and mediastinum to the open neck incision, where the anastomosis between gastric fundus and the remaining cervical esophageal segment is performed. Although the cardia is the stomach's most proximal anatomic component, the fundus of the stomach actually lies superior to the cardia and can be extended upward more easily for anastomosis to the proximal esophageal segment. Also, in tumors of the lower esophagus or gastroesophageal junction, the cardia often must be sacrificed to obtain an adequate distal tumor-free margin. Because the stomach can be elongated to reach the upper chest without disrupting its distal continuity with the duodenum, only a single visceral anastomosis (ie, proximal stomach to proximal esophagus) is necessary to restore continuity of the alimentary tract.

Once the stomach is positioned and sutured to proximal esophagus, most of it lies within the thorax. It preferably is positioned in the usual anatomic location of the esophagus (ie, in the posterior mediastinum). If the posterior mediastinum contains residual tumor that may subsequently obstruct the intrathoracic stomach or if it is fibrotic from prior radiation therapy or a surgical procedure, the stomach alternatively may be positioned behind the sternum in the anterior mediastinum (Orringer, 1996).

A transhiatal approach avoids a thoracotomy incision and its potential pulmonary complications and associated postoperative pain. Most important, transhiatal resection of an esophageal tumor does not appear to compromise cancer recurrence rates and patient survival (Inculet, 1998). An esophageal anastomosis in the neck rather than the thorax is advantageous in the event of a postoperative anastomotic disruption. Cervical anastomotic leaks (ie, those that occur in the neck) have less severe consequences and are more easily managed than if the anastomosis is located in the thorax (Gandhi & Naunheim, 1997; Daniel et al., 1992). Manipulation in the neck occasionally injures the recurrent laryngeal nerve.

A transthoracic approach, like a transhiatal approach, includes an upper abdominal incision through which the stomach is mobilized. However, instead of a neck incision, a right thoracotomy is performed. Through the thoracotomy incision, the entire esophagus is exposed and under direct visualization is freed from its mediastinal attachments along with surrounding lymph and fatty tissue. A transthoracic approach provides better exposure, allowing easier mobilization of viscera. It also allows an en bloc esophagectomy (ie, radical excision of regional mediastinal lymph nodes and other tissue surrounding the esophagus).

A transthoracic approach is recommended when an extended or radical en bloc resection of the thoracic esophagus incorporating surrounding mediastinal structures is necessary and when preoperative staging has not conclusively defined the interface between an esophageal tumor and adjacent airway or mediastinal tissues (Casson, 1998). Some surgeons believe that curative resection necessitates an en bloc resection with systematic mediastinal and abdominal lymphadenectomy in all patients with endoscopically visible esophageal tumors to provide the greatest likelihood of removing all potentially involved lymph nodes (Nigro et al., 1999).

With either operative approach, the vagus nerves are divided in the process of performing esophagectomy with esophagogastrostomy. Because vagotomy impairs gastric emptying, many surgeons routinely revise the gastric pylorus to facilitate gastric outflow. A pyloromyotomy (division of serosa and muscle layers of the pylorus) or pyloroplasty (full-thickness division of pylorus and suture reclosure) usually is performed. However, concomitant revision of the pylorus remains controversial because it sometimes results in duodenogastric reflux and the development of gastroesophagitis.

A jejunostomy tube almost always is placed during esophagectomy to provide an alternative means for providing alimentation to the patient during the postoperative period. Esophageal contents must be diverted and oral nourishment withheld for 4 to 6 days to allow adequate healing of the esophageal anastomosis. During this period, adequate nutrition is important to ensure recovery from operation and wound healing in these patients, who usually are malnourished and debilitated because of

the underlying disease. Jejunostomy feedings avoid infectious complications associated with intravenous hyperalimentation and potential gastroesophageal reflux from tube feedings delivered by means of gastrostomy. A nasogastric tube also is placed to divert secretions from the esophagus and prevent distention at the anastomotic site. A contrast swallow study usually is performed 4 to 6 days after surgery to confirm the integrity of the anastomosis. If no leak is present and bowel function has resumed, oral feedings are gradually reinstituted.

Esophagectomy With Colon Interposition

The surgical procedure to substitute colon for resected esophagus is called *esophagectomy with colon interposition* (Fig. 39-6). It also is referred to as a *colon swing* procedure. If colon is to be used as the replacement viscera, a number of preoperative interventions are performed. The patient is restricted to a clear liquid diet to cleanse the bowel of fecal material, and oral antibiotics are administered to reduce bacterial flora in the bowel. A colonoscopy may be performed to inspect the colon visually. In addition, a barium enema may be performed to assess anatomic configuration of the colon and to detect any pathologic process. Because the location of arterial blood vessels to the colon is occasionally anomalous, an angiogram may be performed as well to define vascular anatomy.

Colon interposition may be performed through a transhiatal or a transthoracic approach. Either the right

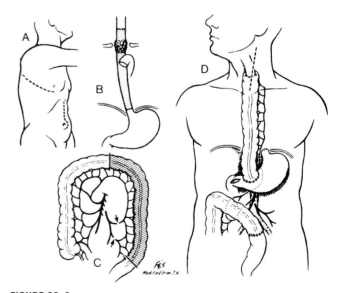

FIGURE 39-6. Esophagectomy with colon interposition using transthoracic approach. (**A**) Incisions. (**B**) Extent of esophageal resection (*shaded area*). (**C**) Segment of left colon to be used for interposition (*shaded area*). (**D**) Colon segment has been anastomosed to the esophagus proximally and stomach distally; remaining bowel segments have been anastomosed to restore bowel continuity; a pyloromyotomy has been performed to facilitate gastric emptying. (Ellis FH Jr, 1980: Esophagogastrectomy for carcinoma: Technical considerations based on anatomic location of lesion. Surg Clin North Amer 60:277)

(proximal) or left (distal) colon may be used to replace the esophagus. The right colon is the easiest to mobilize but has a variable blood supply, shorter vascular pedicle, and disparate size; the left colon is used more commonly because its mesenteric arterial supply is adequate to span longer defects and it is thicker, making it easier to suture (Hiebert, 1996). Esophageal replacement with left colon interposition usually is performed through a left neck incision and a midline laparotomy incision. Through the laparotomy incision, the colon is mobilized extensively, including both hepatic and splenic flexures, the entire descending colon, and the upper sigmoid colon. The necessary length of colon is harvested, ensuring that blood supply to both the resected portion and remaining bowel is adequate. Through the neck incision, a forceps is passed along the spine, corresponding to the bed of the resected esophagus, to grasp the upper end of the colon graft and draw it upward into the neck incision. As an alternative, a substernal tunnel may be created and the colon graft is placed in the retrosternal space. The segment of colon is anastomosed to the esophagus proximally and the stomach distally. The two remaining bowel segments in the abdomen are anastomosed to restore bowel continuity.

Results of Esophageal Resection

The operative mortality rate after surgical resection for esophageal carcinoma is less than 5%, but associated morbidity remains relatively high (Casson, 1998). For early-stage esophageal tumors, complete surgical resection may be curative, with 5-year survival rates approaching 70%; for most patients with locally advanced tumors, however, the overall survival rate remains less than 20% at 5 years (Kennedy & Casson, 1999).

Respiratory and cardiovascular complications are the most common forms of perioperative morbidity. The primary complication specifically related to esophagectomy is failure of the anastomosis to heal properly, resulting in an anastomotic leak. Esophageal anastomoses are more likely to leak than those in other gastrointestinal viscera because of the absence of a serosal covering on the esophagus. Breakdown of an esophageal anastomosis is most serious when the anastomosis is within the thorax. The nonsterile esophageal secretions spill into the mediastinum, causing mediastinitis. Esophageal stricture also can develop at the anastomotic site and lead to postoperative dysphagia (Lam et al., 1992). Possible causes of anastomotic stricture include anastomotic leakage, alkaline or acidic reflux, a technical problem with the anastomosis, and local recurrence of carcinoma (Wang et al., 1992).

None of the substitute viscera functions as well as the native esophagus, in which peristalsis propels food into the stomach (Collard et al., 1992). Although most patients are able to achieve adequate oral alimentation, modifications in the amount and type of food ingested may be necessary to avoid uncomfortable postprandial symptoms. Dumping syndrome is a group of postprandial intestinal vasomotor symptoms (epigastric distention, sweating, palpitations, tachycardia, light-headedness, nausea, increased peristalsis, excessive flatus,

diarrhea, and disorientation) that often occurs during the postoperative period in patients who have undergone esophagogastrectomy; the symptoms are severe in approximately 1% of patients (Bains, 1997; Collard et al., 1992). The complications of esophageal operations are discussed further in Chapter 43, Complications of Thoracic Operations.

Palliative Surgical Interventions

Palliative surgical therapy sometimes is performed to alleviate the disabling and unpleasant symptoms that develop eventually in patients with incurable esophageal cancer. Objectives of palliative procedures include (1) relief of dysphagia, (2) diversion of saliva and prevention of aspiration, (3) prevention of tumor ulceration (with resulting hemorrhage) or infection (with resulting sepsis), and (4) provision of a route for enteral alimentation.

Average survival in patients receiving palliative therapy is less than 10 months (Low & Pagliero, 1996). Therefore, palliative interventions must be carefully planned to enhance rather than detract from the patient's quality of life during this short interval. Surgical procedures designed to achieve palliation may necessitate lengthy hospitalization and cause untoward complications. The most reasonable treatment objective is to restore for as long as possible the patient's ability to swallow with minimal iatrogenic morbidity. Esophagectomy with esophagogastrostomy sometimes is performed as a palliative procedure to relieve dysphagia in severely symptomatic patients with minimal local extension to regional lymphatic tissue. However, many surgeons consider the significant operative risk unacceptable given the short life expectancy.

In patients unable to swallow saliva, a proximal esophagostomy and gastrostomy or jejunostomy may be performed. In this procedure, the esophagus is stapled and divided above the tumor and a fistula is surgically created between the proximal esophageal segment and the skin, allowing saliva to drain into an external esophagostomy pouch. A gastrostomy or jejunostomy feeding tube is placed concomitantly for alimentation. Alternatively, esophageal dilatation (ie, bougienage) may be performed to dilate the obstructed esophageal segment, or the obstructed segment may be intubated with a prosthetic stent (esophageal intubation). Either photodynamic laser therapy or brachytherapy (implantation of radioactive isotopes in the tumor) may be performed through an esophagoscope to destroy tumor that is occluding the esophageal lumen. Unfortunately, only modest success is achieved with any of these measures.

▶ Other Esophageal Disorders

Esophageal Perforation

Esophageal perforation may occur as a consequence of severe vomiting, penetrating trauma, instrumentation, or foreign body ingestion. The resultant leakage of digestive fluids, food, and bacteria into the periesophageal spaces causes diffuse cellulitis. The diagnosis of esophageal perforation is suggested by severe chest pain, fever, and radiographic evidence of mediastinal or subcutaneous air, particularly when these findings are associated with a clinical history of instrumentation, trauma, or vomiting. Definitive diagnosis is achieved by contrast swallow study.

Treatment of esophageal perforation includes intravenous antibiotic therapy and prompt surgical exploration to drain the infected area and repair the esophageal wall. If surgical treatment is delayed or infection is extensive, primary repair of the esophagus may not be possible. Instead, esophageal diversion is performed; the upper esophagus is divided and the proximal esophageal segment is brought out through the skin of the neck as a fistula to drain saliva (Fig. 39-7). The distal esophageal segment is sutured closed, and its upper end is attached to the back of the newly created esophageal stoma. Gastric drainage and enteral feeding tubes are placed to decompress the stomach and provide alimentation, respectively. Esophageal reconstruction is performed after the infection resolves.

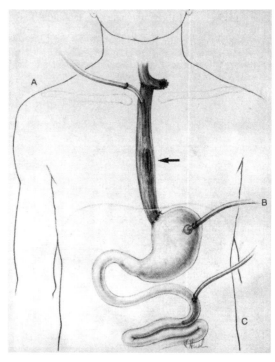

FIGURE 39-7. Esophageal diversion may be necessary for treatment of esophageal rupture (*arrow*) if diagnosis is delayed and infection well established. (**A**) The esophagus is divided at the level of the sternal manubrium, bringing the proximal end out to the skin. The distal esophagus is closed and attached to the back of the esophageal stoma. Distal to this closure line, a drainage catheter is inserted through a pursestring suture in the side of the esophagus and brought out through a small incision on the opposite side of the neck. (**B**) Through a laparotomy incision, the cardia is closed and a gastrostomy tube is inserted. (**C**) A jejunostomy tube is inserted for enteral feeding. (Skinner DB, 1991: Esophageal rupture. In Atlas of Esophageal Surgery, p. 181. New York, Churchill Livingstone)

Esophageal perforation is discussed further in Chapter 32, Cardiac and Thoracic Trauma, and Chapter 34, Esophageal Diseases.

Other Diseases Requiring Esophagectomy

Esophagectomy is recommended by some surgeons for patients with Barrett's esophagus and high-grade dysplasia (ie, markedly abnormal cells). These patients have a high incidence of early adenocarcinoma that cannot be detected by surveillance endoscopic biopsies alone (Hagen, 1997). Esophagectomy performed at this early stage for high-grade dysplasia or intramucosal carcinoma is more likely to be curative. Esophagectomy also is performed occasionally for treatment of severe esophageal damage owing to esophageal motility disorders, caustic injury, or connective tissue disorders (eg, scleroderma). It is indicated in patients whose esophageal function has been destroyed by the underlying disease process or who have already undergone multiple surgical procedures on the esophagus (Stein et al., 1992a).

The most common benign esophageal diseases leading to esophageal replacement are end-stage GERD and advanced motility disorders (Watson et al., 1998). Proper patient selection for esophageal replacement as treatment for nonmalignant disease is difficult and controversial. Typically, patients considered for esophageal resection have failed medical therapy and multiple operative procedures designed to improve foregut function. Although esophageal replacement is a radical surgical procedure, additional nonextirpative (ie, nonremoval of the esophagus) procedures have the potential to (1) cause further tissue damage with additional loss of esophageal function, (2) reduce blood supply to the esophagus with the possibility of ischemic necrosis, and (3) damage the vagus nerves with the possibility of altered foregut motility (Watson et al., 1998).

Some surgeons consider colon to be the replacement conduit of choice in patients with benign disease. Although colon interposition is a more technically difficult procedure, the colon may be preferable as a long-term replacement viscera. It is more durable over time and provides a better quality of deglutition (swallowing) than stomach (Stein et al., 1992a). Esophageal resection and reconstruction for benign disease carries an operative mortality rate of 2% and is associated with an improvement in symptoms in 98% of patients (Watson et al., 1998).

REFERENCES

Allen MS, 1997: The laparoscopic Nissen fundoplication. Operative Techniques in Cardiac and Thoracic Surgery: A Comparative Atlas 2:44

Altorki NK, 1998: Excision of esophageal diverticula. In Kaiser LR, Kron IL, Spray TL (eds): Mastery of Cardiothoracic Surgery. Philadelphia, Lippincott Williams & Wilkins

Altorki NK, Skinner DB, Minsky BD, et al., 1996: Carcinoma of the esophagus. In Baue AE, Geha AS, Hammond GL, et al. (eds): Glenn's Thoracic and Cardiovascular Surgery, ed. 6. Stamford, CT, Appleton & Lange

Bains MS, 1997: Complications of abdominal right-thoracic (Ivor Lewis) esophagectomy. Chest Surg Clin North Am 7:587

Banbury MK, Rice TW, Goldblum JR, 1999: Esophagectomy with gastric reconstruction for achalasia. J Thorac Cardiovasc Surg 117:1077

Block MI, Cooper JD, 1997: The Belsey Mark IV procedure. Operative Techniques in Cardiac and Thoracic Surgery: A Comparative Atlas 2:2

Cameron AJ, 1998: Management of Barrett's esophagus. Mayo Clin Proc 73:457

Casson AG, 1998: Thoracic approaches to esophagectomy. In Kaiser LR, Kron IL, Spray TL (eds): Mastery of Cardiothoracic Surgery. Philadelphia, Lippincott Williams & Wilkins

Collard JM, Otte JB, Reynaert M, Kestens PJ, 1992: Quality of life three years or more after esophagectomy for cancer. J Thorac Cardiovasc Surg 104:391

Cooper JD, 1997: Current role of esophageal function studies. Semin Thorac Cardiovasc Surg 9:157

Cox JL, Sundt TM, 1997: Introduction. Operative Techniques in Cardiac and Thoracic Surgery: A Comparative Atlas 2:1

Daniel TM, Fleisher KJ, Flanagan TL, et al., 1992: Transhiatal esophagectomy: A safe alternative for selected patients. Ann Thorac Surg 54:686

DeMeester TR, 1997: Management of adenocarcinoma arising in Barrett's esophagus. Semin Thorac Cardiovasc Surg 9:290

Duranceau A, 1995: Disorders of the esophagus in the adult. In Sabiston DC Jr, Spencer FC (eds): Surgery of the Chest, ed. 6. Philadelphia, WB Saunders

Duranceau A, 1996: Esophageal dysmotility. In Baue AE, Geha AS, Hammond GL, et al. (eds): Glenn's Thoracic and Cardiovascular Surgery, ed. 6. Stamford, CT, Appleton & Lange

Ferguson MK, 1998: Antireflux procedures. In Kaiser LR, Kron IL, Spray TL (eds): Mastery of Cardiothoracic Surgery. Philadelphia, Lippincott Williams & Wilkins

Ferguson MK, 1991: Achalasia: Current evaluation and therapy. Ann Thorac Surg 52:336

Gandhi SK, Naunheim KS, 1997: Complications of transhiatal esophagectomy. Chest Surg Clin North Am 7:601

Hagen JA, 1997: Management of Barrett's esophagus with dysplasia. Semin Thorac Cardiovasc Surg 9:285

Heitmiller RF, 1998: Surgery of achalasia and other motility disorders. In Kaiser LR, Kron IL, Spray TL (eds): Mastery of Cardiothoracic Surgery. Philadelphia, Lippincott Williams & Wilkins

Hiebert CA, 1996: Surgical options for esophageal excision replacement: Colonic interposition. In Baue AE, Geha AS, Hammond GL, et al. (eds): Glenn's Thoracic and Cardiovascular Surgery, ed. 6. Stamford, CT, Appleton & Lange

Hill LD, Mazza DE, Aye RW, 1997: The Hill repair. Operative Techniques in Cardiac and Thoracic Surgery: A Comparative Atlas 2:16

Huang GJ, 1994: Replacement of the esophagus with the stomach. In Shields TW (ed): General Thoracic Surgery, ed. 4. Baltimore, Williams & Wilkins

Inculet RI, 1998: Transhiatal esophagectomy. In Kaiser LR, Kron IL, Spray TL (eds): Mastery of Cardiothoracic Surgery. Philadelphia, Lippincott Williams & Wilkins

Kennedy R, Casson AG, 1999: Esophageal cancer: Surgery. In Casson AG, Johnston MR (eds): Key Topics in Thoracic Surgery. Oxford, Bios

Koshy SS, Nostrant TT, 1997: Pathophysiology and endoscopic/balloon treatment of esophageal motility disorders. Surg Clin North Am 77:971

Lam TC, Fok M, Cheng SW, Wong J, 1992: Anastomotic complications after esophagectomy for cancer. J Thorac Cardiovasc Surg 104:395

Low DE, Pagliero KM, 1996: Palliative treatment of carcinoma of the esophagus. In Baue AE, Geha AS, Hammond GL, et al. (eds): Glenn's Thoracic and Cardiovascular Surgery, ed. 6. Stamford, CT, Appleton & Lange

Naunheim KS, Baue AE, 1996: Medical and surgical treatment of hiatal hernia and gastroesophageal reflux. In Baue AE, Geha AS, Hammond GL, et al. (eds): Glenn's Thoracic and Cardiovascular Surgery, ed. 6. Stamford, CT, Appleton & Lange

Naunheim KS, Petruska PJ, Roy TS, et al., 1992: Preoperative chemotherapy and radiotherapy for esophageal carcinoma. J Thorac Cardiovasc Surg 103:887

Nigro JJ, Hagen JA, DeMeester TR, et al., 1999: Prevalence and location of nodal metastases in distal esophageal adenocarcinoma confined to the wall: Implications for therapy. J Thorac Cardiovasc Surg 177:16

Orringer MB, 1996: Surgical options for esophageal resection and reconstruction with stomach. In Baue AE, Geha AS, Hammond GL, et al. (eds): Glenn's Thoracic and Cardiovascular Surgery, ed. 6. Stamford, CT, Appleton & Lange

Orringer MB, 1997: Tumors of the esophagus. In Sabiston DC Jr (ed): Textbook of Surgery: The Biological Basis of Modern Surgical Practice, ed. 15. Philadelphia, WB Saunders

Pearson FG, 1997. Hiatus hernia and gastroesophageal reflux: Indications for surgery and selection of operation. Semin Thorac Cardiovasc Surg 9:163

Pera M, Trastek VF, Carpenter HA, et al., 1992: Barrett's esophagus with high-grade dysplasia: An indication for esophagectomy. Ann Thorac Surg 54:199

Ribet M, Debrueres B, Lecomte-Houcke M, 1992: Resection for advanced cancer of the thoracic esophagus: Cervical or thoracic anastomosis. J Thorac Cardiovasc Surg 103:784

Rice TW, Gagner M, 1997. Laparoscopic antireflux surgery. Semin Thorac Cardiovasc Surg 9:173

Scott M, Gelhot AR, 1999: Gastroesophageal reflux disease: Diagnosis and management. Am Fam Physician 59:1161

Skinner DB, 1994: Gastroesophageal reflux. In Shields TW (ed): General Thoracic Surgery, ed. 4. Baltimore, Williams & Wilkins

Skinner DB, 1995: The Belsey Mark IV antireflux repair. In Sabiston DC Jr, Spencer FC (eds): Surgery of the Chest, ed. 6. Philadelphia, WB Saunders

Stein HJ, DeMeester TR, Hinder RA, 1992a: Evaluation and surgical management of motor disorders of the esophageal body and lower esophageal sphincter. Curr Probl Surg 24:447

Stein HJ, DeMeester TR, Hinder RA, 1992b: Evaluation and surgical management of pharyngoesophageal swallowing disorders. Curr Probl Surg 24:429

Trastek VF, 1994: Esophageal diverticula. In Shields TW (ed): General Thoracic Surgery, ed. 4. Baltimore, Williams & Wilkins

Wang LS, Huang MH, Huang BS, Chien KY, 1992: Gastric substitution for resectable carcinoma of the esophagus: An analysis of 368 cases. Ann Thorac Surg 53:289

Watson TJ, DeMeester TR, Kauer WKH, et al., 1998: Esophageal replacement for end-stage benign esophageal disease. J Thorac Cardiovasc Surg 115:1241

Wilkins EW, 1994: Motor disturbances of deglutition. In Shields TW (ed): General Thoracic Surgery, ed. 4. Baltimore, Williams & Wilkins

40

Surgery of the Pleura, Trachea, Chest Wall, and Mediastinum

By far, most thoracic operations are performed for treatment of pulmonary or esophageal diseases, as discussed in Chapter 38, Surgical Treatment of Pulmonary Diseases, and Chapter 39, Surgical Treatment of Esophageal Diseases. In this chapter, the focus is on less commonly performed types of thoracic surgery—operations that involve the pleura, trachea, chest wall, or structures in the mediastinum.

▶ Operations on the Pleura

Pleural Abrasion

Pleural abrasion, also called pleurodesis or pleural scarification, is an operation in which the visceral and parietal pleural surfaces are mechanically abraded. The most common reason for performing pleural abrasion is to prevent recurrent pneumothorax and lung collapse in patients with a predilection for spontaneous pneumothoraces. These patients, who typically are slender, young adults with otherwise normal lungs, have a propensity for development of pneumothoraces owing to idiopathic rupture of air-filled blebs on the lung's surface. Patients who have experienced an initial episode of

spontaneous pneumothorax have an approximately 20% risk of recurrence after the first episode and an even greater recurrence risk after the second episode; most recurrences are on the ipsilateral (same) side.

An initial episode of spontaneous pneumothorax most commonly is treated with chest tube drainage of the pleural space. Pleural abrasion usually is reserved for patients who experience a second or third spontaneous pneumothorax. Certain situations, however, dictate pleural abrasion after a single episode. For example, surgical therapy is performed after the first pneumothorax in patients in whom a recurrent episode could be life threatening, such as airline pilots, scuba divers, and people who spend time in areas remote from available medical care. Sometimes, surgical therapy becomes necessary after an initial pneumothorax because the visceral pleura fails to seal and an air leak persists beyond 7 to 10 days. An operation also is recommended in patients who experience spontaneous pneumothorax after a previous pneumothorax on the contralateral side or in the rare circumstance of simultaneous bilateral pneumothoraces.

Pleural abrasion usually is performed using video-assisted thoracoscopy. Alternatively, a small axillary thoracotomy incision may be used. A dry gauze sponge is used to abrade the parietal pleura. The resulting cap-

507

illary bleeding, erythema, and pleural inflammation cause adhesion formation and pleural symphysis (ie, a fusing together of the pleural surfaces). Blebs are detected in as many as 85% of patients undergoing operative procedures for spontaneous pneumothorax (Cohen et al., 1995). Identified blebs are resected, most commonly with a stapling device (Fig. 40-1). At the conclusion of the procedure, the surgeon examines the lung for residual air leakage by instilling saline in the pleural space while the operative lung is inflated.

Pleural abrasion is highly successful in preventing recurrent pneumothoraces. In the event of subsequent bleb rupture, the pleural symphysis prevents accumulation of air in the pleural space and collapse of the lung. Rarely, pleural abrasion is inadequate to prevent portions of the lung from collapsing. In this case, a reoperation may be necessary to abrade further the pleural surface and staple the portion of lung tissue from which air is leaking.

Talc Poudrage

Patients with malignant pleural effusion occasionally undergo a surgical procedure to prevent recurrent fluid accumulation. *Talc poudrage* is a form of pleurodesis in which an irritating powder (talc) is applied to promote adhesion between the visceral and parietal pleura. Because talc is insoluble, it usually is administered as a powder by insufflation (blowing the powder into the pleural space) at thoracoscopy or thoracotomy (Rusch, 1995). This is in contrast to soluble sclerosing agents (eg, bleomycin or doxycycline) that typically are instilled through a chest tube. Talc also can be administered through a chest tube as a slurry (ie, watery mixture of insoluble matter).

Most often, talc poudrage is performed using video-assisted thoracoscopy. The pleural space is entered and the pleural effusion is drained by aspiration. Sterile talc powder is then insufflated diffusely into the pleural space

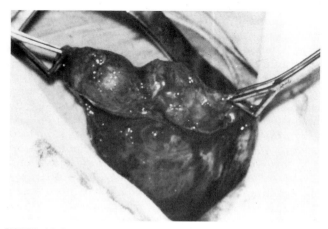

FIGURE 40-1. Operative photograph demonstrating well-circumscribed subpleural blebs at the apex of the lung. (Deslauriers J, Leblanc P, 1994: Bullous and bleb diseases of the lung. In Shields TW [ed]: General Thoracic Surgery, ed. 4, p. 908. Baltimore, Williams & Wilkins)

to coat visceral and parietal pleural surfaces throughout the space. Talc poudrage is an effective method of preventing fluid reaccumulation and may be used if more conservative therapy fails. However, patients with malignant pleural effusion have a very limited life expectancy; approximately one half of patients die within 3 months of therapy (Rusch, 1995). Given the grim prognosis associated with malignant pleural effusion, the morbidity of an operation often is thought to outweigh the benefit.

Pleurectomy

A *pleurectomy*, or removal of the parietal pleura, is another surgical technique for causing adhesion formation and pleural symphysis. Through a small thoracotomy incision, the intercostal muscles are divided and the pleural space is entered. When performed to treat pneumothorax, the parietal pleura is abraded or stripped from the endothoracic fascia in the area over the apex of the lung (LoCicero, 1996). As during pleural abrasion, identified apical blebs are excised with a stapling instrument.

Pleurectomy is performed less commonly than pleural abrasion for treatment of spontaneous pneumothorax. It probably is no more effective than pleurodesis, is associated with a higher incidence of morbidity, and makes subsequent thoracotomy for unrelated disease more difficult (Cohen et al., 1995). A more extensive pleurectomy can be an effective operation for preventing recurrent malignant pleural effusions. As with pleural abrasion and talc poudrage, however, the palliative benefits of pleurectomy seldom are thought to outweigh the associated morbidity of the operation in patients with limited life expectancy due to terminal illness.

Pleurectomy occasionally is performed for treatment of diffuse malignant mesothelioma, a type of cancer that arises in the pleura and often is associated with asbestos exposure. Diffuse malignant mesothelioma usually is fatal. Median survival time after diagnosis is only 6 to 14 months (LoCicero, 1996). No available form of therapy has proven clearly superior, and the role of surgical therapy remains controversial. However, pleurectomy nearly always limits recurrence of pleural effusions, and some surgeons have reported marginally extended survival (LoCicero, 1996).

An alternative surgical approach for treatment of mesothelioma is pleural resection combined with removal of the ipsilateral lung, an operation known as *extrapleural pneumonectomy*. Trimodal therapy, consisting of extrapleural pneumonectomy followed by combination chemotherapy and radiation therapy, may prolong survival in patients with resectable mesothelioma tumors of an epithelial cell type (Sugarbaker & Garcia, 1998). Because neither pleurectomy nor extrapleural pneumonectomy has been shown to increase survival time significantly, many physicians advocate only supportive therapy for patients with malignant mesothelioma.

Decortication

Decortication is the surgical removal of a restrictive, fibrous membrane or layer of tissue from the pleural surface of the lung and, if necessary, from the chest wall and diaphragm (Shields, 1994a). The purpose of the operation is to free lung that has become entrapped by abnormal fibrous tissue, sometimes called a *fibrous peel.* Most commonly, decortication is performed to remove a fibrous peel that has developed secondary to an inadequately drained hemothorax or as a result of empyema.

Both hemothorax and empyema initially are treated with chest tube thoracostomy drainage. If a significant hemothorax is undetected or inadequately drained, the blood remaining in the pleural space eventually becomes organized and cannot be evacuated with tube drainage. When this occurs, operative evacuation of the blood and decortication of the fibrous peel overlying the lung become necessary to achieve lung reexpansion. Similarly, decortication may become necessary in patients with empyema if the cavity is unusually thick walled and does not decrease in size over time (Cohen et al., 1995).

Decortication typically is performed through a posterolateral thoracotomy incision in the fifth or sixth intercostal space. A rib may be resected to provide better exposure of the pleural space. A small incision is made in the visceral pleura. By using blunt dissection primarily and sharp dissection as necessary, the visceral peel covering the lung is removed, allowing underlying lung to expand (Fig. 40-2). When decortication includes removal of both the visceral and parietal peels that form an empyema sac, the operation is called an *empyemectomy.* The primary postoperative problems associated with decortication are persistent air leak, bleeding, and sepsis (Shields, 1994a).

► Operations on the Trachea

Tracheal Resection

Tracheal resection may be indicated in the treatment of various pathologic conditions affecting the trachea, including tracheal tumors, damage to the trachea from intubation or trauma, and tracheoesophageal fistulae. Surgery of the trachea has evolved more slowly than other types of thoracic surgery owing to the rarity of tracheal tumors, the anatomic complexities of tracheal reconstruction, and the biologic incompatibilities that have occurred with prosthetic materials used for tracheal replacement (Grillo, 1994).

Primary tumors of the trachea are rare. Most are malignant and are either squamous cell carcinoma or adenoid cystic carcinoma. Tracheal tumors frequently are not diagnosed until the patient has symptoms of progressive airway obstruction. Even then, symptoms, such as dyspnea, stridor, wheezing, and cough, may be attributed initially to asthma or bronchitis; furthermore, when these symptoms are evaluated with plain chest radiography, there may be no, or only a subtle, abnormality in the mediastinum or tracheal air column (Pearson et al., 1995).

Traumatic damage to the trachea may result from prolonged or traumatic intubation, traumatic laceration, radiation therapy, tracheal burns, aspiration of a caustic substance, or infection. The most common etiology of tracheal damage is injury caused by intubation of the trachea with an endotracheal or tracheostomy tube. Postintubation stricture currently is the most common indication for tracheal resection (Keshavjee & Pearson, 1995). It typically occurs at the level of a tracheostomy stoma or of a tracheostomy or endotracheal tube cuff.

Damage to the trachea less commonly causes tracheal malacia or development of a tracheoesophageal fistula (ie, communication between the trachea and esophagus). Tracheal malacia is the collapse of a segment of tracheal wall. It may be caused by endotracheal tube cuff injury or may develop secondary to chronic compression from a lesion external to the trachea (Mathisen & Grillo, 1996). Tracheoesophageal fistula can occur as a complication of prolonged intubation of the trachea or secondary to esophageal perforation and resultant infection.

Depending on the area of tracheal disease, operations to resect and reconstruct the trachea may be performed through a cervical incision, a median sternotomy, or a posterolateral thoracotomy. The various surgical approaches are based on knowledge of the trachea's anatomic position in the thorax. When viewed laterally, the trachea in an erect person courses backward and downward at an angle from a nearly subcutaneous position at the infracricoid level to rest against the esophagus and vertebral column at the carina (Grillo, 1994). Consequently, resection of a lesion in the upper half of the trachea is best performed through an anterior collar incision with or without a partial vertical division of the sternum (Grillo, 1995). A posterolateral thoracotomy incision is more suitable for a lesion in the lower trachea. Operations on the trachea necessitate special techniques to ensure adequate ventilation. Principles of airway management during tracheal resection and reconstruction include (1) full control of the airway at all times, (2) bronchoscopic examination of the airway by both the surgeon and anesthesiologist, (3) slow and gentle induction of anesthesia, and (4) spontaneous ventilation during and after the operation (Grillo, 1994).

Particularly in patients with postintubation injury, it is preferable to delay resection and reconstruction until active inflammatory changes beyond the margins of the stricture have subsided (Keshavjee & Pearson, 1995). To date, no prosthetic graft has proved successful for replacement of resected trachea. Inflammation with resultant granulation tissue and stricture formation typically develops after prosthesis implantation in the trachea. Consequently, tracheal reconstruction usually is performed by direct anastomosis of the tracheal segments above and below the area of circumferential resection. The trachea in the average adult is approximately 11 cm in length. Usually, it is possible to remove up to one half

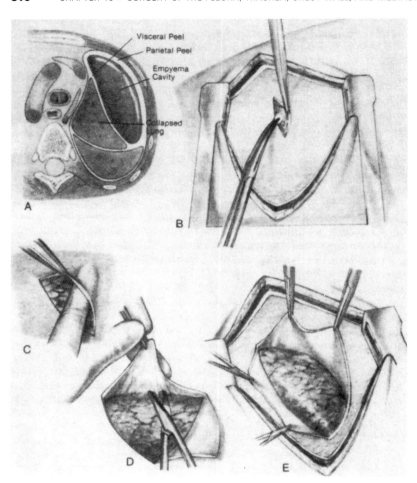

FIGURE 40-2. Decortication of the pleura. (**A**) Cross-sectional diagram of thorax demonstrating the relationship of the empyema cavity and its walls to the chest wall and underlying lung. (**B**) The chest has been opened and the empyema space entered; the thick parietal peel has been incised and retracted; dissection of the visceral peel from underlying lung is begun through a small incision in the visceral peel. (**C**) Sometimes the peel can be separated from the lung with gentle blunt dissection. (**D**) Sharp dissection may be necessary. (**E**) The area of decorticated lung is now able to expand from its partially collapsed state. (Hood MR, 1993: Operations for trauma. In Techniques in General Thoracic Surgery, ed. 2, p. 54. Philadelphia, Lea & Febiger)

the length of the trachea and successfully reconstruct it with primary anastomosis of the remaining segments.

Initially, the patient is intubated in a normal fashion. The trachea is exposed and mobilized carefully to preserve adequate blood supply (Fig. 40-3). Traction sutures are placed in the trachea above and below the lesion. After making an incision in the anterior surface of the trachea distal to the lesion, the endotracheal tube is withdrawn so that its tip is above the incision. A sterile, specially designed, flexible endotracheal tube is inserted through the incision into the distal trachea to continue ventilation while tracheal integrity is disrupted. Diseased or damaged segments of trachea are surgically removed with circumferential resection of the involved portion of trachea. The resection is performed through healthy trachea because reconstruction with inflamed tissue would compromise success of the primary anastomosis (Keshavjee & Pearson, 1995).

After resecting the diseased or damaged section, the traction sutures are used to approximate the remaining proximal and distal tracheal segments and a primary anastomosis is performed. To achieve a satisfactory result with tracheal reconstruction, it is important to avoid undue tension at the anastomotic site. At the conclusion of the operation, heavy sutures may be placed between the patient's chin and chest to maintain the head in a for-

ward position. These so-called *guardian sutures* prevent tension on the tracheal anastomosis that would occur with hyperextension of the neck. The sutures are left in place for 5 to 7 days.

Patients usually are extubated in the operating room to allow the surgeon to assess the airway and to be certain that the anastomosis is satisfactory (Donahue & Mathisen, 1998). Providing adequate postoperative pulmonary hygiene necessitates special considerations. Coughing and deep-breathing regimens are essential to prevent atelectasis. Endotracheal suctioning and reintubation are avoided if at all possible because of potential injury to or disruption of the tracheal anastomosis. If endotracheal suctioning does become necessary, it is performed by the surgeon, using a bronchoscope to provide visual guidance. Potential complications of tracheal operations include anastomotic dehiscence, infection, and tracheal stenosis at the anastomotic site. Anastomotic dehiscence usually is a fatal complication.

Tracheostomy

Tracheostomy, also called *tracheotomy*, is performed to overcome upper airway obstruction or to provide a secure airway to facilitate secretion removal or long-term

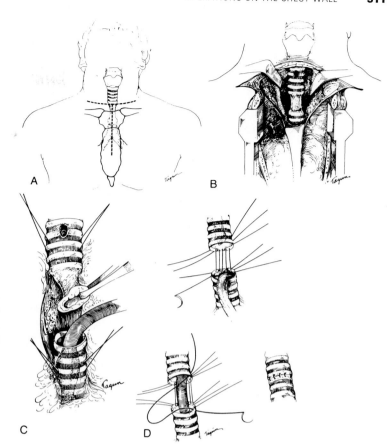

FIGURE 40-3. Resection and reconstruction of the upper trachea. (**A**) Collar incision is often sufficient, but median sternotomy improves access to mediastinum. (**B**) Retraction of innominate vein and artery to expose trachea adequately. (**C**) Division of trachea and intubation of distal trachea across operative field. (**D**) Tracheal segment has been resected; posterolateral sutures are placed to begin anastomosis of proximal and distal trachea (*top*). Proximal endotracheal tube is advanced into distal trachea (*bottom left*) and anterior sutures are placed (*bottom right*). (Grillo HC, 1972: Tracheal reconstruction: Indications and techniques. Arch Otolaryngol 96:37. Copyright © 1972, American Medical Association)

ventilatory support in patients with respiratory insufficiency. Most commonly, it is performed for the latter indication, typically in critically ill patients who require mechanical ventilation for more than 10 to 14 days. Tracheostomy reduces the likelihood of complications associated with prolonged intubation with an endotracheal tube. It also frees the patient's nose or mouth of the tube and allows resumption of oral feedings if the patient's level of consciousness and swallowing mechanism are not impaired.

Tracheostomy preferably is performed as a planned procedure in an operating room with an endotracheal tube in place and with the assistance of anesthesia personnel (Boyd et al., 1995). Most often, general anesthesia is used. The patient is placed in a supine position with the head extended to place a maximal amount of trachea above the sternal notch. A short horizontal skin incision is made 1 to 2 cm below the cricoid cartilage. The strap muscles are separated and the thyroid isthmus is divided or retracted to expose the trachea. A vertical incision is created in the anterior surface of the trachea in the area of the third tracheal ring. A tracheostomy tube with a high-volume, low-pressure cuff is inserted through the opening and ventilation through the tube is begun. The tracheostomy tube is secured with tapes passed through the flanges of the tube and then tied around the patient's neck. Complications related to tracheostomy occur uncommonly. Early postoperative complications include

bleeding, wound infection, subcutaneous emphysema, tube obstruction or displacement, and swallowing problems. Late complications include granuloma formation; tracheal stenosis; and trachea-innominate artery, tracheoesophageal, or tracheocutaneous fistula (Golde et al., 1995).

A *minitracheostomy* may be performed in patients who are self-ventilating but who require frequent suctioning for retained secretions. Minitracheostomy consists of percutaneous insertion of a small-diameter, flanged cannula through the cricothyroid membrane into the trachea. The procedure can be performed at the bedside and is associated with minimal morbidity. The minitracheostomy cannula can remain in place for days or weeks and is used for intermittent suctioning. When the minitracheostomy cannula is removed, the stoma closes, usually within 48 hours.

▶ Operations on the Chest Wall

Chest Wall Resection

Chest wall resection most often is performed to treat primary neoplasms of the chest wall. Chest wall tumors may arise from any of a variety of cell types and may involve the soft tissues of the thorax, the bony structures, or both. Approximately one half of chest wall tumors are malignant, and of the malignant tumors, approximately one half are primary tumors originating in the bone, soft tissue, nerves, or muscle of the chest wall (Compeau & Johnston, 1999). Chest wall tumors usually occur as slowly enlarging masses that are asymptomatic; with continued growth, nearly all malignant tumors and two thirds of benign tumors become painful (Pairolero, 1995). Computed tomography or magnetic resonance imaging is used to define the extent of the tumor and to delineate involvement of adjacent structures. Definitive diagnosis is achieved with needle, incisional, or excisional biopsy. The issue of which form of biopsy is most appropriate for diagnosis of a chest wall tumor remains somewhat controversial; most surgeons now recommend either incisional or needle biopsy to establish a definitive diagnosis before surgical resection of the tumor (Miller, 1998).

The treatment of choice for most benign and malignant chest wall tumors is surgical resection. Benign tumors often become painful if not resected, and some benign tumors undergo malignant degeneration. Malignant tumors of the chest wall are treated with wide surgical resection; the tumor is removed en bloc (as a whole) along with any contiguous structures invaded by the tumor. To allow adequate tumor-free margins, several centimeters of tumor-free soft tissue, a normal rib above and below the tumor, and 5 cm of tumor-free rib are included in the resection (McCormack, 1996). Occasionally, palliative resection of a malignant chest wall tumor is performed to reduce pain or to remove a tumor that is infected, ulcerated, or bleeding.

If the removal of a chest wall neoplasm necessitates resection of a significant amount of rib segments, the resulting defect may need to be covered with prosthetic material or muscle to provide stabilization of the chest wall. Both the extent of resection and the method of reconstruction must be designed so that the thorax maintains adequate support of respiration and protection of underlying organs (Pairolero, 1995). The primary complications of chest wall resection and reconstruction are respiratory insufficiency produced by instability of the chest wall and infection.

Thoracoplasty

Thoracoplasty is an operation in which a portion of the bony structure of the chest wall is resected. Removal of the skeletal support allows that portion of the chest wall to sink in toward the mediastinum, thus reducing the size of the hemithorax and partially collapsing underlying lung (Shields, 1994b). Before the availability of effective pharmacologic agents for the treatment of tuberculosis, thoracoplasty was one of several methods used to put the lung to rest with the hope of inactivating the disease (Deslauriers & Jacques, 1995). Today, the procedure is performed in selected patients with chronic infection of the pleural space. However, thoracoplasty is cosmetically disfiguring and can lead to chronic spine and shoulder problems. Because muscle transposition offers an alterna-

tive treatment that is much less debilitating, thoracoplasty is performed infrequently (Webb & Harrison, 1996). Nevertheless, it remains a therapeutic option for selected patients with chronically infected apical spaces and no remaining lung or a lung that cannot be expanded because of intrinsic disease (Deslauriers & Jacques, 1995).

Window Thoracostomy

A *window thoracostomy* describes a surgically created, epithelial-lined opening in the chest wall. The purpose of a window thoracostomy is to provide permanent, dependent drainage of the pleural space for conditions such as tuberculous or pyogenic empyema, malignant pleural effusion, and chronic bronchopleural fistula (Boyd & Glassman, 1998). Short segments of two adjacent ribs are removed and the overlying flap of skin and subcutaneous tissue is inserted into the pleural space and fixed to the chest wall to prevent closure of the opening. Examples of window thoracostomies are a *Clagett window thoracostomy*, illustrated in Chapter 33, Pulmonary, Tracheal, and Pleural Diseases (Fig. 33-4) and an *Eloesser flap*, depicted in Chapter 43, Complications of Thoracic Operations (Fig. 43-1).

▶ Operations Involving Mediastinal Structures

Thymectomy for Myasthenia Gravis

Thymectomy, or removal of the thymus gland, is performed most often for the treatment of myasthenia gravis, a disease characterized by progressive weakness and easy fatigability of voluntary muscles. Myasthenia gravis is an autoimmune disorder in which antibodies are produced against acetylcholine receptors of the muscle endplate, resulting in impaired neuromuscular transmission (Krucylak & Naunheim, 1999). Because muscles innervated by the cranial nerves are involved more often and at an earlier stage, presenting symptoms typically include ptosis, ophthalmoplegia, dysarthria, and dysphagia (DeCamp et al., 1996).

For reasons that are incompletely understood, surgical resection of the thymus gland usually produces significant clinical improvement in patients with myasthenia gravis. Precise indications and timing for thymectomy in patients with myasthenia gravis, however, are somewhat controversial. Surgical resection is recommended in all patients with myasthenia gravis and a thymoma (tumor of the thymus gland). Ten to 15% of patients with myasthenia gravis have an associated thymoma and 30% or more patients with thymoma have myasthenia gravis (Trastek, 1998). In patients without thymoma, surgical therapy typically is performed in those with generalized symptoms of myasthenia gravis, including ptosis, dysarthria, dysphagia, and weakness of respiratory muscles.

Thymectomy may be performed through one of several

incisions, including a partial upper sternal-splitting incision, a transverse cervical incision, or a median sternotomy incision with cervical extension (Trastek & Pairolero, 1991). A transcervical approach often is used because it offers the advantages of lower morbidity, a briefer hospitalization, and a faster patient recovery with comparable long-term clinical outcomes (Bril et al., 1998). A median sternotomy is used if a thymoma is present.

The thymus gland is a bilobular structure with an H-shaped configuration. Most of the thymus is in the anterior mediastinum, overlying the pericardium and great vessels at the base of the heart; the upper poles of each lobe extend into the neck and are attached to the thyroid gland (Trastek & Shields, 1994). After entering the mediastinal cavity, the thymus is carefully freed from attaching tissue (Fig. 40-4). Both pleural cavities may be opened to expose the phrenic nerves adequately and avoid injuring them during the dissection.

Patients who undergo thymectomy for myasthenia gravis require careful monitoring of postoperative respiratory status. In patients with disease of relatively short duration and mild symptoms, extubation is considered several hours after operation; patients with more severe myasthenia gravis may require intubation for longer periods (Wechsler, 1995). Long-term results of thymectomy in patients with myasthenia gravis are difficult to evaluate because of the uncertain natural history of untreated myasthenia gravis, the unpredictable rate of disease progression, and the unpredictable occurrence of spontaneous remission (Hagen & Cooper, 1997). Nevertheless, most patients demonstrate clinical improvement after thymectomy and complete remission is reported in 44% of patients (Bril et al., 1998).

Resection of Primary Mediastinal Neoplasms and Cysts

Surgical resection of mediastinal masses is the major modality for treatment of neoplasms and cysts that originate in the mediastinum. Although most mediastinal masses represent metastatic spread of malignant disease and are not treated surgically, a variety of primary neoplasms or cysts can originate in the mediastinum. Most common are neurogenic tumors, primary cysts, thymomas, lymphomas, and germ cell tumors (Davis et al., 1995). Approximately two thirds of primary mediastinal masses are benign (Strollo et al., 1997).

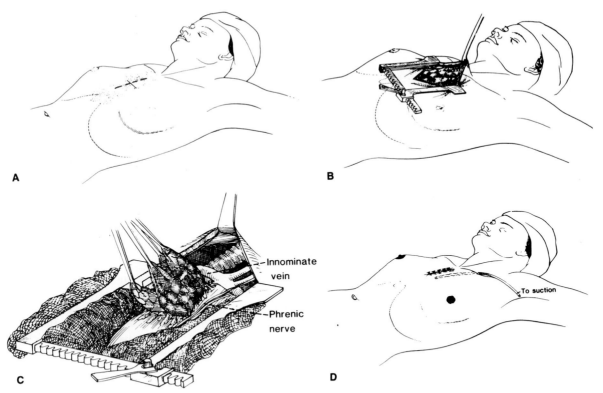

FIGURE 40-4. Thymectomy. (**A**) A short midline incision is made. (**B**) Manubrium and sternum are divided, and mediastinum is exposed by spreading sternum and retracting incision cephalad. (**C**) After ligation and division of its blood supply, the entire thymus is freed from adjacent pericardium and mediastinal pleura by blunt and sharp dissection. Care is taken to remove all thymic tissue, including cervical extensions, while carefully preserving phrenic nerves. (**D**) Incision has been closed. A small catheter is placed for suction drainage if pleural spaces have not been violated. A chest tube is necessary if the pleura has been entered. (Trastek VF, Shields TW, 1994: Surgery of the thymus gland. In Shields TW [ed]: General Thoracic Surgery, ed. 4, p. 1778. Baltimore, Williams & Wilkins)

A mediastinal mass usually is detected because of an abnormal shadow or configuration on a chest roentgenogram. A presumptive diagnosis often can be established because most mediastinal masses have a predilection for specific age groups and anatomic locations in the mediastinum (Pearson, 1992). Masses in the anterior mediastinum are most common and include thymoma, lymphoma, and germ cell tumors. Masses in the visceral, or middle, mediastinal subdivision most often are lymphomas or cysts, and those in the posterior mediastinum usually are neurogenic tumors. These neoplasms are discussed in greater detail in Chapter 35, Diseases of the Mediastinum and Chest Wall.

Nearly one half of patients with mediastinal masses are asymptomatic and have a normal physical examination (Darling, 1999). Malignant masses are more likely to cause symptoms of compression or obstruction because malignant disease often is accompanied by distortion and fixation of vital structures that are otherwise mobile enough to conform to distortion from pressure (Shields, 1991). The most common symptoms of mediastinal tumors are chest or back pain, cough, and dyspnea. Tumor location affects the type of symptoms that occur.

Definitive diagnosis of a mediastinal mass before surgical exploration is important. Although many benign and malignant mediastinal masses are best treated with surgical resection, other modalities may be preferable for specific tumors. For example, combination chemotherapy and large-volume radiation therapy is the primary form of therapy for seminoma, a malignant germ cell tumor (Darling, 1999). Tissue for histologic examination may be obtained through mediastinoscopy, mediastinotomy, or, less commonly, thoracoscopy or thoracotomy. In some instances, a cytologic diagnosis can be made from fluid obtained with fine-needle aspiration of a mediastinal mass.

Depending on the location and extent of a mediastinal tumor, surgical resection may be performed using a median sternotomy or right or left posterolateral thoracotomy incision. Neurogenic tumors with intraspinal extension may be approached using a thoracotomy incision that is extended vertically upward along the vertebrae. After entering the mediastinal cavity and exposing the lesion, the surgeon excises all of the mass or as much as is technically possible without injuring nearby vital structures. Even if all malignant disease cannot be totally excised, surgical "debulking" of a mediastinal tumor may be an important component of multimodal therapy. In other cases, adjunctive surgical excision may be performed to remove small residual masses after primary treatment with chemotherapy.

Postoperative care after removal of a mediastinal mass is similar to that of patients who undergo other noncardiac thoracic operations. If a median sternotomy incision has been used, patients typically experience less postoperative pain and pulmonary morbidity than after thoracotomy, in which major chest wall muscles are divided. Mediastinal tube drainage is usually necessary for 24 to 48 hours.

Surgical Bypass of the Superior Vena Cava

Surgical bypass of the superior vena cava (SVC) may be performed in selected patients for treatment of the clinical entity known as SVC syndrome. The SVC is the major blood vessel draining venous blood from the head, neck, upper extremities, and upper thorax; it is confined in a tight compartment in the anterosuperior mediastinum. SVC syndrome develops when the vessel is obstructed either as a result of extrinsic compression or internal occlusion from intraluminal thrombus or a foreign body. It is characterized by swelling of the face, neck, and upper extremities; distention of veins in the neck, shoulder, and chest wall; dyspnea; and cough.

Surgical therapy sometimes is performed in patients with severe SVC syndrome caused by a benign process. Patients with nearly complete to complete SVC obstruction benefit most from an operation to bypass the SVC, particularly when cerebral or airway symptoms of obstruction are present (Doty et al., 1999). The most commonly performed type of SVC bypass consists of placing a vein graft between the innominate or jugular vein and the right atrial appendage of the heart. The operation is performed through a median sternotomy incision, which may be extended onto the neck if the jugular vein is to be used. A biopsy of the obstructing process in the mediastinum is performed, and the upper pericardium is opened to expose the right atrial appendage. The innominate or jugular vein is exposed and mobilized.

Although a number of conduits have been used to bypass the SVC, autologous vein is used most commonly (DeCamp et al., 1996). A composite, or spiral, vein graft often is created to avoid potential venous drainage problems associated with harvesting a vein of similar size to the SVC. The composite graft is fashioned from a segment of autologous saphenous vein harvested from the leg. The vein segment is divided longitudinally and wrapped in spiral fashion around a plastic thoracostomy tube similar in diameter to the vein to which the graft will be anastomosed. The saphenous vein edges are sutured, and an end-to-end anastomosis is created between the innominate or jugular vein and the composite graft. The plastic tube is then removed from within the graft. The proximal end of the graft is sutured to the right atrial appendage.

Spiral vein bypass grafting for SVC obstruction resulting from benign disease is associated with a long-term graft patency rate of 88%; approximately 90% of patients experience total resolution of symptoms related to SVC syndrome (Doty et al., 1999). Early graft thrombosis is the primary complication of the operation (Hartz & Shields, 1991).

REFERENCES

Boyd AD, Glassman LR, 1998: Thoracic incisions. In Kaiser LR, Kron IL, Spray TL (eds): Mastery of Cardiothoracic Surgery. Philadelphia, Lippincott Williams & Wilkins
Boyd AD, Ribakove GH, Sparaco RJ, 1995: Tracheal intubation and mechanical ventilation: The surgeon's viewpoint.

In Sabiston DC Jr, Spencer FC (eds): Surgery of the Chest, ed. 6. Philadelphia, WB Saunders

Bril V, Kojic J, Ilse WK, et al., 1998: Long-term clinical outcome after transcervical thymectomy for myasthenia gravis. Ann Thorac Surg 65:1520

Cohen RG, DeMeester TR, Lafontaine E, 1995: The pleura. In Sabiston DC Jr, Spencer FC (eds): Surgery of the Chest, ed. 6. Philadelphia, WB Saunders

Compeau C, Johnston MR, 1999: Chest-wall tumors. In Casson AG, Johnston MR (eds): Key Topics in Thoracic Surgery. Oxford, Bios

Darling G, 1999: Mediastinum and mediastinal masses. In Casson AG, Johnston MR (eds): Key Topics in Thoracic Surgery. Oxford, Bios

Davis RD Jr, Oldham HN Jr, Sabiston DC Jr, 1995: The mediastinum. In Sabiston DC Jr, Spencer FC (eds): Surgery of the Chest, ed. 6. Philadelphia, WB Saunders

DeCamp MM, Swanson SJ, Sugarbaker DJ, 1996: The mediastinum. In Baue AE, Geha AS, Hammond GL, et al. (eds): Glenn's Thoracic and Cardiovascular Surgery, ed. 6. Stamford, CT, Appleton & Lange

Deslauriers J, Jacques LF, 1995: Surgical techniques: Thoracoplasty. In Pearson FG, Deslauriers J, Ginsberg RJ, et al. (eds): Thoracic Surgery. New York, Churchill Livingstone

Donahue DM, Mathisen DJ, 1998: Tracheal resection and reconstruction. In Kaiser LR, Kron IL, Spray TL (eds): Mastery of Cardiothoracic Surgery. Philadelphia, Lippincott Williams & Wilkins

Doty JR, Flores JH, Doty DB, 1999: Superior vena cava obstruction: Bypass using spiral vein graft. Ann Thorac Surg 67:1111

Golde AR, Irish JC, Gullane PJ, 1995: Surgical techniques: Tracheotomy. In Pearson FG, Deslauriers J, Ginsberg RJ, et al. (eds): Thoracic Surgery. New York, Churchill Livingstone

Grillo HC, 1994: Surgical anatomy of the trachea and techniques of resection. In Shields TW (ed): General Thoracic Surgery, ed. 4. Baltimore, Williams & Wilkins

Grillo HC, 1995: Congenital lesions, neoplasms, inflammation, infections, injuries, and other lesions of the trachea. In Sabiston DC Jr, Spencer FC (eds): Surgery of the Chest, ed. 6. Philadelphia, WB Saunders

Hagen JA, Cooper JD, 1997: Surgical management of myasthenia gravis. In Sabiston DC Jr (ed): Textbook of Surgery: The Biological Basis of Modern Surgical Practice, ed. 15. Philadelphia, WB Saunders

Hartz RS, Shields TW, 1991: Vein grafts and prosthetic grafts for replacement of the superior vena cava. In Shields TW (ed): The Mediastinum. Philadelphia, Lea & Febiger

Keshavjee S, Pearson FG, 1995: Surgical techniques: Tracheal resection. In Pearson FG, Deslauriers J, Ginsberg RJ, et al. (eds): Thoracic Surgery. New York, Churchill Livingstone

Krucylak PE, Naunheim KS, 1999: Preoperative preparation and anesthetic management of patients with myasthenia gravis. Semin Thorac Cardiovasc Surg 11:47

LoCicero J, 1996: Benign and malignant disorders of the pleura. In Baue AE, Geha AS, Hammond GL, et al. (eds): Glenn's Thoracic and Cardiovascular Surgery, ed. 6. Stamford, CT, Appleton & Lange:

Mathisen DJ, Grillo HC, 1996: The trachea: Tracheostomy, tumors, strictures, tracheomalacia, and tracheal resection and reconstruction. In Baue AE, Geha AS, Hammond GL, et al. (eds): Glenn's Thoracic and Cardiovascular Surgery, ed. 6. Stamford, CT, Appleton & Lange

McCormack PM, 1996: Chest wall tumors. In Baue AE, Geha AS, Hammond GL, et al. (eds): Glenn's Thoracic and Cardiovascular Surgery, ed. 6. Stamford, CT, Appleton & Lange

Miller JI, 1998: Surgical resection of the chest wall including the sternum. In Kaiser LR, Kron IL, Spray TL (eds): Mastery of Cardiothoracic Surgery. Philadelphia, Lippincott Williams & Wilkins

Pairolero PC, 1995: Surgical management of neoplasms of the chest wall. In Sabiston DC Jr, Spencer FC (eds): Surgery of the Chest, ed. 6. Philadelphia, WB Saunders

Pearson FG, 1992: Mediastinal tumors. Semin Thorac Cardiovasc Surg 4:1

Pearson FG, Cardoso P, Keshavjee S, 1995: Upper airway tumors: Primary tumors. In Pearson FG, Deslauriers J, Ginsberg RJ, et al. (eds): Thoracic Surgery. New York, Churchill Livingstone

Rusch VW, 1995: Pleural effusion: Benign and malignant. In Pearson FG, Deslauriers J, Ginsberg RJ, et al. (eds): Thoracic Surgery. New York, Churchill Livingstone

Shields TW, 1991: Primary mediastinal tumors and cysts and their diagnostic investigation. In Shields TW (ed): The Mediastinum. Philadelphia, Lea & Febiger

Shields TW, 1994a: Decortication of the lung. In Shields TW (ed): General Thoracic Surgery, ed. 4. Baltimore, Williams & Wilkins

Shields TW, 1994b: Thoracoplasty. In Shields TW (ed): General Thoracic Surgery, ed. 4. Baltimore, Williams & Wilkins

Strollo DC, Rosado de Christenson ML, Jett JR, 1997: Primary mediastinal tumors: Part I. Tumors of the anterior mediastinum. Chest 112:511

Sugarbaker DJ, Garcia JP, 1998: Multimodality therapy for malignant pleural mesothelioma. Chest 112(Suppl 4):272S

Trastek VF, 1998: Thymectomy. In Kaiser LR, Kron IL, Spray TL (eds): Mastery of Cardiothoracic Surgery. Philadelphia, Lippincott Williams & Wilkins

Trastek VF, Pairolero PC, 1991: Standard thymectomy. In Shields TW (ed): The Mediastinum. Philadelphia, Lea & Febiger

Trastek VF, Shields TW, 1994: Surgery of the thymus gland. In Shields TW (ed): General Thoracic Surgery, ed. 4. Baltimore, Williams & Wilkins

Webb WR, Harrison LH, 1996: Pleural space problems and thoracoplasty. In Baue AE, Geha AS, Hammond GL, et al. (eds): Glenn's Thoracic and Cardiovascular Surgery, ed. 6. Stamford, CT, Appleton & Lange

Wechsler AS, 1995: Surgical management of myasthenia gravis. In Sabiston DC Jr, Spencer FC (eds): Surgery of the Chest, ed. 6. Philadelphia, WB Saunders

POSTOPERATIVE
MANAGEMENT

41

Postoperative Management of Thoracic Surgical Patients

Kimberly Wilder, RN, MSN, ACNP
and Betsy Finkelmeier, RN, MS, MM

Thoracic surgery may be performed as treatment for diseases of the lungs, esophagus, or mediastinum. Pulmonary resection is the most frequently performed thoracic operation, usually in patients with carcinoma of the lung. It is the treatment of choice for lung cancer because it provides the best chances of survival. Although the postoperative regimen varies somewhat depending on the specific disease and type of operation, many components of postoperative care are similar for all types of noncardiac thoracic surgery. Most patients follow a predictable course of recovery. Typically, patients undergoing a routine lobectomy or pneumonectomy remain in an intensive or intermediate care unit for 24 hours after surgery and then continue their convalescence on a general postoperative unit. Many patients can be discharged after 4 to 6 days (Table 41-1).

► The Postoperative Regimen

Early Management

Transfer from the operating room to the recovery room or intensive care unit is performed when the operation is concluded and the patient's vital signs demonstrate hemodynamic stability. The anesthesiologist or surgeon accompanies the patient and communicates information to the nurse regarding (1) the operation performed and type of anesthesia used, (2) any significant intraoperative findings or complications, (3) the amount of intraoperative blood products and fluids administered, and (4) any current medication or fluid infusions.

The nurse's first priority on patient arrival is reestablishment of monitoring capabilities, appropriate chest tube management, and, if the patient is still intubated, mechanical ventilation. Vital signs are measured to confirm hemodynamic stability, and an overall assessment of the patient's condition is performed. Intravenous catheters are assessed for patency and proper infusion rates. The arterial catheter, chest tubes, urethral catheter, and nasogastric tube are examined for proper functioning.

Continuous electrocardiographic, arterial pressure, and pulse oximetry monitoring usually are performed while the patient is in the recovery room or intensive care unit. Vital signs, including heart rate, respiratory rate, blood pressure, and temperature, are recorded every 1 to 2 hours, or more frequently if the patient's condition is unstable (Table 41-2).

Breath sounds are auscultated every 2 to 4 hours, and the presence of diminished or adventitious sounds is noted. Many patients can be extubated in the operating room or shortly after admission to the recovery area. If so, supplemental oxygen using a high-humidity delivery system is administered for several days. In patients who have undergone airway or lung surgery, early extubation is particularly desirable because extended mechanical

TABLE 41-1

Clinical Pathway for Patients Undergoing Thoracotomy

Interventions	DOS:ICU	POD #1	POD #2	POD #3	POD #4
Tests	CBC/platelets, BCP ABG per protocol BG q6h if diabetic Portable CXR	CBC/platelets, BCP Glucometer q6h if diabetic Portable CXR	PA/lateral CXR (1 in AM and 1 after D/C chest tubes)	PA/lateral CXR	PA/lateral CXR
Treatments	Cardiac monitor VS per protocol Initiate weaning protocol, I&O q1h Chest tube −20 cm suction Foley catheter	Telemetry, RT Chest tubes to water-seal drainage Transfer to floor VS q8h, IS q1h w/a I&O q4h, PIL Daily weight, Foley	VS qs Incision care Wean oxygen IS q1h w/a Daily weight D/C telemetry, chest tubes, epidural, Foley	VS qs Daily weight IS q1h w/a Incision care	VS qs IS q1h w/a Incision care Daily weight
Medications	ATB × 3 doses Epidural analgesia	Resume preoperative medications	PO analgesia after D/C epidural	PO analgesia	PO analgesia
Diet	NPO, clear liquids 4 h after extubation	Advance to preoperative diet	Preoperative diet	Preoperative diet	Preoperative diet
Activity	Bedrest, consult PT if needed	OOB to chair Ambulate in room	Ambulate × 3 PT	Ambulate × 5 PT	Ambulate × 6 PT
Education and Discharge Planning	Discuss plan of care with family Orient to ICU	Discuss plan of care Functional assessment Pastoral care prn	Consult HHS, SW prn	Discharge instructions Discharge plan finalized Prescriptions reviewed	Review discharge instructions and prescriptions Discharge home

DOS, day of surgery; ICU, intensive care unit, POD, postoperative day; CBC, complete blood count; BCP, blood chemistry panel; ABG, arterial blood gas; BG, blood glucose; CXR, chest roentgenogram; PA, posteroanterior; D/C, discontinue; VS, vital signs; I&O, intake and output; RT, respiratory therapy; IS, incentive spirometry; w/a, while awake; PIL, peripheral intravenous heparin lock; qs, every shift; ATB, antibiotics; PO, orally; NPO, nothing by mouth; PT, physical therapy; OOB, out of bed; HHS, home health service; SW, social worker.

ventilation may cause barotrauma and contribute to bronchopleural fistula development (Quill, 1992). Data demonstrate that patients requiring prolonged postoperative intubation have a higher mortality and morbidity rate and prolonged hospitalization (Desiderio & Downey, 1998).

If mechanical ventilation is required, an intermittent mandatory ventilation mode usually is used and the patient is weaned during the first 24 hours. Continuous pulse oximetry monitoring is performed and arterial blood gases are measured after changes are made in ventilatory parameters or as warranted by changes in the patient's condition. While the patient is ventilated, a nasogastric tube is usually in place to prevent gastric distention from swallowed air. Weaning and extubation are performed when the patient demonstrates adequate respiratory parameters for self-ventilation (eg, arterial oxygen tension > 60 mm Hg, arterial carbon dioxide tension < 50 mm Hg, respiratory rate < 30 breaths per minute, negative inspiratory force > −25 cm H_2O, and vital capacity > 15 mL/kg) (Sandler, 1995). The patient's level of mentation also influences the timing of weaning and extubation. The most common causes of ventilatory weaning failure are pneumo-

nia, bronchopleural fistula, bronchial spasm, and respiratory muscle fatigue (Todd & Ralph-Edwards, 1995).

Patients usually are normovolemic with electrolytes in balance when leaving the operating room (Deschamps et al., 1992a). Maintenance intravenous fluids are administered until the patient is alert enough to take liquids orally. Patients who have undergone lung resection should not receive excessive intravenous fluid either during or after surgery. Intraoperative lung manipulation and collapse may impair pulmonary lymphatic drainage and lead to increased extravasation of fluid; excessive fluid administration during the operation may result in pulmonary edema, decreased alveolar gas permeability, and decreased pulmonary compliance, which fosters atelectasis and further hypoxia (Todd & Ralph-Edwards, 1995). Patients who have undergone pneumonectomy are particularly sensitive to volume overload because one half of the pulmonary vascular bed has been removed (Amar, 1997). Consequently, fluid status is carefully monitored after pneumonectomy, maintenance fluid repletion is reduced, and blood transfusion is avoided if possible (Deschamps et al., 1992b). In patients with a history of cardiac dis-

TABLE 41-2

Desirable Parameters in Postoperative Thoracic Surgical Patients

Parameter	Desired Values
Heart rate	60–100 beats per minute
Blood pressure	100–140 mm Hg (systolic)
Respiratory rate	16–24 breaths per minute
Oxygen saturation	> 90%
Temperature	< 37.5°C
Urine output	> 30 mL/h
Chest tube output	< 100 mL/h

ease, a central venous or pulmonary artery catheter may be in place to guide perioperative fluid administration. Intake and output from the urinary drainage catheter are recorded hourly.

Chest tubes are assessed frequently during the early postoperative hours to ensure patency, record blood loss, and to check for an air leak. The rate of bleeding usually is 100 mL/h or less and decreases over the first few postoperative hours. In addition to monitoring chest tube output, postoperative bleeding is assessed by serial hematocrit evaluations, examination of a postoperative chest roentgenogram for detection of hemothorax, and observation of the patient for clinical manifestations of hypovolemia.

A chest roentgenogram, complete blood cell count, arterial blood gas, and blood chemistry survey are obtained shortly after patient arrival in the recovery area. The chest roentgenogram demonstrates the position of intrathoracic tubes and catheters and allows early detection of pathophysiologic events, such as pneumothorax, hemothorax, atelectasis, or mediastinal shift. It also provides a baseline for comparison with subsequent roentgenograms when evaluating clinical problems that arise during the postoperative period. Ideally, the initial postoperative chest roentgenogram demonstrates full lung expansion (ie, no pneumothorax) and minimal or no hemothorax. The roentgenogram in a patient who has undergone pneumonectomy demonstrates an empty hemithorax on the operative side with only a small amount of fluid in the space. After removal of the entire lung, the pleural space fills gradually with serosanguineous fluid until the hemithorax is full and the air is absorbed (Cohen et al., 1995).

While the patient is on bed rest, repositioning is performed every 2 hours. Repositioning the patient at regular intervals lessens ventilation–perfusion mismatching that occurs because pulmonary arterial blood flow is directed preferentially to dependent portions of lung and remaining segments are better ventilated. Intermittent repositioning also lessens retention of bronchial secretions in dependent portions of the lungs and facilitates drainage of accumulated blood from the pleural space.

The head of the bed usually is maintained in a slightly elevated position (45 degrees) to enhance effectiveness of deep breathing and clearing of secretions. Particularly in

obese patients, elevating the head of the bed avoids impingement of abdominal viscera on diaphragmatic movement. After pneumonectomy, the patient is positioned either on the back or with the operative side down to avoid retention of secretions and hypoventilation in the remaining lung.

Continued Management

In patients who have undergone pulmonary resection, an oral diet usually is resumed on the first postoperative day and advanced gradually. Medications that the patient has been taking before surgery are reinstituted with the diet. An NPO status is maintained for longer periods after esophageal resection or repair procedures, as discussed later in the chapter. Daily weights are obtained throughout the postoperative period to assist in evaluation of the patient's fluid status.

The patient usually can sit in a chair and ambulate across the room on the first postoperative day, unless prolonged mechanical ventilation is necessary. Getting the patient out of bed is one of the most important postoperative lung expansion maneuvers; it increases functional residual capacity as much as 10% to 20% (Ronan & Murray, 1992). Ambulation in the corridor at least three to four times per day begins on the second postoperative day if the hemodynamic and ventilatory status are stable. Activity should progress so that each day walking is performed more frequently and for longer periods. By the third and fourth postoperative day, the patient is usually spending most of the day out of bed and ambulating in the corridor four to five times daily. The patient is also encouraged to increase gradually the range of motion to the arm on the operative side.

After the first 24 hours, the sterile dressing covering the surgical incision is removed and the incision remains uncovered. The incision is cleansed daily and inspected for drainage or erythema of surrounding tissue. The need for perioperative antibiotic prophylaxis in patients who undergo thoracic operations remains controversial. Many surgeons administer two to three doses during the postoperative period with no preoperative dose. A cephalosporin (vancomycin in penicillin-allergic patients) typically is chosen for prophylaxis against infection because of its broad antibiotic spectrum and low incidence of associated toxicity and side effects (Kaiser, 1995).

▶ Pulmonary Hygiene Interventions

Attention to the patient's *pulmonary status* is one of the most important components of postoperative nursing management in thoracic surgical patients. Observation of the patient's respirations and careful auscultation may reveal early evidence of atelectasis, pneumothorax, or pulmonary edema before clinical deterioration of the patient (Table 41-3).

A number of factors associated with thoracic operations impair the efficiency of respiratory gas exchange

TABLE 41-3

Clinical Indicators of Respiratory Insufficiency

PATIENT APPEARANCE
Agitation
Confusion
Anxiety
Somnolence
Ashen color
Diaphoresis

VITAL SIGNS
Tachypnea
Tachycardia
Elevated temperature

ARTERIAL BLOOD GAS MEASUREMENTS
Decreasing PaO_2
Decreasing oxygen saturation
Increasing $PaCO_2$

PULMONARY AUSCULTATION
Diminished breath sounds
Rhonchi
Rales

PaO_2, partial pressure of arterial oxygen; $PaCO_2$, partial pressure of arterial carbon dioxide.

and ventilation during the postoperative period. Some degree of atelectasis is always present because of the decrease in functional residual capacity that accompanies a thoracotomy (Joob & Hartz, 1994). Incisional discomfort, immobility, and pain medications contribute to continued atelectasis. In addition, many operations on the thorax are performed using single-lung anesthesia, in which one lung is maintained in a deflated state for the duration of the operation. After operations on the esophagus, a nasogastric tube remains in place for several postoperative days and impairs effective coughing and clearing of secretions.

The postoperative changes in pulmonary function are present immediately after a thoracic operation, slowly worsen during the next 1 to 2 days and, in most patients, then return to normal (Anderson & Bartlett, 1991). Patients who undergo pulmonary resection are at particular risk for respiratory complications because the loss of functional lung tissue is often superimposed on underlying obstructive pulmonary disease. Consistent pulmonary hygiene interventions are necessary to evacuate retained pulmonary secretions and eliminate atelectasis. Although pneumonia after thoracotomy is less common than in the past, it remains an important source of perioperative morbidity and mortality (Nelson & Moran, 1992).

Respiratory maneuvers that facilitate maximal lung inflation are important because shallow breathing, the lack of spontaneous deep breaths, and alveolar collapse are the steps that lead to postoperative deterioration of pulmonary function (Anderson & Bartlett, 1991). As soon as

consciousness is regained, the patient is assisted in deep breathing and coughing maneuvers every 1 to 2 hours to ensure that pulmonary secretions are cleared and atelectatic segments are reexpanded. Typically, the patient uses an incentive spirometry device intermittently to take and sustain a series of deep inspirations. After several cycles of deep breathing, the patient coughs forcefully. A pillow or blanket is usually placed against the incisional area to brace the chest wall and reduce discomfort.

Some thoracic surgeons also advocate routine chest physiotherapy (eg, postural drainage, chest percussion, and vibration) (Fig. 41-1). However, these procedures produce a fair amount of discomfort in the presence of a thoracotomy incision. Unless significant underlying pulmonary impairment is present, many patients can clear secretions effectively and maintain full lung expansion with incentive spirometry, coughing, and early ambulation alone. More aggressive interventions, including chest physiotherapy or aerosolized bronchodilator treatments, are instituted promptly in (1) patients with tenacious secretions or marginal pulmonary function, or (2) those with fever and auscultatory or radiographic evidence of atelectasis.

Nasotracheal suctioning is performed in patients who are unable to clear secretions with coughing. With the patient in an upright position, a catheter is inserted through the nose until it reaches the pharynx, where a gagging reflex is produced. As the patient takes slow, deep breaths, the catheter is advanced at the beginning of a deep inspiration through the vocal cords and into the trachea (Allen & Pairolero, 1996). Once the catheter is in the trachea, it can be intermittently attached to low suction for 5 to 10 seconds at a time. A small amount of

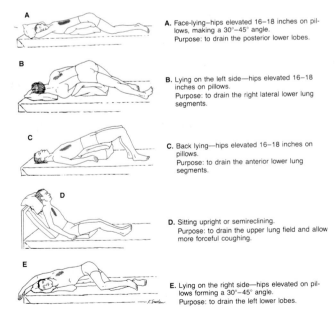

A. Face-lying—hips elevated 16–18 inches on pillows, making a 30°–45° angle.
Purpose: to drain the posterior lower lobes.

B. Lying on the left side—hips elevated 16–18 inches on pillows.
Purpose: to drain the right lateral lower lung segments.

C. Back lying—hips elevated 16–18 inches on pillows.
Purpose: to drain the anterior lower lung segments.

D. Sitting upright or semireclining.
Purpose: to drain the upper lung field and allow more forceful coughing.

E. Lying on the right side—hips elevated on pillows forming a 30°–45° angle.
Purpose: to drain the left lower lobes.

FIGURE 41-1. Positioning of patient for postural lung drainage. (Hudak CM, Gallo BM, Morton PG, 1998: Patient management: Respiratory system. In Critical Care Nursing: A Holistic Approach, ed. 7. Philadelphia, Lippincott Williams & Wilkins)

saline may be instilled through the catheter to induce coughing and loosen tenacious secretions. A high concentration of oxygen is administered throughout the suctioning procedure and the patient is closely observed for evidence of cardiac arrhythmias or profound hypoxemia. Nasotracheal suctioning usually is quite uncomfortable for the patient. It is made easier if patient cooperation is elicited at the beginning of the procedure and the catheter is well lubricated and inserted gently.

Infrequently, a patient retains copious amounts of secretions that cannot be evacuated with nasotracheal suctioning. Serial bronchoscopy with deep lavage and suctioning may be required to prevent respiratory failure and the need for intubation and mechanical ventilation. In patients receiving aggressive pulmonary hygiene therapy, adequate rest periods must be provided between treatments. Otherwise, fatigue and increased oxygen consumption associated with the interventions can worsen hypoinflation or hypoxemia (Hawthorne, 1992). Minitracheostomy is an effective surgical technique to provide assistance in the removal of airway secretions (Callaghan et al., 1994). Minitracheostomy is achieved by inserting a flanged, small-diameter cannula through the cricothyroid membrane into the trachea to be used for frequent suctioning in patients with copious secretions (Fig. 41-2). The procedure can be performed at the bedside, presents minimal risk to the patient, and helps to prevent postoperative sputum retention, atelectasis, and complications that are common in patients with poor lung function. The catheter may stay in place for the duration of the hospitalization and removal of the cannula results in stoma closure within 48 hours (Wain et al., 1990).

Prolonged mechanical ventilation may be required in the postoperative period for a number of reasons, including prolonged anesthesia, fluid overload, potential space problems after pulmonary resection (ie, when spontaneous ventilation does not result in expansion of the operative lung to fill the entire hemithorax), hemodynamic instability, myocardial ischemia or infarction, or acute respiratory failure (Todd, 1989). Underlying chronic obstructive pulmonary disease and chest wall splinting secondary to inadequate pain control also may contribute to the need for prolonged ventilatory support.

▶ Drainage of the Pleural Space

Most noncardiac thoracic operations are performed through a thoracotomy incision. At the conclusion of the operation, chest drainage tubes are placed in the pleural

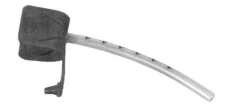

FIGURE 41-2. Minitracheostomy tube. (Courtesy of SIMS Portex, Inc., Keene, NH)

space for postoperative evacuation of blood and air from the thorax. Usually, two large-bore chest tubes are placed in the operative hemithorax. The tubes are inserted through separate small skin incisions in the anterolateral chest wall so that the patient can lie comfortably in a supine position without compressing the chest tubes (Deschamps et al., 1992a). One chest tube usually is directed anteriorly toward the apex to evacuate air that rises to the top of the pleural space; the other tube is directed posteriorly to drain fluid that collects in dependent areas.

Postoperative drainage of the pleural space is unique because of the negative pressure that normally exists within the thorax. Chest tubes are connected to a sterile drainage system with the capability of underwater seal and suction drainage. A controlled amount of continuous suction (-20 cm H_2O is the conventional amount) commonly is applied to the pleural space during the early postoperative period. Applying suction helps achieve full expansion of the lung so that visceral and parietal pleural surfaces appose; cessation of both air leakage and bleeding is enhanced by apposition of the pleural surfaces. Except when excessive amounts of lung tissue have been removed, the remaining lung tissue usually expands to fill the entire hemithorax. Once the lung is fully expanded, the chest drainage system often is converted to water seal drainage without suction.

The surgeon achieves hemostasis and seals leaking alveolar surfaces of the lung before closing a thoracotomy incision. Nevertheless, some degree of bleeding and (after pulmonary resection operations) air leakage can be anticipated in the postoperative period. Bleeding usually originates from oozing surfaces of incised pulmonary parenchyma or from areas where pleural adhesions have been divided. Adequate chest tube drainage prevents accumulation of blood in the pleural space. A hemothorax prevents full expansion of the ipsilateral lung. It also provides an excellent medium for growth of bacteria and may lead to empyema and possible entrapment of the lung in a collapsed state. Sometimes blood pools in the pleural space while the patient is lying in one position for a prolonged time; if so, a large quantity of blood (400 to 500 mL) may drain rapidly into the chest tube drainage system when the patient is repositioned.

Chest drainage is also important to evacuate air from the pleural space. Patients who have had a portion of a lung removed normally have air leakage that persists for several days. After lobectomy, air leakage usually originates from areas where incomplete fissures were divided. Air leaks after wedge resection or segmentectomy arise from raw parenchymal surfaces produced through creation of intersegmental planes (Duhaylongsod & Wolfe, 1992). Air may also leak from denuded parenchyma in areas where the lung was adherent to the undersurface of the chest wall.

Occasionally, an air leak persists for more than a week. In most instances, such prolonged air leaks represent inadequate healing or closure of distal bronchioles or alveoli (ie, a bronchoalveolar-pleural fistula) (Rice & Kirby, 1992). If a vigorous air leak is present, it is advisable to maintain negative suction to the chest tubes at all times. Extension tubing may be added to the suction source to allow the patient to ambulate freely in the room. Once the lung is fully expanded and the air leak is small, suction is often discontinued and the tubes are maintained with underwater seal drainage. This allows the patient to ambulate more freely. Most persistent air leaks eventually seal with continued thoracostomy drainage. It is important that each nurse caring for the patient regularly check for the presence of an air leak and for secure attachment of the chest tube to the patient and a tight connection between the chest tube and drainage system tubing. Breaks in integrity of the closed drainage system allow air entry into the system, causing a false air leak and possible delay in chest tube removal.

The severity of an air leak is evaluated by the proportion of the respiratory cycle during which bubbling is observed in the water seal chamber of the chest drainage system. Large air leaks produce continuous bubbling, whereas small to moderate leaks produce bubbling only during expiration in self-ventilating patients and during inspiration in those who are mechanically ventilated (Elefteriades et al., 1996). Sometimes, an air leak persists that is slight enough that it produces only intermittent bubbling in the water seal chamber and thus remains undetected. If there is any uncertainty about whether a slight air leak remains, the surgeon may choose to obtain a chest roentgenogram while the chest tube is clamped. If the chest roentgenogram reveals a pneumothorax or the patient experiences symptoms, the tube is promptly unclamped. This maneuver, which is the only indication for clamping a chest tube, reveals the need for continued pleural drainage and spares the patient the discomfort of having a tube removed, only to require insertion of another tube several hours later.

While chest tubes are in place, chest roentgenograms usually are obtained on a daily basis to evaluate lung expansion and the presence of pleural air or fluid. Chest tubes are removed when there is no leakage of air and when bleeding has ceased or is less than 100 to 150 mL/24 hours. In patients in whom an esophageal resection has been performed, chest tubes usually remain until the absence of leakage from the esophageal anastomosis is confirmed by contrast esophagography. Chest tubes also may remain in place in patients requiring prolonged mechanical ventilation with high levels of positive end-expiratory pressure because of the likelihood of barotrauma with resultant tension pneumothorax.

Removal of a pleural chest tube requires careful adherence to technique to prevent iatrogenic pneumothorax. In mechanically ventilated patients, one person delivers and sustains a deep inspiration with a self-inflating bag while a second person removes the chest tube and applies an occlusive dressing. In self-ventilating patients, thoracic surgeons usually advocate one of two techniques. The rationale guiding both techniques is to minimize the likelihood of the patient gasping as the tube is removed and thereby drawing air into the pleural space through the subcutaneous tube tract. The tube is removed quickly from the chest either (1) while the patient is performing a Valsalva maneuver after a deep inspira-

tion, or (2) during a full exhalation. With either technique, an occlusive dressing is applied to the chest tube site as the tube is withdrawn.

Operations performed through median sternotomy incisions (eg, mediastinal tumor resection) necessitate tube thoracostomy drainage of blood from the mediastinum. Mediastinal tubes are inserted through small incisions below the xiphoid process. Patients who have undergone pneumonectomy usually have no chest tube placed or a chest tube is placed and clamped for the first 12 to 24 hours after surgery. During a pneumonectomy, the entire lung is removed from the hemithorax and the remaining bronchial segment is securely closed with suture. Application of continuous negative suction to the empty hemithorax could produce undesirable shifting of the mediastinum toward the operative side.

If no chest tube is placed (or a tube is placed and clamped), pressure within the operative hemithorax is adjusted at the conclusion of the operation to approximate a negative pressure of 2 to 4 cm H_2O during inspiration and a positive pressure of 2 to 4 cm H_2O during expiration (Shields, 1994). Adjusting pressure in the empty hemithorax maintains the mediastinum in a midline position. It is usually accomplished after closing the thoracic incision by aspiration of air through thoracentesis. A chest tube may be inserted at the time of pneumonectomy and placed to water seal drainage *without suction* if the pleural space is infected or unusual bleeding is anticipated. Management of chest tubes is discussed in more detail in Chapter 42, Pleural Thoracostomy Drainage.

► Postoperative Pain Management

Pain management is an integral part of the postoperative recovery for the patient undergoing a thoracic surgical procedure. Research has shown that thoracic surgical procedures cause more and longer-lasting pain than most other incisions, including sternotomy. The pain associated with a thoracotomy (chest wall) incision, division of the chest wall musculature, and the presence of drainage tubes, results from the neural activation of somatic fibers (Jain & Datta, 1997). Thus, it is normal for patients to have a great deal of postoperative discomfort, particularly when moving about and when performing deep breathing and coughing exercises. Excessive pain and splinting can result in a decrease in vital capacity, retention of secretions, atelectasis, ventilation–perfusion mismatch, and deterioration of arterial blood oxygenation (Deschamps et al., 1992a). Postoperative pain has several other detrimental effects, including (1) an increase in cardiac work that may provoke cardiac arrhythmias or myocardial ischemia; (2) an increase in vagal tone, resulting in a propensity for nausea and vomiting; and (3) elevated hormonal tone leading to water retention and hyperglycemia (Joob & Hartz, 1994). Adequate pain relief has been shown to reduce morbidity and mortality rates and shorten hospitalization by reducing the stress response (Jain & Datta, 1997).

One of the most common methods of pain management in thoracic surgical patients is *epidural anesthesia* (ie, delivery of analgesic agents through a catheter positioned in the epidural space) (Fig. 41-3). The catheter may be inserted in the operating or recovery room and usually remains in place for 1 to 3 days. The direct application of narcotics into the epidural space produces effective pain relief without the heavy sedation and respiratory depression associated with intravenous or intramuscular narcotics (Bragg, 1989). As a result, patients arrive in the recovery area alert and relatively pain free, thus reducing the likelihood of hypoventilation (Hawthorne, 1992).

Agents commonly used for epidural analgesia include the opioids fentanyl, morphine, methadone, and meperidine and the local anesthetic bupivacaine (Marcaine) (Piccione & Faber, 1991). The analgesia, dosing guidelines, management of side effects, and catheter care are managed by a member of the postoperative analgesia service, but the nurse must be aware of the desired and adverse effects of the medications being given. The level of analgesia and degree of respiratory depression or somnolence must be continuously assessed so that adjustments can be made to maintain an adequate level of pain control without excessive sedation (Lubenow et al., 1994).

A disadvantage of epidural analgesia is that an infusion pump is necessary for dosage titration. A urethral catheter usually remains in place as well because of possible associated urinary retention. Patient mobility is somewhat curtailed by these attachments, and assistance must be given to the patient to ensure progressive mobility. Common side effects of epidural analgesia include pruritus, nausea and vomiting, and urinary retention.

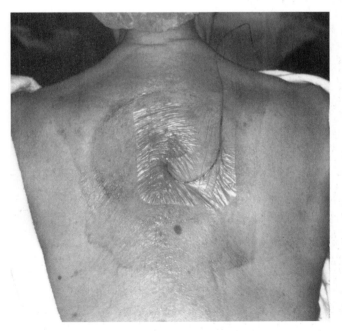

FIGURE 41-3. Epidural catheter has been placed just before anesthesia induction in this patient who is about to undergo a thoracotomy for pulmonary resection.

Epidural analgesia also may be complicated by dural puncture and spinal headache, total spinal blockade, hypotension, and tachyphylaxis (Jain & Datta, 1997).

Postoperative pain control may be achieved alternatively with parenteral administration of opioids. Morphine sulfate commonly is used. During the early postoperative period, opioids usually are administered intravenously if the patient is mechanically ventilated or under continuous observation in an intensive care unit. When the patient is moved to a general nursing unit, an intramuscular route is used for narcotic administration. A disadvantage of intramuscular narcotics is the varying level of analgesia, with excessive pain at low narcotic levels and possible respiratory depression or confusion at high levels.

Alternatively, intravenous narcotics may be administered on the general nursing unit using a patient-controlled system (ie, *patient-controlled analgesia*). Commercially designed pump systems allow the patient to self-administer predetermined doses of pain medication intravenously. A lockout interval prevents the patient from administering medication too frequently. Devices typically allow delivery of a continuous infusion of medication that can be supplemented with patient-controlled boluses; the devices also record a profile of the drug administration (Lubenow et al., 1994). Morphine or meperidine is used commonly.

An infrequently used method of postoperative pain management is *interpleural regional analgesia*. A catheter is placed percutaneously through the chest wall directly into the pleural space. Pain medication is then infused continuously or intermittently into the space between the visceral and parietal pleura. Local anesthetics infused into the pleural space diffuse through the parietal pleura to the intercostal neurovascular bundle, producing a unilateral nerve block at multiple levels (Lubenow et al., 1994). In patients with persistent chest wall pain, the surgeon may perform intercostal nerve blockade. Bupivacaine solution is injected percutaneously into the area of the intercostal nerve (subcostal groove on the undersurface of the rib) of several subsequent rib segments. If successful pain relief is achieved, the procedure may be repeated.

Regardless of the system used for pain control, it is necessary to medicate the patient adequately so that deep breathing, coughing, and ambulation can be performed without a great deal of discomfort. However, toxic effects may result from overzealous pain control. Probably the most commonly seen deleterious effects are oversedation, confusion, and psychosis. Development of any neurologic changes should prompt reassessment and reduction of medication dosing. Because patients tend to require prolonged use of narcotics during the first week after thoracotomy, constipation is almost routine and ileus can occur. Daily assessment of bowel function is important, and administration of laxatives may be necessary. Signs of developing ileus include abdominal distention, absence of bowel sounds, and lack of bowel movements or flatus. In the late postoperative period and by the time of discharge, the patient usually is taking only oral analgesics. Acetaminophen (Tylenol) with codeine or hydrocodone bitartrate (Vicodin) may be prescribed when the patient is discharged.

► Potential Postoperative Problems

The major problems that can arise in the postoperative period are arrhythmias, myocardial infarction, respiratory insufficiency, and hemorrhage. *Postoperative arrhythmias* occur in 9% to 33% of patients who undergo thoracic operations, usually within 1 to 5 days after surgery (Amar, 1997). Despite extensive experimental and clinical investigation, the etiology of most arrhythmias that occur after thoracotomy is multifactorial and incompletely understood (Ferguson, 1992). Supraventricular tachycardia (SVT), especially atrial fibrillation or atrial flutter, is particularly common in postoperative patients (Fig. 41-4).

Supraventricular arrhythmias develop in an estimated 20% of patients who undergo pulmonary resection (Kaiser, 1998). The extent of resection and age of the patient are the most important risk factors for development of arrhythmias. Digoxin and diltiazem usually are used for treatment; digoxin also may be given prophylactically to patients with an increased risk for postoperative supraventricular arrhythmias. Other antiarrhythmic agents used to treat postoperative SVT include quinidine, procainamide, and verapamil (Amar, 1997). Beta-blocking medications are used infrequently in thoracic surgical patients because of the prevalence of obstructive pulmonary disease and of congestive heart failure; both conditions are contraindications to the use of beta-blocking agents because of the potential for bronchospasm and worsening of heart failure. The most important component of treating postoperative SVT is control of the ventricular rate.

Postoperative ventricular arrhythmias are less common and almost always occur transiently. They are often the result of a precipitating factor, such as hypoxemia or hypokalemia. Less commonly, ventricular arrhythmias develop secondary to acute myocardial ischemia or infarction. Intravenous lidocaine is administered if premature ventricular contractions are multifocal, occur in couplets or at a frequency greater than six per minute, or fall on the T wave of the preceding complex.

Perioperative myocardial infarction occurs in a small number of patients who undergo thoracic operations. Patients at greatest risk are those with underlying coronary artery disease and unstable angina, recent myocardial infarction, congestive heart failure, uncontrolled hypertension, or critical aortic stenosis (Hillis et al., 1995). Perioperative myocardial ischemia is most likely during the first 48 hours when major alterations occur in adrenergic activity, plasma catecholamine levels, body temperature, pulmonary function, fluid balance, and pain (Mathisen & Wain, 1992).

Respiratory insufficiency occurs occasionally during the postoperative period. Patients at greatest risk are those with marginal pulmonary function who undergo lobectomy or pneumonectomy and debilitated patients who undergo esophageal resection. Respiratory failure almost always necessitates prolonged intubation and mechanical ventilation, which can lead to a number of deleterious consequences. The presence of an indwelling endotracheal tube provides a route for tracheobronchial contamination that can lead to pneumonia. Also, mechanical ventilation can produce barotrauma, possible rupture of bronchial anastomoses, and continuation of parenchymal air leaks.

Excessive bleeding is uncommon after noncardiac thoracic operations. It can originate from oozing blood vessels in the parenchyma or chest wall muscles or occur secondary to a coagulation abnormality. Rarely, disruption of a pulmonary artery or vein ligature causes massive hemorrhage. Sustained blood loss greater than 150 mL/h in the absence of abnormal coagulation usually necessitates reexploration of the thorax. Manifestations of excessive bleeding are less obvious in patients who have undergone pneumonectomy without chest tube placement. Because blood accumulates in the empty hemithorax, other indicators of bleeding, such as hematocrit level, radiographic evidence of an increasing fluid level in the operative hemithorax, and clinical signs of hypovolemia, are used to detect significant blood loss. Complications are discussed in more detail in Chapter 43, Complications of Thoracic Operations.

► Special Considerations

Considerations After Esophageal Surgery

Patients who have undergone an esophageal surgical procedure almost always have a nasogastric tube placed at the time of operation. Maintaining proper function of the

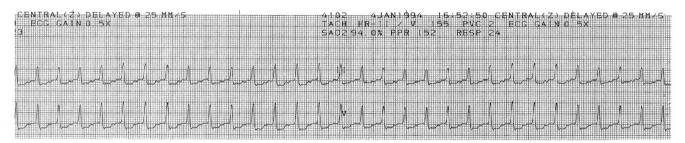

FIGURE 41-4. Postoperative supraventricular tachycardia; rhythm tracing on postoperative day 2 in patient who underwent lobectomy demonstrates atrial flutter with a ventricular rate of 152 beats per minute.

nasogastric tube is particularly important in the early period after general anesthesia when the patient has not yet regained the cough reflex; regurgitation and aspiration can occur if the tube is not functioning properly (Orringer, 1991a). Also, because the nasogastric tube interferes with the patient's ability to cough and clear secretions effectively, pulmonary hygiene interventions are essential to avoid retention of secretions and atelectasis.

The length of time that a nasogastric tube remains in place depends on two factors: (1) the return of normal bowel function, and (2) the likelihood of postoperative esophageal disruption. Operations that require only a partial-thickness incision or the placement of sutures in the esophagus are less often associated with esophageal disruption than are procedures that necessitate surgical division and anastomosis of the esophagus (Table 41-4). However, esophageal perforation can occur after any operation on the esophagus. For example, during antireflux operations, the esophagus may be perforated during intraoperative esophagoscopy, secondary to stricture disruption during esophageal dilatation, or at the site of gastric or esophageal sutures placed during the repair (Orringer, 1991b). Consequently, esophageal integrity usually is evaluated by contrast esophagogram before beginning postoperative oral nourishment; an esophagogram is repeated if unexplained fever, mental status changes, or chest pain develop after a diet is resumed.

After operations in which esophageal disruption is unlikely, the nasogastric tube remains in place for 24 to 48 hours and oral feedings usually can be resumed when the patient begins passing flatus or has a bowel movement. After operations in which the esophagus has been surgically divided, nasogastric suction is continued for approximately 4 to 5 days. The nasogastric tube is secured with tape and the patient restrained, if necessary, to prevent tube dislodgment. Reinsertion or manipulation of a nasogastric tube after esophageal resection is performed by the surgeon. If a proximal esophageal anastomosis is present,

TABLE 41-4

Risk of Esophageal Disruption After Esophageal Operations

OPERATIONS WITH LESS RISK*
Esophagomyotomy
Antireflux procedures
  Nissen fundoplication
  Belsey mark IV operation
  Hill posterior gastropexy

OPERATIONS WITH GREATER RISK†
Esophagectomy or esophagogastrectomy
  With esophagogastrostomy
  With colon interposition
Repair of esophageal perforation

*Procedures include partial-thickness incision or placement of sutures in esophagus.
†Procedures include surgical division and anastomosis of the esophagus.

endotracheal suctioning is avoided or performed with caution because of the potential for disrupting the anastomosis if the catheter is introduced into the esophagus.

Malnourishment is a common problem in patients who require esophageal resection. The underlying disease is often esophageal cancer with associated dysphagia and a compromised nutritional status. A feeding jejunostomy usually is placed during surgery so that adequate nutrition can be maintained throughout the postoperative period. If the gastrointestinal tract is functional, enteral feedings are preferable because of the risk of sepsis associated with central venous hyperalimentation. Enteral feedings also are thought to maintain gut integrity, thus reducing translocation or the movement of enteric pathogens across the bowel mucosa and into the systemic circulation (Berry & Braunschweig, 1998). The potential for enteral feedings to prevent sepsis of bowel origin is one of the major reasons why enteral nutrition has become favored over parenteral nutrition in critically ill patients (Marino, 1998).

Enteral alimentation through a feeding jejunostomy is initiated when bowel sounds are present and the patient is passing flatus. A number of commercial enteral feedings are available. Typically, a feeding solution is selected that (1) is isotonic, (2) provides at least one calorie per milliliter so that large volumes need not be infused, and (3) is unlikely to produce diarrhea. If persistent diarrhea occurs with enteral feedings or if the patient acquires a postoperative ileus, enteral feedings are temporarily discontinued. Intravenous hyperalimentation may be instituted alternatively.

A contrast esophagogram is performed 4 to 6 days after surgery to assess integrity of the esophageal wall. If no leak is demonstrated (ie, no contrast medium leaks into the mediastinum), feedings are resumed gradually, beginning with clear liquids and progressing according to the patient's tolerance. If a leak is present, an NPO status is maintained and enteral or intravenous alimentation is continued. Unless residual tumor or infection remains in the area of the anastomosis, a postoperative anastomotic leak usually heals spontaneously, although it may take several weeks. Oral nourishment is resumed when an intact esophagus is demonstrated by esophagogram.

Esophageal resection for cancer usually necessitates removal of most of the esophagus and substitution of the stomach or a segment of colon in its place. After esophagectomy, gastric emptying may be delayed and patients may experience some difficulty in resuming oral feedings. Neither of the substitute viscera (ie, stomach or colon) functions as well as native esophagus in which peristalsis propels food into the stomach (Collard et al., 1992). A histamine H_2-receptor antagonist (eg, cimetidine) and metoclopramide may be prescribed (Wolfe & Sebastian, 1992). Several other interventions may also be helpful. First, the patient is maintained on a mechanically soft diet to enhance passage of the food through the replacement viscera. Second, the patient is instructed to take small bites and to chew food thoroughly. Often, six small meals are tolerated better than three larger ones. Finally, the patient is instructed to maintain an upright position during and after meals. Gastric emptying usually improves gradually.

Considerations in Patients With Malignant Disease

The diagnosis and prognosis of a malignant disease carries tremendous stress and devastation for the patient and family. Lung cancer and esophageal cancer, the two most common thoracic malignancies, both are associated with a grim prognosis unless detected early in the disease. It has been estimated that over 900,000 deaths are associated with lung cancer worldwide (Pisani et al., 1999). For patients with esophageal carcinoma, cure is possible in fewer than 10% of patients (Ginsberg & Waters, 1994).

Sometimes the patient has had some clinical manifestations of malignant disease, but in other cases the patient may have had no warning symptoms that a tumor was present until the time of diagnosis. If the definitive diagnosis is made during an operative procedure, the nurse at the bedside may be confronted with the patient, on awakening from general anesthesia, requesting information about the diagnosis. The family also may seek assistance from the nurse in discussing operative findings with the patient during the initial postoperative visit. Their initial visit with the patient may be particularly stressful when an exploratory thoracotomy has been performed and plans for surgical resection abandoned because of tumor location or metastatic spread.

Provision of adequate emotional support to the patient and family during this period depends on the nurse and physician working together to provide appropriate information and counseling. Although it is the surgeon's responsibility and prerogative to determine when and what information about the diagnosis is communicated to the patient, it is somewhat unpredictable when the patient will awaken fully from general anesthesia and become alert enough to ask for and retain information. Consequently, the patient may request information when the surgeon is unavailable to come to the patient's bedside. If the patient is persistently asking for information, the surgeon may delegate another physician or an advanced practice nurse to talk with the patient.

A nurse who assumes responsibility for providing a patient or family with preliminary information about a malignant diagnosis should (1) feel comfortable with the responsibility, (2) be knowledgeable enough about the disease and operative findings to impart the information accurately, (3) have a clear understanding of the precise information to be communicated, and (4) defer questions about the prognostic implications or projected therapy to the appropriate physician. This type of responsibility usually is reserved for an advanced practice nurse or those clinical nurses with expert knowledge who have a close, collaborative working relationship with the thoracic surgeon and well-developed communication and interpersonal skills.

More frequently, it is the physician who provides information about a malignant diagnosis and the nurse who remains at the bedside and intervenes with the patient and family as they begin to cope with implications of the diagnosis. Several obstacles must be overcome for the nurse to provide adequate emotional support. First, the patient remains in the postoperative setting only during the acute phase of the illness. A limited amount of time is available before the patient is discharged or transferred to another setting. Second, cardiothoracic nurses spend most of their time developing acute or critical care nursing skills. Providing counseling for patients who face chronic illness due to malignancy calls on skills that the cardiothoracic surgical nurse uses less frequently. Finally, there are usually legitimate time constraints that preclude the nurse from either sitting down to spend time talking with the patient or ensuring that there will be a period of time to talk without multiple interruptions.

In view of these constraints, it is important to build into the plan of care interventions for meeting the patient's emotional needs. Staff nurses can play a crucial role in supporting the patient and family, even if they cannot realistically set aside blocks of time specifically for this purpose. There is a particular intimacy that develops between patient and nurse as a result of the physical care that the nurse provides. This helps to counteract the aforementioned constraints and fosters open communication, if the nurse actively observes and listens for cues from the patient. Frequently, all that is necessary to begin the process are such simple signals to the patient as sitting down in the room, maintaining eye contact, and asking questions in a manner that conveys an interest in more than a cursory answer. Whether or not the patient chooses to discuss the illness and its implications, these nursing interventions demonstrate to the patient that the nurse is available to discuss feelings and concerns. Appropriate consultations for supportive therapy are initiated before discharging the patient.

► Discharge Preparations

Anticipatory planning for discharge is begun before surgery so that arrangements for special circumstances can be handled efficiently and without delaying discharge from the hospital. Discharge preparation of a postoperative thoracic surgical patient is usually straightforward. Some patients, however, have more complex discharge needs. If the patient goes home with enteral feedings, a tracheostomy, or an open wound, visits from a community-based nursing service may be indicated. Even if there are no skilled nursing needs, homemaker services for shopping, meal preparation, or assistance with bathing may be necessary if the patient is elderly, lives alone, or has other disabilities. The nurse at the bedside is usually in the best position to assess the patient's functional capacity and the need for special assistance at home.

By the day of discharge, most patients are ambulatory and performing all self-care activities. The amount and type of prescribed activity at discharge is somewhat variable, depending on the patient's underlying condition and the type of operative procedure performed. Patients are encouraged to remain out of bed for most of the day and to take short walks at least three times daily; stair climbing may be performed as well. Fatigue and mild dyspnea with exertion are common. Sexual activity can be resumed as soon as the patient is ambulating for several blocks and climbing stairs without dyspnea. The patient should be advised that normal sexual drive may be diminished because of the physical and emotional fatigue associated with a major operation.

The patient is usually the best judge of how much activity can be performed without excessive fatigue. Most patients who undergo major pulmonary resection procedures continue to experience some dyspnea with exertion for the first few postoperative weeks. However, shortness of breath that worsens after discharge from the hospital or that develops precipitously is not typical and should be reported promptly to the physician.

Lifting and vigorous upper extremity physical activities are usually prohibited for 1 to 2 months. Patients are instructed to avoid carrying heavy items, such as groceries, children, or laundry, and also activities such as golf or swimming during this period. Most surgeons recommend that the patient refrain from driving for 1 month after a major thoracic operation. However, the patient can ride in a car and usually can travel by train or plane. Long car trips should include intermittent opportunities for the patient to get out of the car and ambulate. Return to work depends on the type of work and the patient's stamina. If the job does not involve lifting or strenuous physical exertion, the patient can usually return within 4 to 6 weeks.

If the patient has a lateral thoracotomy incision, chest wall discomfort usually persists for 2 to 3 months. An oral pain medication, such as acetaminophen with codeine, is prescribed for the first few weeks at home. A heating pad or warm baths or showers may also be helpful. The patient may be reluctant to use the affected arm. Exercises such as brushing one's hair or "climbing" the affected hand up a wall are helpful in restoring the patient's range of motion to the shoulder.

Insomnia and anorexia are common complaints during the first few weeks at home. As the patient increasingly resumes normal activities of daily living, the sleeping pattern usually improves. Also, as the patient becomes more active, appetite begins to increase. The patient is encouraged to eat a diet that is high in protein and calories. Smaller, more frequent meals may be better tolerated than three large meals. The patient's weight may continue to drift downward several pounds during the first postoperative month. However, the physician should be notified if the weight loss is more than 5 pounds or if weight loss continues more than a month after surgery. This is particularly true in patients who have undergone surgical resection of a malignant tumor.

Medications that the patient was taking before the operation usually are continued. Digoxin may be prescribed for 4 to 6 weeks in patients who have had postoperative atrial fibrillation or other supraventricular ar-

rhythmias. Usually, no other special medications are necessary after a thoracic operation. The patient is instructed to cleanse the incision daily while showering or bathing and to report any evidence of infection (eg, incisional erythema or drainage or temperature more than 101°F [38.3°C]). If the patient was smoking before the operation, counseling is provided about smoking cessation. Smoking is harmful because of its vasoconstrictive effects on blood vessels and its irreversible damage to the lungs. Patients with lung cancer also are at greater risk for development of a second primary lung tumor if cigarette smoking is continued. Motivation to discontinue smoking is usually high after a thoracic operation, and the likelihood of success is enhanced by the patient's abstinence from smoking during the hospitalization.

If the patient has had surgical resection of a malignant tumor, adjunctive radiation or chemotherapy may be recommended. Usually, treatments are initiated several weeks after the operation, when the patient has recovered from the initial stress of the surgery. These treatments often can be performed during outpatient visits. Before discharge, the nurse ascertains that all necessary arrangements for adjuvant therapy have been made and that the patient understands the plan for therapy. Often, multiple physicians have been involved in the patient's care, and the nurse can help clarify for the patient the plan for ongoing medical supervision.

REFERENCES

Allen MS, Pairolero PC, 1996: Postoperative care and complications in the thoracic surgery patient. In Baue AE, Geha AS, Hammond GL, et al. (eds): Glenn's Thoracic and Cardiovascular Surgery, ed. 6. Stamford, CT, Appleton & Lange

Amar D, 1997: Prevention and management of dysrhythmias following thoracic surgery. Chest Surg Clin North Am 7:818

Anderson HL III, Bartlett RH, 1991: Respiratory care of the surgical patient. In Burton GG, Hodgkin JE, Ward JJ (eds): Respiratory Care: A Guide to Clinical Practice, ed. 3. Philadelphia, JB Lippincott

Berry JK, Braunschweig CA, 1998: Nutritional assessment of the critically ill patient. Critical Care Nursing Quarterly 21:33

Bragg CL, 1989: Practical aspects of epidural and intrathecal narcotic analgesia in the intensive care setting. Heart Lung 18:599

Callaghan SP, Doremus KA, Wilson DJ, O'Donnell MM, 1994: Minitracheostomy: An alternative to "blind" endotracheal suctioning. Dimensions of Critical Care Nursing 13:38

Cohen RG, DeMeester TR, Lafontaine E, 1995: The pleura. In Sabiston DC Jr, Spencer FC (eds): Surgery of the Chest, ed. 6. Philadelphia, WB Saunders

Collard JM, Otte JB, Reynaert M, Kestens PJ, 1992: Quality of life three years or more after esophagectomy for cancer. J Thorac Cardiovasc Surg 104:391

Deschamps C, Allen MS, Trastek VF, Pairolero PC, 1992a: Postoperative management. Chest Surg Clin North Am 2:713

Deschamps C, Pairolero PC, Allen MS, Trastek VF, 1992b: Postpneumonectomy pulmonary edema. Chest Surg Clin North Am 2:785

Desiderio D, Downey R, 1998: Critical issues in early extubation and hospital discharge in thoracic oncology surgery. J Cardiothorac Vasc Anesth 12(Suppl 2):3

Duhaylongsod FG, Wolfe WG, 1992: Complications of pulmonary resection. In Wolfe WG (ed): Complications in Thoracic Surgery. St. Louis, Mosby–Year Book

Elefteriades JA, Geha AS, Cohn LS, 1996: Chest tubes. In House Officer Guide to ICU Care: Fundamentals of Management of the Heart and Lungs, ed. 2. Philadelphia, Lippincott-Raven

Ferguson TB, 1992: Arrhythmias associated with thoracotomy. In Wolfe WG (ed): Complications in Thoracic Surgery. St. Louis, Mosby–Year Book

Ginsberg RJ, Waters PF, 1994: Surgical palliation of inoperable carcinoma of the esophagus. In Shields TW (ed): General Thoracic Surgery, ed. 4. Baltimore, Williams & Wilkins

Hawthorne MH, 1992: Recognition of thoracic surgical complications: A nursing perspective. In Wolfe WG (ed): Complications in Thoracic Surgery. St. Louis, Mosby–Year Book

Hillis LD, Lange RA, Winniford MD, Page RL, 1995: Noncardiac surgery in patients with coronary artery disease. In Manual of Clinical Problems in Cardiology, ed. 5. Boston, Little, Brown

Jain S, Datta S, 1997: Postoperative pain management. Chest Surg Clin North Am 7:773

Joob AW, Hartz RS, 1994: General principles of postoperative care. In Shields TW (ed): General Thoracic Surgery, ed. 4. Baltimore, Williams & Wilkins

Kaiser AB, 1995: Use of antibiotics in cardiac and thoracic surgery. In Sabiston DC Jr, Spencer FC (eds): Surgery of the Chest, ed. 6. Philadelphia, WB Saunders

Kaiser LR, 1998: Right-sided pulmonary resections. In Kaiser LR, Kron IL, Spray TL (eds): Mastery of Cardiothoracic Surgery. Philadelphia Lippincott Williams & Wilkins

Lubenow TR, Faber LP, McCarthy RJ, et al., 1994: Post-thoracotomy pain management using continuous epidural analgesia in 1,324 patients. Ann Thorac Surg 58:924

Marino PL, 1998: Enteral nutrition. In The ICU Book, ed. 2. Baltimore, Williams & Wilkins

Mathisen DJ, Wain JC Jr, 1992: Cardiac complications following pulmonary resection. Chest Surg Clin North Am 2:793

Nelson ME, Moran JF, 1992: Post-thoracotomy pneumonia. In Wolfe WG (ed): Complications in Thoracic Surgery. St. Louis, Mosby–Year Book

Orringer MB, 1991a: Complications of esophageal resection and reconstruction. In Waldhausen JA, Orringer MB (eds): Complications in Cardiothoracic Surgery. St. Louis, Mosby–Year Book

Orringer MB, 1991b: Complications of hiatus hernia surgery. In Waldhausen JA, Orringer MB (eds): Complications in Cardiothoracic Surgery. St. Louis, Mosby–Year Book

Piccione W Jr, Faber LP, 1991: Management of complications related to pulmonary resection. In Waldhausen JA, Orringer MB (eds): Complications in Cardiothoracic Surgery. St. Louis, Mosby–Year Book

Pisani P, Parkin DM, Bray F, Ferlay J, 1999: Estimates of the worldwide mortality from 25 cancers in 1990. Int J Cancer 83:18

Quill TJ, 1992: Anesthetic complications in thoracic surgery. In Wolfe WG (ed): Complications in Thoracic Surgery. St. Louis, Mosby–Year Book

Rice TW, Kirby TJ, 1992: Prolonged air leak. Chest Surg Clin North Am 2:803

Ronan KP, Murray MJ, 1992: Perioperative assessment and mechanical ventilation. Chest Surg Clin North Am 2:745

Sandler AN, 1995: Anesthesia. In Pearson GF, Deslauriers J, Ginsberg RJ, et al. (eds): Thoracic Surgery. New York, Churchill Livingstone

Shields TW, 1994: General features and complications of pulmonary resections. In Shields TW (ed): General Thoracic Surgery, ed. 4. Baltimore, Williams & Wilkins

Todd TR, 1989: The respiratory intensive care unit. In Grillo HC, Austen WG, Wilkins EW, et al. (eds): Current Therapy in Cardiothoracic Surgery. Toronto, Canada, BC Decker

Todd TR, Ralph-Edwards AC, 1995: Perioperative management. In Pearson GF, Deslauriers J, Ginsberg RJ, et al. (eds): Thoracic Surgery. New York, Churchill Livingstone

Wain JC, Wilson DJ, Mathisen DJ, 1990: Clinical experience with minitracheostomy. Ann Thorac Surg 49:881

Wolfe WG, Sebastian MW, 1992: Complications following esophagectomy and esophagogastrostomy. In Wolfe WG (ed): Complications in Thoracic Surgery. St. Louis, Mosby–Year Book

42

Pleural Thoracostomy Drainage

*T*horacostomy drainage is an integral component in the care of thoracic surgical patients. In the United States, more than 1.3 million chest catheters are used annually (Munnell, 1997). Chest tubes may be placed to drain fluid or air from any of the three distinct compartments that compose the thorax (ie, the mediastinum and the right and left pleural spaces). Mediastinal chest tubes are placed routinely at the conclusion of cardiac operations or other procedures performed through a median sternotomy incision (eg, mediastinal tumor resection). The discussion in this chapter focuses on thoracostomy drainage of the pleural spaces.

The pleural space in each hemithorax lies between the visceral pleura, a thin sheet of tissue that covers the surfaces of the lungs, and the parietal pleura, the tissue lining that covers the undersurfaces of the ribs, the diaphragm, and the structures of the mediastinum (Munnell, 1991). Under normal conditions, each lung is fully expanded and completely fills the hemithorax. Consequently, the visceral and parietal pleural surfaces are apposed and the so-called pleural space is a potential space only, containing no air and only 5 to 10 mL of fluid. Pressure within the space is slightly negative in comparison to atmospheric pressure. It varies from approximately -6 to -12 cm H_2O on inspiration and from -4 to -8 cm H_2O on expiration (Hudak et al., 1998).

▶ Indications for Pleural Drainage

Postoperative Drainage

Most noncardiac thoracic operations are performed through a thoracotomy incision and thus necessitate opening one of the pleural spaces. At the conclusion of a thoracotomy, chest tubes are placed in the operative hemithorax to achieve two objectives: (1) evacuation of blood and air from the pleural space, and (2) maintenance of lung expansion in the presence of visceral pleural disruption. Usually, two large-bore tubes are inserted through separate incisions in the operative side of the thorax.

One tube is positioned posteriorly and toward the base of the lung for drainage of blood that collects in dependent areas. Blood loss into the chest drainage system usually occurs at a rate of 75 to 100 mL/h for the first several postoperative hours and gradually subsides. Adequate postoperative evacuation of blood is important; fluid that accumulates in the pleural space impedes expansion of the ipsilateral lung. An undrained hemothorax also may lead to infection of the pleural space (empyema) and potential entrapment of the lung in a collapsed state.

The second chest tube placed at the time of thoracotomy is positioned anteriorly near the apex of the lung for evacuation of air. In patients who have undergone partial lung resection (ie, lobectomy, segmentectomy, or wedge resection), air can leak for several days from remaining parenchymal tissue in areas where incomplete fissures were divided or adhesions were freed. Evacuation of air from the pleural space is essential to allow full expansion of remaining lung tissue. The portion of lung remaining after pulmonary resection (usually one or two lobes) almost always expands fully to obliterate the pleural space.

Several compensatory mechanisms that occur after pulmonary resection facilitate postoperative pleural space obliteration, including shift of the mediastinum toward the operative side, narrowing of the ipsilateral intercostal spaces, and elevation of the ipsilateral hemidiaphragm (Joob & Hartz, 1994). Once the lung fills the hemithorax, apposition of the pleural surfaces results in cessation of air leakage in most patients within 24 to 48 hours (Duhaylongsod & Wolfe, 1992). Less frequently, persistent air leakage necessitates prolonged chest tube drainage or, in rare cases, surgical intervention. In other cases, air leakage stops but the remaining lung fails to fill the hemithorax fully. If so, an air-filled space remains. Usually, a persistent air space causes no clinical sequelae and gradually disappears over months (Shields, 1994a). Infrequently, a residual air space becomes infected.

In patients who undergo pneumonectomy, a chest tube often is not placed unless infection is present or excessive bleeding is suspected. Intrapleural pressure is adjusted at the conclusion of the operation by aspirating air from the pleural space with a syringe after the operative hemithorax is closed. Equalizing pressure in the empty hemithorax prevents shifting of mediastinal contents to the nonoperative side with resultant respiratory impairment. The empty hemithorax eventually fills with gelatinous fluid. If a chest tube is placed at the time of pneumonectomy, it is clamped or connected to passive drainage without suction because the application of suction would cause undesirable mediastinal shifting toward the operative hemithorax.

Pleural Drainage in Nonsurgical Patients

Pneumothorax

Pneumothorax in nonsurgical patients most often results from idiopathic rupture of a pseudocyst, or air-filled bleb, in the peripheral lung tissue. Primary spontaneous pneumothorax usually occurs in young adults with lungs that are otherwise normal. Secondary spontaneous pneumothorax most often occurs in older people with chronic obstructive lung disease or bullous emphysema. Approximately 20% of patients with spontaneous pneumothorax experience a recurrent pneumothorax, usually on the same side. After a second spontaneous pneumothorax, the risk for a third is even greater.

Pneumothorax also can result from iatrogenic perforation of the lung during invasive procedures, such as subclavian vein catheter insertion or transthoracic needle

biopsy. Pneumothorax associated with trauma usually is due to lung injury caused by fractured rib segments or a penetrating object. In patients receiving mechanical ventilation with high levels of positive end-expiratory pressure, pneumothorax can occur due to overdistention and rupture of alveoli (Ronan & Murray, 1992). The highest risk of pneumothorax is in patients with adult respiratory distress syndrome, where the incidence of pneumothorax approaches 60% (Marino, 1998).

Pneumothorax reduces pulmonary volumes, pulmonary compliance, and diffusing capacity; the pathophysiologic consequences depend on its size, the presence of tension, and the condition of the underlying lung (Cohen et al., 1995). Because the chest wall is relatively noncompliant, air accumulating in the pleural space causes the ipsilateral lung to collapse. If air leakage continues without drainage of the pleural space, the increasing intrapleural pressure causes shifting of mediastinal contents toward the contralateral hemithorax, a condition known as *tension pneumothorax* (Fig. 42-1).

If untreated, tension pneumothorax can cause severe hemodynamic compromise or even death. Displacement of the heart toward the opposite side impairs venous return through the superior and inferior venae cavae; because the heart cannot fill adequately, stroke volume and cardiac output fall and shock ensues (Elefteriades et al., 1996a). Treatment of tension pneumothorax is emergent chest tube thoracostomy, which may be performed without a confirmatory chest roentgenogram if warranted by findings on physical examination and by the patient's clinical condition (Fry & Paape, 1994). If necessary, a 14- or 16-gauge needle or angiocatheter can be inserted quickly

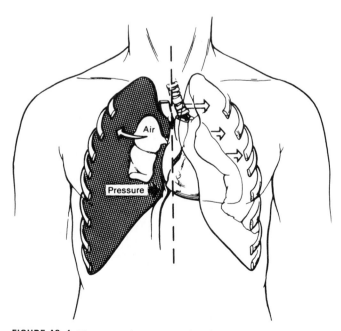

FIGURE 42-1. Diagrammatic representation of tension pneumothorax with total collapse of lung and shifting of mediastinum to contralateral side. (Hudak CM, Gallo BM, Benz JJ, 1990: Intervention alternatives: Respiratory system. In Critical Care Nursing, ed. 5, p. 337. Philadelphia, JB Lippincott)

in the midclavicular line in the second intercostal space for management of a life-threatening tension pneumothorax.

Fluid Collections

Fluid in the pleural space may be blood (hemothorax), serous fluid (pleural effusion), pus (empyema), or chyle (chylothorax). *Hemothorax* in nonsurgical patients most often is the result of chest trauma. Although some degree of bleeding occurs with almost all cases of chest trauma, significant hemothorax usually represents injury to the heart, great vessels, or intercostal or pulmonary parenchymal blood vessels. In patients with traumatic hemothorax and significant bleeding, blood shed into the thoracostomy drainage system may be salvaged, filtered, and reinfused using a drainage system with autotransfusion capabilities.

Pleural effusion occurs when the equilibrium of fluid entering and leaving the pleural space is disturbed. Under normal conditions, fluid flows into the pleural space from systemic capillaries in the parietal pleura. Pulmonary capillaries and lymphatics rapidly absorb the fluid, leaving only a small residual amount in the pleural space. A variety of conditions can cause an imbalance in the normal movement of pleural fluid, resulting in fluid accumulation in the pleural space and compression of the ipsilateral lung. These conditions include increased capillary permeability from inflammation or tumor implants, increased hydrostatic pressure due to congestive heart failure, decreased oncotic pressure caused by hypoalbuminemia, increased negative intrapleural pressure due to atelectasis, and decreased lymphatic drainage due to lymphatic obstruction caused by tumor (Rusch, 1995). Malignant disease is the most common cause of pleural effusion.

Empyema occurs when the normally sterile pleural space becomes infected. An empyema can develop as a complication of a prior thoracic procedure, chest trauma, or pulmonary infection. The infectious process causes accumulation of suppurative fluid in the pleural space and can lead to sepsis if the space is not adequately drained. *Chylothorax* occurs when chyle (lymph fluid originating primarily in the intestinal tract) enters the pleural space as a result of disruption or obstruction of the thoracic duct, a large intrathoracic lymphatic channel located near the esophagus. The primary cause of chylothorax is cancer (Yeam & Sassoon, 1997). Laceration of the thoracic duct most often occurs as a complication of a thoracic operation, such as esophagectomy, but the duct also can be injured by trauma or during placement of a left subclavian venous catheter (Rodgers, 1998). Chylous pleural drainage is distinguished from other types of pleural effusions by its characteristic milky appearance.

▶ Principles of Pleural Drainage

Chest Tube Insertion

Thoracic drainage tubes are made from silicone or plastic, with multiple drainage holes and a radiopaque line for radiographic localization (Compeau & Johnston,

1999). A smaller-diameter tube (24 to 28 French) is adequate for evacuation of air or a transudative effusion. A larger bore tube (28 to 32 French) is advantageous for drainage of blood or suppurative material. The tubes are made of pliable material to avoid lung injury during insertion or while the tube is in place. They must be rigid enough, however, so that the lumen is not compromised by kinking or pressure (Hood, 1989).

Chest tubes typically are inserted through skin incisions located on the anterolateral aspect of the thorax (Deschamps et al., 1992). The specific insertion site is determined by the nature of the material to be drained. Air, a low-density gas, tends to collect in the upper half of the pleural space, and fluid, because of its higher density, accumulates inferiorly when the patient is upright and posteriorly when the patient is supine (Courad et al., 1990). In most patients, a chest tube inserted into any location in the pleural space effectively evacuates either air or fluid. However, specific placement of the tube makes drainage of the pleural space more efficient.

A chest tube designed to evacuate pneumothorax typically is inserted in the third interspace in the anterior or midaxillary line and is directed anteriorly and toward the apex of the lung so that its drainage holes lie between the lung apex and the anterior chest wall. A tube placed in this location is less likely to injure great vessels, the subclavian artery or vein, or the pulmonary hilum during insertion. Conversely, a tube placed to drain fluid is inserted in the fifth or sixth intercostal space in the midaxillary line and directed posteriorly, because fluid can be expected to collect dependently in the costophrenic and costovertebral angles. Tubes rarely are placed in the posterior chest because of resultant inability of the patient to recline in a supine position without discomfort or occlusion of the tube.

Chest tube insertion is a painful procedure; if time and the patient's condition permit, a parenteral dose of narcotic medication is administered 20 to 30 minutes before insertion of the tube. The skin in the area of the chosen insertion site is cleansed with an antiseptic solution (eg, povidone-iodine) and a sterile drape is applied. Local anesthesia is achieved by infiltrating the skin, subcutaneous tissue, intercostal tissue, and parietal pleura with 1% lidocaine solution. Using sterile technique, a small transverse skin incision is made at the intercostal space below that selected for insertion of the tube. A hemostat is used to dissect bluntly subcutaneous tissue overlying the rib, thereby creating a tract before separating intercostal muscle on the superior margin of the rib and penetrating the parietal pleura (Fig. 42-2). Creation of a subcutaneous tract prevents air leakage at the tube insertion site while the tube is in place. It also provides a more occlusive soft tissue closure of the chest wall at the time of chest tube removal (Munnell, 1991).

The tube is passed over the top of the rib to avoid injury to the intercostal neurovascular bundle (intercostal nerves and blood vessels) that run in a groove on the inferior aspect of each rib; the parietal pleura is punctured with the clamp, and an efflux of air or fluid usually is en-

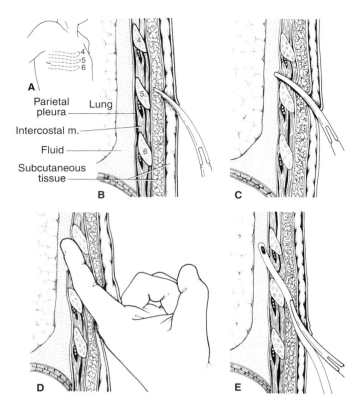

Parietal pleura Lung

Intercostal m.

Fluid

Subcutaneous tissue

FIGURE 42-2. Schematic demonstrating steps of chest tube insertion. (**A**) Using local anesthesia, a small transverse skin incision is made in the mid-axillary line of the fifth intercostal space. (**B**) A tract is developed through subcutaneous tissue using blunt dissection with hemostat. (**C**) The intercostal muscles are separated over the edge of the fifth rib, and the parietal pleura is gently penetrated. (**D**) A fingertip is inserted to confirm entry into the pleural space and ensure that lung is not adherent to the parietal pleura. (**E**) The tip of the chest tube is inserted through the subcutaneous tract and advanced into appropriate position so that all drainage holes are within the pleural space. (Symbas PN, 1989: Initial general management. In Cardiothoracic Trauma, p. 8. Philadelphia, WB Saunders)

countered (Mutch & Allen, 1999). Before inserting the tube into the pleural space, a fingertip is inserted to ensure that it is the pleural space that has been entered and that the lung is not adherent to parietal pleura. After digital exploration, the chest tube is clamped near its tip and advanced into the pleural space in the appropriate direction to maximize drainage. All drainage holes are positioned within the pleural space so that air evacuated from the pleural space does not enter the subcutaneous tissue (Munnell, 1991). After proper positioning, the tube is secured to the skin at the insertion site with heavy silk sutures to avoid dislodgment, and a petrolatum gauze occlusive dressing is applied to provide an airtight seal.

Typically, the chest tube is connected by 6 feet of latex tubing to a prepared drainage system placed below the level of the chest. This length of tubing allows the patient to turn and move about comfortably and minimizes the likelihood that drainage will be drawn back into the chest with deep inspirations (Erickson, 1989a). All connections are secured with tape to prevent disconnection. A chest

roentgenogram is obtained to confirm proper tube position and to ensure that the most proximal side hole, as identified by a short interruption in the radiopaque line on the tube, is clearly within the pleural space.

Most thoracic surgeons prefer not to advance or manipulate a chest tube once it is in place because of the risk of infecting the pleural space and producing an empyema. Consequently, if the position of a tube is inadequate to evacuate pleural air or fluid effectively, placement of an additional tube through a separate incision may be necessary. In some patients, air or fluid cannot move freely within the pleural space because of adhesions (ie, areas in which visceral and parietal pleura are adherent to one another). In such cases, the air or fluid is said to be *loculated*.

Patients who have had previous thoracic operations, radiation therapy, pulmonary infection, or inflammatory processes are more likely to have loculated fluid collections. In these patients, more precise tube placement is required for air or fluid evacuation. In certain cases, it may be necessary to place the tube under ultrasound or computed tomographic guidance. Alternatively, video-assisted thoracoscopy may be performed. During thoracoscopy, the pleural surfaces are visualized and adhesions can be mechanically disrupted to allow free drainage of fluid or air from the pleural space.

Chest tube insertion can be associated with major complications if intrathoracic or intra-abdominal structures are injured. The incidence of significant technical complications secondary to chest tube insertion is 1% to 2% (Douglas, 1992). Injury to intrathoracic or intra-abdominal structures is more likely when (1) a trocar is used during chest tube insertion, or (2) a tube is inserted without digital exploration of the insertion site to ensure that the subcutaneous tract leads into the pleural space and to determine whether any tissue or organ is adherent to pleura at the insertion site (Symbas, 1989).

Forceful insertion in an area where lung is adherent to the chest wall may lacerate pulmonary parenchyma. If the tube is not inserted directly over the top of the chosen rib, the intercostal artery or vein that lies on the inferior surface of the rib can be lacerated (Keagy & Wilcox, 1989). A chest tube that is placed too low can perforate the diaphragm and lacerate the liver, spleen, or stomach (Munnell, 1997; Miller & Sahn, 1987). Rarely, the internal thoracic artery, the heart, or one of the great vessels is lacerated by a chest tube, causing significant hemothorax. Subcutaneous emphysema may occur if one or more of the drainage holes are located outside the pleural space.

Maintenance of Pleural Drainage

The Drainage System

A variety of commercial chest drainage systems are available. All are designed using basic principles that provide a sterile system for passive or suction drainage of air and fluid while preventing outside air from entering the thoracic cavity. The classic "three-bottle" system, described by Howe in 1952, was used for many years to provide thoracostomy drainage and serves as the basis for almost all thoracic drainage systems in use today (Howe, 1952; Munnell, 1997) (Fig. 42-3). The design of current drainage systems varies according to the specific manufacturer. Disposable systems, such as the Pleur-evac (Genzyme Surgical Products, Fall River, MA), consist of a single plastic circuit compartmentalized into three chambers. This type of chest drainage system is described here.

The first chamber of the drainage system (ie, the chamber nearest the chest tube) is for collection of fluid.

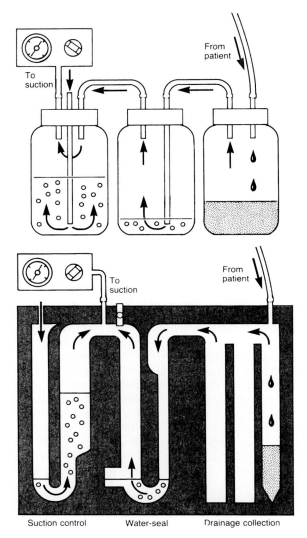

Suction control   Water-seal   Drainage collection

FIGURE 42-3. (**Top**) Classic "three-bottle" chest drainage system. The first chamber (*right*) collects fluid evacuated from the pleural space. The second chamber, containing a small amount of sterile water or saline, provides a water seal that prevents atmospheric air from entering the pleural space through the chest tube. The third chamber, filled with 20 cm of sterile water or saline, allows regulation of the amount of suction. (**Bottom**) Disposable chest drainage system designed using principles of the three-bottle system. (Luce JM, Tyler ML, Pierson DJ, 1984: Drainage, obliteration, and decortication of the pleural space. In Intensive Respiratory Care, p. 166. Philadelphia, WB Saunders)

Graded labeling on the chamber allows quantification of the amount of fluid drainage. The second, or water-seal, chamber controls flow of air through the system so that it can move in one direction only; that is, out of the pleural space. A small amount (2 cm) of sterile water or saline is placed in the second chamber to create a water-seal or one-way valve. When air trapped in the pleural space exceeds 2 cm H_2O pressure, it bubbles through the water in the second chamber and out through the atmospheric vent. However, outside air that enters the second chamber through the vent cannot penetrate the water seal to enter the first chamber.

The third, or suction, chamber regulates the amount of negative suction applied to the pleural space. Usually, 20 cm of sterile water or saline is placed in the third chamber. To establish suction, tubing from the chamber is connected to a wall suction unit that creates negative pressure by removing air from the drainage system. Outside air can enter the third chamber through an atmospheric vent that is separated from the suction source by the column of water in the third chamber. Therefore, the degree of negative pressure in the drainage system is controlled by the amount of water in the chamber. When negative pressure reaches an amount equal to the height of the water column, outside air begins to bubble through the water, preventing negative pressure from exceeding this amount.

A "waterless" disposable drainage system has become available that provides a one-way seal and controlled suction without the addition of fluid to the system (Pleur-evac Sahara, Genzyme Surgical Products) (Fig. 42-4).

Assessment and Maintenance of the System

When a chest tube is in place, the chest drainage system to which it is attached must be viewed as an extension of the pleural space. Periodic assessment of the system for proper functioning is essential. The tubing and drainage chambers always are maintained in a position beneath the level of the chest to prevent siphoning of fluid from the drainage chamber into the pleural space (Bojar, 1989). If water-seal drainage without suction is used, the tubing to the wall suction unit is disconnected because this segment of tubing serves as the atmospheric vent for the second chamber. Because fluid evaporates over time, water levels in the water-seal and suction chambers are assessed daily and replenished as necessary. The system is inspected regularly to identify cracks in the plastic housing.

When suction is applied to the drainage system, vigorous bubbling is not necessary. As long as continuous, gentle bubbling occurs, the prescribed amount of suction is present. The amount of suction necessary to evacuate the pleural space is variable but must exceed the intrapleural vacuum created during each inspiration (Joob & Hartz, 1994). Recall that negative pressure in the pleural space normally varies between −4 and −12 cm H_2O pressure. Consequently, −20 cm H_2O is sufficient to evacuate most gaseous and liquid effusions from the space (Courad et al., 1990). Higher levels of suction (−25 to −40 cm H_2O pressure) may be required in se-

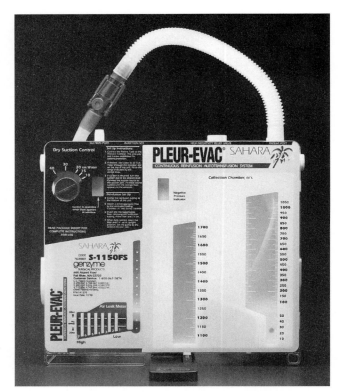

FIGURE 42-4. Pleur-evac Sahara chest drainage system. Controlled suction and a one-way valve mechanism are provided without the use of fluid in the system. The waterless one-way valve mechanism opens on expiration, allowing air to exit the pleural space, then closes rapidly to prevent atmospheric air from entering during inspiration; an optional air leak indicator, which does require the addition of water, may be used to assess and quantitate air leakage. (Courtesy of Genzyme Surgical Products, Fall River, MA)

trapleural pressures, often associated with atelectasis or incomplete lung reexpansion (Grégoire & Deslauries, 1995). It may be observed after pulmonary resection or in the presence of atelectasis or incomplete lung expansion resulting from other reasons (Munnell, 1997).

Bubbling in the water-seal chamber indicates air leakage from the lung into the pleural space or a disrupted connection in the drainage system. The severity of the air leak is reflected by the proportion of the respiratory cycle during which bubbling occurs (Elefteriades, et al., 1996b). If an air leak is small, bubbling does not occur continuously. The patient is instructed to take a deep breath and cough. If air is present in the pleural space, the positive pressure created by coughing causes air to be expelled into the drainage system and through the water in the water-seal chamber. Cessation of an air leak is manifested by an inability to evoke bubbling in the water-seal chamber with suction disconnected and while the patient is coughing.

Infrequently, bubbling in the water-seal chamber represents leakage of outside air into the system through a loose tubing connection or a defect in the drainage unit. If an air leak is noted, the drainage system is assessed. The dressing is removed to determine if air is being drawn in through the chest tube insertion site. Each of the tubing connections is examined to ensure that it is airtight. The location of a leak in the drainage system is identified by applying a clamp on the tubing at progressively distal sites to the chest wall, beginning with the chest tube as it exits the chest and moving distally toward the drainage system (Munnell, 1991). If clamping the tubing results in cessation of air leakage (ie, absence of bubbling in the water-seal chamber), the leak is located proximal to the clamp. Air leakage that continues with a clamp applied to tubing just proximal to the drainage unit itself is indicative of a defect in the drainage unit; the unit should be replaced.

If fluid in the water-seal chamber does not fluctuate when suction is disconnected, the tube is essentially nonfunctional. Absence of respiratory fluctuation may represent full lung expansion and occlusion of drainage holes by the surface of the lung. Alternatively, the tube may be kinked or occluded with fibrinous clot or debris. If the tube lumen is occluded and the patient has residual air or fluid in the pleural space, the tube may be stripped to restore patency. Stripping (also called *milking*) a chest tube consists of occluding the tube proximally with both hands and moving the distal hand in a sweeping motion along the length of the tube (Fig. 42-5). The proximal hand is then removed while the tube is still occluded distally. Stripping a chest tube mechanically dislodges clots or fibrin in the tubing and creates a brief pulse of increased suction (Erickson, 1989b). If chest tube patency is not restored by stripping a nonfunctional tube and pleural drainage is still required, the tube may be removed and replaced with another tube (Hood, 1989).

Protocols for performance of chest tube stripping vary because the procedure is known to create excessive negative suction. Vacuums of up to −400 cm H_2O have been reported to result from stripping a chest tube (Munnell, 1997). Although some thoracic surgeons advocate routine stripping of chest tubes, others believe it should be

lected situations, such as a persistent residual space, fibrinous hemothorax, empyema, or profuse air leak.

The tubing is inspected regularly, beginning at the chest wall, to ensure that all connections are tight and that the tubing is not kinked. Tubing between the chest tube and drainage system is adjusted to prevent coiling or loops that would allow fluid accumulation. Fluid in a dependent loop of tubing creates a "water-trap" effect that may inhibit drainage and negate suction (Hood, 1989). If a column of fluid greater than 20 cm (ie, the height of the water column in the third chamber) collects in a dependent loop, no suction is being applied to the pleural space despite continuous bubbling in the third chamber.

Respiratory oscillation and the presence of an air leak are assessed by instructing the patient to inhale and exhale deeply while suction is momentarily disconnected. With passive water-seal drainage, fluid in the water-seal chamber rises and falls in synchrony with the patient's respirations as negative pressure in the thorax increases during inhalation and decreases during exhalation. In patients receiving positive-pressure mechanical ventilation, oscillatory variations are reversed; the water column falls during inhalation and rises during exhalation. Increased amplitude of respiratory oscillations suggests high negative in-

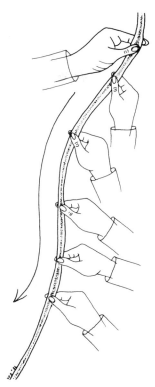

FIGURE 42-5. Stripping a chest tube. The tube is occluded proximally with both hands; one hand is held stationary while the other (still maintaining compression) is moved in a sweeping motion along the tube several times. While the tube is still occluded at the distal location, the proximal hand is released, creating a brief pulse of increased negative suction. The procedure is facilitated by putting lubricant on the hand used to strip the tube. (Courtesy of Genzyme Surgical Products, Fall River, MA)

reserved for restoring patency to tubes that are nonfunctional. The effects of briefly increased suction in the pleural space are unknown, but it is postulated that stripping could injure lung tissue or exacerbate blood loss in patients with active bleeding. Furthermore, in most instances routine stripping does not appear to be necessary to maintain tube patency (Lim-Levy et al., 1986).

Clamps are almost never applied to chest tubes. During patient transport or ambulation, suction is disconnected, converting the system to passive water-seal drainage. If a chest tube becomes accidentally disconnected, it is promptly reconnected to the chest drainage system with suction. The physician is notified and a chest roentgenogram is obtained to ensure that the lung remains expanded. The disconnected tube should not be clamped before reconnecting the chest drainage system.

Any tipping that causes spillage of contents of the drainage system from one chamber to another requires replacement of the drainage system. Replacement of the system also may be required if the collection chamber becomes filled. After preparing a new system for use, tape securing the chest tube to the connecting tubing is removed carefully. The chest tube is momentarily clamped while the connecting tubing of the system in use is dis-

connected and that of the new drainage system is connected to the chest tube. The clamp is then removed and tape is reapplied at the connection site. Replacing the drainage system in a patient with a profuse air leak should be performed with a physician in attendance and is discussed later in the chapter.

Cytologic, microbiologic, or cellular analysis of pleural fluid may be important to establish etiology of a pleural effusion. Pleural fluid for analysis is best obtained by the physician at the time of chest tube insertion. Although most chest drainage systems have a self-sealing diaphragm on the drainage chamber for pleural fluid aspiration, laboratory analysis of fluid that has accumulated in the drainage chamber over a period of days usually is not helpful in making critical clinical decisions. For example, fluid in the drainage chamber is not useful for microbiologic analysis if infection is suspected because it is likely to be colonized with bacteria even if fluid in the pleural space is not infected. Because the chest tube and latex connecting tubing are not self-sealing, it is not advisable to obtain fluid through needle aspiration of the tubing. Consequently, if pleural fluid for microbiologic analysis is required after a chest tube has been inserted, the physician usually clamps the chest tube, disconnects it from the latex tubing, and carefully swabs the inside of the tube distal to the clamp with a sterile applicator.

Patient Management

With properly positioned chest tubes, the pleural space almost always can be drained effectively. Failure to achieve drainage or lung reexpansion with an appropriately positioned tube represents either (1) air or fluid accumulation at a rate greater than can be drained by the chest tube, or (2) underlying lung that is incapable of expanding (Bolling, 1991).

Chest tubes used to drain hemothorax or moderate to large pleural effusions usually are connected to suction drainage. The amount of fluid drainage is measured hourly in patients with active bleeding and at least every 8 hours in patients with lesser amounts of drainage. The character of the drainage is documented. Blood can be characterized as active (bright red) bleeding or old (dark) blood and pleural fluid may be described as serosanguineous, straw colored, purulent, or chylous.

Large, chronic pleural effusions are drained gradually to avoid complications that can result from rapid evacuation of pleural fluid. Unilateral pulmonary edema or sudden hypotension secondary to a vasovagal reaction may occur and appear to be related to the rapidity with which fluid is drained from the pleural space (Douglas, 1992). One method is to drain 1500 mL initially and then clamp the tube for a 2-hour period, repeating the process every 2 hours until drainage slows (Meko & Patterson, 1999). If the collection chamber becomes filled, the drainage system must be replaced. Water-seal, or passive, drainage may be used instead of suction drainage once fluid drainage is minimal.

Routine repositioning of patients on bed rest facilitates fluid drainage. Sometimes, blood or transudative fluid pools in the pleural space as a result of the patient lying in a certain position for an extended period. If so, a large quantity of fluid (eg, 400 to 500 mL) may drain rapidly into the chest drainage system when the patient is moved. When this amount of blood drains into the system, the patient is observed closely to ensure that the blood loss represents accumulated blood in the pleural space and not active bleeding. Sustained bleeding into the pleural space at a rate of greater than 150 mL/h or more than 400 mL in 1 hour usually prompts operative exploration of the chest to identify and control the bleeding source.

A chest tube inserted for pneumothorax usually is connected to suction drainage until the chest radiograph demonstrates full lung expansion. In most instances of spontaneous pneumothorax, the air leak disappears over the course of 1 to 2 days (Meko & Patterson, 1999). Air leaks due to spontaneous pneumothorax occasionally fail to resolve with thoracostomy drainage. Air leaks that persist beyond 2 weeks may require surgical intervention (Chee et al., 1998). After pulmonary resection procedures, air leakage is expected for several days but uncommonly may persist for several weeks.

Suction usually can be discontinued during periods of ambulation unless a large air leak is present. While suction is disconnected, water-seal drainage allows continued egress of pleural air. When the patient returns to the room, suction is resumed. Once the lung is fully expanded, apposition of the visceral and parietal pleurae facilitates cessation of the air leak regardless of whether suction is applied to the space.

Chest discomfort is common while a chest tube is in place. The degree of discomfort often increases when the lung reexpands and the visceral and parietal pleural surfaces are again in apposition. Although the patient may require more analgesia during this period, the pain indicates that the chest tube has been effective in achieving lung reexpansion. The patient should receive adequate analgesic medication to avoid chest wall splinting and hypoventilation.

Chest roentgenograms usually are obtained daily after chest tube placement and then at least every several days. The roentgenogram allows definitive evaluation of the presence of air or fluid in the pleural space. A chest film also is obtained within several hours after converting from suction to water-seal drainage to ensure that the lung remains expanded. In most instances, chest tubes remain in place for less than a week. However, if a chest tube is in place for longer, the occlusive dressing is removed and replaced so that the insertion site can be inspected for evidence of infection. Dressing changes are then performed every 48 to 72 hours until the tube is removed.

Chest Tube Removal

Chest tubes are removed when (1) fluid drainage is less than 100 to 150 mL/d, and (2) there has been no evidence of an air leak after 24 to 48 hours of water-seal drainage. Some thoracic surgeons prefer to clamp a tube for several hours before its removal. This simulates having no tube in place and allows detection of a slow air leak that causes only occasional bubbling in the water-seal chamber. Such a slow air leak may not be detected by intermittent assessment of the water-seal chamber but could result in lung collapse after the tube is removed. A clamp is applied to the chest tube, and a chest roentgenogram is obtained to ensure that the lung remains expanded. If the chest roentgenogram demonstrates continued lung expansion, the tube is removed.

While the chest tube is clamped, tension pneumothorax can occur if an unsuspected air leak is present. During the time that the clamp is in place, the nurse observes the patient for shortness of breath or chest pain that indicates pleural air accumulation (ie, pneumothorax). If symptoms of pneumothorax occur, the clamp is removed to restore water-seal or suction drainage and the physician is notified. If the patient's symptoms represent pneumothorax, bubbling occurs in the water-seal chamber as soon as the clamp is released.

Removal of chest tubes in cardiothoracic surgical settings sometimes is performed by nurses who have been trained to perform the procedure. The optimal technique for chest tube removal in self-ventilating patients is a source of some controversy among thoracic surgeons. The underlying principle is prevention of air entry into the pleural space caused by involuntary patient inspiration in response to pain as the tube is withdrawn from the chest. Some surgeons believe there is less possibility of iatrogenic pneumothorax if the tube is withdrawn while the patient is performing a Valsalva maneuver after a deep inspiration; others advocate chest tube removal during a full exhalation.

With whichever technique is used, the nurse should be familiar with the principles involved and perform steps of the procedure in a consistent fashion. A clamp is applied to the chest tube to be removed. An occlusive dressing is prepared using petrolatum gauze and nonporous tape. The chest tube dressing and the suture holding the tube in place are removed. The patient is instructed to practice performing the chosen breathing technique. When the patient has demonstrated compliance with the breathing routine, he or she again breathes as instructed. The nurse holds the chest tube in one hand and with the other holds the prepared sterile dressing over the insertion site. The tube is removed quickly but smoothly while the chest tube entry site is occluded by manual compression of the dressing over the site. Adhesive tape is applied by a second nurse to form an occlusive dressing. A chest roentgenogram is obtained within several hours to ensure that tube removal has not caused pneumothorax.

If two pleural chest tubes with insertion sites close to one another are to be removed, both tubes are clamped and pulled together. If a second chest tube connected by a "Y" connector to the same drainage system is to remain in the chest, it is clamped and disconnected while the first tube (also clamped) is pulled. The remaining chest tube is then reattached to the drainage system with a straight connector and the clamp is removed.

In mechanically ventilated patients, chest tube removal

is performed by two people. One delivers and sustains an inspiration, using a self-inflating ventilation bag; a second person removes the tube during the sustained inspiration and applies the dressing. In thin, frail patients and in those with impaired healing, a pursestring suture may be used to close the chest tube insertion incision at the time of tube removal. Suture closure of the insertion site ensures that recurrent pneumothorax does not result from air entry through the chest tube tract (Douglas, 1992).

If no pursestring suture has been placed, the occlusive dressing remains in place for 48 hours to prevent air entering into the pleural cavity through the chest tube tract in the subcutaneous tissue. After this time, the tract usually has closed and a dressing is no longer required. Occasionally, small amounts of residual fluid in the pleural space continue to drain through the chest tube insertion site for several days after the occlusive dressing has been removed. If so, the site is covered with a gauze dressing until drainage ceases. The patient is instructed to bathe normally and change the dressing daily or more frequently, depending on the amount of drainage.

▶ Special Situations

Massive Air Leak

A *massive air leak* is said to exist when air is entering the pleural space so rapidly that it causes continuous bubbling in the water-seal chamber with suction drainage. Massive air leaks occur most commonly in patients receiving mechanical ventilation with high levels of positive end-expiratory pressure. When alveolar rupture occurs in these patients, positive-pressure mechanical ventilation and positive end-expiratory pressure facilitate rapid leakage of air through the visceral disruption into the pleural space. Massive air leaks also may occur with traumatic airway disruption, ruptured bullae, pneumothorax associated with *Pneumocystis carinii* pneumonia, and occasionally in patients with barotrauma (Munnell, 1997).

Patients with massive air leaks depend on continuous suction drainage to control the rapid egress of air into the pleural space. If the rate of air leakage is greater than can be evacuated by the chest drainage system, the lung fails to reexpand. The patient also may develop *subcutaneous emphysema* or tracking of air into subcutaneous layers of the face, neck, shoulders, or chest (Fig. 42-6). Subcutaneous emphysema is easily detectable by palpation; the soft tissue feels spongy and crunchy to the touch. Occasionally, air tracks into the fascial layer of the neck, distorting the vocal cords and producing a change in the pitch of the patient's voice. If subcutaneous emphysema is excessive, it also may extend down the abdomen into the scrotum, where it usually is prevented from extending into the thighs by the attachments of the inguinal ligament (Allen & Pairolero, 1996).

Continued lung collapse or development of subcutaneous emphysema indicates a need for better evacuation of air from the pleural space. Increasing air flow through the system (ie, increasing the wall suction setting) may facilitate air evacuation, but may increase the magnitude of the bronchopleural fistula, increase air stealing with resultant hypoxia, and, rarely, trap lung in the chest catheter drainage openings (Munnell, 1997). Additional water may be added to the suction chamber to increase the amount of suction, although this is limited by the size of the chamber. An Emerson pump (J. H. Emerson Co., Cambridge, MA), which can generate higher levels of negative suction, may be used alternatively. The insertion of an additional chest tube also may be required to evacuate air that is accumulating rapidly in the pleural space.

Critically ill patients who require mechanical ventilation and who have a massive air leak often are only marginally stable. Tension pneumothorax can occur despite a patent chest tube. Even momentary lung collapse due to discontinuation of suction or occlusion of the tube can result in hypotension or cardiac arrest. If the drainage system must be changed, it is advisable to have a physician in attendance. The equipment is prepared and a second physician or nurse assists so that the patient is dis-

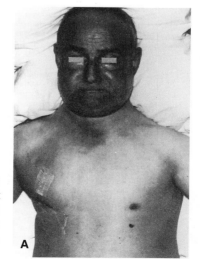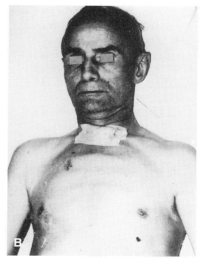

FIGURE 42-6. (**A**) Patient with subcutaneous emphysema; note swollen appearance of face and neck. (**B**) Same patient after subcutaneous emphysema resolved. (Eijgelaar A, 1991: Intrathoracic gas collections. In Webb WR, Besson A [eds]: Thoracic Surgery: Management of Chest Injuries, p. 35. St. Louis, Mosby–Year Book)

connected from suction for only a matter of seconds. The tube is not clamped at any time during the drainage system change.

Chronic Pleural Drainage

Infection of the pleural space occurs most often as a result of pyogenic pneumonia but can also develop as a complication of a thoracic operation, a subphrenic abscess, or chest trauma (Shields, 1994b). The accumulation of pus in the pleural space is termed *empyema thoracis*. Usually, the presence of purulent material causes an inflammatory response that fuses pleural margins around accumulated fluid, localizing the process into a contained pleural abscess (ie, an empyema cavity) (Finkelmeier, 1986).

Empyema often is treated with chronic tube thoracostomy drainage until the cavity fills with granulation tissue, the remaining lung expands, the mediastinum shifts, and the cavity contracts and is obliterated (Alexander & Fetter, 1992). The closed chest drainage system can be converted to open drainage when loculation of the empyema cavity occurs, as evidenced by cessation of respiratory oscillations in the water-seal chamber. Once this occurs, the tube is disconnected from the drainage system and a chest roentgenogram is obtained. If the patient remains without symptoms of pneumothorax and the chest film demonstrates continued lung expansion, the tube is left open to air.

When a chest tube is converted to open drainage in this manner, it is referred to as an *empyema tube*. The tube typically is severed so that only 2 to 3 inches extend outside the skin. After the tube has been cut, a large safety pin is inserted through the exposed portion of the tube and secured by tape to the chest wall so that the tube cannot migrate completely into the chest with respiratory pressure variations. The tube also remains sutured to the skin so that it does not slide out of the empyema cavity. Depending on the amount of drainage, an empyema tube is covered with a glove, ostomy pouch, or dressing.

If an empyema tube adequately drains the infected space, the patient remains afebrile and usually can be discharged from the hospital. If drainage from the tube is thick and purulent, it may be necessary for a family member or visiting nurse to irrigate the tube intermittently with saline solution so that it does not become occluded. The patient is instructed to reinsert the tube if it falls out to prevent closure of the skin opening. Over a period of weeks, the tube is withdrawn gradually from the cavity, an inch or so at a time. Tube repositioning prevents the tube from eroding the lung and permits cavity closure (Lawrence, 1989). A sinogram (ie, roentgenogram of cavity following injection of contrast medium) sometimes is obtained to document the size of the remaining cavity.

Pleural Sclerosis

A common reason for placement of a chest tube is to evacuate a malignant pleural effusion. Several forms of advanced carcinoma are associated with recurring effusions. Approximately 75% of malignant pleural effusions are associated with lung cancer (30%), breast cancer (25%), or lymphoma (20%) (Light, 1997). As fluid accumulates in the pleural space, the patient experiences increasing shortness of breath. The fluid may be evacuated by a thoracentesis or chest tube thoracostomy, but it is likely to reaccumulate.

If chest tube thoracostomy drainage is performed, it often is accompanied by *pleural sclerosis* to obliterate the pleural space. The inflammatory reaction produced by pleural sclerosis causes visceral and parietal pleural surfaces to adhere to one another so that fluid cannot collect between them. If this is successful, the patient does not experience recurring effusion in the pleural space. Pleural sclerosis is performed when the effusion has been completely drained, as evidenced by less than 100 mL of drainage per day. Removal of the fluid allows reexpansion of the lung and apposition of the parietal and visceral pleural surfaces.

A sclerosing agent, such as doxycycline, bleomycin, or talc, is administered through the chest tube into the pleural space, the tube is clamped, and the patient is instructed to change position every 15 minutes for 2 hours (Meko & Patterson, 1999). Repositioning allows the sclerosing agent to cover all the pleural surfaces. The chest tube clamp is then released, and the tube is left in place for several more days to prevent reaccumulation of fluid, maintain lung expansion, and allow the pleural surfaces to become adherent as a result of the induced chemical pleuritis. Chemical sclerosis is often painful. Parenteral narcotic analgesia is administered before introduction of the sclerosing agent and while the sclerosing agent is in the pleural space. In addition, lidocaine is added to the sclerosing solution to provide topical anesthesia. Chemical pleurodesis effectively controls pleural

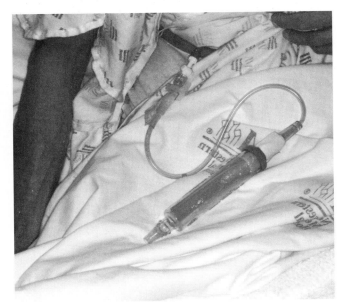

FIGURE 42-7. Chest drainage catheter in this patient with a persistent air leak has been connected to a Heimlich valve.

effusions in 70% to 90% of properly selected patients with malignant effusions (Light, 1997).

Prolonged Air Leak

In some patients, healing processes are impaired and air leaks persist, necessitating continued chest drainage for several weeks. For example, prolonged air leaks often develop in patients with acquired immunodeficiency syndrome and *P. carinii* pneumonia. If the air leak is small, a Heimlich valve may be substituted for the water-seal chest drainage system. A *Heimlich valve* (Becton Dickinson, Franklin Lakes, NJ) is a rigid extension tube designed to be connected to the chest tube. It contains a one-way flutter valve that allows air to escape from the chest tube to the atmosphere but prevents atmospheric air from entering the pleural space (Fig. 42-7). The chest tube and Heimlich valve are taped to the chest wall. The patient can be discharged from the hospital, ambulate freely, and wear clothing that obscures the chest tube from view. The use of Heimlich valves to allow outpatient chest tube management has been expanded in some centers to include patients with primary spontaneous pneumothorax and selected patients with prolonged air leak after pulmonary resection (Ponn et al., 1997).

REFERENCES

Alexander JC, Fetter JE, 1992: Postresectional empyema and bronchopleural fistula. In Wolfe WG (ed): Complications in Thoracic Surgery. St. Louis, Mosby–Year Book

Allen MS, Pairolero PC, 1996: Postoperative care and complications in the thoracic surgery patient. In Baue AE, Geha AS, Hammond GL, et al. (eds): Glenn's Thoracic and Cardiovascular Surgery, ed. 6. Stamford, CT, Appleton & Lange

Bojar RM, 1989: Postoperative care. In Bojar RM (ed): Manual of Perioperative Care in Cardiac and Thoracic Surgery. Boston, Blackwell

Bolling SF, 1991: The management of complications of venous access monitoring and chest tubes. In Waldhausen JA, Orringer MB (eds): Complications in Cardiothoracic Surgery. St. Louis, Mosby–Year Book

Chee CB, Abisheganaden J, Yeo JK, et al., 1998: Persistent airleak in spontaneous pneumothorax—clinical course and outcome. Respir Med 92:757

Cohen RG, DeMeester TR, Lafontaine E, 1995: The pleura. In Sabiston DC Jr, Spencer FC (eds): Surgery of the Chest, ed. 6. Philadelphia, WB Saunders

Compeau C, Johnston MR, 1999: Chest tubes. In Casson AG, Johnston MR (eds): Key Topics in Thoracic Surgery. Oxford, Bios

Courad LL, Velly JF, N'Diaye M, 1990: Principles and techniques of chest drainage and suction. In Deslauriers J, Lacquet LK (eds): Thoracic Surgery: Surgical Management of Pleural Diseases. St. Louis, CV Mosby

Deschamps C, Allen MS, Trastek VF, Pairolero PC, 1992: Postoperative management. Chest Surg Clin North Am 2:713

Douglas JM Jr, 1992: Complications related to patient positioning, thoracic incisions, and chest tube placement. In Wolfe WG (ed): Complications in Thoracic Surgery. St. Louis, Mosby–Year Book

Duhaylongsod FG, Wolfe WG, 1992: Complications of pulmonary resection. In Wolfe WG (ed): Complications in Thoracic Surgery. St. Louis, Mosby–Year Book

Elefteriades JA, Geha AS, Cohn LS, 1996a: Chest trauma. In House Officer Guide to ICU Care: Fundamentals of Management of the Heart and Lungs, ed. 2. Philadelphia, Lippincott-Raven

Elefteriades JA, Geha AS, Cohn LS, 1996b: Chest tubes. In House Officer Guide to ICU Care: Fundamentals of Management of the Heart and Lungs, ed. 2. Philadelphia, Lippincott-Raven

Erickson RS, 1989a: Mastering the ins and outs of chest drainage—1. Nursing 89 19:37

Erickson RS, 1989b: Mastering the ins and outs of chest drainage—2. Nursing 89 19:47

Finkelmeier BA, 1986: Difficult problems in postoperative management. Critical Care Quarterly 9:3

Fry WA, Paape K, 1994: Pneumothorax. In Shields TW (ed): General Thoracic Surgery, ed. 4. Baltimore, Williams and Wilkins

Grégoire J, Deslauriers J, 1995: Closed drainage and suction systems. In Pearson FG, Deslauries J, Ginsberg RJ, et al (eds): Thoracic Surgery. New York, Churchill Livingstone

Hood RM, 1989: Post-injury and postoperative care of thoracic trauma. In Hood RM, Boyd AD, Culliford AT (eds): Thoracic Trauma. Philadelphia, WB Saunders

Howe BE Jr, 1952: Evaluation of chest suction with artificial thorax. Surg Forum 2:1

Hudak CM, Gallo BM, Morton PG, 1998: Patient management: Respiratory system. In Critical Care Nursing, ed. 7. Philadelphia, Lippincott Williams & Wilkins

Joob AW, Hartz RS, 1994: General principles of postoperative care. In Shields TW (ed): General Thoracic Surgery, ed. 4. Baltimore, Williams & Wilkins

Keagy BA, Wilcox BR, 1989: Spontaneous pneumothorax. In Grillo HC, Austen WG, Wilkins EW, et al. (eds): Current Therapy in Cardiothoracic Surgery. Toronto, Canada, BC Decker

Lawrence GH, 1989: Empyema and bronchopleural fistula. In Grillo HC, Austen WG, Wilkins EW, et al. (eds): Current Therapy in Cardiothoracic Surgery. Toronto, Canada, BC Decker

Light RW, 1997: Pleural diseases, pleural effusions. In Khan MG, Lynch JP (eds): Pulmonary Disease Diagnosis and Therapy: A Practical Approach. Baltimore, Williams & Wilkins

Lim-Levy F, Babler SA, DeGroot-Kosolcharoen J, et al., 1986: Is milking and stripping chest tubes really necessary? Ann Thorac Surg 42:77

Marino PL, 1998: The ventilator-dependent patient. In The ICU Book, ed. 2. Baltimore, Williams & Wilkins

Meko JB, Patterson GA, 1999: General thoracic surgery. In Doherty GM, Meko JB, Olson JA, et al. (eds): The Washington Manual of Surgery, ed. 2. Philadelphia, Lippincott Williams & Wilkins

Miller KS, Sahn SA, 1987: Chest tubes: Indications, technique, management, and complications. Chest 91:258

Munnell ER, 1991: Chest drainage in the traumatized patient. In Webb WR, Besson A (eds): Thoracic Surgery: Surgical Management of Chest Injuries. St. Louis, Mosby–Year Book

Munnell ER, 1997: Thoracic drainage. Ann Thorac Surg 63:1497

Mutch MG, Allen BT, 1999: Common surgical procedures. In Doherty GM, Meko JB, Olson JA, et al. (eds): The Washington Manual of Surgery, ed. 2. Philadelphia, Lippincott Williams & Wilkins

Ponn RB, Silverman HJ, Federico JA, 1997: Outpatient chest tube management. Ann Thorac Surg 64:1437

Rodgers BM, 1998: The thoracic duct and the management of chylothorax. In Kaiser LR, Kron IL, Spray TL (eds): Mastery of Cardiothoracic Surgery. Philadelphia, Lippincott Williams & Wilkins

Ronan KP, Murray MJ, 1992: Perioperative assessment and mechanical ventilation. Chest Surg Clin North Am 2: 745

Rusch VW, 1995: Pleural effusion: Benign and malignant. In

Pearson FG, Deslauriers J, Ginsberg RJ, et al. (eds): Thoracic Surgery. New York, Churchill Livingstone

Shields TW, 1994a: General features and complications of pulmonary resections. In Shields TW (ed): General Thoracic Surgery, ed. 4. Baltimore, Williams & Wilkins

Shields TW, 1994b: Parapneumonic empyema. In Shields TW (ed): General Thoracic Surgery, ed. 4. Baltimore, Williams & Wilkins

Symbas PN, 1989: Chest drainage tubes. Surg Clin North Am 69:41

Yeam I, Sassoon C, 1997: Hemothorax and chylothorax. Curr Opin Pulm Med 3:310

43

Complications of Thoracic Operations

Significant complications after thoracic operations are relatively uncommon. The low incidence of morbidity and mortality may be attributed to a number of factors associated with contemporary perioperative management, including thorough preoperative evaluation of pulmonary, cardiac, and nutritional states; careful candidate selection for operative intervention; sophisticated perioperative hemodynamic monitoring; meticulous handling of tissue by the surgeon with preservation of adequate blood supply to areas of resection; and the availability of specialized nursing care in the postoperative period (Finkelmeier, 1986). Furthermore, the advent of limited pulmonary resections, thoracoscopic surgical techniques, and postoperative epidural analgesia has made thoracic surgical procedures possible in some patients who formerly would have been excluded from surgery because of a prohibitive risk (Reilly et al., 1993).

Nevertheless, a variety of complications can occur, some of which have lethal or debilitating consequences. More than two thirds of complications after thoracic operations involve the cardiopulmonary systems; cardiac complications tend to be minor, such as arrhythmias, whereas pulmonary complications are associated with greater morbidity and account for more deaths (Ginsberg, 1995). The most important determinant of postoperative morbidity is the preoperative condition of the patient, particularly the patient's pulmonary and cardiac status.

Thoracic operations most often are performed for resection of malignant neoplasms. Because smoking is a risk factor for both lung cancer and squamous cell esophageal cancer, many surgical candidates have a long smoking history and underlying chronic obstructive pulmonary disease. Associated major medical diseases, such as coronary artery disease or diabetes, also are often present because lung cancer and esophageal cancer typically occur in middle-aged or elderly people. Patients with esophageal cancer often have dysphagia and some degree of esophageal obstruction. Unless the tumor is detected early, weight loss and debilitation may have occurred. In addition, because alcohol abuse is a risk factor for squamous cell esophageal cancer, patients with squamous cell esophageal tumors may have hepatic dysfunction or cardiomyopathy.

► Respiratory Complications

Respiratory complications are one of the most common sources of morbidity in thoracic surgical patients. Postoperative deterioration in pulmonary function and gas exchange can be expected after any major surgical procedure as a result of (1) a reduction in vital capacity, tidal volume, and functional residual capacity; (2) a diminution of the normal sighing mechanism that helps to maintain lung volume and pulmonary compliance; (3) an alteration in the central respiratory drive secondary to narcotic administration; and (4) restricted ventilation due to immobility and pain (Todd, 1994). Although pulmonary dysfunction can complicate any thoracic operation, it is most likely after pulmonary resection operations (ie, when a portion or all of a lung is removed). Pulmonary complications occur most frequently in the first 2 to 4 days after operation (Todd & Ralph-Edwards, 1995). Specific factors that predispose to postoperative respiratory impairment are displayed in Table 43-1.

Atelectasis

Atelectasis is the most common type of postoperative pulmonary dysfunction, with a reported incidence ranging from 10% to 70% (Piccione & Faber, 1991). Some degree of atelectasis is inevitable because of a decrease in functional residual capacity after thoracotomy (Joob & Hartz, 1994). The use of general anesthesia, division of chest wall musculature, immobility, and administration of narcotics for pain control all compromise the patient's ability intermittently to hyperexpand the lungs, as would occur normally. In addition, many thoracic operations are performed using single-lung ventilation, in which the ipsilateral lung is maintained in a deflated state during the operation to improve exposure.

TABLE 43-1

Factors Contributing to Respiratory Complications in Patients Who Undergo Thoracic Operations

Underlying obstructive pulmonary disease
Single-lung ventilation*
Physiologic consequences of thoracotomy incision
Excessive lung resection†
Acute injury to remaining lung†
Prolonged intubation
Inadequate pain control
Indwelling nasogastric tube‡
Excessive sedation
Fluid overload
Aspiration
Multiple transfusions of blood products

*Anesthetic technique used in many thoracic operations.
†Pulmonary resection operations.
‡Esophageal resection operations.

Postoperative atelectasis usually occurs in a lobar or segmental pattern. The presence of collapsed portions of lung tissue decreases pulmonary compliance, increases the work of breathing, and produces areas of poor ventilation with resultant ventilation–perfusion mismatch (Bojar et al., 1989a). Clinical manifestations of atelectasis include fever, tachypnea, and diminished breath sounds on auscultation. Acute shortness of breath and a variable degree of cyanosis may occur with massive atelectasis (Shields, 1994).

Consistent performance of prescribed pulmonary hygiene interventions is essential to minimize postoperative atelectasis. In most cases, incentive spirometry, coughing, and deep breathing are sufficient to clear secretions and expand atelectatic airways. Atelectasis associated with respiratory insufficiency must be treated with more aggressive interventions, such as nasotracheal suctioning, endotracheal intubation, mechanical ventilation, or intermittent bronchoscopy for lavage and deep suctioning. Minitracheostomy may be useful in patients with continued copious secretions to allow frequent tracheal suctioning.

Pneumonia

Pneumonia remains a significant cause of morbidity after thoracic operations. It is most common in patients who require prolonged intubation or who are immunocompromised. Esophageal resection for cancer and chest wall resection are thoracic operations associated with a higher incidence of pneumonia. Patients who undergo esophageal resection may have a poor preoperative nutritional status, chronic low-grade aspiration, poor gastric emptying, and operative disruption of normal esophageal sphincter mechanisms; major chest wall resections place the patient at greater risk by significantly compromising postoperative ventilatory function (Nelson & Moran, 1992).

Postoperative pneumonia also may occur because of unrelieved atelectasis or aspiration of liquid gastric contents into the lungs (Allen & Pairolero, 1996). It is usually bacterial in origin. Common causative organisms include *Hemophilus influenzae,* pneumococcus, and *S. aureus* (Kaiser, 1995). Treatment consists of organism-specific antibiotic therapy, pulmonary hygiene interventions, and respiratory support as indicated by the patient's condition.

Acute Respiratory Failure

Acute respiratory failure is defined as a clinical state in which oxygen delivery and alveolar gas exchange are inadequate to support tissue oxygenation. The most common cause of postoperative respiratory failure is retention of pulmonary secretions secondary to shallow breathing, ineffective cough, and splinting of the chest wall. Other, less common etiologic factors include pneumonia and pulmonary edema. Acute respiratory failure is most common after major pulmonary resection operations in patients with underlying obstructive pulmonary disease. Despite preoperative clinical assessment and pulmonary function testing, it is not possible to predict with certainty a patient's ability to withstand removal of a portion or all of a lung.

Acute respiratory failure often develops insidiously over hours or days. Clinical signs of a deteriorating respiratory status include (1) tachypnea; (2) dyspnea and the use of accessory muscles of respiration; (3) decreasing arterial oxygen tension and decreasing, then increasing, arterial carbon dioxide tension; (4) tachycardia; (5) pallor and diaphoresis; and (6) anxiety, disorientation, or obtundation (Hawthorne, 1992).

Once acute respiratory distress develops, endotracheal intubation and institution of mechanical ventilation usually are necessary. Frequent endotracheal suctioning is instituted to clear secretions and reexpand airways. Etiologic factors, such as pneumonia or pulmonary edema, are treated appropriately, and enteral alimentation is begun. Ventilatory support is continued until the patient demonstrates pulmonary function adequate for self-ventilation. If respiratory failure persists for more than 2 weeks, a tracheostomy usually is performed to avoid potential complications of prolonged endotracheal intubation.

The most severe form of respiratory failure is *adult respiratory distress syndrome (ARDS)*. The condition is characterized by refractory hypoxemia, noncompliant lungs, and diffuse and sometimes homogeneous infiltrates throughout both lungs (Mehta & Pae, 1997). ARDS usually follows an episode of sepsis or shock that produces changes in capillary membrane permeability and the release of bronchoconstricting mediators. The pathophysiology remains unknown, although multiple theories exist on how the alveolar capillary membrane injury occurs (Multz & Dantzker, 1997).

The primary therapy for ARDS is mechanical ventilatory support. A high fraction of inspired oxygen (FiO_2) and positive end-expiratory pressure level usually are necessary to sustain adequate oxygenation. Bronchodilators are used to relieve bronchospasm, secretions are removed by frequent suctioning, and broad-spectrum antibiotics are administered to prevent infection (Mehta & Pae, 1997). Contributing factors, such as pneumonia, atelectasis, pulmonary edema, or anemia, are identified and corrected with appropriate therapy. ARDS is associated with a 40% or greater mortality rate, and patients who do survive require prolonged intensive care (Todd, 1992).

Patients who have undergone pneumonectomy may acquire a unique clinical entity known as *postpneumonectomy edema*. The complication occurs in 3% to 5% of patients undergoing pneumonectomy and does not appear to be related to fluid administration or fluid balance (Deslauriers et al., 1999). Postpneumonectomy edema, which has an unknown etiology, is distinct from pulmonary edema resulting from more common postoperative causes, such as heart failure, aspiration, sepsis, or ARDS (Klemperer & Ginsberg, 1999). It is characterized by progressive dyspnea, hypoxemia, and radiologic evidence of infiltrations in the remaining lung. Treatment includes diuretics, supplemental oxygen, fluid restriction, and ventilatory support. However, once the process of postpneumonectomy edema has begun, no conventional therapy seems to improve the patient's condition; death occurs in 80% to 100% of patients (Deslauriers et al., 1999).

▶ Cardiovascular Complications

Hemorrhage

Hemorrhage is uncommon after thoracic operations if adequate hemostasis is achieved in the operating room before closing the chest. In patients who undergo pulmonary resection, significant bleeding sometimes arises from oozing small blood vessels in areas of denuded lung parenchyma, especially when incomplete fissures have been divided by blunt dissection or when inflamed pleural adhesions have been manually separated (Elefteriades et al., 1996). Postoperative hemorrhage also can occur from a coagulopathy caused by an underlying coagulation abnormality or liver failure (Allen & Pairolero, 1996). Rarely, disruption of a pulmonary artery or vein ligature occurs, causing precipitous, massive hemorrhage.

The degree of postoperative blood loss is evaluated by frequent observation of chest tube output, as well as by serial hematocrit levels and radiographic evidence of hemothorax. If no chest tube is in place (after pneumonectomy), excessive bleeding is detected by roentgenographic demonstration of an abnormally large fluid collection in the operative hemithorax or by clinical signs of hypovolemia. Postoperative coagulopathy is treated with administration of platelets, fresh frozen plasma, or cryoprecipitate to restore adequate coagulation.

In patients with normal coagulation, continued blood loss of greater than 150 mL/h usually prompts operative reexploration to identify and control the source of bleeding. In the rare case of massive hemorrhage, the surgeon may need to reopen the chest incision in the intensive care unit and digitally compress the bleeding vessel to save the patient's life. The patient then is transported to the operating room for exploration and closure of the incision under sterile conditions. Adequate evacuation of a hemothorax is important. Blood accumulating in the chest can compromise respiratory function. In addition, residual hemothorax provides an excellent medium for growth of bacteria and may lead to empyema and entrapment of the lung in a collapsed state.

Cardiac Arrhythmias

Cardiac arrhythmias occur in 9% to 33% of patients who undergo thoracic operations (Amar, 1997). Postoperative arrhythmias develop most often in patients who are older than 50 years of age, who have preexisting cardiovascular disease, and who undergo pneumonectomy or esophageal surgery (Allen & Pairolero, 1996). More than 95% of arrhythmias occur within the first postoperative week, with a peak incidence between the second and fourth postoperative day (Naunheim, 1999; Todd & Ralph-Edwards, 1995). The most frequently occurring arrhythmia is supraventricular tachycardia, in particular, atrial fibrillation. Atrial fibrillation occurs in as many as 20% to 30% of patients who undergo pneumonectomy (Klemperer & Ginsberg, 1999).

Supraventricular tachycardia usually is easily treated with standard pharmacologic agents. Digoxin typically is selected as the agent of choice. Other antiarrhythmic medications that may be used to treat postoperative supraventricular tachycardia include procainamide, verapamil, or diltiazem. Propranolol or other beta-blocking medications that may produce bronchospasm are used less commonly because of the prevalence of obstructive lung disease in patients who require thoracic surgery.

Sinus tachycardia is another common postoperative arrhythmia. It is usually provoked by a hypermetabolic state, such as occurs with fever, anxiety, pain, or anemia. Once the precipitating factor is corrected, the arrhythmia usually subsides. Ventricular arrhythmias are less common after thoracic operations. They usually indicate an acute problem requiring treatment, such as hypoxemia, hypokalemia, or myocardial ischemia. Lidocaine may be used to suppress ventricular ectopy while the causative factor is identified and treated.

Other Cardiovascular Complications

Perioperative myocardial infarction occurs in approximately 3% of patients who undergo thoracotomy (Bojar et al., 1989a). At greatest risk are patients with underlying coronary artery disease and unstable angina, recent myocardial infarction, congestive heart failure, uncontrolled hypertension, or critical aortic stenosis (Hillis et al., 1995). Ischemic events are most likely during the early postoperative period when major alterations occur in adrenergic activity, plasma catecholamine levels, body temperature, pulmonary function, fluid balance, and pain (Mathisen & Wain, 1992). Perioperative myocardial infarction is suggested by characteristic chest discomfort or electrocardiographic abnormalities. A 12-lead electrocardiogram and serial creatine kinase isoenzyme measurements are obtained to confirm the diagnosis. Appropriate pharmacologic and supportive therapy is instituted.

Congestive heart failure can occur as a result of excessive perioperative intravenous hydration or because of underlying heart disease. Congestive heart failure typically occurs soon after mechanical ventilation is discontinued or 24 to 48 hours after the operation, when fluid administered during surgery that has entered interstitial tissue (ie, the "third space") returns to the vascular system (Goldman, 1997). Patients who have undergone pneumonectomy may have right-sided heart failure secondary to the suddenly reduced pulmonary vascular bed and the subsequent elevation of pulmonary arterial pressure (Zwischenberger et al., 1999). In patients

with underlying ventricular dysfunction, the increased afterload to right ventricular ejection may cause the right ventricle to fail.

Cardiogenic pulmonary edema represents an imbalance in hydrostatic and oncotic fluid pressures, along with altered capillary wall permeability. Pulmonary edema develops when fluid entering the peribronchial spaces exceeds the capacity of the lymphatic channels to drain the fluid. Pulmonary compliance decreases, increasing the work of respiration. Fluid moves into the interstitial tissue of the lungs, collapsing or flooding alveoli. Blood flowing through capillaries adjacent to nonventilated alveoli passes without an exchange of oxygen, thus producing a right-to-left intrapulmonary shunt (Allen & Pairolero, 1996). Patients who have undergone pneumonectomy are particularly susceptible because one lung is absent and the entire cardiac output from the right side of the heart travels through the pulmonary vasculature of the remaining lung only.

Cardiogenic pulmonary edema is manifested by tachypnea, anxiety, restlessness, and acute respiratory insufficiency. Treatment includes administration of diuretic agents to remove excess fluid and supplemental oxygen to enhance oxygenation. Intubation and mechanical ventilation with positive end-expiratory pressure may be necessary, depending on the degree of associated respiratory failure.

Pulmonary embolism occurs rarely in patients undergoing thoracic operations. The most common presentation consists of sudden-onset dyspnea and tachypnea (present in more than 90% of patients), tachycardia, or low-grade fever (Zwischenberger et al., 1999). A pulmonary angiogram is used to diagnose pulmonary embolism definitively. Mortality associated with pulmonary embolism is high (50% to 100%), most likely because of the poor cardiopulmonary reserve in patients undergoing thoracic operations (Todd & Ralph-Edwards, 1995).

▶ Incisional Complications

Wound infection is uncommon after thoracotomy because of the excellent blood supply to the thoracic cage and the immunologic competence of the pleural space (Douglas, 1992). Infections that do occur usually result from contamination during operation or develop in patients with risk factors for infection, such as diabetes, chronic corticosteroid therapy, an immunocompromised state, or obesity (Trastek et al., 1992).

The most frequent causative organism for infection of surgical wounds is *S. aureus* (Kaiser, 1995). Incisional infections most often are superficial and are manifested by incisional drainage, erythema, swelling, and tenderness of surrounding subcutaneous tissue. Fever and an elevated white blood cell count are other typical findings. Fluid expressed from the incision is cultured to identify the causative organism. Treatment consists of intravenous antibiotic therapy and local wound care. The subcutaneous layer of the infected segment of the incision may be opened to allow adequate drainage. Necrotic tissue is débrided as necessary, and the wound is cleansed and redressed several times daily.

Rarely, deep wound infection occurs and causes dehiscence, or separation, of the entire wound. In extreme cases, the muscle and ribs may separate, leading to collapse of the underlying lung and acute respiratory insufficiency. Emergent operative exploration is necessary to débride nonviable tissue, irrigate the pleural cavity, and reclose the ribs, chest wall, and usually the skin (McLaughlin, 1991).

Occasionally, complications develop that are related secondarily to a surgical incision. Complications specifically associated with lateral thoracotomy incisions include (1) traction injury to the brachial plexus from overextension of the shoulder, (2) neurovascular injury at the elbow from inadequate padding of the elbow, (3) a "winged scapula" (abnormal protrusion of the scapula) from division of the long thoracic nerve or from excessive posterior retraction, and (4) numbness in the medial aspect of the upper arm and axilla from intercostobrachial nerve injury (Warren, 1989).

▶ Complications of Pulmonary Resection

Persistent Air Space

A *persistent air space* is a potential complication of pulmonary resection operations. When a large portion, but not all, of a lung is removed, the volume of remaining lung may be inadequate to fill the hemithorax completely and an air space remains. Persistent air spaces are unusual because of several compensatory mechanisms that help obliterate a residual space after lobectomy or bilobectomy. The remaining lobe or lobes overexpand, the diaphragm on the operative side moves up, the ipsilateral intercostal spaces narrow, and the mediastinum shifts toward the operative hemithorax (Joob & Hartz, 1994).

Postoperative interventions that help avoid a persistent air space include deep breathing exercises and other pulmonary hygiene measures that promote expansion of atelectatic segments. In some cases, endotracheal suctioning and serial bronchoscopy may be necessary to expand fully collapsed portions of lung. Maintaining suction to the pleural space also promotes full lung expansion. Apposition of the visceral and parietal pleura over as great an area as possible facilitates adherence between the two surfaces (Townsend & Westaby, 1989).

Occasionally, an air space persists despite these compensatory mechanisms and preventive interventions. Factors that contribute to a residual air space include a large or persistent air leak, a resection that includes two lobes on the right or that leaves only the basal segments of the lower lobe, pulmonary fibrosis, disease in the remaining lung that limits expansion, incomplete decortication, postoperative atelectasis, and a fixed mediastinum due to irradiation or prior inflammation (Piccione & Faber, 1991). A persistent air space causes no clinical sequelae in most patients and gradually disappears over a period of months (Shields, 1994). However, the presence of a resid-

ual space is worrisome because of the potential for development of an empyema.

Empyema

An *empyema* (ie, an infection of the pleural space) is a potential complication of any thoracic operation but is most likely after pneumonectomy or when a residual air space remains after a partial lung resection. Empyema occurs in 2% to 16% of patients who undergo pulmonary resection operations (Deschamps et al., 1999). It occurs in 5% of patients after standard pneumonectomy and in 10% of patients who undergo completion pneumonectomy (Gharagozloo et al., 1998). Empyemas are more common after pulmonary resection performed for inflammatory disease than after operations for tumor resection (Shields, 1994). The most frequent causative organisms are *S. aureus* and *Pseudomonas aeruginosa* (Deschamps et al., 1999; Pairolero et al., 1990). A prolonged air leak or bronchopleural fistula may contribute to development of postoperative empyema (Alexander & Fetter, 1992). A bronchopleural fistula is present in more than 80% of patients with postpneumonectomy empyema, particularly in those in whom the empyema develops within the first month of operation (Gharagozloo et al., 1998).

Signs of pleural space infection include fever, purulent chest tube drainage, elevated white blood cell count, and roentgenographic evidence of an air-fluid level. Symptoms include lethargy and anorexia. If empyema is suspected, a thoracentesis is performed and fluid from the pleural space is cultured to identify the causative pathogen. The primary therapy for empyema is effective drainage of the infected space by chest tube thoracostomy. Bronchoscopy is performed to ensure that a bronchopleural fistula has not developed (Todd & Ralph-Edwards, 1995). Organism-specific antimicrobial therapy also is instituted. Further treatment modalities vary depending on the etiology of the empyema, the presence of remaining lung and its ability to reexpand to fill the space, and the presence or absence of a bronchopleural fistula.

Empyema occurring in the early postoperative period after pneumonectomy may be treated with a Clagett procedure. A thoracotomy is performed to débride the empyema cavity and close the bronchopleural fistula that almost always is present. Chest tubes are left in place until the space is adequately drained and cultures are negative; the cavity is then filled with an antibiotic solution that remains in the hemithorax to obliterate the space.

If antibiotics and closed chest tube drainage do not successfully eradicate the infection, chronic drainage of the cavity with one or more chest tubes may be necessary to achieve its obliteration. As the infective process in the pleural space evolves, the inflammatory response fuses pleural margins around accumulated fluid, localizing the process into a contained pleural abscess (ie, an empyema cavity) (Finkelmeier, 1986). Once areas of pleural fusing around the cavity develop sufficiently to keep the lung adherent to the chest wall, the chest tube or tubes may be disconnected from the water-seal drainage system. A chest roentgenogram is obtained to ensure that the lung remains expanded with the cavity open to air. If so, the chest tube is severed 1 to 2 inches from the skin surface and sutured in place. Depending on the amount of drainage, a dressing or ostomy pouch is applied over the tube.

Empyema tubes usually remain in place for several weeks or months. The size of the cavity may be evaluated intermittently by sinogram (ie, the injection of a small amount of contrast material into the cavity followed by radiographic examination). As cavity size diminishes, the tube is advanced gradually to prevent its erosion into the lung and to allow closure of the cavity. A tube remains in the cavity until the intrapleural space is nearly eradicated to prevent leaving a closed cavity that is likely to become reinfected. In the case of a very large cavity or if a drainage tube cannot be adequately secured, a portion of rib may be resected to create a larger opening. A larger tube can then be placed through the bed of the resected rib. Alternatively, an epithelial-lined drainage tract (ie, Eloesser flap or Clagett window) may be surgically created (Fig. 43-1).

Depending on the specific circumstances, a surgical procedure sometimes is necessary to facilitate eradication of an empyema cavity. In patients with empyema after partial lung resection, the inflammatory fibrin reac-

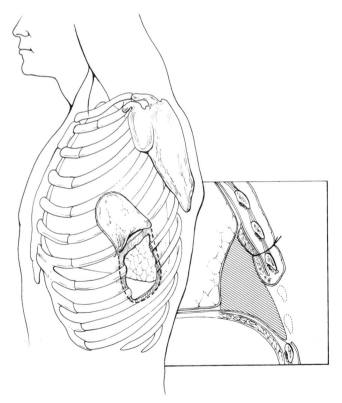

FIGURE 43-1. Eloesser flap. (**Left**) Flap formed and segment of chest wall resected. (**Right**) Flap inserted and fixed to chest wall. (Boyd AD, Glassman LR, 1998: Thoracic incisions. In Kaiser LR, Kron IL, Spray TL [eds]: Mastery of Cardiothoracic Surgery. p. 35. Philadelphia, Lippincott Williams & Wilkins)

tion around the cavity can compress and entrap lung tissue, preventing the lung from expanding to obliterate the cavity (Alexander & Fetter, 1992). If so, decortication (ie, removal of a restricting fibrotic membrane from the visceral pleural surface) may be necessary to allow the underlying lung to reexpand fully.

If the remaining lung is inadequate to fill the space or if parenchymal fibrosis prevents lung reexpansion, a vascularized muscle flap may be translocated to the empyema cavity to obliterate the cavity. The chest wall muscles (eg, pectoralis major or latissimus dorsi) usually are used to create a muscle flap. These muscles all have a single dominant blood supply, and their proximity to the pulmonary hilus makes it possible for them to be rotated and transposed to most intrathoracic locations (Pairolero et al., 1992). Rarely, a thoracoplasty may be necessary to reduce the volume of an empyema cavity and facilitate healing. A thoracoplasty consists of removal of the skeletal support of a portion of the chest wall.

Prolonged Air Leak and Bronchopleural Fistula

Air leakage almost always is present after operations in which a portion of a lung is removed. Air leaks usually originate in areas where incomplete fissures were divided or from denuded parenchyma that has been separated from areas where it adhered to the undersurface of the chest wall. Air leaks typically cease after several days but uncommonly persist for more than a week.

Most *prolonged air leaks* represent inadequate or failed closure of distal bronchioles or alveolar spaces and are termed *bronchoalveolar-pleural fistulae* (Rice & Kirby, 1992). They usually are associated with incomplete lung reexpansion and a residual pleural space. Prolonged air leakage is treated with continued chest tube drainage. Suction usually is maintained until the lung is fully expanded. Once this occurs, the chest tube may be converted to water-seal drainage without suction until the air leak ceases.

Less commonly, a *bronchopleural fistula*, or persistent air leak from a proximal bronchus into the pleural space, occurs after pulmonary resection. Two pathophysiologic concepts help explain failure of a bronchial anastomosis to heal properly. First, blood supply to the bronchus is variable and may be compromised during the operative dissection; second, the tubular cartilaginous structure of the bronchus causes it to have a normal tendency to spring open (Allen et al., 1992). Bronchopleural fistulae are more likely after pneumonectomy than after lesser pulmonary resections; most common is a bronchopleural fistula after right pneumonectomy (Shields, 1994). Postpneumonectomy bronchopleural fistula is a difficult problem to manage and is a strong predictor of subsequent death, which occurs in as many as 70% of patients in whom the complication develops (Klemperer & Ginsberg, 1999).

Factors that increase the risk for development of a bronchopleural fistula include more extensive resection, residual carcinoma in the bronchial stump, preoperative irradiation, bronchial devascularization due to radical mediastinal lymphadenectomy, and diabetes (Todd & Ralph-Edwards, 1995). Careful intraoperative bronchial dissection, meticulous closure, and coverage of the bronchial stump with pericardium, pericardial fat, pleura, or intercostal muscle are surgical techniques that lessen the likelihood of bronchopleural fistula development (Bojar et al., 1989b).

An early bronchopleural fistula (within the first or second postoperative day) usually represents a technical problem with the surgical closure of the remaining bronchial segment; late bronchopleural fistula (8 to 10 days after operation) can occur because of (1) failed bronchial healing secondary to a lack of viable tissue coverage overlying the anastomotic site, or (2) rupture of the anastomosis caused by infection of the pleural space (Shields, 1994). The incidence of bronchopleural fistula has decreased, but the mortality rate associated with the complication remains high (Allen et al., 1992).

A bronchopleural fistula is manifest by a persistent, large air leak. If the rate of air leakage exceeds that which can be evacuated through the chest tubes, subcutaneous emphysema develops as air tracks through subcutaneous tissue planes in the neck, shoulders, and chest. In severe cases, subcutaneous emphysema may extend into the arms, abdomen, and groins. The presence of subcutaneous emphysema indicates for better evacuation of pleural air, either by increasing the amount of suction to existing chest tubes or by placing an additional tube. No specific treatment is required for subcutaneous emphysema itself, which gradually dissipates over the course of several days.

Patients who have undergone pneumonectomy may not have a chest tube in place after surgery. Consequently, the development of a bronchopleural fistula causes a decrease in the postpneumonectomy space fluid level and progressive subcutaneous emphysema. The patient typically expectorates moderate or large amounts of gelatinous, serosanguineous material that has accumulated in the postpneumonectomy space during the days after the operation.

The immediate consequence of a postpneumonectomy bronchopleural communication may be flooding of the remaining lung with fluid expectorated from the operative hemithorax. Emergent chest tube thoracostomy is performed to drain the hemithorax. The chest tube is placed with the patient in an upright position, leaning forward to avoid fluid draining into the remaining lung when the chest wall is entered. Intubation and mechanical ventilation also may be necessary. If so, the bronchus to the remaining lung is selectively intubated and the endotracheal tube cuff is inflated. This allows single-lung mechanical ventilation, isolating the remaining lung from purulent material in the operative hemithorax and eliminating air leakage through the fistula in the contralateral bronchial stump. An associated empyema often develops because the postpneumonectomy space provides an excellent medium for growth of pathogenic organisms introduced into the space through the fistula.

The diagnosis of bronchopleural fistula is confirmed during bronchoscopy. Management of a bronchopleural fistula is complex and depends on timing of fistula development, degree of infection in the pleural space, and presence of remaining pulmonary parenchyma (ie, whether bronchopleural fistula occurs after pneumonectomy or lobectomy). Despite these variables, therapy is guided by three basic principles: (1) adequate pleural drainage, (2) closure of the fistula, and (3) obliteration of the residual pleural space (Allen et al., 1992).

Bronchopleural fistulae sometimes heal spontaneously, requiring only chest tube drainage of the pleural space. Surgical intervention may be necessary for a large or persistent fistula. The bronchial stump is closed and covered with transposed muscle, omentum, or pericardial fat. A concomitant surgical procedure, such as a chest wall muscle flap or thoracoplasty, may be necessary to obliterate an associated empyema cavity.

Other Complications

Cardiac herniation is mechanical displacement and entrapment of the heart through an iatrogenic defect in the pericardium. The pericardial defect is created during pulmonary resection procedures that necessitate opening the pericardial sac to ligate pulmonary hilar blood vessels. Cardiac herniation is a rare complication, most commonly associated with intrapericardial pneumonectomy (Piccione & Faber, 1991). It produces acute hemodynamic instability because mechanical compression of the great vessels decreases cardiac filling and cardiac output. The onset is sudden and is marked by hypotension, tachycardia, and cyanosis, usually within 24 hours of operation (Todd & Ralph-Edwards, 1995).

When cardiac herniation is diagnosed, the patient is positioned immediately on the side opposite the pneumonectomy in an attempt to return the heart to the pericardial sac and relieve the cardiac malposition (Mathisen & Wain, 1992). Emergent surgical reexploration is then performed to reduce the herniation and repair the defect in the pericardium. There are two surgical options for management of the pericardial defect: (1) enlarging the defect so that strangulation will not occur even if the heart is displaced, and (2) closing the defect (eg, using a Gore-Tex [W. L. Gore, Flagstaff, AZ] patch) so that the heart will not be displaced (Zwischenberger et al., 1999).

Lobar torsion, or rotation of a remaining lobe on its bronchovascular pedicle, is a rare complication of lobectomy. Lobar torsion may develop secondary to excessive intraoperative traction or may occur spontaneously. The diagnosis is suggested by radiographic findings and is confirmed during bronchoscopy by the appearance of the twisted lobar bronchus (Wagner & Nesbitt, 1992). Urgent surgical exploration is performed to relieve the torsion and, if necessary, resect the affected lobe. If lobar torsion is unrecognized, the lobar artery or vein may be injured, leading to lobar infarction and gangrene. Clinical manifestations of lobar gangrene include a persistent air leak, fever, and foul-smelling sputum (Bojar et al., 1989b). Surgical reexploration is performed urgently to resect the necrotic lung tissue.

▶ Complications of Esophageal Surgery

The various types of esophageal operations are each associated with specific complications, which are displayed in Table 43-2. The remaining discussion focuses on complications related to esophageal resection procedures.

Anastomotic Leak

Operations in which a part or all of the esophagus must be removed necessitate replacement of the resected esophageal segment with stomach or, less commonly, colon or small

TABLE 43-2

Procedure-Specific Complications of Esophageal Surgery

Operative Procedure	Complications
Esophagomyotomy (cricopharyngeus)	Recurrent laryngeal nerve injury Wound infection/fistula formation
Esophagomyotomy (distal esophagus)	Gastroesophageal reflux
Antireflux operations (Nissen, Dor, Belsey, Toupet, Hill, Collis-Nissen, Collis-Belsey procedures)	Esophageal or gastric perforation Paraesophageal herniation Splenic injury Disruption of gastric wrap Dysphagia Recurrent gastroesophageal reflux "Gas-bloat" syndrome* Excessive intestinal gas Acute gastric dilatation
Esophagectomy with esophago-gastrostomy	Recurrent laryngeal nerve injury Chylothorax Tracheobronchial injury Anastomotic leak Dysphagia Stricture Dumping syndrome Delayed gastric emptying Gastroesophageal reflux Intrathoracic herniation of abdominal viscera Necrosis of gastric conduit
Esophagectomy with colon interposition	Recurrent laryngeal nerve injury Chylothorax Tracheobronchial injury Ischemic graft (colon) necrosis Anastomotic leak Stricture of esophagocolonic anastomosis Graft redundancy Gastrocolic reflux with peptic colitis Early satiety, dysphagia

*Symptom complex including inability to belch and vomit, bloating, and abdominal pain.

intestine. Depending on the visceral substitute chosen, the surgical procedure requires either one or three anastomoses to restore continuity to the gastrointestinal tract.

Esophagectomy with esophagogastrostomy (resection of the esophagus and replacement with stomach) is the most commonly performed esophageal resection operation. It includes repositioning of the stomach in the thorax to replace the resected esophagus. Because the stomach can be elongated to reach the upper chest without disrupting its distal continuity with the duodenum, only a single visceral anastomosis is necessary. This anastomosis, between the proximal stomach and the esophageal remnant, may be either in the mediastinum (intrathoracic) or neck (cervical).

When a segment of colon is used for esophageal replacement (esophagectomy with colon interposition), it must be removed completely from its normal anatomic position to be translocated to the thorax. Consequently, three anastomoses are required to perform the procedure: (1) colon to proximal esophagus, (2) colon to stomach, and (3) reanastomosis of the two remaining bowel segments from which the colon was harvested.

The principal complication specifically related to esophageal resection is *disruption of the esophageal anastomosis* with leakage of nonsterile esophageal contents into the surrounding tissues. Esophageal anastomoses are particularly susceptible to disruption because, in contrast to other viscera, the esophageal wall has no serosal layer but consists only of mucosa, submucosa, and muscularis. In addition, the arterial blood supply is variable and can be segmental; if blood flow to an esophageal anastomosis is compromised, ischemic necrosis can result (Wolfe & Sebastian, 1992). Other factors that increase the risk of anastomotic disruption include preoperative irradiation, residual tumor at the anastomotic site, a poor nutritional status, and distal blockage (gastric outlet obstruction). The reported incidence of anastomotic leak after esophagectomy varies considerably, typically ranging from 5% to 15% (Bains, 1997; Gandhi & Naunheim, 1997; Loinaz & Altorki, 1997).

Because of the potential for postoperative anastomotic disruption, nasogastric suction is maintained and oral nourishment is withheld for 4 to 5 days after esophageal resection. Nutrition is provided enterally during this period through a jejunostomy tube. To protect integrity of the anastomosis, the nasogastric tube usually is not manipulated and, if a proximal anastomosis is present, endotracheal suctioning is avoided. Before removing the nasogastric tube and instituting oral nourishment, a contrast esophagogram is performed to rule out esophageal disruption and leakage. Also, a pleural chest tube is left in place until integrity of the anastomosis is demonstrated by the postoperative contrast study. After confirmation of esophageal integrity, a diet is resumed slowly, beginning with liquids and a mechanical soft diet before advancing to regular foods.

If anastomotic disruption does occur, nonsterile digestive fluids, saliva, and bacteria leak into the periesophageal spaces, causing diffuse cellulitis. Cervical anastomotic leaks usually cause only local inflammation and tenderness with or without subcutaneous crepitation but without constitutional symptoms (Huang, 1994). The localized infection often can be managed with local drainage, nasogastric suction, maintenance of NPO status, and organism-specific antibiotics. The morbidity and mortality associated with a leak in a cervical anastomosis is less than if the anastomosis is located in the chest (Gandhi & Naunheim, 1997).

Intrathoracic esophageal anastomotic disruption that occurs within the first days after operation is most serious and may cause acute tension pyopneumothorax, high fever, dyspnea, or shock; leaks that develop after 4 to 5 days usually cause a more localized empyema or pyopneumothorax manifest by chest pain, fever, tachycardia, and general constitutional symptoms (Huang, 1994). Infection in the thorax is more difficult to manage because of resultant mediastinitis and sepsis. Surgical exploration of the chest usually is necessary to establish adequate drainage of the infection. Disruption of an intrathoracic anastomosis is fatal in 50% of the patients in whom it occurs (Orringer, 1997).

Other Complications

Chylothorax is the accumulation of fat-rich lymphatic fluid in the pleural space as a result of disruption of the thoracic duct or one of its branches. The thoracic duct is the largest lymphatic channel, conveying most of the lymph (chyle) in the body into the circulatory system (Fig. 43-2). Chyle is composed primarily of lymphatic drainage of the intestine but also includes lymph from the lungs, liver, abdominal wall, and extremities (Rodgers, 1998). Thus, lymphatic fluid contained in the thoracic duct is rich in fat and protein (Miller, 1994). Most often, lymphatic disruption occurs in the thorax, but it also can occur in the abdomen as a result of mobilization of the intra-abdominal esophagus and stomach.

Injury to the thoracic duct may occur during almost any thoracic operation, but proximity of the duct to the esophagus makes the complication more common after procedures that necessitate mobilization of the esophagus. Chylothorax is manifest by drainage of large amounts of milky fluid through the chest tubes after resumption of oral nourishment in the postoperative period. The primary consequence of the complication is nutritional depletion, particularly hypoproteinemia. Chylothorax is of most concern in patients with underlying nutritional depletion due to preoperative esophageal obstruction (Orringer, 1991).

Treatment consists of reducing chyle production by dietary restriction of long-chain fatty acids. Nourishment is provided in the form of a clear liquid or low-residue, elemental diet or intravenous hyperalimentation. Total parenteral nutrition with complete enteral rest is the most effective means of reducing thoracic duct flow and facilitating cessation of a chylous leak (Vallieres et al., 1999). Chest tube drainage is maintained until drainage is less than 100 mL/d. Chylothorax usually

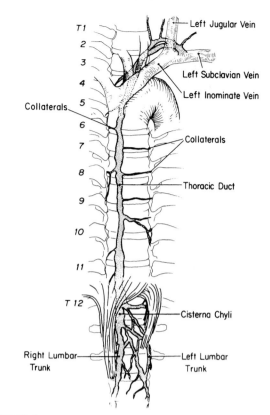

FIGURE 43-2. The most common course and position of the thoracic duct. (Cohen RG, DeMeester TR, Lafontaine E, 1995: The pleura. In Sabiston DC Jr, Spencer FC [eds]: Surgery of the Chest, ed. 6, p. 536. Philadelphia, WB Saunders)

resolves with dietary fat restriction and chest tube drainage. If it persists, operative ligation of the disrupted lymphatic channel is performed. A preoperative saline flush lymphangiogram is obtained to ascertain whether the lymphatic disruption is in the thorax or the abdomen. A thoracotomy approach is used if the thoracic duct disruption is intrathoracic, the most common location. The thoracic duct usually is not visible to the surgeon and it often is impossible to identify the fistula location. Consequently, repair usually consists of a mass ligation of tissue containing the thoracic duct at the supradiaphragmatic level.

Intraoperative *injury to the recurrent laryngeal nerve* can occur as a complication of esophagectomy. It usually occurs during dissection of the esophagus in the neck, but also can occur during intrathoracic mobilization and dissection of the superior mediastinal and thoracic inlet lymph nodes (Bains, 1997). Laryngeal nerve injury occurs more frequently during transhiatal esophagectomy than with esophageal resection through a thoracotomy incision. It usually is manifest by persistent hoarseness and is confirmed with laryngoscopic examination (Inculet, 1998). Postoperative hoarseness is reported in approximately 9% of patients and usually resolves spontaneously (Gandhi & Naunheim, 1997). Injury of the recurrent laryngeal nerve uncommonly leads to significant pulmonary complications due to impaired coughing and a lessened ability to protect the airway from aspiration.

Esophageal resection may be associated with *postoperative dysphagia* resulting from the loss of normal peristaltic function of the esophagus. Neither stomach nor colon functions as effectively in the chest as does the native esophagus in transporting food. Dumping syndrome is a group of postprandial intestinal vasomotor symptoms (epigastric distention, sweating, palpitations, tachycardia, light-headedness, nausea, increased peristalsis, excessive flatus, diarrhea, and disorientation) that often occurs during the postoperative period in patients who have undergone esophagogastrectomy; the symptoms are severe in approximately 1% of patients (Bains, 1997; Collard, 1992). Delayed gastric emptying or gastroesophageal reflux also can occur. Modifications in the amount and type of food ingested may be required to avoid dysphagia and other unpleasant symptoms. The patient is instructed to eat smaller meals, chew food thoroughly, and maintain an upright position during and after meals. These modifications also decrease the likelihood of postoperative aspiration.

Postoperative dysphagia sometimes results from the development of an esophageal stricture at the anastomotic site. Anastomotic strictures may be observed in the early postoperative period or may present several months or even years later (Bains, 1997). Factors contributing to stricture formation include anastomotic leakage, tumor recurrence, tension on the suture line, and esophagitis (Bojar et al., 1989b). Strictures are treated with bougienage (ie, mechanical dilatation) of the anastomosis. It may be necessary to perform dilatation several times or chronically to relieve symptoms.

REFERENCES

Alexander JC, Fetter JE, 1992: Postresectional empyema and bronchopleural fistula. In Wolfe WG (ed): Complications in Thoracic Surgery. St. Louis, Mosby–Year Book

Allen MS, Deschamps C, Trastek VF, Pairolero PC, 1992: Bronchopleural fistula. Chest Surg Clin North Am 2:823

Allen MS, Pairolero PC, 1996: Postoperative care and complications in thoracic surgery. In Baue AE, Geha AS, Hammond GL, et al. (eds): Glenn's Thoracic and Cardiovascular Surgery, ed. 6. Stamford, CT, Appleton & Lange

Amar D, 1997: Prevention and management of dysrhythmias following thoracic surgery. Chest Surg Clin North Am 7:818

Bains MS, 1997: Complications of abdominal right-thoracic (Ivor Lewis) esophagectomy. Chest Surg Clin North Am 7:587

Bojar RM, Murphy RE, Payne DD, Diehl JT, 1989a: Postoperative care. In Manual of Perioperative Care in Cardiac and Thoracic Surgery. Boston, Blackwell

Bojar RM, Murphy RE, Payne DD, Diehl JT, 1989b: Management of postoperative complications. In Manual of Perioperative Care in Cardiac and Thoracic Surgery. Boston, Blackwell

Collard JM, Otte JB, Reynaert M, Kestens PJ, 1992: Quality of life three years or more after esophagectomy for cancer. J Thorac Cardiovasc Surg 104:391

Deschamps C, Pairolero PC, Allen MS, et al., 1999: Early complications: Bronchopleural fistula and empyema. Chest Surg Clin North Am 9:587

Deslauriers J, Aucoin A, Gregoire J, 1999: Early complications: Postpneumonectomy edema. Chest Surg Clin North Am 9:565

Douglas JM, 1992: Complications related to patient positioning, thoracic incisions, and chest tube placement. In Wolfe WG (ed): Complications in Thoracic Surgery. St. Louis, Mosby–Year Book

Elefteriades JA, Geha AS, 1996: Problems following noncardiac thoracic surgery. In House Officer Guide to ICU Care: Fundamentals of Management of the Heart and Lungs, ed. 2. Philadelphia, Lippincott-Raven

Finkelmeier BA, 1986: Difficult problems in postoperative management. Critical Care Quarterly 9:3

Gandhi SK, Naunheim KS, 1997: Complications of transhiatal esophagectomy. Chest Surg Clin North Am 7:601

Gharagozloo F, Trachiotis G, Wolfe A, et al., 1998: Pleural space irrigation and modified Clagett procedure for the treatment of early postpneumonectomy empyema. J Thorac Cardiovasc Surg

Ginsberg RJ, 1995: Preoperative assessment of the thoracic surgical patient: A surgeon's viewpoint. In Pearson FG, Deslauriers J, Ginsberg RJ et al. (eds): Thoracic Surgery. New York, Churchill Livingstone

Goldman L, 1997: General anesthesia and noncardiac surgery in patients with heart disease. In Braunwald E (ed): Heart Disease: A Textbook of Cardiovascular Medicine, ed. 5. Philadelphia, WB Saunders

Hawthorne MH, 1992: Recognition of thoracic surgical complications: A nursing perspective. In Wolfe WG (ed): Complications in Thoracic Surgery. St. Louis, Mosby–Year Book

Hillis LD, Lange RA, Winniford MD, Page RL, 1995: Noncardiac surgery in patients with coronary artery disease. In Manual of Clinical Problems in Cardiology, ed. 5. Boston, Little, Brown

Huang GJ, 1994: Replacement of the esophagus with the stomach. In Shields TW (ed): General Thoracic Surgery, ed. 4. Baltimore, Williams & Wilkins

Inculet RI, 1998: Transhiatal esophagectomy. In Kaiser LR, Kron IL, Spray TL (eds): Mastery of Cardiothoracic Surgery. Philadelphia, Lippincott Williams & Wilkins

Joob AW, Hartz RS, 1994: General principles of postoperative care. In Shields TW (ed): General Thoracic Surgery, ed. 4. Baltimore, Williams & Wilkins

Kaiser AB, 1995: Use of antibiotics in cardiac and thoracic surgery. In Sabiston DC Jr, Spencer FC (eds): Surgery of the Chest, ed. 6. Philadelphia, WB Saunders

Klemperer J, Ginsberg RJ, 1999: Morbidity and mortality after pneumonectomy. Chest Surg Clin North Am 9:515

Loinaz C, Altorki NK, 1997: Pitfalls and complications of colon interposition. Chest Surg Clin North Am 7:533

Mathisen DJ, Wain JC Jr, 1992: Cardiac complications following pulmonary resection. Chest Surg Clin North Am 2:793

McLaughlin JS, 1991: Positional and incisional complications of thoracic surgery. In Waldhausen JA, Orringer MB (eds): Complications in Cardiothoracic Surgery. St. Louis, Mosby–Year Book

Mehta SM, Pae WE, 1997: Complications of cardiac surgery. In Edmunds LH Jr (ed): Cardiac Surgery in the Adult. New York, McGraw-Hill

Miller JI, 1994: Chylothorax. In Shields TW (ed): General Thoracic Surgery, ed. 4. Baltimore, Williams & Wilkins

Multz AS, Dantzker DR, 1997: Adult respiratory distress syndrome. In Parrillo JE (ed): Current Therapy in Critical Care Medicine, ed. 3. St. Louis, Mosby

Naunheim KS, 1999: Postoperative care and monitoring. Chest Surg Clin North Am 9:501

Nelson ME, Moran JF, 1992: Post-thoracotomy pneumonia. In Wolfe WG (ed): Complications in Thoracic Surgery. St. Louis, Mosby–Year Book

Orringer MB, 1991: Complications of esophageal resection and reconstruction. In Waldhausen JA, Orringer MB (eds): Complications in Cardiothoracic Surgery. St. Louis, Mosby–Year Book

Orringer MB, 1997: Tumors of the esophagus. In Sabiston DC Jr (ed): Textbook of Surgery: The Biological Basis of Modern Surgical Practice, ed. 15. Philadelphia, WB Saunders

Pairolero PC, Arnold PG, Trastek VF, et al., 1990: Postpneumonectomy empyema. J Thorac Cardiovasc Surg 99:958

Pairolero PC, Deschamps C, Allen MS, Trastek VF, 1992: Postoperative empyema. Chest Surg Clin North Am 2:813

Piccione W Jr, Faber LP, 1991: Management of complications related to pulmonary resection. In Waldhausen JA, Orringer MB (eds): Complications in Cardiothoracic Surgery. St. Louis, Mosby–Year Book

Reilly JJ, Mentzer SJ, Sugarbaker DJ, 1993: Preoperative assessment of patients undergoing pulmonary resection. Chest 103:342S

Rice TW, Kirby TJ, 1992: Prolonged air leak. Chest Surg Clin North Am 2:803

Rodgers BM, 1998: The thoracic duct and the management of chylothorax. In Kaiser LR, Kron IL, Spray TL (eds): Mastery of Cardiothoracic Surgery. Philadelphia, Lippincott Williams & Wilkins

Shields TW, 1994: General features and complications of pulmonary resections. In Shields TW (ed): General Thoracic Surgery, ed. 4. Baltimore, Williams & Wilkins

Todd TR, 1992: The adult respiratory distress syndrome. Chest Surg Clin North Am 2:769

Todd TR, 1994: Ventilatory support of postoperative surgical patients. In Shields TW (ed): General Thoracic Surgery, ed. 4. Baltimore, Williams & Wilkins

Todd TR, Ralph-Edwards AC, 1995: Perioperative management. In Pearson FG, Deslauriers J, Ginsberg RJ et al. (eds): Thoracic Surgery. New York, Churchill Livingstone

Townsend ER, Westaby S, 1989: Space problems during and after lung resection. In Grillo HC, Austen WG, Wilkins EW, et al. (eds): Current Therapy in Cardiothoracic Surgery. Toronto, Canada, BC Decker

Trastek VF, Pairolero PC, Allen MS, Deschamps C, 1992: Unusual complications of pulmonary resection. Chest Surg Clin North Am 2:853

Vallieres E, Karmy-Jones R, Wood DE, 1999: Early complications: Chylothorax. Chest Surg Clin North Am 9:609

Wagner RB, Nesbitt JC, 1992: Pulmonary torsion and gangrene. Chest Surg Clin North Am 2:839

Warren WH, 1989: Lateral thoracotomy: Technique, indications, and complications. In Grillo HC, Austen WG, Wilkins EW, et al. (eds): Current Therapy in Cardiothoracic Surgery. Toronto, Canada, BC Decker

Wolfe WG, Sebastian MW, 1992: Complications following esophagectomy and esophagogastrectomy. In Wolfe WG (ed): Complications in Thoracic Surgery. St. Louis, Mosby–Year Book

Zwischenberger JB, Alpard SK, Bidani A, 1999: Early complications: Respiratory failure. Chest Surg Clin North Am 9:543

44

Postoperative Chest Roentgenogram Interpretation

The *chest roentgenogram* is an invaluable diagnostic tool in the daily care of cardiothoracic surgical patients. In acutely ill patients, it remains the gold standard for initial evaluation of the lungs, heart, mediastinum, and aorta (Elefteriades et al., 1996a). A preoperative chest roentgenogram is obtained shortly before every elective cardiac or thoracic operation to detect abnormalities that might alter the planned surgical therapy. This preoperative film also provides a baseline for comparison with postoperative films. During the postoperative period, chest roentgenograms typically are obtained (1) immediately after the operation is concluded, (2) daily while the patient is critically ill, (3) after placement of intrathoracic catheters or tubes, (4) to detect pneumothorax after chest tube removal, and (5) if there is an unexplained deterioration in the patient's cardiopulmonary status.

Postoperative chest roentgenograms often are available for review by nurses who work in cardiothoracic surgical nursing units. The nurse at the bedside may be the first to view a chest roentgenogram that demonstrates new clinical information. A basic knowledge of the radiographic appearance of normal anatomic structures, intrathoracic catheters and tubes, and common postoperative abnormalities provides nurses in these settings with additional information that can enhance patient management. With appropriate physician consultation, the nurse can facilitate timely modifications in therapy based on radiographic findings. The ability to correlate radiographic findings with the patient's clinical status also increases the nurse's understanding of intrathoracic anatomy and pathophysiology. This chapter provides general information about chest roentgenograms as well as guidelines for recognizing normal postoperative alterations and common intrathoracic abnormalities of acute clinical significance.

▶ The Portable Chest Roentgenogram

Technique and Patient Positioning

Most chest roentgenograms available for viewing by nurses are obtained at the patient's bedside using portable equipment. An anteroposterior (AP) projection is used; that is, the x-ray tube is positioned in front of the patient's chest and the film cassette behind the patient's back. The x-ray beam passes through the patient from front to back. An AP projection is opposite that used for standard posteroanterior (PA) chest roentgenograms taken in a radiology department in which the x-ray beam passes through the patient from back to front.

A portable chest roentgenogram is of lesser quality than one obtained using equipment available in a radiology department. Also, AP and PA roentgenograms in the same patient are not comparable because an AP technique enlarges the shadow of the anteriorly positioned heart. Despite these limitations, a portable AP chest film provides a useful radiographic view of the thorax for clinical decision making in patients too ill to be transported away from the nursing unit.

To provide the maximal amount of diagnostic information from a portable roentgenogram, consistent attention to technique and patient position is essential because it significantly influences the appearance of intrathoracic structures. Portable roentgenograms in hemodynamically stable patients are taken with the patient sitting fully upright in the bed. The hemidiaphragms appear lower when the patient is upright and the lungs appear more fully expanded than when the patient is in a supine position and the diaphragm is pushed upward by abdominal viscera (Matthay & Sostman, 1990). Ideally, the patient's chest is perfectly perpendicular to the x-ray tube; if not, a lordotic projection is obtained in which the heart appears larger and indistinct and the height of the lung fields is decreased (Huseby, 1995). It may not be possible to position a patient whose condition is unstable in an upright position; if so, the roentgenogram is obtained with the patient supine.

Chest roentgenograms usually are taken at the end of a full inspiration to demonstrate most clearly the intrathoracic structures, particularly the lungs. If the inspiratory effort is not good, the elevated diaphragm may cause a transverse appearance of the heart and give the pulmonary vasculature a falsely engorged appearance. Rotation of the patient also can distort the appearance of the heart and hilar areas and cause the lung fields to appear different in density. The degree of rotation is assessed by the appearance of the trachea, the clavicular heads, and the relationship of the anterior ends of the ribs with the thoracic spine. In a straight PA view, the trachea should be projected over the spinous processes of the cervical and upper thoracic vertebrae, the lengths of the two clavicles are equal, and the distances between the ends of the anterior ribs and the lateral margins of the thoracic spine are equal (Boxt, 1998).

Guidelines for Review

Chest roentgenogram interpretation begins with knowledge of the appearance of the normal anatomic structures as viewed on a PA and lateral chest roentgenogram (Fig. 44-1, A and B). A properly penetrated chest roentgenogram should allow differentiation of the four basic radiographic densities: air, bone, soft tissue, and fat (Boxt, 1998). The various structures are reviewed in a sequential fashion, examining each for abnormalities. The observed radiographic findings must be correlated with clinical information about the patient. For example, when comparing a roentgenogram obtained after extubation with a prior film obtained during mechanical ventilation, the decreased quantity of air in the lungs may make the roentgenographic appearance worse, whereas physiologically the patient is actually better (Milne, 1980).

A roentgenogram of the adult chest displays the heart, lungs, bony thorax, and soft tissues of the chest wall, all of which produce different radiographic densities. Bone, which is densest, creates the lightest, or most radiodense, shadow; lung, which is largely air, appears lucent, or black (Huseby, 1995). Examination of thoracic bony structures (ribs, sternum, vertebrae, clavicles, and scapulae) is not particularly relevant for cardiothoracic surgical nurses. Except in victims of chest trauma, it is unusual to detect an abnormality of acute clinical significance. The soft tissues, which create a radiodense shadow surrounding the bony thorax, also usually are normal. The most common soft tissue abnormality, subcutaneous emphysema, occurs infrequently and is described later in the chapter.

The *mediastinal shadow* is the radiodense area between the right and left lung fields. The heart and great vessels are the primary structures that create the mediastinal shadow. Portions of the cardiac chambers, aorta, and pulmonary artery create the borders of what is termed the *cardiac silhouette* (Boxt, 1998). The right heart border, which extends slightly to the right of the thoracic spine, is formed predominantly by the right atrium. The left heart border comprises the aortic arch, main pulmonary artery, left atrial appendage, and left ventricle. Most of the cardiac mass lies in the left hemithorax.

The *trachea* usually can be seen in the mediastinal shadow as an air-filled structure located slightly to the right of the midline. The main bronchi are somewhat smaller in diameter than the trachea; the right mainstem bronchus continues downward from the trachea more vertically than the left in adults and divides into two main branches (Juhl, 1993). The shadows of other mediastinal structures, such as the esophagus, thymus, and lymph nodes, merge with one another and are superimposed on the shadows of the spine, heart, and sternum (Squire & Novelline, 1988).

Mediastinal width cannot be assessed accurately on AP roentgenograms because of mediastinal widening that occurs secondary to technique. On a PA roentgenogram, the simplest method of estimating mediastinal width is to determine the cardiothoracic ratio (ie, the width of the cardiac silhouette at its widest diameter near the diaphragm compared with the width of the chest). The normal cardiac silhouette on a PA roentgenogram is no more than one half the width of the thoracic cavity.

Mediastinal shift (ie, shifting of the trachea and other midline structures) is an important radiologic finding that can be caused by a variety of pathologic conditions. For example, an abnormality associated with volume loss, such as atelectasis, produces shifting of midline structures toward the affected side of the thorax. Conversely, space-occupying abnormalities (eg, pneumothorax or pleural effusion) may shift the trachea and mediastinal shadow away from the affected side.

The *lung fields* occupy most of the right and left hemithorax. The lungs are examined primarily for areas of abnormally increased density or lucency. The normally expanded lungs appear predominantly translucent, or black. The interstitium of the lung (a continuum of loose connective tissue throughout the lung) normally is not visible radiographically, but becomes visible when disease (eg, tumor, edema, fibrosis) increases its volume and attenuation (Collins & Stern, 1999a). Interlobar fissures, created by the visceral pleura that lines each lobe, usually are not apparent on an AP roentgenogram unless fluid has collected in the fissure or a lobe is collapsed and therefore opacified (Freundlich & Bragg, 1992a).

Fine, white, linear shadows, known as *lung markings,* normally are evident throughout the lung fields and

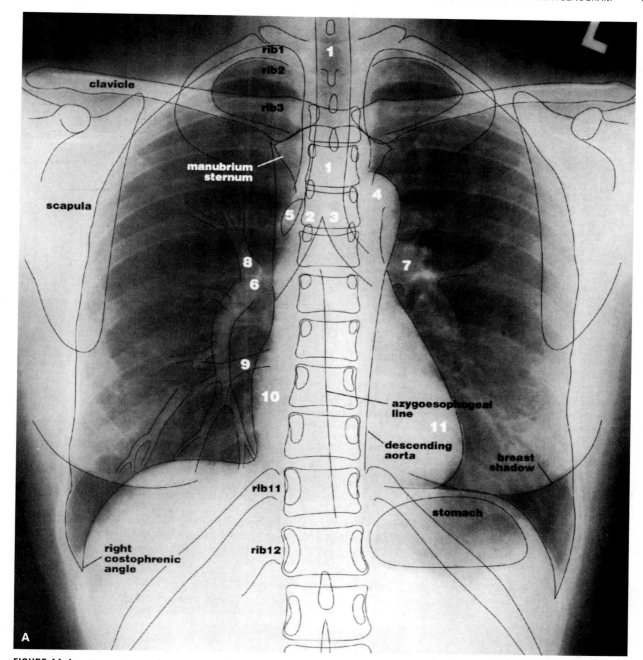

FIGURE 44-1. (**A**) Normal anatomic structures on the PA chest radiograph: trachea (1), right mainstem bronchus (2), left mainstem bronchus (3), aortic "knob" or arch (4), azygos vein emptying into superior vena cava (5), right interlobar pulmonary artery (6), left pulmonary artery (7), right upper lobe pulmonary artery (8), right inferior pulmonary vein (9), right atrium (10), left ventricle (11), and other structures as labeled. *(continued)*

represent pulmonary blood vessels. Lung markings should be visible extending to all edges of the thorax. In an upright film, these pulmonary vascular markings appear primarily in the bases with scant vascular markings in the upper lung fields. Although the distribution of pulmonary vessels is uniform between upper and lower lung zones, the intrapulmonary vessels of the lower lobes carry greater pulmonary blood flow and thus appear larger radiographically when the patient is upright;

when the patient is supine, pulmonary vessels in the upper lung fields appear larger with respect to lower lobe vessels (Boxt, 1998).

The heaviest and widest lung markings on either side of the heart shadow are created by the major pulmonary arteries and veins. These large pulmonary arteries and veins, and to a lesser extent nearby bronchi, form the complex shadow on either side of the heart known as the *pulmonary hilum* (Westra, 1990). Most right and left hi-

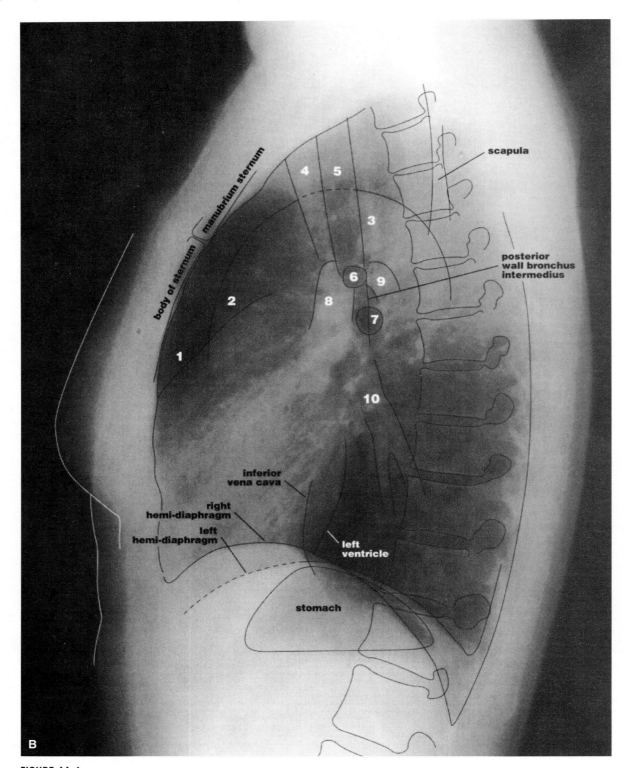

FIGURE 44-1. (CONTINUED) (B) Normal structures on the lateral chest radiograph: pulmonary outflow tract (1), ascending aorta (2), aortic arch (3), brachiocephalic vessels (4), trachea (5), right upper lobe bronchus (6), left upper lobe bronchus (7), right pulmonary artery (8), left pulmonary artery (9), confluence of pulmonary veins (10), and other structures as labeled. (Collins J, Stern EJ, 1999: Normal anatomy of the chest. In Chest Radiology: The Essentials, p. 3. Philadelphia, Lippincott Williams & Wilkins)

lar opacities are formed by the right and left pulmonary arteries, respectively (Boxt, 1998). Hilar densities should be symmetric in size and density (Collins & Stern, 1999b). The left hilum is higher than the right.

The right and left hemidiaphragms appear on the roentgenogram as smooth, dome-shaped structures that are in sharp contrast to the radiolucent lungs above (Juhl, 1993). In most people, the right hemidiaphragm is 1.5 to 2.0 cm higher than the left (Collins & Stern, 1999b). The junction of the diaphragm and chest wall on either side of the thorax is known as the *costophrenic angle* or *sulcus* and should appear as a sharply defined angle. Beneath the left hemidiaphragm is a lucent area representing air in the stomach (ie, the stomach bubble).

▶ Intrathoracic Catheters, Tubes, and Devices

Postoperative cardiothoracic surgical patients typically have several intrathoracic catheters and tubes. Each plays an important role in postoperative monitoring or facilitating recovery from the operation. Radiopaque markings make these catheters and tubes visible on the chest roentgenogram and allow confirmation of proper positioning (Fig. 44-2). Implanted prosthetic devices, such as cardiac valves or pacemakers, also may be identifiable on the postoperative roentgenogram.

An endotracheal tube is identified by a radiopaque line at the distal end of the tube. When the head and neck are in a neutral position, the tip of the endotracheal tube should lie in the midtrachea, approximately 4 to 7 cm above the carina (Collins & Stern, 1999c). The carina is located on the roentgenogram by following the inferior wall of the left mainstem bronchus medially until it joins the right mainstem bronchus (Goodman, 1983a). With flexion of the neck, the tip of the endotracheal tube moves slightly downward in the trachea; when the neck is extended, it moves upward (Khan & Settle, 1996). If the tube is positioned so that the end is distal to the carina, extending into the right mainstem bronchus, the left lung or right upper lobe is not ventilated and becomes atelectatic. If the distal end of an endotracheal tube is too high, accidental extubation is more likely.

A pulmonary artery catheter can be traced on the roentgenogram through the superior vena cava, right atrium, and right ventricle. The tip of the catheter, positioned in a branch of the right or left main pulmonary artery, is apparent overlying the lung shadow on that side. If the tip is coiled in the right ventricle, pulmonary artery pressures cannot be measured and ventricular arrhythmias may develop from mechanical irritation of the ventricle. If the tip is positioned too far peripherally in one of the pulmonary artery branches, it can totally occlude the vessel, leading to pulmonary ischemia or infarction. A central venous catheter usually is positioned so that the catheter tip is in the right atrium or superior vena cava. It should appear on the roentgenogram on the right side of the mediastinal shadow approximately halfway down the right heart border.

Temporary pacing leads, usually placed on the atrial and ventricular epicardium during cardiac operations, appear as thin, coiled wires superimposed over the heart shadow. An intra-aortic balloon catheter usually is inserted into the femoral artery and advanced retrograde through the descending thoracic aorta so that its tip is positioned just distal to the left subclavian artery. The radiopaque marker defining the tip of the catheter should appear to the left of the thoracic spine, just below the aortic knob. A nasogastric tube is identified by the radiodense marking demonstrating the tip and side hole of the tube below the diaphragm and within or past the gastric lumen (Umali & Smith, 1991).

A mediastinal chest tube is identified by a radiodense line superimposed on the mediastinal shadow. A tube placed in the anterior mediastinum is visible parallel to the sternum; a posterior tube lies between the inferior heart border and diaphragm (Goodman, 1980). A pleural chest tube placed to evacuate pneumothorax is positioned so that its drainage holes lie between the apex of the lung and the anterior chest wall. A pleural tube placed to drain fluid is positioned inferiorly and posteriorly in the pleural space. All drainage holes should be positioned within the pleural cavity (Munnell, 1991). The last, or most proximal, side hole is identified on the chest roentgenogram by a short interruption in the radiodense line on the chest tube. It should appear medial to the inner margin of the ribs (Collins & Stern, 1999c).

Implanted cardiac valve prostheses may or may not

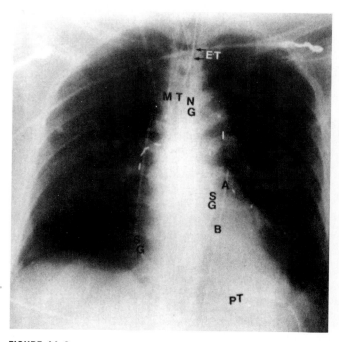

FIGURE 44-2. Portable chest roentgenogram taken after coronary artery bypass operation demonstrating position of endotracheal tube (ET), mediastinal chest tube (MT), nasogastric tube (NG), pulmonary artery catheter (SG), intra-aortic balloon catheter (A-B), and pericardial chest tube (PT). (Sider L, 1986: Interpretation of the postoperative chest radiograph. Critical Care Quarterly 9:73)

be visible on the chest roentgenogram, depending on the specific prosthesis. In most instances, the orientation of a radiodense valvular prosthesis reveals its position within the heart. The intracardiac position of cardiac valve prostheses also can be recognized by drawing an imaginary line from the right cardiophrenic border to the upper third of the left heart border (Sider, 1986). Prostheses implanted to replace atrioventricular (mitral or tricuspid) valves appear below this line, and those that replace semilunar (aortic or pulmonic) valves are visible above the line (Fig. 44-3).

A permanent pacemaker and pacing leads are easily visualized on a chest roentgenogram. A permanent pacemaker connected to transvenous leads is visible superimposed over the right or left upper lung field. A transvenous ventricular lead can be traced through the right side of the heart to its tip at the apex of the right ventricle, and an atrial lead appears superimposed on the right atrial shadow (Fig. 44-4). Permanent epicardial pacing leads are used rarely; an epicardial lead attached to the right atrium appears at the edge of the right heart border, a right ventricular lead appears superimposed over the heart shadow, and a left ventricular lead appears at the edge of the left heart border. A pacemaker connected to epicardial leads usually is visible in the subcutaneous tissue of the upper abdomen.

▶ Typical Postoperative Alterations

Thoracic Operations

Patients who have undergone thoracotomy usually have two pleural chest tubes, one directed toward the apex of the lung and one toward the base (Fig. 44-5). An endotracheal tube may also be present during the early post-

operative hours. Areas where ribs have been surgically divided or resected are often apparent in the rib cage of the operative hemithorax. After partial lung resection (ie, wedge resection, segmentectomy, or lobectomy) the chest roentgenogram ideally demonstrates full lung expansion on the operative side and minimal or no pleural fluid accumulation. Although small air leaks typically are present after pulmonary resection, there may be no radiographic evidence of pneumothorax because the chest drainage system usually prevents air accumulation in the pleural space. Often, a row of metallic staples, used to seal lung tissue that has been incised, is visible in the area of pulmonary resection.

After wedge resection or segmentectomy, an infiltrate representing hemorrhage, contusion, or atelectasis may be apparent in the involved lobe. After lobectomy, the remaining lobe or lobes overexpands to fill the space left vacant by the resected lobe. The roentgenogram may demonstrate other compensatory changes as well that facilitate expansion of remaining lung to fill the operative hemithorax, including shifting of the mediastinum toward the operative side, narrowing of ipsilateral (same side) intercostal spaces, and elevation of the ipsilateral hemidiaphragm (Joob & Hartz, 1994) (Fig. 44-6). A small air space sometimes remains at the top of the operative hemithorax.

A chest roentgenogram in the early hours after pneumonectomy demonstrates a vacant hemithorax with little or no fluid, a fully expanded contralateral (opposite) lung, and an approximately midline trachea (Goodman, 1983b). Often, no chest tube is in place or a clamped tube may be positioned in the empty pleural space. During the first several days after pneumonectomy, the roentgenogram provides an important means of assessing mediastinal position. Mediastinal shift toward either the operative or nonoperative side may occur (Elefteriades et al., 1996b).

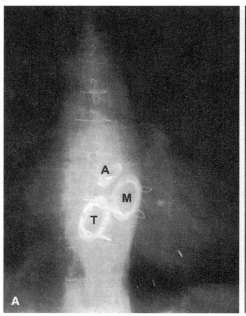
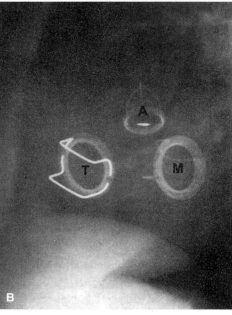

FIGURE 44-3. (**A**) AP radiograph demonstrating projection of prosthetic valves in the aortic (A), mitral (M), and tricuspid (T) positions. (**B**) Radiographic appearance in the lateral projection of aortic (A), mitral (M), and tricuspid (T) prosthetic valves. (Garcia JM, 1998: Prosthetic valve disease. In Topol EJ [ed]: Comprehensive Cardiovascular Medicine, p. 612. Philadelphia, Lippincott Williams & Wilkins)

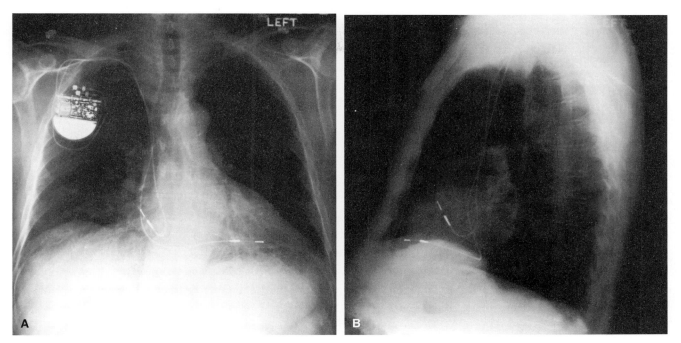

FIGURE 44-4. Posteroanterior (**A**) and lateral (**B**) chest roentgenograms illustrating the pulse generator and atrial and ventricular leads of a dual-chamber, transvenous permanent pacemaker. (Courtesy of Arthur Palmer, MD)

Gradual mediastinal shift toward the nonoperative side may indicate either atelectasis of the remaining lung or fluid accumulation in the operative hemithorax faster than air in the space can be resorbed (Goodman, 1980). Conversely, if air is resorbed more quickly than fluid is secreted into the empty space, the mediastinum may shift toward the operative side. Normally, the vacant hemithorax gradually fills with fluid over weeks or months until the pneumonectomy space is completely opacified by fluid or only a small air space at the top of the hemithorax remains (Fig. 44-7).

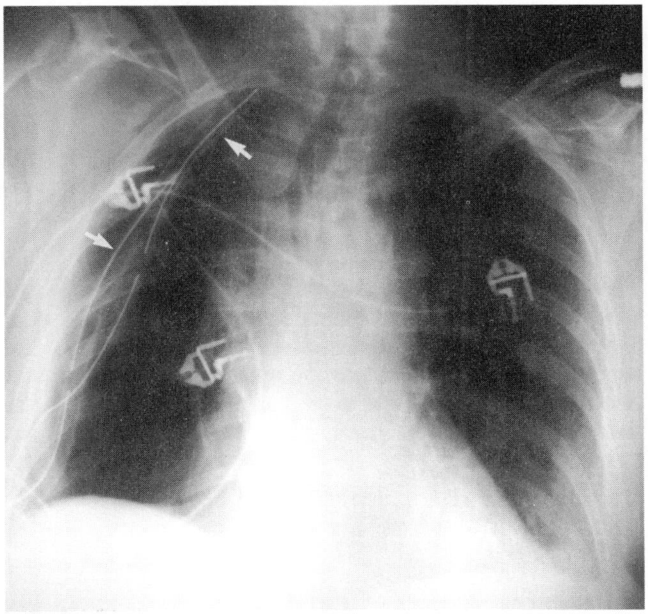

Cardiac Operations

After cardiac operations, patients typically have an endotracheal tube, a pulmonary artery catheter, a central venous catheter, two mediastinal chest tubes, epicardial pacing wires, and a nasogastric tube. In patients with perioperative low cardiac output, an intra-aortic balloon catheter may have been placed. A pleural chest tube may be present if one of the pleural spaces was opened. Rib fractures, particularly of the first or second rib, sometimes occur during median sternotomy and may be apparent on the postoperative roentgenogram (Chiles, 1992). Approximately 75% of patients have some degree of atelectasis in the left lower lobe of the lung; another 10% to 20% have bilateral atelectasis (Goodman, 1983b).

▶ Common Abnormalities

Densities in the Pulmonary Parenchyma

FIGURE 44-5. Portable chest roentgenogram obtained in early postoperative hours after right upper lobectomy. Two chest tubes have been positioned in the right pleural space (*arrows*). The loss of one lobe on the right side has caused tracheal deviation and narrowing of right-sided intercostal spaces. (Courtesy of Axel W. Joob, MD)

The most common cause of a parenchymal (ie, lung tissue) density in postoperative cardiothoracic surgical patients is *atelectasis;* that is, loss of lung volume due to collapse of the normally air-filled alveoli. Because the at-

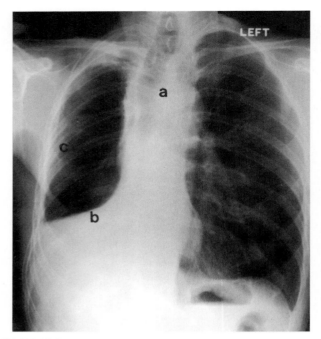

FIGURE 44-6. Posteroanterior roentgenogram after lobectomy of the right middle and lower lobes. Compensatory changes that facilitate expansion of the remaining upper lobe to fill the space include mediastinal shift (a) toward the operative hemithorax (note deviation of trachea to the right), elevation of right diaphragm (b), and narrowing of intercostal spaces on the right side (c). (Courtesy of Robert M. Vanecko, MD)

assist in localizing a pulmonary opacity. It is present when a parenchymal abnormality obliterates the border of contiguous structures, such as the heart, aorta, or diaphragm (Juhl, 1993). For example, right middle lobe atelectasis obscures the right heart border, whereas right lower lobe atelectasis obscures the right hemidiaphragm.

When a main bronchus is obstructed, the entire lung may become atelectatic. Complete collapse of either lung results in opacification of the hemithorax and shift of mediastinal structures to the affected side (Collins & Stern, 1999d). Compensatory hyperexpansion of the contralateral lung causes it to appear excessively lucent.

An abnormal parenchymal density also may represent *alveolar consolidation;* that is, flooding of alveoli with fluid or material to the virtual exclusion of air (Freundlich & Bragg, 1992b). Alveolar consolidation may result from a variety of pathophysiologic entities, including pneumonia, pulmonary edema, aspiration, or intrapulmonary hemorrhage. Pneumonia is probably the most frequently observed cause of pulmonary consolidation in postoperative patients. Like atelectasis, pneumonia causes a focal opacity in the lung field. Depending on the stage of infection and organism involved, pneumonia can vary in appearance from a streaky, hazy area in the lung to a dense consolidation (Sider, 1986). Differentiation of pneumonia

electatic area of lung no longer contains air, it appears as a white shadow in the lung field. Knowledge of the location of the various lung lobes as projected on frontal and lateral roentgenograms is essential in identifying what portion of the lung is affected (Fig. 44-8).

The amount of atelectasis may be confined to several segments or may extend to an entire lobe or lung. Opacification of atelectatic lung may not be seen until a considerable amount of volume loss has occurred (Collins & Stern, 1999d). A common form of atelectasis in postoperative patients is discoid, or plate-like, atelectasis caused by collapse of small subsegmental areas of lung due to hypoventilation. Discoid atelectasis is named for its characteristic appearance as a linear, plate-shaped opacification in the lung field. It usually abuts the pleura, is perpendicular to the pleural surface, and ranges in thickness from a few millimeters to a centimeter or more (Collins & Stern, 1999d).

Sometimes, a lobar bronchus becomes obstructed with secretions causing opacification of an entire lobe (Fig. 44-9). Lobar atelectasis often can be detected by displacement of interlobar fissures in association with increased density of the collapsed lobe (Miller, 1994). An air bronchogram also may be visible in areas of parenchymal consolidation. An air bronchogram is a branching, tubular lucency representing a bronchus passing through airless parenchyma; it indicates that the underlying opacity must be parenchymal rather than mediastinal or pleural (Collins & Stern, 1999e). A silhouette sign may

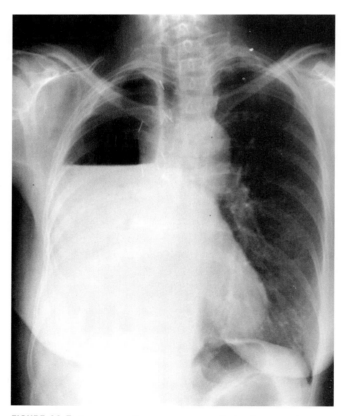

FIGURE 44-7. Posteroanterior roentgenogram obtained 1 week after right pneumonectomy demonstrates typical fluid accumulation in operative hemithorax. A subsequent roentgenogram several months later revealed further fluid accumulation with only a small residual air space at the top of the hemithorax. (Courtesy of Robert M. Vanecko, MD)

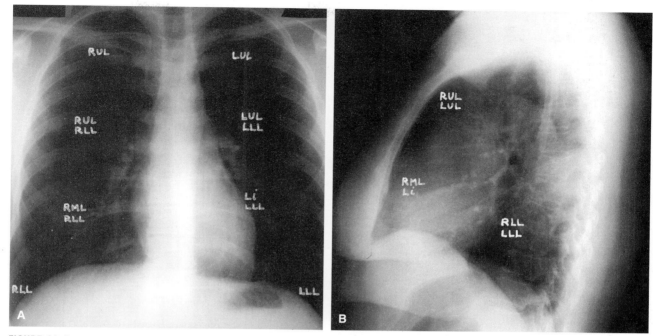

FIGURE 44-8. Location of the lung lobes on frontal (**A**) and PA (**B**) chest radiographs. RUL, right upper lobe; RLL, right lower lobe; RML, right middle lobe; LUL, left upper lobe; LLL, left lower lobe; Li, lingula. (Huseby JS, 1995: Radiologic examination of the chest. In Woods SL, Froelicher ES, Halpenny CJ, Motzer SU [eds]: Cardiac Nursing, ed. 3, p. 281. Philadelphia, JB Lippincott)

and atelectasis can be difficult, and sometimes both are present. Except in patients who require prolonged intubation and mechanical ventilation, most postoperative parenchymal densities represent atelectasis.

Pulmonary infarction occurs rarely in patients who undergo cardiac and thoracic operations, as a result of pulmonary embolism or as a complication of a pulmonary artery catheter. Pulmonary infarction secondary to pulmonary embolism usually produces multifocal opacities, predominantly in the lower lung zones (Collins & Stern, 1999f). However, chest roentgenograms lack the sensitivity to differentiate definitively opacities due to parenchymal infarction from those due to other causes. Although computed tomographic (CT) imaging also cannot definitively establish the diagnosis. However, pulmonary infarction is suggested by the presence on lung window CT images of areas of parenchymal consolidation adjacent to a pleural surface that are wedge shaped or that have convex, bulging borders (Sagel & Slone, 1998).

Fluid Collections

Hemorrhage in postoperative patients is always a concern and is one reason that patients undergoing cardiac or thoracic operations have portable chest roentgenograms on arrival in the postoperative intensive care or recovery unit. The degree of postoperative bleeding is best evaluated by quantification of blood loss in the chest drainage system. However, if the rate of bleeding is excessive or the tubes become occluded by clotted blood, blood accumulates in

the chest. The roentgenogram may assist in establishing a diagnosis of postoperative hemorrhage by demonstrating mediastinal widening or hemothorax before clinical manifestations of hypovolemia develop. The chest roentgenogram is particularly important in detecting postoperative hemorrhage after pneumonectomy because a chest tube may not be placed.

In patients undergoing cardiac operations, undrained blood collects in the mediastinal space, producing a widening of the mediastinal shadow on the chest film. Although mediastinal widths on the preoperative PA and postoperative AP films are not comparable, comparison of two serial postoperative films may reveal an increasing mediastinal width. This finding, particularly if supported by clinical findings, is suggestive of mediastinal hemorrhage. A hemothorax, or blood in the pleural space, also may be present if one or both of the pleural spaces was opened during the operation.

In patients who have undergone pulmonary resection operations, blood that accumulates in the pleural space appears radiographically as a homogeneous opacity in a dependent position in the pleural cavity (Miller, 1994). Although a pleural fluid density appears the same whether it is blood (hemothorax), serous fluid (pleural effusion), pus (empyema), or chyle (chylothorax), a new pleural fluid collection in the early postoperative hours after a thoracic operation can be assumed to be a hemothorax.

In most cases of acute hemothorax, the fluid moves freely in the pleural space with changes in the patient's position. Roentgenograms obtained for initial evaluation of a patient with chest trauma or in the early post-

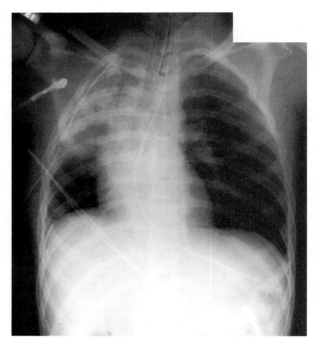

FIGURE 44-9. Right upper lobe atelectasis. Note opacification of right upper lung field and mediastinal shift (tracheal deviation) toward right hemithorax. Also apparent on the roentgenogram are a right pleural chest tube, an endotracheal tube, and a nasogastric tube. (Courtesy of Robert M. Vanecko, MD)

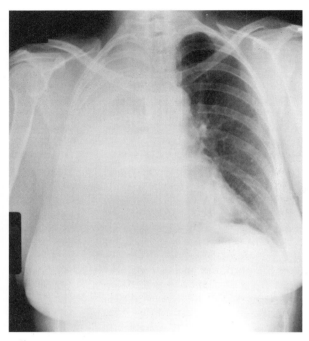

FIGURE 44-10. Supine chest roentgenogram demonstrating massive right hemothorax. With the patient in a supine position, the blood in the pleural space has layered out, opacifying the entire right lung field. (Courtesy of Robert M. Vanecko, MD)

operative period after a thoracic operation usually are taken with the patient in a supine position; blood in the pleural space layers out over the posterior surface of the lung field, producing a diffuse shadow that makes the affected lung appear denser than the lung on the opposite side (Fig. 44-10). If an upright roentgenogram is taken, the blood appears at the base of the lung, causing blunting of the normally sharply defined costophrenic angle. Excessive bleeding after pneumonectomy is manifested radiographically by a rapid increase in the fluid level in the operative hemithorax. The mediastinum and heart may be shifted toward the contralateral side.

In patients who undergo coronary artery revascularization, serous *pleural effusions* frequently develop during the early postoperative period, particularly on the left side (Fig. 44-11). Large pleural effusions, especially if bilateral, may be overlooked on a supine film because they create diffuse opacifications of both hemithoraces (Moreno-Cabral et al., 1988). On an upright film, the fluid is easily apparent at the bases of the lungs. A lateral decubitus projection, taken with the patient lying on the right or left side, also may be helpful in diagnosing the presence and mobility of fluid in the pleural space (Freundlich & Bragg, 1992c). In the lateral decubitus view, the fluid forms a shadow parallel to the thoracic wall (Umali & Smith, 1991). Pleural fluid occasionally collects and is loculated in an interlobar fissure, causing the fissure to appear as a cigar-shaped opacity (Miller, 1994).

An unusual cause of postoperative pleural fluid accumulation is operative injury of the thoracic duct with re-

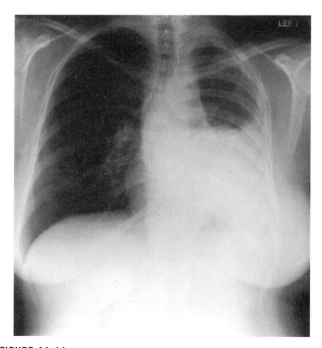

FIGURE 44-11. A moderate left-sided pleural effusion is apparent on this roentgenogram obtained with the patient in an upright position. (Courtesy of Robert M. Vanecko, MD)

sultant chylothorax. It is most likely after esophageal or pulmonary resection. Although not radiographically distinguishable from a transudative pleural effusion, chylothorax is diagnosed easily with thoracentesis or chest tube thoracostomy because of the characteristic milky appearance of the chylous fluid.

Air Collections

Pleural air accumulation, or *pneumothorax*, produces a dark space devoid of the thin white lung markings that normally are present throughout the lung fields. The pleural air displaces the visceral pleura away from the parietal pleura lining the chest wall. The visceral pleura, which normally is not visualized, becomes visible as a thin opacity separating the vessel-containing lung and the avascular, air-filled space (Collins & Stern, 1999g).

A pneumothorax usually appears in nondependent areas of the pleural space unless the air is trapped or loculated beneath the lung. Consequently, in an upright chest roentgenogram, pneumothorax typically is seen at the apex of the lung. If the patient is in a supine position, air collects medially and anteriorly. A medial pneumothorax produces a lucent line next to the mediastinal shadow; an anterior air collection may not be visible without a cross-table lateral roentgenogram. If the pleural space contains fluid as well as air, the roentgenogram demonstrates an air-fluid level (ie, a straight line separating the radiopaque fluid from the radiolucent air).

Pneumothorax is categorized according to the estimated amount of the hemithorax that it occupies. A small cap of air above the apex of the lung is termed a 5% to 10% pneumothorax. A 100% pneumothorax is present if the entire lung is collapsed by pleural air; the lung appears

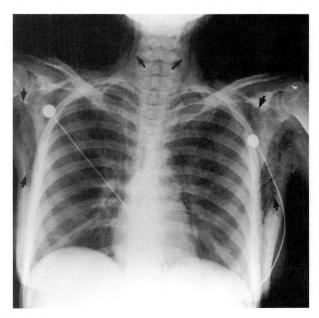

FIGURE 44-13. Chest roentgenogram in a patient with significant subcutaneous emphysema. Note translucent streaking in the subcutaneous tissue of the chest wall and neck (*arrows*). (Courtesy of Robert M. Vanecko, MD)

as a small, opaque structure abutting the mediastinum, and the remaining hemithorax is radiolucent (Fig. 44-12). A tension pneumothorax exists if mediastinal structures are shifted toward the opposite side. On the side of the tension pneumothorax, the lung appears compressed, the cardiac contour is flattened, and the hemidiaphragm may be inverted (Chiles, 1992).

Air occasionally accumulates in the subcutaneous tissues because a large air leak is present or because drainage of the pleural space is inadequate. Termed *subcutaneous emphysema,* air dissecting interstitial tissue appears radiographically as irregular radiolucent mottling and linear shadows in the soft tissues (Khan & Settle, 1996) (Fig. 44-13). Uncommonly, air may enter and collect in the mediastinum, producing a *pneumomediastinum*. Pneumomediastinum produces streaky lucencies in the mediastinum that highlight the contours of the aorta and pulmonary artery (Collins & Stern, 1999h).

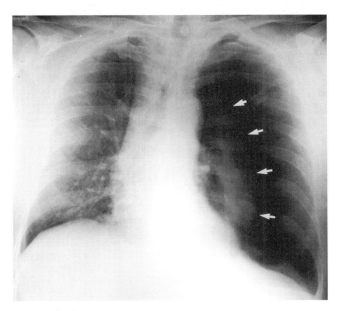

FIGURE 44-12. Roentgenogram demonstrating 100% left pneumothorax. Note edge of collapsed lung (*arrows*) and absence of lung markings beyond. (Courtesy of Robert M. Vanecko, MD)

REFERENCES

Boxt LM, 1998: Plain film examination of the chest. In Topol EJ (ed): Comprehensive Cardiovascular Medicine. Philadelphia, Lippincott Williams & Wilkins

Chiles C, 1992: Radiologic recognition of complications of thoracic surgery. In Wolfe WG (ed): Complications in Thoracic Surgery. St. Louis, Mosby–Year Book

Collins J, Stern EJ, 1999a: Interstitial lung disease. In Chest Radiology: The Essentials. Philadelphia, Lippincott Williams & Wilkins

Collins J, Stern EJ, 1999b: Normal anatomy of the chest. In Chest Radiology: The Essentials. Philadelphia, Lippincott Williams & Wilkins

Collins J, Stern EJ, 1999c: Monitoring and support devices. In

Chest Radiology: The Essentials. Philadelphia, Lippincott Williams & Wilkins

Collins J, Stern EJ, 1999d: Atelectasis. In Chest Radiology: The Essentials. Philadelphia, Lippincott Williams & Wilkins

Collins J, Stern EJ, 1999e: Signs in chest radiology. In Chest Radiology: The Essentials. Philadelphia, Lippincott Williams & Wilkins

Collins J, Stern EJ, 1999f: Peripheral lung disease. In Chest Radiology: The Essentials. Philadelphia, Lippincott Williams & Wilkins

Collins J, Stern EJ, 1999g: Chest wall, pleura, and diaphragm. In Chest Radiology: The Essentials. Philadelphia, Lippincott Williams & Wilkins

Collins J, Stern EJ, 1999h: Acute chest trauma. In Chest Radiology: The Essentials. Philadelphia, Lippincott Williams & Wilkins

Elefteriades JA, Geha AS, Cohen LS, 1996a: Thoracic imaging in acute disease. In House Officer Guide to ICU Care: Fundamentals of Management of the Heart and Lungs, ed. 2. Philadelphia, Lippincott-Raven

Elefteriades JA, Geha AS, Cohen LS, 1996b: Problems following noncardiac thoracic surgery. In House Officer Guide to ICU Care: Fundamentals of Management of the Heart and Lungs, ed. 2. Philadelphia, Lippincott-Raven

Freundlich IM, Bragg DG, 1992a: Anatomy. In Radiologic Approach to Diseases of the Chest. Baltimore, Williams & Wilkins

Freundlich IM, Bragg DG, 1992b: Alveolar consolidation. In Radiologic Approach to Diseases of the Chest. Baltimore, Williams & Wilkins

Freundlich IM, Bragg DG, 1992c: Introduction. In Radiologic Approach to Diseases of the Chest. Baltimore, Williams & Wilkins

Goodman LR, 1980: Postoperative chest radiograph: II. Alterations after major intrathoracic surgery. Am J Roentgenol 134:803

Goodman LR, 1983a: Pulmonary support and monitoring apparatus. In Goodman LR, Putman CE (eds): Intensive Care Radiology: Imaging of the Critically Ill, ed. 2. Philadelphia, WB Saunders

Goodman LR, 1983b: The post-thoracotomy radiograph. In Goodman LR, Putman CE (eds): Intensive Care Radiology: Imaging of the Critically Ill, ed. 2. Philadelphia, WB Saunders

Huseby JS, 1995: Radiologic examination of the chest. In Woods SL, Froelicher ES, Halpenny CJ, Motzer SU (eds): Cardiac Nursing, ed. 3. Philadelphia, JB Lippincott

Khan A, Settle, DF, 1996: Critical care radiology. In Kvetan V, Dantzker DR (eds): The Critically Ill Cardiac Patient: Multisystem Dysfunction and Management. Philadelphia, Lippincott-Raven

Joob AW, Hartz RS, 1994: General principles of postoperative care. In Shields TW (ed): General Thoracic Surgery, ed. 4. Baltimore, Williams & Wilkins

Juhl JH, 1993: Methods of examination, anatomy, and congenital malformations of the chest. In Juhl JH, Crummy AB (eds): Paul and Juhl's Essentials of Radiologic Imaging. Philadelphia, JB Lippincott

Matthay RA, Sostman HD, 1990: Chest imaging. In George RB, Light RW, Matthay MA, Matthay RA (eds): Chest Medicine, ed. 2. Baltimore, Williams & Wilkins

Miller WT, 1994: Roentgenographic evaluation of the lungs and chest. In Shields TW (ed): General Thoracic Surgery, ed. 4. Baltimore, Williams & Wilkins

Milne EN, 1980: Chest radiology in the surgical patient. Surg Clin North Am 60:1503

Moreno-Cabral CE, Mitchell RS, Miller DC, 1988: Perioperative care. In Manual of Postoperative Management of Adult Cardiac Surgery. Baltimore, Williams & Wilkins

Munnell ER, 1991: Chest drainage in the traumatized patient. In Webb WR, Besson A (eds): Thoracic Surgery: Surgical Management of Chest Injuries. St. Louis, Mosby–Year Book

Sagel SS, Slone RM, 1998: Lung. In Lee JK, Sagel SS, Stanley RJ, Heiken JP (eds): Computed Body Tomography With MRI Correlation, ed. 3. Philadelphia, Lippincott Williams & Wilkins

Sider L, 1986: Interpretation of the postoperative chest radiograph. Critical Care Quarterly 9:71

Squire LF, Novelline RA, 1988: Study of the mediastinal structures. In Fundamentals of Radiology, ed. 4. Cambridge, MA, Harvard University Press

Umali CB, Smith EH, 1991: The chest radiographic examination. In Rippe JM, Irwin RS, Alpert JS, Fink MP (eds): Intensive Care Medicine, ed. 2. Boston, Little, Brown

Westra D, 1990: Conventional chest radiography. In Sperber M (ed): Radiologic Diagnosis of Chest Disease. New York, Springer-Verlag

Index

NOTE: A *t* following a page number indicates tabular material and an *f* following a page number indicates a figure. Drugs are listed under their generic names. When a drug trade name is listed, the reader is referred to the generic name.